Essentials of Anaesthetic Equipment

FOURTH EDITION

Baha Al-Shaikh FCARCSI, FRCA

Consultant Anaesthetist, William Harvey Hospital, Ashford, Kent, UK

Honorary Senior Lecturer, King's College London, University of London, UK

Visiting Professor, Canterbury Christ Church University, UK

Simon Stacey FRCA

Consultant Anaesthetist, Barts and The London NHS Trust, London, UK

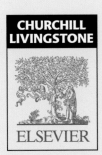
CHURCHILL LIVINGSTONE

ELSEVIER

Edinburgh   London   New York   Oxford   Philadelphia   St Louis   Sydney   Toronto   2013

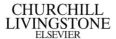

First edition 1995
Second edition 2002
Third edition 2007
Fourth edition 2013
 Reprinted 2013, 2014

ISBN: 978-0-7020-4954-5

British Library Cataloguing in Publication Data
A catalogue record for this book is available from the British Library

Library of Congress Cataloging in Publication Data
A catalog record for this book is available from the Library of Congress

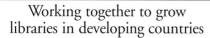

Working together to grow
libraries in developing countries

www.elsevier.com | www.bookaid.org | www.sabre.org

ELSEVIER   BOOK AID International   Sabre Foundation

ELSEVIER   your source for books, journals and multimedia in the health sciences

www.elsevierhealth.com

Printed in China

The publisher's policy is to use **paper manufactured from sustainable forests**

Acknowledgements

We are extremely grateful to the many manufacturers and others who have supplied the necessary information and images for this edition. Without their help, this fourth edition could not have gone ahead in its current format.

Special mention goes to Andy Coughlan of Smiths Medical for his unflagging help with all things photographic. Below is a list of the people and their companies who helped us by providing images during the preparation of the book.

We are also grateful to the association of Anaesthetists of Great Britain and Ireland for granting permission to reproduce their equipment checklist and monitoring recommendations.

Molly Bruton (Vygon)

Tony Calvo (Olympus)

Emma Christmas (Gambro)

Andy Coughlan (Smith's Medical)

Inga Dolezar (Chart BioMedical)

Bjrake Frank-Duab (Radiometer)

Andrew Garnham (Penlon)

John Jones (MAQUET)

John van Kessel (B Braun)

Vanessa Light (Philips Health Care)

Sharon Maris (Teleflex)

Lucy Martin-Davis (Verathon Medical)

Anne Pattinson (Draeger)

Mark Pedley (Blue Box Medical)

Lee Pettitt (Rimer Alco)

Ciska Proos (B Braun)

Malcolm Pyke (Philips Heath Care)

Siama Rafiq (BD Medical)

Emma Richardson (Argon Medical)

Rachel Stein (I-Flow)

Frank Toal (B Braun)

Jill Garratt (Zoll Medical)

Contents

Preface

Over 20 years ago, we conspired to write our colour equipment textbook *'Essentials of Anaesthetic Equipment'*. It is now in its fourth edition and hopefully as relevant to anaesthetic practice as ever.

We have tried to keep the book concise, however due to the sheer number of new anaesthetic equipment products used in the clinical practice today, the size of the book has increased slightly. We have tried to freshen up the photography/diagrams wherever possible. The text has been updated too and single best answer questions have been included.

We hope this book will continue to be the equipment book of choice for both the trainees sitting FRCA exams and their trainers and a useful reference tool for our Nursing and Operating Department Practitioner colleagues.

BA-S   Ashford, Kent
SGS   London
2013

Chapter 1

Medical gas supply

Gas supply

Medical gas supply takes the form of either cylinders or a piped gas system, depending on the requirements of the hospital.

Cylinders

Components

1. Cylinders are made of thin-walled seamless molybdenum steel in which gases and vapours are stored under pressure. They are designed to withstand considerable internal pressure.
2. The top end of the cylinder is called the neck, and this ends in a tapered screw thread into which the valve is fitted. The thread is sealed with a material that melts if the cylinder is exposed to intense heat. This allows the gas to escape so reducing the risk of an explosion.
3. There is a plastic disc around the neck of the cylinder. The year when the cylinder was last examined can be identified from the shape and colour of the disc.
4. Cylinders are manufactured in different sizes (A to J). Sizes A and H are not used for medical gases. Cylinders attached to the anaesthetic machine are usually size E (Figs 1.1–1.4), while size J cylinders are commonly used for cylinder manifolds. Size E oxygen cylinders contain 680 L, whereas size E nitrous oxide cylinders can release 1800 L. The smallest sized cylinder, size C, can hold 1.2 L of water, and size E can hold 4.7 L while the larger size J can hold 47.2 L of water.
5. Lightweight cylinders can be made from aluminium alloy with

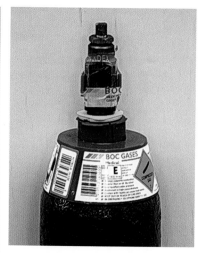

Fig. 1.1 Nitrous oxide cylinder with its wrapping and labels.

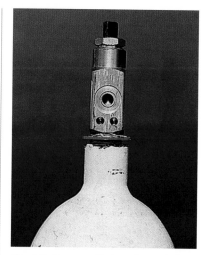

Fig. 1.2 Oxygen cylinder valve and pin index.

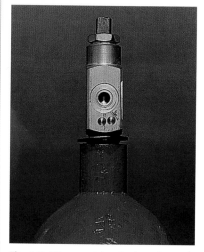

Fig. 1.3 Nitrous oxide cylinder valve and pin index.

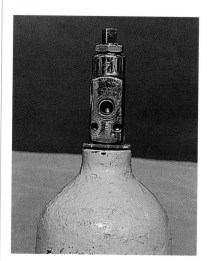

Fig. 1.4 Carbon dioxide cylinder valve and pin index.

a fibreglass covering in epoxy resin matrix. These can be used to provide oxygen at home, during transport or in magnetic resonance scanners. They have a flat base to help in storage and handling.

- **Gas** exits in the gaseous state at room temperature. Its liquefaction at room temperature is impossible, since the room temperature is above its critical temperature.
- **Vapour** is the gaseous state of a substance below its critical temperature. At room temperature and atmospheric pressure, the substance is liquid.
- **Critical temperature** is the temperature above which a substance cannot be liquefied no matter how much pressure is applied. The critical temperatures for nitrous oxide and oxygen are 36.5 and −118°C respectively.

Oxygen is stored as a gas at a pressure of 13 700 kPa whereas nitrous oxide is stored in a liquid phase with its vapour on top at a pressure of 4400 kPa. As the liquid is less compressible than the gas, this means that the cylinder should only be partially filled. The amount of filling is called the **filling ratio**. Partially filling the cylinders with liquid minimizes the risk of dangerous increases in pressure with any increase in the ambient temperature that can lead to an explosion. In the UK, the filling ratio for nitrous oxide and carbon dioxide is 0.75. In hotter climates, the filling ratio is reduced to 0.67.

> **The filling ratio** is the weight of the fluid in the cylinder divided by the weight of water required to fill the cylinder.

A full oxygen cylinder at atmospheric pressure can deliver 130 times its capacity of oxygen. A typical size E full oxygen cylinder delivering 4 L per minute will last for 2 hours and 50 minutes but will last only 45 minutes when delivering 15 L/min.

A full oxygen cylinder at atmospheric pressure can deliver 130 times its capacity of oxygen.

At constant temperature, a gas-containing cylinder shows a linear and proportional reduction in cylinder pressure as it empties. For a cylinder that contains liquid and vapour, initially the pressure remains constant as more vapour is produced to replace that used. Once all the liquid has been evaporated, the pressure in the cylinder decreases. The temperature in such a cylinder can decrease because of the loss of the latent heat of vaporization leading to the formation of ice on the outside of the cylinder.

Cylinders in use are checked and tested by manufacturers at regular intervals, usually 5 years. Test details are recorded on the plastic disc between the valve and the neck of the cylinder. They are also engraved on the cylinder:

1. Internal endoscopic examination.
2. Flattening, bend and impact tests are carried out on at least one cylinder in every 100.
3. Pressure test: the cylinder is subjected to high pressures of about 22 000 kPa, which is more than 50% above their normal working pressure.
4. Tensile test where strips of the cylinder are cut and stretched. This test is carried out on at least one cylinder in every 100.

The marks engraved on the cylinders are:

1. Test pressure.
2. Dates of test performed.
3. Chemical formula of the cylinder's content.
4. Tare weight (weight of nitrous oxide cylinder when empty).

Labelling
The cylinder label includes the following details:
- Name, chemical symbol, pharmaceutical form, specification of the product, its licence number and the proportion of the constituent gases in a gas mixture.
- Substance identification number and batch number.
- Hazard warnings and safety instructions.
- Cylinder size code.
- Nominal cylinder contents (litres).
- Maximum cylinder pressure (bars).
- Filling date, shelf life and expiry date.
- Directions for use.
- Storage and handling precautions.

Problems in practice and safety features

1. The gases and vapours should be free of water vapour when stored in cylinders. Water vapour freezes and blocks the exit port when the temperature of the cylinder decreases on opening.
2. The outlet valve uses the pin-index system to make it almost impossible to connect a cylinder to the wrong yoke (Fig. 1.5).
3. Cylinders are colour-coded to reduce accidental use of the wrong gas or vapour. In the UK, the colour-coding is a two-part colour, shoulder and body (Table 1.1). To improve safety, there are plans to change the colours of the bodies of cylinders using medical gas to white while

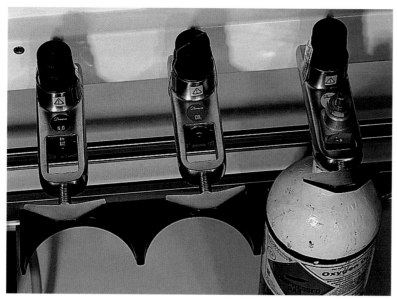

Fig. 1.5 Anaesthetic machine cylinder yokes. For the sake of comparison, the Bodok seal is absent from the nitrous oxide yoke (left).

keeping the colours of the shoulders according to the European Standard EN 1089-3.

4. Cylinders should be checked regularly while in use to ensure that they have sufficient content and that leaks do not occur.

5. Cylinders should be stored in a purpose built, dry, well-ventilated and fireproof room, preferably inside and not subjected to extremes of heat. They should not be stored near flammable materials such as oil or grease or near any source of heat. They should not be exposed to continuous dampness, corrosive chemicals or fumes. This can lead to corrosion of cylinders and their valves.

6. To avoid accidents, full cylinders should be stored separately from empty ones. F, G and J size cylinders are stored upright to avoid damage to the valves. C, D and E size cylinders can be stored horizontally on shelves made of a material that does not damage the surface of the cylinders.

7. Overpressurized cylinders are hazardous and should be reported to the manufacturer.

Table 1.1 Colour coding of medical gas cylinders, their pressure when full and their physical state in the cylinder

	Body colour	Shoulder colour	Pressure, kPa (at room temperature)	Physical state in cylinder
Oxygen	Black (green in USA)	White	13 700	Gas
Nitrous oxide	Blue	Blue	4400	Liquid/vapour
Carbon dioxide	Grey	Grey	5000	Liquid/vapour
Air	Grey (yellow in USA)	White/black quarters	13 700	Gas
Entonox	Blue	White/blue quarters	13 700	Gas
Oxygen/helium (Heliox)	Black	White/brown quarters	13 700	Gas

Oxygen

Nitrous oxide

Entonox
(50% N_2O/50%O_2)

Air

Carbon dioxide

Helium/oxygen mixture
(79% He/21% O_2)

Cylinders

- Cylinders are made of thin-walled molybdenum steel to withstand high pressures, e.g. 13 700 kPa and 4400 kPa for oxygen and nitrous oxide respectively. Lightweight aluminium is also available.
- They are made in different sizes: size E cylinders are used on the anaesthetic machine; size J cylinders are used in cylinder banks.
- Oxygen cylinders contain gas whereas nitrous oxide cylinders contain a mixture of liquid and vapour. In the UK, nitrous oxide cylinders are 75% filled with liquid nitrous oxide (filling ratio); this is 67% in hotter climates.
- At a constant temperature, the pressure in a gas cylinder decreases linearly and proportionally as it empties. This is not true in cylinders containing liquid/vapour.
- They are colour-coded (shoulder and body).

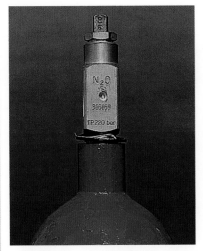

Fig. 1.6 Chemical formula (N_2O) engraved on a nitrous oxide cylinder valve.

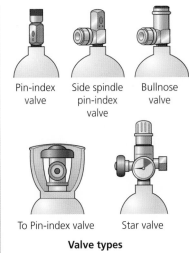

Pin-index valve   Side spindle pin-index valve   Bullnose valve

To Pin-index valve   Star valve

Valve types

Fig. 1.7 Cylinder valves.

Cylinder valves

These valves seal the cylinder contents. The chemical formula of the particular gas is engraved on the valve (Fig. 1.6). Other types of valves, the bull nose, the hand wheel and the star, are used under special circumstances (Fig. 1.7).

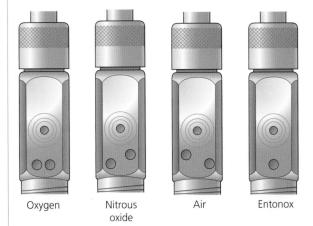

Oxygen   Nitrous oxide   Air   Entonox

Fig. 1.8 Pin-index system. Note the different configuration for each gas.

Components

1. The valve is mounted on the top of the cylinder, screwed into the neck via a threaded connection. It is made of brass and sometimes chromium plated.
2. An on/off spindle is used to open and close the valve by opposing a plastic facing against the valve seating.

3. The exit port for supplying gas to the apparatus (e.g. anaesthetic machine).
4. A safety relief device allows the discharge of cylinder contents to the atmosphere if the cylinder is overpressurized.
5. The non-interchangeable safety system (pin-index system) is used on cylinders of size E or smaller as well as on F- and G-size Entonox cylinders. A specific pin configuration exists for each medical gas on the yoke of the anaesthetic machine. The matching configuration of holes on the valve block allows only the correct gas cylinder to be

fitted in the yoke (Figs 1.8 and 1.9). The gas exit port will not seal against the washer of the yoke unless the pins and holes are aligned.
6. A more recent modification is where the external part of the valve is designed to allow manual turning on and off of the cylinder without the need for a key (Fig. 1.10).

Mechanism of action

1. The cylinder valve acts as a mechanism for opening and closing the gas pathway.

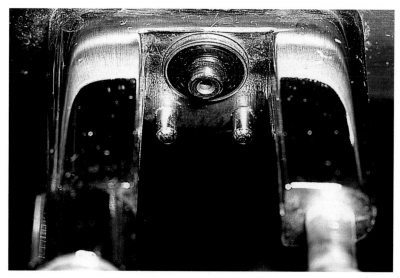
Fig. 1.9 A cylinder yoke and pin-index system. Note that a Bodok seal is in position.

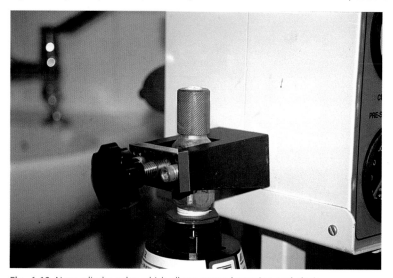
Fig. 1.10 New cylinder valve which allows manual opening and closing.

2. A compressible yoke-sealing washer (**Bodok seal**) must be placed between valve outlet and the apparatus to make a gas-tight joint (Fig. 1.11).

Problems in practice and safety features

1. The plastic wrapping of the valve should be removed just before use. The valve should be slightly opened and closed (cracked) before connecting the

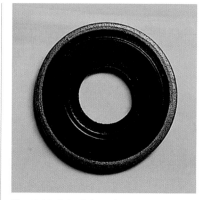
Fig. 1.11 A Bodok seal.

cylinder to the anaesthetic machine. This clears particles of dust, oil and grease from the exit port, which would otherwise enter the anaesthetic machine.

2. The valve should be opened slowly when attached to the anaesthetic machine or regulator. This prevents the rapid rise in pressure and the associated rise in temperature of the gas in the machine's pipelines. The cylinder valve should be fully open when in use (the valve must be turned two full revolutions).

3. During closure, overtightening of the valve should be avoided. This might lead to damage to the seal between the valve and the cylinder neck.

4. The Bodok seal should be inspected for damage prior to use. Having a spare seal readily available is advisable.

Cylinder valves
- They are mounted on the neck of the cylinder.
- Act as an on/off device for the discharge of cylinder contents.
- Pin-index system prevents cylinder identification errors.
- Bodok sealing washer must be placed between the valve and the yoke of the anaesthetic machine.
- A newly designed valve allows keyless manual turning on and off.

Piped gas supply (piped medical gas and vacuum – PMGV)

PMGV is a system where gases are delivered from central supply points to different sites in the hospital at a pressure of about 400 kPa. Special outlet valves supply the various needs throughout the hospital.

Oxygen, nitrous oxide, Entonox, compressed air and medical vacuum are commonly supplied through the pipeline system.

Components

1. Central supply points such as cylinder banks or liquid oxygen storage tank.
2. Pipework made of special high-quality copper alloy, which both prevents degradation of the gases it contains and has bacteriostatic properties. The fittings used are made from brass and are brazed rather than soldered.
3. The size of the pipes differs according to the demand that they carry. Pipes with a 42 mm diameter are usually used for leaving the manifold. Smaller diameter tubes, such as 15 mm, are used after repeated branching.
4. Outlets are identified by gas colour coding, gas name and by shape (Fig. 1.12). They accept matching quick connect/ disconnect probes, Schrader sockets (Fig. 1.13), with an indexing collar specific for each gas (or gas mixture).
5. Outlets can be installed as flush-fitting units, surface-fitting units, on booms or pendants, or suspended on a hose and gang mounted (Fig. 1.14).
6. Flexible colour-coded hoses connect the outlets to the anaesthetic machine (Fig. 1.15). The anaesthetic machine end should be permanently fixed using a nut and liner union where the thread is gas specific and non-interchangeable (non-interchangeable screw thread, **NIST**, is the British Standard).
7. Isolating valves behind break glass covers are positioned at strategic points throughout the

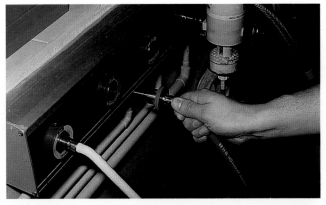

Fig. 1.12 Inserting a remote probe into its matching wall-mounted outlet socket.

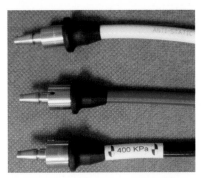

Fig. 1.13 Gas probes for oxygen (top), nitrous oxide (middle) and air (bottom). Note the locking groove on the probe to ensure connectivity.

pipeline network. They are also known as area valve service units (AVSUs) (Fig. 1.16). They can be accessed to isolate the supply to an area in cases of fire or other emergency

Problems in practice and safety features

1. A reserve bank of cylinders is available should the primary supply fail. Low-pressure alarms detect gas supply failure (Fig. 1.17).
2. Single hose test is performed to detect cross-connection.
3. Tug test is performed to detect misconnection.
4. Regulations for PMGV installation, repair and modification are enforced.

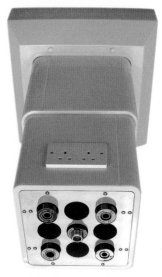

Fig. 1.14 Outlet sockets mounted in a retractable ceiling unit. (Courtesy of Penlon Ltd, Abingdon, UK (www.penlon. com).)

5. Anaesthetists are responsible for the gases supplied from the terminal outlet through to the anaesthetic machine. Pharmacy, supplies and engineering departments share the responsibility for the gas pipelines 'behind the wall'.
6. There is a risk of fire from worn or damaged hoses that are designed to carry gases under pressure from a primary source such as a cylinder or wall-mounted terminal to medical

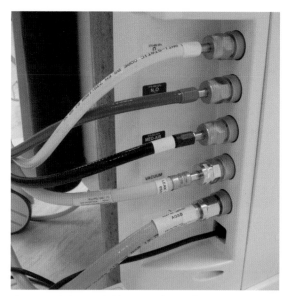

Fig. 1.15 Colour-coded hoses with NIST fittings attached to an anaesthetic machine.

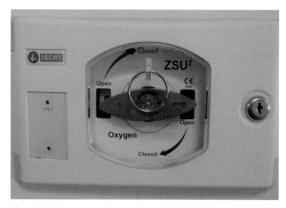

Fig. 1.16 An area valve service unit (AVSU).

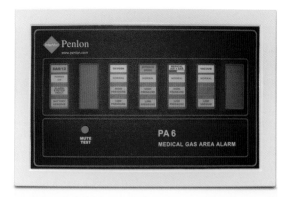

Fig. 1.17 Medical gas alarm panel. (Courtesy of Penlon Ltd, Abingdon, UK (www.penlon.com).)

devices such as ventilators and anaesthetic machines. Because of heavy wear and tear, the risk of rupture is greatest in oxygen hoses used with transport devices. Regular inspection and replacement, every 2–5 years, of all medical gas hoses is recommended.

Piped gas supply

- There is a network of copper alloy pipelines throughout the hospital from central supply points.
- The outlets are colour- and shape-coded to accept matching 'Schrader' probes.
- Flexible and colour-coded pipelines run from the anaesthetic machine to the outlets.
- Single hose and tug tests are performed to test for cross-connection and misconnection respectively.
- There is risk of fire from worn and damaged hoses.

Sources of gas supply

The source of supply can be cylinder manifold(s) and, in the case of oxygen, a liquid oxygen storage tank or oxygen concentrator (Fig. 1.18).

CYLINDER MANIFOLD

Manifolds are used to supply nitrous oxide, Entonox and oxygen.

Components

1. Large cylinders (e.g. size J each with 6800 L capacity) are usually divided into two equal groups, primary and secondary. The two groups alternate in supplying the pipelines (Fig. 1.19). The number of cylinders depends on the expected demand.

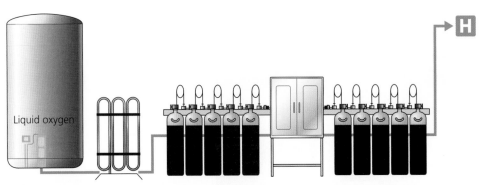

Fig. 1.18 Sources of oxygen supply in a hospital. A vacuum-insulated evaporator (left) and a cylinder manifold (right).

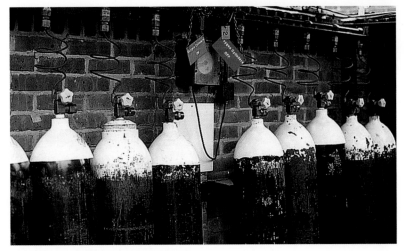

Fig. 1.19 An oxygen cylinder manifold.

2. All cylinders in each group are connected through non-return valves to a common pipe. This in turn is connected to the pipeline through pressure regulators.
3. As nitrous oxide is only available in cylinders (in contrast to liquid oxygen), its manifold is larger than that of oxygen. The latter usually acts as a back up to liquid oxygen supply (see later).

Mechanism of action

1. In either group, all the cylinders' valves are opened. This allows them to empty simultaneously.
2. The supply is automatically changed to the secondary group when the primary group is nearly empty. The changeover is achieved through a pressure-sensitive device that detects when the cylinders are nearly empty.
3. The changeover activates an electrical signalling system to alert staff to the need to change the cylinders.

Problems in practice and safety features

1. The manifold should be housed in a well-ventilated room built of fireproof material away from the main buildings of the hospital.
2. The manifold room should not be used as a general cylinder store.
3. All empty cylinders should be removed immediately from the manifold room.

LIQUID OXYGEN

A vacuum-insulated evaporator (VIE) (Fig. 1.20) is the most economical way to store and supply oxygen.

Components

1. A thermally insulated double-walled steel tank with a layer of perlite in a vacuum is used as the insulation (Fig. 1.21). It can be described as a giant thermos flask, employing the same principles.
2. A pressure regulator allows gas to enter the pipelines and maintains the pressure through the pipelines at about 400 kPa.
3. A safety valve opens at 1700 kPa allowing the gas to escape when there is a build-up of pressure within the vessel. This can be caused by underdemand for oxygen.
4. A control valve opens when there is an excessive demand on the system. This allows liquid oxygen to evaporate by passing through superheaters made of uninsulated coils of copper tubing.

Mechanism of action

1. Liquid oxygen is stored (up to 1500 L) at a temperature of −150° to −170°C (lower than

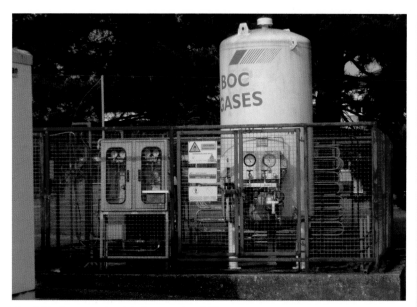

Fig. 1.20 A vacuum-insulated evaporator (VIE).

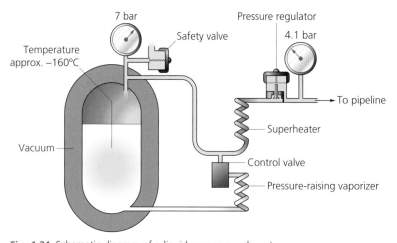

Fig. 1.21 Schematic diagram of a liquid oxygen supply system.

the critical temperature) and at a pressure of 10.5 bars.

2. The temperature of the vessel is maintained by the high-vacuum shell. Evaporation of the liquid oxygen requires heat (latent heat of vaporization). This heat is taken from the liquid oxygen, helping to maintain its low temperature.

3. The storage vessel rests on a weighing balance to measure

the mass of the liquid. More recently, a differential pressure gauge which measures the pressure difference between the bottom and top of the liquid oxygen can be used instead. The information obtained is sent to the hospital alarm system. As liquid oxygen evaporates, its mass decreases, reducing the

pressure at the bottom. By measuring the difference in pressure, the contents of the VIE can be calculated. When required, fresh supplies of liquid oxygen are pumped from a tanker into the vessel.

4. The cold oxygen gas is warmed once outside the vessel in a coil of copper tubing. The increase in temperature causes an increase in pressure.

5. At a temperature of 15°C and atmospheric pressure, liquid oxygen can give 842 times its volume as gas.

Problems in practice and safety features

1. Reserve banks of cylinders are kept in case of supply failure.

2. A liquid oxygen storage vessel should be housed away from main buildings due to the fire hazard. The risk of fire is increased in cases of liquid spillage.

3. Spillage of cryogenic liquid can cause cold burns, frostbite and hypothermia.

OXYGEN CONCENTRATORS

Oxygen concentrators, also known as *pressure swing adsorption systems*, extract oxygen from air by differential adsorption. These devices may be small, designed to supply oxygen to a single patient (Fig. 1.22), supply oxygen to an anaesthetic machine (Fig. 1.23) or they can be large enough to supply oxygen for a medical gas pipeline system (Fig. 1.24).

Components

A zeolite molecular sieve is used. Zeolites are hydrated aluminium silicates of the alkaline earth metals in a powder or granular form. Many zeolite columns are used.

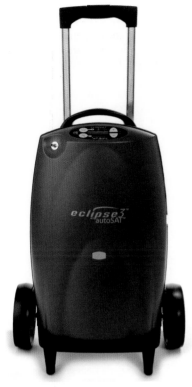

Fig. 1.22 The portable Eclipse 3 home oxygen concentaror. (Courtesy of Chart BioMedical Ltd.)

Mechanism of action (Fig. 1.25)

1. Ambient air is filtered and pressurized to about 137 kPa by a compressor.

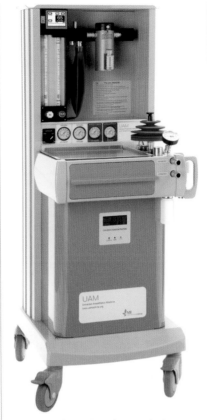

Fig. 1.23 The universal anaesthetic machine (UAM) which has a built-in oxygen concentrator (see Ch. 2 for more details). (Courtesy of UAM Global.)

2. Air is exposed to a zeolite molecular sieve column, forming a very large surface area, at a certain pressure.

3. The sieve selectively retains nitrogen and other unwanted components of air. These are released into the atmosphere after heating the column and applying a vacuum.

4. The changeover between columns is made by a time switch, typically cycles of around 20 seconds, allowing for a continuous supply of oxygen.

5. The maximum oxygen concentration achieved is 95% by volume. Argon is the main remaining constituent.

6. The life of the zeolite crystal can be expected to be at least 20 000 hours (which is about 10 years of use). Routine maintenance consists of changing filters at regular intervals.

Problems in practice and safety features

Although the oxygen concentration achieved is sufficient for the vast majority of clinical applications, its use with the circle system leads to argon accumulation. To avoid this, higher fresh gas flows are required.

Source of supply

- Cylinder manifold: banks of large cylinders, usually size J, are used.
- Liquid oxygen: a thermally insulated vessel at a temperature of −150° to −170°C and at a pressure of 5–10 atmospheres is used.
- Oxygen concentrator: a zeolite molecular sieve is used.

Entonox (BOC Medical)

This is a compressed gas mixture containing 50% oxygen and 50% nitrous oxide by volume. It is commonly used in the casualty and labour ward settings to provide

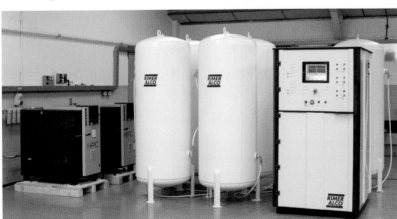

Fig. 1.24 The RA40/D/M hospital oxygen concentrator. It produces 80 L/min of oxygen. (Courtesy of Rimer Alco Ltd.)

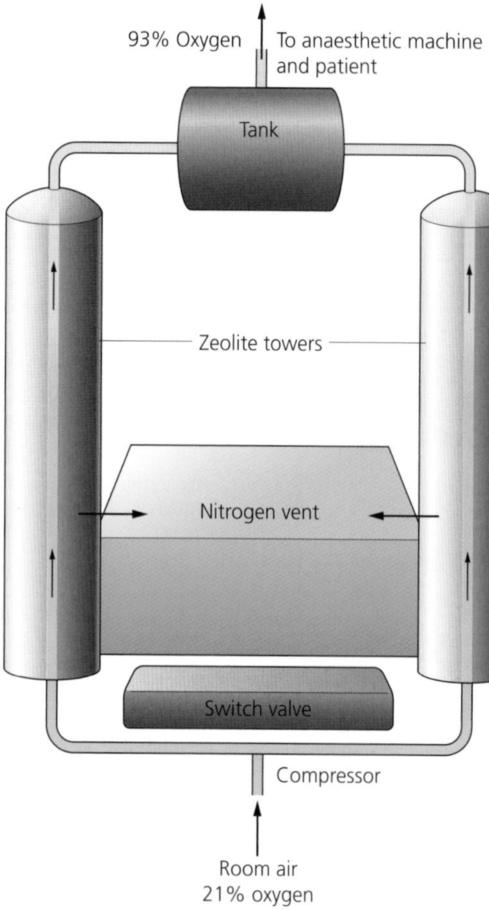

93% Oxygen | To anaesthetic machine and patient

Tank

Zeolite towers

Nitrogen vent

Switch valve

Compressor

Room air
21% oxygen

Fig. 1.25 Mechanism of action of a concentrator.

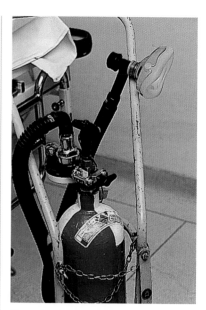

Fig. 1.26 An Entonox cylinder and delivery system.

- above the liquid, a gas mixture of high oxygen concentration.

   This means that when used at a constant flow rate, a gas with a high concentration of oxygen is supplied first. This is followed by a gas of decreasing oxygen concentration as the liquid evaporates. This may lead

analgesia. A two-stage pressure demand regulator is attached to the Entonox cylinder when in use (Figs 1.26 and 1.27). As the patient inspires through the mask or mouth piece, gas flow is allowed to occur. Gas flow ceases at the end of an inspiratory effort. Entonox is compressed into cylinders to a pressure of 13 700 kPa. Entonox cylinders should be stored at 10°C for 24 hours before use.

   If the temperature of the Entonox cylinder is decreased to below −5.5°C, liquefaction and separation of the two components occur (**Poynting effect**). This results in:

- a liquid mixture containing mostly nitrous oxide with about 20% oxygen dissolved in it

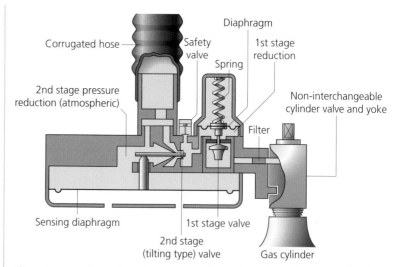

Fig. 1.27 The Entonox two-stage pressure demand regulator. (From Aitkenhead AR, Smith G, Rowbotham DJ (2007) Textbook of Anaesthesia, 5th edn. Churchill Livingstone, with permission.)

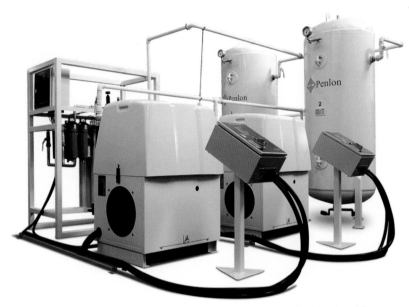

Fig. 1.28 Compressed medical air plant. (Courtesy of Penlon Ltd, Abingdon, UK (www.penlon.com).)

Centralized vacuum or suction system (Fig. 1.29)

Suction devices play a crucial part in the care of patients in the operating theatre, intensive care unit and other parts of the hospital.

Components

1. A pump or a power source that is capable of continuously generating a negative pressure of −500 mmHg.
2. A suction controller with a filter.
3. A receiver or a collection vessel.
4. A suction tubing and suction nozzle (e.g. a Yankaeur sucker) or catheter.

To determine the efficiency of central-piped vacuum systems

- A negative pressure of at least −53 kPa (−400 mmHg) should be maintained at the outlet.
- Each central-piped vacuum outlet should be able to withstand a flow of free air of at least 40 L/min.
- A unit should take no longer than 10 seconds to generate a vacuum (500 mmHg) with a displacement of air of 25 L/min.

Mechanism of action

1. Negative pressure is generated by an electric motor and pneumatic-driven pumps using the Venturi principle.
2. The amount of vacuum generated can be manually adjusted by the suction controller. This device has a variable orifice with a float assembly, a back-up filter to prevent liquid entering the system and ports to connect to a

---

to the supply of hypoxic mixtures, with less than 20% oxygen, as the cylinder is nearly empty.

Rewarming and mixing of both the cylinder and its contents reverses the separation and liquefaction.

Problems in practice and safety features

Liquefaction and separation of the components can be prevented by:

1. Cylinders being stored horizontally for about 24 hours at temperatures of or above 5°C before use. The horizontal position increases the area for diffusion. If the contents are well mixed by repeated inversion, cylinders can be used earlier than 24 hours.
2. Large cylinders are equipped with a dip tube with its tip ending in the liquid phase. This results in the liquid being used first, preventing the delivery of an oxygen concentration of less than 20%. Prolonged use of Entonox

should be avoided because of the effect of nitrous oxide on the bone marrow especially in the critically ill patient. Adequate facilities for scavenging should be provided to protect hospital staff.

Compressed air

Medical air is supplied in a hospital for clinical uses or to drive power tools. The former is supplied at a pressure of 400 kPa and the latter at 700 kPa. The anaesthetic machines and most intensive care ventilator blenders accept a 400 kPa supply. The terminal outlets for the two pressures are different to prevent misconnection.

Air may be supplied from cylinder manifolds, or more economically from a compressor plant with duty and back-up compressors (Fig. 1.28). Oil-free medical air is cleaned by filters and separators and then dried before use.

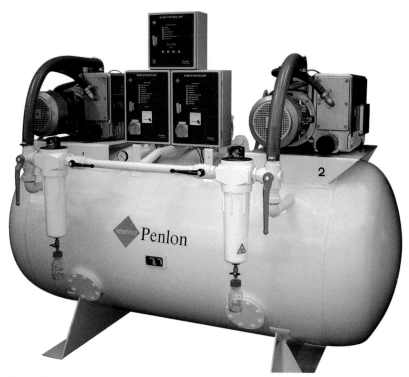

Fig. 1.29 Medical vacuum plant. (Courtesy of Penlon Ltd, Abingdon, UK (www.penlon.com).)

FURTHER READING

Health Technical Memorandum 2022, 1997. Medical gas pipeline systems. The Stationery Office, London

Health Technical Memorandum 02-01, 2006. Medical gas pipeline systems, part A; design, installation, validation and verification. The Stationery Office, London.

Health Technical Memorandum 02-01, 2006. Medical gas pipeline systems, part B; operational management. The Stationery Office, London.

Highly, D., 2009. Medical gases, their storage and delivery. Anaesthesia and Intensive Care Medicine 10 (11), 523–527.

MHRA, 2011. Medical device alert: anaesthetic machine: auxillary common gas outlet (ACGO) manufactured by GE Healthcare (MDA/2011/118). Online. Available at: http://www.mhra.gov.uk/Publications/Safetywarnings/MedicalDeviceAlerts/CON137664

National Health Service, 2009. Oxygen safety in hospitals. Online. Available at: http://www.nrls.npsa.nhs.uk/resources/?entryid45=62811&p=7

Poolacherla, R., Nickells, J., 2006. Suction devices. Anaesthesia and Intensive Care Medicine 7 (10), 354–355.

collection vessel or reservoir through flexible tubing.
3. The reservoir must have sufficient capacity to receive the aspirated material. Too large a capacity will make the system cumbersome and will take a long time to generate adequate negative pressure.
4. The suction tubing should be flexible and firm to prevent collapse. Also it should be transparent so that the contents aspirated can be visualized, and of sufficient internal diameter and length for optimal suction.
5. The negative pressure (or degree of suctioning) can be adjusted to suit its use; e.g. a lesser degree of suctioning is required to clear oral secretions in a child than in an adult.

6. Bacterial filters are used to prevent spread of infectious bacteria, with a removal of 99.999% of bacteria. Filters are also used to prevent fluids, condensate and smoke from contaminating the system.
7. It is recommended that there are at least two vacuum outlets per each operating theatre, one per anaesthetic room and one per recovery or intensive care unit bed.

Problems in practice and safety features

To prevent trauma to the tissues during suction, the nozzles should taper, be smooth and have multiple holes, so that if one is blocked the others will continue suction.

MCQs

In the following lists, which of the statements (a) to (e) are true?

1. Concerning cylinders:
   a) Oxygen is stored in cylinders as a gas.
   b) The pressure in a half-filled oxygen cylinder is 13 700 kPa.
   c) The pressure in a half-full nitrous oxide cylinder is 4400 kPa.
   d) Nitrous oxide is stored in the cylinder in the gas phase.
   e) Pressure in a full Entonox cylinder is 13 700 kPa.

2. Entonox:
   a) Entonox is 50:50 mixture by weight of O_2 and N_2O.
   b) Entonox has a critical temperature of 5.5°C.
   c) Entonox cylinders should be stored upright.
   d) At room temperature, Entonox cylinders contain only gas.
   e) Entonox cylinders have blue bodies and white and blue quarters on the shoulders.

3. Oxygen:
   a) For medical use, oxygen is usually formed from fractional distillation of air.
   b) Long-term use can cause bone marrow depression.
   c) In hyperbaric concentrations, oxygen may cause convulsions.
   d) At constant volume, the absolute pressure of oxygen is directly proportional to its absolute temperature.
   e) The critical temperature of oxygen is −118°C.

4. Oxygen concentrators:
   a) Oxygen concentrators concentrate O_2 that has been delivered from an oxygen cylinder manifold.
   b) Argon accumulation can occur when oxygen concentrators are used with the circle system.
   c) They are made of columns of a zeolite molecular sieve.
   d) They can achieve O_2 concentrations of up to 100%.
   e) They can only be used in home oxygen therapy.

5. Oxygen:
   a) Oxygen is stored in cylinders at approximately 140 bars.
   b) It has a critical temperature of 36.5°C.
   c) It is a liquid in its cylinder.
   d) It may form an inflammable mixture with oil.
   e) It obeys Boyle's law.

6. Concerning cylinders:
   a) The filling ratio = weight of liquid in the cylinder divided by the weight of water required to fill the cylinder.
   b) The tare weight is the weight of the cylinder plus its contents.
   c) Nitrous oxide cylinders have a blue body and blue and white top.
   d) A full oxygen cylinder has a pressure of approximately 137 bars.
   e) At 40°C, a nitrous oxide cylinder contains both liquid and vapour.

7. Concerning piped gas supply in the operating theatre:
   a) Compressed air is supplied only under one pressure.
   b) The NIST system is the British Standard.
   c) Only oxygen and air are supplied.
   d) E-size cylinders are normally used in cylinder manifolds.
   e) Liquid oxygen is stored at temperatures above −100°C.

8. True or false:
   a) There is no need for cylinders to undergo regular checks.
   b) The only agent identification on the cylinder is its colour.
   c) When attached to the anaesthetic machine, the cylinder valve should be opened slowly.
   d) When warmed, liquid oxygen can give 842 times its volume as gas.
   e) Cylinders are made of thick-walled steel to withstand the high internal pressure.

SINGLE BEST ANSWER (SBA)

9. Concerning piped medical gas and vacuum (PMGV):
   a) Outlets are only colour-coded.
   b) Outlets are shape- and colour-coded.
   c) All the supplies can be interrupted using a single AVSU.
   d) Copper sulphate pipes are used to carry oxygen throughout the hospital.
   e) Back-up cylinders for the oxygen supply are undesirable.

Answers

1. Concerning cylinders:
   a) *True.* Oxygen is stored in the cylinder as a gas.
   b) *False.* Oxygen is stored as a gas in the cylinder where gas laws apply. The pressure gauge accurately reflects the contents of the cylinder. A full oxygen cylinder has a pressure of 13 700 kPa. Pressure in a half-full oxygen cylinder is therefore 6850 kPa.
   c) *True.* Nitrous oxide is stored in the cylinder in the liquid form. The pressure of a full nitrous oxide cylinder is about 4400 kPa. As the cylinder is used, the vapour above the liquid is used first. This vapour is replaced by new vapour from the liquid. Therefore the pressure is maintained. So the cylinder is nearly empty before the pressure starts to decrease. For this reason, the pressure gauge does not accurately reflect the contents of the cylinder.
   d) *False.* Nitrous oxide is stored in the cylinder as a liquid. The vapour above the liquid is delivered to the patient.
   e) *True.* Entonox is a compressed gas mixture containing 50% oxygen and 50% nitrous oxide by volume.

2. Entonox:
   a) *False.* Entonox is a 50:50 mixture of O_2 and N_2O by volume and not by weight.
   b) *False.* The critical temperature of Entonox is −5.5°C. At or below this temperature, liquefaction and separation of the two components occurs. This results in a liquid mixture of mainly nitrous

oxide and about 20% oxygen. Above the liquid is a gaseous mixture with a high concentration of oxygen.
   c) *False.* This increases the risk of liquefaction and separation of the components. To prevent this, Entonox cylinders should be stored horizontally for about 24 hours at temperatures at or above 5°C. This position increases the area for diffusion. With repeated inversion, Entonox cylinders can be used earlier than 24 hours.
   d) *True.* Liquefaction and separation of nitrous oxide and oxygen occurs at or below −5.5°C.
   e) *True.*

3. Oxygen:
   a) *True.* Except for oxygen concentrators which use zeolites.
   b) *False.* Long-term use of oxygen has no effect on the bone marrow. Long-term use of N_2O can cause bone marrow depression especially with high concentrations in critically ill patients.
   c) *True.*
   d) *True.* This is Gay–Lussac's law where pressure = constant × temperature. Oxygen also obeys the other gas laws (Dalton's law of partial pressures, Boyle's and Charles's laws).
   e) *True.* At or below −118°C, oxygen changes to the liquid phase. This is used in the design of the vacuum insulated evaporator where oxygen is stored in the liquid phase at temperatures of −150 to −170°C.

4. Oxygen concentrators:
   a) *False.* Oxygen concentrators extract oxygen from air using a zeolite molecular sieve. Many columns of zeolite are used. Zeolites are hydrated aluminium silicates of the alkaline earth metals.
   b) *True.* The maximum oxygen concentration achieved by oxygen concentrators is 95%. The rest is mainly argon. Using low flows with the circle breathing system can lead to the accumulation of argon. Higher fresh gas flows are required to avoid this.
   c) *True.* The zeolite molecular sieve selectively retains nitrogen and other unwanted gases in air. These are released into the atmosphere. The changeover between columns is made by a time switch.
   d) *False.* Oxygen concentrators can deliver a maximum oxygen concentration of 95%.
   e) *False.* Oxygen concentrators can be small, delivering oxygen to a single patient, or they can be large enough to supply oxygen to hospitals.

5. Oxygen:
   a) *True.* Molybdenum steel or aluminium alloy cylinders are used to store oxygen at pressures of approximately 14 000 kVa (140 bars).
   b) *False.* The critical temperature of O_2 is −118°C. Above that temperature, oxygen cannot be liquefied however much pressure is applied.
   c) *False.* Oxygen is a gas in the cylinder as its critical temperature is −118°C.
   d) *True.* Oil is flammable while oxygen aids combustion.

Oxygen cylinders should be stored away from oil.

e) *True.* At a constant temperature, the volume of a given mass of oxygen varies inversely with the absolute pressure (volume = constant × 1/pressure). Oxygen obeys other gas laws.

6. Concerning cylinders:

a) *True.* The filling ratio is used when filling cylinders with liquid, e.g. nitrous oxide. As the liquid is less compressible than the gas, the cylinder should be only partially filled. Depending on the ambient temperature, the filling ratio can be from 0.67 to 0.75.

b) *False.* The tare weight is the weight of the empty cylinder. This is used to estimate the amount of the contents of the cylinder. It is one of the marks engraved on the cylinders.

c) *False.* Nitrous oxide cylinders have a blue body and top. Entonox cylinders have a blue body and blue and white top.

d) *True.*

e) *False.* At 40°C, nitrous oxide exists as a gas only. This is above its critical temperature, 36.5°C, so it cannot be liquefied above that.

7. Concerning piped gas supply in the operating theatre:

a) *False.* Air is supplied at two different pressures; at 400 kVa when it is delivered to the patient and at 700 kPa when used to operate power tools in the operating theatre.

b) *True.* This stands for non-interchangeable screw thread. This is one of the safety features present in the piped gas supply system. Flexible colour-coded hoses connect the outlets to the anaesthetic machine. The connections to the anaesthetic machine should be permanently fixed using a nut and liner union where the thread is gas-specific and non-interchangeable.

c) *False.* Oxygen, nitrous oxide, air and vacuum can be supplied by the piped gas system.

d) *False.* Larger cylinders, e.g. J size, are normally used in a cylinder manifold. E-size cylinders are usually mounted on the anaesthetic machine.

e) *False.* Liquid oxygen has to be stored at temperatures below its critical temperature, −118°C. So oxygen stored at temperatures above −100°C (above its critical temperature) exists as a gas.

8. True or false:

a) *False.* Cylinders should be checked regularly by the manufacturers. Internal endoscopic examination, pressure testing, flattening, bending and impact testing and tensile testing are done on a regular basis.

b) *False.* To identify the agent, the name, chemical symbol, pharmaceutical form and specification of the agent, in addition to the colour of the cylinder are used.

c) *True.* When attached to an anaesthetic machine, the cylinder valve should be opened slowly to prevent the rapid rise in pressure within the machine's pipelines.

d) *True.* It is more economical to store oxygen as liquid before supplying it. At a temperature of 15°C and atmospheric pressure, liquid oxygen can give 842 times its volume as gas.

e) *False.* For ease of transport, cylinders are made of thin-walled seamless molybdenum steel. They are designed to withstand considerable internal pressures and tested up to pressures of about 22 000 kPa.

9. b)

Chapter 2

The anaesthetic machine

The anaesthetic machine receives medical gases (oxygen, nitrous oxide, air) under pressure and accurately controls the flow of each gas individually. A gas mixture of the desired composition at a defined flow rate is created before a known concentration of an inhalational agent vapour is added. Gas and vapour mixtures are continuously delivered to the common gas outlet of the machine, as fresh gas flow (FGF), and to the breathing sytem and patient (Figs 2.1 and 2.2). It consists of:

1. gas supplies (see Chapter 1)
2. pressure gauges
3. pressure regulators (reducing valves)
4. flowmeters
5. vaporizers
6. common gas outlet
7. a variety of other features, e.g. high-flow oxygen flush, pressure relief valve and oxygen supply failure alarm and suction apparatus
8. most modern anaesthetic machines or stations incorporate a circle breathing system (see Chapter 4) and a bag-in-bottle type ventilator (see Chapter 8).

Safety features of a modern anaesthetic machine to ensure the delivery of a safe gas mixture should include the following:

- Colour-coded pressure gauges.
- Colour-coded flowmeters.
- An oxygen flowmeter controlled by a single touch-coded knob.
- Oxygen is the last gas to be added to the mixture.
- Oxygen concentration monitor or analyser.
- Nitrous oxide is cut off when the oxygen pressure is low.
- Oxygen : nitrous oxide ratio monitor and controller.
- Pin index safety system for cylinders and non-interchangeable screw thread (NIST) for pipelines.
- Alarm for failure of oxygen supply.
- Ventilator disconnection alarm.
- At least one reserve oxygen cylinder should be available on machines that use pipeline supply.

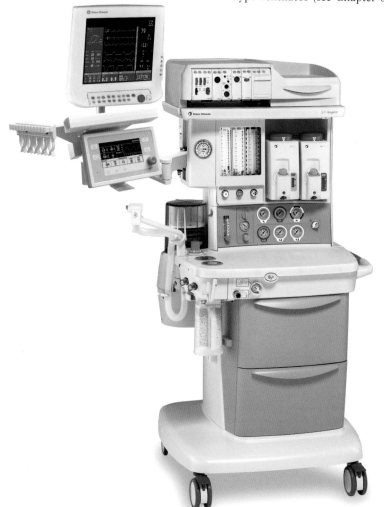

Fig. 2.1 The Datex-Ohmeda Aestiva S/5 anaesthetic machine.

Pressure gauge

This measures the pressure in the cylinder or pipeline. The pressure gauges for oxygen, nitrous oxide and medical air are mounted in a front-facing panel on the anaesthetic machine (Fig. 2.3).

Some modern anaesthetic machine designs have a digital display of the gas supply pressures (Fig. 2.4).

Components

1. A robust, flexible and coiled tube which is oval in cross-section (Fig. 2.5). It should be able to withstand the sudden high pressure when the cylinder is switched on.

2. The tube is sealed at its inner end and connected to a needle pointer which moves over a dial.
3. The other end of the tube is exposed to the gas supply.

Mechanism of action

1. The high-pressure gas causes the tube to uncoil (Bourdon gauge).

2. The movement of the tube causes the needle pointer to move on the calibrated dial indicating the pressure.

Problems in practice and safety features

1. Each pressure gauge is colour-coded and calibrated for a particular gas or vapour. The pressure measured indicates the contents available in an oxygen cylinder. Oxygen is

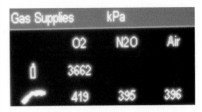

Fig. 2.4 Digital display of pressure gauges for oxygen (cylinder and pipeline), nitrous oxide (pipeline) and air (pipeline).

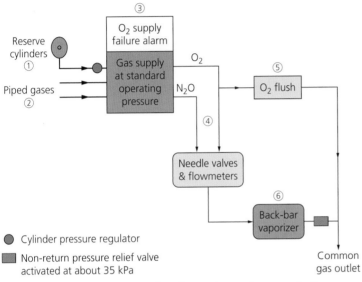

● Cylinder pressure regulator

▨ Non-return pressure relief valve activated at about 35 kPa

Fig. 2.2 Diagrammatic representation of a continuous flow anaesthetic machine. Pressures throughout the system: 1. O_2: 13 700 kPa, N_2O: 4400 kPa; 2. pipeline: about 400 kPa; 3. O_2 supply failure alarm activated at <250 kPa; 4. regulated gas supply at about 400 kPa; 5. O_2: flush 45 L/min at a pressure of about 400 kPa; 6. back-bar pressure 1–10 kPa (depending on flow rate and type of vaporizer).

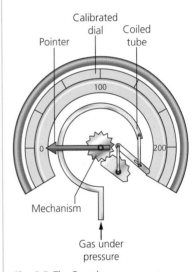

Fig. 2.5 The Bourdon pressure gauge.

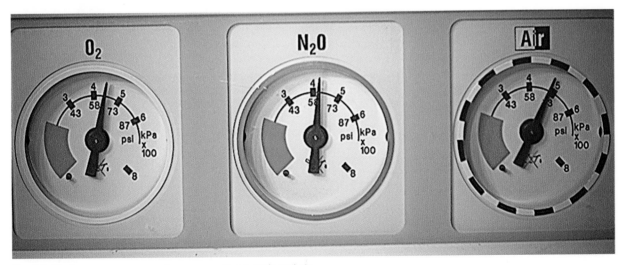

Fig. 2.3 Pipeline pressure gauges for oxygen, nitrous oxide and air.

stored as a gas and obeys Boyle's gas law (pressure × volume = constant). This is not the case in a nitrous oxide cylinder since it is stored as a liquid and vapour.

2. A pressure gauge designed for pipelines should not be used to measure cylinder pressure and vice versa. This leads to inaccuracies and/or damage to the pressure gauge.

3. Should the coiled tube rupture, the gas vents from the back of the pressure gauge casing. The face of the pressure gauge is made of heavy glass as an additional safety feature.

> ### *Pressure gauge*
> - Measures pressure in cylinder or pipeline.
> - Pressure acts to straighten a coiled tube.
> - Colour-coded and calibrated for a particular gas or vapour.

Pressure regulator (reducing valve)

Pressure regulators are used because:

- Gas and vapour are stored under high pressure in cylinders. A regulator reduces the variable cylinder pressure to a constant safer operating pressure of about 400 kPa (just below the pipeline pressure) (Fig. 2.6).
- The temperature and pressure of the cylinder contents decrease with use. In order to maintain flow, constant adjustment is required in the absence of regulators.
- Regulators protect the components of the anaesthetic machine against pressure surges.

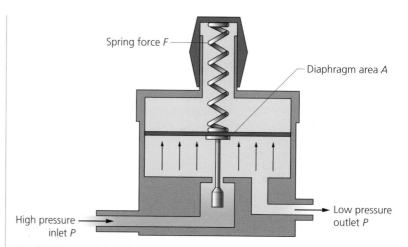

Fig. 2.6 The principles of a pressure regulator (reducing valve).

- The use of pressure regulators allows low-pressure piping and connectors to be used in the machine. This makes the consequences of any gas leak much less serious.

They are positioned between the cylinders and the rest of the anaesthetic machine (Figs 2.7 and 2.8).

Components

1. An inlet, with a filter, leading to a high-pressure chamber with a valve.
2. This valve leads to a low-pressure chamber and outlet.
3. A diaphragm attached to a spring is situated in the low-pressure chamber.

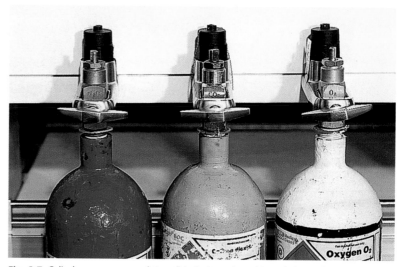

Fig. 2.7 Cylinder pressure regulators (black domes) positioned above the cylinder yokes in the Datex-Ohmeda Flexima anaesthetic machine.

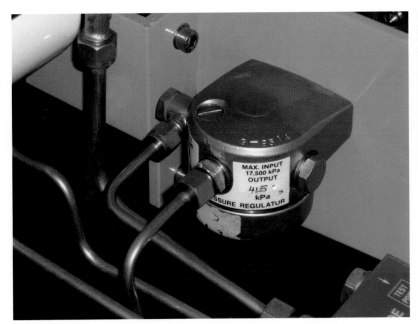

Fig. 2.8 Cylinder pressure regulator (the machine's tray has been removed).

Mechanism of action

1. Gas enters the high-pressure chamber and passes into the low-pressure chamber via the valve.
2. The force exerted by the high-pressure gas tries to close the valve. The opposing force of the diaphragm and spring tries to open the valve. A balance is reached between the two opposing forces. This maintains a gas flow under a constant pressure of about 400 kPa.

Problems in practice and safety features

1. Formation of ice inside the regulator can occur. If the cylinder contains water vapour, this may condense and freeze as a result of the heat lost when gas expands on entry into the low-pressure chamber.
2. The diaphragm can rupture.
3. Relief valves (usually set at 700 kPa) are fitted downstream

of the regulators and allow the escape of gas should the regulators fail.
4. A one-way valve is positioned within the cylinder supply line. This prevents backflow and loss of gas from the pipeline supplies should a cylinder not be connected. This one-way valve may be incorporated into the design of the pressure regulator.

Pressure regulator
- Reduces pressure of gases from cylinders to about 400 kPa (similar to pipeline pressure).
- Allows fine control of gas flow and protects the anaesthetic machine from high pressures.
- A balance between two opposing forces maintains a constant operating pressure.

Second-stage regulators and flow restrictors

The control of pipeline pressure surges can be achieved either by using a second-stage pressure regulator or a flow restrictor (Fig. 2.9) – a constriction, between the pipeline supply and the rest of the anaesthetic machine. A lower pressure (100–200 kPa) is achieved. If there are only flow restrictors and no regulators in the pipeline supply, adjustment of the flowmeter controls is usually necessary whenever there is change in pipeline pressure.

Flow restrictors may also be used downstream of vaporizers to prevent back pressure effect (see later).

One-way valve or backflow check valves

These valves are usually placed next to the inlet yoke. Their function is to prevent loss or leakage of gas from an empty yoke. They also prevent accidental transfilling between paired cylinders.

Flow control (needle) valves

These valves control the flow through the flowmeters by manual

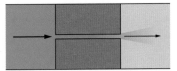

Fig. 2.9 A flow restrictor. The constriction causes a significant pressure drop when there is a high gas flow rate.

adjustment. They are positioned at the base of the associated flowmeter tube (Fig. 2.10). Increasing the flow of a gas is achieved by turning the valve in an anticlockwise direction.

Components

1. The body, made of brass, screws into the base of the flowmeter.
2. The stem screws into the body and ends in a needle. It has screw threads allowing fine adjustment.
3. The flow control knobs are labelled and colour-coded.
4. A flow control knob guard is fitted in some designs to protect against accidental adjustment in the flowmeters.

Flowmeters

Flowmeters measure the flow rate of a gas passing through them. They are individually calibrated for each gas. Calibration occurs at room temperature and atmospheric pressure (sea level). They have an accuracy of about ±2.5%. For flows above 1 L/min, the units are L/min, and for flows below that, the units are 100 mL/min (Fig. 2.11).

Components

1. A flow control (needle) valve.
2. A tapered (wider at the top), transparent plastic or glass tube.
3. A lightweight rotating bobbin or ball. Bobbin-stops at either end of the tube ensure that it is always visible to the operator at extremes of flow.

Mechanism of action

1. When the needle valve is opened, gas is free to enter the tapered tube.

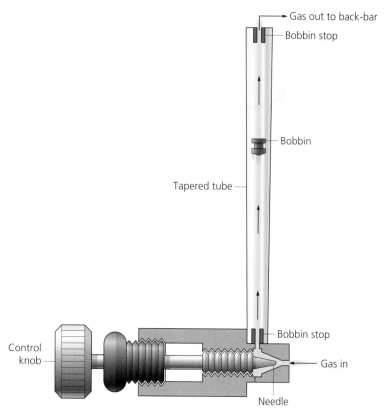

Fig. 2.10 A flow control (needle) valve and flowmeter.

2. The bobbin is held floating within the tube by the gas flow passing around it. The higher the flow rate, the higher the bobbin rises within the tube.
3. The effect of gravity on the bobbin is counteracted by the gas flow. A constant pressure difference across the bobbin exists as it floats.
4. The clearance between the bobbin and the tube wall widens as the gas flow increases (Fig. 2.12).
5. At low flow rates, the clearance is longer and narrower, thus acting as a tube. Under these circumstances, the flow is laminar and a function of gas viscosity (Poiseuille's law).
6. At high flow rates, the clearance is shorter and wider, thus acting

as an orifice. Here, the flow is turbulent and a function of gas density.
7. The top of the bobbin has slits (flutes) cut into its side. As gas flows past it, the slits cause the bobbin to rotate. A dot on the bobbin indicates to the operator that the bobbin is rotating and not stuck.
8. The reading of the flowmeter is taken from the top of the bobbin (Fig. 2.13). When a ball is used, the reading is generally taken from the midpoint of the ball.
9. When very low flows are required, e.g. in the circle breathing system, an arrangement of two flowmeters in series is used. One flowmeter reads a maximum of 1 L/min allowing fine adjustment of the

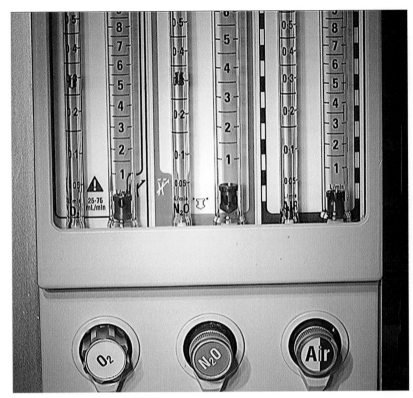

Fig. 2.11 A flowmeter panel.

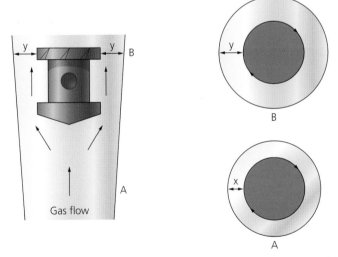

Fig. 2.12 Mechanism of action of the flowmeter. As the bobbin rises from A to B, the clearance increases (from x to y).

flow. One flow control per gas is needed for both flowmeters (Fig. 2.14).

10. There is a stop on the oxygen flow control valve to ensure a minimum oxygen flow of 200–300 mL/min past the needle valve. This ensures that the oxygen flow cannot be discontinued completely.

Problems in practice and safety features

1. The flow control knobs are colour-coded for their respective gases. The oxygen control knob is situated to the left (in the UK) and, in some designs, is larger with larger ridges and has a longer stem than the other control knobs, making it easily recognizable (Fig. 2.15). In the USA and Canada, the oxygen control knob is situated to the right.

2. The European Standard for anaesthetic machines (EN 740) requires them to have the means to prevent the delivery of a gas mixture with an oxygen concentration below 25%. Current designs make it impossible for nitrous oxide to be delivered without the addition of a fixed percentage of oxygen. This is achieved by using interactive oxygen and nitrous oxide controls. This helps to prevent the possibility of delivering a hypoxic mixture to the patient. In the mechanical system, two gears are connected together by a precision stainless steel link chain. One gear with 14 teeth is fixed on the nitrous oxide flow control valve spindle. The other gear has 29 teeth and can rotate the oxygen flow control valve spindle, rather like a nut rotating on a bolt. For every 2.07 revolutions of the nitrous oxide flow control knob, the oxygen knob and spindle set to the lowest oxygen flow will rotate once. Because the gear on the oxygen flow control is mounted like a nut on a bolt, oxygen flow can be adjusted independently of nitrous oxide flow.

3. A crack in a flowmeter may result in a hypoxic mixture (Fig. 2.16). To avoid this, oxygen

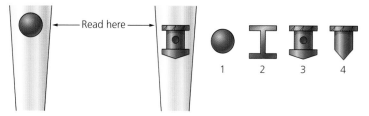

Fig. 2.13 Reading a flowmeter (top). Different types of bobbin: 1. ball; 2. non-rotating H float; 3. skirted; 4. non-skirted.

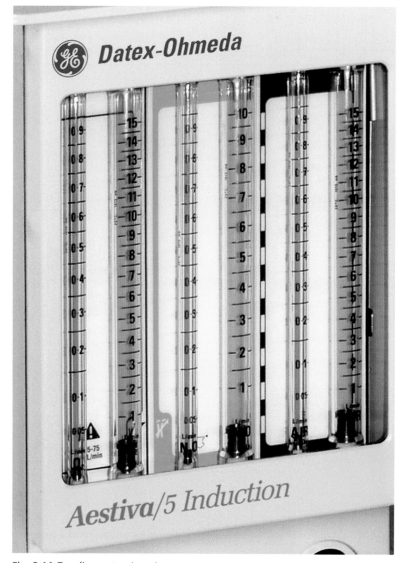

Fig. 2.14 Two flowmeters in series.

is the last gas to be added to the mixture delivered to the back bar.

4. Flow measurements can become inaccurate if the bobbin sticks to the inside wall of the flowmeter. The commonest causes are:
   a) dirt: this is a problem at low flow rates when the clearance is narrow. The source of the dirt is usually a contaminated gas supply. Filters, acting before gas enters the flowmeters, will remove the dirt
   b) static electricity: the charge usually builds up over a period of time, leading to inaccuracies of up to 35%. Using antistatic materials in flowmeter construction helps to eliminate any build-up of charge. Application of antistatic spray removes any charge present.
5. Flowmeters are designed to be read in a vertical position, so any change in the position of the machine can affect the accuracy.
6. Pressure rises at the common gas outlet are transmitted back to the gas above the bobbin. This results in a drop in the level of the bobbin with an inaccurate reading. This can happen with minute volume divider ventilators as back pressure is exerted as they cycle with inaccuracies of up to 10%. A flow restrictor is fitted downstream of the flowmeters to prevent this occurring.
7. Accidents have resulted from failure to see the bobbin clearly at the extreme ends of the tube. This can be prevented by illuminating the flowmeter bank and installing a wire stop at the top to prevent the bobbin reaching the top of the tube.
8. If facilities for the use of carbon dioxide are fitted to the machine, the flowmeter is designed to allow a maximum of 500 mL/min to be added to the FGF. This ensures that dangerous levels of hypercarbia are avoided.
9. Highly accurate computer controlled gas mixers are available.

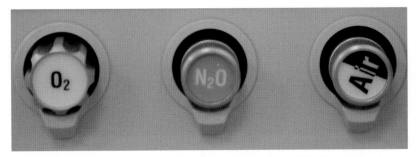

Fig. 2.15 Flow control knobs. Note the colour-coding and the distinctive-shape oxygen control knob.

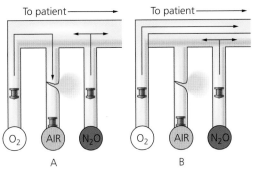

Fig. 2.16 (A) A broken air flowmeter allows oxygen to escape and a hypoxic mixture to be delivered from the back bar. (B) A possible design measure to prevent this.

Flowmeter
- Both laminar and turbulent flows are encountered, making both the viscosity and density of the gas relevant.
- The bobbin should not stick to the tapered tube.
- Oxygen is the last gas to be added to the mixture.
- It is very accurate with an error margin of ±2.5%.

Vaporizers

A vaporizer is designed to add a controlled amount of an inhalational agent, after changing it from liquid to vapour, to the FGF. This is normally expressed as a percentage of saturated vapour added to the gas flow.

Characteristics of the ideal vaporizer

1. Its performance is not affected by changes in FGF, volume of the liquid agent, ambient temperature and pressure, decrease in temperature due to vaporization and pressure fluctuation due to the mode of respiration.
2. Low resistance to flow.
3. Light weight with small liquid requirement.
4. Economy and safety in use with minimal servicing requirements.
5. Corrosion- and solvent-resistant construction.

Vaporizers can be classified according to location:

1. Inside the breathing system. Gases pass through a very low resistance, draw-over vaporizer due to the patient's respiratory efforts (e.g. Goldman, Oxford Miniature Vaporizer; OMV). Such vaporizers are simple in design, light in weight, agent non-specific, i.e. allowing the use of any volatile agent, small and inexpensive. For these reasons, they are used in the 'field' or in otherwise difficult environments. However, they are not as efficient as the plenum vaporizers as their performance is affected as the temperature of the anaesthetic agent decreases due to loss of latent heat during vaporization.
2. Outside the breathing system. Gases are driven through a plenum (high resistance, unidirectional and agent specific) vaporizer due to gas supply pressure.

PLENUM VAPORIZER (FIG. 2.17)

Components

1. The case with the filling level indicator and a port for the filling device.
2. Percentage control dial on top of the case.
3. The bypass channel and the vaporization chamber. The latter has wicks or baffles to increase the surface area available for vaporization (Fig. 2.18).
4. The splitting ratio is controlled by a temperature-sensitive valve utilizing a bimetallic strip (Fig. 2.19). The latter is made of two strips of metal with different coefficients of thermal expansion bonded together. It is positioned inside the vaporization chamber in the Tec Mk 2 whereas in Tec Mk 3, 4 and 5, it is outside the vaporization chamber. An ether-filled bellows is the temperature compensating device in the M&IE Vapamasta Vaporizer 5 and 6. The bellows

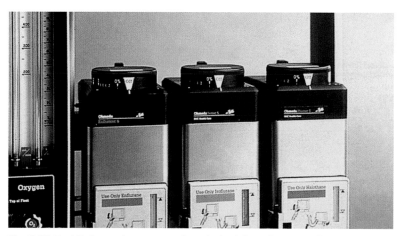

Fig. 2.17 Tec Mk 5 vaporizers mounted on the back bar of an anaesthetic machine.

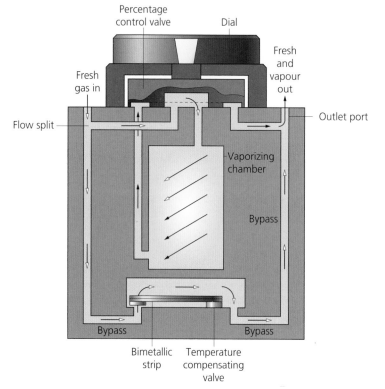

Fig. 2.18 A schematic diagram of the Tec Mk 5, an example of a plenum vaporizer.

vaporizer when it is switched on (Fig. 2.22).

Mechanism of action

1. The calibration of each vaporizer is agent-specific.
2. Fresh gas flow is split into two streams on entering the vaporizer. One stream flows through the bypass channel and the other, smaller stream, flows through the vaporizing chamber. The two gas streams reunite as the gas leaves the vaporizer.
3. The vaporization chamber is designed so that the gas leaving it is always fully saturated with vapour before it rejoins the bypass gas stream. This should be achieved despite changes in the FGF.
4. Full saturation with vapour is achieved by increasing the surface area of contact between the carrier gas and the anaesthetic agent. This is achieved by having wicks saturated by the inhalational agent, a series of baffles or by bubbling the gas through the liquid.
5. The desired concentration is obtained by adjusting the percentage control dial. This alters the amount of gas flowing through the bypass channel to that flowing through the vaporization chamber.
6. In the modern designs, the vapour concentration supplied by the vaporizer is virtually independent of the FGFs between 0.5 and 15 L/min.
7. During vaporization, cooling occurs due to the loss of latent heat of vaporization. Lowering the temperature of the agent makes it less volatile. In order to compensate for temperature changes:
   a) the vaporizer is made of a material with high density and

contracts as the temperature of the vaporizer decreases.
5. The vaporizers are mounted on the back bar (Fig. 2.20) using the interlocking Selectatec system (Fig. 2.21). The percentage control dial cannot be moved unless the locking lever of the system is engaged (in Mk 4 and 5). The interlocking extension rods prevent more than one vaporizer being used at any one time, preventing contamination of the one downstream (in Mk 4 and 5). The FGF only enters the

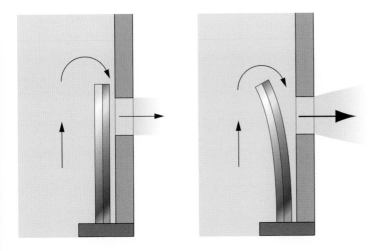

Fig. 2.19 Mechanism of action of a bimetallic strip.

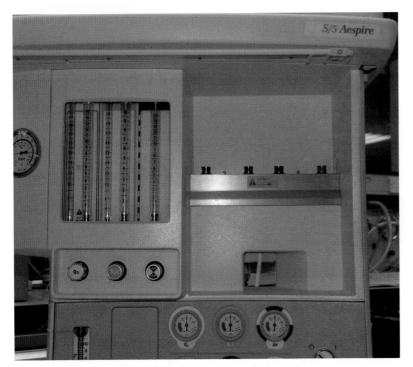

Fig. 2.20 An empty Selectatec back bar of an anaesthetic machine.

high specific heat capacity with a very high thermal conductivity, e.g. copper. Copper acts as a heat sink, readily giving heat to the anaesthetic agent and maintaining its temperature

b) a temperature sensitive valve (e.g. bimetallic strip or bellows) within the body of the vaporizer automatically adjusts the splitting ratio according to the temperature. It allows more flow into the vaporizing chamber as the temperature decreases.

8. The amount of vapour carried by the FGF is a function of both the saturated vapour pressure (SVP) of the agent and the atmospheric pressure. At high altitudes, the atmospheric pressure is reduced whereas the SVP remains the same. This leads to an increased amount of vapour whereas the saturation of the agent remains the same. The opposite occurs in hyperbaric chambers. This is of no clinical relevance as it is the partial pressure of the agent in the alveoli that determines the clinical effect of the agent.

Problems in practice and safety features

1. In modern vaporizers (Tec Mk 5), the liquid anaesthetic agent does not enter the bypass channel even if the vaporizer is tipped upside down due to an antispill mechanism. In earlier designs, dangerously high concentrations of anaesthetic agent could be delivered to the patient in cases of agent spillage into the bypass channel. Despite that, it is recommended that the vaporizer is purged with a FGF of 5 L/min for 30 min with the percentage control dial set at 5%.

2. The Selectatec system increases the potential for leaks. This is due to the risk of accidental removal of the O-rings with changes of vaporizers.

3. Minute volume divider ventilators exert back pressure as they cycle. This pressure forces some of the gas exiting the outlet port back into the vaporizing chamber, where more vapour is added. Retrograde flow may also contaminate the bypass channel. These effects cause an increase in the inspired concentration of the agent which may be toxic. These pressure fluctuations can be compensated for by:

a) long inlet port into the vaporizing chamber as in

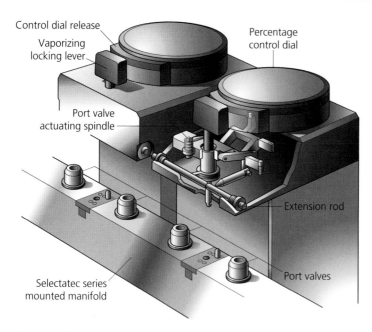

Fig. 2.21 The Selectatec vaporizer interlock mechanism. See text for details. (Reproduced with permission from Datex-Ohmeda.)

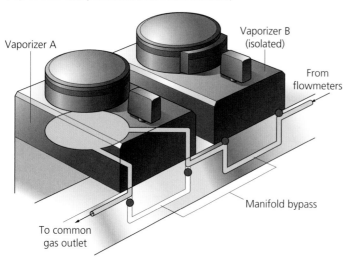

Fig. 2.22 The Selectatec series mounted manifold bypass circuit. Only when a vaporizer is locked in position and turned on can fresh gas enter. Vaporizer B is turned off and is isolated from the fresh gas which only enters vaporizer A which is turned on. If no vaporizer is fitted, the port valves are closed. (Reproduced with permission from Datex-Ohmeda.)

Tec Mk 3. This ensures that the bypass channel is not contaminated by retrograde flow from the vaporizing chamber

b) downstream flow restrictors: used to maintain the vaporizer at a pressure greater than any pressure required to operate commonly used ventilators

c) both the bypass channel and the vaporizing chamber are of equal volumes so gas expansion and compression are equal.

4. Preservatives, such as thymol in halothane, accumulate on the wicks of vaporizers with time. Large quantities may interfere with the function of the vaporizer. Thymol can also cause the bimetallic strip in the Tec Mk 2 to stick. Enflurane and isoflurane do not contain preservative.

5. A pressure relief valve downstream of the vaporizer opens at about 35 kPa. This prevents damage to flowmeters or vaporizers if the common gas outlet is blocked.

6. The bimetallic strip has been situated in the bypass channel since the Tec Mk 3. It is possible for the chemically active strip to corrode in a mixture of oxygen and the inhalational agent within the vaporizing chamber (Tec Mk 2).

Vaporizers
- The case is made of copper which is a good heat sink.
- Consists of a bypass channel and vaporization chamber. The latter has wicks to increase the surface area available for vaporization.
- A temperature-sensitive valve controls the splitting ratio. It is positioned outside the vaporizing chamber in Tec Mk 3, 4 and 5.
- The gas leaving the vaporizing chamber is fully saturated.
- The effect of back pressure is compensated for.

Vaporizer filling devices

These are agent-specific being geometrically coded (keyed) to fit the safety filling port of the correct vaporizer and anaesthetic agent supply bottle (Fig. 2.23). They prevent the risk of adding the wrong agent to the wrong vaporizer and decrease the extent of spillage. The safety filling system, in

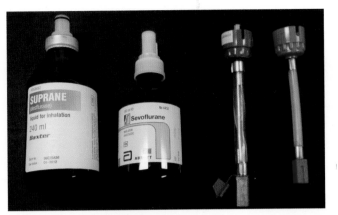

Fig. 2.23 Agent-specific, colour-coded filling devices; (left to right) desflurane, sevoflourane, isoflurane and enflurane.

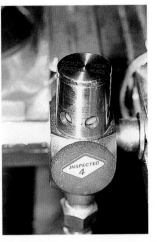

Fig. 2.24 A non-return pressure relief valve situated at the end of the back bar.

addition, ensures that the vaporizer cannot overflow. Fillers used for desflurane and sevoflurane have valves that are only opened when fully inserted into their ports. This prevents spillage.

The fillers are colour-coded:

Red   Halothane
Orange Enflurane
Purple   Isoflurane
Yellow Sevoflurane
Blue   Desflurane

A more recent design feature is the antipollution cap allowing the filler to be left fitted to the bottle between uses to prevent the agent from vaporizing. It also eliminates air locks, speeding up vaporizer filling, and ensures that the bottle is completely emptied, reducing wastage.

Non-return pressure relief safety valve

This is situated downstream of the vaporizers either on the back bar itself or near the common gas outlet (Fig. 2.24).

1. Its non-return design helps to prevent back pressure effects

commonly encountered using minute volume divider ventilators.
2. It opens when the pressure in the back bar exceeds about 35 kPa. Flowmeter and vaporizer components can be damaged at higher pressures.

Emergency oxygen flush

This is usually activated by a non-locking button (Fig. 2.25).

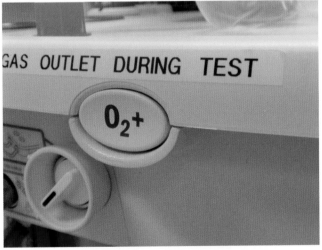

GAS OUTLET DURING TEST

O₂+

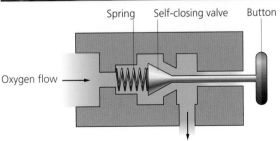

Fig. 2.25 The emergency oxygen flush button (above); its mechanism of action (below).

When pressed, pure oxygen is supplied from the outlet of the anaesthetic machine. The flow bypasses the flowmeters and the vaporizers. A flow of about 35–75 L/min at a pressure of about 400 kPa is expected. The emergency oxygen flush is usually activated by a non-locking button and using a self-closing valve. It is designed to minimize unintended and accidental operation by staff or other equipment. The button is recessed in a housing to prevent accidental depression.

Problems in practice and safety features

1. The high operating pressure and flow of the oxygen flush puts the patient at a higher risk of barotrauma.
2. When the emergency oxygen flush is used inappropriately, it leads to dilution of the anaesthetic gases and possible awareness.
3. It should not be activated while ventilating a patient using a minute volume divider ventilator.

Compressed oxygen outlet(s)

One or more compressed oxygen outlets used to provide oxygen at about 400 kPa (Fig. 2.26). It can be used to drive ventilators or a manually controlled jet injector.

Oxygen supply failure alarm

There are many designs available (Fig. 2.27) but the characteristics of the ideal warning device are:

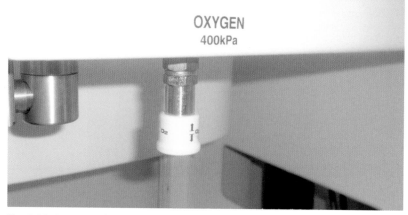

Fig. 2.26 Compressed oxygen outlet.

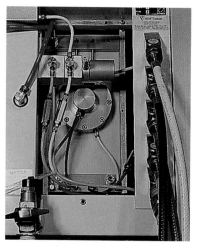

Fig. 2.27 The oxygen supply failure alarm in the Datex-Ohmeda Flexima anaesthetic machine.

1. Activation depends on the pressure of oxygen itself.
2. It requires no batteries or mains power.
3. It gives an audible signal of a special character and of sufficient duration and volume to attract attention.
4. It should give a warning of impending failure and a further alarm that failure has occurred.
5. It should have pressure-linked controls which interrupt the flow of all other gases when it comes into operation. Atmospheric air is allowed to be delivered to the patient, without carbon dioxide accumulation. It should be impossible to resume anaesthesia until the oxygen supply has been restored.
6. The alarm should be positioned on the reduced pressure side of the oxygen supply line.
7. It should be tamper proof.
8. It is not affected by backpressure from the anaesthetic ventilator.

In modern machines, if the oxygen supply pressure falls below 200 kPa, the low-pressure supply alarm sounds. With supply pressures below 137 kPa, the 'fail safe' valve will interrupt the flow of other gases to their flowmeters so that only oxygen can be delivered (Fig. 2.28). The oxygen flow set on the oxygen flowmeter will not decrease until the oxygen supply pressure falls below 100 kPa.

Anti-hypoxic safety features

These features are designed to prevent the delivery of gaseous mixtures with oxygen concentrations of less than 25%. This can be achieved by:

- *Mechanical means*: a chain links the oxygen and nitrous oxide flow control valves. Increasing the flow rate of nitrous oxide leads to a proportional increase in oxygen flow rate.
- *Pneumatic means*: a pressure-sensitive diaphragm measuring the changes in oxygen and nitrous oxide concentrations.
- *A paramagnetic oxygen analyser* continuously measuring the oxygen concentration. Nitrous oxide flow is switched off automatically when oxygen concentration falls under 25%.

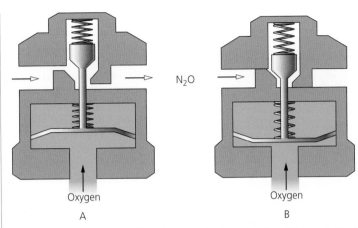

Fig. 2.28 Oxygen supply failure alarm mechanism of action. (A) O_2 pressure is higher than 200 kPa so allowing N_2O flow (blue). (B) O_2 pressure is lower than 200 kPa so cutting off N_2O flow.

Common gas outlet (Fig. 2.29)

This is where the anaesthetic machine 'ends'. At the common gas outlet, the gas mixture made at the flowmeters, plus any inhaled anaesthetic agent added by the vaporizer, exits the machine and enters the fresh gas tubing that conducts it to the breathing system. The common gas outlet is a conically tapered pipe with a 22 mm male/15 mm female. It can be fixed or on a swivelling connector. The connector of the common gas outlet should be strong enough to withstand a torque of up to 10 Nm because of the heavy equipment that may be attached.

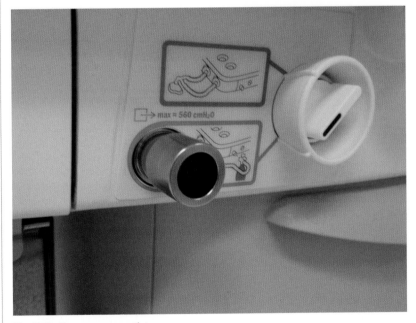

Fig. 2.29 Common gas outlet.

Other modifications and designs

1. Desflurane vaporizer (Figs 2.30 and 2.31). Desflurane is an inhalational agent with unique physical properties making it extremely volatile. Its SVP is 664 mmHg at 20°C and, with a boiling point of 23.5°C at atmospheric pressure which is only slightly above normal room temperature, precludes the use of a normal variable-bypass type vaporizer. In order to overcome these physical properties, vaporizers with a completely different design from the previous Tec series are used despite the similar appearance.

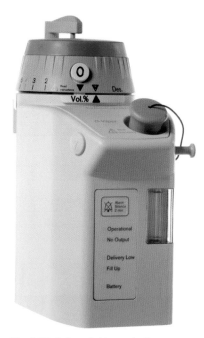

Fig. 2.30 Dräger D Vapor desflurane vaporizer. (Courtesy of Dräger.)

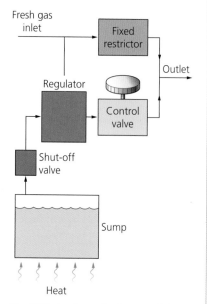

Fig. 2.31 A schematic diagram of the Tec Mk 6 vaporizer. (Reproduced with permission from Datex-Ohmeda.)

They are mounted on the Selectatec system.

a) An electrically heated desflurane vaporization chamber (sump) with a capacity of 450 mL. The chamber requires a warm-up period of 5–10 minutes to reach its operating temperature of 39°C (i.e. above its boiling point) and a SVP of more than 1550 mmHg (about two atmospheric pressures). The vaporizer will not function below this temperature and pressure.

b) A fixed restriction/orifice is positioned in the FGF path. The FGF does not enter the vaporization chamber. Instead, the FGF enters the path of the regulated concentration of desflurane vapour before the resulting gas mixture is delivered to the patient.

c) A differential pressure transducer adjusts a pressure-regulating valve at the outlet of the vaporization chamber. The transducer senses pressure at the fixed restriction on one side and the pressure of desflurane vapour upstream to the pressure-regulating valve on the other side. This transducer ensures that the pressure of desflurane vapour upstream of the control valve equals the pressure of fresh gas flow at the fixed restriction.

d) A percentage control dial with a rotary valve adjusts a second resistor which controls the flow of desflurane vapour into the FGF and thus the output concentration. The dial calibration is from 0% to 18%.

e) The fixed restriction/orifice ensures that the pressure of the carrier gas within the vaporizer is proportional to gas flow. The transducer ensures that the pressure of desflurane vapour upstream of the resistor equals pressure of FGF at the orifice. This means that the flow of desflurane out of the vaporizing chamber is proportional to the FGF, so enabling the output concentration to be made independent of FGF rate.

f) The vaporizer incorporates malfunction alarms (auditory and visual). There is a back-up 9-volt battery should there be a mains failure.

2. Since most of the anaesthetic machine is made from metal, it should not be used close to magnetic resonance imaging (MRI) scanner. Distorted readings and physical damage to the scanner are possible because of the attraction of the strong magnetic fields. Newly designed anaesthetic machines made of totally non-ferrous material solve this problem (Fig. 2.32).

3. Newly designed anaesthetic machines are more sophisticated than that described above. Many important components have become electrically or electronically controlled as an integrated system (Fig. 2.33). Thermistors can be used to measure the flow of gases. Gas flow causes changes in temperature which are measured by the thermistors. Changes in temperature are calibrated to measure flows of gases. Other designs measure flows using electronic flow sensors based on the principle of the pneumotachograph. Pressure difference is measured across a laminar flow resistor through which the gas flows. Using a differential pressure transducer, flow is measured and displayed on a screen in the form of a virtual graduated flowmeter, together with a digital display.

In the Dräger Zeus IE workstation, the anaesthetist

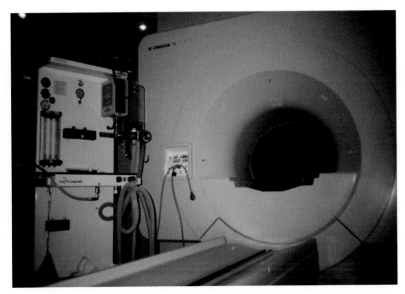

Fig. 2.32 A non-ferrous MRI compatible anaesthetic machine.

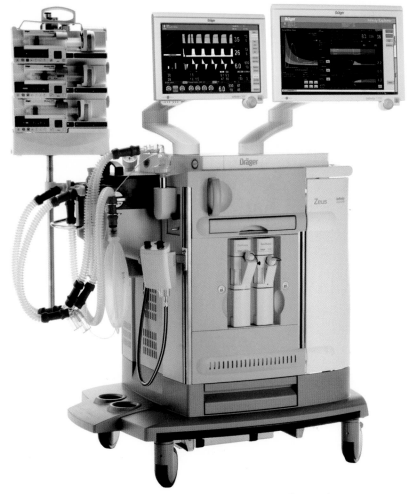

Fig. 2.33 Dräger Zeus IE anaesthetic workstation. (Courtesy of Dräger.)

sets the FiO_2 and end-tidal anaesthetic agent concentration. The system then works to achieve these targets in the quickest and safest way. Direct injectors are used instead of the traditional vaporizers. This allows direct injection of the inhalational agent into the breathing system. This in turn allows for rapid changes in the inhalational agent concentration independent of the FGF. The workstation also has a number of pumps allowing intravenous infusion when required.

4. Quantiflex Anaesthetic Machine (Fig. 2.34). This machine has the following features:
   a) Two flowmeters, one for oxygen and one for nitrous oxide, with one control knob for both flowmeters.
   b) The oxygen flowmeter is situated to the right, whereas the nitrous oxide flowmeter is situated to the left.
   c) The relative concentrations of oxygen and nitrous oxide are adjusted by a mixture control wheel. The oxygen concentration can be adjusted

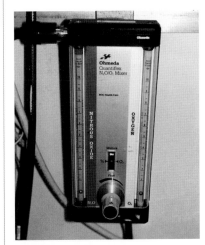

Fig. 2.34 Quantiflex Anaesthetic Machine.

in 10% steps from 30% to 100%.
d) This design prevents the delivery of hypoxic mixtures.
e) It is mainly used in dental anaesthesia.
Some newly designed anaesthetic machines have an extra outlet with its own flowmeter to deliver oxygen to conscious or lightly sedated patients via a face mask. This can be used in patients undergoing surgery under regional anaesthesia with sedation.

5. Universal Anaesthesia Machine (UAM) (Figs 1.23 and 2.35). This was developed to enable the provision of anaesthesia in poorly resourced countries where compressed gases and electricity supplies are unreliable.

The UAM differs from standard anaesthetic machines by the use of an electrically powered oxygen concentrator (producing 10 L/min of 95% oxygen), drawover vaporizer, bellows and balloon valve. The UAM can function in both continuous flow and drawover modes, entraining air as necessary (e.g. if electricity supply to the concentrator fails), with the vaporizer functioning as normal. Alternatively, oxygen can be provided via cylinder, pipeline or the side emergency inlet. The UAM has two flowmeters, one for oxygen and the other for either nitrous oxide or air. A 2-L reservoir bag is positioned distal to the flowmeters on the back bar. A negative pressure valve allows entrainment of air (if the FGF is

less than the patient's minute ventilation) and a positive pressure relief valve prevents overpressure of the bag.

A low-resistance vaporizer is fitted downstream of the positive pressure valve. Vaporizers calibrated for the use of isoflurane or halothane are available. Distally, the set of silicone bellows (up to 1600 mL) allows manual ventilation through a standard dual limb breathing system. The expiratory valve is sited on the side of the machine, and comprises a long-life silicone balloon housed in a clear plastic tube.

A fuel cell oxygen concentration monitor with a touch-screen display, as well as a safety anti-hypoxic feature, are included in the design.

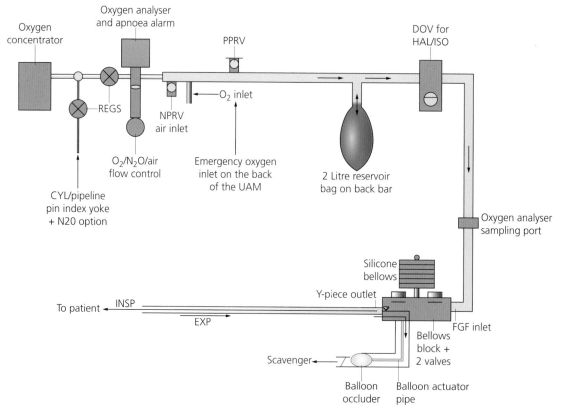

Fig. 2.35 Diagramatic representation of UAM. (Courtesy of UAM Global.)

Anaesthesia in remote areas

The apparatus used must be compact, portable and robust. The Triservice apparatus is suitable for use in remote areas where supply of compressed gases and vapours is difficult (Figs 2.36 and 2.37). The Triservice anaesthetic apparatus name derives from the three military services: Army, Navy and Air Force.

Components

1. A face mask with a non-rebreathing valve fitted.
2. A short length of tubing leading to a self-inflating bag.
3. A second length of tubing leading from the self-inflating bag to two Oxford Miniature Vaporizers (OMV).
4. An oxygen cylinder can be connected upstream of the vaporizers. A third length of tubing acts as an oxygen reservoir during expiration.

Mechanism of action

1. The Triservice apparatus can be used for both spontaneous and controlled ventilation.
   a) The patient can draw air through the vaporizers. The exhaled gases are vented out via the non-rebreathing valve.
   b) The self-inflating bag can be used for controlled or assisted ventilation.
2. The OMV is a draw-over vaporizer with a capacity for 50 mL of anaesthetic agent. The wick is made of metal with no temperature compensation features. There is an ethylene glycol jacket acting as a heat sink to help to stabilize the vaporizer temperature. The calibration scale on the vaporizer can be detached allowing the use of different inhalational agents. A different inhalational agent can be used after blowing air for 10 minutes and rinsing the wicks with the new agent. The vaporizer casing has extendable feet fitted.
3. The downstream vaporizer is traditionally filled with trichloroethylene to compensate for the absence of the analgesic effect of nitrous oxide.

Problems in practice and safety features

1. The vaporizers' heat sink (ethylene glycol jacket) is not suitable for prolonged use at high gas flows. The vapour concentration decreases as the temperature decreases.
2. During use, accidental tipping of the vaporizer can spill liquid agent into the breathing system. The vaporizer is spillproof when turned off.

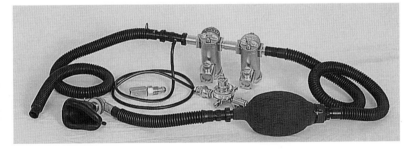

Fig. 2.36 The Triservice apparatus.

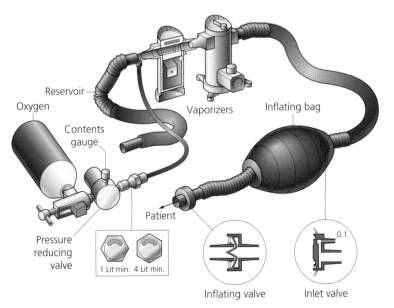

Fig. 2.37 Mechanism of action of the Triservice apparatus.

> ### *Triservice apparatus*
> - Consists of two OMVs, self-inflating bag and non-rebreathing valve.
> - The apparatus is suitable for both spontaneous and controlled breathing.
> - OMV is a draw-over vaporizer with no temperature compensation. It has a heat sink. It can be used with different inhalational agents.

FURTHER READING

Eisenkraft, J.B., 2005. Anaesthesia machine basics. Seminars in Anaesthesia. Perioperative Medicine and Pain 24, 138–146.

MHRA, 2010. Medical device alert: anaesthetic vaporizers – all manufacturers (MDA/2010/052). Online. Available at: http://www.mhra.gov.uk/Publications/Safetywarnings/MedicalDeviceAlerts/CON085024.

MHRA, 2010. Medical device alert: various models of anaesthetic carestations manufactured by GE Healthcare (MDA/2010/058). Online. Available at: http://www.mhra.gov.uk/Publications/Safetywarnings/MedicalDeviceAlerts/CON087755.

MHRA, 2010. Anaesthetic machine e-learning module. Online. Available at: http://www.mhra.gov.uk/ConferencesLearningCentre/LearningCentre/Deviceslearningmodules/Anaestheticmachines/index.htm.

NHS, 2011. Airway suction equipment. Online. Available at: http://www.nrls.npsa.nhs.uk/resources/?entryid45=94845.

MCQs

In the following lists, which of the following statements (a) to (e) are true?

1. Flowmeters in an anaesthetic machine:
   a) N_2O may be used in an O_2 flowmeter without a change in calibration.
   b) Flowmeters use a tube and bobbin.
   c) They are an example of a variable orifice device.
   d) They have a linear scale.
   e) Both laminar and turbulent flows are encountered.

2. Vaporizers:
   a) Manual ventilation using a vaporizer in circle (VIC) causes a reduction in the inspired concentration of the inhalational agent.
   b) A Tec Mark 3 vaporizer can be used as a VIC.
   c) Gas flow emerging from the vaporizing chamber should be fully saturated with the inhalational agent.
   d) The bimetallic strip valve in Tec Mark 5 is in the vaporizing chamber.
   e) The inhalational agent concentration delivered to the patient gradually decreases the longer the vaporizer is used due to cooling of the agent.

3. Pressure gauges on an anaesthetic machine:
   a) Use the Bourdon pressure gauge principle.
   b) The pressure reflects accurately the cylinders' contents for both oxygen and nitrous oxide.
   c) Can be interchangeable between oxygen and nitrous oxide.
   d) The same pressure gauge can be used for both cylinder and pipeline gas supply.
   e) They are colour-coded for a particular gas or vapour.

4. Laminar flow:
   a) It is directly proportional to the square root of pressure.
   b) Halving the radius results in a flow equivalent to a 16th of the original laminar flow.
   c) It is related to the density of the fluid.
   d) The flow is greatest in the centre.
   e) Laminar flow changes to turbulent when Reynold's number exceeds 2000.

5. Flowmeters on an anaesthetic machine:
   a) They have an accuracy of ±2.5%.
   b) They have a tapered tube with a narrow top.
   c) Oxygen is the first gas to be added to the mixture at the back bar.
   d) At high flows, the density of the gas is important in measuring the flow.
   e) The reading of the flow is from the top of the bobbin.

6. Concerning the Triservice apparatus:
   a) Two plenum vaporizers are used.
   b) It can be used for both spontaneous and controlled ventilation.
   c) An inflating bag and a one-way valve are used.
   d) The Oxford Miniature Vaporizer has a metal wick and a heat sink.
   e) Supplementary oxygen can be added to the system.

7. Pressure regulators:
   a) They are only used to reduce the pressure of gases.
   b) They maintain a gas flow at a constant pressure of about 400 kPa.
   c) Their main purpose is to protect the patient.
   d) Relief valves open at 700 kPa in case of failure.
   e) Flow restrictors can additionally be used in pipeline supply.

8. The safety features found in an anaesthetic machine include:
   a) Oxygen supply failure alarm.
   b) Colour-coded flowmeters.
   c) Vaporizer level alarm.
   d) Ventilator disconnection alarm.
   e) Two vaporizers can be safely used at the same time.

9. The non-return valve on the back bar of an anaesthetic machine between the vaporizer and common gas outlet:
   a) Decreases the pumping effect.
   b) Often is incorporated with a pressure relief valve on modern machines.
   c) Is designed to protect the patient.
   d) Is designed to protect the machine.
   e) Opens at a pressure of 70 kPa.

10. The oxygen emergency flush on an anaesthetic machine
    a) Operates at 20 L/min.
    b) Is always safe to use during anaesthesia.
    c) Operates at 40 L/min.
    d) Increases risk of awareness during anaesthesia.
    e) Can be safely used with a minute volume divider ventilator.

SINGLE BEST ANSWER (SBA)

11. Concerning a desflurane vaporizer:
    a) Is ready for use immediately.
    b) Can be used with other inhalational agents.
    c) Needs an electrical supply to function.
    d) Fresh gas flow enters the vaporization chamber.
    e) Is colour-coded red.

Answers

1. Flowmeters in an anaesthetic machine:
   a) *False. The flowmeters in an anaesthetic machine are calibrated for the particular gas(es) used taking into consideration the viscosity and density of the gas(es). N_2O and O_2 have different viscosities and densities so unless the flowmeters are recalibrated, false readings will result.*
   b) *True. They are constant pressure, variable orifice flowmeters. A tapered transparent tube with a lightweight rotating bobbin. The bobbin is held floating in the tube by the gas flow. The clearance between the bobbin and the tube wall widens as the flow increases. The pressure across the bobbin remains constant as the effect of gravity on the bobbin is countered by the gas flow.*
   c) *True. See above.*
   d) *False. The flowmeters do not have a linear scale. There are different scales for low and high flow rates.*
   e) *True. At low flows, the flowmeter acts as a tube, as the clearance between the bobbin and the wall of the tube is longer and narrower. This leads to laminar flow which is dependent on the viscosity (Poiseuille's law). At high flows, the flowmeter acts as an orifice. The clearance is shorter and wider. This leads to turbulent flow which is dependent on density.*

2. Vaporizers:
   a) *False. During manual (or controlled) ventilation using a VIC vaporizer, the inspired concentration of the inhalational agent is increased. It can increase to dangerous concentrations. Unless the concentration of the inhalational agent(s) is measured continuously, this technique is not recommended.*
   b) *False. As the patient is breathing through a VIC vaporizer, it should have very low internal resistance. The Tec Mark 3 has a high internal resistance because of the wicks in the vaporizing chamber.*
   c) *True. This can be achieved by increasing the surface area of contact between the carrier gas and the anaesthetic agent. Full saturation should be achieved despite changes in fresh gas flow. The final concentration is delivered to the patient after mixing with the fresh gas flow from the bypass channel.*
   d) *False. The bimetallic strip valve in the Tec Mk 5 is in the bypass chamber. The bimetallic strip has been positioned in the bypass chamber since the Tec Mk 3. This was done to avoid corrosion of the strip in a mixture of oxygen and inhalational agent when positioned in the vaporizing chamber.*

   e) *False. The concentration delivered to the patient stays constant because of temperature compensating mechanisms. This can be achieved by:*
   - *using a material with high density and high specific thermal conductivity (e.g. copper) which acts as a heat sink readily giving heat to the agent and maintaining its temperature*
   - *a temperature-sensitive valve within the vaporizer which automatically adjusts the splitting ratio according to the temperature, so if the temperature decreases due to loss of latent heat of vaporization, it allows more flow into the vaporizing chamber.*

3. Pressure gauges on an anaesthetic machine:
   a) *True. A pressure gauge consists of a coiled tube that is subjected to pressure from the inside. The high-pressure gas causes the tube to uncoil. The movement of the tube causes a needle pointer to move on a calibrated dial indicating the pressure.*
   b) *False. Oxygen is stored as a gas in the cylinder hence it obeys the gas laws. The pressure changes in an oxygen cylinder accurately reflect the contents. Nitrous oxide is stored as a liquid and vapour so it does not obey Boyle's gas law. This means that the pressure changes in a nitrous oxide cylinder do not accurately reflect the contents of the cylinder.*

c) *False.* The pressure gauges are calibrated for a particular gas or vapour. Oxygen and nitrous oxide pressure gauges are not interchangeable.

d) *False.* Cylinders are kept under much higher pressures (13 700 kPa for oxygen and 5400 kPa for nitrous oxide) than the pipeline gas supply (about 400 kPa). Using the same pressure gauges for both cylinders and pipeline gas supply can lead to inaccuracies and/or damage to pressure gauges.

e) *True.* Colour-coding is one of the safety features used in the use and delivery of gases in medical practice. In the UK, white is for oxygen, blue for nitrous oxide and black for medical air.

4. Laminar flow:
a) *False.* Laminar flow is directly proportional to pressure. Hagen–Poiseuille equation: Flow $\propto$ pressure $\times$ radius^4/ viscosity $\times$ length.

b) *True.* From the above equation, the flow $\propto$ radius^4.

c) *False.* Laminar flow is related to viscosity. Turbulent flow is related to density.

d) *True.* Laminar flow is greatest in the centre at about twice the mean flow rate. The flow is slower nearer to the wall of the tube. At the wall the flow is almost zero.

e) *True.* Reynold's number is the index used to predict the type of flow, laminar or turbulent. Reynold's number = velocity of fluid $\times$ density $\times$ radius of tube/viscosity. In laminar flow, Reynold's number is <2000. In turbulent flow, Reynold's number is >2000.

5. Flowmeters on an anaesthetic machine:
a) *True.* The flowmeters on the anaesthetic machine are very accurate with an accuracy of ±2.5%.

b) *False.* The flowmeters on an anaesthetic machine are tapered tubes. The top is wider than the bottom.

c) *False.* Oxygen is the last gas to be added to the mixture at the back bar. This is a safety feature in the design of the anaesthetic machine. If there is a crack in a flowmeter, a hypoxic mixture may result if oxygen is added first to the mixture.

d) *True.* At high flows, the flow is turbulent which is dependent on density. At low flows, the flow is laminar which is dependent on viscosity.

e) *True.* When a ball is used, the reading is taken from the midpoint.

6. Concerning the Triservice apparatus:
a) *False.* In the Triservice apparatus, two Oxford Miniature, draw-over, Vaporizers (OMV) are used. Plenum vaporizers are not used due to their high internal resistance. The OMV is light weight and, by changing its calibration scale, different inhalational agents can be used easily.

b) *True.* The system allows both spontaneous and controlled ventilation. The resistance to breathing is low allowing spontaneous ventilation. The self-inflating bag provides the means to control ventilation.

c) *True.* As above.

d) *True.* The OMV has a metal wick to increase area of vaporization within the vaporization chamber. The heat sink consists of an ethylene glycol jacket to stabilize the vaporizer temperature.

e) *True.* Supplementary oxygen can be added to the system from an oxygen cylinder. The oxygen is added to the reservoir proximal to the vaporizer(s).

7. Pressure regulators:
a) *False.* Pressure regulators are used to reduce pressure of gases and also to maintain a constant flow. In the absence of pressure regulators, the flowmeters need to be adjusted regularly to maintain constant flows as the contents of the cylinders are used up. The temperature and pressure of the cylinder contents decrease with use.

b) *True.* Pressure regulators are designed to maintain a gas flow at a constant pressure of about 400 kPa irrespective of the pressure and temperature of the contents of the cylinder.

c) *False.* Pressure regulators offer no protection to the patient. Their main function is to protect the anaesthetic machine from the high pressure of the cylinder and to maintain a constant flow of gas.

d) *True.* In situations where the pressure regulator fails, a relief valve that opens at 700 kPa prevents the build up of excessive pressure.

e) *True.* Flow restrictors can be used in a pipeline supply. They are designed to protect the anaesthetic machine from pressure surges in the system. They consist of a constriction between the pipeline supply and the anaesthetic machine.

8. The safety features found in an anaesthetic machine include:

a) *True. This is an essential safety feature in the anaesthetic machine. The ideal design should operate under the pressure of oxygen itself, give a characteristic audible signal, be capable of warning of impending failure and give a further alarm when failure has occurred, be capable of interrupting the flow of other gases and not require batteries or mains power to operate.*

b) *True. The flowmeters are colour-coded and also the shape and size of the oxygen flowmeter knob is different from the nitrous oxide knob. This allows the identification of the oxygen knob even in a dark environment.*

c) *False. The vaporizer level can be monitored by the anaesthetist. This is part of the anaesthetic machine checklist. There is no alarm system.*

d) *True. A ventilator disconnection alarm is essential when a ventilator is used. They are also used to monitor leaks, obstruction and malfunction. They can be pressure and/or volume monitoring alarms. In addition, clinical observation, end-tidal carbon dioxide concentration and airway pressure are also 'disconnection alarms'.*

e) *False. Only one vaporizer can be used at any one time. This is due to the interlocking Selectatec system where interlocking extension rods prevent more than one vaporizer being used at any one time. These rods prevent the percentage control dial from moving, preventing contamination of the downstream vaporizer.*

9. The non-return valve on the back bar of an anaesthetic machine between the vaporizer and common gas outlet:

a) *True. Minute volume divider ventilators exert back pressure as they cycle. This causes reversal of the fresh gas flow through the vaporizer. This leads to an uncontrolled increase in the concentration of the inhalational agent. Also the back pressure causes the fluctuation of the bobbins in the flowmeters as the ventilator cycles. The non-return valve on the back bar prevents these events from happening.*

b) *True. The non-return valve on the back bar opens when the pressure in the back bar exceeds 35 kPa. Flowmeters and vaporizer components can be damaged at higher pressures.*

c) *True. By preventing the effects of back pressure on the flowmeters and vaporizer as the minute volume divider ventilator cycles, the non-return valve on the back bar provides some protection to the patient. The flows on the flowmeters and the desired concentration of the inhalational agent can be accurately delivered to the patient.*

d) *True. See b).*

e) *False. The non-return valve on the back bar of the anaesthetic machine opens at a pressure of 35 kPa.*

10. The oxygen emergency flush on an anaesthetic machine:

a) *False. 35–75 L/min can be delivered by activating the oxygen emergency flush on the anaesthetic machine.*

b) *False. The inappropriate use of the oxygen flush during anaesthesia increases risk of awareness (a 100% oxygen can be delivered) and barotrauma to the patient (because of the high flows delivered).*

c) *True. See a).*

d) *True. This can happen by diluting the anaesthetic mixture; see b).*

e) *False. Because of the high FGF (35–70 L/min), the minute volume divider ventilator does not function appropriately.*

11. c)

Chapter 3

Pollution in theatre and scavenging

Since the late 1960s, there has been speculation that trace anaesthetic gases/vapours may have a harmful effect on operating theatre personnel. It has been concluded from currently available studies that there is no association between occupational exposure to trace levels of waste anaesthetic vapours in scavenged operating theatres and adverse health effects. However, it is desirable to vent out the exhaled anaesthetic vapours and maintain a vapour-free theatre environment. A prudent plan for minimizing exposure includes maintenance of equipment, training of personnel and routine exposure monitoring. Although not universally agreed upon, the recommended maximum accepted concentrations in the UK (issued in 1996), over an 8-hour, time-weighted average (see Table 3.1 for main causes), are as follows:

- 100 particles per million (ppm) for nitrous oxide
- 50 ppm for enflurane
- 50 ppm for isoflurane
- 10 ppm for halothane
- 20 ppm for sevoflurane (recommended by Abbot Laboratories)
- no limit set for desflurane although a 50 ppm target is advisable due to its similarity to enflurane. .

These levels were chosen because they are well below the levels at which any significant adverse effects occurred in animals and represent levels at which there is no evidence to suggest human health would be affected.

In the United States, the maximum accepted concentrations of any halogenated agent should be less than 2 ppm. When such agents are used in combination with nitrous oxide, levels of less than 0.5 ppm should be achieved. Nitrous oxide, when used as the sole anaesthetic agent,

Table 3.1 Causes of operating theatre pollution

Anaesthetic techniques	Incomplete scavenging of the gases from ventilator and/or adjustable pressure limiting (APL) valve Poorly fitting face mask Paediatric breathing systems, e.g. T-piece Failure to turn off fresh gas and/or vaporizer at the end of an anaesthetic Uncuffed tracheal tubes Filling of the vaporizers Exhalation of the gases/vapours during recovery
Anaesthetic machine	Leaks from the various connections used, e.g. 'O' rings, soda lime canister
Others	Cryosurgery units and cardiopulmonary bypass circuit if a vapour is used

at 8-hour time-weighted average concentrations should be less than 25 ppm during the administration of an anaesthetic.

Holland has a limit of 25 ppm for nitrous oxide, whereas Italy, Sweden, Norway and Denmark set 100 ppm as their limit for exposure to nitrous oxide. The differences illustrate the difficulty in setting standards without adequate data.

Methods used to decrease theatre pollution are listed below:

1. Adequate theatre ventilation and air conditioning, with frequent and rapid changing of the circulating air (15–20 times per hour). This is one of the most important factors in reducing pollution. Theatres that are unventilated are four times as contaminated with anaesthetic gases and vapours compared to those with proper ventilation. A non-recirculating ventilation system is usually used. A recirculating ventilation system is not recommended. In labour wards, where anaesthetic agents including Entonox are used, rooms should be well ventilated with a minimum of five air changes per hour.
2. Use of the circle breathing system. This system recycles the exhaled anaesthetic vapours, absorbing CO_2. It requires a very low fresh gas flow, so reducing the amount of inhalational agents used. This decreases the level of theatre environment contamination.
3. Total intravenous anaesthesia.
4. Regional anaesthesia.
5. Avoiding spillage and using fume cupboards during vaporizer filling. This used to be a significant contributor to the hazard of pollution in the operating theatre. Modern vaporizers use special agent-specific filling devices as a safety feature and to reduce spillage and pollution.
6. Scavenging.

Sampling procedures for evaluating waste anaesthetic vapour concentrations in air should be conducted for nitrous oxide and halogenated agents on a yearly basis in the UK and on a quarterly basis in the USA in each location where anaesthesia is administered. Monitoring should include:

a) leak testing of equipment
b) sampling air in the theatre personnel breathing zone.

Anaesthetic equipment, gas scavenging, gas supply, flowmeters and ventilation systems must be subject to a planned preventative maintenance (PPM) programme. At least once annually, the general ventilation system and the scavenging equipment should be examined and tested by a responsible person.

Scavenging

In any location in which inhalation anaesthetics are administered, there should be an adequate and reliable system for scavenging waste anaesthetic gases. A scavenging system is capable of collecting the waste anaesthetic gases from the breathing system and discarding them safely. Unscavenged operating theatres can show N_2O levels of 400–3000 ppm.

A well-designed scavenging system should consist of a collecting device for gases from the breathing system/ventilator at the site of overflow, a ventilation system to carry waste anaesthetic gases from the operating theatre and a method for limiting both positive and negative pressure variations in the breathing system.

The performance of the scavenging system should be part of the anaesthetic machine check.

Scavenging systems can be divided into passive and active systems.

PASSIVE SYSTEM

The passive system is simple to construct with zero running cost.

Components

1. The collecting and transfer system which consists of a shroud connected to the adjustable pressure limiting (APL) valve (or expiratory valve of the ventilator). A 30-mm connector attached to transfer tubing leads to a receiving system (Fig. 3.1). The 30-mm wide-bore connector is designed as a safety measure in order to prevent accidental misconnection to other ports of the breathing system (Fig. 3.2).
2. A receiving system (reservoir bag) can be used. Two spring-loaded valves guard against excessive positive pressures (1000 Pa) in case of a distal obstruction or negative pressures (−50 Pa) in case of increased demand in the scavenging system. Without these valves, excessive positive pressure increases the risk of barotrauma should there be an obstruction beyond the receiving system. Excessive negative pressure could lead to the collapse of the reservoir bag of the breathing system and the risk of rebreathing.
3. The disposal system is a wide-bore copper pipe leading to the atmosphere directly or via the theatre ventilation system.

Mechanism of action

1. The exhaled gases are driven by either the patient's respiratory efforts or the ventilator.
2. The receiving system should be mounted on the anaesthetic machine to minimize the length of transfer tubing and resistance to flow.

Problems in practice and safety features

1. Connecting the scavenging system to the exit grille of the theatre ventilation is possible. Recirculation or reversing of the flow is a problem in this situation.

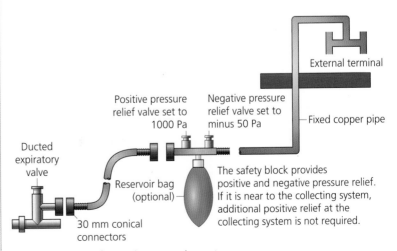

Positive pressure relief valve set to 1000 Pa

Negative pressure relief valve set to minus 50 Pa

External terminal

Fixed copper pipe

Ducted expiratory valve

Reservoir bag (optional)

30 mm conical connectors

The safety block provides positive and negative pressure relief. If it is near to the collecting system, additional positive relief at the collecting system is not required.

Fig. 3.1 Diagram of a passive scavenging system.

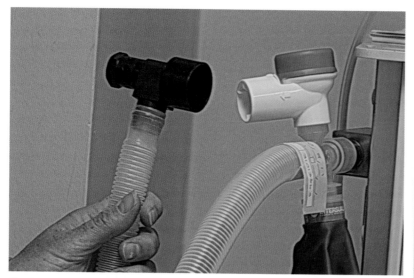

Fig. 3.2 Attaching a 30-mm connecter to the APL valve of the breathing system. The 30-mm wide bore is designed as safety measure.

Mechanism of action

1. The vacuum drives the gases through the system. Active scavenging systems are able to deal with a wide range of expiratory flow rates (30–130 L/min).
2. A motorized fan, a pump or a Venturi system is used to generate the vacuum or negative pressure that is transmitted through the pipes.
3. The receiving system is capable of coping with changes in gas flow rates. Increased demands (or excessive negative pressure) allow ambient air to be entrained so maintaining the pressure. The opposite occurs during excessive positive pressure. As a result, a uniform gas flow is passed to the disposal system.

Problems in practice and safety features

1. The reservoir is designed to prevent excessive negative or positive pressures being applied

2. Excess positive or negative pressures caused by the wind at the outlet might affect the performance and even reverse the flow.
3. The outlet should be fitted with a wire mesh to protect against insects.
4. Compressing or occluding the passive hose may lead to the escape of gases/vapours into the operating theatre so polluting it. The disposal hose should be made of non-compressible materials and not placed on the floor.

ACTIVE SYSTEM

Components

1. The collecting and transfer system which is similar to that of the passive system (Fig. 3.3).
2. The receiving system (Fig 3.4) is usually a valveless, open-ended reservoir positioned between the receiving and disposal components. A bacterial filter situated downstream and a visual flow indicator positioned

between the receiving and disposal systems can be used. A reservoir bag with two spring-loaded safety valves can also be used as a receiving system.
3. The active disposal system consists of a fan or a pump used to generate a vacuum (Fig. 3.5).

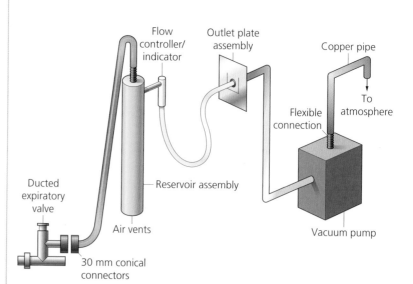

Fig. 3.3 Diagram of an active scavenging system.

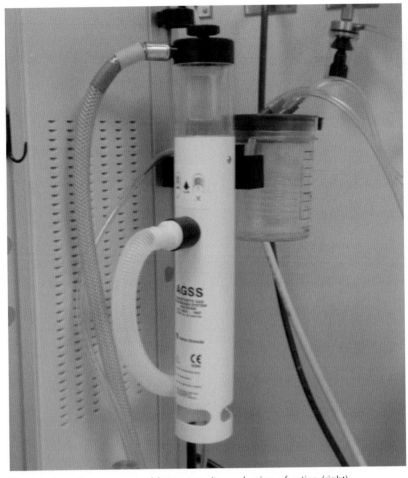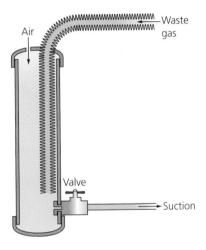

Fig. 3.4 Anaesthetic gases receiving system. Its mechanism of action (right).

to the patient. Excessive negative pressure leads to the collapse of the reservoir bag of the breathing system and the risk of rebreathing. Excessive positive pressure increases the risk of barotrauma should there be an obstruction beyond the receiving system.

2. An independent vacuum pump should be used for scavenging purposes.

Scavenging
- Active or passive systems.
- Consists of a collecting and transfer system, a receiving system and a disposal system.

- Both excessive positive and negative pressure variations in the system are limited.
- Other methods used to reduce theatre pollution: theatre ventilation, circle system, total intravenous and regional anaesthesia.

Charcoal canisters (Cardiff Aldasorber)

The canister is a compact passive scavenging system (Fig. 3.6).

Components

1. A canister.
2. Charcoal particles.
3. Transfer tubing connecting the canister to the APL valve of the breathing system or the expiratory valve of the ventilator.

Mechanism of action

1. The charcoal particles absorb the halogenated inhalational agents (halothane, enflurane and isoflurane).
2. The increasing weight of the canister is the only indication that it is exhausted.

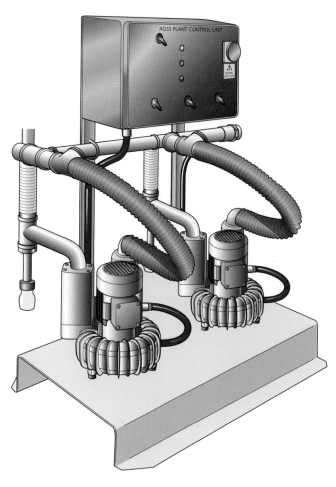

Fig. 3.5 Anaesthetic gases scavenging system (AGSS) vacuum pumps used in an active scavenging system. (Courtesy of Penlon Ltd, Abingdon, UK (www.penlon.com).)

3. It is usually replaced after every 12 hours of use.

Problems in practice and safety features

1. It cannot absorb nitrous oxide.
2. Heating the canister causes the release of the inhalational agents.

Charcoal canisters

- A canister with charcoal granules used to absorb halogenated agents.
- Does not absorb nitrous oxide.
- Its weight indicates the degree of exhaustion. Usually replaced after every 12 hours of use.
- When heated, the agents escape back into the atmosphere.

FURTHER READING

American Institute of Architects, 1992. Guidelines for construction and equipment of hospitals and medical facilities. AIA, Washington DC.

Department of Health, 1996. Advice on the implementation of the Health and Safety Commission's occupational exposure standards for anaesthetic agents. DoH, London.

Health Service Advisory Committee, 1996. Anaesthetic agents: controlling exposure under the Control of Substances Hazardous to Health Regulations (COSHH). HSAC, London.

Henderson, K.A., Raj, A., Hall, J.E., 2002. The use of nitrous oxide in anaesthetic practice: a questionnaire survey. Anaesthesia 57 (12), 1155–1158.

MHRA, 2010. Medical device alert: anaesthetic gas scavenging systems (AGSS) – all manufacturers (MDA/2010/021). Online. Available at: http://www.mhra.gov.uk/Publications/Safetywarnings/MedicalDeviceAlerts/CON076104.

United States Department of Labor, 1999. Anaesthetic gases: guidelines for workplace exposures. Online. Available at: http://www.osha.gov/dts/osta/anestheticgases/index.html.

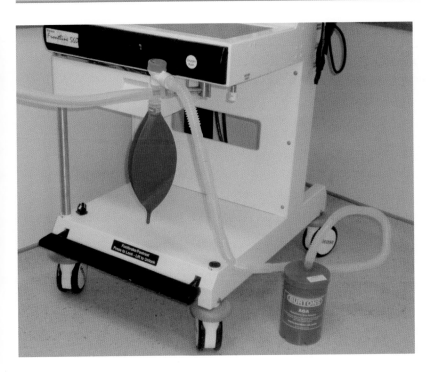

Fig. 3.6 Charcoal canister connected to the APL valve of the breathing system.

MCQs

In the following lists, which of the statements (a) to (e) are true?

1. Pollution in theatre:
   a) The Cardiff Aldasorber can absorb N_2O and the inhalational agents.
   b) The circulating air in theatre should be changed 15–20 times per hour.
   c) In the scavenging system, excessive positive and negative pressures should be prevented from being applied to the patient.
   d) In the active scavenging system, an ordinary vacuum pump can be utilized.
   e) The maximum accepted concentration of nitrous oxide is 100 ppm.

2. Important factors in reducing pollution in the operating theatre:
   a) Scavenging.
   b) Low-flow anaesthesia using the circle system.
   c) Adequate theatre ventilation.
   d) The use of fume cupboards when filling vaporizers.
   e) Cardiff Aldasorber.

3. Passive scavenging system:
   a) Is easy to build and maintain.
   b) Is efficient.
   c) There is no need to have positive or negative relief valves in the collecting system.
   d) The exhaled gases are driven by the patient's respiratory effort or the ventilator.
   e) Commonly uses 15-mm connectors in the United Kingdom.

4. Concerning anaesthetic agents pollution:
   a) There is an international standard for the concentrations of trace inhalational agents in the operating theatre environment.
   b) In the UK, monitoring of inhalational agent concentration in the operating theatre is done annually.
   c) PPM stands for particles per million.
   d) An unscavenged operating theatre would have less than 100 particles per million of nitrous oxide.
   e) A T-piece paediatric breathing system can cause theatre pollution.

SINGLE BEST ANSWER (SBA)

5. Operating theatre pollution:
   a) Does not exist.
   b) Only occurs in anaesthetic rooms.
   c) Can be detected by analysing a sample from the theatre's atmosphere.
   d) Can be eliminated by regular monitoring alone.
   e) Can be eliminated by using the laryngeal mask more often.

Answers

1. Pollution in theatre:
   a) *False.* Cardiff Aldasorber can only absorb the inhalational agents but not nitrous oxide. This limits its use in reducing pollution in the operating theatre.
   b) *True.* Changing the circulating air in the operating theatre 15–20 times per hour is one of the most effective methods of reducing pollution. An unventilated theatre is about four times more polluted compared to a properly ventilated one.
   c) *True.* The patient should be protected against excessive positive and negative pressures being applied by the scavenging system. Excessive positive pressure puts the patient under the risk of barotrauma. Excessive negative pressure causes the reservoir in the breathing system to collapse thus leading to incorrect performance of the breathing system.

   d) *False.* Because of the nature of the flow of the exhaled gases, the scavenging system should be capable of tolerating high and variable gas flows. The flow of exhaled gases is very variable during both spontaneous and controlled ventilation. An ordinary vacuum pump might not be capable of coping with such variable flows, from 30 to 120 L/min. The active scavenging system is a high-flow, low-pressure system. A pressure of -0.5 cm H_2O to the patient breathing system is needed. This cannot be achieved with an ordinary vacuum pump (low-flow, high-pressure system).
   e) *True.* In the UK, the maximum accepted concentration of nitrous oxide is 100 ppm over an 8-hour time-weighted average.

2. Important factors in reducing pollution in the operating theatre:
   a) *True.* In any location in which inhalation anaesthetics are administered, there should be an adequate and reliable system for scavenging waste anaesthetic gases. Unscavenged operating theatres can show 400–3000 ppm of N_2O, which is much higher than the maximum acceptable concentration.
   b) *True.*
   c) *True.* One of the most important factors in reducing pollution is adequate theatre ventilation. The circulating air is changed 15–20 times per hour. Unventilated theatres are four times more contaminated than properly ventilated theatres.
   d) *False.* Modern vaporizers use agent-specific filling keys which limit spillage.
   e) *False.* Cardiff Aldasorber absorbs the inhalational agents but not nitrous oxide.

3. Passive scavenging system:
   a) *True.* A passive scavenging system is easy and cheap to build and costs nothing to maintain. There is no need for a purpose-built vacuum pump system with the necessary maintenance required.
   b) *False.* The passive system is not an efficient system. Its efficiency depends on the direction of the wind blowing at the outlet. Negative or positive pressure might affect the performance and even reverse the flow.
   c) *False.* The positive pressure relief valve protects the patient against excessive pressure build up in the breathing system and barotrauma. The negative pressure relief valve prevents the breathing system reservoir from being exhausted, ensuring correct performance of the breathing system.
   d) *True.* The driving forces for gases in the passive system are the patient's respiratory effort or the ventilator. For this reason, the transfer tubing should be made as short as possible to reduce resistance to flow.
   e) *False.* 30-mm connectors are used in the UK as a safety feature to prevent misconnection.

4. Concerning anaesthetic agents pollution:
   a) *False.* There is not an international standard for the concentrations of trace inhalational agents in the operating theatre environment. This is mainly because of unavailability of adequate data. Different countries set their own standards but there is an agreement on the importance of maintaining a vapour-free environment in the operating theatre.
   b) *True.* Monitoring of inhalational agent concentration in the operating theatre is done annually in the UK and on a quarterly basis in the USA in each location where anaesthesia is administered.
   c) *False.* PPM (capitals) stands for planned preventative maintenance, whereas ppm (small letters) stands for particles per million.
   d) *False.* An unscavenged operating theatre would have 400–3000 ppm of nitrous oxide. In the UK, the recommended maximum accepted concentration over an 8-hour time-weighted average is 100 ppm of nitrous oxide.
   e) *True.* A T-piece paediatric breathing system can cause theatre pollution because of the open-ended reservoir. A modified version has an APL valve allowing scavenging of the anaesthetic vapours (see Chapter 4).

5. c)

Chapter 4

Breathing systems

Breathing systems must fulfil three objectives:

1. Delivery of oxygen.
2. Removal of carbon dioxide from the patient.
3. Delivery of inhaled anaesthetic agents. These agents are predominantly eliminated by the lungs also, so the breathing system must be able to expel them as necessary.

There are several breathing systems used in anaesthesia. Mapleson classified them into A, B, C, D and E. After further revision of the classification, a Mapleson F breathing system was added (Fig. 4.1). Currently, only systems A, D, E and F and their modifications are commonly used during anaesthesia. Mapleson B

and C systems are used more frequently during the recovery period and in emergency situations.

> The fresh gas flow (FGF) rate required to prevent rebreathing of alveolar gas is a measure of the efficiency of a breathing system.

Properties of the ideal breathing system

1. Simple and safe to use.
2. Delivers the intended inspired gas mixture.
3. Permits spontaneous, manual and controlled ventilation in all age groups.

4. Efficient, requiring low FGF rates.
5. Protects the patient from barotrauma.
6. Sturdy, compact and lightweight in design.
7. Permits the easy removal of waste exhaled gases.
8. Easy to maintain with minimal running costs.

Components of the breathing systems

ADJUSTABLE PRESSURE LIMITING (APL) VALVE

This is a valve which allows the exhaled gases and excess FGF to leave the breathing system (Fig. 4.2). It does not allow room air to enter the breathing system. Synonymous terms for the APL valve are expiratory valve, spill valve and relief valve.

Components

1. Three ports: the inlet, the patient and the exhaust ports. The latter can be open to the atmosphere or connected to the scavenging system using a shroud.
2. A lightweight disc rests on a knife-edge seating. The disc is held onto its seating by a spring. The tension in the spring, and therefore the valve's opening pressure, are controlled by the valve dial.

Mechanism of action

1. This is a one-way, adjustable, spring-loaded valve. The spring is used to adjust the pressure required to open the valve. The disc rests on a knife-edge seating in order to minimize its area of contact.

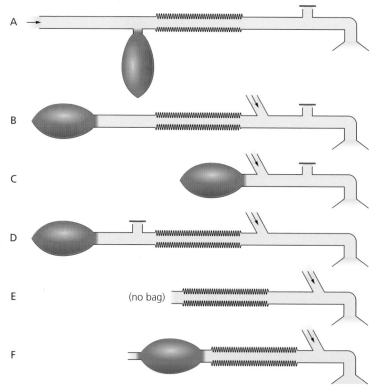

Fig. 4.1 Mapleson classification of anaesthetic breathing systems. The arrow indicates entry of fresh gas to the system.

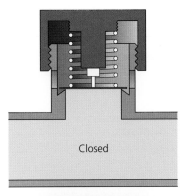

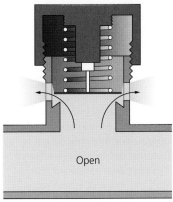

Fig. 4.2 Diagram of an adjustable pressure limiting (APL) valve.

2. The valve allows gases to escape when the pressure in the breathing system exceeds the valve's opening pressure.
3. During spontaneous ventilation, the patient generates a positive pressure in the system during expiration, causing the valve to open. A pressure of less than 1 cm H_2O (0.1 kPa) is needed to actuate the valve when it is in the open position.
4. During positive pressure ventilation, a controlled leak is produced by adjusting the valve dial during inspiration. This allows control of the patient's airway pressure.

Problems in practice and safety features

1. Malfunction of the scavenging system may cause excessive negative pressure. This can lead to the APL valve remaining open throughout respiration. This leads to an unwanted enormous increase in the breathing system's dead space.
2. The patient may be exposed to excessive positive pressure if the valve is closed during assisted ventilation. A pressure relief safety mechanism actuated at a pressure of about 60 cm H_2O is present in some designs (Fig. 4.3).
3. Water vapour in exhaled gas may condense on the valve. The surface tension of the condensed water may cause the valve to stick. The disc is usually made of a hydrophobic (water repelling) material, which prevents water condensing on the disc.

> ### Adjustable pressure limiting (APL) valve
> - One-way spring-loaded valve with three ports.
> - The spring adjusts the pressure required to open the valve.

RESERVOIR BAG

The reservoir bag is an important component of most breathing systems.

Components

1. It is made of anti-static rubber or plastic. Latex-free versions also exist. Designs tend to be ellipsoidal in shape.
2. The standard adult size is 2 L. The smallest size for paediatric use is 0.5 L. Volumes from 0.5 to 6 L exist. Bigger size reservoir bags are useful during inhalational induction, e.g. adult induction with sevoflurane.

Mechanism of action

1. Accommodates the FGF during expiration acting as a reservoir available for the following inspiration. Otherwise, the FGF

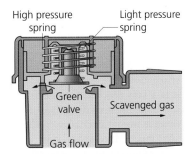

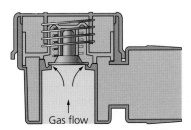

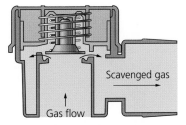

Fig. 4.3 Intersurgical APL valve. In the open position (left), the valve is actuated by pressures of less than 0.1 kPa (1 cm H_2O) with minimal resistance to flow. A 3/4 clockwise turn of the dial takes the valve through a range of pressure limiting positions to the closed position (centre). In the closed position, the breathing system pressure, and therefore the intrapulmonary pressure, is protected by a pressure relief mechanism (right) actuated at 6 kPa (60 cm H_2O). This safety relief mechanism cannot be overridden.

must be at least the patient's peak inspiratory flow to prevent rebreathing. As this peak inspiratory flow may exceed 30 L/min in adults, breathing directly from the FGF will be insufficient.

2. It acts as a monitor of the patient's ventilatory pattern during spontaneous breathing. It serves as a very inaccurate guide to the patient's tidal volume.
3. It can be used to assist or control ventilation.
4. When employed in conjunction with the T-piece (Mapleson F), a 0.5 L double-ended bag is used. The distal hole acts as an expiratory port (Fig. 4.4).

Problems in practice and safety features

1. Because of its compliance, the reservoir bag can accommodate rises in pressure in the breathing system better than other parts. When grossly overinflated, the rubber reservoir bag can limit

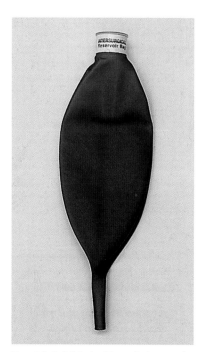

Fig. 4.4 A 0.5-L double-ended reservoir.

the pressure in the breathing system to about 40 cm H_2O. This is due to the law of Laplace dictating that the pressure (P) will fall as the bag's radius (r) increases: $P = 2(\text{tension})/r$.

2. The size of the bag depends on the breathing system and the patient. A small bag may not be large enough to provide a sufficient reservoir for a large tidal volume.
3. Too large a reservoir bag makes it difficult for it to act as a respiratory monitor.

Reservoir bag
- Made of rubber or plastic.
- 2-L size commonly used for adults. Bigger sizes can be used for inhalational induction in adults.
- Accommodates FGF.
- Can assist or control ventilation.
- Limits pressure build-up in the breathing system.

TUBINGS

These connect one part of a breathing system to another. They also act as a reservoir for gases in certain systems. They tend to be made of plastic, but other materials such as silicone rubber and silver-impregnated bactericidal plastics are available.

The length of the breathing tubing is variable depending on the configuration of the breathing system used. They must promote laminar flow wherever possible and this is achieved by their being of a uniform and large diameter. The size for adults is 22 mm wide. However, paediatric tubing is 15 mm wide, to reduce bulk. The corrugations resist kinking and increase flexibility, but they produce greater turbulence than smooth-bore tubes.

Specific configurations are described below.

Magill system (Mapleson A)

This breathing system is popular and widely used in the UK.

Components

1. Corrugated rubber or plastic tubing (usually 110–180 cm in length) and an internal volume of at least 550 mL.
2. A reservoir bag, mounted at the machine end.
3. APL valve situated at the patient end.

Mechanism of action

1. During the first inspiration, all the gases are fresh and consist of oxygen and anaesthetic gases from the anaesthetic machine.
2. As the patient exhales (Fig. 4.5C), the gases coming from the anatomical dead space (i.e. they have not undergone gas exchange so contain no CO_2) are exhaled first and enter the tubing and are channelled back towards the reservoir bag which is being filled continuously with FGF.
3. During the expiratory pause, pressure built up within the system allows the FGF to expel the alveolar gases first out through the APL valve (Fig. 4.5D).
4. By that time the patient inspires again (Fig. 4.5B), getting a mixture of FGF and the rebreathed anatomical dead space gases.
5. It is a very efficient system for spontaneous breathing. Because there is no gas exchange in the anatomical dead space, the FGF requirements to prevent rebreathing of alveolar gases are theoretically equal to the patient's alveolar minute volume (about 70 mL/kg/min).

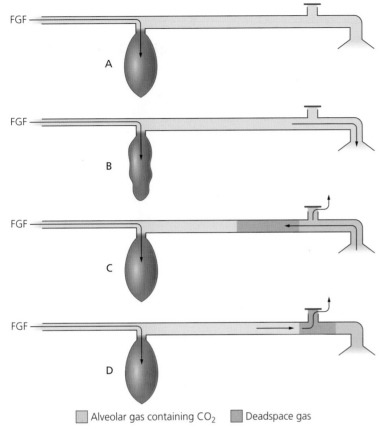

Alveolar gas containing CO_2 Deadspace gas

Fig. 4.5 Mechanism of action of the Magill breathing system during spontaneous ventilation; see text for details (FGF: fresh gas flow).

6. The Magill system is not an efficient system for controlled ventilation. A FGF rate of three times the alveolar minute volume is required to prevent rebreathing.

Problems in practice and safety features

It is not suitable for use with children of less than 25–30 kg body weight. This is because of the increased dead space caused by the system's geometry at the patient end. Dead space is further increased by the angle piece and face mask.

One of its disadvantages is the heaviness of the APL valve at the patient's end, especially if connected to a scavenging system. This places a lot of drag on the connections at the patient end.

Magill (Mapleson A) breathing system

- Efficient for spontaneous ventilation. FGF required is equal to alveolar minute volume (about 70 mL/kg/min).
- Inefficient for controlled ventilation. FGF three times alveolar minute volume.
- APL valve is at the patient's end.
- Not suitable for paediatric practice.

Lack system (Mapleson A)

This is a coaxial modification of the Magill Mapleson A system.

Components

1. 1.8 m length coaxial tubing (tube inside a tube). The FGF is through the outside tube, and the exhaled gases flow through the inside tube (Fig. 4.6A).
2. The inside tube is wide in diameter (14 mm) to reduce resistance to expiration. The outer tube's diameter is 30 mm.
3. The reservoir bag is mounted at the machine end.
4. The APL valve is mounted at the machine end eliminating the drag on the connections at the patient end, which is a problem with the Magill system.

Mechanism of action

1. A similar mechanism to the Magill system except the Lack system is a coaxial version. The fresh gas flows through the outside tube whereas the exhaled gases flow through the inside tube.
2. A FGF rate of about 70 mL/kg/min is required in order to prevent rebreathing. This makes it an efficient breathing system for spontaneous ventilation.
3. Since it is based on the Magill system, it is not suitable for controlled ventilation.

Instead of the coaxial design, a parallel tubing version of the system exists (Fig. 4.6B). This has separate inspiratory and expiratory tubing, and retains the same flow characteristics as the coaxial version.

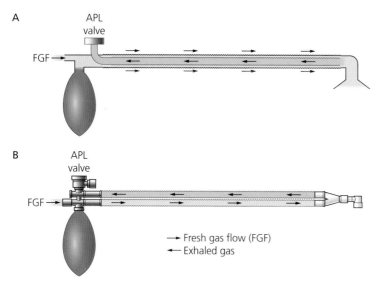

Fig. 4.6 (A) The coaxial Lack breathing system. (B) The parallel Lack breathing system.

Lack breathing system

- Coaxial version of Mapleson A, making it efficient for spontaneous ventilation. FGF rate of about 70 mL/kg/min is required.
- FGF is delivered along the outside tube and the exhaled gases flow along the inner tube.
- APL valve is at the machine end.
- Not suitable for controlled ventilation.

Mapleson B and C systems (see Fig. 4.1)

Components

1. A reservoir bag. In the B system, corrugated tubing is attached to the bag and both act as a reservoir.
2. An APL valve at the patient's end.
3. FGF is added just proximal to the APL.

Mechanism of action

Both systems are not efficient during spontaneous ventilation. A FGF of 1.5–2 times the minute volume is required to prevent rebreathing.

During controlled ventilation, the B system is more efficient due to the corrugated tubing acting as a reservoir. A FGF of more than 50% of the minute ventilation is still required to prevent rebreathing.

Mapleson B and C breathing systems

- B system has a tubing and bag reservoir.
- Both B and C systems are not efficient for spontaneous and controlled ventilation.
- B system is more efficient than A system during controlled ventilation.

Bain system (Mapleson D)

The Bain system is a coaxial version of the Mapleson D system (Fig. 4.7). It is lightweight and compact at the patient end. It is useful where access to the patient is limited, such as during head and neck surgery.

A Manley ventilator which has been switched to spontaneous ventilation mode is an example of a non-coaxial Mapleson D system.

Components

1. A length of coaxial tubing (tube inside a tube). The usual length is 180 cm, but it can be supplied at 270 cm (for dental or ophthalmic surgery) and 540 cm (for magnetic resonance imaging (MRI) scans where the anaesthetic machine needs to be kept outside the scanner's magnetic field). Increasing the length of the tubing does not affect the physical properties of the breathing system.
2. The fresh gas flows through the inner tube while the exhaled gases flow through the outside tube (Fig. 4.8). The internal lumen has a swivel mount at the patient end. This ensures that the internal tube cannot kink, so ensuring delivery of fresh gas to the patient.
3. The reservoir bag is mounted at the machine end.

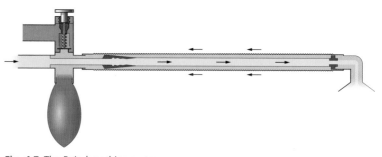

Fig. 4.7 The Bain breathing system.

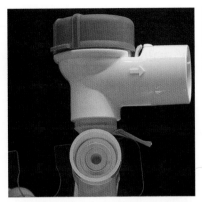

Fig. 4.8 The proximal (machine's) end of coaxial Bain's breathing system. The FGF flows through the narrow inner tube.

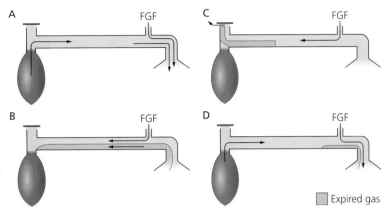

Expired gas

Fig. 4.9 Mechanism of action of the Mapleson D breathing system during spontaneous ventilation.

4. The APL valve is mounted at the machine end.

Mechanism of action

1. During spontaneous ventilation, the patient's exhaled gases are channelled back to the reservoir bag and become mixed with fresh gas (Fig. 4.9B). Pressure build-up within the system will open the APL valve allowing the venting of the mixture of the exhaled gases and fresh gas (Fig. 4.9C).
2. The FGF required to prevent rebreathing (as seen in Fig. 4.9D) during spontaneous ventilation is about 1.5–2 times the alveolar minute volume. A flow rate of 150–200 mL/kg/min is required. This makes it an inefficient and uneconomical system for use during spontaneous ventilation.
3. It is a more efficient system for controlled ventilation. A flow of 70–100 mL/kg/min will maintain normocapnia. A flow of 100 mL/kg/min will cause moderate hypocapnia during controlled ventilation.
4. Connection to a ventilator is possible (Fig. 4.10). By

removing the reservoir bag, a ventilator such as the Penlon Nuffield 200 can be connected to the bag mount using a 1-m length of corrugated tubing (the volume of tubing must exceed 500 mL if the driving gas from the ventilator is not to enter the breathing system). The APL valve must be fully closed.

5. A parallel version of the D system is available.

Problems in practice and safety features

1. The internal tube can kink, preventing fresh gas being delivered to the patient.
2. The internal tube can become disconnected at the machine end causing a large increase in the

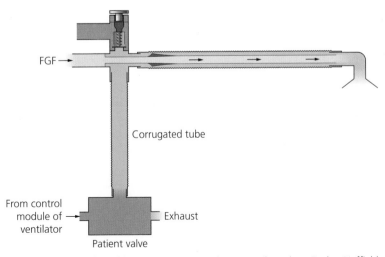

Fig. 4.10 The Bain breathing system connected to a ventilator (e.g. Penlon Nuffield 200) via tubing connected to the bag mount.

dead space, resulting in hypoxaemia and hypercapnia. Movement of the reservoir bag during spontaneous ventilation is not therefore an indication that the fresh gas is being delivered to the patient.

Bain breathing system
- Coaxial version of Mapleson D. A parallel version exits.
- Fresh gas flows along the inner tube and the exhaled gases flow along the outer tube.
- Not efficient for spontaneous ventilation. FGF rate required is 150–200 mL/kg/min.
- Efficient during controlled ventilation. FGF rate required is 70–100 mL/kg/min.

T-piece system (Mapleson E and F)

This is a valveless breathing system used in anaesthesia for children up to 25–30 kg body weight (Fig. 4.11). It is suitable for both spontaneous and controlled ventilation.

Components

1. A T-shaped tubing with three open ports (Fig. 4.12).
2. Fresh gas from the anaesthetic machine is delivered via a tube to one port.
3. The second port leads to the patient's mask or tracheal tube. The connection should be as short as possible to reduce dead space.
4. The third port leads to reservoir tubing. Jackson-Rees added a double-ended bag to the end of the reservoir tubing (making it Mapleson F).
5. A recent modification exists where an APL valve is included before a closed-ended 500 mL reservoir bag. A pressure relief safety mechanism in the APL valve is actuated at a pressure of 30 cm H_2O (Fig. 4.13). This design allows effective scavenging.

Mechanism of action

1. The system requires an FGF of 2.5–3 times the minute volume to prevent rebreathing with a minimal flow of 4 L/min.
2. The double-ended bag acts as a visual monitor during spontaneous ventilation. In addition, the bag can be used for assisted or controlled ventilation.
3. The bag can provide a degree of continuous positive airway pressure (CPAP) during spontaneous ventilation.
4. Controlled ventilation is performed either by manual squeezing of the double-ended bag (intermittent occlusion of the reservoir tubing in the Mapleson E) or by removing the bag and connecting the reservoir tubing to a ventilator such as the Penlon Nuffield 200.
5. The volume of the reservoir tubing determines the degree of rebreathing (too large a tube) or entrainment of ambient air (too small a tube). The volume of the reservoir tubing should approximate to the patient's tidal volume.

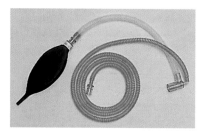

Fig. 4.11 A T-piece breathing system.

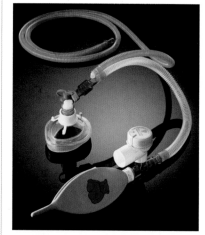

Fig. 4.13 Intersurgical T-piece incorporating an APL valve and closed reservoir bag to enable effective scavenging.

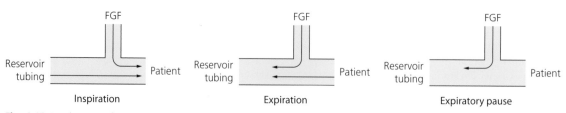

Inspiration	Expiration	Expiratory pause

Fig. 4.12 Mechanism of action of the T-piece breathing system.

Problems in practice and safety features

1. Since there is no APL valve used in this breathing system, scavenging is a problem.
2. Patients under 6 years of age have a low functional residual capacity (FRC). Mapleson E was designed before the advantages of CPAP were recognized for increasing the FRC. This problem can be partially overcome in the Mapleson F with the addition of the double-ended bag.

T-piece E and F breathing system
- Used in paediatric practice up to 25–30 kg body weight.
- Requires a high FGF during spontaneous ventilation.
- Offers minimal resistance to expiration.
- Valveless breathing system.
- Scavenging is difficult.
- A recent design with an APL valve and a closed-ended reservoir allows effective scavenging.

The Humphrey ADE breathing system

This is a very versatile breathing system which combines the advantages of Mapleson A, D and E systems. It can therefore be used efficiently for spontaneous and controlled ventilation in both adults and children. The mode of use is determined by the position of one lever which is mounted on the Humphrey block (Fig. 4.14). Both parallel and coaxial versions exist with similar efficiency. The parallel version will be considered here.

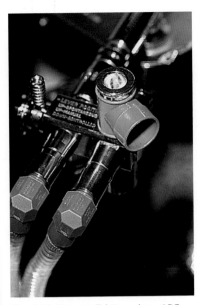

Fig. 4.14 The parallel Humphrey ADE breathing system.

Components

1. Two lengths of 15 mm smooth-bore tubing (corrugated tubing is not recommended). One delivers the fresh gas and the other carries away the exhaled gas. Distally they are connected to a Y-connection leading to the patient. Proximally they are connected to the Humphrey block.
2. The Humphrey block is at the machine end and consists of:
   a) an APL valve featuring a visible indicator of valve performance
   b) a 2-L reservoir bag
   c) a lever to select either spontaneous or controlled ventilation
   d) a port to which a ventilator can be connected, e.g. Penlon Nuffield 200
   e) a safety pressure relief valve which opens at pressure in excess of 60 cm H_2O
   f) a new design incorporating a soda lime canister.

Mechanism of action

1. With the lever up (Fig. 4.15A) in the spontaneous mode, the reservoir bag and APL valve are connected to the breathing system as in the Magill system.
2. With the lever down (Fig. 4.15B) in the ventilator mode, the reservoir bag and the APL valve are isolated from the breathing system as in the Mapleson E system. The expiratory tubing channels the exhaled gas via the ventilator port. Scavenging occurs at the ventilator's expiratory valve.
3. The system is suitable for paediatric and adult use. The tubing is rather narrow, with a low internal volume. Because of its smooth bore, there is no significant increase in resistance to flow compared to the 22-mm corrugated tubing used in other systems. Small tidal volumes are possible during controlled ventilation and less energy is needed to overcome the inertia of gases during spontaneous ventilation.
4. The presence of an APL valve in the breathing system offers a physiological advantage during paediatric anaesthesia, since it is designed to offer a small amount of PEEP (1 cm H_2O).
5. During spontaneous ventilation:
   a) an FGF of about 50–60 mL/kg/min is needed in adults
   b) the recommended initial FGF for children weighing less than 25 kg body weight is 3 L/min. This offers a considerable margin for safety.
6. During controlled ventilation:
   a) an FGF of 70 mL/kg is needed in adults
   b) the recommended initial FGF for children weighing less than 25 kg body weight is 3 L/min. However, adjustment may be necessary to maintain normocarbia.

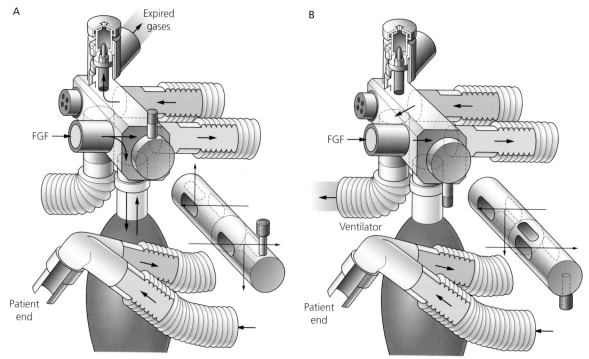

A

Expired gases

FGF

Patient end

B

FGF

Ventilator

Patient end

Fig. 4.15 Mechanism of action of the parallel Humphrey ADE breathing system. With the lever up (A), the system functions in its Mapleson A mode for spontaneous ventilation. For mechanical ventilation, the lever is down (B) and the system functions in its Mapleson E mode. (Reproduced with permission from Dr D Humphrey.)

Humphrey ADE breathing system
- Can be used efficiently for spontaneous and controlled ventilation.
- Can be used in both adult and paediatric anaesthetic practice.
- Both parallel and coaxial versions exist.
- A ventilator can be connected.

Soda lime and the circle breathing system

Over 80% of the anaesthetic gases are wasted when FGF of 5.0 L/min is used. Typically, the reduction of FGF from 3.0 L/min

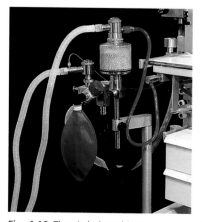

Fig. 4.16 The circle breathing system.

to 1.0 L/min results in a saving of about 50% of the total consumption of any volatile anaesthetic agent.

In this breathing system, soda lime is used to absorb the patient's exhaled carbon dioxide (Fig. 4.16).

FGF requirements are low, making the circle system very efficient and causing minimal pollution. As a result, there has been renewed interest in low-flow anaesthesia due to the cost of new, expensive inhalational agents, together with the increased awareness of the pollution caused by the inhalational agents themselves (see Table 3.1).

Depending on the FGF, the system can either be:

- **Closed circle anaesthesia.** The FGF is just sufficient to replace the volume of gas and vapour taken up by the patient. No gas leaves via the APL valve and the exhaled gases are rebreathed after carbon dioxide is absorbed. Significant leaks from the breathing system are eliminated. In practice, this is possible only if the gases sampled by the gas analyser are returned back to the system.

- **Minimal flow anaesthesia.** The FGF is reduced to 0.5 L/min.
- **Low-flow anaesthesia.** The FGF used is less than the patient's alveolar ventilation (usually below 1.5 L/min). Excess gases leave the system via the APL valve.

Components

1. A vertically positioned canister containing soda lime. The canister has two ports, one to deliver inspired gases to the patient and the other to receive exhaled gases from the patient.
2. Inspiratory and expiratory tubings connected to the canister. Each port incorporates a unidirectional valve.
3. FGF from the anaesthetic machine is positioned distal to the soda lime canister, but proximal to the inspiratory valve.
4. An APL valve is positioned between the expiratory valve and canister and connected to a 2-L reservoir bag.
5. A vaporizer mounted on the anaesthetic machine back bar (*vaporizer outside circle* – VOC) or a vaporizer positioned on the expiratory limb within the system (*vaporizer inside circle* – VIC).
6. Soda lime consists of 94% calcium hydroxide and 5% sodium hydroxide with a small amount of potassium hydroxide (less than 0.1%). It has a pH of 13.5 and a moisture content of 14–19%. Some modern types of soda lime have no potassium hydroxide. Soda lime granules are prone to powder formation, especially during transport. Disintegrated granules increase resistance to breathing. Because of this, silica (0.2%) is added to harden the absorbents and reduce powder formation. A dye or colour indicator is added to change the granules' colour when the soda lime is exhausted. Colour changes can be from white to violet/purple (ethyl violet dye), from pink to white (titan yellow dye) or from green to violet. Colour changes occur when the pH is less than 10. Newer types of soda lime have a low concentration of a zeolite added. This helps to maintain the pH at a high level for longer and retains moisture so improving carbon dioxide absorption and reducing the formation of carbon monoxide and compound A.

7. The size of soda lime granules is 4–8 mesh. Strainers with 4–8 mesh have four and eight openings per inch respectively. Therefore, the higher the mesh number, the smaller the particles are. Recently produced soda lime made to a uniform shape of 3–4-mm spheres allows more even flow of gases and a reduction in channelling. This results in a longer life with lower dust content and lower resistance to flow: 1 kg can absorb more than 120 L of CO_2.

8. Barylime, which consists of barium hydroxide (80%) and calcium hydroxide (20%), is widely used in the USA. Another absorber is Amsorb® that consists of $CaCl_2$ and $Ca(OH)_2$.

Mechanism of action

1. High FGF of several L/min is needed in the initial period to denitrogenate the circle system and the functional residual capacity (FRC). This is important to avoid the build up of unacceptable levels of nitrogen in the system. In closed circle anaesthesia, a high FGF is needed for up to 15 minutes. In low-flow anaesthesia, a high FGF of up to 6 minutes is required. The FGF can be later reduced to 0.5–1 L/min. If no N_2O is used during anaesthesia (i.e. an oxygen/air mix is used), it is not necessary to eliminate nitrogen because air contains nitrogen. A short period of high flow is needed to prime the system and the patient with the inhalational agent.

2. Exhaled gases are circled back to the canister, where carbon dioxide absorption takes place and water and heat (exothermic reaction) are produced. The warmed and humidified gas joins the FGF to be delivered to the patient (Fig. 4.17).

then

$$K_2CO_3 + Ca(OH)_2 \rightarrow CaCO_3 + 2KOH$$

or

$$CO_2 + 2NaOH \rightarrow Na_2CO_3 + H_2O + heat$$

then

$$Na_2CO_3 + Ca(OH)_2 \rightarrow 2NaOH + CaCO_3$$

3. Chemical sequences for the absorption of carbon dioxide by soda lime:
   a) Note how both NaOH and KOH are regenerated at the expense of $Ca(OH)_2$. This explains soda lime's mix – only a little Na(OH) and K(OH) and a lot of $Ca(OH)_2$:

$$H_2O + CO_2 \rightarrow H_2CO_3$$

then

$$H_2CO_3 + 2KOH \rightarrow K_2CO_3 + 2H_2O$$

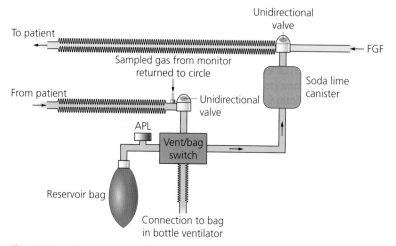

Fig. 4.17 Mechanism of action of the circle breathing system.

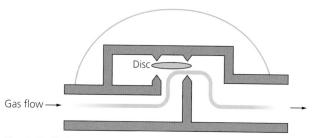

Fig. 4.18 Circle system unidirectional valve.

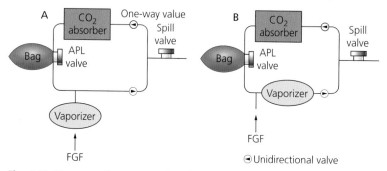

Fig. 4.19 Diagrammatic representation of the circle system with (A) vaporizer outside the circle (VOC) and (B) vaporizer inside the circle (VIC).

b) As can be seen above, this is an exothermic reaction, which alters the pH of the whole system. The reaction also produces water. One mole of water is produced for each mole of CO_2 absorbed.

c) The direction of gas flow is controlled via the unidirectional valves made of discs that rest on a 'knife-edge' (Fig. 4.18). They allow gas to flow in one direction only and prevent the mixing of inspired and expired gases, thus preventing rebreathing. These are mounted in see-through plastic domes so that they can be seen to be working satisfactorily.

4. The canister is positioned vertically to prevent exhaled gas channelling through unfilled portions. Larger canisters are more efficient than smaller ones because of the higher litres of CO_2/kg weight capacity. Double absorbers with two cartridges used simultaneously are more efficient than single absorbers.

5. The lower the FGF used, the more rapidly soda lime granules are consumed. This is because most of the exhaled gases pass through the absorber with very little being discarded through the APL valve. For a 70–80 kg patient with a tidal volume of 500 mL, respiratory rate of 12/min and CO_2 production of 250 mL/min, using an FGF of 1 L/min, the soda lime will be exhausted after 5–7 hours of use. For the same patient but using an FGF of 3 L/min, the soda lime will be exhausted after 6–8 hours of use.

6. The circle system can be used for both spontaneous and controlled ventilation.

7. Disposable circle breathing systems exist. They feature coaxial inspiratory tubing. The inner tubing delivers the FGF from the anaesthetic machine and the outer tubing delivers the recircled gas flow. Both gas flows mix distally. This allows a more rapid change in the inhalational gas and vapour concentration at the patient end.

USE OF VAPORIZERS IN THE CIRCLE BREATHING SYSTEM

VOC vaporizers (Fig. 4.19) are positioned on the back bar of the anaesthetic machine. They are high-efficiency vaporizers that can deliver high-output concentrations at low flows. They have high internal resistance.

1. The vaporizer should be able to deliver accurate concentrations of inhalational agent with both high and low FGFs. This is easily achieved by most modern vaporizers, e.g. the Tec series.

2. The volume of the circle system is large in relation to the low FGF used. Rapid changes in the concentration of the inspired vapour can be achieved by increasing the FGF to the circle system. Delivering the FGF distally, using a coaxial inspiratory tubing design, allows faster changes in inspired vapour concentration compared to conventional circle systems at low flows.

VIC vaporizers (see Fig. 4.19) are designed to offer minimal resistance to gas flow and have no wicks on which water vapour might condense (e.g. Goldman vaporizer). The VIC is a low-efficiency vaporizer adding only small amounts of vapour to the gas recirculating through it.

1. FGF will be vapour free and thus dilutes the inspired vapour concentration.

2. During spontaneous ventilation, respiration is depressed with deepening of anaesthesia. Uptake of the anaesthetic agent is therefore reduced. This is an example of a feedback safety mechanism. The safety mechanism is lost during controlled ventilation.

Problems in practice and safety features

1. Adequate monitoring of inspired oxygen, end-tidal carbon dioxide and inhalational agent concentrations is essential.

2. The unidirectional valves may stick and fail to close because of water vapour condensation. This leads to an enormous increase in dead space.

3. The resistance to breathing is increased especially during spontaneous ventilation. The main cause of resistance to breathing is due to the unidirectional valves. Dust formation can increase resistance to breathing further. It can also lead to clogging and channelling, so reducing efficiency. Newer soda lime designs claim less dust formation.

4. Compound A (a penta-fluoroisoproprenyl fluoro-methyl ether, which is nephrotoxic in rats) is produced when sevoflurane is used in conjunction with soda lime. This is due to the degradation of sevoflurane (dehydrohalogenation) as a result of the alkali metal hydroxide present in soda lime.

   Factors that increase the production of compound A are:
   a) increasing temperature
   b) high sevoflurane concentrations
   c) use of barylime rather than soda lime
   d) low fresh gas flow
   e) newer designs of soda lime, being non-caustic (no KOH and only very low levels of NaOH), claim less or no production of compound A. For substance A production, barylime is worse than soda lime and Amsorb® is the safest.

5. Carbon monoxide production can occur when volatile agents containing the CHF_2 moiety (enflurane, isoflurane and desflurane) are used with very dry granules when the water content is less than 1.5% in soda lime or less than 5% in barylime. This can occur when the system is left unused for a long length of time, e.g. overnight or at weekends, or when a small basal flow from the anaesthetic machine occurs. Carbon monoxide accumulation and subsequent carboxyhaemoglobin formation is said to occur at less than 0.1% per hour, so may become significant in smokers when ultra-low flows are used; oxygen flushes of the system (e.g. once an hour) will prevent this.

   More recent designs of soda lime claim less or no production of carbon monoxide. The association of strong alkalis such as KOH and NaOH to the production of carbon monoxide has led to the subsequent removal of KOH and reduction in amounts of NaOH used. Some absorbers (e.g. Amsorb®) do not use strong alkalis at all.

6. Other substances can accumulate such as methane, acetone, ethanol and hydrogen. However, they do not generally become clinically significant.

7. Uneven filling of the canister with soda lime leads to channelling of gases and decreased efficiency.

8. The circle system is bulkier, less portable and more difficult to clean.

9. Soda lime is corrosive. Protective clothing, gloves and eye/face protection can be used.

10. Because of the many connections, there is an increased potential for leaks and disconnection.

The circle breathing system

- Soda lime canister with two unidirectional valves attached to inspiratory and expiratory tubings. An APL valve and a reservoir bag are connected to the system.
- Soda lime consists of 94% calcium hydroxide, 5% sodium hydroxide and a small amount of potassium hydroxide.
- Soda lime absorbs the exhaled carbon dioxide and produces water and heat (so humidifies and warms inspired gases).
- Very efficient breathing system using low FGF and reducing pollution.
- A high initial flow is required.
- Vaporizers can be VIC or VOC.

Waters canister ('to-and-fro') bidirectional flow breathing system

Currently, this system is not widely used in anaesthetic practice. It consists of a Mapleson C system with a soda lime canister positioned between the APL valve and the reservoir. A filter is positioned in the canister to prevent the soda lime granules 'entering' the breathing system and the risk of inhaling them. It is not an efficient system as the granules nearest to the patient are exhausted first, so increasing the dead space. It is also a cumbersome system as the canister has to be positioned horizontally and packed tightly with the soda lime granules to prevent channelling of the gases (Fig. 4.20).

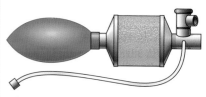

Fig. 4.20 The Waters canister breathing system.

FURTHER READING

Department of Health, 2004. Protecting the breathing circuit in anaesthesia. DoH, London.

Miller, R.D., Eriksson, L.I., Lee, A., et al, 2009. Miller's anaesthesia, seventh ed. Churchill Livingstone, Edinburgh.

MCQs

In the following lists, which of the statements (a) to (e) are true?

1. APL valve in a breathing system:
 a) In the open position, a pressure of less than 1 cm H_2O (0.1 kPa) is needed to actuate the valve.
 b) A pressure relief mechanism is activated at a pressure of 60 cm H_2O.
 c) Is incorporated in the T-piece breathing system.
 d) The dead space of the breathing system is reduced during spontaneous ventilation when excessive negative pressure from the scavenging system is applied through the APL valve.
 e) Should be closed during controlled ventilation using a Bain breathing system and an intermittent blower ventilator.

2. Breathing systems:
 a) The FGF rate required to prevent rebreathing of alveolar gas in the breathing system is a measure of the efficiency of a breathing system.
 b) The reservoir bag limits the pressure build-up in a breathing system to about 40 cm H_2O.
 c) A FGF of 150 mL/kg/min is needed in the Mapleson A system during spontaneous ventilation.
 d) The inner tube in the Bain system delivers the FGF.
 e) The Humphrey ADE system can be used for spontaneous ventilation only.

3. Dead space:
 a) The face mask in the Mapleson A breathing system has no effect on the dead space.
 b) Disconnection of the inner tube at the patient's end in the Bain system results in an increase in dead space.
 c) Failure of the unidirectional valves to close in the circle system has no effect on the system's dead space.
 d) The anatomic dead space is about 150 mL.
 e) Bohr's equation is used to measure the physiological dead space.

4. Concerning soda lime:
 a) 20% volume for volume of soda lime is sodium hydroxide.
 b) 90% is calcium carbonate.
 c) 1 kg of soda lime can absorb about 120 mL of CO_2.
 d) The reaction with carbon dioxide is exothermic.
 e) Soda lime fills half of the canister.

5. The Bain breathing system:
 a) Is an example of a Mapleson A system.
 b) Requires a FGF of 70 mL/kg during spontaneous ventilation.
 c) Is made of standard corrugated tubing.
 d) Can be used in a T-piece system.
 e) Can be used for both spontaneous and controlled ventilation.

6. T-piece breathing system:
 a) Can be used in paediatric practice only.
 b) Mapleson F system is the E system plus an open-ended reservoir bag.
 c) Is an efficient system.
 d) With a constant FGF, a too small reservoir has no effect on the performance of the system.
 e) The reservoir bag in Mapleson F provides a degree of CPAP during spontaneous ventilation.

7. Which of the following are true and which are false?
 a) The Magill classification is used to describe anaesthetic breathing systems.
 b) Modern anaesthetic breathing systems are constructed using anti-static materials.
 c) Efficiency of a breathing system is determined by the mode of ventilation of the patient.
 d) As long as the valve is present in a breathing system, its position is not important.
 e) Circle systems must only be used with very low FGFs.

8. The circle breathing system:
   a) With low flow rates, substance A can be produced when sevoflurane is used.
   b) The Goldman vaporizer is an example of a VOC.
   c) Failure of the unidirectional valves to close leads to an enormous increase in the dead space.
   d) Patients should not be allowed to breathe spontaneously, because of the high resistance caused by the soda lime.
   e) Exhaustion of the soda lime can be detected by an end-tidal CO_2 rebreathing waveform.

9. Regarding the circle system:
   a) A high FGF is needed in the first 15 minutes to wash out any CO_2 remaining in the breathing system.
   b) The pH of soda lime is highly acidic.
   c) The lower the FGF, the slower the exhaustion of soda lime granules.
   d) The Waters to-and-fro system is very efficient.
   e) Partially harmful substances can be produced when using soda lime.

SINGLE BEST ANSWER (SBA)

10. The APL valve:
    a) Is present in all breathing systems.
    b) Is actuated at only very high pressures when in the open position.
    c) Can act as a scavenging system.
    d) Scavenging systems can usually be attached to it.
    e) Is coloured bright yellow for safety reasons.

Answers

1. APL valve in a breathing system
   a) *True. The valve is designed to offer minimal resistance to exhalation and to prevent build-up of positive pressure in the breathing system in cases of malfunction or obstruction. A very low pressure of less than 1 cm H_2O is needed to actuate it. This is designed for the safety of the patient.*
   b) *True. This is a safety feature in the design of the APL valve. If the APL valve is closed, a build-up of pressure within the breathing system puts the patient at the risk of barotrauma. A pressure relief mechanism is activated at a pressure of 60 cm H_2O, allowing the reduction of pressure within the system.*
   c) *False. There are no valves in the standard T-piece system. This is to keep resistance to a minimum. A recent modification exists where an APL valve is included before a closed-ended 500-mL reservoir bag. A pressure relief safety mechanism in the APL valve is actuated at a pressure of 30 cm H_2O. This design allows for effective scavenging.*
   d) *False. There is a huge increase in the dead space resulting in rebreathing. This is because excessive negative pressure can lead the APL valve to remain open throughout breathing.*
   e) *True. When ventilation is controlled using a Bain breathing system and an intermittent blower ventilator, the APL valve must be closed completely. This is to prevent the escape of inhaled gases*

through the APL valve leading to inadequate ventilation.

2. Breathing systems:
   a) *True. The FGF rate required to prevent rebreathing is a measure of the efficiency of a breathing system; e.g. in spontaneous breathing, the circle system is the most efficient system whereas the Bain system is the least efficient.*
   b) *True. This is a safety feature to protect the patient from overpressure. Because of its high compliance, the reservoir bag can accommodate rises in pressure within the system better than other parts. Due to the law of Laplace (pressure = 2(tension)/radius), when the reservoir is overinflated, it can limit the pressure in the breathing system to about 40 cm H_2O.*
   c) *False. Mapleson A system is an efficient system during spontaneous breathing needing a FGF of about 70 mL/kg/min. Mapleson D needs an FGF of 150– 200 mL/kg/min.*
   d) *True. The inner tube delivers the FGF as close as possible to the patient. The outer tube, which is connected to the reservoir bag, takes the exhaled gases.*
   e) *False. The Humphrey ADE system is a very versatile system and can be used for both spontaneous and controlled ventilation both for adults and in paediatrics.*

3. Dead space:
   a) *False. The face mask increases the dead space in the*

Mapleson A breathing system. The dead space can increase up to 200 mL in adults.
   b) *True. Disconnection of the inner tube, which delivers the FGF, at the patient's end in the Bain system leads to an increase in dead space and rebreathing.*
   c) *False. The unidirectional valves are essential for the performance of the circle system. Failure to close leads to a significant increase in the dead space.*
   d) *True. The anatomic dead space is that part of the respiratory system which takes no part in the gas exchange.*
   e) *True. $V_D/V_T = P_ACO_2 - P_ECO_2/P_ACO_2$ where V_D is dead space; V_T is tidal volume; P_ACO_2 is alveolar CO_2 tension; P_ECO_2 is mixed expired CO_2 tension. Normally $V_D/V_T = 0.25–0.35$.*

4. Concerning soda lime:
   a) *False. Sodium hydroxide constitutes about 5% of the soda lime.*
   b) *False. Calcium carbonate is a product of the reaction between soda lime and carbon dioxide.*
   $CO_2 + 2NaOH$
   $\rightarrow Na_2CO_3 + H_2O + heat$
   $Na_2CO_3 + Ca(OH)_2$
   $\rightarrow 2NaOH + CaCO_3$
   c) *False. 1 kg of soda lime can absorb 120 L of CO_2.*
   d) *True. Heat is produced as a byproduct of the reaction between CO_2 and sodium hydroxide.*
   e) *False. In order to achieve adequate CO_2 absorption, the canister should be well packed*

to avoid channelling and incomplete CO_2 absorption.

---

5. The Bain breathing system:
   a) False. The Bain breathing system is an example of a Mapleson D system.
   b) False. A FGF of about 150–200 mL/kg/min is required to prevent rebreathing in the Bain system during spontaneous ventilation. This makes it an inefficient breathing system.
   c) False. The Bain system is usually made of a coaxial tubing. A more recent design, a pair of parallel corrugated tubings, is also available.
   d) False. The Bain breathing system is a Mapleson D whereas the T-piece system is an E system. The Bain system has an APL valve whereas the T-piece is a valveless system.
   e) True. The Bain system can be used for spontaneous ventilation requiring an FGF of 150–200 mL/kg. It can also be used for controlled ventilation requiring an FGF of 70–100 mL/kg. During controlled ventilation, the APL valve is fully closed, the reservoir bag is removed and a ventilator like the Penlon Nuffield 200 with a 1 m length of tubing is connected instead.

---

6. T-piece breathing system:
   a) False. Although the T-piece breathing system is mainly used in paediatrics, it can be used in adults with a suitable FGF and reservoir volume. An FGF of 2.5–3 times the minute volume and a reservoir approximating the tidal volume are needed. Such a system is usually used in recovery and for intensive care patients.

b) True. Jackson-Rees added a double-ended bag to the reservoir tubing of the Mapleson E thus converting it to a Mapleson F. The bag acts as a visual monitor during spontaneous ventilation and can be used for assisted or controlled ventilation.
c) False. The T-piece system is not an efficient system as it requires an FGF of 2.5–3 times the minute volume to prevent rebreathing.
d) False. If the reservoir is too small, entrainment of ambient air will occur resulting in dilution of the FGF.
e) True. Patients under the age of 6 years have a small FRC. General anaesthesia causes a further decrease in the FRC. The reservoir bag in the Mapleson F provides a degree of CPAP during spontaneous ventilation, helping to improve the FRC.

---

7. Which of the following are true or false?
   a) False. Mapleson classification is used. The Mapleson A breathing system was described by Magill.
   b) False. As modern anaesthetic agents are not flammable, modern breathing systems are not constructed using anti-static materials. They are normally made of plastic.
   c) True. Efficiency of a breathing system differs during spontaneous and controlled ventilation; e.g. the Mapleson A system is more efficient during spontaneous than controlled ventilation whereas the opposite is true of the D system.
   d) False. The position of the valve in the breathing system is crucial in the function and efficiency of a breathing system.

e) False. The circle system can be used with low flows (e.g. 2–3 L/min) as well as very low flows (e.g. 0.5–1.5 L/min). This can be achieved safely with adequate monitoring of the inspired and exhaled concentration of the gases and vapours used.

---

8. The circle breathing system:
   a) True. Substance A can be produced when sevoflurane is used with soda lime under low flow rates. Newer designs of soda lime claim lesser production of substance A.
   b) False. The Goldman vaporizer is a VIC. It is positioned on the expiratory limb with minimal resistance to flow and no wicks.
   c) True. The function of the unidirectional valves in the circle system is crucial for its function. Failure of the valve to close causes rebreathing resulting from the huge increase in the dead space of the system. This usually happens because of water vapour condensing on the valve.
   d) False. The circle system can be used for both spontaneous and controlled ventilation. Soda lime increases the resistance to flow but is clinically insignificant.
   e) True. As the soda lime gets exhausted, a rebreathing end-tidal CO_2 waveform can be detected. A dye is added that changes the granules' colour as they become exhausted.

---

9. Regarding circle system:
   a) False. High FGF (several L/min) is needed initially to denitrogenate the system and the functional residual capacity (FRC) to avoid the build-up of unacceptable

levels of nitrogen in the system. In closed circle anaesthesia, a high FGF for up to 15 minutes, and in low-flow anaesthesia, a high FGF of up to 6 minutes are required and these can later be reduced to 0.5–1 L/min. If no N_2O is used during anaesthesia, it is not necessary to eliminate nitrogen. A short period of high flow is needed to prime the system and the patient with the inhalational agent.

b) *False.* The pH of soda lime is highly alkaline, 13.5, because of the presence of calcium hydroxide, sodium hydroxide and small amounts, if any, of potassium hydroxide. This makes the soda lime a corrosive substance. Colour changes occur when the pH is less than 10.

c) *False.* The lower the FGF, the more rapidly soda lime granules are exhausted because most of the exhaled gases pass through the absorber with very little being discarded through the APL valve. For a 70–80-kg patient with a tidal volume of 500 mL, respiratory rate of 12/min and CO_2 production of 250 mL/min, using an FGF of 1 L/min, the soda lime will be exhausted in 5–7 h of use. For the same patient but using an FGF of 3 L/min, the soda lime will be exhausted in 6–8 h of use.

d) *False.* It is not an efficient system as the granules nearest to the patient are exhausted first so increasing the dead space.

e) *True.* Substance A, nephrotoxic in rats, can be produced when sevoflurane is used with soda lime although newer designs claim less or no substance A production. Carbon monoxide can occur when dry soda lime is used. Newer designs claim less or no carbon monoxide production.

10. d)

Chapter 5

Tracheal and tracheostomy tubes and airways

Tracheal tubes

Tracheal tubes provide a means of securing the patient's airway. These disposable plastic tubes are made of polyvinyl chloride (PVC) which could be clear, ivory or siliconized. As plastic is not radio-opaque, tracheal tubes have a radio-opaque line running along their length, which enables their position to be determined on chest X-rays. The siliconized PVC aids the passage of suction catheters through the tube. In the past, tracheal tubes used to be made of rubber allowing them to be reused after cleaning and autoclaving.

FEATURES OF TRACHEAL TUBES (FIG. 5.1)

Size

1. The 'size' of a tracheal tube refers to its **internal diameter** which is marked on the outside of the tube in millimetres. Narrower tubes increase the resistance to gas flow, therefore the largest possible internal diameter should be used. This is especially important during spontaneous ventilation where the patient's own respiratory effort must overcome the tube's resistance. A size 4-mm tracheal tube has 16 times more resistance to gas flow than a size 8-mm tube. Usually, a size 8.5–9-mm internal diameter tube is selected for an average size adult male and a size 7.5–8-mm internal diameter tube for an average size adult female. Paediatric sizes are determined on the basis of age and weight (Table 5.1). Tracheal tubes have both internal diameter (ID) and outside diameter (OD) markings. There are various methods or formulae used to

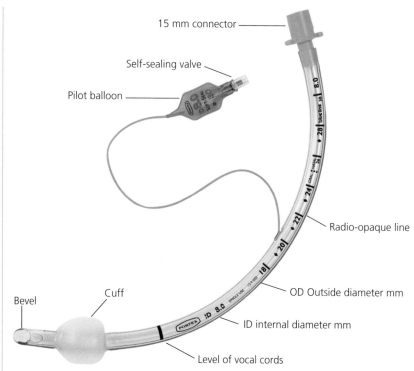

Fig. 5.1 Features of a cuffed tracheal tube. Some designs have the markings of IT (implantation tested) and Z–79 stands (the Z–79 Committee of the American National Standards Institute). (Courtesy of Smiths Medical.)

Table 5.1 A guide to the size and length of oral tracheal tubes used in paediatric practice

Age	Weight (kg)	Size (ID mm)	Length (cm)
Neonate	2–4	2.5–3.5	10–12
1–6 months	4–6	4.0–4.5	12–14
6–12 months	6–10	4.5–5.0	14–16
1–3 years	10–15	5.0–5.5	16–18
4–6 years	15–20	5.5–6.5	18–20
7–10 years	25–35	6.5–7.0	20–22
10–14 years	40–50	7.0–7.5	22–24

determine the size of paediatric tracheal tubes. A commonly used formula is:

$$\text{Internal diameter in mm} = \frac{\text{age in years}}{4} + 4$$

2. The **length** (taken from the tip of the tube) is marked in centimetres on the outside of the tube. The tube can be cut down to size to suit the individual patient. If the tube is cut too long, there is a significant risk of it advancing into one of the main bronchi (usually the right one, see Fig. 5.2). Black intubation depth markers located 3 cm proximal to the cuff can be seen in some designs (Fig. 5.1). These assist the accurate placement of

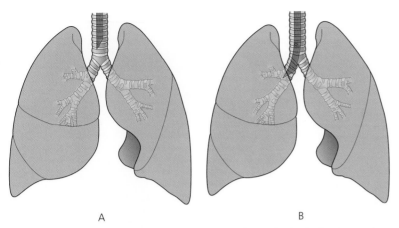

A   B

Fig. 5.2 (A) Correctly positioned tracheal tube. (B) The tracheal tube has been advanced too far, into the right main bronchus.

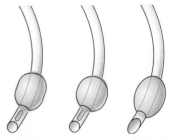

Fig. 5.4 Different types of tracheal tube cuffs. High volume (left), intermediate volume (centre), low volume (right).

the tracheal tube tip within the trachea. The vocal cords should be at the black mark in tubes with one mark, or should be between marks if there are two such marks. However, these are only rough estimates and correct tracheal tube position depth should always be confirmed by auscultation.

The bevel

1. The bevel is left-facing and oval in shape in most tube designs. A left-facing bevel improves the view of the vocal cords during intubation.
2. Some designs have a side hole just above and opposite the bevel, called a Murphy eye. This enables ventilation to occur should the bevel become occluded by secretions, blood or the wall of the trachea (Fig. 5.3).

The cuff

Tracheal (oral or nasal) tubes can be either cuffed or uncuffed. The cuff, when inflated, provides an air-tight seal between the tube and the tracheal wall (Fig. 5.4). This air-tight seal protects the patient's airway from aspiration and allows efficient ventilation during IPPV.

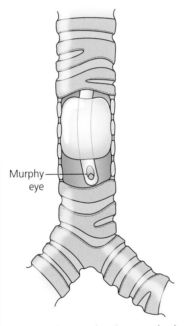

Murphy eye

Fig. 5.3 Diagram showing a tracheal tube with an obstructed bevel against the trachea wall but a patent Murphey's eye so allowing ventilation.

1. The cuff is connected to its pilot balloon which has a self-sealing valve for injecting air. The pilot balloon also indicates whether the cuff is inflated or not. After intubation, the cuff is inflated until no gas leak can be heard during intermittent positive pressure ventilation (IPPV).

2. The narrowest point in the adult's airway is the glottis (which is hexagonal). In order to achieve an air-tight seal, cuffed tubes are used in adults.
3. The narrowest point in a child's airway is the cricoid cartilage. Since this is essentially circular, a correctly sized uncuffed tube will fit well. Because of the narrow upper airway in children, post-extubation subglottic oedema can be a problem. In order to minimize the risk, the presence of a small leak around the tube at an airway pressure of 15 cm H_2O is desirable.
4. Cuffs can either be:
   a) high pressure/low volume
   b) low pressure/high volume.

High-pressure/low-volume cuffs

1. These can prevent the passing of vomitus, secretions or blood into the lungs.
2. At the same time, they exert a high pressure on the tracheal wall. If left in position for long periods, they may cause necrosis of the tracheal mucosa (Fig. 5.5).

Low-pressure/high-volume cuffs

1. These exert minimal pressure on the tracheal wall as the pressure equilibrates over a wider area (Fig. 5.6). This allows the cuff to remain inflated for longer periods.

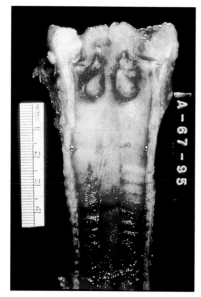

Fig. 5.5 A postmortem tracheal specimen. Note the black necrotic area which was caused by long-term intubation with a high-pressure cuffed tube.

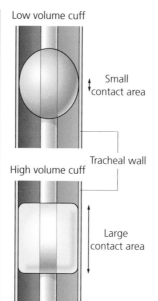

Low volume cuff

Small contact area

Tracheal wall

High volume cuff

Large contact area

Fig. 5.6 Diagram illustrating how a low-volume cuff (top) maintains a seal against a relatively small area of tracheal wall compared to a high-volume cuff (bottom).

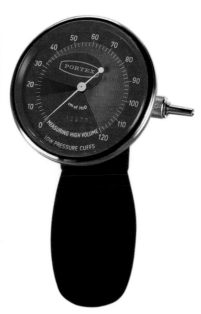

Fig. 5.7 Cuff pressure gauge. (Courtesy of Smiths Medical.)

2. They are less capable of preventing the aspiration of vomitus or secretions. This is due to the possibility of wrinkles forming in the cuff.

The pressure in the cuff should be checked at frequent and regular intervals (Fig. 5.7 and 5.8). The pressure may increase mainly because of diffusion of nitrous oxide into the cuff. Expansion of the air inside the cuff due to the increase in its temperature from room to body temperature and the diffusion of oxygen from the anaesthetic mixture (about 33%) into the air (21%) in the cuff can also lead to increase in the intracuff pressure. An increase in pressure of about 10–12 mmHg is expected after 30 minutes of anaesthesia with 66% nitrous oxide. A more recent design cuff material (Soft Seal, Portex) allows minimum diffusion of nitrous oxide into the cuff with a pressure increase of 1–2 mmHg only. The pressure may decrease because of a leak in the cuff or pilot balloon's valve.

Route of insertion

1. Tubes can be inserted orally or nasally (Fig. 5.9).
2. The indications for nasal intubation include:
   a) surgery where access via the mouth is necessary, e.g. ENT or dental operations
   b) long-term ventilated patients on intensive care units. Patients tolerate a nasal tube

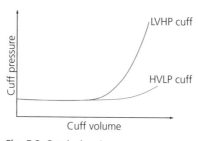

Cuff pressure

LVHP cuff

HVLP cuff

Cuff volume

Fig. 5.8 Graph showing pressure changes in low-volume/high-pressure (LVHP) cuff and high-volume/low-pressure (HVLP) cuff. Note the steep rise in cuff pressure in the LVHP cuff when the cuff volume reaches a critical volume. A more gradual increase in pressure is seen in the HVLP cuff.

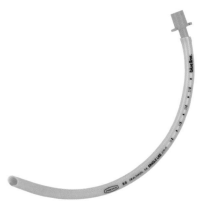

Fig. 5.9 A non-cuffed oral/nasal tracheal tube. (Courtesy of Smiths Medical.)

better, and cannot bite on the tube. However, long-term nasal intubation may cause sinus infection.

3. Nasal intubation is usually avoided, if possible, in children up to the age of 8–11 years. Hypertrophy of the adenoids in this age group increases the risk of profuse bleeding if nasal intubation is performed.
4. Ivory PVC nasotracheal tubes cause less trauma to the nasal mucosa.

Connectors

These connect the tracheal tubes to the breathing system (or catheter mount). There are various designs and modifications (Fig. 5.10). They are made of plastic or metal and should have an adequate internal diameter to reduce the resistance to gas flow.

On the breathing system end, the British Standard connector has a 15-mm diameter at the proximal end. An 8.5-mm diameter version exists for neonatal use. On the tracheal tube end, the connector has a diameter that depends on the size of the tracheal tube. Connectors designed for use with nasal tracheal tubes have a more acute angle than the oral ones (e.g. Magill's connector). Some designs have an extra port for suction.

Problems in practice and safety features

1. Obstruction of the tracheal tube by kinking, herniation of the cuff, occlusion by secretions, foreign body or the bevel lying against the wall of the trachea.
2. Oesophageal or bronchial intubation.
3. Trauma and injury to the various tissues and structures during and after intubation.

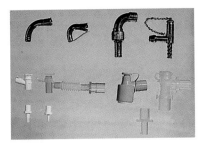

Fig. 5.10 A range of tracheal tube connectors. Top row from left to right: Magill oral, Magill nasal, Nosworthy, Cobb suction. (Note the Magill nasal connector has been supplied with a piece of wire threaded through it to demonstrate its patency.) Bottom row: Paediatric 8.5-mm connectors (left), standard 15-mm connectors (right).

> **Tracheal tubes**
> - Usually made of plastic.
> - Oral or nasal (avoid nasal intubation in children).
> - Cuffed or uncuffed.
> - The cuff can be low pressure/high volume, high pressure/low volume.

Specially designed tracheal tubes

OXFORD TRACHEAL TUBE

This anatomically L-shaped tracheal tube is used in anaesthesia for head and neck surgery because it is non-kinking (Fig. 5.11). The tube can be made of rubber or plastic and can be cuffed or uncuffed. The bevel is oval in shape and faces posteriorly and an introducing stylet is supplied to aid the insertion of the tube. Its thick wall adds to the tube's external diameter making it wider for a given internal diameter. This is undesirable especially in paediatric anaesthesia.

The distance from the bevel to the curve of the tube is fixed. If the tube is too long, the problem cannot be corrected by withdrawing the tube and shortening it because this means losing its anatomical fit.

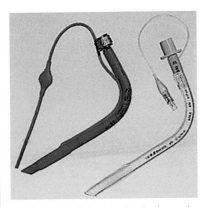

Fig. 5.11 The Oxford tracheal tube, red rubber (left) and plastic (right).

ARMOURED TRACHEAL TUBE

Armoured tracheal tubes are made of plastic or silicone rubber (Fig. 5.12). The walls of the armoured tube are thicker than ordinary tracheal tubes because they contain an embedded spiral of metal wire or tough nylon. They are used in anaesthesia for head and neck surgery. The spiral helps to prevent the kinking and occlusion of the tracheal tube when the head and/or neck is rotated or flexed so giving it strength and flexibility at the same time. An introducer stylet is used to aid intubation.

Because of the spiral, it is not possible to cut the tube to the desired length. This increases the risk of bronchial intubation. Two markers, situated just above the cuff, are present on some designs. These indicate the correct position for the vocal cords.

POLAR AND RAE TRACHEAL TUBES

The **polar tube** is a north- or south-facing preformed nasal cuffed or uncuffed tracheal tube

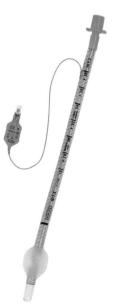

Fig. 5.12 Armoured cuffed tracheal tube. (Courtesy of Smiths Medical.)

(Fig. 5.13). It is used mainly during anaesthesia for maxillofacial surgery as it does not impede surgical access. Because of its design and shape, it lies over the nose and the forehead. It can be converted to an ordinary tracheal tube by cutting it at the scissors mark just proximal to the pilot tube and reconnecting the 15-mm connector. An oral version of the polar tube exists.

The **RAE (Ring, Adair and Elwyn) tube** has a preformed shape to fit the mouth or nose without kinking. It has a bend located just as the tube emerges, so the connections to the breathing system are at the level of the chin or forehead and not interfering with the surgical access. RAE tubes can be either north- or south-facing, cuffed or uncuffed.

Because of its preformed shape, there is a higher risk of bronchial intubation than with ordinary tracheal tubes. The cuffed RAE tracheal tube has one Murphy eye whereas the uncuffed version has two eyes. Since the uncuffed version is mainly used in paediatric practice, two Murphy eyes ensure adequate ventilation should the tube prove too long.

The tube can be temporarily straightened to insert a suction catheter.

LASER RESISTANT TRACHEAL TUBES

These tubes are used in anaesthesia for laser surgery on the larynx or trachea (Fig. 5.14). They are designed to withstand the effect of carbon dioxide and potassium-titanyl-phosphate (KTP) laser beams, avoiding the risk of fire or damage to the tracheal tube. One design has a flexible stainless steel body. Reflected beams from the tube are defocused to reduce the accidental laser strikes to healthy tissues (Fig. 5.15). Other designs

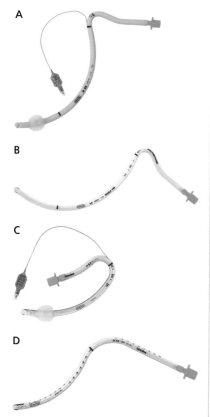

Fig. 5.13 Polar and RAE tracheal tubes: (A) cuffed nasal north facing; (B) non-cuffed nasal north facing; (C) cuffed oral south-facing; (D) non-cuffed oral north-facing. (Coutresy of Smiths Medical.)

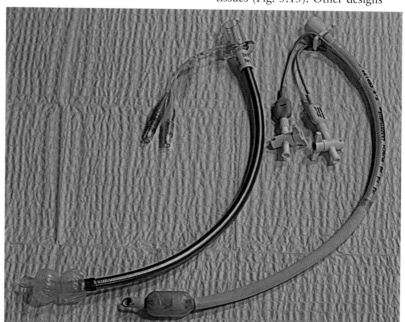

Fig. 5.14 Laser resistant tracheal tubes. Note the stainless steel tube (left) with two cuffs. The tube on the right is covered with laser protective wrapping. Laser beam

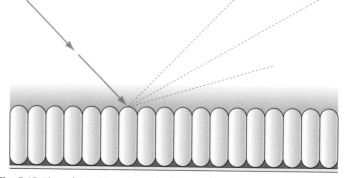

Fig. 5.15 The reflected laser beam is defocused.

have a laser resistant metal foil wrapped around the tube for protection. The cuff is filled with methylene blue coloured saline. If the laser manages to damage the cuff, the colouring will help identify rupture and the saline will help prevent an airway fire.

Some designs have two cuffs. This ensures a tracheal seal should the upper cuff be damaged by laser. An air-filled cuff, hit by the laser beam, may ignite and so it is recommended that the cuffs are filled with saline instead of air.

EVOKED POTENTIALS TRACHEAL TUBES (FIG. 5.16)

These tubes are used in a number of surgical procedures that have the risks of damage to nerves, e.g thyroid surgery. Bipolar stainless steel contact electrical electrodes are embebded in the tracheal tubes above the cuff where they are in contact with the vocal cords. These electrodes are connected to a nerve stimulator. An additional earth electrode is attached to the skin of the patient.

The use of such tubes allows continuous nerve monitoring throughout surgery providing visual and audible warnings.

MICROLARYNGEAL TUBE

This tube allows better exposure and surgical access to the larynx. It has a small diameter (usually 5-mm ID) with an adult sized cuff (Fig. 5.17). Its length is sufficient to allow nasal intubation if required. The tube is made of ivory PVC to reduce trauma to the nasal mucosa.

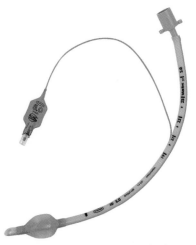

Fig. 5.17 Microlaryngeal tracheal tube. (Courtesy of Smiths Medical.)

Tracheostomy tracheal tubes

These are curved plastic tubes usually inserted through the second, third and fourth tracheal cartilage rings (Fig. 5.18).

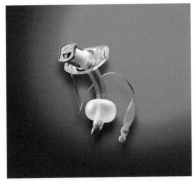

Fig. 5.18 Cuffed tracheostomy tube. (Courtesy of Smiths Medical.)

Components

1. An introducer used for insertion.
2. Wings attached to the proximal part of the tube to fix it in place with a ribbon or suture. Some designs have an adjustable flange to fit the variable thickness of the subcutaneous tissues (Fig. 5.19).
3. They can be cuffed or uncuffed. The former have a pilot balloon.
4. The proximal end can have a standard 15-mm connector.

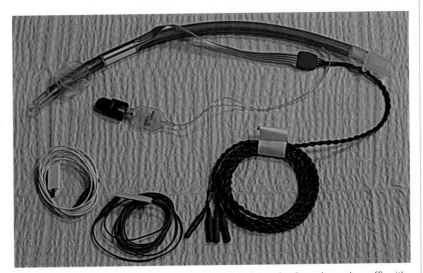

Fig. 5.16 Evoked potential tracheal tube. Note the electrodes (just above the cuff) with their cables. The other cable is earth.

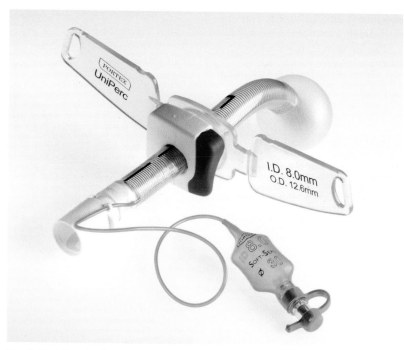

Fig. 5.19 Adjustable flange tracheostomy tube. (Courtesy of Smiths Medical.)

5. The tip is usually cut square, rather than bevelled. This is to decrease the risk of obstruction by lying against the tracheal wall.

6. A more recent design with an additional suctioning lumen which opens just above the cuff exists. The cuff shape is designed to allow the secretions above it to be suctioned effectively through the suctioning lumen (Fig. 5.20).

7. Some tubes have an inner cannula. Secretions can collect and dry out on the inner lumen of the tube leading to obstruction. The internal cannula can be replaced instead of changing the complete tube in such cases. The cannula leads to a slight reduction of the internal diameter of the tube.

8. There are different sizes of tracheostomy tubes to fit neonates to adults.

9. Older uncuffed metal tracheostomy tubes made of a non-irritant and bactericidal silver are rarely used in current practice. Some designs have a one-way flap valve and a

window at the angle of the tube to allow the patient to speak.

Tracheostomy tubes are used for the following

1. Long-term intermittent positive pressure ventilation.
2. Upper airway obstruction that cannot be bypassed with an oral/nasal tracheal tube.
3. Maintenance of an airway and to protect the lungs in patients with impaired pharyngeal or laryngeal reflexes and after major head and neck surgery (e.g. laryngectomy).
4. Long-term control of excessive bronchial secretions especially in patients with a reduced level of consciousness.
5. To facilitate weaning from a ventilator. This is due to a reduction in the sedation required, as the patients tolerate tracheostomy tubes better than tracheal tubes. Also, there is a reduction in the anatomical dead space.

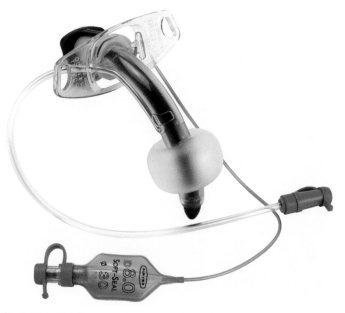

Fig. 5.20 Smith's Portex tracheostomy tube with an above-cuff suction facility.

Benefits of tracheostomy

- Increased patient comfort.
- Less need for sedation.
- Improved access for oral hygiene.
- Possibility of oral nutrition.
- Bronchial suctioning aided.
- Reduced dead space.
- Reduced airway resistance.
- Reduced risk of glottic trauma.

Problems in practice and safety features

Surgical tracheostomy has a mortality rate of <1% but has a total complications rate as high as 40%. The complications rate is higher in the intensive care unit and emergency patients.

The complications can be divided into:

1. Immediate:
   a) haemorrhage
   b) tube misplacement (e.g. into a main bronchus)
   c) occlusion of tube by cuff herniation
   d) occlusion of the tube tip against carina or tracheal wall
   e) pneumothorax.
2. Delayed:
   a) blockage of the tube by secretions which can be sudden or gradual; this is rare with adequate humidification and suction
   b) infection of the stoma
   c) overinflation of the cuff leads to ulceration and distension of the trachea
   d) mucosal ulceration because of excessive cuff pressures, asymmetrical inflation of the cuff or tube migration.
3. Late:
   a) granulomata of the trachea may cause respiratory difficulty after extubation
   b) persistent sinus at the tracheostomy site

c) tracheal dilatation
d) tracheal stenosis at the cuff site
e) scar formation.

THE FENESTRATED TRACHEOSTOMY TUBE (FIG. 5.21)

1. The fenestration (window) in the greater curvature channels air to the vocal cords allowing the patient to speak.
2. After deflation of the cuff, the patient can breathe around the cuff and through the fenestration as well as through the stoma. This reduces airway resistance and assists in weaning from

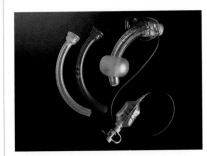

Fig. 5.21 A Portex unfenestrated inner cannula (left), fenestrated inner cannula (middle) and Blue Line Ultra fenestrated tracheostomy tube with Soft-Seal cuff (right).

tracheostomy in spontaneously breathing patients.
3. Some tubes have a fenestrated inner cannula.

LARYNGECTOMY (MONTANDON) TUBE

This is a cuffed tube inserted through a tracheostomy to facilitate intermittent positive pressure ventilation during neck surgery (Fig. 5.22). It has the advantage of offering better surgical access by allowing the breathing system to be connected well away from the surgical field. Usually, it is replaced with a tracheostomy, tube at the end of operation.

Tracheostomy tubes

- Can be plastic or metal, cuffed or uncuffed.
- The tip is cut horizontally.
- Used for long-term intubation.
- Percutaneous tracheostomy tubes are becoming more popular and have fewer complications than the surgical technique.
- Speaking versions exist.

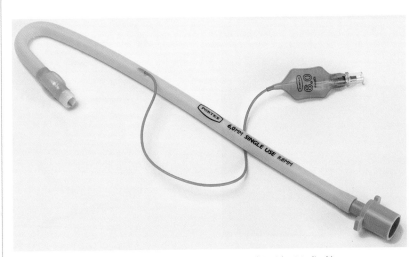

Fig. 5.22 Montandon laryngectomy tube. (Courtesy of Smiths Medical.)

TRACHEOSTOMY SPEAKING VALVE (FIG. 5.23)

This is a one-way speaking valve. It is fitted to the uncuffed tracheostomy tube or to the cuffed tracheostomy tube with its cuff deflated.

Tracheostomy button (Fig. 5.24)

Once a tracheostomy is removed after long-term use, this device is inserted into the stoma to maintain patency of the tract and also act as a route for tracheal suction.

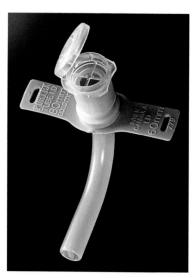

Fig. 5.23 A tracheostomy speaking valve mounted on an uncuffed tracheostomy tube.

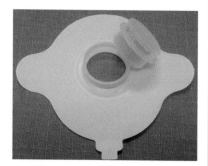

Fig. 5.24 Tracheostomy button and its skin dressing.

PERCUTANEOUS TRACHEOSTOMY TUBES

These tubes are inserted between the first and second or second and third tracheal rings, usually at the bedside in the intensive care unit.

1. If the patient is intubated, the tracheal tube is withdrawn until the tip is just below the vocal cords. Then the cuff is inflated and rested on the vocal cords. A laryngeal mask can be used instead.
2. Through an introducing needle, a Seldinger guidewire is inserted into the trachea. A fibreoptic bronchoscope should be used throughout the procedure. It helps to ensure the initial puncture of the trachea is in the midline and free of the tracheal tube. It can also ensure that the posterior tracheal wall is not damaged during the procedure. Finally, it can assess the position of the tracheostomy tube relative to the carina.
3. A pair of specially designed Griggs forceps are inserted over the guidewire. These forceps are used to dilate the trachea. A tracheostomy tube is threaded over the guidewire and advanced into the trachea. The guidewire is then removed (Fig. 5.25).
4. A series of curved dilators can be used instead of the dilating forceps. The diameter of the stoma is serially increased until the desired diameter is achieved. A single curved dilator of a graduated diameter can be used instead (Fig. 5.26). A tracheostomy tube can then be inserted.
5. An adjustable flange percutaneous tracheostomy is available. The flange can be adjusted to suit the patient's anatomy, e.g. in the obese patient. The flange can be moved away from the stoma site to aid in cleaning around the stoma.
6. The procedure can be performed in the intensive care unit with a lower incidence of complications

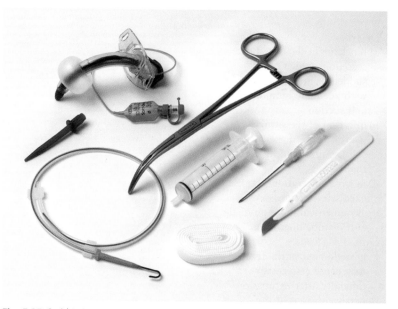

Fig. 5.25 Smith's Portex Griggs percutaneous tracheostomy set.

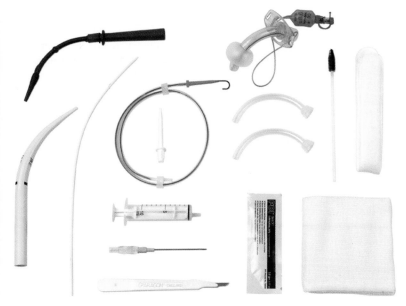

Fig. 5.26 Smith's Portex Ultraperc single dilator percutaneous tracheostomy set.

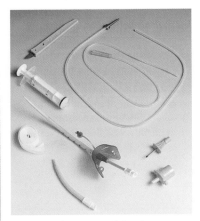

Fig. 5.27 The Portex minitracheostomy set inserted using the Seldinger technique.

than the conventional open surgical method (infection rate, subglottic stenosis and bleeding problems). The operative time is about half that of a formal surgical procedure.

7. Percutaneous tracheostomy can be performed faster using the dilating forceps technique compared to the dilator technique.

8. There is an increased risk of surgical emphysema due to air leaks from the trachea to the surrounding tissues. Loss of the airway, bleeding and incorrect placement of the needle are potential difficulties during the procedure. The risk of aspiration is increased when the tracheal tube has to be withdrawn at the start of the procedure.

9. Relative contraindications include enlarged thyroid gland, non-palpable cricoid cartilage, paediatric application, previous neck surgery and positive end expiratory pressure (PEEP) of more than 15 cm H_2O. The latter is because of the difficulty

in applying a high PEEP during the process of insertion.

10. Reinsertion of a percutaneously fashioned tube can be more difficult than the surgical one as the stoma may close immediately. A track is formed after long-term intubation and the tracheostomy tube can be removed. In order to protect the patency of the tract, a tracheostomy button is inserted into the stoma. It also acts as a route for tracheal suction. Tracheostomy buttons are made of straight rigid plastic.

Minitracheostomy tube

This tube is inserted percutaneously into the trachea through the avascular cricothyroid membrane (Fig. 5.27).

Components

1. A siliconized PVC tube 10 cm in length with an internal diameter

of 4 mm. Some designs have lengths ranging from 3.5 to 7.5 cm with internal diameters from 2 to 6 mm.

2. The proximal end of the tube has a standard 15-mm connector that allows attachment to breathing systems. The proximal end also has wings used to secure the tube with the ribbon supplied.

3. A 2-cm, 16-G needle is used to puncture the cricothyroid cartilage. A 50-cm guidewire is used to help in the tracheal cannulation. A 10-mL syringe is used to aspirate air to confirm the correct placement of the needle.

4. A 7-cm curved dilator and a curved introducer are used to facilitate the insertion of the cricothyrotomy tube in some designs.

Mechanism of action

1. The Seldinger technique is used to insert the tube.

2. It is an effective method to clear tracheobronchial secretions in patients with an inefficient cough.

3. In an emergency, it can be used in patients with upper airway obstruction that cannot be bypassed with a tracheal tube.

Problems in practice and safety features

Percutaneous insertion of minitracheostomy has the risk of:

1. pneumothorax
2. perforation of the oesophagus
3. severe haemorrhage
4. ossification of the cricothyroid membrane
5. incorrect placement.

> **Minitracheostomy**
> - Tube inserted into the trachea through the cricothyroid membrane using the Seldinger technique.
> - Used for clearing secretions and maintaining an airway in an emergency.

Cricothyrotomy tube (Fig. 5.28)

This tube is used to maintain the airway in emergency situations such as on the battlefield. It is inserted into the trachea through the cricothyroid cartilage.

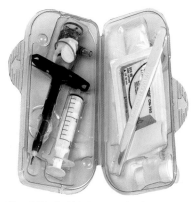

Fig. 5.28 Smith's Portex cricothyrotomy set.

Components

1. A scalpel and syringe
2. A needle with a veress design and a dilator. The needle has a 'red flag' indicator. This helps in locating the tissues.
3. 6-mm cuffed tube.

Mechanism of action

1. After a 2-cm horizontal skin incision has been made, the needle is inserted perpendicular to the skin.
2. As the needle enters the trachea, the red indicator disappears. The needle is advanced carefully until the red reappears, indicating contact with the posterior wall of the trachea.
3. As the cricothyrotomy tube is advanced into the trachea, the needle and the dilator are removed.

Problems in practice and safety features

The cricothyrotomy tube has complications similar to the minitracheostomy tube.

> **Cricothyrotomy**
> - A cuffed 6-mm tube is inserted into the trachea through the cricothyroid cartilage.
> - A veress needle is designed to locate the trachea.
> - Used in emergencies to establish an airway.

Double lumen endobronchial tubes

During thoracic surgery, there is a need for one lung to be deflated. This offers the surgeon easier and better access within the designated hemithorax. In order to achieve this, double lumen tubes are used which allow the anaesthetist to selectively deflate one lung while maintaining standard ventilation of the other.

Components

1. The Mallinckrodt Bronchocath double lumen tube has two separate colour-coded lumens, each with its own bevel (Fig. 5.29). One lumen ends in the trachea and the other lumen ends in either the left or right main bronchus.
2. Each lumen has its own cuff (tracheal and bronchial cuffs) and colour-coded pilot balloons. Both lumens and pilot balloons are labelled.
3. There are two curves to the tube: the standard anterior curve to fit into the oropharyngeal laryngeal tracheal airway and the second curve, either to the right or left, to fit into the right or left bronchus respectively.
4. The proximal end of these tubes is connected to a Y-shaped catheter mount attached to the breathing system.

Mechanism of action

1. Because of the differing anatomy of the main bronchi and their branches, both right and left versions of any particular double lumen tube must exist.
2. Once the tubes are correctly positioned, the anaesthetist can selectively ventilate one lung. So, for operations requiring that the right lung is deflated, a left-sided double lumen tube would be used that enabled selective ventilation of the left lung alone and vice versa.
3. It is desirable, when possible, to insert a left double lumen tube instead of a right one. This reduces the risk of upper lobe bronchus obstruction by the

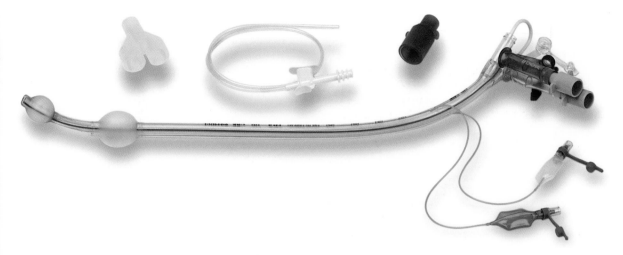

Fig. 5.29 Double lumen endobronchial tube (left sided).

bronchial cuff in the right-sided version.

4. The right-sided version has an eye in the bronchial cuff to facilitate ventilation of the right upper lobe. The distance between the right upper lobe bronchus and the carina in an adult is only 2.5 cm, so there is a real risk of occluding it with the bronchial cuff. There is no eye in the left-sided version because the distance between the carina and the left upper lobe bronchus is about 5 cm, which is adequate to place the cuff.

5. The tubes come in different sizes to fit adult patients, but not in paediatric sizes.

Tube positioning

1. The position of the tube should be checked by auscultation immediately after intubation and after positioning the patient for the operation. It is also recommended to use a fibreoptic bronchoscope to confirm correct positioning of the double lumen tube.

2. The tracheal cuff is inflated first until no leak is heard. At this

point, both lungs can be ventilated. Next, the tracheal limb of the Y-catheter mount is clamped and disconnected from the tracheal lumen tube. Then, the bronchial cuff is inflated with only a few millilitres of air until no leak is heard from the tracheal tube. At this stage, only the lung ventilated via the bronchial lumen should be ventilated. The ability to selectively ventilate the other lung should also be checked by clamping the bronchial limb of the Y-catheter mount and disconnecting it from the bronchial lumen having already reconnected the tracheal lumen. At this stage, only the lung ventilated via the tracheal lumen should be ventilated.

The commonly used double lumen bronchial tubes are:

1. **Robertshaw** (rubber) tubes (Fig. 5.30).
2. **Single-use plastic** tubes. These tubes require an introducer for insertion. A more recent version of the single use has the facility of applying continuous positive airway pressure (CPAP) to the

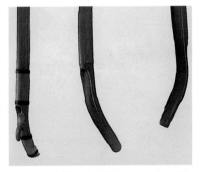

Fig. 5.30 White double lumen tube with carinal hook (left). Left and right versions of the Robertshaw double lumen tube (centre and right).

deflated lung to improve arterial oxygenation (Fig. 5.31).

3. **Carlens** (left-sided version) and **White** (right-sided version) tubes that use a carinal hook to aid final positioning of the tube (Fig. 5.30). The hook can cause trauma to the larynx or carina. Because of the relatively small lumens (6 and 8 mm), the Carlens tube causes an increase in airway resistance and difficulty in suctioning thick secretions.

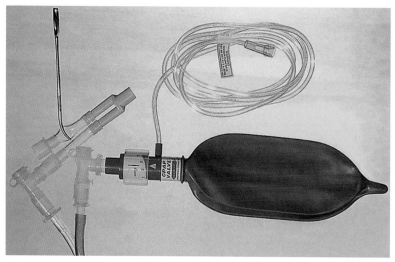

Fig. 5.31 Bronchocath double lumen tube with the bronchial lumen connected to a CPAP valve assembly. The disconnected limb of the Y-shaped catheter mount has been clamped.

Double lumen endobronchial tubes
- Two separate lumens each with its own cuff and pilot tube.
- There are two curves, anterior and lateral.
- The right-sided version has an eye in the bronchial cuff to facilitate ventilation of the right upper lobe.
- Commonly used ones are Robertshaw, Bronchocath and Carlens (and White). The latter has a carinal hook.

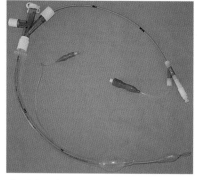

Fig. 5.32 The Arndt endobronchial blocker set.

Endobronchial blocker

The endobronchial blocker is an alternative means to the double lumen tube for providing one-lung ventilation (Fig. 5.32).

Components

1. The blocker catheter. This is a 9-FG, 78-cm catheter that has a distal cuff inflated via a pilot balloon. A guide loop emerges from its tip (Fig. 5.33).
2. Multiport adapter.

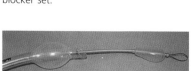

Fig. 5.33 Detail of the blocker emerging from a standard endotracheal tube. The guide loop is used to advance the blocker over a paediatric fibreoptic bronchoscope into the desired main bronchus.

Mechanism of action

The patient is intubated with a standard endotracheal tube. A specially designed multiport adapter is connected to the tube's standard 15-mm connector. The blocker can be advanced over a paediatric fibreoptic bronchoscope into the desired main bronchus while maintaining ventilation.

When the blocker's position is satisfactory, the balloon can be inflated, sealing off the desired main bronchus. Ventilation of the contralateral lung is maintained via the tracheal tube.

Oropharyngeal airway

This anatomically shaped airway is inserted through the mouth into the oropharynx above the tongue to maintain the patency of the upper airway (Fig. 5.34) in cases of upper airway obstruction caused by a decreased level of consciousness in a patient. Decreased consciousness can lead to loss of pharyngeal tone that can result in airway obstruction by the tongue, epiglottis, soft palate or pharyngeal tissues. There are various regularly used types of oropharyngeal airway. The most common type is the Guedel airway, named after its developer Arthur Guedel, an American anaesthetist who served in France during the First World War. It is available in up to nine sizes, which have a standardized number coding (the smallest '000' to the largest '6').

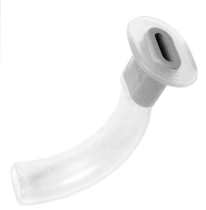

Fig. 5.34 An oropharyngeal (Guedel) airway. (Courtesy of Smiths Medical.)

Components

1. The curved body of the oropharyngeal airway contains the air channel. It is flattened anteroposteriorly and curved laterally.
2. There is a flange at the oral end to prevent the oropharyngeal airway from falling back into the mouth so avoiding further posterior displacement into the pharynx.
3. The bite portion is straight and fits between the teeth. It is made of hard plastic to prevent occlusion of the air channel should the patient bite the oropharyngeal airway.

Mechanism of action

1. The patient's airway is kept patent by preventing the tongue and epiglottis from falling backwards.
2. Oropharyngeal airways are designed in different sizes to fit the majority of patients from neonates to adults.
3. The air channel should be as large as possible in order to pass suction catheters.
4. As a good indication, a suitable Guedel airway size can be equivalent to either distance from the patient's incisors to the angle of the mandible, or corner of the patient's mouth to the tragus.
5. In adults, the Guedel airway is initially inserted upside down, with the curvature facing caudad. Once partially inserted, it is then rotated through 180° and advanced until the bite block rests between the incisors. This method prevents the tongue being pushed back into the pharynx, causing further obstruction.
6. In children, it is often recommended that the Guedel airway is inserted the right way round, using a tongue depressor or laryngoscope to depress the tongue. This is done to minimize

the risk of trauma to the oropharyngeal mucosa. The same technique can also be used in adults.
7. Bermann airway is another type of oropharyngeal airway, designed to assist with oral fibreoptic intubation (Fig. 5.35). It acts to guide the fibrescope around the back of the tongue to the larynx, with the purpose of both maintaining the patient's airway and acting as a bite block, thus preventing damage to the fibrescope. Unlike a Guedel airway, it has a side opening which allows it to be removed from the fibrescope, prior to the railroading of the tracheal tube into the trachea.

Problems in practice and safety features

1. Trauma to the different tissues during insertion.
2. Trauma to the teeth, crowns/caps if the patient bites on it.
3. If inserted in a patient whose pharyngeal reflexes are not depressed enough, the gag reflex can be induced that might lead to vomiting and laryngospasm.
4. They confer no protection against aspiration.
5. The degree to which airway patency has been increased after insertion of a Guedel airway should be assessed, not assumed. It should also always be

remembered that a badly inserted Guedel airway can make airway patency worse rather than better.

> **Oropharyngeal airway**
> - Anatomically shaped.
> - Inserted through the mouth above the tongue into the oropharynx.
> - Maintains the patency of the upper airway.
> - Can cause trauma and injury to different structures.
> - Risk of gag reflex stimulation and vomiting.
> - Bermann airway is designed to assist with oral fibreoptic intubation.

Nasopharyngeal airway

This airway is inserted through the nose into the nasopharynx, bypassing the mouth and the oropharynx. The distal end is just above the epiglottis and below the base of the tongue (Fig. 5.36).

Components

1. The rounded curved body of the nasopharyngeal airway.
2. The bevel is left-facing.

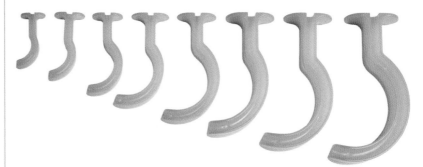

Fig. 5.35 A range of Bermann airway. (Courtesy of Smiths Medical.)

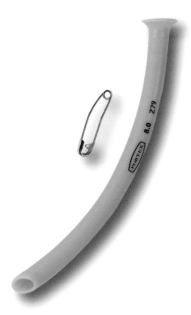

Fig. 5.36 Nasopharyngeal airway. The safety pin is to prevent the airway from migrating into the nose. (Courtesy of Smiths Medical.)

3. The proximal end has a flange. A 'safety pin' is provided to prevent the airway from migrating into the nose.

Mechanism of action

1. It is an alternative to the oropharyngeal airway when the mouth cannot be opened or an oral airway does not relieve the obstruction.
2. Nasotracheal suction can be performed using a catheter passed through the nasal airway.
3. It is better tolerated by semi-awake patients than the oral airway.
4. A lubricant is used to help in its insertion.
5. The size inserted can be estimated as size 6 for an average height female and size 7 for an average height male.
6. Once lubricated, it can be inserted through either nares, although the left-facing bevel is designed to ease insertion into the right nostril. On insertion, it should be passed backwards through the nasopharynx, such that its distal end lies beyond the pharyngeal border of the soft palate but not beyond the epiglottis.

Problems in practice and safety features

1. Its use is not recommended when the patient has a bleeding disorder, is on anticoagulants, has nasal deformities or sepsis.
2. Excess force should not be used during insertion as a false passage may be created.
3. An airway that is too large can result in pressure necrosis of the nasal mucosa, while an airway that is too small may be ineffective at relieving airway obstruction.

Nasopharyngeal airway
- Inserted through the nose into the nasopharynx.
- A useful alternative to the oropharyngeal airway.
- Not recommended in coagulopathy, nasal sepsis and deformities.

Supraglottic (or extraglottic) airway devices

The introduction of the laryngeal mask airway heralded an era of hands-free airway maintenance without the need for tracheal intubation. Many other airway devices that lie outside the trachea and attempt to provide a leak-free seal for spontaneous ventilation, while some provide an adequate seal for positive pressure ventilation under normal conditions, have been used. These devices are collectively known as supraglottic or extraglottic airways devices.

These devices provide the following:

1. The ability to be placed without direct visualization of the larynx.
2. Increased speed and ease of placement when compared with tracheal intubation, both by experienced and less experienced operators.
3. Increased cardiovascular stability on insertion and emergence.
4. During emergence, improved oxygen saturation and lower frequency of coughing.
5. Minimal rise in intraocular pressure on insertion.
6. When the device is properly placed, it can act as a conduit for oral tracheal intubation due to the anatomical alignment of its aperture with the glottic opening.
7. In the 'can't intubate, can't ventilate' scenario, the decision to use such devices should be made early to gain time while attempts are made to secure a definite airway.
8. Such devices normally provide little or no protection against aspiration of refluxed gastric contents, and are therefore contraindicated in patients with full stomachs or prone to reflux. However, second-generation devices (e.g. LMA-ProSeal™, LMA-Supreme™, and i-gel (see later)) offer many improvements such as high cuff seal, second seal, gastric access and drain tube. These allow for rapid drainage of gastric fluids or secretions and reduce the risk of gastric gas insufflation during ventilation. Future indications might even be in emergency medicine, where gastric vacuity is unknown, and in cases of increased risk of regurgitation.

9. Extraglottic airways would normally elicit airway reflexes such as the gag reflex, and therefore require depression of pharyngeal reflexes by general or topical anaesthesia.

10. These devices are increasingly used in a variety of settings, including routine anaesthesia, emergency airway management and as an aid to intubation.

Laryngeal mask

This very useful device is frequently used as an alternative to either the face mask or tracheal tube during anaesthesia (Fig. 5.37).

Components

1. A transparent tube of wide internal diameter. The proximal end is a standard 15-mm connection.

2. An elliptical cuff at the distal end. The cuff resembles a small face mask to form an air-tight seal around the posterior perimeter of the larynx and is inflated via a pilot balloon with a self-sealing valve. A non-metallic self-sealing valve is available for use during magnetic resonance imaging (MRI) scans.

3. The original design (Intavent Classic LMA™) had two slits or bars at the junction between the tube and the cuff to prevent the epiglottis from obstructing the lumen of the laryngeal mask. Newer designs, such as Portex SoftSeal™ and Intersurgical Solus™, omit the bars with no adverse clinical effects.

4. A modified design (LMA-ProSeal™) has an additional lumen (drain tube) lateral to the airway tube and traverses the floor of the mask to open in the mask tip opposite the upper oesophageal sphincter allowing blind passage of an orogastric tube and helps in the drainage of gastric air or secretions. Both tubes are contained within an integrated bite block. The cuff inflates in a three-dimensional manner with the elliptical cuff augmented by a second cuff behind the bowl, known as the rear boot or dorsal cuff. This design improves the seal pressure. A single-use version, LMA Supreme™, is available which combines the best features of previous LMA versions, and contains an elliptical and anatomically shaped curve, which facilitates insertion success and provides a double seal. A first seal is important for adequacy of gas exchange, better known as the oropharyngeal seal (Fig. 5.38). It also incorporates a second seal, designed to reduce the risk of stomach insufflation during ventilation, to provide a passive conduit for (unexpected) regurgitation or active suctioning of gastric content and enhances the effectiveness of the first seal.

5. Low-cost disposable laryngeal masks have been introduced and are widely used (Fig. 5.39).

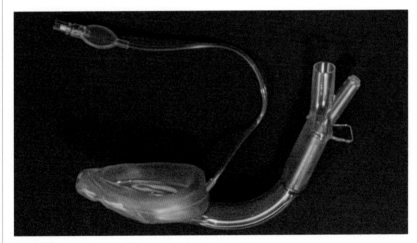

Fig. 5.38 LMA-Supreme™. Note the drainage lumen.

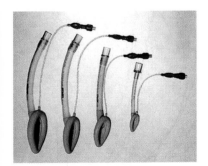

Fig. 5.37 A range of different sized laryngeal masks (non-reinforced).

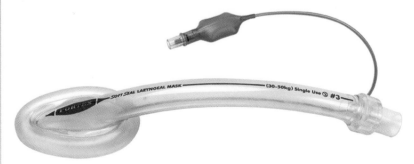

Fig. 5.39 Smith's Portex single-use Soft-Seal laryngeal mask.

Table 5.2 The recommended sizes and cuff inflation volumes

	Size of patient	Cuff inflation volume
Size 1	Neonates, infants up to 5 kg	Up to 4 mL
Size 1.5	Infants 5–10 kg	Up to 7 mL
Size 2	Infants/children 10–20 kg	Up to 10 mL
Size 2.5	Children 20–30 kg	Up to 14 mL
Size 3	Paediatric 30–50 kg	Up to 20 mL
Size 4	Adult 50–70 kg	Up to 30 mL
Size 5	Adult 70–100 kg	Up to 40 mL
Size 6	Large adult over 100 kg	Up to 60 mL

Mechanism of action

1. A variety of techniques have been described for the insertion of the laryngeal mask. It should provide an adequate seal for spontaneous and mechanical ventilation with a minimal leak, at a pressure of 20–25-cm H_2O. A seal pressure of up to 35 cm H_2O can be achieved with the LMA-Proseal™.
2. The cuff is deflated and lubricated before use. It is inserted through the mouth. The cuff lies over the larynx.
3. Once the cuff is in position, it is inflated (Table 5.2).
4. Partial inflation of the cuff before insertion is used by some anaesthetists.
5. The laryngeal masks have wide internal diameters in order to reduce the flow resistance to a minimum (e.g. the internal diameters of sizes 2, 3, 4 and 5 are 7, 10, 10 and 11.5 mm respectively). This makes them suitable for long procedures using a spontaneous ventilation technique.
6. It also has a role as an aid in difficult intubation. Once in position, it can be used to introduce a bougie or a narrow lumen tracheal tube into the trachea. Alternatively, the laryngeal mask may be used to guide passage of a fibreoptic bronchoscope into the trachea, thus allowing intubation of the trachea.

The **reinforced version** of the laryngeal mask is used for head and neck surgery (Fig. 5.40).

1. The tubes, although flexible, are kink and crush resistant, because of a stainless steel wire spiral in their wall. The tube can be moved during surgery without loss of the cuff's seal against the larynx. The breathing system can easily be connected at any angle from the mouth.
2. A throat pack can be used with the reinforced version.
3. The reinforced laryngeal masks have smaller internal diameters and longer lengths than the standard versions, causing an increase in flow resistance. This makes their use with spontaneous ventilation for prolonged periods less suitable.

Currently there is a trend to use disposable single-use laryngeal masks. Some have similar designs to the original Classic LMA™ such as Portex Soft Seal™ and Silicone LM™, Intavent Unique™ and Intersurgical Solus™ laryngeal masks. Some have different designs such as the Ambu laryngeal mask and the Cobra-PLA™ airway device. Their clinical performance is similar to the original Classic LMA™ with some achieving even better results and with fewer traumas. They are

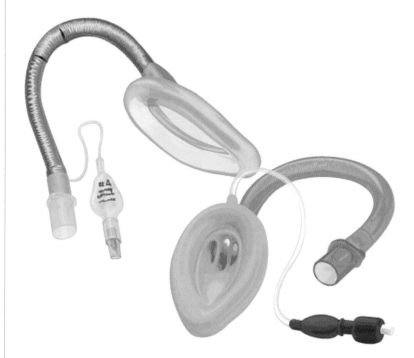

Fig. 5.40 Reinforced laryngeal mask, single use (left) and reusable (right).

made of PVC apart from the Portex Silicone LM™, which is made of silicone rubber.

The recommended safety checks before the use of laryngeal masks

- Inflate the cuff and look for signs of herniation.
- Check that the lumen of the tube is patent.
- The tube can be bent to 180° without kinking or occlusion.
- Inspect the device for signs of dehiscence of the tube or mask aperture bars, and cuff separations. In the reusable devices, look for signs of damage or weakness where the teeth were in contact with the tube.
- The device should also be inspected after removal from the patient for signs of bleeding.

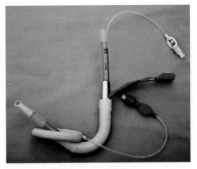

Fig. 5.41 The intubating LMA.

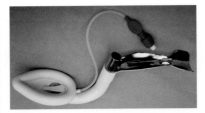

Fig. 5.42 The intubating LMA.

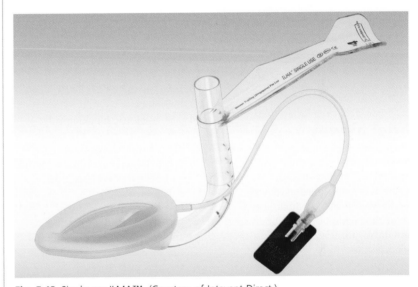

Fig. 5.43 Single-use ILMA™. (Courtesy of Intavent Direct.)

The intubating laryngeal mask airway (ILMA™)

This is a modification of the laryngeal mask designed to facilitate tracheal intubation with a tracheal tube either blindly or in conjunction with a fibrescope while minimizing the requirements for head and neck manipulation. The specially designed laryngeal mask is inserted first (Fig. 5.41). A specially designed tracheal tube is then passed through the laryngeal mask through the vocal cords into the trachea (Fig. 5.42). Single-use ILMA™ is available (Fig. 5.43).

Problems in practice and safety features

1. The laryngeal mask does not protect against the aspiration of gastric contents.

2. Despite the presence of the slits or bars, about 10% of patients develop airway obstruction because of down-folding of the epiglottis. Although clinically often insignificant, a higher proportion of obstructions by the epiglottis can be observed endoscopically.

3. The manufacturers recommend using the laryngeal masks for a maximum of 40 times. The cuff is likely to perish after autoclaving. A record card that accompanies the laryngeal mask registers the number of autoclaving episodes.

4. Unlike the tracheal tube, rotation of the laryngeal mask may result in complete airway obstruction. In order to assess the laryngeal mask's orientation when inserted, a black line is present on the tube. This should face the upper lip of the patient when the laryngeal mask is in position.

5. Cricoid pressure may prevent correct placement of the laryngeal mask.

6. A common cause of airway obstruction during laryngeal mask anaesthesia is down-folding of the epiglottis, which occurs in 20–56% of patients.

I-gel airway

The i-gel airway is a single-use extraglottic airway that uses an anatomically designed mask to fit the perilaryngeal and hypopharyngeal structures without the use of an inflatable cuff (Fig. 5.44). It also incorporates a second drain tube.

Components

1. The large lumen is for ventilation with a proximal 15-mm connector. Distally, it ends in a non-inflatable gel-like cuff with a ridge at the superior anterior edge.

2. Two separate ventilation and gastric channels or lumens. The distal end of the integrated gastric lumen is positioned in the upper oesophagus.
3. The body is a wide oval in cross section.

Mechanism of action

1. The soft, gel-like plastic from which the i-gel is manufactured is intended to mould into place without the use of an inflatable cuff.
2. The gastric channel allows direct suctioning or passage of a gastric tube.
3. The wide oval-in-cross-section body is designed to prevent rotation and to act as an integral bite block.
4. The epiglottic blocking ridge is intended to reduce the possibility of epiglottic down-folding.
5. It is available in adult, paediatric and neonatal sizes (1, 1.5, 2, 2.5, 3, 4, and 5).
6. It is intended for use with fasted patients, with both spontaneous and controlled ventilation, and can be used as a conduit for tracheal intubation.

Problems in practice and safety features

Despite its gastric channel, the i-gel does not offer absolute protection from aspiration of gastric contents.

COBRA perilaryngeal airway (PLA™)

The COBRA-PLA™ consists of a large ventilation tube with a distal circumferential inflatable cuff, designed to reside in the hypopharynx at the base of the tongue, sealing off the upper oropharynx. It differs from other extraglottic airway devices as the distal tip lies proximal to the oesophageal inlet.

The distal end consists of softened plastic slotted openings designed to hold the soft tissues and epiglottis out of the way of the laryngeal inlet, while the slotted openings direct inspiratory gas into the trachea. The openings are flexible enough to allow the passage of a tracheal tube.

The COBRA-PLA™ allows both spontaneous and controlled ventilation but provides no effective protection against aspiration. The tube has a wider diameter than usual making the device suitable to be used as a rescue airway through which tracheal intubation can then be attempted. An internal ramp in the COBRA head is designed to help guide a tracheal tube into the larynx when the device is used as an intubation conduit. The cuff is inflated using an integrated pilot balloon.

It is available in eight sizes. Paediatric models have a distal gas sampling port in the COBRA head, which minimizes sampling dead space increasing the accuracy of capnometry. COBRA Plus models include a temperature probe on the lateral posterior part of the cuff for core temperature monitoring (Fig. 5.45).

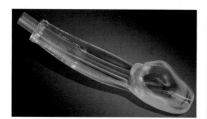

Fig. 5.44 The i-gel airway. (Courtesy of Intersurgical.)

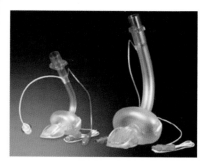

Fig. 5.45 COBRA PLA Plus™ device. Note the temperature probe used for core temperature monitoring.

FURTHER READING

Brimacombe, J., 2004. Laryngeal mask anesthesia: principles and practice, second ed. WB Saunders, Philadelphia.

Gothard, J.W.W., 2005. Anaesthetic equipment for thoracic surgery. Anaesthesia and Intensive Care Medicine 6 (12), 425–427.

MHRA, 2011. Medical device alert: endotracheal (ET) tubes, adult and paediatric sizes manufactured by Unomedical (a ConvaTec company) (MDA/2011/025). Online. Available at: http://www.mhra.gov.uk/Publications/Safetywarnings/MedicalDeviceAlerts/CON111625?tabName=Device

MCQs

In the following lists, which of the statements (a) to (e) are true?

1. Concerning tracheal tubes:
   a) The RAE tracheal tube is ideal for microlaryngeal surgery.
   b) Preformed tracheal tubes have a higher risk of bronchial intubation.
   c) Laryngeal masks can be used in nasal surgery.
   d) RAE tubes stand for reinforced anaesthetic endotracheal tubes.
   e) The Oxford tracheal tube has a left-facing bevel.

2. Laryngeal masks:
   a) They can prevent aspiration of gastric contents.
   b) The bars at the junction of the cuff and the tube prevent foreign bodies from entering the trachea.
   c) Because of its large internal diameter, it can be used in spontaneously breathing patients for long periods of time.
   d) It can be autoclaved and used repeatedly for an unlimited number of times.
   e) The standard design can be used in MRI.

3. Double lumen endobronchial tubes:
   a) Robertshaw double lumen tubes have carinal hooks.
   b) The left-sided tubes have an eye in the bronchial cuff to facilitate ventilation of the left upper lobe.
   c) Carlens double lumen tubes have relatively small lumens.
   d) CPAP can be applied to the deflated lung to improve oxygenation.
   e) Fibreoptic bronchoscopy can be used to ensure correct positioning of the tube.

4. Concerning the tracheal tube cuff during anaesthesia:
   a) Low-pressure/high-volume cuffs prevent aspiration of gastric contents.
   b) The intracuff pressure can rise significantly because of the diffusion of the anaesthetic inhalational vapour.
   c) High-pressure/low-volume cuffs may cause necrosis of the tracheal mucosa if left in position for long periods.
   d) Low-volume cuffs have a smaller contact area with the tracheal wall than high-volume cuffs.
   e) The pressure in the cuff may decrease because of the diffusion of nitrous oxide.

5. Concerning tracheal tubes:
   a) The ID diameter is measured in centimetres.
   b) Red rubber tubes never have cuffs.
   c) Armoured tubes need to be cut to length.
   d) Tubes should have a Murphy eye to allow suction.
   e) The tip is cut square.

SINGLE BEST ANSWER (SBA)

6. Bronchial blockers
   a) Can be used only with a nasal tracheal tube.
   b) Should be used without a fibreoptic scope for guidance.
   c) Can be used for blocking only the right main bronchus.
   d) Can be used to easily suck out blood and secretions.
   e) Can have a 'hockey stick' design to aid directing placement.

Answers

1. Concerning tracheal tubes:
   a) *False. An RAE tube is a normal size preformed tracheal tube. It does not allow good visibility of the larynx because of its large diameter. A microlaryngeal tracheal tube of 5–6 mm ID is more suitable for microlaryngeal surgery, allowing good visibility and access to the larynx.*
   b) *True. Because the shape of these tubes is fixed, they might not fit all patients of different sizes and shapes; e.g. a small, short-necked patient having an RAE tube inserted is at risk of an endobronchial tube position.*
   c) *True. Some anaesthetists use the laryngeal mask in nasal surgery with a throat pack. This technique has a higher risk of aspiration.*
   d) *False. RAE stands for the initials of the designers (Ring, Adair and Elwyn).*
   e) *False. The Oxford tube is one of the few tracheal tubes with a front-facing bevel. This might make intubation more difficult as it obscures the larynx.*

2. Laryngeal masks:
   a) *False. Laryngeal masks do not protect the airway from the risks of aspiration.*
   b) *False. The bars in the cuff are designed to prevent the epiglottis from blocking the lumen of the tube.*
   c) *True. The laryngeal mask has a large internal diameter, in comparison with a tracheal tube. This reduces the resistance to breathing which is of more importance during spontaneous breathing. This makes the laryngeal mask more suitable for use in spontaneously breathing patients for long periods of time.*
   d) *False. The laryngeal mask can be autoclaved up to 40 times. The cuff is likely to perish after repeated autoclaving. A record should be kept of the number of autoclaves.*
   e) *False. The standard laryngeal mask has a metal component in the one-way inflating valve. This makes it unsuitable for use in MRI. A specially designed laryngeal mask with no metal parts is available for MRI use.*

3. Double lumen endobronchial tubes:
   a) *False. The Robertshaw double lumen tube does not have a carinal hook. The Carlens double lumen tube has a carinal hook.*
   b) *False. Left-sided tubes do not have an eye in the bronchial cuff to facilitate ventilation of the left upper lobe. This is because the distance between the carina and the upper lobe bronchus is about 5 cm, which is enough for the bronchial cuff. Right-sided tubes have an eye to facilitate ventilation of the right upper lobe because the distance between the carina and the upper lobe bronchus is only 2.5 cm.*
   c) *True. Carlens double lumen tubes have relatively small lumens in comparison to the Robertshaw double lumen tube.*
   d) *True. CPAP can be applied to the deflated lung to improve oxygenation during one lung anaesthesia.*
   e) *True. It is sometimes difficult to ensure correct positioning of the double lumen endobronchial tube. By using a fibreoptic bronchoscope, the position of the tube can be adjusted to ensure correct positioning.*

4. Concerning the tracheal tube cuff during anaesthesia:
   a) *False. The design of the low-pressure/high-volume cuff allows wrinkles to be formed around the tracheal wall. The presence of the wrinkles allows aspiration of gastric contents to occur.*
   b) *False. The rise in the intracuff pressure is mainly due to the diffusion of N_2O. Minimal changes are due to diffusion of oxygen (from 21% to say 33%) and because of increase in the temperature of the air in the cuff (from 21° to 37°C). The diffusion of inhalational agents causes minimal changes in pressure due to the low concentrations used (1–2%). New design material cuffs prevent the diffusion of gases thus preventing significant changes in pressure.*
   c) *True. The high pressures achieved by the high-pressure/low-volume cuffs, especially during nitrous oxide anaesthesia, can cause necrosis to the mucosa of the trachea if left in position for a long period.*
   d) *True. Because of the design of the low-volume cuffs, a seal can be maintained against a relatively small area of the tracheal wall. In the case of the high-volume/low-pressure cuffs, a large contact area on the tracheal wall is achieved.*

e) *False. The pressure in the cuff may decrease because of a leak in the cuff or pilot balloon's valve.*

---

5. Concerning tracheal tubes:
   a) *False. The ID is measured in millimetres.*

b) *False.*
c) *False. An armoured tube should not be cut, as that will cut the spiral present in its wall. This increases the risk of tube kinking.*
d) *False. A Murphy eye allows pulmonary ventilation in the*

situation where the bevel of the tube is occluded.
e) *False. The bevel of the tube is usually left-facing to allow easier visualization of the vocal cords. The tracheostomy tube has a square-cut tip.*

---

6. e)

Chapter 6

Masks and oxygen delivery devices

Face masks and angle pieces

The face mask is designed to fit the face anatomically. It comes in different sizes to fit patients of different age groups (from neonates to adults). It is connected to the breathing system via the angle piece.

Components

1. The body of the mask which rests on an air-filled cuff (Fig. 6.1). Some paediatric designs do not have a cuff, e.g. Rendell–Baker (Fig. 6.2).
2. The proximal end of the mask has a 22-mm inlet connection to the angle piece.
3. Some designs have clamps for a harness to be attached.
4. The angle piece has a 90° bend with a 22-mm end to fit into a catheter mount or a breathing system.

Mechanism of action

1. They are made of transparent plastic. Previously, masks made of silicon rubber were used. The transparent plastic allows the detection of vomitus or secretions. It is also more acceptable to the patient during inhalational induction. Some masks are 'flavoured', e.g. strawberry flavour.
2. The cuff helps to ensure a snug fit over the face covering the mouth and nose. It also helps to minimize the mask's pressure on the face. Cuffs can be either air-filled or made from a soft material.
3. The design of the interior of the mask determines the size of its contribution to apparatus dead space. The dead space may increase by up to 200 mL in adults. Paediatric masks are designed to reduce the dead space as much as possible.

Problems in practice and safety features

1. Excessive pressure by the mask may cause injury to the branches of the trigeminal or facial nerves.
2. Sometimes it is difficult to achieve an air-tight seal over the face. Edentulous patients and those with nasogastric tubes pose particular problems.
3. Imprecise application of the mask on the face can cause trauma to the eyes.

> **Face masks**
> - Made of silicone rubber or plastic.
> - Their design ensures a snug fit over the face of the patient.
> - Cause an increase in dead space (up to 200 mL in adults).
> - Can cause trauma to the eyes and facial nerves.

Nasal masks (inhalers)

1. These masks are used during dental chair anaesthesia.
2. An example is the Goldman inhaler (Fig. 6.3) which has an inflatable cuff to fit the face and an adjustable pressure limiting (APL) valve at the proximal end. The mask is connected to tubing which delivers the fresh gas flow.

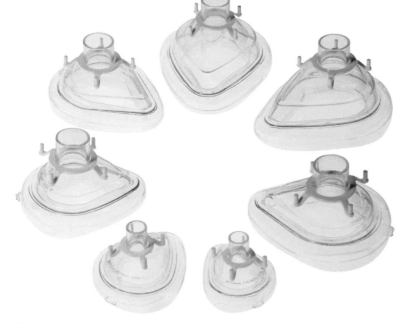

Fig. 6.1 A range of sizes of transparent face masks with air-filled cuffs.

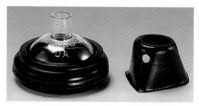

Fig. 6.2 Paediatric face masks. Ambu design (left) and Rendell–Baker design (right).

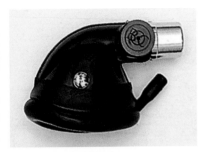

Fig. 6.3 The Goldman nasal inhaler.

3. Other designs have an inlet for delivering the inspired fresh gas flow and an outlet connected to tubing with a unidirectional valve for expired gases.

Catheter mount

This is the flexible link between the breathing system tubing and the tracheal tube, face mask, supraglottic airway device or tracheostomy tube (Fig. 6.4). The length of the catheter mount varies from 45 to 170 mm.

Components

1. A corrugated disposable plastic tubing. Some catheter mounts have a concertina design allowing their length to be adjusted.
2. The distal end is connected to either a 15-mm standard

tracheal tube connector, usually in the shape of an angle piece, or a 22-mm mask fitting.
3. The proximal end has a 22-mm connector for attachment to the breathing system.
4. Some designs have a condenser humidifier built into them.
5. A gas sampling port is found in some designs.

Mechanism of action

1. The mount minimizes the transmission of accidental movements of the breathing system to the tracheal tube. Repeated movements of the tracheal tube can cause injury to the tracheal mucosa.
2. Some designs allow for suction or the introduction of a fibreoptic bronchoscope. This is done via a special port.

Problems in practice and safety features

1. The catheter mount contributes to the apparatus dead space. This is of particular importance in paediatric anaesthesia. The concertina design allows adjustment of the dead space from 25 to 60 mL.
2. Foreign bodies can lodge inside the catheter mount causing an unnoticed blockage of the breathing system. To minimize

this risk, the catheter mount should remain wrapped in its sterile packaging until needed.

Catheter mount

- Acts as an adapter between the tracheal tube and breathing system in addition to stabilizing the tracheal tube.
- Can be made of rubber or plastic with different lengths.
- Some have a condenser humidifier built in.
- Its length contributes to the apparatus dead space.
- Can be blocked by a foreign body.

Oxygen delivery devices

Currently, a variety of delivery devices are used. These devices differ in their ability to deliver a set fractional inspired oxygen concentration (FiO_2). The delivery devices can be divided into variable and fixed performance devices. The former devices deliver a fluctuating FiO_2 whereas the latter devices deliver a more constant and predictable FiO_2 (Table 6.1). The FiO_2 delivered to the patient is dependent on device- and patient-related factors. The FiO_2 delivered can be calculated by measuring the end-tidal oxygen fraction in the nasopharynx using oxygraphy.

Variable performance masks (medium concentration; MC)

These masks are used to deliver oxygen-enriched air to the patient (Fig. 6.5). They are also called

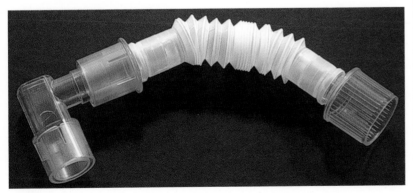

Fig. 6.4 Catheter mount.

low-flow delivery devices. They are widely used in the hospital because of greater patient comfort, low cost, simplicity and the ability to manipulate the FiO_2 without changing the appliance. Their performance varies between patients and from breath to breath within the same patient. These systems have a limited reservoir capacity, so in order to function appropriately, the patient must inhale some ambient air to meet the inspiratory demands. The FiO_2 is determined by the oxygen flow rate, the size of the oxygen reservoir and the respiratory pattern (Table 6.2).

Components

1. The plastic body of the mask with side holes on both sides.
2. A port connected to an oxygen supply.
3. Elastic band(s) to fix the mask to the patient's face.

Mechanism of action

1. Ambient air is entrained through the holes on both sides of the mask. The holes also allow exhaled gases to be vented out.
2. During the expiratory pause, the fresh oxygen supplied helps in venting the exhaled gases through the side holes. The body of the mask (acting as a reservoir) is filled with fresh oxygen supply and is available for the start of the next inspiration.
3. The final concentration of inspired oxygen depends on:
   a) the oxygen supply flow rate
   b) the pattern of ventilation. If there is a pause between expiration and inspiration, the mask fills with oxygen and a high concentration is available at the start of inspiration
   c) the patient's inspiratory flow rate. During inspiration, oxygen is diluted by the air drawn in through the holes

Table 6.1 Classification of the oxygen delivery systems

Variable performance devices	Fixed performance devices
Hudson face masks and partial rebreathing masks Nasal cannulae (prongs or spectacles) Nasal catheters	Venturi-operated devices Anaesthetic breathing systems with a suitably large reservoir

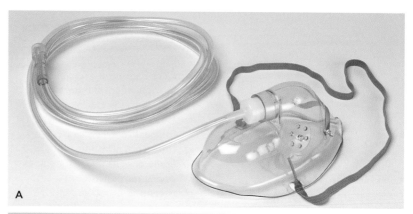

A

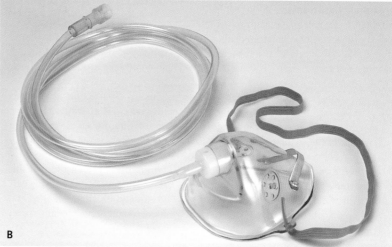

B

Fig. 6.5 (A) Adult variable performance face mask. (B) Paediatric variable performance face mask.

Table 6.2 Factors that affect the delivered FiO_2 in the variable performance masks

High FiO_2 delivered	Low FiO_2 delivered
Low peak inspiratory flow rate Slow respiratory rate High fresh oxygen flow rate Tightly fitting face mask	High peak inspiratory flow rate Fast respiratory rate Low fresh oxygen flow rate Less tightly fitting face mask

when the inspiratory flow rate exceeds the flow of oxygen supply. During normal tidal ventilation, the peak inspiratory flow rate is 20–30 L/min, which is higher than the oxygen supplied to the patient and the oxygen that is contained in the body of the mask, so some ambient air is inhaled to meet the demands thus diluting the fresh oxygen supply. The peak inspiratory flow rate increases further during deep inspiration and during hyperventilation.

d) how tight the mask's fit is on the face.

4. If there is no expiratory pause, alveolar gases may be rebreathed from the mask at the start of inspiration.

5. The rebreathing of carbon dioxide from the body of the mask (apparatus dead space of about 100 mL) is usually of little clinical significance in adults but may be a problem in some patients who are not able to compensate by increasing their alveolar ventilation. Carbon dioxide elimination can be improved by increasing the fresh oxygen flow and is inversely related to the minute ventilation. The rebreathing is also increased when the mask body is large and when the resistance to flow from the side holes is high (when the mask is a good fit). The patients may experience a sense of warmth and humidity, indicating significant rebreathing.

6. A typical example of 4 L/min of oxygen flow delivers an FiO_2 of about 0.35–0.4 providing there is a normal respiratory pattern.

7. Adding a 600–800 mL bag to the mask will act as an extra reservoir (Fig. 6.6). Such masks are known as 'partial rebreathing masks'. The inspired oxygen is derived from the

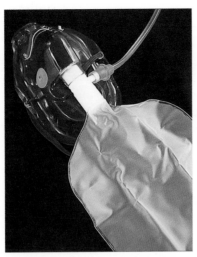

Fig. 6.6 A variable performance mask with a reservoir bag.

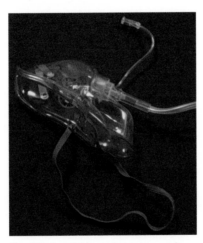

Fig. 6.7 A variable performance mask with an end-tidal CO_2 monitoring port.

continuous fresh oxygen supply, oxygen present in the reservoir (a mixture of the fresh oxygen and exhaled oxygen) and ambient air. Higher variable FiO_2 can be achieved with such masks. A one-way valve is fitted between mask and reservoir to prevent rebreathing.

8. Some designs have an extra port attached to the body of the mask allowing it to be connected to a side-stream CO_2 monitor (Fig. 6.7). This allows it to sample the exhaled CO_2 so

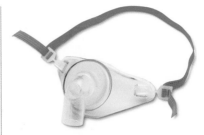

Fig. 6.8 Variable performance tracheostomy mask.

monitoring the patient's respiration during sedation.

9. Similar masks can be used in patients with tracheostomy (Fig. 6.8). As with the face mask, similar factors will affect its performance. Care must be taken to humidify the inspired dry oxygen as the gases delivered bypass the nose and its humidification.

Problems in practice and safety features

These devices are used only when delivering a fixed oxygen concentration is not critical. Patients whose ventilation is dependent on a hypoxic drive must not receive oxygen from a variable performance mask.

Variable performance mask, MC mask

- Entrains ambient air.
- The inspired oxygen concentration depends on the oxygen flow rate, pattern and rate of ventilation, maximum inspiratory flow rate and how well the mask fits the patient's face.

Nasal cannulae

Nasal cannulae are ideal for patients on long-term oxygen therapy (Fig. 6.9). A flow rate of 2–4 L/min

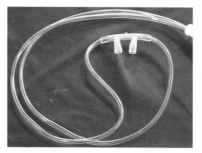

Fig. 6.9 Oxygen nasal cannula.

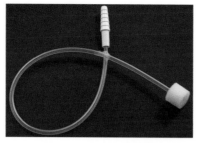

Fig. 6.10 Oxygen nasal catheter.

delivers an FiO$_2$ of 0.28–0.36 respectively. Higher flow rates are uncomfortable.

Components

1. Two prongs which protrude about 1 cm into the nose.
2. These are held in place by an adjustable head strap.

Mechanism of action

1. There is entrainment of ambient air through the nostrils. The nasopharynx acts as a reservoir.
2. The FiO$_2$ achieved is proportional to:
   a) the flow rate of oxygen
   b) the patient's tidal volume, inspiratory flow and respiratory rate
   c) the volume of the nasopharynx.
3. Mouth breathing causes inspiratory air flow. This produces a Venturi effect in the posterior pharynx entraining oxygen from the nose.
4. There is increased patient compliance with nasal cannulae compared to facial oxygen masks. The patient is able to speak, eat and drink.

Problems in practice and safety features

The cannulae and the dry gas flow cause trauma and irritation to the nasal mucosa. They are not appropriate in patients with blocked nasal passages.

Nasal cannulae
- Entrainment of ambient air through the nostrils and during mouth breathing.
- The FiO$_2$ depends on the oxygen flow rate, tidal volume, inspiratory flow rate, respiratory rate and the volume of the nasopharynx.
- Better compliance compared with facial masks.

Nasal catheters

Nasal catheters comprise a single lumen catheter, which is lodged into the anterior naris (nostril) by a foam collar (Fig. 6.10). Oxygen flows of 2–3 L/min can be used. The catheter can be secured to the patient's face by using tape. It should not be used when a nasal

mucosal tear is suspected because of the risk of surgical emphysema.

Open oxygen delivery systems

These are designed to offer the maximum comfort to patients while delivering variable FiO$_2$ concentrations. They fit around the patient's head like head phones, so making minimal physical contact (Fig. 6.11). Such systems are suitable for both nasal and mouth breathing patients. They may be more suitable for patients on long-term oxygen therapy.

A wide range of fresh oxygen flows can be used, so delivering a variable performance. As with the other devices of this kind, similar factors will affect its performance.

Fixed performance devices

VENTURI MASK

These masks are fixed performance devices (sometimes called *high-air-flow oxygen enrichment*, or HAFOE).

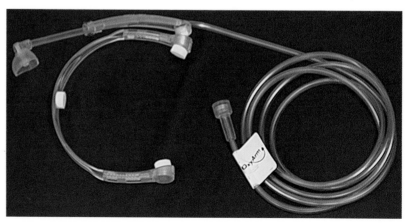

Fig. 6.11 Open oxygen supply system.

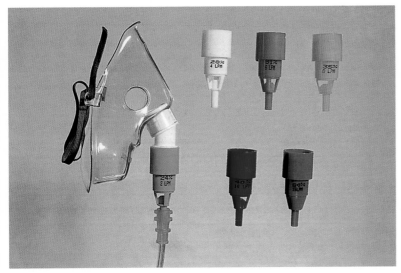

Fig. 6.12 Fixed performance mask with a range of Venturi devices.

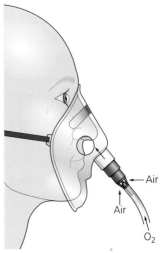

Fig. 6.14 Mechanism of action of the fixed performance Venturi mask.

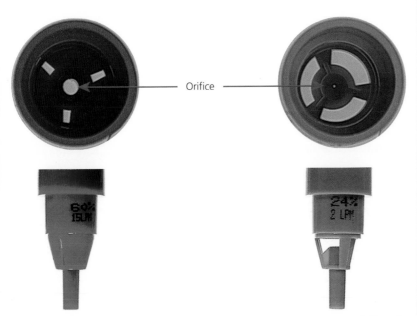

Fig. 6.13 Detail of the Venturi device. Design for administering 60% oxygen (left) and 24% (right). Note the difference in the recommended oxygen flow rates and the size of orifice and air entrainment apertures.

Components

1. The plastic body of the mask with holes on both sides.
2. The proximal end of the mask consists of a Venturi device. The Venturi devices are colour-coded and marked with the recommended oxygen flow rate to provide the desired oxygen concentration (Figs 6.12 and 6.13).
3. Alternatively, a calibrated variable Venturi device can be used to deliver the desired FiO_2.

Mechanism of action

1. The Venturi mask uses the Bernoulli principle, described in 1778, in delivering a predetermined and fixed concentration of oxygen to the patient. The size of the constriction determines the final concentration of oxygen for a given gas flow. This is achieved in spite of the patient's respiratory pattern by providing a higher gas flow than the peak inspiratory flow rate.
2. As the flow of oxygen passes through the constriction, a negative pressure is created. This causes the ambient air to be entrained and mixed with the oxygen flow (Fig. 6.14). The FiO_2 is dependent on the degree of air entrainment. Less entrainment ensures a higher FiO_2 is delivered. This can be achieved by using smaller entrainment apertures or bigger 'windows' to entrain ambient air. The smaller the orifice is, the greater the negative pressure generated, so the more ambient air entrained, the lower the FiO_2. The oxygen concentration

can be 0.24, 0.28, 0.31, 0.35, 0.4 or 0.6.

3. The Bernoulli effect can be written as:

$$P + \frac{1}{2}\rho v^2 = \kappa$$

where κ is the density, v is the velocity, P is the pressure.

4. The total energy during a fluid (gas or liquid) flow consists of the sum of kinetic and potential energy. The kinetic energy is related to the velocity of the flow whereas the potential energy is related to the pressure. As the flow of fresh oxygen passes through the constricted orifice into the larger chamber, the velocity of the gas increases distal to the orifice causing the kinetic energy to increase. As the total energy is constant, there is a decrease in the potential energy so a negative pressure is created. This causes the ambient air to be entrained and mixed with the oxygen flow. The FiO_2 is dependent on the degree of air entrainment. Less entrainment ensures higher FiO_2 is delivered and smaller entrainment apertures are one method of achieving this (Fig. 6.8). The devices must be driven by the correct oxygen flow rate, calibrated for the aperture size if a predictable FiO_2 is to be achieved.

4. Because of the high fresh gas flow rate, the exhaled gases are rapidly flushed from the mask, via its holes. Therefore there is no rebreathing and no increase in dead space.

5. These masks are recommended when a fixed oxygen concentration is desired in patients whose ventilation is dependent on the hypoxic drive.

6. For example, a 24% oxygen Venturi mask has an air:oxygen entrainment ratio of 25:1. This means an oxygen flow of 2 L/min delivers a total flow of

50 L/min, well above the peak inspiratory flow rate.

7. The mask's side holes are used to vent the exhaled gases only (as above) in comparison to the side holes in the variable performance mask where the side holes are used to entrain inspired air in addition to expel exhaled gases.

8. The Venturi face masks are designed for both adult and paediatric use (Fig. 6.14).

9. The Venturi attachments, with a reservoir tubing, can be attached to a tracheal tube or a supraglottic airway device as part of a T-piece breathing system (Fig. 6.15). This arrangement is usually used in recovery wards to deliver oxygen-enriched air to patents.

Problems in practice and safety features

1. These masks are recommended when a fixed oxygen concentration is desired in patients whose ventilation is dependent on their hypoxic drive, such as those with chronic

obstructive pulmonary disease. However, caution should be exercised as it has been shown that the average FiO_2 delivered in such masks is up to 5% above the expected value.

2. The Venturi mask with its Venturi device and the oxygen delivery tubing is often not well tolerated by patients because it is noisy and bulky.

Anaesthetic breathing systems are other examples of the fixed performance devices. The reservoir bag acts to deliver a fresh gas flow that is greater than the patient's peak inspiratory flow rate.

Venturi mask
- Fixed performance device (HAFOE).
- Uses the Venturi principle to entrain ambient air.
- No rebreathing or increase in dead space.
- Changes in kinetic and potential energy during gas flow lead to negative pressure and air entrainment.

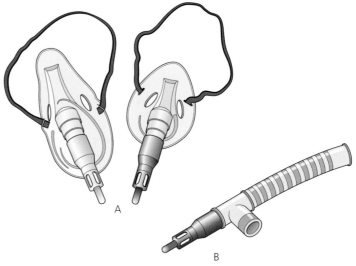

Fig. 6.15 (A) Adult and paediatric Venturi masks. (B) Venturi device as part of a breathing system.

FURTHER READING

Agusti, A.G., Carrera, M., Barbe, F., et al., 1999. Oxygen therapy during exacerbations of chronic obstructive pulmonary disease. European Respiratory Journal 14, 934–939.

British Thoracic Society. Online. Available at: http://www.brit-thoracic.org.uk

Khakhar, M., Heah, T., Al-Shaikh, B., 2002. Oxygen delivery systems for the spontaneously breathing patient. CPD Anaesthesia 4 (1), 27–30.

MHRA, 2011. Medical device alert: oxygen masks manufactured by Lifecare Hospital Supplies Ltd (MDA/2011/015). Online. Available at: http://www.mhra.gov.uk/Publications/Safetywarnings/MedicalDeviceAlerts/CON108738

Stausholm, K., Rosenberg-Adamsen, S., Skriver, M., et al., 1995. Comparison of three devices for oxygen administration in the late postoperative period. British Journal of Anaesthesia 74 (5), 607–609.

Waldau, T., Larsen, V.H., Bonde, J., 1998. Evaluation of five oxygen delivery devices in spontaneously breathing subjects by oxygraphy. Anaesthesia 53, 256–263.

MCQs

In the following lists, which of the statements (a) to (e) are true?

1. Concerning the Venturi mask:
   a) Gas flow produced should be more than 20 L/min.
   b) Reducing the flow of oxygen from 12 to 8 L/min results in a reduction in oxygen concentration.
   c) With a constant oxygen supply flow, widening the orifice in the Venturi device increases the oxygen concentration delivered to the patient.
   d) There is rebreathing in the mask.
   e) The mask is a fixed performance device.

2. High-air-flow oxygen enrichment face masks:
   a) Use the Venturi principle to deliver a fixed O_2 concentration to the patient.
   b) The size of the constriction of the Venturi has no effect on the final O_2 concentration delivered to the patient.
   c) The holes on the side of the mask are used to entrain ambient air.
   d) The gas flow delivered to the patient is more than the peak inspiratory flow rate.
   e) There is significant rebreathing.

3. Face masks used during anaesthesia:
   a) The rubber mask is covered by carbon particles which act as an anti-static measure.
   b) Masks have no effect on the apparatus dead space.
   c) The mask's cuff has to be checked and inflated before use.
   d) The dental nasal masks are also known as nasal inhalers.
   e) Masks have a 15-mm end to fit the catheter mount.

4. Concerning the oxygen nasal cannula:
   a) Is a fixed performance device.
   b) Is a variable performance device.
   c) There is a Venturi effect in the posterior pharynx.
   d) An oxygen flow of 8 L/min is usually used in an adult.
   e) Has increased patient compliance.

5. Variable performance masks:
   a) During slow and deep breathing, a higher FiO_2 can be achieved.
   b) Ambient air is not entrained into the mask.
   c) Alveolar gas rebreathing is not possible.
   d) Normal inspiratory peak flow rate is 20–30 L/min for an adult.
   e) Can be used safely on all patients.

6. Regarding variable performance devices:
   a) They can offer greater patient compliance.
   b) They can deliver an FiO_2 that can vary from breath to breath in the same patient.
   c) The size of the medium concentration oxygen face mask has no effect on rebreathing and CO_2 elimination.
   d) Capnography can be used to measure the FiO_2 delivered to the patient.
   e) With a variable performance mask, the FiO_2 is higher when the face mask is a tight fit.

7. Concerning fixed performance devices:
   a) Anaesthetic breathing systems with reservoirs are fixed performance devices.
   b) Distal to the constriction of a Venturi, there an increase in potential energy.
   c) In a Venturi mask, the higher the entrainment ratio, the higher the FiO_2.
   d) A nasal oxygen catheter is a fixed performance device.
   e) Venturi masks are very well tolerated by patients.

SINGLE BEST ANSWER (SBA)

8. Catheter mounts:
   a) Should have a 22-mm connector at the distal (patient) end.
   b) Should have a 15-mm connector at the proximal (machine) end.
   c) Gas sampling ports should always be built into the structure.
   d) Should never incorporate an angle piece.
   e) Should have a 15-mm connector at the distal (patient) end.

Answers

1. Concerning the Venturi mask:
   a) *True. The Venturi mask is a fixed performance device. In order to achieve this, the flow delivered to the patient should be more than the peak inspiratory flow rate. A flow of more than 20 L/min is adequate.*
   b) *True. It is the flow rate of oxygen through the orifice that determines the final FiO_2 the patient receives. With a constant orifice, the amount of air entrained remains constant. So by reducing the oxygen flow rate from 12 to 8 L/min, there will be less oxygen in the final mixture.*
   c) *True. The wider the orifice, the less the drop in pressure across the orifice and the less the entrainment of the ambient air, hence the less the dilution of the O_2, resulting in an increase in oxygen concentration delivered to the patient. The opposite is also correct.*
   d) *False. There is no rebreathing in the mask because of the high fresh gas flow rates causing the exhaled gases to be flushed from the mask through the side holes.*
   e) *True. The Venturi mask is a fixed performance device that delivers a constant concentration of oxygen in spite of the patient's respiratory pattern, by providing a higher gas flow than the peak inspiratory flow rate.*

2. High-air-flow oxygen enrichment face masks:
   a) *True. Laminar flow through a constriction causes a decrease in pressure at the constriction. This leads to entrainment of ambient air leading to mixture of fixed oxygen concentration.*
   b) *False. It is the size of the orifice that determines the degree of decrease in pressure at the constriction. This determines the amount of ambient air being entrained, hence the final concentration of oxygen.*
   c) *False. In such a mask, the holes are used to expel the exhaled gases. There is no entrainment of ambient air in such a mask because of the high gas flows. The holes in a variable performance mask are used to entrain ambient air.*
   d) *True. The gas flow generated is higher than the peak inspiratory flow rate. This allows the delivery of a fixed oxygen concentration to the patient regardless of the inspiratory flow rate. It also prevents rebreathing.*
   e) *False. There is no rebreathing because of the high flows delivered to the patient. The exhaled gases are expelled through the holes in the mask.*

3. Face masks used during anaesthesia:
   a) *True. Carbon particles prevent the build up of static electricity. The rubber face masks and the rubber tubings used in anaesthesia are covered with carbon. With modern anaesthetic practice where no flammable drugs are used, its significance has all but disappeared.*
   b) *False. Face masks can have a significant effect on the apparatus dead space if the wrong size is chosen. In an adult, the dead space can increase by about 200 mL. It is of more importance in paediatric practice.*
   c) *True. The cuff of the face mask is designed to ensure a snug fit over the patient's face and also to minimize the mask's pressure on the face. Ensuring that the cuff is inflated before use is therefore important.*
   d) *True. Nasal inhalers are nasal masks used during dental anaesthesia allowing good surgical access to the mouth. The Goldman nasal inhaler is an example.*
   e) *False. The face masks have a 22-mm end to fit the angle piece or catheter mount.*

4. Concerning the oxygen nasal cannula:
   a) *False. It is not a fixed performance device. The final FiO_2 depends on the flow rate of oxygen, tidal volume, inspiratory flow, respiratory rate and the volume of the nasopharynx.*
   b) *True. See above.*
   c) *True. During mouth breathing, the inspiratory air flow produces a Venturi effect in the posterior pharynx entraining oxygen from the nose.*
   d) *False. It is uncomfortable for the patient to have higher flows than 1–4 L/min.*
   e) *True. Patients tolerate the nasal cannula for much longer periods than a face mask. Patients are capable of eating, drinking and speaking despite the cannula.*

5. Variable performance masks:
   a) *True. This allows fresh gas flow (FGF) during the expiratory pause to fill the mask ready for the following inspiration. In tachypnoea (fast and shallow breathing), the opposite occurs where there is not enough time for the FGF to fill the mask.*
   b) *False. The maximum inspiratory flow rate is much higher than the FGF, so ambient air is entrained into the mask through the side holes.*
   c) *False. During tachypnoea, there is not enough time for the FGF to fill the mask and expel the exhaled gases. This leads to rebreathing of the exhaled gases.*
   d) *True.*
   e) *False. As their performance is variable, the FiO$_2$ the patient is getting is uncertain. Patients who are dependent on their hypoxic drive require a fixed performance mask.*

6. Regarding variable performance devices:
   a) *True. These devices are better tolerated by patients because they are more comfortable. They also offer simplicity, low cost and the ability to manipulate the FiO$_2$ without changing the appliance.*
   b) *True. The FiO$_2$ delivered can vary from one breath to another in the same patient. This is because of changes in the inspiratory flow rate and respiratory pattern. These lead to changes in the amount of air entrained so altering the FiO$_2$.*
   c) *False. Rebreathing is increased when the mask body is large. In addition, the high inspiratory resistance of the side holes increases the rebreathing. CO$_2$ elimination can be improved by increasing the fresh oxygen flow and is inversely related to the minute ventilation.*
   d) *False. Oxygraphy can be used to measure the FiO$_2$ by measuring the end-tidal oxygen fraction in the nasopharynx.*
   e) *True. The tighter the fit of the face mask, the higher the FiO$_2$. Low peak inspiratory flow rate, slow respiratory rate and a higher oxygen flow rate can also increase the FiO$_2$.*

7. Concerning fixed performance devices:
   a) *True. Anaesthetic breathing systems are fixed performance devices. The reservoir bag acts to deliver an FGF that is greater than the patient's peak inspiratory flow rate.*
   b) *False. The potential energy is related to the pressure, whereas the kinetic energy is related to the velocity of the flow. As the flow of fresh oxygen supply passes through the constricted orifice into the larger chamber, the velocity of the gas increases distal to the orifice causing the kinetic energy to increase. As the total energy is constant, there is a decrease in the potential energy so a negative pressure is created. This causes the ambient air to be entrained and mixed with the oxygen flow.*
   c) *False. The higher the entrainment ratio, the lower the FiO$_2$ delivered. This is because of the 'dilution' of the 100% oxygen fresh flow by ambient air.*
   d) *False. Nasal catheters are variable performance devices.*
   e) *False. Venturi masks are not very well tolerated by patients because of the noise and bulkiness of the masks and the attachments.*

8. e)

Chapter 7

Laryngoscopes and tracheal intubation equipment

Laryngoscopes

These devices are used to perform direct laryngoscopy and to aid in tracheal intubation (Fig. 7.1).

Components

1. The handle houses the power source (batteries) and is designed in different sizes.
2. The blade is fitted to the handle and can be either curved or straight. There is a wide range of designs for both curved and straight blades (Fig. 7.2).

Mechanism of action

1. Usually the straight blade is used for intubating neonates and infants. The blade is advanced over the posterior border of the relatively large, floppy V-shaped epiglottis which is then lifted directly in order to view the larynx (Fig. 7.3B). There are larger size straight blades that can be used in adults.
2. The curved blade (**Macintosh blade**) is designed to fit into the

oral and oropharyngeal cavity. It is inserted through the right angle of the mouth and advanced gradually, pushing the tongue to the left and away from the view until the tip of the blade reaches the vallecula. The blade has a small bulbous tip to help lift the larynx (Fig. 7.3A). The laryngoscope is lifted upwards elevating the larynx

and allowing the vocal cords to be seen. The Macintosh blade is made in four sizes.
3. In the standard designs, the light source is a bulb screwed on to the blade and an electrical connection is made when the blade is opened ready for use. In more recent designs, the bulb is placed in the handle and the light is transmitted to the tip of

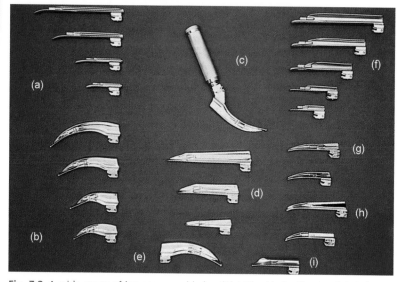

Fig. 7.2 A wide range of laryngoscope blades. (A) Miller blades (large, adult, infant, premature); (B) Macintosh blades (large, adult, child, baby); (C) Macintosh polio blade; (D) Soper blades (adult, child, baby); (E) left-handed Macintosh blade; (F) Wisconsin blades (large, adult, child, baby, neonate); (G) Robertshaw's blades (infant, neonatal); (H) Seward blades (child, baby); (I) Oxford infant blade.

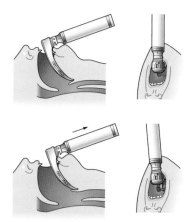

Fig. 7.1 Performing direct laryngoscopy. The vocal cords are visualized by lifting the laryngoscope in an upwards and forwards direction (see arrow).

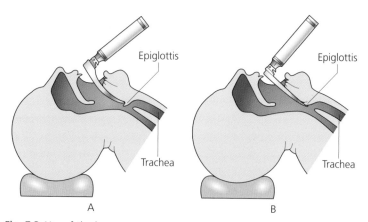

Fig. 7.3 Use of the laryngoscope.

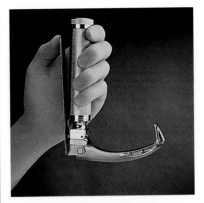

Fig. 7.6 Demonstrating the McCoy laryngoscope's hinged blade tip.

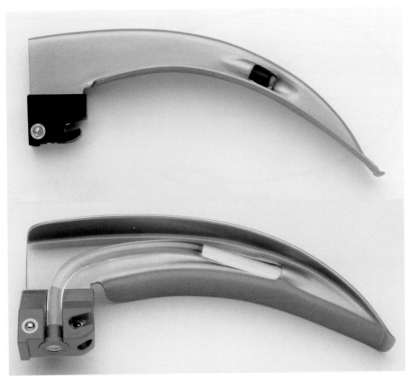

Fig. 7.4 Standard disposable laryngoscope blade (top) with the light bulb mounted on the blade; fibreoptic disposable laryngoscope blade (bottom). (Courtesy of Smiths Medical.)

the blade by means of fibreoptics (Fig. 7.4). Opening the blade turns the light on by forcing the bulb down to contact the battery terminal.

4. A left-sided Macintosh blade is available. It is used in patients with right-sided facial deformities making the use of the right-sided blade difficult.

5. The **McCoy laryngoscope** is based on the standard Macintosh blade. It has a hinged tip which is operated by the lever mechanism present on the back of the handle. It is suited for both routine use and in cases of difficult intubation (Figs 7.5 and 7.6). A more recent McCoy design has a straight blade with a hinged tip. Both the curved and the straight McCoy laryngoscopes use either a traditional bulb in the blade or a

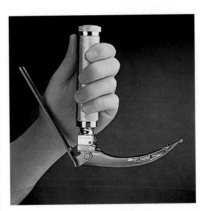

Fig. 7.5 The McCoy laryngoscope, based on a standard Macintosh blade.

lamp mounted in the handle which fibreoptically transmits the light to the blade.

6. A more recent design called the Flexiblade exists, where the whole distal half of the blade can be manoeuvred rather than

just the tip, as in the McCoy. This can be achieved using a lever on the front of the handle.

7. The blades are designed to be interchangeable between different manufacturers and laryngoscope handles. Two international standards are used: ISO 7376/2009 (green system) and ISO 7376/1 (red system) with a coloured marking placed on the blade and handle. The two systems have different dimension hinges and with different light source positions. The 'green system' is the most commonly used fitting standard.

Problems in practice and safety features

1. The risk of trauma and bruising to the different structures (e.g. epiglottis) is higher with the straight blade.

2. It is of vital importance to check the function of the laryngoscope before anaesthesia has commenced. Reduction in power or total failure due to the corrosion at the electrical contact point is possible.

3. Patients with large amounts of breast tissue present difficulty during intubation. Insertion of the blade into the mouth is restricted by the breast tissue

impinging on the handle. To overcome this problem, specially designed blades are used such as the polio blade. The polio blade is at about 120° to the handle allowing laryngoscopy without restriction. The polio blade was first designed to intubate patients ventilated in the iron lung during the poliomyelitis epidemic in the 1950s. A Macintosh laryngoscope blade attached to a short handle can also be useful in this situation.

4. To prevent cross-infection between patients, a disposable blade (Fig. 7.4) is used. A PVC sheath can also be put on the blade of the laryngoscope. The sheath has low light impedance allowing good visibility.

5. Laryngoscope handles must be decontaminated between patients to prevent cross-infection.

Laryngoscopes
- Consist of a handle and a blade. The latter can be straight or curved.
- The bulb is either in the blade or in the handle.
- Different designs and shapes exist.

Fibreoptic intubating laryngoscope

These devices have revolutionized airway management in anaesthesia and intensive care (Fig. 7.7). They are used to perform oral or nasal tracheal intubation (Figs 7.8 and 7.9), to evaluate the airway in trauma, tumour, infection and inhalational injury, to confirm tube placement (tracheal, endobronchial, double lumen or tracheostomy tubes) and to perform tracheobronchial toilet.

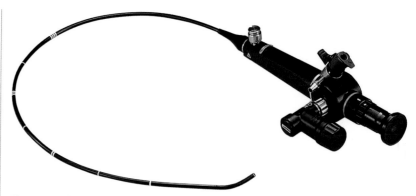

Fig. 7.7 Intubating fibreoptic scope. (Courtesy of Olympus.)

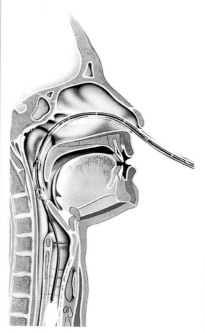

Fig. 7.8 Performing fibreoptic nasal intubation.

Components

1. Control unit which consists of the following:
   a) tip deflection control knob (the bending angle range is 60–180° in the vertical plane)
   b) eye piece
   c) diopter adjustment ring (focusing)
   d) suction channel which can also be used to insufflate oxygen and administer local anaesthetic solutions.

2. The flexible insertion cord consists of bundles of glass fibres. Each bundle consists of 10 000–15 000 fibres nearly identical in diameter and optical characteristics.

3. Light-transmitting cable to transmit light from an external source.

4. Other equipment may be needed, e.g. endoscopic face mask, oral airway, bite block, defogging agent.

Mechanism of action

1. The fibreoptic laryngoscope uses light transmitted through glass fibres. The fibres used have diameters of 5–20 μm, making them capable of transmitting light and being flexible at the same time.

2. The fibres are coated with a thin external layer of glass (of lower refractive index) thus providing optical insulation of each fibre in the bundle. A typical fibreoptic bundle is composed of up to 10 000 individual glass fibres.

3. Light enters the fibre at a specific angle of incidence. It travels down the fibre, repeatedly striking and being reflected from the external layer of glass at a similar angle of incidence until it emerges from the opposite end.

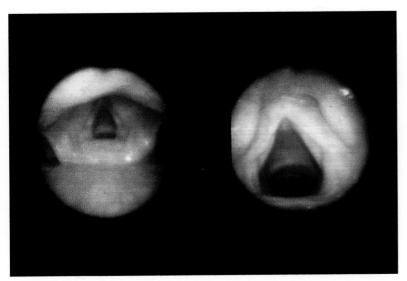

Fig. 7.9 Views of the vocal cords as seen through a fibreoptic laryngoscope.

4. The fibres are 'coherently' arranged throughout the bundle. As each fibre carries a very small part of the overall picture, it is essential for the clear transmission of an image that the arrangement of fibres is the same at both ends of the fibreoptic cable.

5. The insertion cords vary in length and diameter. The latter determines the size of the tracheal tube that can be used. Smaller scopes are available for intubating children. The outer diameter ranges from 1.8 to 6.4 mm allowing the use of tracheal tubes of 3.0–7.0-mm internal diameter.

Problems in practice and safety features

1. The intubating fibreoptic laryngoscope is a delicate instrument that can easily be damaged by careless handling. Damage to the fibre bundles results in loss of the image and light in individual fibres which cannot be repaired.

2. The laryngoscope should be cleaned and dried thoroughly as soon as possible after use.

> **Fibreoptic intubating laryngoscope**
> - The insertion cord consists of glass fibres arranged in bundles.
> - Light is transmitted through the glass fibres.
> - Used for tracheal intubation, airway evaluation and tracheobronchial toilet.
> - Damage to the fibres causes loss of image.

Videolaryngoscopes

Recent advances in miniaturized, high-resolution, digital camera and fibreoptic technology have led to a new generation of 'crossover' devices. These videolaryngoscopes, offering indirect laryngoscopy, combine features of both the flexible fibreoptic scopes and the standard rigid laryngoscopes (Fig. 7.10). The images are transmitted using fibreoptics or lenses and prisms with the light pathways encased in a rigid device. The cameras used offer wide views so allowing the user to see around corners, similar to the fibreoptic scopes. Certain designs have a channel that guides the tracheal tube into the trachea.

Videolaryngoscopes improve the view of the glottis, as the camera eye is only centimetres away from the glottis. Some designs use direct viewing through an eyepiece or an attached or remote screen. Their use requires minimal neck movement and can make laryngoscopy and hopefully successful tracheal intubation easier. Such devices may well supersede the classic laryngoscopes.

Magill forceps

These forceps are designed for ease of use within the mouth and oropharynx. Magill forceps come in small or large sizes (Fig. 7.11). During tracheal intubation, they can be used to direct the tracheal tube towards the larynx and vocal cords.

Care should be taken to protect the tracheal tube cuff from being damaged by the forceps.

Other uses include the insertion and removal of throat packs and removal of foreign bodies in the oropharynx and larynx.

Introducer, bougie, bite guard, local anaesthetic spray, Endotrol tube and Nosworthy airway

1. A local anaesthetic spray is used to coat the laryngeal and tracheal mucosa, usually with lidocaine. This decreases the stimulus of intubation.

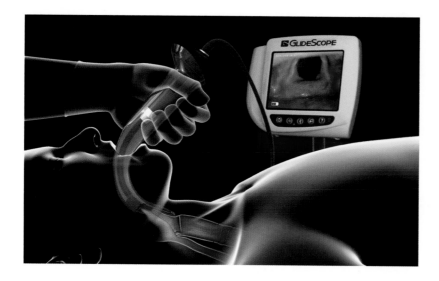

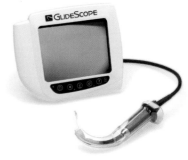

Fig. 7.10 The Glidescope videolaryngoscope. (Courtesy of Verathon Medical UK Ltd.)

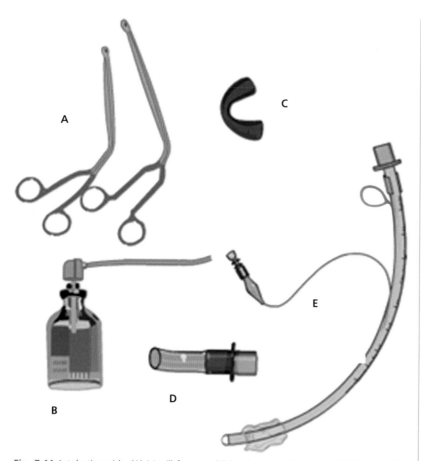

Fig. 7.11 Intubation aids. (A) Magill forceps; (B) local anaesthetic spray; (C) bite guard; (D) Nosworthy airway; (E) Endotrol tube.

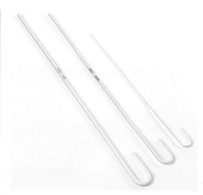

Fig. 7.12 Introducers or stylets. (Courtesy of Smiths Medical.)

2. A bite guard protects the front upper teeth during direct laryngoscopy.
3. The Endotrol tube has a ring-pull on its inner curvature connected to the distal end of the tube. During intubation, the ring-pull can be used to adjust the curvature of the tube.
4. The Nosworthy airway is an example of the many modifications that exist in oropharyngeal airway design. This airway allows the connection of a catheter mount and a breathing system.
5. An introducer or stylet (Fig. 7.12) is used to adjust the curvature of

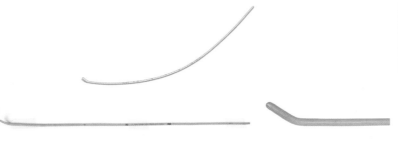

Fig. 7.13 Intubating bougie. Above is a single use bougie. Below is a reusable bougie with its curved tip. (Courtesy of Smiths Medical.)

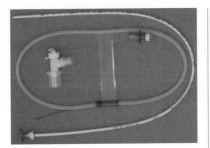

Fig. 7.14 The airway exchange catheter.

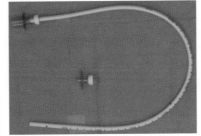

Fig. 7.15 The Aintree intubation catheter.

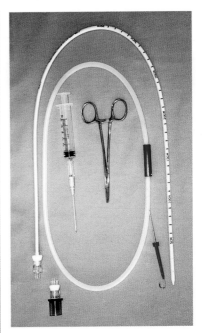

Fig. 7.16 The Cook retrograde intubation set.

a tracheal tube to help direct it through the vocal cords.

6. A gum elastic bougie is used when it is difficult to visualize the vocal cords. First, the bougie is inserted through the vocal cords, then the tracheal tube is railroaded over it. Single use intubating bougies are available (Fig. 7.13).

7. The airway exchange catheter (AEC) (Fig. 7.14) allows the exchange of tracheal tubes. It is a long hollow tube that can be inserted through a tracheal tube. This can then be withdrawn and another tracheal tube is inserted over it. Specially designed detachable 15-mm male taper fit and Luer-Lok connectors can be used to provide temporary oxygenation.

8. The Aintree intubation catheter (Fig. 7.15). This catheter is designed to be used with a fibrescope being passed through a laryngeal mask or other supraglottic airway device. It allows any appropriate size of tracheal tube to be inserted into the trachea which would otherwise be limited by the size of tube that could be passed through the supraglottic airway.

Retrograde intubation set (Fig. 7.16)

This set is used to assist in placement of a tracheal tube when a difficult intubation is encountered.

Components

1. An introducer needle (18 G and 5 cm in length).
2. A guidewire with a J-shaped end.
3. A 14-G 70-cm hollow guiding catheter with distal sideports.

The proximal end has a 15-mm connector.

Mechanism of action

1. The introducer needle is inserted through the cricothyroid membrane.
2. The guidewire is advanced in a retrograde (cephalic) direction to exit orally or nasally.
3. The hollow guiding catheter is then introduced in an antegrade direction into the trachea. The proximal end of the catheter can be connected to an oxygen supply.
4. A tracheal tube (5 mm or larger) can be introduced over the guiding catheter into the trachea.

Problems in practice and safety features

1. Pneumothorax.
2. Haemorrhage.
3. Failure.

FURTHER READING

Cooper, R.J., 2004. Laryngoscopy – its past and future. Canadian Journal of Anaesthesia 51, R1–R5. Online. Available at: http://www.springerlink.com/content/y8k03q8966rj8878/

MHRA, 2011. Medical device alert: reusable laryngoscope handles – all models and manufacturers (MDA/2011/0096). Online. Available at: http://www.mhra.gov.uk/Publications/Safetywarnings/MedicalDeviceAlerts/CON129213

Thong, S.Y., Lim, Y., 2009. Video and optic laryngoscopy assisted tracheal intubation – the new era. Anaesthesia and Intensive Care 37, 219–233. Online. Available at: http://xa.yimg.com/kq/groups/14982767/1890596062/name/Video+and+optic+laryngoscopy+assisted+tracheal+intubation+%C2%96+the+new+era.pdf

MCQs

In the following lists, which of the statements (a) to (e) are true?

1. Laryngoscopes:
   a) Straight blade laryngoscopes are only used in neonates and infants.
   b) The left-sided Macintosh blade is designed for a left-handed anaesthetist.
   c) The Macintosh blade is designed to elevate the larynx.
   d) The Macintosh polio blade can be used in patients with large breasts.
   e) The McCoy laryngoscope can improve the view of the larynx.

2. Light failure during laryngoscopy can be caused by:
   a) Battery failure.
   b) A loose bulb.
   c) The wrong-sized blade having been used.
   d) A blown bulb.
   e) Inadequate connection due to corrosion.

3. Concerning retrograde intubation:
   a) The introducer needle is inserted at the level of second and third tracheal cartilages.
   b) It is a very safe procedure with no complications.
   c) A guidewire is inserted in a cephalic direction.
   d) Supplemental oxygen can be administered.
   e) A tracheal tube (5 mm or larger) can be introduced over the guiding catheter into the trachea.

SINGLE BEST ANSWER (SBA)

4. Videolaryngoscopes:
   a) Are designed for retrograde intubation.
   b) Utilise a screen to display the larynx.
   c) Ensure safe intubation.
   d) Cannot be used in paediatric patients.
   e) Need no power supply.

Answers

1. Laryngoscopes:
   a) *False. Straight blade laryngoscopes can be used for adults, neonates and infants. Because of the shape and size of the larynx in small children, it is usually easier to intubate with a straight blade laryngoscope. The latter can be used in adults, but the curved blade laryngoscope is usually used.*
   b) *False. The left-sided Macintosh blade is designed to be used in cases of difficult access to the right side of the mouth or tongue, e.g. trauma or tumour.*
   c) *True. The Macintosh curved blade is designed to elevate the larynx thus allowing better visualization of the vocal cords.*
   d) *True. The polio blade was designed during the polio epidemic in the 1950s to overcome the problem of intubating patients who were in an 'iron lung'. In current practice, it can be used in patients with large breasts where the breasts do not get in the way of the handle.*
   e) *True. By using the hinged blade tip, the larynx is further elevated. This improves the view of the larynx.*

2. Light failure during laryngoscopy can be caused by:
   a) *True.*
   b) *True.*
   c) *False. This should not cause light failure. It may, however, cause a worse view of the larynx.*
   d) *True.*
   e) *True. This usually happens in the traditional laryngoscope design where the handle needs good contact with the blade for the current to flow from the batteries to the bulb in the blade. Corrosion at that junction can cause light failure. Laryngoscopes using fibreoptics do not suffer from this problem as the bulb is situated in the handle.*

3. Concerning retrograde intubation:
   a) *False. The needle is inserted through the cricothyroid membrane.*
   b) *False. Retrograde intubation can cause haemorrhage or pneumothorax.*
   c) *True. The guidewire is inserted in a retrograde cephalic direction to exit through the mouth or nose.*
   d) *True. Oxygen can be given through the proximal end of the guiding catheter.*
   e) *True.*

4. b)

Chapter 8

Ventilators

Ventilators are used to provide controlled ventilation (intermittent positive pressure ventilation; IPPV). Some have the facilities to provide other ventilatory modes. They can be used in the operating theatre, intensive care unit, during transport of critically ill patients and also at home (e.g. for patients requiring nocturnal respiratory assistance).

Classification of ventilators

There are many ways of classifying ventilators (Table 8.1).
1. The *method of cycling* is used to change over from inspiration to exhalation and vice versa:
   a) *volume* cycling: when the predetermined tidal volume is reached during inspiration, the ventilator changes to exhalation
   b) *time* cycling: when the predetermined inspiratory duration is reached, the ventilator changes to exhalation. The cycling is not affected by the compliance of the patient's lungs. Time cycling is the most commonly used method
   c) *pressure* cycling: when the predetermined pressure is reached during inspiration, the ventilator changes over to exhalation. The duration needed to achieve the critical pressure depends on the compliance of the lungs. The stiffer the lungs are, the quicker the pressure is achieved and vice versa. The ventilator delivers a different tidal volume if compliance or resistance changes
   d) *flow* cycling: when the predetermined flow is reached during inspiration, the ventilator changes over to exhalation. This method is used in older design ventilators.
2. *Inspiratory phase gas control*:
   a) *volume*: a preset volume is delivered
   b) *pressure*: a preset pressure is not exceeded.
3. *Source of power* – can be electric or pneumatic.
4. *Suitability for use* in theatre and/or intensive care.
5. *Suitability for paediatric practice*.
6. *Method of operation* (pattern of gas flow during inspiration):
   a) *pressure* generator: the ventilator produces inspiration by generating a constant and predetermined pressure. Bellows or a moderate weight produce the pressure. The inspiratory flow changes with changes in lung compliance (Table 8.2)
   b) *flow* generator: the ventilator produces inspiration by delivering a predetermined flow of gas. A piston, heavy weight or compressed gas produce the flow. The flow remains unchanged by changes in lung compliance, although pressures will change (see Table 8.2). These ventilators have a high internal resistance to protect the patient from high working pressures.
7. *Sophistication*: new ventilators can function in many of the above modes. They have other modes, e.g. SIMV, PS and CPAP (see pp 224–225).
8. *Function*:
   a) *minute volume dividers*: fresh gas flow (FGF) powers the ventilator. The minute volume equals the FGF divided into preset tidal volumes thus determining the frequency
   b) *bag squeezers* replace the hand ventilation of a Mapleson D or circle system. They need an external source of power
   c) *lightweight portable*: powered by compressed gas and consists of the control unit and patient valve.

Table 8.1 Summary of the methods used in classifying ventilators

Method of cycling	Volume cycling Time cycling Pressure cycling Flow cycling
Inspiratory phase gas control	Volume Pressure
Source of power	Electric Pneumatic
Suitability for use	Operating theatre Intensive care unit Both
Paediatrics use	Yes/no
Method of operation	Pressure generator Flow generator
Sophistication	SIMV, PS, CPAP
Function	Minute volume divider Bag squeezer Lightweight portable

CPAP, continuous positive airway pressure; PS, pressure support; SIMV, synchronized intermittent mandatory ventilation

Table 8.2 Differences between the pressure generator and flow generator ventilators

	Changes in lung compliance	Leak in the system
Pressure generator	Can not compensate	Can compensate (to a degree)
Flow generator	Can compensate (to a degree)	Can not compensate

Characteristics of the ideal ventilator

1. The ventilator should be simple, portable, robust and economical to purchase and use. If compressed gas is used to drive the ventilator, a significant wastage of the compressed gas is expected. Some ventilators use a Venturi to drive the bellows, to reduce the use of compressed oxygen.
2. It should be versatile and supply tidal volumes up to 1500 mL with a respiratory rate of up to 60/min and variable I:E ratio. It can be used with different breathing systems. It can deliver any gas or vapour mixture. The addition of positive end expiratory pressure (PEEP) should be possible.
3. It should monitor the airway pressure, inspired and exhaled minute and tidal volume, respiratory rate and inspired oxygen concentration.
4. There should be facilities to provide humidification. Drugs can be nebulized through it.
5. Disconnection, high airway pressure and power failure alarms should be present.
6. There should be the facility to provide other ventilatory modes, e.g. SIMV, CPAP and pressure support.
7. It should be easy to clean and sterilize.

Some of the commonly used ventilators are described below.

Manley MP3 ventilator

This is a minute volume divider (time cycled, pressure generator). All the FGF (the minute volume) is delivered to the patient divided into readily set tidal volumes (Fig. 8.1).

Components

1. Rubber tubing delivers the FGF from the anaesthetic machine to the ventilator.
2. Two sets of bellows. A smaller time-cycling bellows receives the FGF directly from the gas source and then empties into the main bellows.
3. Three unidirectional valves.
4. An adjustable pressure limiting (APL) valve with tubing and a reservoir bag used during spontaneous or manually controlled ventilation.
5. The ventilator has a pressure gauge (up to 100 cm H_2O), inspiratory time dial, tidal volume adjuster (up to 1000 mL), two knobs to change the mode of ventilation from and to controlled and spontaneous (or manually controlled) ventilation. The inflation pressure is adjusted by sliding the weight to an appropriate position along its rail. The expiratory block is easily removed for autoclaving.

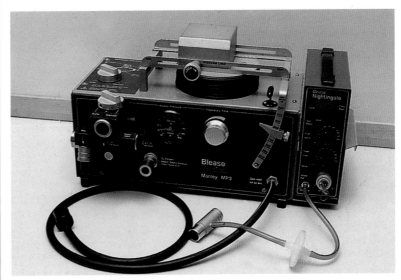

Fig. 8.1 The Blease Manley MP3 with ventilator alarm (right).

Mechanism of action

1. The FGF drives the ventilator.
2. During inspiration, the smaller bellows receives the FGF, while the main bellows delivers its contents to the patient. The inspiratory time dial controls the extent of filling of the smaller bellows before it empties into the main bellows.
3. During expiration, the smaller bellows delivers its contents to the main bellows until the predetermined tidal volume is reached to start inspiration again.
4. Using the ventilator in the spontaneous (manual) ventilation mode changes it to a Mapleson D breathing system.

Problems in practice and safety features

1. The ventilator ceases to cycle and function when the FGF is disconnected. This allows rapid detection of gas supply failure.
2. Ventilating patients with poor pulmonary compliance is not easily achieved.
3. It generates back pressure in the back bar as it cycles.
4. The emergency oxygen flush in the anaesthetic machine should not be activated while ventilating a patient with the Manley.

Manely MP3 ventilator
- It is a minute volume divider.
- Consists of two sets of bellows, three unidirectional valves, an APL valve and a reservoir bag.
- Acts as a Mapleson D breathing system during spontaneous ventilation.

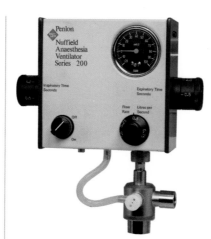

Fig. 8.2 The Penlon Nuffield 200 ventilator. (Courtesy of Penlon Ltd, Abingdon, UK (www.penlon.com).)

Penlon Anaesthesia Nuffield Ventilator Series 200

This is an intermittent blower ventilator. It is small, compact, versatile and easy to use with patients of different sizes, ages and lung compliances. It can be used with different breathing systems (Fig. 8.2). It is a volume-preset, time-cycled, flow generator in adult use. In paediatric use, it is a pressure-preset, time-cycled, flow generator.

Components

1. The control module, consisting of an airway pressure gauge (cm H_2O), inspiratory and expiratory time dials (seconds), inspiratory flow rate dial (L/s) and an on/off switch. Underneath the control module there are connections for the driving gas supply and the valve block. Tubing connects the valve block to the airway pressure gauge.
2. The valve block has three ports:
   a) a port for tubing to connect to the breathing system reservoir bag mount

---

b) an exhaust port which can be connected to the scavenging system
   c) a pressure relief valve which opens at 60 cm H_2O.
3. The valve block can be changed to a paediatric (Newton) valve.

Mechanism of action

1. The ventilator is powered by a driving gas independent from the FGF. The commonly used driving gas is oxygen (at about 400 kPa) supplied from the compressed oxygen outlets on the anaesthetic machine. The driving gas should not reach the patient as it dilutes the FGF, lightening the depth of anaesthesia.
2. It can be used with different breathing systems such as Bain, Humphrey ADE, T-piece and the circle. In the Bain and circle systems, the reservoir bag is replaced by the tubing delivering the driving gas from the ventilator. The APL valve of the breathing system must be fully closed during ventilation.
3. The inspiratory and expiratory times can be adjusted to the desired I/E ratio. Adjusting the inspiratory time and inspiratory flow rate controls determines the tidal volume. The inflation pressure is adjusted by the inspiratory flow rate control.
4. With its standard valve, the ventilator acts as a time-cycled flow generator to deliver a minimal tidal volume of 50 mL. When the valve is changed to a paediatric (Newton) valve, the ventilator changes to a time-cycled pressure generator capable of delivering tidal volumes between 10 and 300 mL. This makes it capable of ventilating premature babies and neonates. It is recommended that the Newton valve is used

for children of less than 20 kg body weight.

5. A PEEP valve may be fitted to the exhaust port.

Problems in practice and safety features

1. The ventilator continues to cycle despite breathing system disconnection.
2. Requires high flows of driving gas.

Penlon Nuffield Anaesthesia Ventilator Series 200

- An intermittent blower with a pressure gauge, inspiratory and expiratory time and flow controls.
- Powered by a driving gas.
- Can be used for both adults and paediatric patients.
- Can be used with different breathing systems.

Bag in bottle ventilator

Modern anaesthetic machines often incorporate a bag in bottle ventilator.

Components

1. A driving unit consisting of:
   a) a chamber (Fig. 8.3) with a tidal volume range of 0–1500 mL (a paediatric version with a range of 0–400 mL exists)
   b) an ascending bellows accommodating the FGF.
2. A control unit with a variety of controls, displays and alarms: the tidal volume, respiratory rate (6–40/min), I/E ratio, airway pressure and power supply (Figs 8.3 and 8.4).

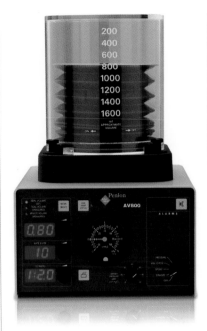

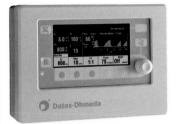

Fig. 8.4 Control panel of the Datex-Ohmeda 7900 ventilator.

Fig. 8.3 Bag in bottle AV800 ventilator. (Courtesy of Penlon Ltd, Abingdon, UK (www.penlon.com).)

Mechanism of action

1. It is a time-cycled ventilator.
2. Compressed air is used as the driving gas (Fig. 8.5). On entering the chamber, the compressed air forces the bellows down, delivering the fresh gas to the patient (the fresh gas is accommodated in the bellows).
3. The driving gas and the fresh gas remain separate.
4. The volume of the driving gas reaching the chamber is equal to the tidal volume.
5. Some designs feature a descending bellows instead.

Problems in practice and safety features

1. Positive pressure in the standing bellows causes a PEEP of 2–4 cm H_2O.
2. The ascending bellows collapses to an empty position and remains stationary in cases of disconnection or leak.

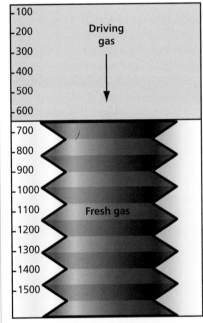

Fig. 8.5 Mechanism of action of the bag in bottle ventilator.

3. The descending bellows hangs down to a fully expanded position in a case of disconnection and may continue to move almost normally in a case of leakage.

Bag in bottle ventilator

- It is a time-cycled ventilator.
- Consists of driving and control units.
- Fresh gas is within the bellows whereas the driving gas is within the chamber.

Servo-*i* ventilator

The Servo-*i* is a versatile intensive care ventilator, capable of being used for paediatric and adult patients. It is fully transportable, utilizing 12 V battery power when mains electricity is not available. It is not intended for use with inhalational anaesthetics, however it can be used with intravenous anaesthetics in the theatre setting if required. It can be used to 'non-invasively' ventilate patients with a tight fitting nasal mask or face mask instead of an endotracheal tube or tracheostomy. Facilities to deliver Heliox also exist.

The most modern versions have advanced tools to safely perform lung recruitment utilizing software that regulates PEEP and aims to maintain lung compliance.

Neurally Adjusted Ventilatory Assist (NAVA) uses a specially adapted nasogastric tube that detects the phrenic nerve impulses to the diaphragm. This enhances the ability of the ventilator to match the respiratory efforts of the patient by timing its assisted breaths.

Components (Fig. 8.6)

1. 'Patient unit' where gases are mixed and administered.
2. 'Graphical user interface' where settings are made and ventilation monitored.

Mechanism of action

1. Gas flow from the oxygen and air inlets is regulated by their respective gas modules.
2. Oxygen concentration is measured by an oxygen cell.
3. The pressure of the delivered gas mixture is measured by the inspiratory pressure transducer.
4. The patient's expiratory gas flow is measured by ultrasonic transducers and the pressure

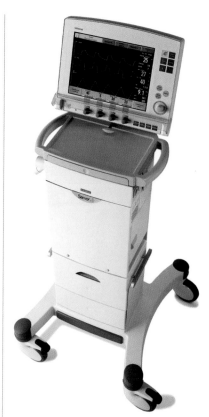

Fig. 8.6 Servo-*i* ventilator.

measured by the expiratory pressure transducer.
5. PEEP in the patient system is regulated by the expiratory valve.

There are various modes of ventilation available:

1. *Synchronized intermittent mandatory ventilation* (SIMV). The ventilator provides mandatory breaths, which are synchronized with the patient's respiratory effort (if present). The type of mandatory breath supplied depends on the setting selected. Usually one of the following is selected:
 a) *pressure-regulated volume control* (PRVC): a preset tidal volume is delivered but limited to 5 cm H_2O below the set upper pressure limit. This automatically limits

barotrauma if the upper pressure limit is appropriately set. The flow during inspiration is decelerating. The patient can trigger extra breaths
 b) *volume control*: a preset tidal volume and respiratory rate are selected. The breath is delivered with constant flow during a preset inspiratory time. The set tidal volume will always be delivered despite high airway pressures if the patient's lungs are not compliant. To prevent excessive pressures being generated in this situation, the upper pressure limit must be set to a suitable level to prevent barotrauma
 c) *pressure control*: a pressure control level above PEEP is selected. The delivered tidal volume is dependent upon the patient's lung compliance and airway resistance together with the tubing and endotracheal tube's resistance. Pressure control ventilation is preferred when there is a leak in the breathing system (e.g. uncuffed endotracheal tube) or where barotrauma is to be avoided (e.g. acute lung injury). If the resistance or compliance improves quickly, there is a risk of excessive tidal volumes being delivered (volutrauma) unless the pressure control setting is reduced.
2. *Supported ventilation modes*: once the patient has enough respiratory drive to trigger the ventilator, usually one of the following modes is selected in addition to the PEEP setting:
 a) *volume support*: assures a set tidal volume by supplying the required pressure support needed to achieve that tidal volume. It allows patients to wean from ventilatory support

themselves as their lungs' compliance and inspiratory muscle strength improves. This is shown by a gradual reduction in the peak airway pressure measured by the ventilator. Once the support is minimal, extubation can be considered

b) *pressure support* (PS): the patient's breath is supported with a set constant pressure above PEEP. This will give a tidal volume that is dependent on the lung compliance and patient's inspiratory muscle strength. The pressure support setting needs reviewing regularly to allow the patient to wean from respiratory support

c) *continuous positive airway pressure* (CPAP): a continuous positive pressure is maintained in the airways similar to that developed with a conventional CPAP flow generator (see Chapter 13). This differs from the conventional CPAP flow generator by allowing measurement of tidal volume, minute volume and respiratory rate, and trends can be observed also.

Problems in practice and safety features

1. A comprehensive alarm system is featured.
2. A mainstream carbon dioxide analyser is available which allows continuous inspiratory and expiratory monitoring of CO_2 to be displayed if required.
3. A single battery module offers 30 minutes of ventilator use. Multiple battery modules (up to 6) can be loaded on the ventilator if a long transport journey is anticipated, allowing extended use. It is recommended

at least two battery modules are loaded for even the shortest transport.

4. The ventilator is heavier (20 kg) than a dedicated transport ventilator.

Servo-i ventilator
- Versatile intensive care ventilator suitable for both paediatric and adult use.
- Wide range of controls, displays and alarms.
- Portable with battery power.

High-frequency jet ventilator

This ventilator reduces the extent of the side-effects of conventional IPPV. There are lower peak airway pressures with better maintenance of the cardiac output and less anti-diuretic hormone production and fluid retention. It is better tolerated by alert patients than conventional IPPV (Fig. 8.7).

Components

1. A Venturi injector is used: a cannula positioned in a tracheal tube (Fig. 8.8B), a cannula positioned in the trachea via the cricothyroid membrane or a modified tracheal tube with two additional small lumens opening distally (Figs 8.8A and 8.9).
2. Solenoid valves are used to deliver the jet gas.
3. Dials and display for driving pressure, frequency and inspiratory time.
4. Built-in peristaltic pump for nebulizing drugs or distilled water for humidifying the jet gas.
5. High-flow air/oxygen or nitrous oxide/oxygen blender determines the mix of the jet gas.

Mechanism of action

1. Frequencies of 20–500 cycles/min can be selected, with minute volumes ranging from 5 to 60 L/min.
2. It is a time-cycled ventilator delivering gas in small jet pulsations. The inspiratory time is adjustable from 20% to 50% of the cycle.
3. The fresh gas leaving the narrow injector at a very high velocity causes entrainment of gas. The amount of entrained gas is uncertain making measurement of tidal volume and FiO_2 difficult.

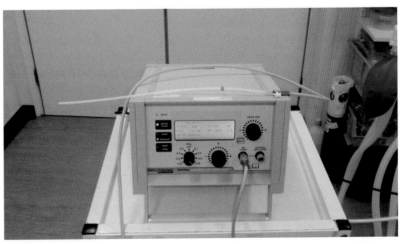

Fig. 8.7 High-frequency jet ventilator with a jet catheter attached.

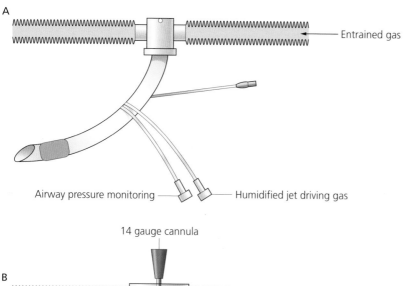

A

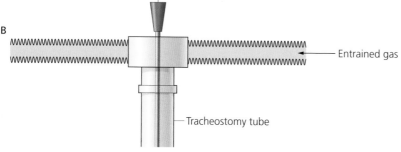

Airway pressure monitoring — Humidified jet driving gas

14 gauge cannula

B

Entrained gas

Tracheostomy tube

Fig. 8.8 (A) A jet tracheal tube with two additional lumens for the jet driving gas and airway pressure monitoring. (B) A 14-gauge cannula positioned within a tracheostomy tube, through which the jet driving gas can be administered.

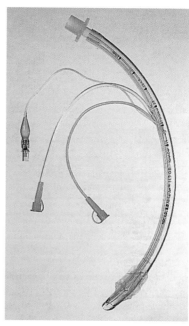

Fig. 8.9 The Mallinckrodt Hi-Lo Jet cuffed tracheal tube. An uncuffed version also exists.

4. The jet and entrained gases impact into the much larger volume of relatively immobile gases in the airway, causing them to move forward.
5. Expiration is passive. PEEP occurs automatically at a respiratory rate of over 100/min. Additional PEEP can be added by means of a PEEP valve.

> **High-frequency jet ventilator**
> - Time-cycled ventilator.
> - A Venturi injector is used.
> - Built-in peristaltic pump for humidification.
> - Frequencies of 20–500 cycles/min. Minute volumes of 5–60 L/min.

Problems in practice and safety features

1. Barotrauma can still occur as expiration is dependent on passive lung and chest wall recoil driving the gas out through the tracheal tube.
2. High-pressure (35–40 cm H_2O) and system malfunction alarms are featured.

VentiPAC

This is a portable ventilator used during the transport of critically ill patients (Fig. 8.10). It is a flow generator, time cycled, volume preset and pressure limited. It also acts as a pressure generator at flows below 0.25 L/s in air mix setting. ParaPAC ventilator allows

synchronization of ventilation with external cardiac massage during cardiopulmonary resuscitation. A neonatal/paediatric version exists.

Components

1. A variety of controls including:
   a) inspiratory flow (6–60 L/min)
   b) inspiratory time (0.5–3.0 s)
   c) expiratory time (0.5–6.0 s)
   d) adjustable inspiratory relief pressure with an audible alarm (20–80 cm H_2O)
   e) air mix/no air mix control
   f) a 'demand' and 'CMV/demand' control (CMV = controlled mandatory ventilation).
2. Inflation pressure monitor to measure the airway pressure.
3. 120-cm polyester or silicone 15-mm tubing with a one-way valve to deliver gases to the patient.
4. Tubing to deliver the oxygen to the ventilator.

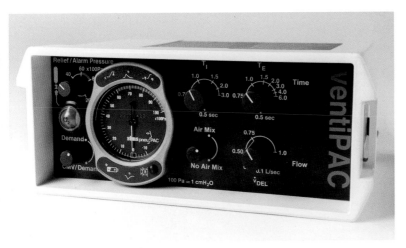

Fig. 8.10 The VentiPAC ventilator.

> **VentiPAC**
> - Portable ventilator powered by pressurized gas.
> - Controls include flow rate, inspiratory time and expiratory time.
> - An FiO_2 of 0.45 or 1.0 can be delivered.
> - It has a demand valve.
> - MRI compatible.

Mechanism of action

1. The source of power is dry, oil-free pressurized gas (270–600 kPa) at 60 L/min. Using air mix mode reduces gas consumption by the ventilator by almost 70%.
2. The frequency is set by adjusting the inspiratory and expiratory times.
3. The tidal volume is set by the adjustment of the flow and inspiratory time.
4. A choice of an FiO_2 of 1.0 (no air mix) or 0.45 (air mix).
5. The demand mode provides 100% oxygen to a spontaneously breathing patient. A visual indicator flashes when a spontaneous breath is detected.
6. CMV/demand mode provides continuous mandatory ventilation. If the patient makes a spontaneous breath, this causes the ventilator to operate in a synchronized minimum mandatory ventilation (SMMV) mode. Any superimposed mandatory ventilatory attempts are synchronized with the breathing pattern.
7. A PEEP valve can be added generating a PEEP of up to 20 cm H_2O.

Problems in practice and safety features

1. There is an adjustable inspiratory pressure relief mechanism with a range of 20–80 cm H_2O to reduce the risk of overpressure and barotruma.
2. There are audible and visual low-pressure (disconnection) and high-pressure (obstruction) alarms.
3. A supply gas failure alarm.
4. The ventilator is magnetic resonance imaging (MRI) compatible.

Pneupac VR1 Emergency Ventilator (Fig. 8.11)

This is a lightweight hand-held, time-cycled, gas-powered flow generator ventilator. It is designed for use in emergency and during transport. It is MRI compatible up to 3 Tesla.

Components

1. Tidal volume/frequency control.
2. Auto/manual control with a manual trigger and push button.
3. Air mix switch allowing the delivery of oxygen at 100% or 50% concentrations.

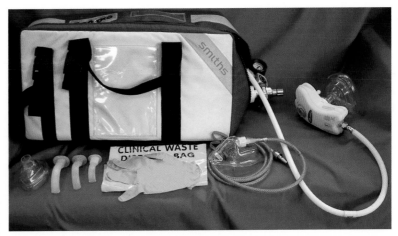

Fig. 8.11 Pneupac VR1 Emergency Ventilator.

4. Patient valve connecting to catheter mount/filter or face mask.
5. Gas supply input.

Mechanism of action

1. The source of power is pressurized oxygen (280–1034 kPa). Using air mix prolongs the duration of use from an oxygen cylinder.
2. A constant I:E ratio of 1:2 with flow rates of 11–32 L/min.
3. An optional patient demand facility is incorporated allowing synchronization between patient and ventilator.
4. The linked manual controls allow the manual triggering of a single controlled ventilation. This allows the ventilator to be used in a variety of chest compression/ventilation options in cardiac life support.
5. Suitable for children (above 10 kg body weight) and adults.

Problems in practice and safety features

1. Pressure relief valve designed to operate at 40 cm H_2O.
2. The manual control triggers a single ventilation equivalent to the volume of ventilation delivered in automatic ventilation. It is not a purge action so it cannot stack breaths and is therefore inherently much safer for the patient.

Pneupac VR1 Emergency Ventilator
- Hand-held, time-cycled, gas-powered flow generator ventilator.
- Used in emergency and transport.
- MRI compatible up to 3 Tesla.
- Various controls.
- Can be used in children and adults.

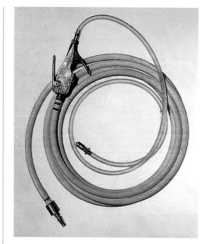

Fig. 8.12 The manually controlled injector. In practice this is connected to a rigid bronchoscope.

Venturi injector device

A manually controlled Venturi ventilation device used during rigid bronchoscopy (Fig. 8.12). The anaesthetist and the operator share the airway. General anaesthesia is maintained intravenously.

Components

1. A high-pressure oxygen source at about 400 kPa (from the anaesthetic machine or direct from a pipeline).
2. An on/off trigger.
3. Connection tubing that can withstand high pressures.
4. A needle of suitable gauge, which allows good air entrainment without creating excessive airway pressures.

Mechanism of action

1. The high-pressure oxygen is injected intermittently through the needle placed at the proximal end of the bronchoscope.
2. This creates a Venturi effect, entraining atmospheric air and

inflating the lungs with oxygen-enriched air.
3. Oxygenation and carbon dioxide elimination are achieved with airway pressures of 25–30 cm H_2O.

Problems in practice and safety features

1. Barotrauma is possible. Airway pressure monitoring is not available.
2. Gastric distension can occur should ventilation commence before the distal end of the bronchoscope is beyond the larynx.

Venturi injector device
- Manually controlled Venturi used during rigid bronchoscopy.
- High-pressure oxygen injected through a needle entraining air.

Self-inflating bag and mask

This is a means of providing manual IPPV. It is portable and is used during resuscitation, transport and short-term ventilation (Fig. 8.13).

Components

1. Self-inflating bag with a connection for added oxygen.
2. A one-way valve with three ports:
   a) inspiratory inlet allowing the entry of fresh gas during inspiration
   b) expiratory outlet allowing the exit of exhaled gas
   c) connection to the face mask or tracheal tube, and marked 'patient'.
3. A reservoir for oxygen to increase the FiO_2 delivered to the patient.

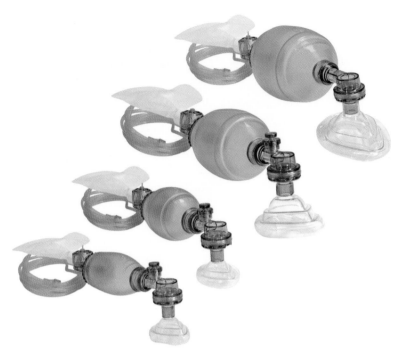

Fig. 8.13 A range of self-inflating resuscitation bags with oxygen reservoirs.

Mechanism of action

1. The non-rebreathing valve (Ambu valve) incorporates a silicone rubber membrane (Fig. 8.14). It has a small dead space and low resistance to flow. At a flow of 25 L/min, an inspiratory resistance of 0.4 cm H_2O and an expiratory resistance of 0.6 cm H_2O are achieved. The valve can easily be dismantled for cleaning and sterilization.

2. The valve acts as a spillover valve allowing excess inspiratory gas to be channelled directly to the expiratory outlet, bypassing the patient port.

3. The valve is suitable for both IPPV and spontaneous ventilation.

4. The shape of the self-inflating bag is automatically restored after compression. This allows fresh gas to be drawn from the reservoir.

5. A paediatric version exists with a smaller inflating bag and a pressure relief valve.

6. Disposable designs for both the adult and paediatric versions exist.

Self-inflating bag
- Compact, portable, self-inflating bag with a one-way valve.
- Oxygen reservoir can be added to increase FiO_2.
- Paediatric version exists.

PEEP valve

This valve is used during IPPV to increase the functional residual capacity (FRC) to improve the patient's oxygenation.

It is a spring-loaded unidirectional valve positioned on the expiratory side of the ventilator breathing system with a standard 22-mm connector. By adjusting the valve knob, a PEEP of between zero and 20 cm H_2O can be achieved (Fig. 8.15).

Fig. 8.14 An Ambu valve disassembled. (Reproduced with permission from AMBU International (UK) Ltd.)

Valve housing

Expiratory connector

Valve membrane

Inspiratory connector

Patient connector

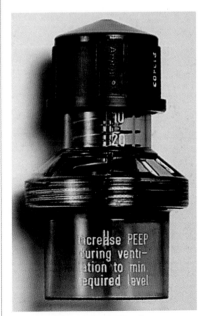

Fig. 8.15 The Ambu PEEP valve.

The valve provides almost constant expiratory resistance over a very wide range of flow rates.

FURTHER READING

Bersten, A.D., 2003. Mechanical ventilation. In: Bersten, A., Soni, N., Oh, T.E. (Eds), Oh's intensive care manual, fifth ed. Butterworth-Heinemann, Edinburgh.

Merck, 2007. Overview of mechanical ventilation. Online. Available at: http://www.merckmanuals.com/professional/critical_care_medicine/respiratory_failure_and_mechanical_ventilation/overview_of_mechanical_ventilation.html.

MHRA, 2010. Medical device alert: all Oxylog 3000 emergency/transport ventilators manufactured by Draeger (MDA/2010/092). Online. Available at: http://www.mhra.gov.uk/Publications/Safetywarnings/MedicalDeviceAlerts/CON100176.

MCQs

In the following lists, which of the following statements (a) to (e) are true?

1. Bag in bottle ventilator:
   a) The FGF is the driving gas at the same time.
   b) Is a minute volume divider.
   c) The bellows can be either ascending or descending.
   d) With a leak, the ascending bellows may continue to move almost normally.
   e) Can be used only for adult patients.

2. Manley ventilator:
   a) Is a minute volume divider.
   b) Has one set of bellows.
   c) During controlled ventilation, it is safe to activate the emergency oxygen flush device of the anaesthetic machine.
   d) A pressure-monitoring ventilator alarm is attached to the expiratory limb.
   e) It acts as a Mapleson D system during spontaneous ventilation mode.

3. Bag in bottle ventilator:
   a) It is a time-cycled ventilator.
   b) There is some mixing of the fresh gas and driving gas.
   c) For safety reasons, the descending bellows design is preferred.
   d) A small PEEP is expected.
   e) The driving gas volume in the chamber equals the tidal volume.

4. Regarding classification of ventilators:
   a) A pressure generator ventilator can compensate for changes in lung compliance.
   b) A flow generator ventilator cannot compensate for leaks in the system.
   c) A time-cycling ventilator is affected by the lung compliance.
   d) The duration of inspiration in a pressure-cycling ventilator is not affected by the compliance of the lungs.
   e) A pressure generator ventilator can compensate, to a degree, for leaks in the system.

5. High-frequency jet ventilation:
   a) The FiO_2 can easily be measured.
   b) Frequencies of up to 500 Hz can be achieved.
   c) The cardiac output is better maintained than conventional IPPV.
   d) Can be used both in anaesthesia and intensive care.
   e) Because of the lower peak airway pressures, there is no risk of barotrauma.

SINGLE BEST ANSWER (SBA)

6. Concerning pressure-control versus volume-control ventilation:
   a) Volume control will provide a set tidal volume.
   b) Pressure control will provide a set tidal volume.
   c) Lung compliance is irrelevant with pressure control.
   d) Paediatric ventilation never uses pressure control ventilation.
   e) Barotrauma is prevented by volume control ventilation.

Answers

1. Bag in bottle ventilator:
   a) *False.* The driving gas is separate from the FGF. The driving gas is usually either oxygen or, more economically, air. There is no mixing between the driving gas and the FGF. The volume of the driving gas reaching the chamber is equal to the tidal volume.
   b) *False.* The tidal volume and respiratory rate can be adjusted separately in a bag in bottle ventilator.
   c) *True.* Most of the bag in bottle ventilators use ascending bellows. This adds to the safety of the system as the bellows will collapse if there is a leak.
   d) *False.* See c).
   e) *False.* The ventilator can be used for both adults and children. A different size bellows can be used for different age groups.

2. Manley ventilator:
   a) *True.* The tidal volume can be set in a Manley ventilator. The whole FGF (minute volume) is delivered to the patient according to the set tidal volume, thus dividing the minute volume.
   b) *False.* There are two sets of bellows in a Manley ventilator, the time-cycling bellows and the main bellows.
   c) *False.* As it is a minute volume divider and the FGF is the driving gas (see a) above), activating the emergency oxygen flush will lead to considerable increase in the minute volume.
   d) *False.* The pressure-monitoring alarm should be

attached to the inspiratory limb and not the expiratory limb. A Wright spirometer can be attached to the expiratory limb to measure the tidal volume.
   e) *True.* During the spontaneous (manual) breathing mode, the Manley ventilator acts as a Mapleson D system.

3. Bag in bottle ventilator:
   a) *True.* The inspiratory and expiratory periods can be determined by adjusting the I : E ratio and the respiratory rate. So, for example, with a rate of 10 breaths/min and an I : E ratio of 1 : 2, each breath lasts for 6 seconds with an inspiration of 2 seconds and expiration of 4 seconds.
   b) *False.* There is no mixing between the fresh gas and the driving gas as they are completely separate.
   c) *False.* In case of a leak in the system, the descending bellows will not collapse. The opposite occurs with the ascending bellows.
   d) *True.* A PEEP of 2–4 cm H_2O is expected due to the compliance of the bellows.
   e) *True.*

4. Regarding classification of ventilators:
   a) *False.* A pressure generator ventilator cannot compensate for changes in lung compliance. It cycles when the set pressure has been reached. This can be a larger or smaller tidal volume depending on the lung compliance.
   b) *True.* It will deliver the set flow whether there is a leak or not.

   c) *False.* The ventilator will cycle with time regardless of the compliance.
   d) *False.* In a lung with low compliance, the inspiration will be shorter because the pressure will be reached more quickly leading the ventilator to cycle and vice versa.
   e) *True.* The ventilator will continue to deliver gases, despite the leak, until a preset pressure has been reached.

5. High-frequency jet ventilation:
   a) *False.* The ventilator uses the Venturi principle to entrain ambient air. The amount of entrainment is uncertain, making the measurement of the FiO_2 difficult.
   b) *False.* Frequencies of up to 500/min (not Hz; i.e. per second) can be achieved with a high-frequency jet ventilator.
   c) *True.* Because of the lower intrathoracic pressures generated during high-frequency jet ventilation, causing a lesser effect on the venous return, the cardiac output is better maintained.
   d) *True.* It can be used both in anaesthesia and intensive care, e.g. in the management of bronchopleural fistula.
   e) *False.* Although the risk is reduced, there is still a risk of barotrauma.

6. a)

Chapter 9

Humidification and filtration

Inhaling dry gases can cause damage to the cells lining the respiratory tract, impairing ciliary function. Within a short period of just 10 min of ventilation with dry gases, cilia function will be disrupted. This increases the patient's susceptibility to respiratory tract infection. A decrease in body temperature (due to the loss of the latent heat of vaporization) occurs as the respiratory tract humidifies the dry gases.

Air fully saturated with water vapour has an absolute humidity of about 44 mg/L at 37°C. During nasal breathing at rest, inspired gases become heated to 36°C with a relative humidity of about 80–90% by the time they reach the carina, largely because of heat transfer in the nose. Mouth breathing reduces this to 60–70% relative humidity. The humidifying property of soda lime can achieve an absolute humidity of 29 mg/L when used with the circle breathing system.

The *isothermic boundary point* is where 37°C and 100% humidity have been achieved. Normally it is a few centimetres distal to the carina. Insertion of a tracheal or tracheostomy tube bypasses the upper airway and moves the isothermic boundary distally.

Characteristics of the ideal humidifier

- Capable of providing adequate levels of humidification.
- Has low resistance to flow and low dead space.
- Provides microbiological protection to the patient.
- Maintenance of body temperature.
- Safe and convenient to use.
- Economical.

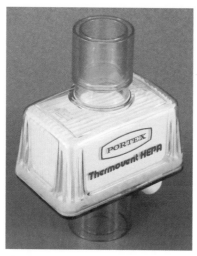

Fig. 9.1 The Thermovent heat and moisture exchanger with hydrophobic filtration properties. (Courtesy of Smiths Medical.)

Heat and moisture exchanger (HME) humidifiers

These are compact, inexpensive, passive and effective humidifiers for most clinical situations (Figs 9.1 and 9.2). The British Standard describes them as 'devices intended to retain a portion of the patient's expired moisture and heat, and return it to the respiratory tract during inspiration'.

The efficiency of an HME is gauged by the proportion of heat and moisture it returns to the patient. Adequate humidification is achieved with a relative humidity of 60–70%. Inspired gases are warmed to temperatures of between 29° and 34°C. HMEs should be able to deliver an absolute humidity of a minimum of 30 g/m³ water vapour at 30°C. HMEs are easy and convenient to use with no need for an external power source.

Components

1. Two ports, designed to accept 15- and 22-mm size tubings and

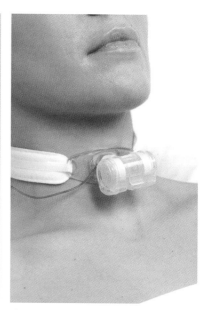

Fig. 9.2 The Thermovent T tracheostomy heat and moisture exchanger. (Courtesy of Smiths Medical.)

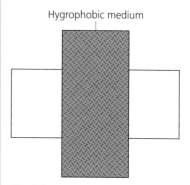

Hygrophobic medium

Fig. 9.3 Heat and moisture exchanger.

connections. Some designs have provision for connection of a sampling tube for gas and vapour concentration monitoring.

2. The head which contains a medium with hygrophobic properties in the form of a mesh with a large surface area (Fig. 9.3). It can be made of ceramic fibre, corrugated aluminium or paper, cellulose, metalized polyurethane foam or stainless-steel fibres.

Mechanism of action

1. Warm humidified exhaled gases pass through the humidifier, causing water vapour to condense on the cooler HME medium. The condensed water is evaporated and returned to the patient with the next inspiration of dry and cold gases, humidifying them. There is no addition of water over and above that previously exhaled.
2. The greater the temperature difference between each side of the HME, the greater the potential for heat and moisture to be transferred during exhalation and inspiration.
3. The HME humidifier requires about 5–20 min before it reaches its optimal ability to humidify dry gases.
4. Some designs with a pore size of about 0.2 µm can filter out bacteria, viruses and particles from the gas flow in either direction, as discussed later. They are called heat and moisture exchanging filters (HMEF).
5. Their volumes range from 7.8 mL (paediatric practice) to 100 mL. This increases the apparatus dead space.
6. The performance of the HME is affected by:
   a) water vapour content and temperature of the inspired and exhaled gases
   b) inspiratory and expiratory flow rates affecting the time the gas is in contact with the HME medium hence the heat and moisture exchange
   c) the volume and efficiency of the HME medium – the larger the medium, the greater the performance. Low thermal conductivity, i.e. poor heat conduction, helps to maintain a greater temperature difference across the HME

increasing the potential performance.

Problems in practice and safety features

1. The estimated increase in resistance to flow due to these humidifiers ranges from 0.1 to 2.0 cm H_2O depending on the flow rate and the device used. Obstruction of the HME with mucus or because of the expansion of saturated heat exchanging material may occur and can result in dangerous increases in resistance.
2. It is recommended that they are used for a maximum of 24 h and for single patient use only. There is a risk of increased airway resistance because of the accumulation of water in the filter housing if used for longer periods.
3. The humidifying efficiency decreases when large tidal volumes are used.
4. For the HME to function adequately, a two-way gas flow is required.
5. For optimal function, HME must be placed in the breathing system close to the patient.

Heat and moisture exchanger (HME) humidifiers

- Water vapour present in the exhaled gases is condensed on the medium. It is evaporated and returned to the patient with the following inspiration.
- A relative humidity of 60–70% can be achieved.
- Some designs incorporate a filter.
- There is an increase in apparatus dead space and airway resistance.
- The water vapour content and temperature of gases, flow rate of gases and the volume of the medium affect performance of HME.

Hot water bath humidifier

This humidifier is used to deliver relative humidities higher than the heat moisture exchange humidifier. It is usually used in intensive care units (Fig. 9.4).

Components

1. A disposable reservoir of water with an inlet and outlet for inspired gases. Heated sterile water partly fills the container.
2. A thermostatically controlled heating element with temperature sensors, both in the

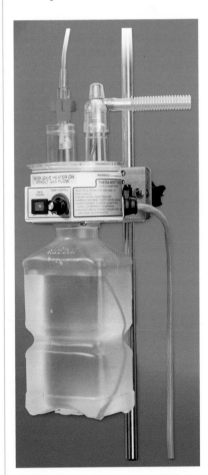

Fig. 9.4 The Aquinox hot water bath humidifier. (Courtesy of Smiths Medical.)

reservoir and in the breathing system close to the patient.

3. Tubing is used to deliver the humidified and warm gases to the patient. It should be as short as possible. A water trap is positioned between the patient and the humidifier along the tubing. The trap is positioned lower than the level of the patient.

Mechanism of action

1. Powered by electricity, the water is heated to between 45°C and 60°C (Fig. 9.5).
2. Dry cold gas enters the container where some passes close to the water surface, gaining maximum saturation. Some gas passes far from the water surface, gaining minimal saturation and heat.
3. The container has a large surface area for vaporization. This is to ensure that the gas is fully saturated at the temperature of the water bath. The amount of gas effectively bypassing the water surface should be minimal.

4. The tubing has poor thermal insulation properties causing a decrease in the temperature of inspired gases. This is partly compensated for by the release of the heat of condensation.
5. By raising the temperature in the humidifier above body temperature, it is possible to deliver gases at 37°C and fully saturated. The temperature of gases at the patient's end is measured by a thermistor. Via a feedback mechanism, the thermistor controls the temperature of water in the container.
6. The temperature of gases at the patient's end depends on the surface area available for vaporization, the flow rate and the amount of cooling and condensation taking place in the inspiratory tubing.
7. Some designs have heated elements placed in the inspiratory and expiratory limb of the breathing system to maintain the temperature and prevent rain out (condensation) within the tube.

Problems in practice and safety features

1. The humidifier, which is electrically powered, should be safe to use with no risk of scalding, overhydration and electric shock. A second backup thermostat cuts in should there be malfunction of the first thermostat.
2. The humidifier and water trap(s) should be positioned below the level of the tracheal tube to prevent flooding of the airway by condensed water.
3. Colonization of the water by bacteria can be prevented by increasing the temperature to 60°C. This poses greater risk of scalding.
4. The humidifier is large, expensive and can be awkward to use.
5. There are more connections in a ventilator set up and so the risk of disconnections or leaks increases.

> ### Hot water bath humidifier
> - Consists of a container with a thermostatically controlled heating element and tubing with water traps.
> - The temperature of water in the container, via a feedback mechanism, is controlled by a thermistor at the patient's end.
> - Full saturation at 37°C can be achieved.
> - Colonization by bacteria is a problem.

Nebulizers (Fig. 9.6)

These produce a mist of microdroplets of water suspended in a gaseous medium. The quantity of water droplets delivered is not limited by gas temperature (as is the

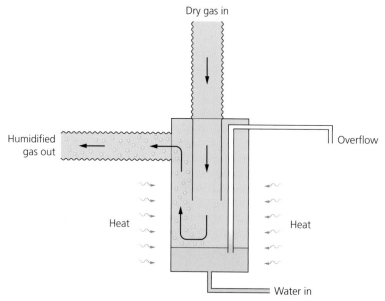

Fig. 9.5 Mechanism of action of the hot water bath humidifier.

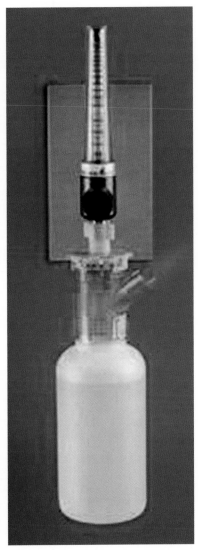

Fig. 9.6 Smith's medical gas-driven nebulizer.

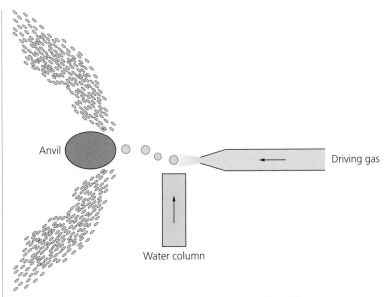

Fig. 9.7 Mechanism of action of a gas-driven nebulizer humidifier.

case with vapour). The smaller the droplets, the more stable they are. Droplets of 2–5 μm deposit in the tracheobronchial tree, whereas 0.5–1 μm droplets deposit in the alveoli. In addition to delivering water, nebulizers are used to deliver medications to peripheral airways and radioactive isotopes in diagnostic lung ventilation imaging.

There are three types: gas driven, spinning disc and ultrasonic.

GAS-DRIVEN (JET) NEBULIZER

Components

1. A capillary tube with the bottom end immersed in a water container.
2. The top end of the capillary tube is close to a Venturi constriction (Fig. 9.7).

Mechanism of action

1. A high-pressure gas flows through the Venturi, creating a negative pressure.
2. Water is drawn up through the capillary tube and broken into a fine spray. Even smaller droplets can be achieved as the spray hits an anvil or a baffle.
3. The majority of the droplets are in the range of 2–4 μm. These droplets tend to deposit on the pharynx and upper airway with a small amount reaching the bronchial level. This nebulizer is also capable of producing larger droplets of up to 20 μm in size. Droplets with diameters of 5 μm or more fall back into the container leaving droplets of 4 μm or less to float out with the fresh gas flow.
4. The device is compact, making it easy to place close to the patient.

SPINNING DISC NEBULIZER

This is a motor-driven spinning disc throwing out microdroplets of water by centrifugal force. The water impinges onto the disc after being drawn from a reservoir via a tube over which the disc is mounted.

ULTRASONIC NEBULIZER

A transducer head vibrates at an ultrasonic frequency (e.g. 3 MHz). The transducer can be immersed into water or water can be dropped on to it, producing droplets less than 1–2 μm in size. Droplets of 1 μm or less are deposited in alveoli and lower airways. This is a highly efficient method of humidifying and also delivering drugs to the airway. There is a risk of overhydration especially in children.

Bacterial and viral filters

These minimize the risk of cross-transmission of bacteria and/or viruses between patients using the same anaesthetic breathing systems. The British Standard defines them as 'devices intended to reduce transmission of particulates, including micro-organisms, in breathing systems'. It is thought that the incidence of bleeding after orotracheal intubation is 86%. The filter should be positioned as close to the patient as possible, e.g. on the disposable catheter mount, to protect the rest of the breathing system, ventilator and anaesthetic machine. It is recommended that a new filter should be used for each patient. A humidification element can be added producing a heat and moisture exchanging filter (HMEF) (see Fig. 9.1).

Characteristics of the ideal filter

1. Efficient: the filter should be effective against both air- and liquid-borne micro-organisms. A filtration action of 99.99–99.999% should be achieved. This allows between 100 and 10 micro-organisms to pass through the filter, respectively, after a 10^6 micro-organism challenge. The filter should be effective bidirectionally.

2. Minimal dead space, particularly for paediatric practice.
3. Minimum resistance, especially when wet.
4. Not affected by anaesthetic agents and does not affect the anaesthetic agents.
5. Effective when either wet or dry. It should completely prevent the passage of contaminated body liquids (blood, saliva and other liquids) which may be present or generated in the breathing system.
6. User friendly, lightweight, not bulky and non-traumatic to the patient.
7. Disposable.
8. Provides some humidification if no other methods being used. Adequate humidification can usually be achieved by the addition of a hygroscopic element to the device.
9. Transparent.
10. Cost effective.

Size of micro-organisms

Hepatitis virus	0.02 μm
Adenovirus	0.07 μm
HIV	0.08 μm
Mycobacterium tuberculosis	0.3 μm
Staphylococcus aureus	1.0 μm
Cytomegalovirus	0.1 μm

Components

1. Two ports designed to accept 15- and 22-mm size tubings and connections.
2. A sampling port to measure the gases'/agents' concentrations positioned on the anaesthetic breathing system side.
3. The filtration element can either be a felt-like electrostatic material or a pleated hydrophobic material.

Mechanism of action

There are five main mechanisms by which filtration can be achieved on a fibre:

1. *Direct interception*: large particles (=1 μm), such as dust and large bacteria, are physically prevented from passing through the pores of the filter because of their large size.
2. *Inertial impaction*: smaller particles (0.5–1 μm) collide with the filter medium because of their inertia. They tend to continue in straight lines, carried along by their own momentum rather than following the path of least resistance taken by the gas. The particles are held by Van der Waal's electrostatic forces.
3. *Diffusional interception*: very small particles (<0.5 μm), such as viruses, are captured because they undergo considerable Brownian motion (i.e. random movement) because of their very small mass. This movement increases their apparent diameter so that they are more likely to be captured by the filter element.
4. *Electrostatic attraction*: this can be very important but it is difficult to measure as it requires knowing the charge on the particles and on the fibres. Increasing the charge on either the particles or the fibres increases the filtration efficiency. Charged particles are attracted to oppositely charged fibres by coulombic attraction.
5. *Gravitational settling*: this affects large particles (>5 μm). The rate of settling depends on the balance between the effect of gravity on the particle and the buoyancy of the particle. In filters used in anaesthesia, it has minimal effect as most of the settling occurs before the particles reach the filter.

ELECTROSTATIC FILTERS (FIG. 9.8)

1. The element used is subjected to an electric field producing a felt-like material with high polarity. One type of fibre becomes positively charged and the other type negatively charged. Usually two polymer fibres (modacrylic and polyprolyne) are used.
2. A flat layer of filter material can be used as the resistance to gas flow is lower per unit area.
3. These filters rely on the electrical charge to attract oppositely charged particles from the gas flow. They have a filtration efficiency of 99.99%.
4. The electrical charge increases the efficiency of the filter when the element is dry but can deteriorate rapidly when it is wet. The resistance to flow increases when the element is wet.
5. The electrical charge on the filter fibres decays with time so it has a limited life.
6. A hygroscopic layer can be added to the filter in order to provide humidification. In such an HMEF, the pressure drop across the element and thus the resistance to breathing will also increase with gradual absorption of water.

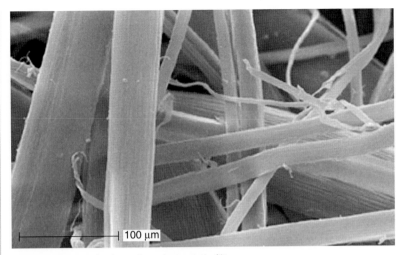

Fig. 9.8 Microscopic view of an electrostatic filter.

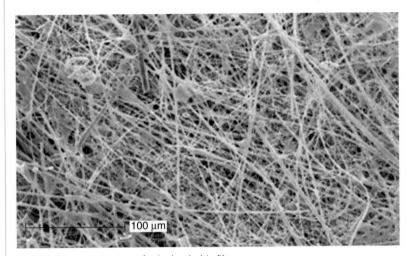

Fig. 9.9 Microscopic view of a hydrophobic filter.

PLEATED HYDROPHOBIC FILTERS (FIG. 9.9)

1. The very small pore size filter membrane provides adequate filtration over longer periods of time. These filters rely on the naturally occurring electrostatic interactions to remove the particles. A filtration efficiency of 99.999% can be achieved.
2. To achieve minimal pressure drop across the device with such a small pore size, so allowing high gas flows while retaining low resistance, a large surface area is required. Pleated paper filters made of inorganic fibres are used to achieve this.
3. The forces between individual liquid water molecules are stronger than those between the water molecules and the hydrophobic membrane. This leads to the collection of water on the surface of the membrane with no absorption. Such a filter can successfully prevent the passage of water under pressures as high as 60 cm H_2O.
4. Although hydrophobic filters provide some humidification, a hygroscopic element can be added to improve humidification.
5. Currently there is no evidence showing any type of filter is clinically superior to another.

Bacterial and viral filters

- Can achieve a filtration efficiency of 99.99–99.999%.
- Electrostatic filters rely on an electrical charge to attract oppositely charged particles. Their efficiency is reduced when wet and they have a limited lifespan.
- Hydrophobic pleated filters can repel water even under high pressures. They have a longer life span.

Further reading

Medical Devices Agency, 1998. Heat and moisture exchangers (HMEs) including those intended for use as breathing system filters. UK Market-Product review. Medical Devices Agency, London, No. 347.

MHRA, 2004. Medical advice alert (MDA/2004/013). Online. Available at: http://www.mhra.gov.uk/home/groups/dts-bs/documents/medicaldevicealert/con008574.pdf.

MHRA, 2004. Medical device alert (MDA/2004/037). Online. Available at: http://www.mhra.gov.uk/home/groups/dts-bs/documents/medicaldevicealert/con008522.pdf.

Turnbull, D., Fisher, P.C., Mills, G.H., et al., 2005. Performance of breathing filters under wet conditions: a laboratory evaluation. British Journal of Anaesthesia 94, 675–682.

Wilkes, A.R., 2002. Breathing system filters. British Journal of Anaesthesia CEPD Reviews 2, 151–154.

Wilkes, A.R., Malan, C.A., Hall, J.E., 2008. The effect of flow on the filtration performance of paediatric breathing system filters. Anaesthesia 63, 71–76.

MCQs

In the following lists, which of the statements (a) to (e) are true?

1. Nebulizers:
   a) The gas-driven nebulizer can deliver much smaller droplets than the ultrasonic nebulizer.
   b) There is a risk of drowning.
   c) The temperature of the gas determines the amount of water delivered.
   d) The smaller the droplets are, the more stable they are.
   e) Droplets of 1 μm or less are deposited in the alveoli and lower airways.

2. Humidity:
   a) Humidity is measured using a hair hygrometer.
   b) Air fully saturated with water vapour has a relative humidity of about 44 mg/L at 37°C.
   c) Using the circle breathing system, some humidification can be achieved despite using dry fresh gas flow.
   d) Relative humidity is the ratio of the mass of water vapour in a given volume of air to the mass of water vapour required to saturate the same volume at the same temperature.
   e) The ideal relative humidity in the operating theatre is about 45–55%.

3. Bacterial and viral filters:
   a) Particles of less than 0.5 μm can be captured by direct interception.
   b) They can achieve a filtration action of 99.999%.
   c) They should be effective when either wet or dry.
   d) The filtration element used can be either an electrostatic or a pleated hydrophobic material.
   e) The hydrophobic filter has a more limited lifespan than the electrostatic filter.

4. Hot water bath humidifiers:
   a) Heating the water improves the performance.
   b) Because of its efficiency, the surface area for vaporization does not have to be large.
   c) There is a risk of scalding to the patient.
   d) Temperature in the humidifier is usually kept below body temperature.
   e) The temperature of water in the container is controlled by a feedback mechanism using a thermistor which measures the temperature of the gases at the patient's end.

5. Heat exchange humidifiers:
   a) Inspired gases are warmed to 29–34°C.
   b) Performance is improved by increasing the volume of the medium.
   c) An absolute humidity of 60–70% can be achieved.
   d) At high flows, the performance is reduced.
   e) Performance is affected by the temperature of the inspired and exhaled gases.

6. Which of the following statements are true:
   a) Mucus can cause obstruction of the heat and moisture exchanger (HME).
   b) 2–5-μm-sized nebulized droplets are deposited in the alveoli.
   c) HMEs should deliver a minimum of 300 g water vapour at 30°C.
   d) A relative humidity of 80% at the carina can be achieved during normal breathing.
   e) HME requires some time before it reaches its optimal ability to humidify dry gases.

Answers

1. Nebulizers:

   a) *False. The ultrasonic nebulizer can deliver very much smaller droplets. 2–4-μm droplets can be delivered by the gas-driven nebulizer. Droplets of less than 1–2 μm in size can be delivered by the ultrasonic nebulizer.*

   b) *True. This is especially so in children using the ultrasonic nebulizer.*

   c) *False. The temperature of the gas has no effect on the quantity of water droplets delivered. The temperature of the gas is of more importance in the humidifier.*

   d) *True. Very small droplets generated by the ultrasonic nebulizer are very stable and can be deposited in the alveoli and lower airways.*

   e) *True. See d).*

2. Humidity:

   a) *True. The hair hygrometer is used to measure relative humidity between 15% and 85%. It is commonly used in the operating theatre. The length of the hair increases with the increase in ambient humidity. This causes a pointer to move over a chart measuring the relative humidity.*

   b) *False. It should be absolute humidity and not relative humidity. Relative humidity is measured as a percentage.*

   c) *True. Water is produced as a product of the reaction between CO_2 and NaOH. An absolute humidity of 29 mg/L at 37°C can be achieved.*

   d) *True.*

   e) *True. A high relative humidity is uncomfortable for the staff in the operating theatre. Too low a relative humidity can lead to the build up of static electricity increasing the risk of ignition.*

3. Bacterial and viral filters:

   a) *False. Such small particles are captured by diffusional interception. Direct interception can capture particles with sizes equal to or more than 1 μm.*

   b) *True. Hydrophobic filters can achieve a filtration action of 99.999%. Electrostatic filters can achieve 99.99% which is thought to be adequate for routine use during anaesthesia.*

   c) *True. Hydrophobic filters are effective both when dry and wet. Electrostatic filters become less effective when wet.*

   d) *True.*

   e) *False. The electrostatic filter has a more limited lifespan than the hydrophobic filter. The efficacy of the electrostatic filter decreases as the electrical charge on the filter fibres decays.*

4. Hot water bath humidifiers:

   a) *True. This is due to the loss of latent heat of vaporization as more water changes into vapour. The lower the water temperature, the less vapour is produced.*

   b) *False. A large surface area is needed to improve efficiency.*

   c) *True. A faulty thermostat can cause overheating of the water. There is usually a second thermostat to prevent this.*

   d) *False. The temperature of the humidifier is usually kept above body temperature. A large amount of heat is lost as the vapour and gases pass through the plastic tubings.*

   e) *True.*

5. Heat exchange humidifiers:

   a) *True.*

   b) *True. The larger the volume of the medium, the better the performance of the HME. This is because of the larger surface area of contact between the gas and the medium.*

   c) *False. A relative, not absolute, humidity of 60–70% can be achieved.*

   d) *True. At high flows, the time the gas is in contact with the medium is reduced so decreasing the performance of the HME. The opposite is also correct.*

   e) *True. The higher the temperature of the gases, the better the performance of the HME.*

6. Which of the following statements are true:

   a) *True. Mucus can cause obstruction of the HME resulting in dangerous increases in resistance.*

   b) *False. 2–5-μm nebulized droplets are deposited in the tracheobronchial tree. Smaller droplets of 0.5–1 μm are deposited in the alveoli.*

   c) *False. HME should deliver a minimum of 30 g water vapour at 30°C.*

   d) *True.*

   e) *True. HME requires 5–20 min before it reaches its optimal ability to humidify dry gases.*

Chapter 10

Non-invasive monitoring

Clinical observation provides vital information regarding the patient. Observations gained from the use of the various monitors should augment that information; skin perfusion, capillary refill, cyanosis, pallor, skin temperature and turgor, chest movement and heart auscultation are just a few examples. The equipment used to monitor the patient is becoming more sophisticated. It is vital that the clinician using these monitors is aware of their limitations and the potential causes of error. Errors can be due to patient, equipment and/or sampling factors.

Monitoring equipment can be invasive or non-invasive. The latter is discussed in this chapter, whereas the former is discussed in Chapter 11.

Integrated monitoring

Until recently, it was common to see the anaesthetic machine adorned with discrete, bulky monitoring devices. Significant advances in information technology have allowed an integrated monitoring approach to occur. Plug-in monitoring modules feed a single visual display on which selected values and waveforms can be arranged and colour-coded (Figs 10.1–10.3).

Although some would argue that such monitoring systems are complex and potentially confusing, their benefits in term of flexibility and ergonomics are undisputed.

More recently, wireless monitoring systems are becoming available. An example is wireless invasive pressure monitoring systems (Fig. 10.4). This reduces the clutter of cables surrounding the patients.

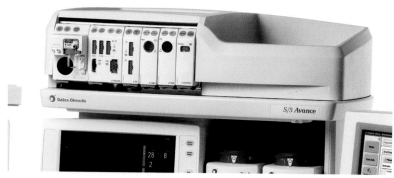

Fig. 10.1 Datex-Ohmeda plug-in monitoring modules mounted on the S/5 Advance anaesthetic machine.

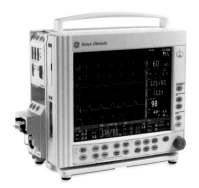

Fig. 10.2 Datex-Ohmeda compact monitor.

Electrocardiogram (ECG)

This monitors the electrical activity of the heart with electrical potentials of 0.5–2 mV at the skin surface. It is useful in determining the heart rate, ischaemia, the presence of arrhythmias and conduction defects. It should be emphasized that it gives no assessment of cardiac output.

The bipolar leads (I, II, III, AVR, AVL and AVF) measure voltage difference between two electrodes. The unipolar leads (V1–6) measure voltage at different electrodes relative to a zero point.

Components

1. Skin electrodes detect the electrical activity of the heart (Fig. 10.5). Silver and silver chloride form a stable electrode combination. Both are held in a cup and separated from the skin by a foam pad soaked in conducting gel.
2. Colour-coded cables to transmit the signal from electrodes to the monitor. Cables are available in 3- and 5-lead versions as snap or grabber design and with a variety of lengths. All the cables of a particular set should have the same length to minimize the effect of electromagnetic interference.
3. The ECG signal is then boosted using an amplifier. The amplifier covers a frequency range of 0.05–150 Hz. It also filters out some of the frequencies considered to be noise. The amplifier has ECG filters that are used to remove the noise/artifacts from ECG and produce a 'clean' signal.
4. An oscilloscope that displays the amplified ECG signal. A high-resolution monochrome or colour monitor is used.

Mechanism of action

1. Proper attachment of ECG electrodes involves cleaning the skin, gently abrading the stratum corneum and ensuring adequate contact using conductive gel. Skin impedance varies at

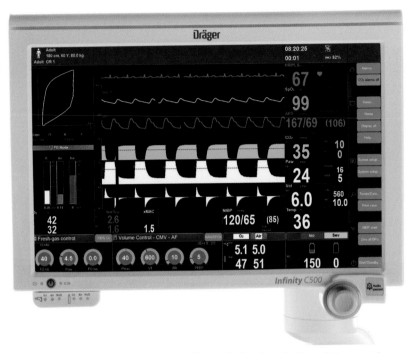

Fig. 10.3 Colour-coded values and waveforms displayed on the Zeus Dräger monitor. (Courtesy of Dräger.)

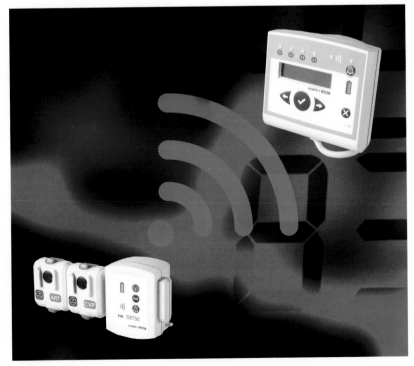

Fig. 10.4 Smiths Medical wireless invasive pressure monitoring system.

different sites and it is thought to be higher in females. The electrodes are best positioned on bony prominences to reduce artifacts from respiration.

2. Modern ECG monitors use multiple filters for signal processing. The filters used should be capable of removing the unwanted frequencies, leaving the signal intact (Fig. 10.6). Two types of filters are used for this purpose:

a) *high-pass filters* attenuate the frequency components of a signal below a certain frequency. They help to remove lower frequency noise from the signal. For example, the respiratory component from ECG can be removed by turning on a 1-Hz high pass filter on the amplifier. The filter will centre the signal around the zero isoline

b) *low-pass filters* attenuate the frequency components of a signal above a certain frequency. They are useful for removing noise from lower frequency signals. So an amplifier with a 35-Hz low-pass filter will remove/ attenuate signals above 35 Hz and help to 'clean' the ECG signal.

3. The ECG monitor can have two modes:

a) the *monitoring mode* has a limited frequency response of 0.5–50 Hz. Filters are used to narrow the bandwidth to reduce environmental artifacts. The high-frequency filters reduce distortions from muscle movement, mains current and electromagnetic interference from other equipment. The low-frequency filters help provide a stable baseline by reducing respiratory and body movement artifacts

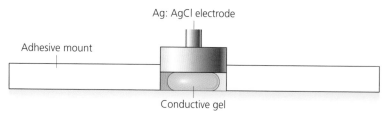

Fig. 10.5 An ECG electrode.

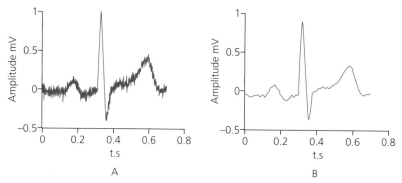

Fig.10.6 ECG filters. (A) Unfiltered signal with noise. (B) Filtered 'clean' signal.

b) the *diagnostic mode* has a wider frequency response of 0.05–150 Hz. The high-frequency limit allows the assessment of the ST segment, QRS morphology and tachyarrhythmias. The low-frequency limit allows representation of P- and T-wave morphology and ST-segment analysis.

4. There are many ECG electrode configurations. Usually during anaesthesia, three skin electrodes are used (right arm, left arm and indifferent leads). The three limb leads used include two that are 'active' and one that is 'inactive' (earth). Sometimes five electrodes are used. Lead II is ideal for detecting arrythmias. CM5 configuration is able to detect 89% of ST-segment changes due to left ventricular ischaemia. In CM5, the right arm electrode is positioned on the manubrium (chest lead from manubrium), the left arm electrode is on V5 position (fifth interspace in the

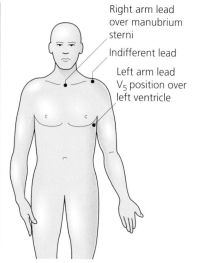

Fig. 10.7 The CM5 ECG lead configuration.

left anterior axillary line) and the indifferent lead is on the left shoulder or any convenient position (Fig. 10.7).

5. The CB5 configuration is useful during thoracic anaesthesia. The right arm electrode is positioned

over the centre of the right scapula and the left arm electrode is over V5.

6. A display speed of 25 mm/s and a sensitivity of 1 mV/cm are standard in the UK.

Problems in practice and safety features

1. Incorrect placement of the ECG electrodes in relation to the heart is a common error, leading to false information.

2. Electrical interference can be a 50-Hz (in UK) mains line interference because of capacitance or inductive coupling effect. Any electrical device powered by AC can act as one plate of a capacitor and the patient acts as the other plate. Interference can also be because of high-frequency current interference from diathermy. Most modern monitors have the facilities to avoid interference. Shielding of cables and leads, differential amplifiers and electronic filters all help to produce an interference-free monitoring system. Differential amplifiers measure the difference between the potential from two different sources. If there is interference common to the two input terminals (e.g. mains frequency), it can be eliminated as only the differences between the two terminals is amplified. This is called *common mode rejection ratio* (CMRR). Amplifiers used in ECG monitoring should have a high CMRR of 100 000 : 1 to 1 000 000 : 1, which is a measurement of capability to reject the noise. They should also have a high input impedance (about 10 MΩ) to minimize the current taken from the electrodes. Table 10.1 shows the various types and sources of interference and how to reduce the interference.

Table 10.1 ECG signal interference

Type of interference	Sources of interference	How to reduce interference
Electromagnetic induction	Any electrical cable or light	Use long ECG and twisted leads (rejecting the induced signal as common mode) Use selective filters in amplifiers
Electrostatic induction and capacitance coupling	Stray capacitances between table, lights, monitors, patients and electrical cables	ECG leads are surrounded by copper screens
Radiofrequency interference (>150 Hz)	Diathermy enters the system by: • mains supply • direct application by probe • radio transmission via probe and wire	High-frequency filters clean up signal before entering input Filtering power supply of amplifiers Double screen electronic components of amplifiers and earth outer screen Newer machines operate at higher frequencies

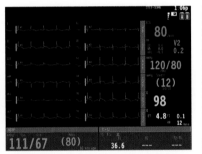

Fig. 10.8 12-lead ECG and ST-segment monitoring.

3. Muscular activity, such as shivering, can produce artifacts. Positioning the electrodes over bony prominences and the use of low-pass filters can reduce these artifacts.
4. High and low ventricular rate alarms and an audible indicator of ventricular rate are standard on most designs. More advanced monitors have the facility to monitor the ST segment (Fig. 10.8). Continuous monitoring and measurement of the height of the ST segment allows early diagnosis of ischaemic changes.

5. Absence of or improperly positioned patient diathermy plate can cause burns at the site of ECG skin electrodes. This is because of the passage of the diathermy current via the electrodes causing a relatively high current density.

ECG

- Silver and silver chloride skin electrodes detect the electrical activity of the heart, 0.5–2 mV at the skin surface.
- The signal is boosted by an amplifier and displayed by an oscilloscope.
- The ECG monitor can have two modes, the monitoring mode (frequency range 0.5–40 Hz) and the diagnostic mode (frequency range 0.05–150 Hz).
- CM5 configuration is used to monitor left ventricular ischaemia.
- Electrical interference can be due either to diathermy or mains frequency.
- Differential amplifiers are used to reduce interference (common mode rejection).

Arterial blood pressure

Oscillometry is the commonest method used to measure blood pressure non-invasively during anaesthesia. The systolic, diastolic and mean arterial pressures and pulse rate are measured, calculated and displayed. These devices give reliable trend information about the blood pressure. They are less reliable in circumstances where a sudden change in blood pressure is anticipated, or where a minimal change in blood pressure is clinically relevant. The term 'device for indirect non-invasive automatic mean arterial pressure' (DINAMAP) is used for such devices.

Components

1. A cuff with a tube used for inflation and deflation. Some designs have an extra tube for transmitting pressure fluctuations to the pressure transducer.
2. The case where the microprocessor, pressure transducer and a solenoid valve which controls the deflation of the arm cuff are housed. It contains the display and a timing mechanism which adjusts the frequency of measurements. Alarm limits can be set for both high and low values.

Mechanism of action

1. The microprocessor is set to control the sequence of inflation and deflation.
2. The cuff is inflated to a pressure above the previous systolic pressure, then it is deflated incrementally. The return of blood flow causes oscillation in cuff pressure (Fig. 10.9).
3. The transducer senses the pressure changes which

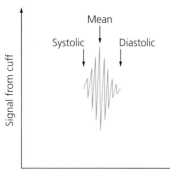

Fig. 10.9 Diagram showing how oscillations in cuff pressure correspond to mean, systolic and diastolic pressures.

are interpreted by the microprocessor. This transducer has an accuracy of ±2%.

4. The output signal from the transducer passes through a filter to an amplifier that amplifies the oscillations. The output from the amplifier passes to the microprocessor through the analogue digital converter (ADC). The microprocessor controls the pneumatic pump for inflation of the cuff and the solenoid valve for deflation of the cuff.

5. The mean arterial blood pressure corresponds to the maximum oscillation at the lowest cuff pressure. The systolic pressure corresponds to the onset of rapidly increasing oscillations.

6. The diastolic pressure corresponds to the onset of rapidly decreasing oscillations. In addition, it is mathematically computed from the systolic and mean pressure values (mean blood pressure = diastolic blood pressure + 1/3 pulse pressure).

7. The cuff must be of the correct size (Table 10.2). It should cover at least two-thirds of the upper arm. The width of the cuff's bladder should be 40% of the mid-circumference of the limb. The middle of the cuff's bladder should be positioned over the brachial artery.

Table 10.2 A guide to the correct blood pressure cuff size

3 cm	Infant
5 cm	Infant
6 cm	Child
9 cm	Small adult
12 cm	Standard adult
15 cm	Large adult

8. Some designs have the ability to apply venous stasis to facilitate intravenous cannulation.

Problems in practice and safety features

1. For the device to measure the arterial blood pressure accurately, it should have a fast cuff inflation and a slow cuff deflation (at a rate of 3 mmHg/s or 2 mmHg/beat). The former is to avoid venous congestion and the latter provides enough time to detect the arterial pulsation.

2. If the cuff is too small, the blood pressure is over-read, while it is under-read if the cuff is too large. The error is greater with too small than too large a cuff.

3. The systolic pressure is over-read at low pressures (systolic pressure less than 60 mmHg) and under-read at high systolic pressures.

4. Atrial fibrillation and other arrhythmias affect performance.

5. External pressure on the cuff or its tubing can cause inaccuracies.

6. Frequently repeated cuff inflations can cause ulnar nerve palsy and petechial haemorrhage of the skin under the cuff.

The Finapres (**fin**ger arterial **pres**sure) device uses a combination of oscillometry and a servo control unit. The volume of blood in the finger varies with the cardiac cycle. A small cuff placed around the finger is used to keep the blood volume of the finger constant. An infrared photo-plethysmograph detects changes in the volume of blood within the finger with each cardiac cycle. A controller system alters the pressure in the cuff accordingly, to keep the volume of blood in the finger constant. The applied pressure waveform correlates with the arterial blood volume and, therefore, with the arterial blood pressure. This applied pressure is then displayed continuously, in real time, as the arterial blood pressure waveform.

THE VON RECKLINGHAUSEN OSCILLOTONOMETER

During the premicroprocessor era, the *Von Recklinghausen Oscillotonometer* was widely used (Fig. 10.10).

Components

1. Two cuffs: the upper, occluding cuff (5 cm wide) overlaps a lower, sensing cuff (10 cm wide). An inflation bulb is attached.

2. The case which contains:
   a) two bellows, one connected to the atmosphere, the other connected to the lower sensing cuff
   b) a mechanical amplification system
   c) the oscillating needle and dial
   d) the control lever
   e) the release valve.

Mechanism of action

1. With the control lever at rest, air is pumped into both cuffs and the air-tight case of the instrument using the inflation bulb to a pressure exceeding systolic arterial pressure. By operating the control lever, the

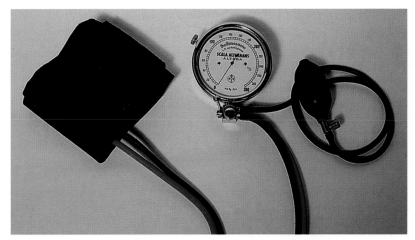

Fig. 10.10 The Von Recklinghausen oscillotonometer.

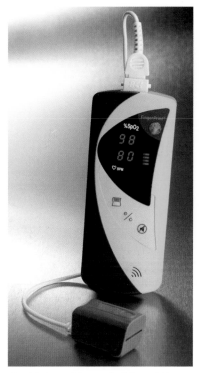

Fig. 10.11 Smiths Medical FingerPrint oximeter.

lower sensing cuff is isolated and the pressure in the upper cuff and instrument case is allowed to decrease slowly through an adjustable leak controlled by the release valve. As systolic pressure is reached, pulsation of the artery under the lower cuff results in pressure oscillations within the cuff and its bellows. The pressure oscillations are transmitted via a mechanical amplification system to the needle. As the pressure in the upper cuff decreases below diastolic pressure, the pulsation ceases.

2. The mean pressure is at the point of maximum oscillation.
3. This method is reliable at low pressures. It is useful to measure trends in blood pressure.

Problems in practice and safety features

1. In order for the device to operate accurately, the cuffs must be correctly positioned and attached to their respective tubes.
2. The diastolic pressure is not measured accurately with this device.

> **Arterial blood pressure**
> - Oscillometry is the method used.
> - Mean arterial pressure corresponds to maximum oscillation.
> - A cuff with a tube(s) is connected to a transducer and a microprocessor.
> - Accurate within the normal range of blood pressure.
> - Arrhythmias and external pressure affect the performance.

Pulse oximetry

This is a non-invasive measurement of the arterial blood oxygen saturation at the level of the arterioles. A continuous display of the oxygenation is achieved by a simple, accurate and rapid method (Fig. 10.11).

Pulse oximetry has proved to be a powerful monitoring tool in the operating theatre, recovery wards, intensive care units, general wards and during the transport of critically ill patients. It is considered to be the greatest technical advance in monitoring of the last decade. It

enables the detection of incipient and unsuspected arterial hypoxaemia, allowing treatment before tissue damage.

Components

1. A probe is positioned on the finger, toe, ear lobe or nose (Fig. 10.12). Two light-emitting diodes (LEDs) produce beams at red and infrared frequencies (660 nm and 940 nm respectively) on one side and there is a sensitive photodetector on the other side. The LEDs operate in sequence at a rate of about 30 times per second (Fig. 10.13).
2. The case houses the microprocessor. There is a display of the oxygen saturation, pulse rate and a plethysmographic waveform of the pulse. Alarm limits can be set for a low saturation value and for both high and low pulse rates.

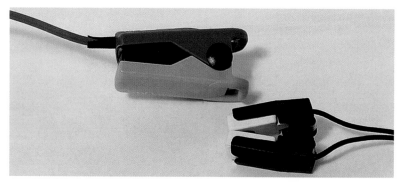

Fig. 10.12 Pulse oximeter probes. Finger probe (top) and ear probe (bottom).

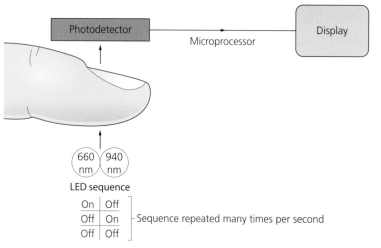

Fig. 10.13 Working principles of the pulse oximeter. The LEDs operate in sequence and when both are off the photodetector measures the background level of ambient light.

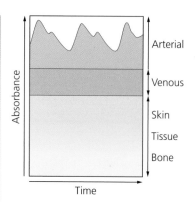

Fig. 10.14 Schematic representation of the contribution of various body components to the absorbance of light.

Mechanism of action

1. The oxygen saturation is estimated by measuring the transmission of light, through a pulsatile vascular tissue bed (e.g. finger). This is based on Beer's law (the relation between the light absorbed and the concentration of solute in the solution) and Lambert's law (relation between absorption of light and the thickness of the absorbing layer).

2. The amount of light transmitted depends on many factors. The light absorbed by non-pulsatile tissues (e.g. skin, soft tissues, bone and venous blood) is constant (DC). The non-constant absorption (AC) is the result of arterial blood pulsations (Fig. 10.14). The sensitive photodetector generates a voltage proportional to the transmitted light. The AC component of the wave is about 1–5% of the total signal.

3. The high frequency of the LEDs allows the absorption to be sampled many times during each pulse beat. This is used to enable running averages of saturation to be calculated many times per second. This decreases the 'noise' (e.g. movement) effect on the signal.

4. The microprocessor is programmed to mathematically analyse both the DC and AC components at 660 and 940 nm calculating the ratio of absorption at these two frequencies (R/IR ratio). The result is related to the arterial saturation. The absorption of oxyhaemoglobin and deoxyhaemoglobin at these two wavelengths is very different. This allows these two wavelengths to provide good sensitivity. 805 nm is one of the isobestic points of oxyhaemoglobin and deoxyhaemoglobin. The OFF part allows a baseline measurement for any changes in ambient light.

5. A more recent design uses multiple wavelengths to eradicate false readings from carboxy haemoglobin and methaemoglobinaemia. Advanced oximeters use more than seven light wavelengths. This has enabled the measurement of haemoglobin value, oxygen content, carboxyhaemoglobin and methaemoglobin concentrations.

6. A variable pitch beep provides an audible signal of changes in saturation.

Problems in practice and safety features

1. It is accurate ($\pm2\%$) in the 70–100% range. Below the saturation of 70%, readings are extrapolated.
2. The absolute measurement of oxygen saturation may vary from one probe to another but with accurate trends. This is due to the variability of the centre wavelength of the LEDs.
3. Carbon monoxide poisoning (including smoking), coloured nail varnish, intravenous injections of certain dyes (e.g. methylene blue, indocyanine green) and drugs responsible for the production of methaemoglobinaemia are all sources of error (Table 10.3).
4. Hypoperfusion and severe peripheral vasoconstriction affect the performance of the pulse oximeter. This is because the AC signal sensed is about 1–5% of the DC signal when the pulse volume is normal. This makes it less accurate during vasoconstriction when the AC component is reduced.
5. The device monitors the oxygen saturation with no direct information regarding oxygen delivery to the tissues.
6. Pulse oximeters average their readings every 10–20 s. They cannot detect acute desaturation. The response time to desaturation is longer with the finger probe (more than 60 s) whereas the ear probe has a response time of 10–15 s.
7. Excessive movement or malposition of the probe is a source of error. Newer designs such as the Masimo oximeter claim more stability despite motion. External fluorescent light can be a source of interference.
8. Inaccurate measurement can be caused by venous pulsation. This can be because of high airway pressures, the Valsalva manoeuvre or other consequences of impaired venous return. Pulse oximeters assume that any pulsatile absorption is caused by arterial blood pulsation only.
9. The site of the application should be checked at regular intervals as the probe can cause pressure sores with continuous use. Some manufacturers recommend changing the site of application every 2 h especially in patients with impaired microcirculation. Burns in infants have been reported.
10. Pulse oximetry only gives information about a patient's oxygenation. It does not give any indication of a patient's ability to eliminate carbon dioxide.

Table 10.3 Sources of error in pulse oximetry

HbF	No significant clinical change (absorption spectrum is similar to the adult Hb over the range of wavelengths used)
MetHb	False low reading
CoHb	False high reading
SulphHb	Not a clinical problem
Bilirubin	Not a clinical problem
Dark skin	No effect
Methylene blue	False low reading
Indocyanine green	False low reading
Nail varnish	May cause false low reading

Pulse oximetry
- Consists of a probe with two LEDs and a photodetector.
- A microprocessor analyses the signal.
- Accurate within the clinical range.
- Inaccurate readings in carbon monoxide poisoning, the presence of dyes and methaemoglobinaemia.
- Hypoperfusion and severe vasoconstriction affect the reading.

End-tidal carbon dioxide analysers (capnographs)

Gases with molecules that contain at least two dissimilar atoms absorb radiation in the infrared region of the spectrum. Using this property, both inspired and exhaled carbon dioxide concentration can be measured directly and continuously throughout the respiratory cycle (Fig. 10.15).

Technical terms used in measuring end-tidal CO_2
1. *Capnograph* is the device that records and shows the graphical display of waveform of CO_2 (measured in kPa or mmHg). It displays the value of CO_2 at the end of expiration, which is known as end-tidal CO_2.
2. *Capnogram* is the graphical plot of CO_2 partial pressure (or percentage) versus time.
3. *Capnometer* is the device which only shows numerical concentration of CO_2 without a waveform.

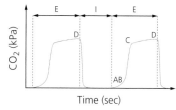

Fig. 10.15 Diagram of an end-tidal carbon dioxide waveform. I = inspiration; E = expiration; A–B represents the emptying of the upper dead space of the airways. As this has not undergone gas exchange, the CO_2 concentration is zero. B–C represents the gas mixture from the upper airways and the CO_2-rich alveolar gas. The CO_2 concentration rises continuously. C–D represents the alveolar gas and is described as the 'alveolar plateau'. The curve rises very slowly. D is the end-tidal CO_2 partial pressure where the highest possible concentration of exhaled CO_2 is achieved at the end of expiration. It represents the final portion of gas which was involved in the gas exchange in the alveoli. Under certain conditions (see text) it represents a reliable index of the arterial CO_2 partial pressure. D–A represents inspiration where the fresh gas contains no CO_2.

The end-tidal CO_2 is less than alveolar CO_2 because the end-tidal CO_2 is always diluted with alveolar dead space gas from unperfused alveoli. These alveoli do not take part in gas exchange and so contain no CO_2. Alveolar CO_2 is less than arterial CO_2 as the blood from unventilated alveoli and lung parenchyma (both have higher CO_2 contents) mixes with the blood from ventilated alveoli. In healthy adults with normal lungs, end-tidal CO_2 is 0.3–0.6 kPa less than arterial CO_2. This difference is reduced if the lungs are ventilated with large tidal volumes. The Greek root kapnos, meaning 'smoke', give us the term capnography (CO_2 can be thought as the 'smoke' of cellular metabolism).

$$End\text{-}tidal\ CO_2 < alveolar\ CO_2 < PaCO_2$$

In reality, the devices used cannot determine the different phases of respiration but simply report the minimum and maximum CO_2

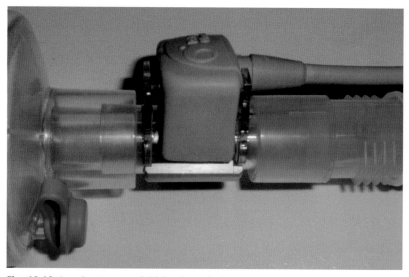

Fig. 10.16 A main-stream end-tidal carbon dioxide analyser.

concentrations during each respiratory cycle.

Components

1. The sampling chamber can either be positioned within the patient's gas stream (main-stream version, Fig. 10.16) or connected to the distal end of the breathing system via a sampling tube (side-stream version, Fig. 10.17).
2. A photodetector measures light reaching it from a light source at the correct infrared wavelength (using optical filters) after passing through two chambers. One acts as a reference whereas the other one is the sampling chamber (Fig. 10.18).

Mechanism of action

1. Carbon dioxide absorbs the infrared radiation particularly at a wavelength of 4.3 μm.
2. The amount of infrared radiation absorbed is proportional to the number of carbon dioxide molecules (partial pressure of carbon dioxide) present in the chamber.
3. The remaining infrared radiation falls on the thermopile detector,

which in turn produces heat. The heat is measured by a temperature sensor and is proportional to the partial pressure of carbon dioxide gas present in the mixture in the sample chamber. This produces an electrical output. This means that the amount of gas present is inversely proportional to the amount of infrared light present at the detector in the sample chamber (Fig 10.19).
4. In the same way, a beam of light passes through the reference chamber which contains room air. The absorption detected from the sample chamber is compared to that in the reference chamber. This allows the calculation of carbon dioxide values.
5. The inspired and exhaled carbon dioxide forms a square wave, with a zero baseline unless there is rebreathing (Fig. 10.20A).
6. A microprocessor-controlled infrared lamp is used. This produces a stable infrared source with a constant output. The current is measured with a current-sensing resistor, the voltage across which is proportional to the current flowing through it. The

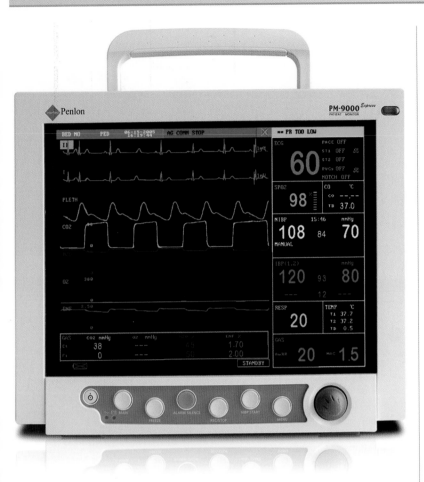

Fig. 10.17 The Penlon PM9000 Express which measures end-tidal CO_2, oximetry and inhalational agent concentration using a side-stream method. (Courtesy of Penlon Ltd, Abingdon, UK (www.penlon.com).)

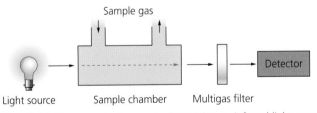

Fig. 10.18 Components of a gas analyser using an infrared light source suitable for end-tidal carbon dioxide measurement. The reference chamber has been omitted for the sake of clarity.

known concentrations of CO_2 to ensure accurate measurement.

Photo-acoustic spectroscopy: in these infrared absorption devices, the sample gas is irradiated with pulsatile infrared radiation of a suitable wavelength. The periodic expansion and contraction produces a pressure fluctuation of audible frequency that can be detected by a microphone.

The advantages of photo-acoustic spectrometry over conventional infrared absorption spectrometry are:

1. The photo-acoustic technique is extremely stable and its calibration remains constant over much longer periods of time.
2. The very fast rise and fall times give a much more accurate representation of any change in CO_2 concentration.

Carbon dioxide analysers can be either side-stream or main-stream analysers.

SIDE-STREAM ANALYSERS

1. This consists of a 1.2-mm internal diameter tube that samples the gases (both inspired and exhaled) at a constant rate (e.g. 150–200 mL/min). The tube is connected to a lightweight adapter near the patient's end of the breathing system (with a pneumotachograph for spirometry) with a small increase in the dead space. It delivers the gases to the sample chamber. It is made of Teflon so it is impermeable to carbon dioxide and does not react with anaesthetic agents.
2. As the gases are humid, there is a moisture trap with an exhaust port, allowing gas to be vented to the atmosphere or returned to the breathing system.

supply to the light source is controlled by the feedback from the sensing resistor maintaining a constant current of 150 mA.
7. Using the rise and fall of the carbon dioxide during the respiratory cycle, monitors are designed to measure the respiratory rate.
8. Alarm limits can be set for both high and low values.
9. To avoid drift, the monitor should be calibrated regularly with

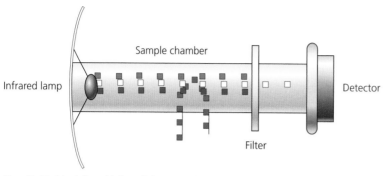

Fig. 10.19 Principles of infrared detector: due to the large amount of infrared absorption in the sample chamber by the carbon dioxide, little infrared finally reaches the detector.

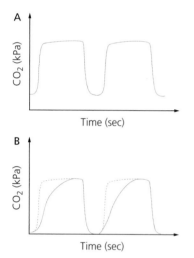

Fig. 10.20 (A) An end-tidal carbon dioxide waveform which does not return to the baseline during inspiration indicating that rebreathing is occurring. (B) An end-tidal carbon dioxide waveform which illustrates the sloping plateau seen in patients with chronic obstructive airways disease. The normal waveform is superimposed (dotted line).

3. In order to accurately measure end-tidal carbon dioxide, the sampling tube should be positioned as close as possible to the patient's trachea.
4. A variable time delay before the sample is presented to the sample chamber is expected. The *transit time* delay depends on the length (which should be as short as possible, e.g. 2 m) and diameter of the sampling tube and the sampling rate. A delay of less than 3.8 s is acceptable. The *rise time* delay is the time for the analyser to respond to the signal and depends upon the size of the sample chamber and the gas flow.
5. Other gases and vapours can be analysed from the same sample.
6. Portable hand-held side-stream analysers are available (Fig. 10.21). They can be used during patient transport and out-of-hospital situations.

MAIN-STREAM ANALYSER

1. The sample chamber is positioned within the patient's gas stream, increasing the dead space. In order to prevent water vapour condensation on its windows, it is heated to about 41°C.
2. Since there is no need for a sampling tube, there is no transport time delay in gas delivery to the sample chamber.
3. Other gases and vapours are not measured simultaneously.

See Table 10.4 for a comparison of side-stream and main-stream analysers.

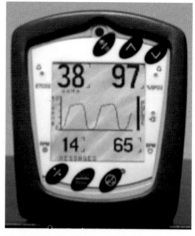

Fig. 10.21 Smith's Medical hand-held side-stream end-tidal carbon dioxide analyser.

Uses (Table 10.5)

In addition to its use as an indicator for the level of ventilation (hypo-, normo- or hyperventilation), end-tidal carbon dioxide measurement is useful:

1. To diagnose oesophageal intubation (no or very little carbon dioxide is detected). Following manual ventilation or the ingestion of carbonated drinks, some carbon dioxide might be present in the stomach. Characteristically, this may result in up to 5–6 waveforms with an abnormal shape and decreasing in amplitude.
2. As a disconnection alarm for a ventilator or breathing system. There is sudden absence of the end-tidal carbon dioxide.
3. To diagnose lung embolism as a sudden decrease in end-tidal carbon dioxide assuming that the arterial blood pressure remains stable.
4. To diagnose malignant hyperpyrexia as a gradual increase in end-tidal carbon dioxide.

Table 10.4 Comparison of various qualities between side-stream and main-stream analysers

	Side stream	Main stream
Disconnection possible	Yes	Yes
Sampling catheter leak common	Yes	No
Calibration gas required	Yes	No
Sensor damage common	No	Some
Multiple gas analysis possible	Yes	No
Use on non-intubated patients	Yes	No

Table 10.5 Summary of the uses of end-tidal CO_2

Increased end-tidal carbon dioxide	Decreased end-tidal carbon dioxide
Hypoventilation	Hyperventilation
Rebreathing	Pulmonary embolism
Sepsis	Hypoperfusion
Malignant hyperpyrexia	Hypometabolism
Hyperthermia	Hypothermia
Skeletal muscle activity	Hypovolaemia
Hypermetabolism	Hypotension

Problems in practice and safety features

1. In patients with chronic obstructive airways disease, the waveform shows a sloping trace and does not accurately reflect the end-tidal carbon dioxide (see Fig. 10.20B). An ascending plateau usually indicates impairment of ventilation: perfusion ratio because of uneven emptying of the alveoli.
2. During paediatric anaesthesia, it can be difficult to produce and interpret end-tidal carbon dioxide because of the high respiratory rates and small tidal volumes. The patient's tidal breath can be diluted with fresh gas.
3. During a prolonged expiration or end-expiratory pause, the gas flow exiting the trachea approaches zero. The sampling line may aspirate gas from the trachea and the inspiratory limb, causing ripples on the expired CO_2 trace (cardiogenic oscillations). They appear during the alveolar plateau in synchrony with the heart beat. It is thought to be due to mechanical agitation of deep lung regions that expel CO_2-rich gas. Such fluctuations can be smoothed over by increasing lung volume using positive end expiratory pressure (PEEP).
4. Dilution of the end-tidal carbon dioxide can occur whenever there are loose connections and system leaks.
5. Nitrous oxide (may be present in the sample for analysis) absorbs infrared light with an absorption spectrum partly overlapping that of carbon dioxide (Fig. 10.22). This causes inaccuracy of the detector, nitrous oxide being interpreted as carbon dioxide. By careful choice of the wavelength using special filters, this can be avoided. This is not a problem in most modern analysers.
6. Collision broadening or pressure broadening is a cause of error. The absorption of carbon dioxide is increased because of the presence of nitrous oxide or nitrogen. Calibration with a gas mixture that contains the same background gases as the sample solves this problem.

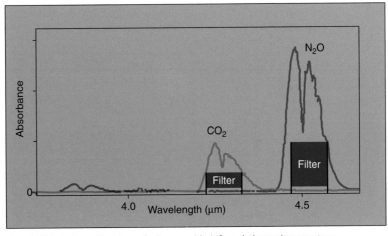

Fig. 10.22 Carbon dioxide and nitrous oxide infrared absorption spectrum.

Oxygen concentration analysers

It is fundamental to monitor oxygen concentration in the gas mixture delivered to the patient during general anaesthesia. The inspired oxygen concentration (FiO_2) is measured using a galvanic, polarographic or paramagnetic method (Fig. 10.23). The galvanic and polarographic analysers have a slow response time (20–30 s) because they are dependent on membrane diffusion. The paramagnetic analyser has a rapid response time. The paramagnetic analyser is currently more widely used. These analysers measure the oxygen partial pressure, displayed as a percentage.

PARAMAGNETIC (PAULING) OXYGEN ANALYSERS

Components

1. Two chambers separated by a sensitive pressure transducer. The gas sample containing oxygen is delivered to the measuring chamber. The reference (room air) is delivered to the other chamber. This is accomplished via a sampling tube.
2. An electromagnet is rapidly switched on and off (a frequency of about 100–110 Hz) creating a changing magnetic field to which the gases are subjected. The electromagnet is designed to have its poles in close proximity, forming a narrow gap.

Mechanism of action (Fig. 10.24)

1. Oxygen is attracted to the magnetic field (paramagnetism) because of the fact that it has two electrons in unpaired orbits. Most of the gases used in anaesthesia are repelled by the magnetic field (diamagnetism).
2. The magnetic field causes the oxygen molecules to be attracted and agitated. This leads to changes in pressure on both sides of the transducer. The pressure difference (about 20–50 μbar) across the transducer is proportional to the oxygen partial pressure difference between the sample and reference gases. The transducer converts this pressure force to an electrical signal that is displayed as oxygen partial pressure or converted to a reading in volume percentage.
3. They are very accurate and highly sensitive. The analyser should function continuously without any service breaks.
4. The recently designed paramagnetic oxygen analysers have a rapid response making it possible to analyse the inspired and expired oxygen concentration on a breath-to-breath basis. The older designs of oxygen analysers had a slow response time (nearly 1 min).
5. The audible alarms can be set for low and high concentration limits (e.g. 28% low and 40% high).

The old version of the paramagnetic analyser consists of a

Polarographic

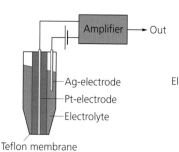

Galvanic (fuel cell)

Paramagnetic

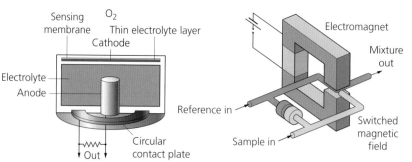

Fig. 10.23 Different types of oxygen analysers.

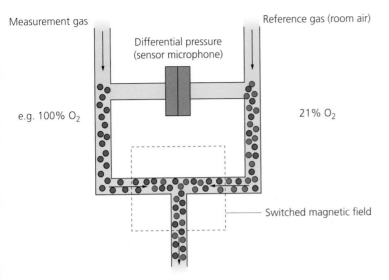

Measurement gas

Differential pressure (sensor microphone)

Reference gas (room air)

e.g. 100% O_2

21% O_2

Switched magnetic field

Fig. 10.24 Paramagnetic oxygen analyser.

container with two spheres filled with nitrogen (a weak diamagnetic gas). The spheres are suspended by a wire allowing them to rotate in a non-uniform magnetic field.

When the sample enters the container, it is attracted by the magnetic field, causing the spheres to rotate. The degree of rotation depends on the number of oxygen molecules present in the sample. The rotation of the spheres displaces a mirror attached to the wire and a light deflected from the mirror falls on a calibrated screen for measuring oxygen concentration.

THE GALVANIC OXYGEN ANALYSER (HERSCH FUEL CELL)

1. It generates a current proportional to the partial pressure of oxygen (so acting as a battery requiring oxygen for the current to flow).
2. It consists of a noble metal cathode and a lead anode in a potassium chloride electrolyte solution. An oxygen-permeable membrane separates the cell from the gases in the breathing system.

3. The oxygen molecules diffuse through the membrane and electrolyte solution to the gold cathode (see Fig. 10.23), generating an electrical current proportional to the partial pressure of oxygen:

$$O_2 + 4e^- + 2H_2O \rightarrow 4(OH)^-\,Pb$$
$$+ 2(OH)^- \rightarrow PbO + H_2O + 2e^-$$

4. Calibration is achieved using 100% oxygen and room air (21% oxygen).
5. It reads either the inspiratory or expiratory oxygen concentration.
6. Water vapour does not affect its performance.
7. It is depleted by continuous exposure to oxygen because of exhaustion of the cell, so limiting its lifespan to about 1 year.
8. The fuel cell has a slow response time of about 20 s with an accuracy of ±3%.

POLAROGRAPHIC (CLARK ELECTRODE) OXYGEN ANALYSERS

1. They have similar principles to the galvanic analysers (see Fig. 10.23). A platinum cathode and

a silver anode in an electrolyte solution are used. The electrodes are polarized by a 600–800 mV power source. An oxygen-permeable Teflon membrane separates the cell from the sample.
2. The number of oxygen molecules that traverse the membrane is proportional to its partial pressure in the sample. An electric current is produced when the cathode donates electrons that are accepted by the anode. For every molecule of oxygen, four electrons are supplied making the current produced proportional to the oxygen partial pressure in the sample.
3. They give only one reading, which is the average of inspiratory and expiratory concentrations.
4. Their life expectancy is limited (about 3 years) because of the deterioration of the membrane.
5. The positioning of the oxygen analyser is debatable. It has been recommended that slow responding analysers are positioned on the inspiratory limb of the breathing system and fast responding analysers are positioned as close as possible to the patient.

Problems in practice and safety features

1. Regular calibration of the analysers is vital.
2. Paramagnetic analysers are affected by water vapour therefore a water trap is incorporated in their design.
3. The galvanic and the polarographic cells have limited lifespans and need regular service.
4. The fuel cell and the polarographic electrode have slow response times of about 20–30 s with an accuracy of ±3%.

Nitrous oxide and inhalational agent concentration analysers

Modern vaporizers are capable of delivering accurate concentrations of the anaesthetic agent(s) with different flows. It is important to monitor the inspired and end-tidal concentrations of the agents. This is of vital importance in the circle system as the exhaled inhalational agent is recirculated and added to the fresh gas flow. In addition, because of the low flow, the inhalational agent concentration the patient is receiving is different from the setting of the vaporizer.

Modern analysers can measure the concentration of all the agents available, halothane, enflurane, isoflurane, sevoflurane and desflurane, on a breath-by-breath basis (Fig. 10.25) using infrared.

Components

1. A sampling tube from an adapter within the breathing system which delivers gas to the analyser.
2. A sample chamber to which gas for analysis is delivered.
3. An infrared light source.
4. Optical filters.
5. A photodetector.

Mechanism of action

1. Infrared absorption analysers are used (Fig. 10.26). The sampled gas enters a chamber where it is exposed to infrared light. A photodetector measures the light reaching it across the correct infrared wavelength band. Absorption of the infrared light is proportional to the vapour concentration. The electrical signal is then analysed and processed to give a measurement of the agent concentration.
2. Optical filters are used to select the desired wavelengths.

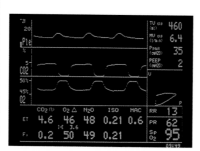

Fig. 10.25 Anaesthetic agent display of the Datex-Ohmeda Capnomac Ultima. Inspired (Fi) and end-tidal (ET) values are displayed for carbon dioxide, oxygen and isoflurane (ISO).

Different analyser designs use different wavelengths for anaesthetic agent analysis. An infrared light of a wavelength of 4.6 μm is used for N_2O. For the inhalational agents, higher wavelengths are used, between 8 and 9 μm. This is to avoid interference from methane and alcohol that happen at the lower 3.3-μm band.

3. Modern sensors can automatically identify and measure concentrations of up to three agents present in a mixture and produce a warning message to the user. Five sensors are used to produce a spectral shape where the five outputs are compared and the shape produced represents the spectral signal of the agent present in the sample. This is compared with the spectral shapes stored in the memory of the sensor and used to identify the agent. Currently, it is possible to detect and measure the concentrations of halothane, enflurane, isoflurane, sevoflurane and desflurane (Figs 10.27 and 10.28).
4. The amplitude of the spectral shape represents the amount of vapour present in the mixture. The amplitude is inversely proportional to the amount of agent present. The output of the infrared lamp is kept constant with a constant supply of current. Optical filters are

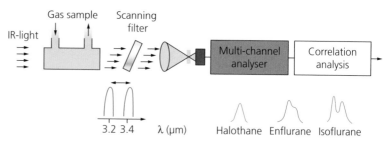

Fig. 10.26 Mechanism of action of an infrared anaesthetic agent monitor with automatic agent identification properties. Agents absorb infrared light differently over a wavelength band of 3.2–3.4 mm. The monitor can therefore identify the agent in use automatically by analysing its unique absorbance pattern.

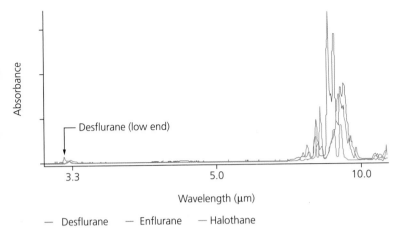

Fig. 10.27 Inhalational agents infrared absorption spectrum.

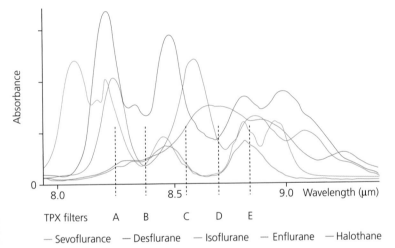

Fig. 10.28 Agent identification and measurement: to measure and identify the agents, all five sensors are used to produce a spectral shape. When the detectors at all five outputs are compared, A, B, C, D and E, a spectral shape is produced, representing the spectral signal of the agent present in the sample.

used to filter the desirable wavelengths. Because of the autodetection, individual calibration for each agent is not necessary.

5. A reference beam is incorporated. This allows the detector software to calculate how much energy has been absorbed by the sample at each wavelength and therefore the concentration of agent in the sample.

6. The sample gas can be returned to the breathing system, making the analysers suitable for use with the circle breathing system.

7. No individual calibration for each agent is necessary.

8. Water vapour has no effect on the performance and accuracy of the analyser.

PIEZOELECTRIC QUARTZ CRYSTAL OSCILLATION

Piezoelectric quartz crystal oscillation can be used to measure the concentration of inhalational agents. A lipophilic-coated piezoelectric quartz crystal undergoes changes in natural resonant frequency when exposed to the lipid-soluble inhalational agents. This change in frequency is directly proportional to the partial pressure of agent. Such a technique lacks agent specificity and sensitivity to water vapour.

Other methods less commonly used for measuring inhalational agent concentration are:

1. *Raman spectroscopy*: the anaesthetic gas sample is illuminated by an intense argon laser. Some light energy is simply reflected but some energy stimulates the sample molecules, causing them to scatter light of a different wavelength from that of the incident light energy (Raman scattering). This scattered light is detected at right angles to the laser beam and the difference in energy level between the incident and reflected light is measured. All molecules in the gas/volatile phase can be identified by their characteristic spectrum of (Raman) scattering.

2. *Ultraviolet absorption*: in the case of halothane, with similar principles to infrared absorption but using ultraviolet absorption.

Problems in practice and safety features

1. Some designs of infrared light absorption analysers are not agent specific. These must be programmed by the user for the specific agent being administered. Incorrect programming results in erroneous measurements.

2. Alarms can be set for inspired and exhaled inhalational agent concentration.

Table 10.6 summarizes the methods used in gas and vapour analysis.

Wright respirometer

This compact and light (weighs less than 150 g) respirometer is used to measure the tidal volume and minute volume (Fig. 10.29).

Components

1. The respirometer consists of an inlet and outlet.
2. A rotating vane surrounded by slits (Fig. 10.30). The vane is attached to a pointer.
3. Buttons on the side of the respirometer to turn the device on and off and reset the pointer to the zero position.

Mechanism of action

1. The Wright respirometer is a one-way system. It allows the measurement of the tidal volume if the flow of the gases is in one direction only. The correct direction for gas flow is indicated by an arrow.
2. The slits surrounding the vane are to create a circular flow in order to rotate the vane. The vane does 150 revolutions for each litre of gas passing through. This causes the pointer to rotate round the respirometer display.
3. The outer display is calibrated at 100 mL per division. The small inner display is calibrated at 1 L per division.

> **Inhalational agent concentration analysers**
> - A sample of gas is used to measure the concentration of inhalational agent using infrared light absorption.
> - By selecting light of the correct wavelengths, the inspired and expired concentrations of the agent(s) can be measured.
> - An infrared light of a wavelength of 4.6 μm is used for N_2O. For other inhalational agents, higher wavelengths are used, between 8 and 9 μm.
> - Ultraviolet absorption, mass spectrometry and quartz crystal oscillation are other methods of measuring the inhalational agents' concentration.

MASS SPECTROMETER

This can be used to identify and measure, on a breath-to-breath basis, the concentrations of the gases and vapours used during anaesthesia. The principle of action is to charge the particles of the sample (bombard them with an electron beam) and then separate the components into a spectrum according to their specific mass:charge ratios – so each has its own 'fingerprint'.

The creation and manipulation of the ions are done in a high vacuum (10^{-5} mmHg) to avoid interference by outside air and to minimize random collisions among the ions and the residual gas. The relative abundance of ions at certain specific mass:charge ratios is determined and is related to the fractional composition of the original gas mixture.

A permanent magnet is used to separate the ion beam into its component ion spectra. Because of the high expense, multiplexed mass spectrometer systems are used with several patient sampling locations on a time-shared basis.

Table 10.6 The various methods used in gas and vapour analysis

Technology	O_2	CO_2	N_2O	Inhalational agent
Infrared		✓	✓	✓
Paramagnetic	✓			
Polarography	✓			
Fuel cell	✓			
Mass spectrometry	✓	✓	✓	✓
Raman spectroscopy	✓	✓	✓	✓
Piezoelectric resonance				✓

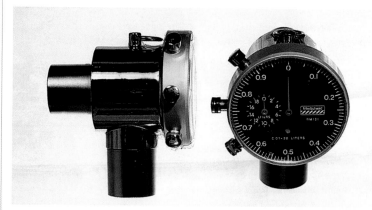

Fig. 10.29 A Wright respirometer. An arrow on the side of the casing indicates the direction of gas flow.

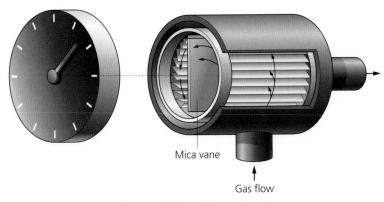

Mica vane

Gas flow

Fig. 10.30 Mechanism of action of the Wright respirometer.

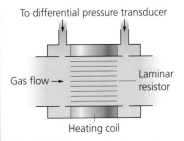

To differential pressure transducer

Gas flow →

Laminar resistor

Heating coil

Fig. 10.31 A pneumotachograph. See text for details.

4. It is usually positioned on the expiratory side of the breathing system, which is at a lower pressure than the inspiratory side. This minimizes the loss of gas volume due to leaks and expansion of the tubing.
5. For clinical use, the respirometer reads accurately the tidal volume and minute volume (±5–10%) within the range of 4–24 L/min. A minimum flow of 2 L/min is required for the respirometer to function accurately.
6. To improve accuracy, the respirometer should be positioned as close to the patient's trachea as possible.
7. The resistance to breathing is very low at about 2 cm H_2O at 100 L/min.
8. A paediatric version exists with a capability of accurate tidal volume measurements between 15 and 200 mL.
9. A more accurate version of the Wright respirometer uses light reflection to measure the tidal volume. The mechanical causes of inaccuracies (friction and inertia) and the accumulation of water vapour are avoided. Other designs use a semiconductive device that is sensitive to changes in magnetic field. Tidal volume and minute volume can be measured by converting these changes electronically. An alarm system can also be added.

Problems in practice and safety features

1. The Wright respirometer tends to over-read at high flow rates and under-read at low flows.
2. Water condensation from the expired gases causes the pointer to stick, thus preventing it from rotating freely.

Wright respirometer
- Rotating vane attached to a pointer.
- Fitted on the expiratory limb to measure the tidal and minute volume with an accuracy of ±5–10%.
- The flow is unidirectional.
- It over-reads at high flows and under-reads at low flows.

Pneumotachograph

This measures gas flow. From this, gas volume can be calculated.

Components

1. A tube with a fixed resistance. The resistance can be a bundle of parallel tubes (Fig. 10.31).
2. Two sensitive pressure transducers on either side of the resistance.

Mechanism of action

1. The principle of its function is sensing the change in pressure across a fixed resistance through which gas flow is laminar.
2. The pressure change is only a few millimetres of water and is linearly proportional, over a certain range, to the flow rate of gas passing through the resistance.
3. The tidal volumes can be summated over a period of a minute to give the minute volume.
4. It can measure flows in both inspiration and expiration (i.e. bidirectional).

Problems in practice and safety features

Water vapour condensation at the resistance will encourage the formation of turbulent flow affecting the accuracy of the measurement. This can be avoided by heating the parallel tubes.

Combined pneumotachograph and Pitot tube

This combination (Fig. 10.32) is designed to improve accuracy and calculate and measure the compliance, airway pressures, gas flow, volume/pressure (Fig. 10.33)

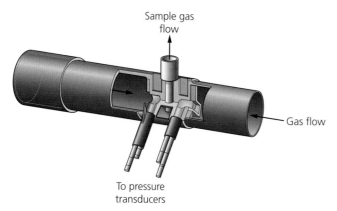

Fig. 10.32 Combined pneumotachograph and Pitot tube. (Courtesy of GE Datex Ohmeda.)

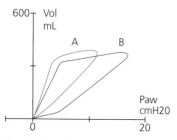

Fig. 10.33 Volume pressure loops in a patient (A) before and (B) during CO_2 insufflation in a laparoscopic operation. Note the decrease in compliance and increase in airway pressure (Paw).

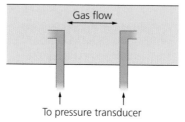

Fig. 10.34 Cross-section of a Pitot tube flowmeter. The two ports are facing in opposite directions within the gas flow.

and flow/volume loops. Modern devices can be used accurately even in neonates and infants.

THE PITOT TUBE

Components

1. Two pressure ports – one facing the direction of gas flow, the other perpendicular to the gas flow. This is used to measure gas flow in one direction only.
2. In order to measure bidirectional flows (inspiration and expiration), two pressure ports face in opposite directions within the gas flow (Fig. 10.34).
3. These pressure ports are connected to pressure transducers.

Mechanism of action

The pressure difference between the ports is proportional to the square of the flow rate.

Problems in practice and safety features

The effects of the density and viscosity of the gas(es) can alter the accuracy. This can be compensated for by continuous gas composition analysis via a sampling tube.

Factors affecting the readings in pnuemotachograph

1. **Location**: should be placed between the breathing system Y-piece and the tracheal tube.
2. **Gas composition**: nominal values of gas composition need to be known with sensors calibrated accordingly.
3. **Gas temperature**: A knowledge gas temperatures is required. Usually, the sensors' software provides default values for a typical patient.
4. **Humidity**: moisture can affect measurement and generation of pressure drop. Have the pressure ports directed upwards to prevent fluid from draining into them.
5. **Apparatus dead space**: Sensors need to have a minimum dead space; <10 ml for the adult flow sensors and <1 ml for the neonatal sensors.
6. **Operating range of flow sensor**: Sensors are designed to function accurately with a very wide range of tidal volumes, I : E ratios, frequencies and flow ranges.
7. **Inter-sensor variability**: Individual sensors can have different performances. There should be no need for individual device calibration of the flow/pressure characteristics

The effects of the density and viscosity of the gas(es) can alter the accuracy. This can be compensated for by continuous gas composition analysis via a sampling tube.

Pneumotachograph
- A bidirectional device to measure the flow rate, tidal and minute volume.
- A laminar flow across a fixed resistance causes changes in pressure which are measured by transducers.
- Condensation at the resistance can cause turbulent flow and inaccuracies.
- Improved accuracy is achieved by adding a Pitot tube(s) and continuous gas composition analysis.

Ventilator alarms

It is mandatory to use a ventilator alarm during intermittent positive pressure ventilation (IPPV) to guard against patient disconnection, leaks, obstruction or malfunction. These can be pressure and/or volume monitoring alarms. Clinical observation, end-tidal carbon dioxide concentration, airway pressure and pulse oximetry are also ventilator monitors.

PRESSURE MONITORING ALARM

Components

1. The case where the pressure alarm limits are set, an automatic on/off switch. A light flashes with each ventilator cycle (Fig. 10.35).
2. The alarm is pressurized by a sensing tube connecting it to the inspiratory limb of the ventilator system.

Mechanism of action

1. In this alarm, the peak inspiratory pressure is usually measured and monitored during controlled ventilation.
2. A decrease in peak inspiratory pressure activates the alarm. This indicates that the ventilator is unable to achieve the preset threshold pressure in the breathing system. Causes can be disconnection, gas leak or inadequate fresh gas flow.
3. An increase in the peak inspiratory pressure usually indicates an obstruction.
4. The low-pressure alarm can be set to 7 cm H_2O, 7 cm H_2O plus time delay or 13 cm H_2O. The high-pressure alarm is set at 60 cm H_2O.

Problems in practice and safety features

Disconnection of the breathing system with partial obstruction of the alarm sensing tube may lead to a condition where the alarm is not activated despite inadequate ventilation.

VOLUME MONITORING ALARM

The expired gas volume can be measured and monitored. Gas volume can be measured either directly using a respirometer or indirectly by integration of the gas flow (pneumotachograph).

These alarms are usually inserted in the expiratory limb with a continuous display of tidal and minute volume. The alarm limits are set for a minimum and maximum tidal and/or minute volume.

Ventilator alarms

- They can be pressure and/or volume monitoring alarms.
- They detect disconnection (low pressure) or obstruction (high pressure) in the ventilator breathing system.
- The pressure alarms are fitted on the inspiratory limb whereas the volume alarms are fitted on the expiratory limb of the breathing system.
- Regular servicing is required.

Peripheral nerve stimulators

These devices are used to monitor transmission across the neuromuscular junction. The depth, adequate reversal and type of neuromuscular blockade can be established (Fig. 10.36).

Components

1. Two surface electrodes (small ECG electrodes) are positioned over the nerve and connected via the leads to the nerve stimulator.

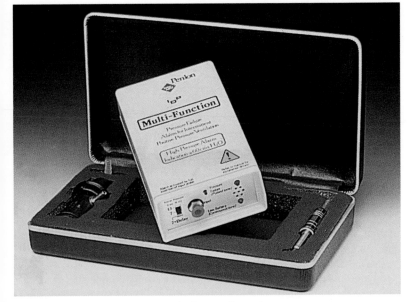

Fig. 10.35 The Penlon pressure monitoring ventilator alarm.

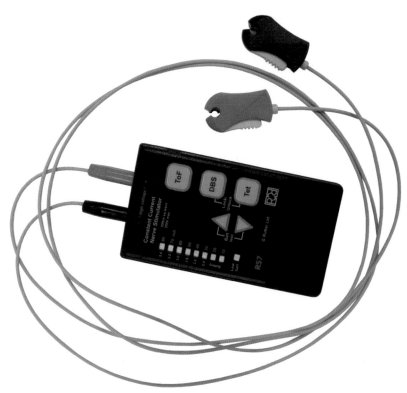

Fig. 10.36 The RS7 peipheral nerve stimulator. (Courtesy of G Rutter Ltd.)

2. Alternatively skin contact can be made via ball electrodes which are mounted on the nerve stimulator casing.
3. The case consists of an on/off switch, facility to deliver a twitch, train-of-four (at 2 Hz) and tetanus (50 Hz). The stimulator is battery operated.

Mechanism of action

1. A supramaximal stimulus is used to stimulate a peripheral nerve. This ensures that all the motor fibres of the nerve are depolarized. The response of the muscle(s) supplied by the nerve is observed. A current of 15–40 mA is used for the ulnar nerve (a current of 50–60 mA may have to be used in obese patients).
2. This device should be battery powered and capable of delivering a constant current.

It is the current magnitude that determines whether the nerve depolarizes or not, so delivering a constant current is more important than delivering a constant voltage as the skin resistance is variable (Ohm's Law).

3. The muscle contraction can be observed visually, palpated, measured using a force transducer, or the electrical activity can be measured (EMG).
4. The duration of the stimulus is less than 0.2–0.3 ms. The stimulus should have a monophasic square wave shape to avoid repetitive nerve firing.
5. Superficial, accessible peripheral nerves are most commonly used for monitoring purposes, e.g. ulnar nerve at the wrist, common peroneal nerve at the neck of the fibula, posterior

tibial nerve at the ankle and the facial nerve.
6. The negative electrode is positioned directly over the most superficial part of the nerve. The positive electrode is positioned along the proximal course of nerve to avoid direct muscle stimulation.
7. Consider the ulnar nerve at the wrist. Two electrodes are positioned over the nerve, with the negative electrode placed distally and the positive electrode positioned about 2 cm proximally. Successful ulnar nerve stimulation causes the contraction of the adductor pollicis brevis muscle.

More advanced devices offer continuous monitoring of the transmission across the neuromuscular junction. A graphical and numerical display of the train-of-four (see below) and the trend provide optimal monitoring. Skin electrodes are used. A reference measurement should be made where the device calculates the supramaximal current needed before the muscle relaxant is given. The device can be used to locate nerves and plexuses with a much lower current (e.g. a maximum of 5.0 mA) during regional anaesthesia. In this mode, a short stimulus can be used, e.g. 40 ms, to reduce the patient's discomfort.

NEUROMUSCULAR MONITORING

There are various methods for monitoring the neuromuscular transmission using a nerve stimulator (Fig. 10.37).

1. *Twitch*: a short duration (0.1–0.2 ms) square wave stimulus of a frequency of 0.1–1 Hz (one stimulus every 10 seconds to one stimulus every 1 second) is applied to a

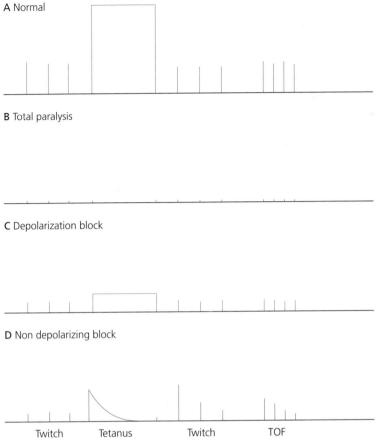

A Normal

B Total paralysis

C Depolarization block

D Non depolarizing block

Twitch   Tetanus   Twitch   TOF

Fig. 10.37 Effects of a single twitch, tetanus and train-of-four (TOF) assessed by a force transducer recording contraction of the adductor pollicis muscle.

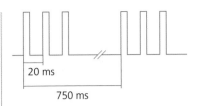

20 ms

750 ms

Fig. 10.38 The pattern of double-burst stimulation. Three impulses of 50 Hz tetanus, at 20-ms intervals, every 750 ms is shown.

peripheral nerve. When used on its own, it is of limited use. It is the least precise method of assessing partial neuromuscular block.

2. *Tetanic stimulation*: a tetanus of 50–100 Hz is used to detect any residual neuromuscular block. Fade will be apparent even with normal response to a twitch. Tetanus is usually applied to anaesthetized patients because of the discomfort caused.

3. *Train-of-four* (TOF): used to monitor the degree of the neuromuscular block clinically. The ratio of the fourth to the first twitch is called the TOF ratio:
   a) four twitches of 2 Hz each applied over 2 s. A gap of 10 s between each TOF
   b) as the muscle relaxant is administered, fade is noticed first, followed by the disappearance of the fourth twitch. This is followed by the disappearance of the third then the second and last by the first twitch
   c) on recovery, the first twitch appears first then the second followed by the third and fourth; reversal of the neuromuscular block is easier if the second twitch is visible
   d) for upper abdominal surgery, at least three twitches must be absent to achieve adequate surgical conditions
   e) the TOF ratio can be estimated using visible or tactile means. Electrical recording of the response is more accurate.

4. *Post-tetanic facilitation or potentiation*: this is used to assess more profound degrees of neuromuscular block.

5. *Double burst stimulation* (Fig. 10.38): this allows a more accurate visual assessment than TOF for residual neuromuscular blockade. Two short bursts of 50 Hz tetanus are applied with a 750-ms interval. Each burst comprises of two or three square wave impulses lasting for 0.2 ms.

Problems in practice and safety features

As the muscles of the hand are small in comparison with the diaphragm (the main respiratory muscle), monitoring the neuromuscular block peripherally does not reflect the true picture of the depth of the diaphragmatic block. The smaller the muscle is, the more sensitive it is to a muscle relaxant.

Peripheral nerve stimulators
- Used to ensure adequate reversal, and to monitor the depth and the type of the block.
- Supramaximal stimulus is used to stimulate the nerve.
- The contraction of the muscle is observed visually, palpated or measured by a pressure transducer.
- The ulnar, facial, posterior tibial and the common peroneal nerves are often used.

Various methods are used to monitor the neuromuscular transmission: twitch, tetanic stimulation, train-of-four, post-tetanic facilitation and double burst stimulation.

Bispectral index (BIS) analysis (Fig. 10.39)

The BIS monitor is a device to monitor the electrical activity and the level of sedation in the brain and to assess the risk of awareness while under sedation/anaesthesia. In addition, it allows titration of hypnotics based on individual

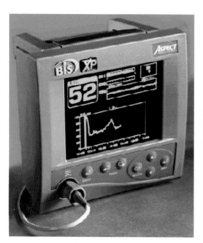

Fig. 10.39 BIS monitor.

requirements to reduce under- and overdosing. BIS has been shown to correlate with measures of sedation/hypnosis, awareness and recall end points likely to be reflected in the cortical EEG. It can provide a continuous and consistent measure of sedation/hypnosis induced by most of the widely used sedative-hypnotic agents. Although BIS can measure the hypnotic components, it is less sensitive to the analgesic/opiate components of an anaesthetic.

Components

1. Display:
   a) BIS (as a single value or trend)
   b) facial electromyogram, EMG (in decibels)
   c) EEG suppression measured
   d) signal quality index (SQI) which indicates the amount of interference from EMG.
2. A forehead sensor with four numbered electrodes (elements) and a smart chip. The sensor uses small tines, which part the outer layers of the skin, and a hydrogel to make electrical contact. It is designed to lower the impedance and to optimize the quality of the signal.
3. A smaller paediatric sensor with three electrodes is available. It has a flexible design to adjust to various head sizes and contours.

Mechanism of action

1. Bispectral analysis is a statistical method that quantifies the level of synchronization of the underlying frequencies in the signal.
2. BIS is a value derived mathematically using information from EEG power and frequency as well as bispectral information. Along with the traditional amplitude and frequency variables, it provides a more complete

description of complex EEG patterns.
3. BIS is an empirical, statistically derived measurement. It uses a linear, dimensionless scale from 0 to 100. The lower the value, the greater the hypnotic effect. A value of 100 represents an awake EEG while zero represents complete electrical silence (cortical suppression). BIS values of 65–85 are recommended for sedation, whereas values of 40–60 are recommended for general anaesthesia. At BIS values of less than 40, cortical suppression becomes discernible in raw EEG as a burst suppression pattern (Fig. 10.40).
4. BIS measures the state of the brain, not the concentration of a particular drug. So a low value for BIS indicates hypnosis irrespective of how it was produced.
5. It has been shown that return of consciousness occurs consistently when the BIS is above 60 and, interestingly, at the same time, changes in blood pressure and heart rate are poor predictors for response.
6. The facial electromyogram (in decibels) is displayed to inform the user of possible interference affecting the BIS value.
7. The sensor is applied on the forehead at an angle. It can be placed on either the right or left side of the head. Element *number 1* is placed at the centre of the forehead, 5 cm above the nose. Element *number 4* is positioned just above and adjacent to the eyebrow. Element *number 2* is positioned between *number 1* and *number 4*. Element *number 3* is positioned on either temple between the corner of the eye and the hairline. The sensor will not function beyond the hairline. Each element should be

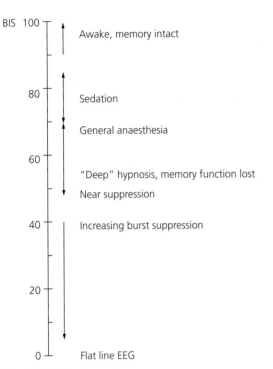

BIS 100 — Awake, memory intact

80 — Sedation

General anaesthesia

60 — "Deep" hypnosis, memory function lost

Near suppression

40 — Increasing burst suppression

20 —

0 — Flat line EEG

Fig. 10.40 BIS values scale.

pressed for 5 seconds with the fingertip.

8. Cerebral ischaemia from any cause can result in a decrease in the BIS value if severe enough to cause a global EEG slowing or outright suppression.

9. BIS is being 'incorporated' as an additional monitoring module that can be added to the existing modular patient monitors such as Datex-Ohmeda S/5, Philips Viridia or GE Marquette Solar 8000M. In addition to its use in the operating theatre, BIS has also been used in the intensive care setting to assess the level of sedation in mechanically ventilated patients.

Problems and safety features

1. Hypothermia of less than 33°C results in a decrease in BIS levels as the brain processes slow. In such situations, e.g. during cardiac bypass procedures, BIS reflects the synergistic effects of hypothermia and hypnotic drugs. A rapid rise in BIS usually occurs during rewarming.

2. Interference from non-EEG electrical signals such as electromyogram. High-frequency facial electromyogram activity may be present in sedated, spontaneously breathing patients and during awakening, causing BIS to increase in conjunction with higher electromyogram. Significant electromyogram interference can lead to a faulty high BIS despite the patient being still unresponsive. EEG signals are considered to exist in the 0.5–30-Hz band whereas electromyogram signals exist in the 30–300-Hz band. Separation is not absolute and low-frequency electromyogram signals can occur in the conventional EEG band range. The more recent BIS XP is less affected by electromyogram.

3. BIS cannot be used to monitor hypnosis during ketamine anaesthesia. This is due to ketamine being a dissociative anaesthetic with excitatory effects on the EEG.

4. Sedative concentrations of nitrous oxide (up to 70%) do not appear to affect BIS.

5. There are conflicting data regarding opioid dose–response and interaction of opioids with hypnotics on BIS.

6. Currently there are insufficient data to evaluate the use of BIS in patients with neurological diseases.

7. When the SQI value goes below 50%, the BIS is not stored in the trend memory. The BIS value on the monitor appears in 'reverse video' to indicate this.

8. Interference from surgical diathermy. A recent version, BIS XP, is better protected from the diathermy.

9. As with any other monitor, the use of BIS does not obviate the need for critical clinical judgement.

BIS

- Monitors the electrical activity in the brain.
- Uses a linear dimensionless scale from 0 to 100. The lower the value, the greater the hypnotic effect. General anaesthesia is at 40–60.
- Interference can be from diathermy or EMG.
- Changes in body temperature and cerebral ischaemia can affect the value.

Entropy of the EEG

This is a more recent technique used to measure the depth of sedation/anaesthesia by measuring the 'regularity' or the amount of disorder of the EEG signal. High levels of entropy during anaesthesia show that the patient is awake, and low levels correlate with deep unconsciousness.

The EEG signal is recorded using electrodes applied to the forehead and side of the head, as with the BIS. The device uses Fourier transformation to calculate the frequencies of voltages for each given time sample (epoch). This is then converted into a normalized frequency spectrum (by squaring the transformed components) for the selected frequency range.

State entropy (SE) index is calculated from a low-frequency range (under 32 Hz) corresponding predominantly to EEG activity.

Response entropy (RE) index uses a higher frequency range (up to 47 Hz) and includes electromyographic (EMG) activity from frontalis muscle.

The concept of *Shannon entropy* is then applied to normalize the entropy values to between zero (total regularity) and 1 (total irregularity).

The commercially available M-entropy module (GE Datex-Ohmeda) converts the entropy scale of zero to 1 into a scale of zero to 100 (similar to the BIS scale). The conversion is not exactly linear to give greater resolution at the most important area to monitor 'depth of anaesthesia' which is between 0.5 and 1.0.

Both RE and SE are displayed with the RE ranges from 100 to zero and the SE ranges from a maximum of 91 to zero (Fig. 10.41). In practice, zero corresponds

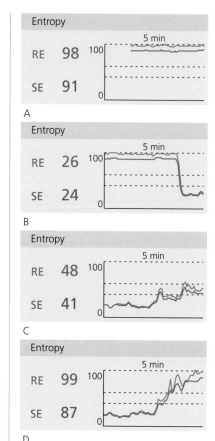

Fig. 10.41 Entropy of EEG. (A) Awake state. Note the difference between the two entropies indicating muscle activity on the face. (B) Immediately after induction of anaesthesia. (C) Maintenance of anaesthesia. (D) Recovery from anaesthesia.

to a very 'deep' level of anaesthesia and values close to 100 correspond to the awake patient. Like BIS, values between 40 and 60 represent clinically desirable depths of anaesthesia. At this level, the SE and RE indexes should be similar if not identical.

As the patient awakens, an increase in the difference between the SE and RE values is seen due to a diminishing effect of drugs on the CNS and an increasing contribution from frontalis EMG.

Entropy of EEG

1. The 'regularity' or the amount of disorder of the EEG signal is used to measure the depth of sedation/anaesthesia.
2. During anaesthesia, low levels correlate with deep unconsciousness.
3. State entropy (SE) index corresponds predominantly to EEG activity.
4. Response entropy (RE) index includes EMG activity from frontalis muscle.

Further reading

McGrath, C.D., Hunter, J.M., 2006. Monitoring of neuromuscular block. Continuing Education in Anaesthesia. Critical Care and Pain 6(1), 7–12.

MHRA, 2010. Medical device alert: Unilect (TM) ECG monitoring electrodes manufactured by Unomedical (MDA/2010/046). Online. Available at: http://www. mhra.gov.uk/Publications/ Safetywarnings/MedicalDeviceAlerts/ CON084595.

MHRA, 2012. Pulse oximeter top tips. Online. Available at: http:// www.mhra.gov.uk/Publications/ Postersandleaflets/CON100224.

Patel, S., Souter, M., 2008. Equipment-related electrocardiographic artifacts: causes, characteristics, consequences, and correction. Anesthesiology 108, 138–148.

MCQs

In the following lists, which of the statements (a) to (e) are true?

1. Concerning capnography:
   a) Capnography is a more useful indicator of ventilator disconnection and oesophageal intubation than pulse oximetry.
   b) Capnography typically works on the absorption of CO_2 in the ultraviolet region of the spectrum.
   c) In side-stream analysers, a delay in measurement of less than 38 s is acceptable.
   d) The main-stream analyser type can measure other gases simultaneously.
   e) In patients with chronic obstructive airways disease, the waveform can show a sloping trace instead of the square shape wave.

2. Concerning oxygen concentration measurement:
   a) An infrared absorption technique is used.
   b) Paramagnetic analysers are commonly used because oxygen is repelled by the magnetic field.
   c) The galvanic (fuel cell) analyser has a slow response time of about 20 s and a lifespan of about 1 year.
   d) The fast responding analysers should be positioned as near the patient as possible.
   e) Paramagnetic analysers can provide breath-to-breath measurement.

3. Pulse oximetry:
   a) The probe consists of two emitting diodes producing beams at red and infrared frequencies.
   b) Accurately reflects the ability of the patient to eliminate CO_2.
   c) The measurements are accurate within the clinical range of 70–100%.
   d) Carbon monoxide in the blood causes a false under-reading.
   e) The site of the probe has to be checked frequently.

4. Arterial blood pressure:
   a) Mean blood pressure is the systolic pressure plus one-third of the pulse pressure.
   b) Too small a cuff causes a false high pressure.
   c) Oscillotonometry is widely used to measure blood pressure.
   d) The Finapres technique uses ultraviolet light absorption to measure the blood pressure.
   e) A slow cuff inflation followed by a fast deflation are needed to improve the accuracy of a non-invasive blood pressure technique.

5. Pneumotachograph:
   a) It is a fixed orifice variable pressure flowmeter.
   b) It consists of two sensitive pressure transducers positioned on either side of a resistance.
   c) It is capable of flowing in one direction only.
   d) A Pitot tube can be added to improve accuracy.
   e) Humidity and water vapour condensation have no effect on its accuracy.

6. Polarographic oxygen electrode:
   a) It can measure oxygen partial pressure in a blood or gas sample.
   b) The electrode acts as a battery requiring no power source.
   c) Oxygen molecules pass from the sample to the potassium chloride solution across a semipermeable membrane.
   d) It uses a silver cathode and a platinum anode.
   e) The amount of electrical current generated is proportional to the oxygen partial pressure.

7. Wright respirometer:
   a) It is best positioned on the inspiratory limb of the ventilator breathing system.
   b) It is a bidirectional device.
   c) It is accurate for clinical use.
   d) It over-reads at high flow rates and under-reads at low flow rates.
   e) It can measure both tidal volume and minute volume.

8. Paramagnetic gases include:
   a) Oxygen.
   b) Sevoflurane.
   c) Nitrous oxide.
   d) Carbon dioxide.
   e) Halothane.

9. Oxygen in a gas mixture can be measured by:
   a) Fuel cell.
   b) Ultraviolet absorption.
   c) Mass spectrometer.
   d) Clark oxygen (polarographic) electrode.
   e) Infrared absorption.

10. The concentrations of volatile agents can be measured using:
    a) Fuel cell.
    b) Piezoelectric crystal.
    c) Ultraviolet spectroscopy.
    d) Infrared spectroscopy.
    e) Clark electrode.

11. A patient with healthy lungs and a $PaCO_2$ of 40 mmHg will have which of the following percentages of CO_2 in the end expiratory mixture?
    a) 4%.
    b) 5%.
    c) 2%.
    d) 1%.
    e) 7%.

12. BIS monitor:
    a) It uses a linear dimensionless scale from 0 to 100 Hz.
    b) Hypothermia can increase the BIS value.
    c) The BIS value is not accurate during ketamine anaesthesia.
    d) Interference can occur due to EMG or diathermy.
    e) BIS can measure the drug concentration of a particular drug.

13. Concerning ECG:
    a) The monitoring mode of ECG has a wider frequency response range than the diagnostic mode.
    b) The electrical potentials have a range of 0.5–2 V.
    c) Interference due to electrostatic induction can be reduced by surrounding ECG leads with copper screens.
    d) Silver and silver chloride electrodes are used.
    e) It is standard in the UK to use a display speed of 25 cm/s and a sensitivity of 1 mV/cm.

14. Infrared spectrometry:
    a) CO_2 absorbs infrared radiation mainly at a wavelength of 4.3 mm.
    b) Photo-acoustic spectrometry is more stable than the conventional infrared spectrometry.
    c) Sampling catheter leak is a potential problem with the side-stream analysers.
    d) A wavelength of 4.6 μm is used for nitrous oxide measurement.
    e) A wavelength of 3.3 μm is used to measure the concentration of inhalational agents.

SINGLE BEST ANSWER (SBA)

15. Regarding the minimum monitoring required for anaesthesia:
    a) Renders bed-side clinical signs obsolete.
    b) ECG monitoring is essential.
    c) Modern ECG monitoring is immune from artefacts.
    d) Non-invasive blood pressure requires two cuffs and a minimum cycle time of 1 minute.
    e) National Institute for Health and Clinical Excellence (NICE) guidelines forbid temperature monitoring.

Answers

1. Concerning capnography:
   a) *True. Capnography gives a fast warning in cases of disconnection or oesophageal intubation. The end-tidal CO_2 will decrease sharply and suddenly. The pulse oximeter will be very slow in detecting disconnection or oesophageal intubation as the arterial oxygen saturation will remain normal for longer periods especially if the patient was preoxygenated.*
   b) *False. CO_2 is absorbed in the infrared region.*
   c) *False. In side-stream analysers, a delay of less than 3.8 s is acceptable. The length of the sampling tubing should be as short as possible, e.g. 2 m, with an internal diameter of 1.2 mm and a sampling rate of about 150 mL/min.*
   d) *False. Only CO_2 can be measured by the main-stream analyser. CO_2, N_2O and inhalational agents can be measured simultaneously with a side-stream analyser.*
   e) *True. In patients with chronic obstructive airways disease, the alveoli empty at different rates because of the differing time constants in different regions of the lung with various degrees of altered compliance and airway resistance.*

2. Concerning oxygen concentration measurement:
   a) *False. Oxygen does not absorb infrared radiation. Only molecules with two differing atoms can absorb infrared radiation.*
   b) *False. Oxygen is attracted by the magnetic field because it has two electrons in unpaired orbits.*
   c) *True. The fuel cell is depleted by continuous exposure to oxygen due to the exhaustion of the cell giving it a lifespan of about 1 year.*
   d) *True. Although the positioning of the oxygen analyser is still debatable, it has been recommended that the fast responding ones are positioned as close to the patient as possible. The slow responding analysers are positioned on the inspiratory limb of the breathing system.*
   e) *True. Modern paramagnetic analysers have a rapid response allowing them to provide breath-to-breath measurement. Older versions have a 1-min response time.*

3. Pulse oximetry:
   a) *True. The probe uses light-emitting diodes (LEDs) that emit light at red (660 nm) and infrared (940 nm) frequencies. The LEDs operate in sequence with an 'off' period when the photodetector measures the background level of ambient light. This sequence happens at a rate of about 30 times per second.*
   b) *False. Pulse oximetry is a measurement of the arterial oxygen saturation.*
   c) *True. Readings below 70% are extrapolated by the manufacturers.*
   d) *False. Using a pulse oximeter, carbon monoxide causes a false high reading of the arterial oxygen saturation.*
   e) *True. The probe can cause pressure sores with continuous use so its site should be checked at regular intervals. Some recommend changing the site every 2 hours.*

4. Arterial blood pressure:
   a) *False. The mean blood pressure is the diastolic pressure plus one-third of the pulse pressure (systolic pressure – diastolic pressure).*
   b) *True. The opposite is also correct.*
   c) *True. Most of the non-invasive blood pressure measuring devices use oscillometry as the basis for measuring blood pressure. Return of the blood flow during deflation causes pressure changes in the cuff. The transducer senses the pressure changes which are interpreted by the microprocessor.*
   d) *False. The Finapres uses oscillometry and a servo control unit is used.*
   e) *False. Slow cuff inflation leads to venous congestion and inaccuracy. A fast cuff deflation might miss the oscillations caused by the return of blood flow (i.e. systolic pressure). A fast inflation and slow deflation of the cuff is needed. A deflation rate of 3 mmHg/s or 2 mmHg/beat is adequate.*

5. Pneumotachograph:
   a) *True.* The pneumotachograph consists of a tube with a fixed resistance, usually as a bundle of parallel tubes, and is therefore a 'fixed orifice' device. As the fluid (gas or liquid) passes across the resistance, the pressure across the resistance changes, therefore it is a 'variable pressure' flowmeter.
   b) *True.* The two pressure transducers measure the pressures on either side of the resistance. The pressure changes are proportional to the flow rate across the resistance.
   c) *False.* It can measure flows in both directions; i.e. it is bidirectional.
   d) *True.* The combined design improves accuracy and allows the measurement and calculation of other parameters: compliance, airway pressure, gas flow, volume/pressure and flow/volume loops.
   e) *False.* A laminar flow is required for the pneumotachograph to measure accurately. Water vapour condensation at the site of the resistance leads to the formation of turbulent flow thus reducing the accuracy of the measurement.

6. Polarographic oxygen electrode:
   a) *True.* The polarographic (Clark) electrode analysers can be used to measure oxygen partial pressure in a gas sample (e.g. on an anaesthetic machine giving an average inspiratory and expiratory concentration) or in blood in a blood gas analyser.
   b) *False.* A power source of about 700 mV is needed in a polarographic analyser. The galvanic analyser (fuel cell) acts as a battery requiring no power source.
   c) *True.* The oxygen molecules pass across a Teflon semipermeable membrane at a rate proportional to their partial pressure in the sample into the sodium chloride solution. The performance of the electrode is affected as the membrane deteriorates or perforates.
   d) *False.* The opposite is correct: the anode is made of silver and the cathode is made of platinum.
   e) *True.* When the oxygen molecules pass across the membrane, very small electrical currents are generated as electrons move from the cathode to the anode.

7. Wright respirometer:
   a) *False.* The Wright respirometer is best positioned on the expiratory limb of the ventilator breathing system. This minimizes the loss of gas volume due to leaks and expansion of the tubing on the inspiratory limb.
   b) *False.* It is a unidirectional device allowing the measurement of the tidal volume if the flow of gases is in one direction only. An arrow on the device indicates the correct direction of the gas flow.
   c) *True.* It is suitable for routine clinical use with an accuracy of ±5–10% within a range of flows of 4–24 L/min.

   d) *True.* Over-reading at high flows and under-reading at low flows is due to the effect of inertia on the rotating vane. Using a Wright respirometer based on light reflection or the use of a semiconductive device, sensitive to changes in magnetic field, instead of the mechanical components, improves the accuracy.
   e) *True.* The Wright respirometer can measure the volume per breath, and if the measurement is continued for 1 minute, the minute volume can be measured as well.

8. Paramagnetic gases include:
   a) *True.* Oxygen is attracted by the magnetic field because it has two electrons in unpaired orbits causing it to possess paramagnetic properties.
   b) *False.*
   c) *False.*
   d) *False.*
   e) *False.*

9. Oxygen in a gas mixture can be measured by:
   a) *True.* The oxygen molecules diffuse through a membrane and electrolyte solution to reach the cathode. This generates a current proportional to the partial pressure of oxygen in the mixture.
   b) *False.* Oxygen does not absorb ultraviolet radiation. Halothane absorbs ultraviolet radiation.

c) *True. Mass spectrometry can be used for the measurement of any gas. It separates the gases according to their molecular weight. The sample is ionized and then the ions are separated. Mass spectrometry allows rapid simultaneous breath-to-breath measurement of oxygen concentration.*

d) *True. Although polarographic analysers are used mainly to measure oxygen partial pressure in a blood sample in blood gas analysers, they can also be used to measure the partial pressure in a gas sample. See Question 6 above.*

e) *False. Gases that absorb infrared radiation have molecules with two different atoms (e.g. carbon and oxygen in CO_2). An oxygen molecule has two similar atoms.*

---

10. The concentrations of volatile agents can be measured using:

a) *False. The fuel cell is used to measure the oxygen concentration.*

b) *True. A piezoelectric quartz crystal with a lipophilic coat undergoes changes in natural frequency when exposed to a lipid-soluble inhalational agent. It lacks agent specificity. It is not widely used in current anaesthetic practice.*

c) *True. Halothane can absorb ultraviolet radiation. It is not used in current anaesthetic practice.*

d) *True. Infrared radiation is absorbed by all the gases with dissimilar atoms in the molecule. Infrared analysers can be either side stream or main stream.*

e) *False. The Clark polarographic electrode is used to measure oxygen concentration.*

---

11. A patient with healthy lungs and a $PaCO_2$ of 40 mmHg will have which of the following percentages of CO_2 in the end expiratory mixture?

a) *False.*

b) *True. In a patient with healthy lungs, the end-tidal CO_2 concentration is a true reflection of the arterial CO_2. A $PaCO_2$ of 40 mmHg (5.3 kPa) is therefore equivalent to an end-tidal CO_2 of about 5 kPa. One atmospheric pressure is 760 mmHg or 101.33 kPa. That makes the end-tidal CO_2 percentage about 5%.*

c) *False.*

d) *False.*

e) *False.*

---

12. BIS monitor:

a) *False. BIS uses a linear dimensionless scale of 0–100 without any units. The lower the BIS value, the greater the hypnotic effect. General anaesthesia is between 40 and 60.*

b) *False. Hypothermia below 33°C decreases the BIS value as the electrical activity in brain is decreased by the low temperature.*

c) *True. The BIS value is not accurate during ketamine anaesthesia. Ketamine is a dissociative anaesthetic with excitatory effects on the EEG.*

d) *True. Newer versions have better protection from diathermy and EMG.*

e) *False. BIS monitors the electrical activity in the brain and not the concentration of a particular drug.*

---

13. Concerning ECG:

a) *False. The monitoring mode has a limited frequency response of 0.5–40 Hz whereas the diagnostic mode has a much wider range of 0.05–100 Hz.*

b) *False. The electrical activity of the heart has an electrical potentials range of 0.5–2 mV.*

c) *True. Surrounding the ECG leads with copper screens reduces interference due to electrostatic induction and capacitance coupling.*

d) *True. Silver and silver chloride form a stable electrode combination. They are held in a cup and separated from the skin by a foam pad soaked in conducting gel.*

e) *False. The standard in the UK is to use a display speed of 25 mm/s and a sensitivity of 1 mV/cm.*

---

14. Infrared spectrometry:

a) *False. CO_2 absorbs infrared radiation mainly at a wavelength of 4.3 μm.*

b) *True. Photo-acoustic spectrometry is more stable than the conventional infrared spectrometry. Its calibration remains constant over much longer periods of time.*

c) *True. This is not the case with the main-stream analysers.*

d) *True. Optical filters are used to select the desired wavelengths to avoid interference from other vapours or gases.*

e) *False. For the inhalational agents, higher wavelengths are used, such as 8–9 μm, to avoid interference from methane and alcohol (at 3.3 μm).*

---

15. b)

Chapter 11

Invasive monitoring

Invasive arterial pressure monitoring

Invasive arterial pressure monitoring provides beat-to-beat real-time information with sustained accuracy.

Components

1. An indwelling Teflon arterial cannula (20 or 22 G) is used (Fig. 11.1). The cannula has parallel walls to minimize the effect on blood flow to the distal parts of the limb. Cannulation can be achieved by directly threading the cannula (either by direct insertion method or a transfixation technique) or by using a modified Seldinger technique with a guidewire to assist in the insertion as in some designs (Fig. 11.2).

2. A column of bubble-free heparinized or plain 0.9% normal saline at a pressure of 300 mmHg, incorporating a flushing device.

3. Via the fluid column, the cannula is connected to a transducer (Figs 11.3–11.5). This in turn is connected to an amplifier and oscilloscope. A strain gauge variable resistor transducer is used.

4. The diaphragm (a very thin membrane) acts as an interface between the transducer and the fluid column.

5. The pressure transducer is a device that changes either electrical resistance or capacitance in response to changes in pressure on a solid-state device. The moving part of the transducer is very small and has little mass.

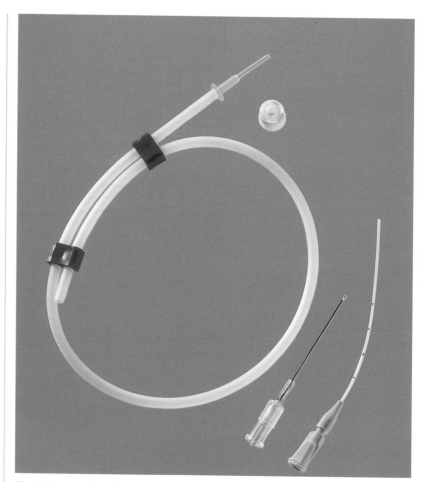

Fig. 11.2 Argon Careflow arterial cannula with its guidewire. (Courtesy of Argon Medical.)

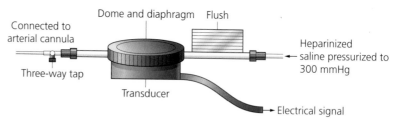

Fig. 11.3 Components of a pressure measuring system.

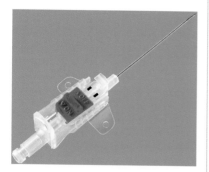

Fig. 11.1 BD Flowswitch arterial cannula. Note the on–off switch valve. (Courtesy of BD.)

Mechanism of action

1. The saline column moves back and forth with the arterial pulsation causing the diaphragm to move. This causes changes in the resistance and current flow through the wires of the transducer.

2. The transducer is connected to a Wheatstone bridge circuit

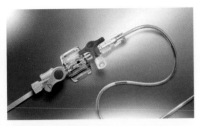

Fig. 11.4 Smith's Medex single-use disposable integrated pressure transducer.

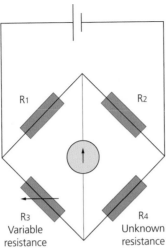

Fig. 11.6 The Wheatstone bridge circuit where null deflection of the galvanometer implies R1/R2 = R3/R4.

R1 R2

R3
Variable resistance

R4
Unknown resistance

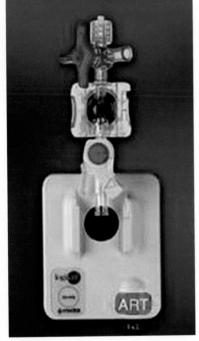

Fig. 11.5 Smith's Medex reusable pressure transducer.

(Fig. 11.6). This is an electrical circuit for the precise comparison of resistors. It uses a null-deflection system consisting of a very sensitive galvanometer and four resistors in two parallel branches: two constant resistors, a variable resistor and the unknown resistor. Changes in resistance and current are measured, electronically converted and displayed as systolic, diastolic and mean arterial pressures. The Wheatstone bridge circuit is ideal for measuring the small changes in resistance found in strain gauges. Most pressure transducers contain four strain gauges that form the four resistors of the Wheatstone bridge.

3. The flushing device allows 3–4 mL per hour of saline (or heparinized saline) to flush the cannula. This is to prevent clotting and backflow through the catheter. Manual flushing of the system is also possible when indicated.

4. The radial artery is the most commonly used artery because the ulnar artery is the dominant artery in the hand. The ulnar artery is connected to the radial artery through the palmar arch in 95% of patients. The brachial, femoral, ulnar or dorsalis pedis arteries are used occasionally.

5. The information gained from invasive arterial pressure monitoring includes heart rate, pulse pressure, the presence of a respiratory swing, left ventricular contractility, vascular tone (SVR) and stroke volume.

The arterial pressure waveform

1. This can be characterized as a complex sine wave that is the summation of a series of simple sine waves of different amplitudes and frequencies.

2. The fundamental frequency (or first harmonic) is equal to the heart rate, so a heart rate of 60 beats per min = 1 beat/s or 1 cycle/s or 1 Hz. The first 10 harmonics of the fundamental frequency contribute to the waveform.

3. The system used to measure arterial blood pressure should be capable of responding to a frequency range of 0.5–40 Hz in order to display the arterial waveform correctly.

4. The dicrotic notch in the arterial pressure waveform represents changes in pressure because of vibrations caused by the closure of the aortic valve.

5. The rate of rise of the upstroke part of the wave (dP/dt) reflects the myocardial contractility. A slow rise upstroke might indicate a need for inotropic support. A positive response to the inotropic support will show a steeper upstroke. The maximum upward slope of the arterial waveform during systole is related to the speed of ventricular ejection.

6. The position of the dicrotic notch on the downstroke of the wave reflects the peripheral vascular resistance. In vasodilated patients, e.g. following an epidural block or in septic patients, the dicrotic notch is positioned lower on the curve. The notch is higher in vasoconstricted patients.

7. The downstroke slope indicates resistance to outflow. A slow fall is seen in vasoconstriction.

8. The stroke volume can be estimated by measuring the area from the beginning of the upstroke to the dicrotic notch. Multiply that by the heart rate and the cardiac output can be estimated.

9. Systolic time indicates the myocardial oxygen demand. Diastolic time indicates myocardial oxygen supply.

10. Mean blood pressure is the average pressure throughout the cardiac cycle. As systole is shorter than diastole, the mean arterial pressure (MAP) is slightly less than the value half way between systolic and diastolic pressures. An estimate of MAP can be obtained by adding a third of the pulse pressure (systolic – diastolic pressure) to the diastolic pressure. MAP can also be determined by integrating a pressure signal over the duration of one cycle, divided by time.

The natural frequency

This is the frequency at which the monitoring system itself resonates and amplifies the signal by up to 20–40%. This determines the frequency response of the monitoring system. The natural frequency should be at least 10 times the fundamental frequency. The natural frequency of the measuring system is much higher than the primary frequency of the arterial waveform which is 1–2 Hz, corresponding to a heart rate of 60–120 beats/min. Stiffer (low compliance) tubing or a shorter length of tubing (less mass) produce higher natural frequencies. This results in the system requiring a much higher pulse rate before amplification.

The natural frequency of the monitoring system is:

1. directly related to the catheter diameter
2. inversely related to the square root of the system compliance
3. inversely related to the square root of the length of the tubing
4. inversely related to the square root of the density of the fluid in the system.

Problems in practice and safety features

1. The arterial pressure waveform should be displayed (Fig. 11.7)

in order to detect damping or resonance. The monitoring system should be able to apply an optimal damping value of 0.64.

a) *Damping* is caused by dissipation of stored energy. Anything that takes energy out of the system results in a progressive diminution of amplitude of oscillations. Increased damping lowers the systolic and elevates the diastolic pressures with loss of detail in the waveform. Damping can be caused by an air bubble (air is more compressible in comparison to the saline column), clot or a highly compliant, soft transducer diaphragm and tube.

b) *Resonance* occurs when the frequency of the driving force coincides with the resonant frequency of the system. If the natural frequency is less than 40 Hz, it falls within the range of the blood pressure and a sine wave will be superimposed on the blood pressure wave. Increased resonance elevates the systolic and lowers the diastolic pressures. The mean pressure should stay unchanged. Resonance can be due to a stiff, non-compliant diaphragm and tube. It is worse with tachycardia.

2. To determine the optimum damping of the system, a square wave test (fast flush test) is used (Fig. 11.8). The system is flushed by applying a pressure of 300 mmHg (compress and release the flush button or pull the lever located near the transducer). This results in a square waveform, followed by oscillations:

a. in an *optimally damped* system, there will be two or three oscillations before settling to zero
b. an *overdamped* system settles to zero without any oscillations.
c. an *underdamped* system oscillates for more than three to four cycles before settling to zero.

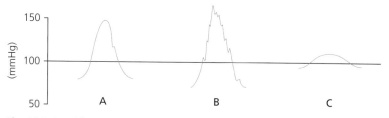

Fig. 11.7 Arterial pressure waveform. (A) Correct, optimally damped waveform. (B) Underdamped waveform. (C) Overdamped waveform.

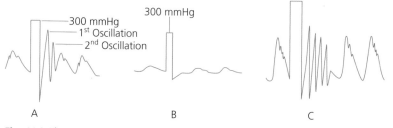

Fig. 11.8 The square wave test (fast flush test). (A) Optimally damped system. (B) Overdamped system. (C) Underdamped system.

3. The transducer should be positioned at the level of the right atrium as a reference point that is at the level of the midaxillary line. Raising or lowering the transducer above or below the level of the right atrium gives error readings equivalent to 7.5 mmHg for each 10 cm.

4. Ischaemia distal to the cannula is rare but should be monitored for. Multiple attempts at insertion and haematoma formation increase the risk of ischaemia.

5. Arterial thrombosis occurs in 20–25% of cases with very rare adverse effects such as ischaemia or necrosis of the hand. Cannulae in place for less than 24 h very rarely cause thrombosis.

6. The arterial pressure wave narrows and increases in amplitude in peripheral vessels. This makes the systolic pressure higher in the dorsalis pedis than in the radial artery. When compared to the aorta, peripheral arteries contain less elastic fibres so they are stiffer and less compliant. The arterial distensibility determines the amplitude and contour of the pressure waveform. In addition, the narrowing and bifurcation of arteries leads to impedance of forward blood flow, which results in backward reflection of the pressure wave.

7. There is risk of bleeding due to disconnection.

8. Inadvertent drug injection causes distal vascular occlusion and gangrene. An arterial cannula should be clearly labelled.

9. Local infection is thought to be less than 20%. Systemic infection is thought to be less than 5%. This is more common in patients with an arterial cannula for more than 4 days with a traumatic insertion.

10. Arterial cannulae should not be inserted in sites with evidence of infection and trauma or through a vascular prosthesis.

11. Periodic checks, calibrations and re-zeroing are carried out to prevent baseline drift of the transducer electrical circuits. Zero calibration eliminates the effect of atmospheric pressure on the measured pressure. This ensures that the monitor indicates zero pressure in the absence of applied pressure, so eliminating the *offset drift* (zero drift). To eliminate the *gradient drift*, calibration at a higher pressure is necessary. The transducer is connected to an aneroid manometer using a sterile tubing, through a three-way stopcock and the manometer pressure is raised to 100 and 200 mmHg. The monitor display should read the same pressure as is applied to the transducer (Fig. 11.9).

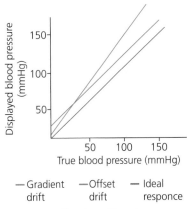

Fig. 11.9 Calibration of invasive pressure monitor.

Central venous catheterization and pressure (CVP)

The CVP is the filling pressure of the right atrium. It can be measured directly using a central venous catheter. The catheter can also be used to administer fluids, blood, drugs, parenteral nutrition and sample blood. Specialized catheters can be used for haemofiltration, haemodialysis (see Chapter 13, Haemofiltration) and transvenous pacemaker placement.

The tip of the catheter is usually positioned in the superior vena cava at the entrance to the right atrium. The internal jugular, subclavian and basilic veins are possible routes for central venous catheterization. The subclavian route is associated with the highest rate of complications but is convenient for the patient and for the nursing care.

The *Seldinger technique* is the common and standard method used for central venous catheterization (Fig. 11.10) regardless of catheter type. The procedure should be done under sterile conditions:

1. Introduce the needle into the vein using the appropriate

Invasive arterial blood pressure
- Consists of an arterial cannula, a heparinized saline column, a flushing device, a transducer, an amplifier and an oscilloscope.
- In addition to blood pressure, other parameters can be measured and estimated such as myocardial contractility, vascular tone and stroke volume.
- The waveform should be displayed to detect any resonance or damping.
- The measuring system should be able to cover a frequency range of 0.5–40 Hz.
- The monitoring system should be able to apply an optimal damping value of 0.64.

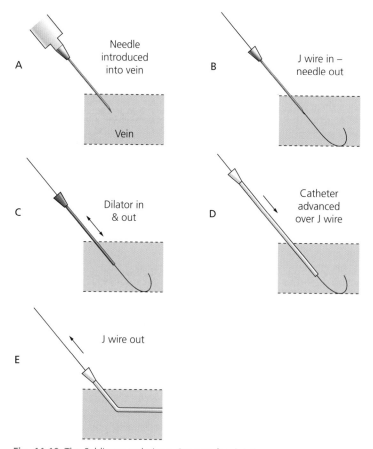

A Needle introduced into vein

Vein

B J wire in – needle out

C Dilator in & out

D Catheter advanced over J wire

E J wire out

Fig. 11.10 The Seldinger technique. See text for details.

landmarks or an ultrasound-locating device.

2. A J-shaped soft tip guidewire is introduced through the needle (and syringe in some designs) into the vein. The needle can then be removed. The J-shaped tip is designed to minimize trauma to the vessels' endothelium.

3. After a small incision in the skin has been made, a dilator is introduced over the guidewire to make a track through the skin and subcutaneous tissues and is then withdrawn.

4. The catheter is then railroaded over the guidewire into its final position before the guidewire is withdrawn.

5. Blood should be aspirated easily from all ports which should then be flushed with saline or heparin solution. All the port sites that are not intended for immediate use are sealed. A port should never be left open to air during insertion because of the risk of air embolism.

6. The catheter is secured onto the skin and covered with a sterile dressing.

7. A chest X-ray is performed to ensure correct positioning of the catheter and to detect pneumo-and/or haemothorax.

8. The use of ultrasound guidance should be routinely considered for the insertion of central venous catheters (Fig. 11.11). There is evidence to show that its use during internal jugular venous catheterization reduces the number of mechanical complications, the number of catheter-placement failures and the time required for insertion.

The CVP is read using either a pressure transducer or a water manometer.

PRESSURE TRANSDUCER

1. A similar measuring system to that used for invasive arterial pressure monitoring (catheter, heparinized saline column, transducer, diaphragm, flushing device and oscilloscope system). The transducer is positioned at the level of the right atrium.

2. A measuring system of limited frequency range is adequate because of the shape of the waveform and the values of the central venous pressure.

FLUID MANOMETER (FIG. 11.12)

1. A giving set with either normal saline or 5% dextrose is connected to the vertical manometer via a three-way tap. The latter is also connected to the central venous catheter.

2. The manometer has a spirit level side arm positioned at the level of the right atrium (zero reference point). The upper end of the column is open to air via a filter. This filter must stay dry to maintain direct connection with the atmosphere.

3. The vertical manometer is filled to about the 20-cm mark. By opening the three-way tap to the patient, a swing of the column should be seen with respiration. The CVP is read in cm H_2O when the fluid level stabilizes.

4. The manometer uses a balance of forces: downward pressure of the fluid (determined by density and height) against pressure of the central venous system (caused by hydrostatic and recoil forces).

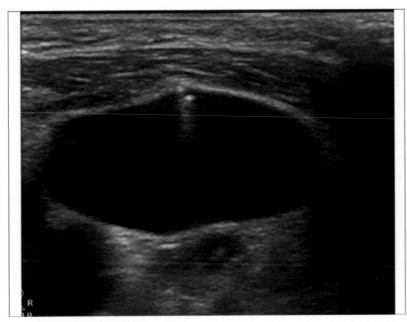

Fig. 11.11 Ultrsound image showing a needle in the internal jugular vein. The carotid artery at the left lower corner.

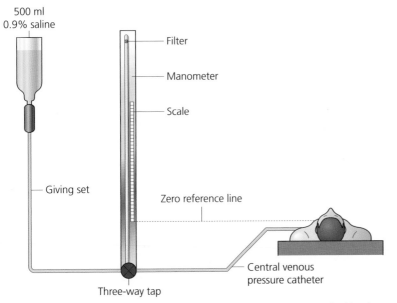

Fig. 11.12 Measurement of CVP using a manometer. The manometer's fluid level falls until the height of the fluid column above the zero reference point is equal to the CVP.

In both techniques, the monitoring system has to be zeroed at the level of the right atrium (usually at the midaxillary line). This eliminates the effect of hydrostatic pressure on the CVP value.

CATHETERS

There are different types of catheters used for central venous cannulation and CVP measurement. They differ in their lumen size, length, number of lumens, the presence or absence of a subcutaneous cuff and the material they are made of. The vast majority of catheters are designed to be inserted using the Seldinger technique although some are designed as 'long' intravenous cannulae (cannula over a needle) (Fig. 11.13).

Antimicrobial-coated catheters have been designed to reduce the incidence of catheter-related bloodstream infection. These can be either antiseptic coated (e.g. chlorhexidine/silver sulfadiazine, benzalkonium chloride, platinum/silver) or antibiotic coated (e.g. minocycline/rifampin) on either the internal or external surface or both. The antibiotic-coated central lines are thought to be more effective in reducing the incidence of infection (Fig. 11.14).

Multilumen catheter

1. The catheter has two or more lumens of different sizes, e.g. 16 G and 18 G (Fig. 11.15). Paediatric sizes also exist (Fig. 11.16).
2. The different lumens should be flushed with heparinized saline before insertion.
3. Single and double lumen versions exist.
4. Simultaneous administration of drugs and CVP monitoring is possible. It does not allow the insertion of a pulmonary artery catheter.
5. These catheters are made of polyurethane. This provides good tensile strength, allowing larger lumens for smaller internal diameter.

LONG CENTRAL CATHETERS/ PERIPHERALLY INSERTED CENTRAL CATHETERS (PICC)

1. These catheters, 60 cm in length, are designed to be inserted through an introducing cannula via an antecubital fossa vein, usually the basilic vein (Fig. 11.17).

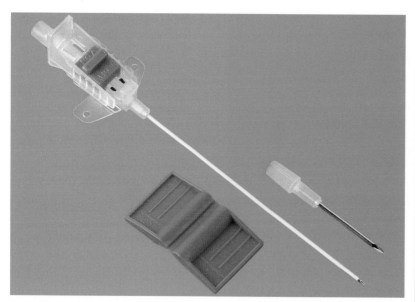

Fig. 11.13 Argon cannula over a needle central line. (Courtesy of Argon Medical Devices.)

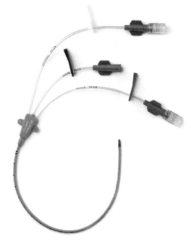

Fig. 11.14 Smith's Medex silver impregnated triple lumen central venous catheter. Both the inside and outside surfaces are impregnated with silver.

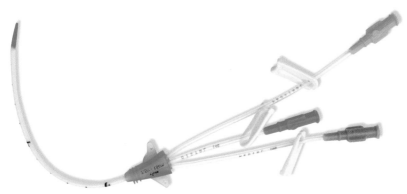

Fig. 11.15 An adult triple lumen catheter. (Courtesy of Vygon (UK) Ltd. © Vygon (UK) Ltd.)

2. They are used when a central catheter is required in situations when it is undesirable to gain access via the internal jugular or the subclavian veins, for example during head and neck surgery or prolonged antibiotic therapy. They are made of soft flexible polyurethane or silicone.

Hickman catheters

1. These central catheters are made of polyurethane or silicone and are usually inserted into the subclavian vein. The catheter can have one, two or three lumens (Fig. 11.18).
2. The proximal end is tunnelled under the skin for a distance of about 10 cm.
3. A Dacron cuff is positioned 3–4 cm from the site of entry into the vein under the skin. It induces a fibroblastic reaction to anchor the catheter in place (Fig. 11.19). The cuff also reduces the risk of infection as it stops the spread of infection from the site of entry to the skin. Some catheters also have a silver impregnated cuff that acts as an anti-microbial barrier.

4. They are used for long-term chemotherapy, parenteral nutrition, blood sampling or as a readily available venous access especially in children requiring frequent anaesthetics during cancer treatment.
5. These lines are designed to remain in situ for several months unless they become infected but require some degree of daily maintenance.

Dialysis catheters

These are large-calibre catheters designed to allow high flow rates of at least 300 mL/min. They are made of silicone or polyurethane. Most of them are dual lumen with staggered end and side holes to prevent admixture of blood at the inflow and outflow portions reducing recirculation.

Problems in practice and safety features

1. Inaccurate readings can be due to catheter blockage, catheter inserted too far or using the wrong zero level.
2. Pneumohaemothorax (with an incidence of 2–10% with

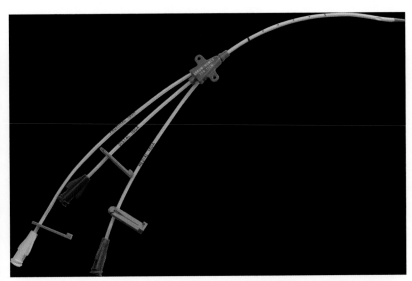

Fig. 11.16 A paediatric triple lumen catheter. (Courtesy of Vygon (UK) Ltd. © Vygon (UK) Ltd.)

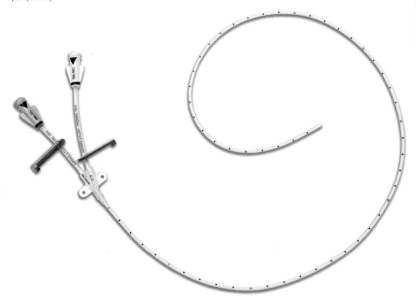

Fig. 11.17 Double lumen PICC line. (Courtesy of Teleflex Medical.)

subclavian vein catheterization and 1–2% with internal jugular catheterization), trauma to the arteries (carotid, subclavian and brachial), air embolism, haematoma and tracheal puncture are complications of insertion.

3. Sepsis and infection are common complications with an incidence of 2.8–20%. *Staphylococcus aureus* and *Enterococcus* are the most common organisms.

Guidelines for reduction in sepsis and infection rates with the use of central venous catheters

- Education and training of staff who insert and maintain the catheters.
- Use the maximum sterile barrier precautions during central venous catheter insertion.

- Use of >0.5% chlorhexidine preparation with alcohol preparations for skin antisepsis. If there is a contraindication to chlorhexidine, tincture of iodine, an iodophor or 70% alcohol can be used as alternative. Antiseptics should be allowed to dry according to the manufacturer's recommendation prior to placing the catheter.
- Use a subclavian site, rather than a jugular or a femoral site, in adult patients to minimize infection risk for non-tunneled CVC placement.
- Use ultrasound guidance to place central venous catheters (if this technology is available) to reduce the number of cannulation attempts and mechanical complications. Ultrasound guidance should only be used by those fully trained in its technique.
- Use a CVC with the minimum number of ports or lumens essential for the management of the patient.
- Promptly remove any intravascular catheter that is no longer essential.
- When adherence to aseptic technique cannot be ensured (i.e. catheters inserted during a medical emergency), replace the catheter as soon as possible, i.e. within 48 h.
- Use either sterile gauze or sterile, transparent, semipermeable dressing to cover the catheter site.
- Use a chlorhexidine/silver sulfadiazine or minocycline/ rifampin-impregnated CVC in patients whose catheter is expected to remain in place >5 days.

(Centers for Disease Control. 2011. Guidelines for the prevention of intravascular catheter-related infections)

4. A false passage may be created if the guidewire or dilator are advanced against resistance. The insertion should be smooth.

5. There may be cardiace complications such as self-limiting arrhythmias due to the irritation caused by the guidewire or catheter. Gradual withdrawal of the device is usually adequate to restore normal rhythm. More serious but unusual complication such as venous or cardiac perforation can be lethal.

6. Catheter-related venous thrombosis is thought to be up to 40% depending on the site, the duration of placement, the technique and the condition of the patient.

7. Microshock. A central venous catheter presents a direct pathway to the heart muscle. Faulty electrical equipment can produce minute electrical currents (less than 1 ampere) which can travel via this route to the myocardium. This can produce ventricular fibrillation (VF) if the tip of the catheter is in direct contact with the myocardium (see Chapter 14). This very small current does not cause any adverse effects if applied to the body surface, but if passed directly to the heart, the current density will be high enough to cause VF, hence the name microshock.

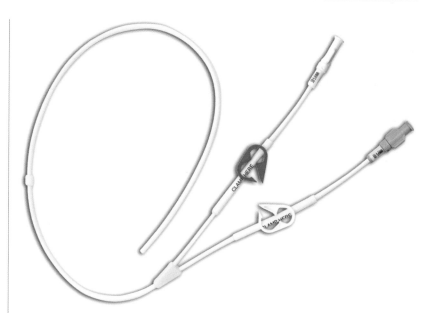

Fig. 11.18 A double lumen long-term Hickman catheter. Note the Dacron cuff. (Courtesy of Vygon (UK) Ltd. © Vygon (UK) Ltd.)

> **Central venous catheterization and pressure**
> - There are different routes of insertion, e.g. the internal jugular, subclavian and basilic veins.
> - The Seldinger technique is the most commonly used.
> - The catheters differ in size, length, number of lumens and material.
> - A pressure transducer or water manometer is used to measure CVP.
> - Sepsis and infection are common.
> - Antibiotic- and/or antiseptic-coated catheters can reduce the incidence of infections.

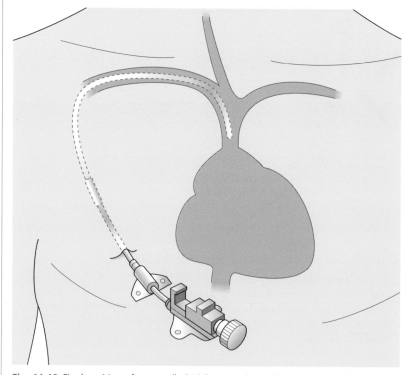

Fig. 11.19 Final position of a tunnelled Hickman catheter. (Reproduced with permission from Viggo-Spectramed, a division of BOC Health Care.)

Invasive electrocardiogram (ECG)

In addition to using skin electrodes to record ECG, other more invasive methods can be used (Fig. 11.20). The following methods can be used:

1. Oesophageal ECG can be recorded by using oesophageal electrodes that are incorporated into an oesophageal stethoscope and temperature probe. It has been found to be useful in detecting atrial arrhythmias. As it is positioned near the posterior aspect of the left ventricle, it can be helpful in detecting posterior wall ischaemia.
2. Intracardiac ECG with electrodes inserted using a multipurpose pulmonary artery flotation catheter. There are three atrial and two ventricular electrodes. In addition to ECG recording, these electrodes can be used in atrial or AV pacing. Such ECG recording has great diagnostic capabilities and can be part of an implantable defibrillator. It is used for loci that cannot be assessed by body surface electrodes, such as the bundle of His or ventricular septal activity,
3. Tracheal ECG using two electrodes embedded into a tracheal tube. It is useful in diagnosing atrial arrhythmias especially in children

Cardiac output

Cardiac output monitoring (the measurement of flow, rather than pressure) has been the subject

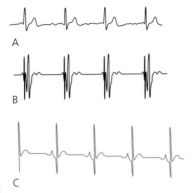

Fig. 11.20 Invasive ECG. (A) Skin electrodes. (B) Oesophageal. (C) Intracardiac.

of a lot of technical development over the last decade. It is helpful to consider the history of this development briefly.

The pulmonary artery (PA) catheter was developed in the 1970s and was the only bed-side piece of equipment available to measure cardiac output. It gained widespread acceptance in the intensive care and anaesthetic community. However, it lost favour due to its technically demanding insertion. Also some papers appeared in journals during the late 1980s and mid 1990s associating its use with an increased mortality in patients. This has now been now refuted, however it remains challenging to insert in some circumstances.

As a result, there was a strong move to adopt less invasive technologies and develop them to replace the PA catheter.

The following techniques exist to provide measurement of cardiac output. Some use a combination of these, for example LiDCO, which uses lithium indicator dilution to calibrate its arterial waveform analysis software. Detailed discussion of each is beyond the

scope of this book and the reader is referred to the further reading section.

1. Arterial waveform analysis either via direct arterial cannulation or 'simulated' via a plethysmographic trace (such as that obtained with the pulse oximeter):
   a) pulse contour analysis
   b) conservation of mass
   c) PRAM Vytech Mostcare (pressure recording analytical method)
   d) pleth variability index (Masimo PVI).
2. Aortic velocimetry using:
   a) Doppler frequency shift (oesophageal and suprasternal Doppler)
   b) electrical velocimetry (Aesculon and Icon).
3. Formal echocardiography:
   a) transoesophageal
   b) transthoracic.
4. Transthoracic impedence.
5. Pulmonary gas clearance.
6. Indicator dilution:
   a) Thermal dilution
   b) Lithium dilution
   c) Dye dilution.
7. Electrical velocimetry (EV) is the technique which non-invasively measures rate-of-change of electrical conductivity of blood in the aorta using four standard ECG surface electrodes.

Balloon-tipped flow-guided pulmonary artery catheter

Pulmonary artery (PA) catheters are usually inserted via the internal jugular or subclavian veins via an introducer. They are floated through the right atrium and ventricle into the pulmonary artery.

Components

PA catheters are available in sizes 5–8 G and are usually 110 cm in length (Fig. 11.21). They have up to five lumens and are marked at 10-cm intervals:

1. The distal lumen ends in the pulmonary artery. It is used to measure PA and pulmonary capillary wedge (PCW) pressures and to sample mixed venous blood.
2. The proximal lumen should ideally open in the right atrium, being positioned about 30 cm from the tip of the catheter. It can be used to continuously monitor the CVP, to administer the injectate to measure the cardiac output (by thermodilution) or to infuse fluids. Depending on the design, a second proximal lumen may be present which is usually dedicated to infusions of drugs.
3. Another lumen contains two insulated wires leading to a thermistor that is about 3.7 cm from the catheter tip. Proximally it is connected to a cardiac output computer.
4. The balloon inflation lumen is used to inflate the balloon which is situated at the catheter tip.

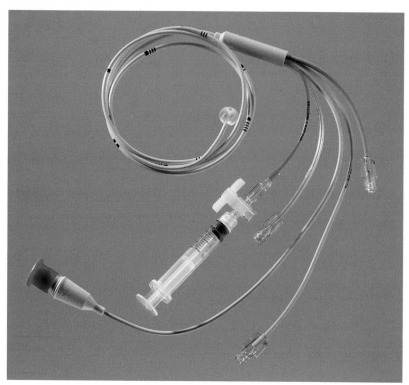

Fig. 11.21 Argon balloon-tipped flow-guided pulmonary artery catheter with five lumens. (Courtesy of Argon Medical Devices.)

Up to 1.5 mL of air is needed. When the balloon is inflated, the catheter floats with the blood flow into a pulmonary artery branch (Fig. 11.22).

Mechanism of action

1. Before insertion, flush all the lines and test the balloon with 1–1.5 mL of air.
2. The distal lumen of the catheter is connected to a transducer pressure measuring system for continuous monitoring as the catheter is advanced. As the catheter passes via the superior vena cava to the right atrium, low pressure waves (mean of 3–8 mmHg normally) are displayed (Fig. 11.23). The distance from the internal jugular or the subclavian vein to the right atrium is about 15–20 cm.
3. The balloon is partly inflated, enabling the blood flow to carry the catheter tip through the tricuspid valve into the right ventricle. Tall pressure waves (15–25 mmHg systolic and 0–10 mmHg diastolic) are displayed.
4. As the balloon tip floats through the pulmonary valve into the PA, the pressure waveform changes with higher diastolic pressure (10–20 mmHg), but similar systolic pressures. The dicrotic notch, caused by the closure of the pulmonary valve, can be noted. The distance from the

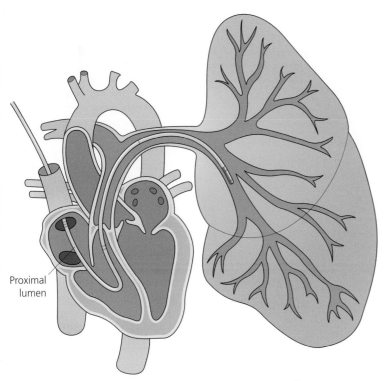

Proximal lumen

Fig. 11.22 Position of the pulmonary artery catheter tip in a pulmonary artery branch. The desired position of the proximal lumen in the right atrium is indicated by an arrow.

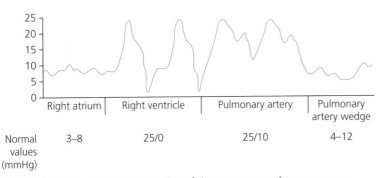

	Right atrium	Right ventricle	Pulmonary artery	Pulmonary artery wedge
Normal values (mmHg)	3–8	25/0	25/10	4–12

Fig. 11.23 Diagrammatic representation of the pressure waveforms seen as a pulmonary artery flotation catheter is advanced until it wedges in a branch of the pulmonary artery.

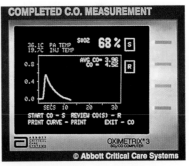

COMPLETED C.O. MEASUREMENT

Fig. 11.24 The Abbott cardiac output computer. Cardiac output is measured using a thermodilution technique which produces a temperature–time curve. Cardiac output is computed from this information. When connected to the appropriate catheter, mixed venous oxygen saturation (SvO_2) can also be monitored.

right ventricle to the pulmonary artery should be less than 10 cm, unless there is cardiomegaly.

5. The balloon is fully inflated enabling the blood flow to carry the tip of the catheter into a pulmonary artery branch, where it wedges. This is shown as a damped pressure waveform (pulmonary capillary wedge pressure (PCWP), mean pressure of 4–12 mmHg). This reflects the left atrial filling pressure. The balloon should then be deflated so the catheter floats back into the PA. The balloon should be kept deflated until another PCWP reading is required.

6. The cardiac output can be measured using thermodilution. Ten mL of cold injectate is administered upstream via the proximal lumen. The thermistor (in the pulmonary artery) measures the change in temperature of the blood downstream. A temperature–time curve is displayed from which the computer can calculate the cardiac output (Fig. 11.24). The volume of injectate should be known accurately and the whole volume injected quickly. Usually the mean of three readings is taken. Because of the relatively high incidence of complications, less invasive techniques are being developed to measure the cardiac output. Thermodilution remains the standard method for measuring the cardiac output.

7. Some designs have the facility to continuously monitor the mixed venous oxygen saturation using

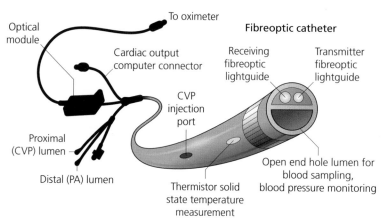

Fibreoptic catheter

Fig. 11.25 Mechanism of action of the Abbott Oximetrix pulmonary artery catheter. This uses fibreoptic technology to measure mixed venous oxygen saturation (SvO_2).

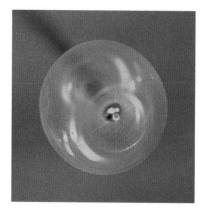

Fig. 11.26 The Abbott Oximetrix pulmonary artery catheter tip.

fibreoptic technology (Figs 11.25 and 11.26). Cardiac pacing capability is present in some designs.

Information gained from PA catheter

The responses to fluid challenges and therapeutic regimens are monitored in preference to isolated individual readings. The following can be measured: CVP, right ventricular (RV) pressure, PA pressure, PCWP, cardiac output, cardiac index, stroke volume, stroke volume index, left and right ventricular stroke work index, systemic vascular resistance, pulmonary vascular resistance, mixed venous oximetry (SvO_2), blood temperature and degree of shunt.

Problems in practice and safety features

The overall morbidity of such catheters is 0.4%.

1. Complications due to central venous cannulation (as above).
2. Complications due to catheter passage and advancement. These include arrhythmias (ventricular ectopics, ventricular tachycardia and others), heart block, knotting/kinking (common in low-flow states and patients with large hearts; a 'rule of thumb' is that the catheter should not be advanced more than 10–15 cm without a change in the pressure waveform), valvular damage and perforation of PA vessel.
3. Complications due to the presence in the PA. These include thrombosis (can be reduced by the use of heparin-bonded catheters), PA rupture (more common in the elderly, may present as haemoptysis and is often fatal), infection, balloon rupture, pulmonary infarction, valve damage and arrhythmias.
4. In certain conditions, the PCWP does not accurately reflect left ventricular filling pressure. Such conditions include mitral stenosis and regurgitation, left atrial myxoma, ball valve thrombus, pulmonary veno-occlusive disease, total anomalous pulmonary venous drainage, cardiac tamponade and acute right ventricular dilatation resulting from right ventricular infarction, massive pulmonary embolism and acute severe tricuspid regurgitation.
5. Catheter whip can occur because of the coursing of the pulmonary catheter through the right heart. Cardiac contractions can produce 'shock transients' or 'whip' artifacts. Negative deflections due to a whip artifact may lead to an underestimation of pulmonary artery pressures.

Balloon-tipped flow-guided pulmonary artery catheter

- Inserted via a large central vein into the right atrium, right ventricle, pulmonary artery and branch with contiguous pressure monitoring.
- Used to measure left ventricular filling pressure in addition to other parameters.
- Complications are due to central venous cannulation, the passage of the catheter through different structures and the presence of the catheter in the circulation.
- PCWP does not accurately reflect left ventricular (LV) filling pressure in certain conditions.

Oesophageal Doppler haemodynamic measurement

An estimate of cardiac output can be quickly obtained using the minimally invasive oesophageal Doppler. Patient response to therapeutic manoeuvres (e.g. fluid challenge) can also be rapidly assessed. The technique has the advantage of the smooth muscle tone of the oesophagus acting as a natural means of maintaining the probe in position for repeated measurements. In addition, the oesophagus is in close anatomical proximity to the aorta so that signal interference from bone, soft tissue and lung is minimized. Over the past three decades, the oesophageal Doppler has evolved from an experimental technique to a relatively simple bed-side procedure with the latest models incorporating both Doppler and echo-ultrasound in a single probe.

The measurement of cardiac output using the oesophageal Doppler method correlates well with that obtained from a pulmonary artery catheter. Oesophageal Doppler ultrasonography has been used for intravascular volume optimization in both the perioperative period and in the critical care setting. Its use in cardiac, general and orthopaedic surgery has been associated with a reduction in morbidity and hospital stay. Because of the mild discomfort associated with placing the probe and maintaining it in a fixed position, patients require adequate sedation.

Components

1. A monitor housing:
   a) a screen for visual verification of correct signal measurement (Fig. 11.27)
   b) technology that enables beat-to-beat calculation of the stroke volume and cardiac output.
2. An insulated, thin, latex-free silicone oesophageal probe containing a Doppler transducer angled at 45° (Fig. 11.27). The probe has a diameter of 6 mm with an internal spring coil to ensure flexibility and rigidity.

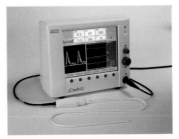

Fig. 11.27 The CardioQ oesophageal Doppler machine and attached probe (foreground).

Mechanism of action

1. The device relies on the Doppler principle. There is an increase in observed frequency of a signal when the signal source approaches the observer and a decrease when the source moves away.
2. The changes in the frequency of the transmitted ultrasound result from the encounter of the wavefront with moving red blood cells. If the transmitted sound waves encounter a group of red cells moving towards the source, they are reflected back at a frequency higher than that at which they were sent, producing a *positive Doppler shift*. The opposite effect occurs when a given frequency sent into tissues encounters red cells moving away. The result is the return of a frequency lower than that transmitted, resulting in a *negative Doppler shift*. Analysis of the reflected frequencies allows determination of velocity of flow.
3. The lubricated probe is inserted via the mouth with the bevel of the tip facing up at the back of the patient's throat into the distal oesophagus to a depth of about 35–40 cm from the teeth.
4. The probe is rotated and slowly pulled back while listening to the audible signal. The ideal probe tip location is at the level between the fifth and sixth

thoracic vertebrae because, at that level, the descending aorta is adjacent and parallel to the distal oesophagus. This location is achieved by superficially landmarking the distance to the third sternocostal junction anteriorly. A correctly positioned probe can measure the blood flow in this major vessel using a high ultrasound frequency of 4 MHz.
5. The Doppler signal waveform is analysed and the stroke volume and total cardiac output are computed using the Doppler equation and a normogram which corrects for variations found with differing patient age, sex and body surface area.

The Doppler equation

$$v = \frac{cf_d}{2f_T \cos\theta}$$

where:
v is flow velocity
c is speed of sound in body tissue (1540 m/s)
f_d is Doppler frequency shift
$\cos\theta$ is cosine of angle between sound beam and blood flow (45°)
f_T is frequency of transmitted ultrasound (Hz).

---

6. The parameters obtained from analysis of the Doppler signal waveform allow the operator to gain an assessment of cardiac output, stroke volume, volaemic status, systemic vascular resistance and myocardial function (Fig. 11.28).

Problems in practice and safety features

1. The probe is fully insulated and safe when diathermy is being used.
2. The probe cannot easily be held in the correct position for long periods. Frequent repositioning

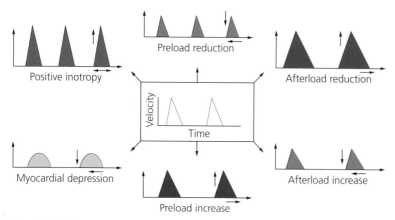

Fig. 11.28 Changes in oesophageal Doppler waveform associated with a variety of clinical situations. (Reproduced with permission from Dr M Singer.)

may be necessary if continuous monitoring is required.

3. Oesophageal Doppler measurement can only be used in an adequately sedated, intubated patient. Its use in awake patients has been described using local anaesthesia. A suprasternal probe is also available and can be used in awake patients.

4. Insertion of the probe is not recommended in patients with pharyngo-oesophageal pathology (e.g. oesophageal varices).

5. The role of the oesophageal Doppler in children is still being evaluated.

Oesophageal Doppler

- Minimally invasive and rapid estimate of cardiac output using the Doppler principle.
- Insulated Doppler probe lies in the distal oesophagus emitting a high ultrasound frequency of 4 MHz.
- Continuous monitoring is possible, although frequent probe repositioning is a problem.

LiDCOrapid

This is a cardiac output monitor that uses arterial pressure waveform analysis software to generate a 'nominal' cardiac output value. Because it does not require calibration, it can be quickly set up and the effects of fluids or inotropes assessed (Fig. 11.29).

Components

1. Monitor housing containing:
   a) screen displaying real-time cardiac output parameters
   b) software technology for computing the cardiac output and other parameters
   c) electrical connection feeding the arterial waveform from the patient's bed-side invasive pressure monitor.

Mechanism of action

1. The patient's existing invasive blood pressure trace is fed by a cable into the LiDCOrapid. From this, the software algorithm generates a nominal stroke volume and cardiac output.

2. The LiDCOrapid displays the following parameters: heart rate, pressures (MAP, systolic and diastolic), stroke volume and cardiac output.

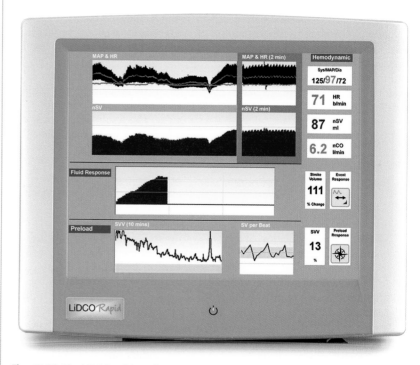

Fig. 11.29 The LiDCOrapid cardiac output monitor.

3. Dynamic preload parameters can also be generated by the software to assess the stroke volume response to a fluid challenge.

Problems in practice and safety features

The performance of the software may be compromised in the following patient groups:

1. Patients with aortic valve regurgitation.
2. Patients being treated with an intra-aortic balloon pump or cardiac arrythmias that will disrupt the usual arterial waveform pattern.
3. Patients with highly damped peripheral arterial lines or with pronounced peripheral arterial vasoconstriction.
4. The Lidco Plus can be calibrated using a single-point lithium indicator dilution process. This offers more accurate cardiac output measurement.

Temperature probes

Monitoring a patient's temperature during surgery is a common and routine procedure. Different types of thermometers are available.

THERMISTOR

Components

1. A small bead of a temperature-dependent semiconductor.
2. Wheatstone bridge circuit.

Mechanism of action

1. The thermistor has electrical resistance which changes non-linearly with temperature.

The response is made linear electronically. This property allows them to accurately measure temperature to an order of 0.1°C.

2. It can be made in very small sizes and is relatively cheap to manufacture.
3. It is mounted in a plastic or stainless steel probe making it mechanically robust, and it can be chemically sterilized.
4. It is used in PA catheters to measure cardiac output.
5. In the negative thermal conductivity thermistors, such as cobalt oxide, copper oxide and manganese oxide, the electrical resistance decreases as the temperature increases. In the positive thermal conductivity thermistors, such as barium titanate, the electrical resistance increases with the temperature.

Problems in practice and safety features

Thermistors need to be stabilized as they age.

INFRARED TYMPANIC THERMOMETER

Components

1. A small probe with a disposable and transparent cover is inserted into the external auditory meatus.
2. The detector (which consists of a series of thermocouples called a thermopile).

Mechanism of action

1. The detector receives infrared radiation from the tympanic membrane.
2. The infrared signal detected is converted into an electrical signal that is processed to

measure accurately the core temperature within 3 s.
3. The rate of radiation by an object is proportional to temperature to the fourth power.

Problems in practice and safety features

1. Non-continuous intermittent readings.
2. The probe has to be accurately aimed at the tympanic membrane. False low readings from the sides of the ear canal can be a problem.
3. Wax in the ear can affect the accuracy.

THERMOCOUPLES

These are devices that make use of the principle that two different metals in contact generate a voltage, which is temperature dependent (Fig. 11.30).

Components

1. Two strips of dissimilar metals (0.4–2-mm diameter) of different specific heats and in contact from both ends. Usually copper-constantan (copper with 40% nickel) junctions are used.
2. A galvanometer.

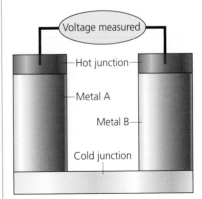

Fig. 11.30 Thermocouple.

Mechanism of action

1. One junction is used as the measuring junction whereas the other one is the reference. The latter is kept at a constant temperature.
2. The metals expand and contract to different degrees with change in temperature producing an electrical potential that is compared to a reference junction. The current produced is directly proportional to the temperature difference between the two junctions, i.e. there is a linear relationship between voltage and temperature.
3. The voltage produced is called the Seebeck effect or thermoelectric effect.
4. The measuring junction produces a potential of 40 μV per °C. This potential is measured by an amplifier.
5. They are stable and accurate to 0.1°C.
6. If multiple thermocouples are linked in series, they constitute a thermopile. This is done to improve their sensitivity

Body core temperature can be measured using different sites:

1. *Rectal* temperature does not accurately reflect the core temperature in anaesthetized patients. During an operation, changes in temperature are relatively rapid and the rectal temperature lags behind.
2. *Oesophageal* temperature accurately reflects the core temperature with the probe positioned in the lower oesophagus (at the level of the left atrium). Here the probe is not affected by the cooler tracheal temperature (Fig. 11.31).
3. *Tympanic membrane* temperature is closely associated with brain temperature. It

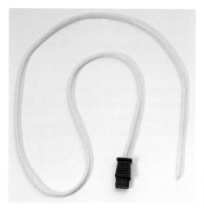

Fig. 11.31 Oesophageal/rectal temperature probe.

accurately reflects core temperature, compared with lower oesophageal temperature. Thermocouple and thermistor probes as well as the infrared probe can be used (Figs 11.32 and 11.33).

4. *Bladder* temperature correlates well with the core temperature when there is a normal urine output (Fig. 11.34).

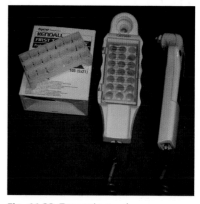

Fig. 11.33 Tympanic membrane thermometer.

5. *Skin* temperature, when measured with the core temperature, can be useful in determining the volaemic status of the patient (Fig. 11.35).

The axilla is the best location for monitoring muscle temperature, making it most suitable for detecting malignant hyperthermia.

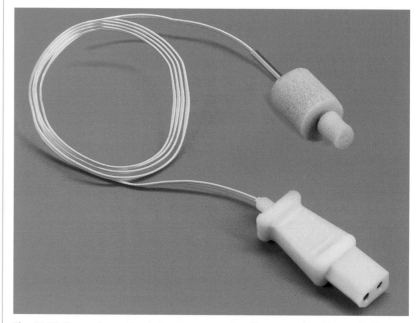

Fig. 11.32 Tympanic membrane temperature probe. (Courtesy of Smiths Medical.)

Temperature probes

- They can be thermistors, thermocouples or infrared thermometers.
- Core and skin temperatures can be measured.
- Core temperature can be measured from the rectum, oesophagus, tympanic membrane or the bladder.

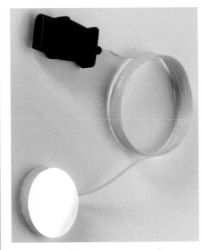

Fig. 11.35 Skin temperature probe.

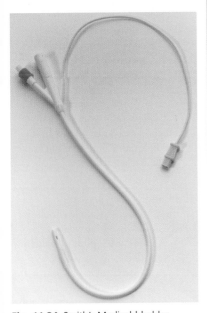

Fig. 11.34 Smith's Medical bladder catheter with a temperature probe.

FURTHER READING

Centers for Disease Control and Prevention, 2011. Guidelines for the prevention of intravascular catheter-related infections. Online. Available at: http://www.cdc.gov/hicpac/pdf/guidelines/bsi-guidelines-2011.pdf.

National Institute for Health and Clinical Excellence, 2008. Inadvertent perioperative hypothermia. The management of inadvertent perioperative hypothermia in adults. Online. Available at: http://www.nice.org.uk/nicemedia/pdf/CG65NICEGuidance.pdf.

NHS, 2008. Infusions and sampling from arterial lines. Online. Available at: http://www.nrls.npsa.nhs.uk/resources/?entryid45=59891&p=10.

Shoemaker, W.C., Velmahos, G.C., Demetriades, D., 2002. Procedures and monitoring for the critically ill. WB Saunders, Philadelphia.

MCQs

In the following lists, which of the statements (a) to (e) are true?

1. Thermometers:
   a) The electrical resistance of a thermistor changes non-linearly with temperature.
   b) Thermocouples are used in measuring cardiac output using the thermodilution method.
   c) The Seebeck effect is used to measure the temperature with thermocouples.
   d) Thermometers can be used to measure core and peripheral temperatures at the same time.
   e) A galvanometer is used to measure the potential in a thermocouple.

2. Concerning direct arterial blood pressure measurement:
   a) A 16-G radial artery cannula is suitable.
   b) The position of the dicrotic notch in the waveform can reflect the vascular tone.
   c) The monitoring system should be capable of responding to a frequency range of up to 40 Hz.
   d) Increased damping of the waveform causes an increase in systolic pressure and a decrease in diastolic pressure.
   e) Air bubbles produce an overdamped waveform.

3. Balloon-tipped flow-guided pulmonary artery catheter:
   a) They can have up to five separate lumens.
   b) They measure the cardiac output using the Doppler technique.
   c) The balloon should be left wedged and inflated in order to get a continuous reading of the left ventricular filling pressure.
   d) Mixed venous blood oxygen saturation can be measured.
   e) They use a thermocouple at the tip to measure the temperature of the blood.

4. If the mean arterial blood pressure is 100 mmHg, pulmonary capillary wedge pressure is 10 mmHg, mean pulmonary artery pressure is 15 mmHg, cardiac output is 5 L/min and CVP is 5 mmHg, which of the following statements are correct?
   a) The unit for vascular resistance is dyne s^{-1} cm^5.
   b) The pulmonary vascular resistance is about 800.
   c) The peripheral vascular resistance is about 1500.
   d) The patient has pulmonary hypertension.
   e) The patient has normal peripheral vascular resistance.

5. Concerning central venous pressure and cannulation:
   a) 10 mmHg is equivalent to 7.5 cm H_2O.
   b) During cannulation, the left internal jugular vein is the approach of choice since the heart lies mainly in the left side of the chest.
   c) Subclavian vein cannulation has a higher incidence of pneumothorax than the internal jugular vein.
   d) The 'J'-shaped end of the guidewire is inserted first.
   e) The Dacron cuff used in a Hickman's line is to anchor the catheter only.

6. In an invasive pressure measurement system, which of the following is/are correct:
   a) A clot causes high systolic and low diastolic pressures.
   b) A transducer diaphragm with very low compliance causes low systolic and high diastolic pressures.
   c) A soft wide lumen catheter causes low systolic and high diastolic pressures.
   d) An air bubble causes low systolic and diastolic pressures.
   e) A short and narrow lumen catheter is ideal.

7. Concerning the oesophageal Doppler:
   a) The ideal probe location is at the level between the fifth and sixth thoracic vertebrae.
   b) It emits a pulsed ultrasound wave of 4 Hz.
   c) Red cells moving towards the ultrasound source reflect the sound back at a frequency lower than that at which it was sent, producing a positive Doppler shift.
   d) The oesophageal probe tip is located at a depth of about 40 cm.
   e) The angle between the ultrasound beam and blood flow is 75°.

SINGLE BEST ANSWER (SBA)

8. Direct arterial pressure monitoring:
   a) A minimum of a 16-G cannula should be used.
   b) Bubbles of air in the transducer aid accuracy.
   c) The first 10 harmonics of the fundamental frequency can be ignored.
   d) The system needs to respond to a frequency range of 0.5–40 Hz.
   e) Vasoconstriction lowers the position of the dicrotic notch.

Answers

1. Thermometers:
   a) *True. The response is non-linear but can be made linear electronically.*
   b) *False. Thermistors are used in measuring the cardiac output by thermodilution. Thermocouples are not used in measuring the cardiac output by thermodilution.*
   c) *True. The Seebeck effect is when the electrical potential produced at the junction of two dissimilar metals is dependent on the temperature of the junction. This is the principle used in thermocouples.*
   d) *True. The gradient between the core and peripheral temperatures is useful in assessing the degree of skin perfusion and the circulatory volume. For example, hypovolaemia causes a decrease in skin perfusion which reduces the peripheral temperature and thus increases the gradient. The normal gradient is about 2–4°C.*
   e) *True. The galvanometer is placed between the junctions of the thermocouple, the reference and the measuring junctions. This allows the current to be measured. Changes in current are calibrated to measure the temperature difference between the two junctions.*

2. Concerning direct arterial blood pressure measurement:
   a) *False. A 16-G cannula is far too big to be inserted into an artery. 20-G or 22-G cannulae are usually used allowing adequate blood flow to pass by the cannula distally.*
   b) *True. The position of the dicrotic notch (which represents the closure of the aortic valve) is on the downstroke curve. A high dicrotic notch can be seen in vasoconstricted patients with high peripheral vascular resistance. A low dicrotic notch can be seen in vasodilated patients (e.g. patients with epidurals or sepsis).*
   c) *True. The addition of the shape of the dicrotic notch to an already simple waveform makes a maximum frequency of 40 Hz adequate for such a monitoring system. Because of the complicated waveform of the ECG, the monitoring system requires a much wider range of frequencies (maximum of 100 Hz).*
   d) *False. Increased damping leads to a decrease in systolic pressure and an increase in diastolic pressure. Decreased damping causes the opposite. The mean pressure remains the same.*
   e) *True. This is due to the difference in the compressibility of the two media, air and saline. Air is more compressible in contrast to the saline column.*

3. Balloon-tipped flow-guided pulmonary artery catheter:
   a) *True. The most distal lumen is in the pulmonary artery. There are one or two proximal lumens in the right atrium: one lumen carries the insulated wires leading to the thermistor proximal to the tip of the catheter and another lumen is used to inflate the balloon at the tip of the catheter.*
   b) *False. The cardiac output is measured by thermodilution. A 'cold' injectate (e.g. saline) is injected via the proximal lumen. The changes in blood temperature are measured by the thermistor in the pulmonary artery. A temperature–time curve is displayed from which the cardiac output can be calculated.*
   c) *False. Leaving the balloon wedged and inflated is dangerous and should not be done. This is due to the risk of ischaemia to the distal parts of the lungs supplied by the pulmonary artery or its branches.*
   d) *True. Using fibreoptics, the mixed venous oxygen saturation can be measured on some designs. This allows the calculation of oxygen extraction by the tissues.*
   e) *False. A thermistor is used to measure the temperature of the blood. Thermistors are made to very small sizes.*

4. If the mean arterial blood pressure is 100 mmHg, pulmonary capillary wedge pressure is 10 mmHg, mean pulmonary artery pressure is 15 mmHg, cardiac output is 5 L/min and CVP is 5 mmHg, which of the following statements are correct?
   a) *False. The unit for vascular resistance is dyne s cm^{-5}.*
   b) *False. The pulmonary vascular resistance = mean pulmonary artery pressure*

– left atrial pressure × 80/ cardiac output (15 − 10 × 80/5 = 80 dyne s cm^{-5}).

c) *True.* The peripheral vascular resistance = mean arterial pressure − right atrial pressure × 80/cardiac output (100 − 5 × 80/5 = 1520 dyne s cm^{-5}.

d) *False.* The normal mean pulmonary artery pressure is about 15 mmHg (systolic pressure of about 25 and a diastolic pressure of about 10 mmHg) and pulmonary vascular resistance is 80–120 dyne s cm^{-5}.

e) *True.* The normal peripheral vascular resistance is 1000–1500 dyne s cm^{-5}.

---

5. Concerning central venous pressure and cannulation:
a) *False.* 10 cm H$_2$O is equivalent to 7.5 mmHg or 1 kPa.
b) *False.* The right internal jugular is usually preferred first as the internal jugular, the brachiocephalic veins and the superior vena cava are nearly in a straight line.
c) *True.* The higher incidence of pneumothorax with the subclavian approach makes the internal jugular the preferred vein.
d) *True.* The 'J'-shaped end of the guidewire is inserted first because it is atraumatic and soft.
e) *False.* In addition to anchoring the catheter, the cuff also reduces the risk of infection by stopping the spread of infection from the site of skin entry. Some catheters have a silver impregnated cuff that acts as an anti-microbial barrier.

---

6. In an invasive pressure measurement system, which of the following is/are correct:
a) *False.* A clot will cause damping of the system as pressure changes are not accurately transmitted. The systolic pressure is decreased and the diastolic pressure is increased.
b) *False.* A too rigid diaphragm will cause the system to resonate. This leads to high systolic and low diastolic pressures.
c) *True.* A soft wide lumen catheter will increase the damping of the system (see a) above).
d) *False.* An air bubble will increase the damping of the system (see a) above).
e) *True.* A catheter that is short and narrow allows transmission of pressure changes accurately. For clinical use, a maximum length of 2 m is acceptable.

---

7. Concerning the oesophageal Doppler:
a) *True.* The ideal probe tip location is at the level between the fifth and sixth thoracic vertebrae. At that level, the descending aorta is adjacent and parallel to the distal oesophagus. This location is achieved by superficially landmarking the distance to the third sternocostal junction anteriorly.
b) *False.* The frequency used is 4 MHz.
c) *False.* Red cells moving towards the ultrasound source reflect the sound back at a frequency higher than that at which they were sent, producing a positive Doppler shift. The opposite produces a negative Doppler shift.
d) *True.* The tip of the probe is positioned in the distal oesophagus at about 40 cm depth.
e) *False.* The angle between the ultrasound beam and blood flow is 45°.

---

8. d)

Chapter 12

Pain management and regional anaesthesia

Patient controlled analgesia (PCA)

PCA represents one of the most significant advances in the treatment of postoperative pain. Improved technology enables pumps to accurately deliver boluses of opioid when a demand button is activated by the patient.

It is the patient who determines the plasma concentration of the opioid, this being a balance between the dose required to control the pain and that which causes side-effects. The plasma concentration of the opioid is maintained at a relatively constant level with the dose requirements being generally smaller.

Components

1. A pump with an accuracy of at least ±5% of the programmed dose (Fig. 12.1).
2. The remote demand button connected to the pump and activated by the patient.
3. An anti-siphon and backflow valve.

Mechanism of action

1. Different modes of analgesic administration can be employed:
   a) patient controlled on-demand bolus administration (PCA)
   b) continuous background infusion and patient controlled bolus administration.
2. The initial programming of the pump must be tailored for the individual patient. The mode of administration, the amount of analgesic administered per bolus, the 'lock-out' time (i.e. the time period during which the patient is prevented from receiving another bolus despite activating the demand button), the duration of the administration of the bolus and the maximum amount of analgesic permitted per unit time are all variable settings on a PCA device.
3. Some designs have the capability to be used as a PCA pump for a particular variable duration then switching automatically to a continuous infusion as programmed.

4. The history of the drug administration including the total dose of the analgesic, the number of boluses and the number of successful and failed attempts can be displayed.
5. The devices have memory capabilities so they retain their programming during syringe changing.
6. Tamper-resistant features are included.
7. Some designs have a safety measure where an accidental triggering of the device is usually prevented by the need for the patient to make two successive presses on the hand control within 1 second.
8. PCA devices operate on mains or battery.
9. Different routes of administration can be used for PCA, e.g. intravenous, intramuscular, subcutaneous or epidural routes.
10. Alarms are included for malfunction, occlusion and disconnection.
11. Ambulatory PCA pumps are available allowing patient's mobilization during use (Fig. 12.2).

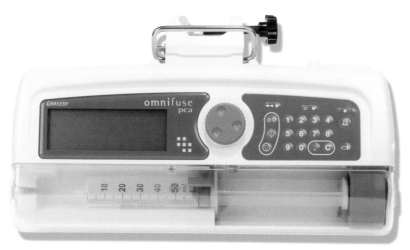

Fig. 12.1 The Graseby Omnifuse PCA pump.

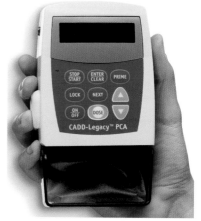

Fig. 12.2 The CADD Legacy portable PCA.

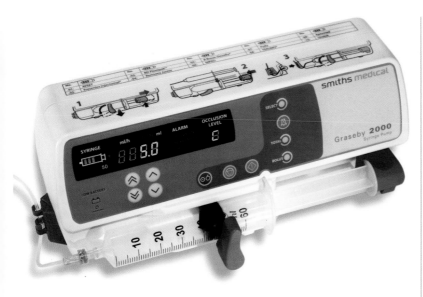

Fig. 12.3 The Graseby 2000 syringe pump.

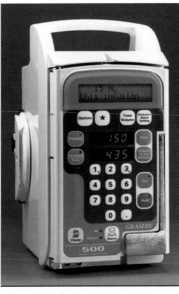

Fig. 12.4 The Graseby volumetric pump.

Problems in practice and safety features

1. The ability of the patient to co-operate and understand is essential.
2. Availability of trained staff to programme the device and monitor the patient is vital.
3. In the PCA mode, the patient may awaken in severe pain because no boluses were administered during sleep.
4. Some PCA devices require special giving sets and syringes.
5. Technical errors can be fatal.

Patient controlled analgesia (PCA)

- The patient has the ability to administer the opioid as required.
- The device is programmed by the anaesthetist.
- Different modes of administration.
- Tamper-resistant designs are featured.
- Ambulatory designs are available.
- Technical errors can be fatal.

SYRINGE PUMPS

These are programmable pumps that can be adjusted to give variable rates of infusion and also bolus administration (Fig. 12.3). They are used to maintain continuous infusions of analgesics (or other drugs). The type of flow is pulsatile continuous delivery and their accuracy is within ±2–5%. Some designs can accept a variety of different size syringes. The power source can be battery and/or mains.

It is important to prevent free flow from the syringe pump. Anti-siphon valves are usually used to achieve this. Inadvertent free flow can occur if the syringe barrel or plunger is not engaged firmly in the pump mechanism. The syringe should be securely clamped to the pump. Syringe drivers should not be positioned above the level of the patient. If the pump is more than 100 cm above the patient, a gravitational pressure can be generated that overcomes the friction between a non-secured plunger and barrel. Siphoning can also occur if there is a crack in the syringe allowing air to enter.

Some pumps have a 'back-off' function that prevents the pump from administering a bolus following an obstruction due to increased pressure in the system. An anti-reflux valve should be inserted in any other line that is connected to the infusion line. Anti-reflux valves prevent backflow up the secondary and often lower pressure line should a distal occlusion occur and they avoid a subsequent inadvertent bolus.

VOLUMETRIC PUMPS

These are programmable pumps designed to be used with specific giving set tubing (Fig. 12.4). They are more suitable for infusions where accuracy of total volume is more important than precise flow rate. Their accuracy is generally within ±5–10%. Volumetric pump accuracy is sensitive to the internal diameter of the giving set tubing. Various mechanisms of action exist. Peristaltic, cassette and reservoir systems are commonly used.

The power source can be battery and/or mains.

TARGET CONTROLLED INFUSION PUMPS

These pumps have advanced software technology where the age and the weight of the patient are entered in addition to the drug's desired plasma concentration. They are mainly used with a propofol and remifentanil infusion technique. The software is capable of estimating the plasma and effect (brain) concentrations allowing the anaesthetist to adjust the infusion rate accordingly.

Elastomeric pumps

These recently designed light, portable and disposable pumps allow continous infusions of local anaesthetic solutions. Continuous incisional infiltration or nerve blocks can be used so allowing the delivery of continuous analgesia (Fig. 12.5).

Components

1. A small balloon-like pump that is filled with local anaesthetic. Variable volumes of 100–600 mL are available.
2. Specially designed catheters with lengths of 7–30 cm and of different gauges.
3. A bacterial filter and a flow restrictor.

Mechanism of action

1. The balloon deflates slowly and spontaneously delivering a set amount of local anaesthetic solution per hour. Rates of 2–14 mL/h can be programmed.
2. Catheters are designed with multiple orifices allowing the infusion of local anaesthetic solution over a large area.

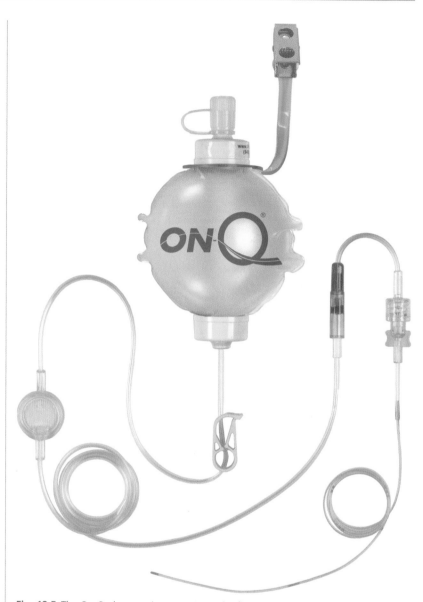

Fig. 12.5 The On-Q elastomeric pump. Note the flow restricter, bacterial filter, anti-syphon valve and the attached catheter. (Courtesy of I-Flow Corporation.)

3. An extra on-demand bolus facility is available in some designs. This allows boluses of 5 mL solution with a lock-out time of 60 min.
4. Some designs allow the simultaneous infusion of two surgical sites.
5. Silver-coated dressing for anti-microbial effect is provided.

Problems in practice and safety features

1. Some of the local anaesthetic may get absorbed into the balloon.
2. The infusion rate profile can vary throughout the infusion. It is thought that the initial rate is higher than expected initially especially if the pump is under

filled. The infusion rates tend to decrease over the infusion period.

3. It is important to follow the manufacturer's instructions regarding positioning of the device in relation to the body and ambient temperature. Changes in temperature can affect the flow rate. A change of 10°C in the temperature of water-based fluids results in altered viscosity, which causes a 20–30% change in flow rate.

Epidural needles

Epidural needles are used to identify and cannulate the epidural space. The Tuohy needle is widely used in the UK (Fig. 12.6).

Components

1. The needle is 10 cm in length with a shaft of 8 cm (with 1-cm markings). A 15-cm version exists for obese patients.

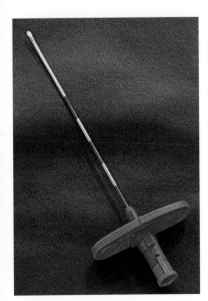

Fig. 12.6 18-G Tuohy needle. Note the 1 cm markings along its shaft.

2. The needle wall is thin in order to allow a catheter to be inserted through it.
3. The needle is provided with a stylet introducer to prevent occlusion of the lumen by a core of tissue as the needle is inserted.
4. The bevel (called a Huber point) is designed to be slightly oblique at 20° to the shaft, with a rather blunt leading edge.
5. Some designs allow the wings at the hub to be added or removed.
6. The commonly used gauges are either 16 G or 18 G.

Mechanism of action

1. The markings on the needle enable the anaesthetist to determine the distance between the skin and the epidural space. Hence the length of the catheter left inside the epidural space can be estimated.
2. The shape and design of the bevel (Fig 12.7) enable the anaesthetist to direct the catheter within the epidural space (either in a cephalic or caudal direction).
3. The bluntness of the bevel also minimizes the risk of accidental dural puncture.
4. Some anaesthetists prefer winged epidural needles for better control and handling of the needle during insertion.
5. A paediatric 19-G, 5-cm long Tuohy needle (with 0.5-cm markings), allowing the passage of a 21-G nylon catheter, is available.

6. A combined spinal–epidural technique is possible using a 26-G spinal needle of about 12 cm length with a standard 16-G Tuohy needle. The Tuohy needle is first positioned in the epidural space then the spinal needle is introduced through it into the subarachnoid space (Fig. 12.7). A relatively high pressure is required to inject through the spinal needle because of its small bore. This might lead to accidental displacement of the tip of the needle from the subarachnoid space leading to a failed or partial block. To prevent this happening, in some designs, the spinal needle is 'anchored' to the epidural needle to prevent displacement (Fig. 12.8).

Problems in practice and safety features

1. During insertion of the catheter through the needle, if it is necessary to withdraw the catheter, the needle must be withdrawn simultaneously. This is because of the risk of the catheter being transected by the oblique bevel.
2. In accidental dural puncture, there is a high incidence of postdural headache due to the epidural needle's large bore (e.g. 16 G or 18 G).
3. Wrong route errors: in order to avoid administering drugs that were intended for intravenous administration, all epidural bolus doses are performed using syringes, needles and other

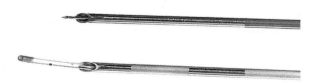

Fig. 12.7 Detail of a spinal needle introduced through a Tuohy needle (top); an epidural catheter passing through a Tuohy needle (bottom).

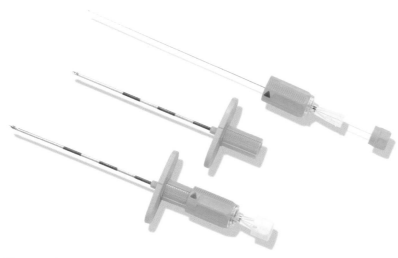

Fig. 12.8 The Portex CSEcure combined spinal-epidural device. The spinal needle (top); the epidural needle (middle); the spinal needle inserted and 'anchored' to the epidural needle (bottom).

devices with safer connectors that cannot connect with intravenous Luer connectors.

Epidural needle
- 10-cm Tuohy needle with the oblique bevel (Huber point) is most popular. Five- and 15-cm lengths exist.
- It has 1-cm markings to measure the depth of the epidural space.
- A stylet introducer is provided with the needle.
- A combined epidural–spinal technique is becoming more popular.

Epidural catheter, filter and loss of resistance device (Fig. 12.9)

THE CATHETER

Components

1. 90-cm transparent, malleable tube made of either nylon or Teflon and biologically inert. The 16-G version has an external diameter of about 1 mm and an internal diameter of 0.55 mm.
2. The distal end has two or three side ports with a closed and rounded tip in order to reduce the risk of vascular or dural puncture (see Fig. 12.7). Paediatric designs, 18 G or 19 G, have closer distal side ports.
3. Some designs have an open end.
4. The distal end of the catheter is marked clearly at 5-cm intervals, with additional 1-cm markings between 5 and 15 cm (Fig. 12.10).
5. The proximal end of the catheter is connected to a Luer lock and a filter (Fig. 12.10).
6. In order to prevent kinking, some designs incorporate a coil-reinforced catheter.
7. Some designs are radio-opaque. These catheters tend to be more rigid than the normal design. They can be used in patients with chronic pain to ensure correct placement of the catheter.

Mechanism of action

1. The catheters are designed to pass easily through their matched gauge epidural needles.
2. The markings enable the anaesthetist to place the desired length of catheter within the epidural space (usually 3–5 cm).
3. There are catheters with a single port at the distal tip. These offer a rather sharp point and increase the incidence of catheter-induced vascular or dural puncture.
4. An epidural fixing device can be used to prevent the catheter falling out. The device clips on the catheter. It has an adhesive flange that secures it to the skin. The device does not occlude the catheter and does not increase the resistance to injection (Fig. 12.11).

Problems in practice and safety features

1. The patency of the catheter should be tested prior to insertion.
2. The catheter can puncture an epidural vessel or the dura at the time of insertion or even days later.
3. The catheter should not be withdrawn through the Tuohy needle once it has been threaded beyond the bevel as that can transect the catheter. Both needle and catheter should be removed in unison.
4. It is almost impossible to predict in which direction the epidural catheter is heading when it is advanced.
5. Once the catheter has been removed from the patient, it should be inspected for any signs of breakage. The side ports are points of catheter weakness where it is possible for the catheter to break. Usually, if a portion of the catheter were to remain in the patient after

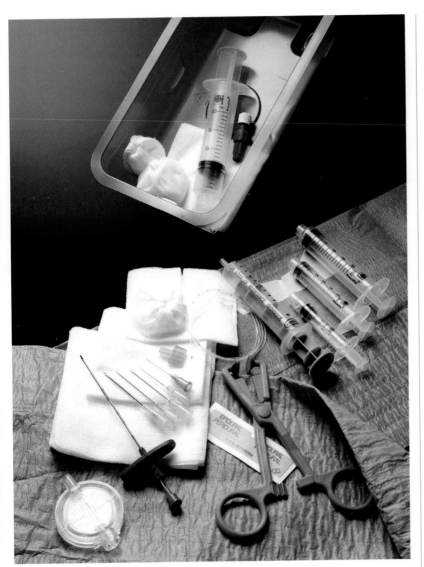

Fig. 12.9 The Portex epidural set containing Tuohy needle, loss of resistance syringe and a range of other syringes and needles, epidural catheter and filter, drape, swabs and epidural catheter label.

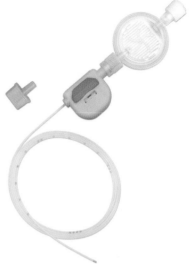

Fig. 12.10 Portex epidural catheter and filter. Note the markings up to 20 cm.

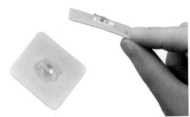

Fig. 12.11 Smith's Portex LockIt Plus epidural catheter fixing device.

Plastic and glass versions are available.

removal, conservative management would be recommended.

6. Advancing the catheter too much can cause knotting (Fig. 12.12).

THE FILTER (SEE FIG. 12.10)

The hydrophilic filter is a 0.22-micron mesh which acts as a bacterial, viral and foreign body (e.g. glass) filter with a priming volume of about 0.7 mL. It is recommended that the filter should be changed every 24 h if the catheter is going to stay in situ for long periods.

LOSS OF RESISTANCE DEVICE OR SYRINGE

The syringe has a special low-resistance plunger used to identify the epidural space by loss of resistance to either air or saline.

Epidural catheter, filter and syringe

- Marked 90-cm catheter with distal side or end ports.
- It should not be advanced for more than 5 cm inside the epidural space.
- The proximal end is connected to a 0.22-micron mesh bacterial, viral and foreign body filter.
- A low-resistance plunger syringe is used to identify the epidural space.

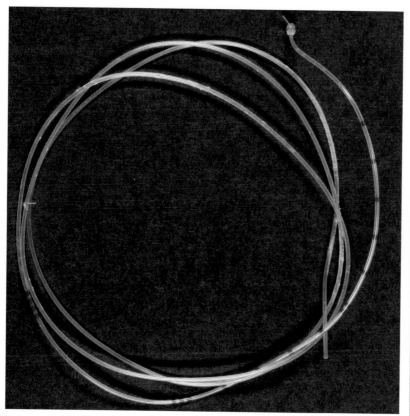

Fig. 12.12 An epidural catheter with a knot near its tip. (Courtesy of Dr MS Rao.)

Spinal needles

These needles are used to inject local anaesthetic(s) and/or opiates into the subarachnoid space. In addition, they are used to sample cerebrospinal fluid (CSF) or for intrathecal injections of antibiotics and cytotoxics (Fig. 12.13).

Components

1. The needle's length varies from 5 to 15 cm; the 10-cm version is most commonly used. They have a transparent hub in order to identify quickly the flow of CSF.
2. A stylet is used to prevent a core of tissue occluding the lumen of the needle during insertion. It also acts to strengthen the shaft.

The stylet is withdrawn once the tip of the needle is (or is suspected to be) in the subarachnoid space.
3. Spinal needles are made in different sizes, from 18 G to 29 G in diameter. 32-G spinal needles have been described but are not widely used.
4. The 25-G and smaller needles are used with an introducer which is usually an 18-G or 19-G needle.
5. There are two designs for the bevel. The cutting, traumatic bevel is seen in the Yale and Quincke needles. The non-cutting, atraumatic pencil point, with a side hole just proximal to the tip, is seen in the Whitacre and Sprotte needles (Figs 12.14 and 12.15).

6. A 28-G nylon, open-ended microcatheter can be inserted through a Crawford spinal needle (23 G). A stylet inside the catheter is removed during the insertion. This allows top-ups to be administered. The priming volume is 0.03 mL with a length of 910 mm. A 0.2-micron filter is attached to the catheter (Fig. 12.16).

Mechanism of action

1. The large 22-G needle is more rigid and easier to direct. It gives a better feedback feel as it passes through the different tissue layers.
2. The CSF is slower to emerge from the smaller sized needles. Aspirating gently with a syringe can speed up the tracking back of CSF.
3. Continuous spinal anaesthesia can be achieved by inserting 3–4 cm of the 28-G spinal microcatheter into the subarachnoid space.

Problems in practice and safety features

1. *Wrong route errors*: in order to avoid administering drugs that were intended for intravenous administration, all spinal (intrathecal) bolus doses and lumbar puncture samples are performed using syringes, needles and other devices with safer connectors that cannot connect with intravenous Luer connectors (Figs 12.17 and 12.18).

Dural headache

1. The incidence of dural headache is directly proportional to the gauge of the needle and the number of punctures made through the dura and indirectly proportional to the age of

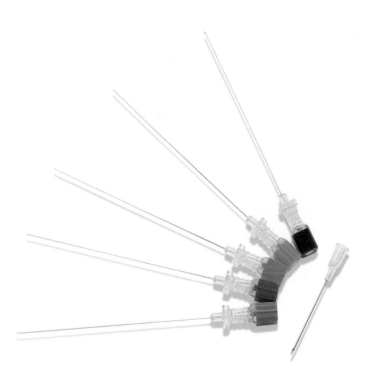

Fig. 12.13 Different size spinal needles with their introducer. From left; 27 G (grey), 26 G (brown), 25 G (orange), 24 G (purple) and 22 G (black). (Courtesy of Smiths Medical.)

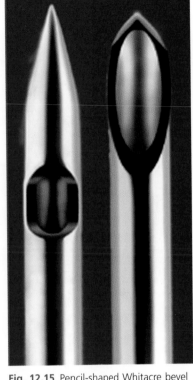

Fig. 12.15 Pencil-shaped Whitacre bevel (left) and cutting Quincke bevel (right).

the patient. There is a 30% incidence of dural headache using a 20-G spinal needle, whereas the incidence is reduced to about 1% when a 26-G needle is used. For this reason, smaller gauge spinal needles are preferred.

2. The Whitacre and Sprotte atraumatic needles separate rather than cut the longitudinal fibres of the dura. The defect in the dura has a higher chance of sealing after the removal of the needles. This reduces the incidence of dural headache.

3. Traumatic bevel needles cut the dural fibres, producing a ragged tear which allows leakage of CSF. Dural headache is thought to be caused by the leakage of CSF.

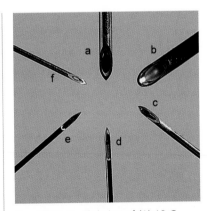

Fig. 12.14 Bevel design of (A) 18-G Quincke; (B) 16-G Tuohy; (C) 22-G Yale; (D) 24-G Sprotte; (E) 25-G Whitacre; (F) 25-G Yale.

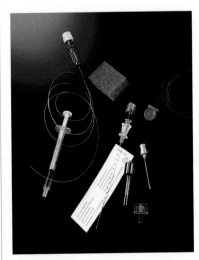

Fig. 12.16 The Portex spinal microcatheter set.

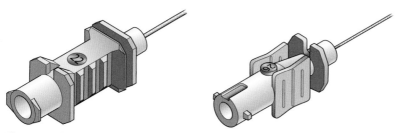

Fig. 12.17 The standard Luer connection spinal needle (left) and the Portex Correct Inject spinal needle designed to avoid wrong route error injections.

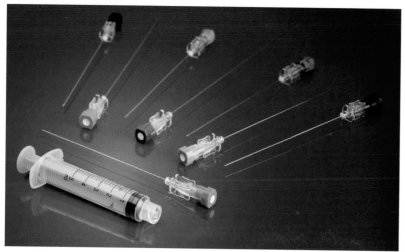

Fig. 12.18 Portex Correct Inject range of spinal needles and syringe designed to avoid wrong route error injections.

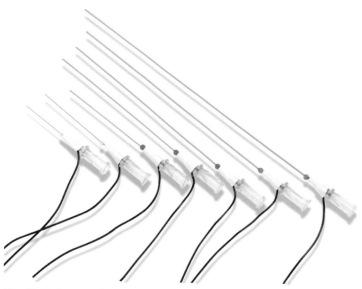

Fig. 12.19 A range of Smiths Medical insulated peripheral nerve block needles of different lengths.

4. The risk of dural headache is higher during pregnancy and labour, day-surgery patients and those who have experienced a dural headache in the past.

Spinal microcatheters

1. They are difficult to advance.
2. There is a risk of trauma to nerves.
3. Cauda equina syndrome is thought to be due to the potential neurotoxicity from the anaesthetic solutions rather than the microcatheter.

> **Spinal needles**
> - They have a stylet and a transparent hub.
> - Different gauges from 18 G to 32 G.
> - The bevel can be cutting (Yale and Quincke) or pencil-like (Whitacre and Sprotte).
> - Can cause dural headache.
> - Continuous spinal block using a 28-G microcatheter is possible.

Nerve block needles

These needles are used in regional anaesthesia to identify a nerve plexus or peripheral nerve (Fig. 12.19).

Components

1. They are made of steel with a Luer-lock attachment.
2. They have short, rather blunt bevels in order to cause minimal trauma to the nervous tissue. The bluntness makes skin insertion more difficult. This can be overcome by a small incision.
3. The needles have transparent hubs which allow earlier recognition of intravascular placement while performing blocks.

4. A side port for injecting the local anaesthetic solution is found in some designs.
5. The needles are connected to a nerve stimulator to aid in localizing the nerve using an insulated cable to prevent leakage of current (see Chapter 14).
6. 22-G size needles are optimal for the vast majority of blocks. There are different lengths depending on the depth of the nerve or plexus. Some suggested length needles for common blocks are:
   a) interscalene block: 25–50 mm
   b) axillary block: 35–50 mm
   c) psoas compartment block: 80–120 mm
   d) femoral nerve block: 50 mm
   e) sciatic nerve block (depending on the approach): 80–150 mm.
7. A pencil-shaped needle tip with a distal side hole for injecting local anaesthetic drugs is available.

Mechanism of action

1. The needle should first be introduced through the skin and subcutaneous tissues and then attached to the lead of the nerve stimulator.
2. An initial high output (e.g. 1–3 mA) from the nerve stimulator is selected. For superficial nerves, a starting current of 1–2 mA should be sufficient in most cases. For deeper nerves, it may be necessary to increase the initial current to 3 mA or even more. The needle is advanced slowly towards the nerve until nerve stimulation is noticed. The output is then reduced until a maximal stimulation is obtained with the minimal output. This current should be 0.2–0.4 mA. Contractions with such a low current mean that the tip of the needle is touching or very close to the nerve. Higher currents suggest that the needle is unlikely to be near the nerve. Contractions at a current less than 0.2 mA may indicate possible intraneural needle placement.
3. The blunt nerve block needle pushes the nerve ahead of itself as it is advanced, whereas a sharp needle is more likely to pierce the nerve. Blunt needles give a better feedback feel as resistance changes as they pass through the different layers of tissues.
4. As the local anaesthetic solution is injected, the stimulation is markedly reduced after only a small volume (about 2 mL) is injected. This is due to displacement of the nerve by the needle tip. Failure of the twitching to disappear (or pain experienced by the awake patient) after injection may indicate intraneural needle placement.
5. The immobile needle technique is used for major nerve and plexus blocks when a large volume of local anaesthetic solution is used. One operator maintains the needle in position, while the second operator, after aspiration, injects the local anaesthetic solution through the side port. This technique reduces the possibility of accidental misplacement and intravascular injection.
6. Catheters can be inserted and left in situ after localizing the nerve or plexus (Fig. 12.20). Repeat bolus or continuous infusion of local anaesthetic solution can then be administered. Catheter techniques can be used to enhance the spread (such as in the axillary block) or to prolong the duration of the block.
7. Stimulating catheters can also be inserted to provide a continuous

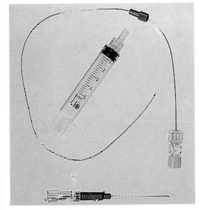

Fig. 12.20 A catheter set for continuous plexus anaesthesia.

block. The catheter body is made from insulating plastic material and usually contains a metallic wire, inside which conducts the current to its exposed tip electrode. Usually, such stimulating catheters are placed using a continuous nerve block needle which is placed first using nerve stimulation. It acts as an introducer needle for the catheter. Once this needle is placed close to the nerve or plexus to be blocked, the stimulating catheter is introduced through it and the nerve stimulator is connected to the catheter. Stimulation through the catheter should reconfirm the catheter tip position in close proximity to the target nerve(s). However, it must be noted that the threshold currents with stimulating catheters may be considerably higher. Injection of local anaesthetic or saline (which is frequently used to widen the space for threading the catheter more easily) should be avoided, as this may increase the threshold current considerably and may even prevent a motor response.

Nerve block needles can either be insulated with an exposed tip or non-insulated.

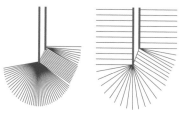

Fig. 12.21 Current density and flow from an insulated needle (left) and non-insulated needle (right). Note the current leakage from the shaft in addition to the bevel of the latter.

INSULATED NEEDLES

These needles are Teflon coated with exposed tips. The current passes through the tip only (Fig. 12.21). The insulated needles have a slightly greater diameter than similar non-insulated needles, which may result in a higher risk of nerve injury. The plexus or nerve can be identified with a smaller current than that required using the non-insulated needles.

NON-INSULATED NEEDLES

These needles allow current to pass through the tip as well the shaft (Fig. 12.21). They are effective in regional anaesthesia because the maximum density of the current is being localized to the tip because of its lower resistance. However, a nerve may be stimulated via the shaft. In this situation, the local anaesthetic solution injected will be placed away from the nerve resulting in an unsuccessful block.

> **Nerve block needles**
> - Made of steel with short blunt bevel to reduce trauma to nerves and improve feedback feel.
> - 22 G is optimal with lengths of 50–150 mm available.
> - Can be insulated or non-insulated.
> - Immobile needle technique is commonly used.

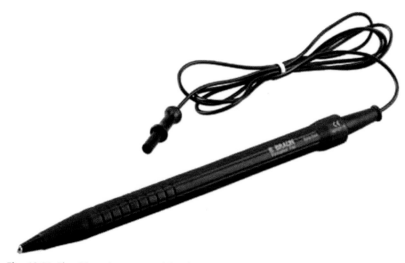

Fig. 12.22 The Stimuplex pen used for the percutaneous localization of nerves. (Courtesy of B Braun.)

Percutaneous localization of nerves

This recent new technique allows rapid, relatively painless and non-invasive localization of superficial nerves using a pen-like device (Fig. 12.22). This technique allows the identification of the optimal angle and needle entry point before introducing the needle into the patient. Such a device can be used to identify nerves up to 3 cm in depth.

Nerve stimulator for nerve blocks

This device is designed to produce visible muscular contractions at a predetermined current and voltage once a nerve plexus or peripheral nerve(s) has been located, without actually touching it, thereby providing a greater accuracy for local anaesthetic deposition (Fig. 12.23).

The ideal peripheral nerve stimulator
- Constant current output despite changes in resistance of the external circuit (tissues, needles, connectors, etc.).
- Clear meter reading (digital) to 0.1 mA.
- Variable output control.
- Linear output.
- Clearly marked polarity.
- Short pulse width.
- Pulse of 1–2 Hz.
- Battery indicator.
- High-quality clips of low resistance.

Components

1. The nerve stimulator case with an on/off switch and a dial selecting the amplitude of the current.
2. Two leads to complete the circuit. One is connected to an ECG skin electrode and the other to the locating needle. The polarity of the leads should be clearly indicated and

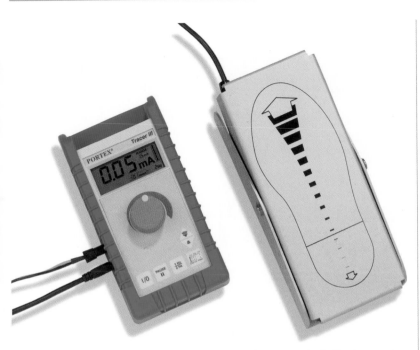

Fig. 12.23 The Portex Tracer III peripheral nerve stimulatort. Note its facility for remote control.

5. Nerve location can be very accurately defined, especially when low currents are used. The success rate of technically difficult nerve blocks can be increased by using a nerve stimulator. A sciatic nerve block with a success rate of over 90% can be achieved in experienced hands, compared to about 50% without using a nerve stimulator.

6. Remote control of the nerve stimulator allows sterile one-hand operation (Figs 12.23 and 12.24).

Problems in practice and safety features

1. Higher currents will stimulate nerve fibres even if the tip of the needle is not adjacent to the nerve. The muscle fibres themselves can also be directly stimulated when a high current is used. In both situations, the outcome will be an unsuccessful block once the local anaesthetic solution has been injected.

2. The positive ground electrode should have good contact with clear dry skin. As the current flows between the two electrodes

colour-coded with the negative lead being attached to the needle.

Mechanism of action

1. A small constant current (0.25–0.5 mA) is used to stimulate the nerve fibres causing the motor fibres to contract. Less current is needed if the needle is connected to the negative lead than to the positive lead. When the negative (cathode) lead is used to locate the nerve, the current causes changes in the resting membrane potential of the cells, producing an area of depolarization and so causing an action potential. If the stimulating electrode is positive (anode), the current causes an area of hyperpolarization near the needle tip and a ring of depolarization distal to the tip. This requires a much higher current.

2. The frequency is set at 1–2 Hz. Tetanic stimuli are not used because of the discomfort caused. Using 2-Hz frequency allows more frequent feedback.

3. The duration of the stimulus should be short (50–100 ms) to generate painless motor contraction.

4. The nerve stimulator is battery operated to improve patient safety.

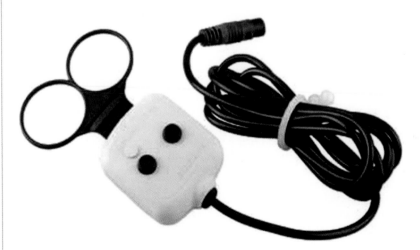

Fig. 12.24 Stimuplex remote control. (Courtesy of B Braun.)

(needle and ground), it is preferable not to position the ground over a superficial nerve. The passage of the current through the myocardium should also be avoided.

3. Most stimulators have a connection/disconnection indicator to ensure that the operator is aware of the delivery or not of stimulus current.

4. It is not recommended to use nerve stimulators designed to monitor the extent of neuromuscular blockade for regional nerve blocks. These are high-output devices which can damage the nervous tissue.

5. It should be remembered that using the nerve stimulator is no excuse for not having the sound knowledge of surface and neuroanatomy required to perform regional anaesthesia.

Peripheral nerve stimulator

• It has two leads, the positive one to the skin and the negative to the needle.
• A small current of 0.5 mA or less is used with a frequency of 1–2 Hz.
• The stimulus is of short duration (1–2 ms).

Ultrasound guidance in regional anaesthesia

This more recent technique uses ultrasound control to locate the nerves/plexuses. It is thought that a higher success rate can be achieved when it is used, with lower complication rates.

More specially designed needles for the use of ultrasound are available allowing a better reflection of the ultrasound waves (Fig. 12.25). The needles have echogenic

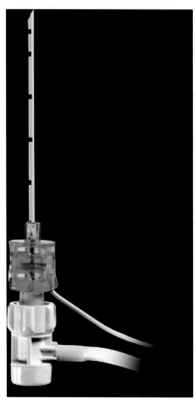

Fig. 12.25 B Braun Contiplex S Ultra designed for improved echogenicity. (Courtesy of B Braun.)

laser markings to facilitate better needle visualization with minimal acoustic shadowing.

Most nerve blocks need ultrasound frequencies in the range of 10–14 MHz. Many broadband ultrasound transducers with a bandwidth of 5–12 or 8–14 MHz can offer excellent resolution of superficial structures in the upper frequency range and good penetration depth in the lower frequency range.

The true echogenicity of a nerve is only captured if the sound beam is oriented perpendicularly to the nerve axis. This can be achieved best with *linear array transducers* with parallel sound beam emission rather than with *sector transducers*. The latter are characterized by diverging sound waves, such that

the echotexture of the nerves will only be displayed in the centre of the image.

The linear probes are most often used for the majority of peripheral blocks. The curved arrays are used for deep nerve structures (lower frequency is required). Smaller footprint probes are useful for smaller infants and children and for certain uses such as very superficial blocks (e.g. ankle blocks).

Portable ultrasound units are available.

Ultrasound is described in more detail in Chapter 13.

FURTHER READING

Dalrymple, P., Chelliah, S., 2006. Electrical nerve locators. Continuing Education in Anaesthesia. Critical Care and Pain 6 (1), 32–36

Keay, S., Callander, C., 2004. The safe use of infusion devices. Continuing Education in Anaesthesia. Critical Care and Pain 4 (3), 81–85

Marhofer, P., Greher, M., Kapral, S., 2005. Ultrasound guidance in regional anaesthesia. British Journal of Anaesthesia 94 (1), 7–17

MHRA, 2007. Intravascular and epidural devices – top tips. Online. Available at: http://www.mhra.gov.uk/Publications/Postersandleaflets/CON2025731

MHRA, 2010. Infusion systems, DB 2003(02) v2.0. Online. Available at: http://www.mhra.gov.uk/Publications/Safetyguidance/DeviceBulletins/CON007321

NHS, 2007. Epidural injections and infusions. Online. Available at: http://www.nrls.npsa.nhs.uk/resources/?entryid45=59807&p=11

NHS, 2010. Safer ambulatory syringe drivers. Online. Available at: http://www.nrls.npsa.nhs.uk/resources/?entryid45=92908&p=2

NHS, 2010. Design for patient safety: a guide to the design of electronic infusion devices. Online. Available at: http://www.nrls.npsa.nhs.uk/resources/?entryid45=68534&p=4

NHS, 2011. Safer spinal (intrathecal), epidural and regional devices. Online. Available at: http://www.nrls.npsa.nhs.uk/resources/?entryid45=94529&p=2

Obstetric Anaesthetists' Association, 2012. Spinal/epidural needle design. Online. Available at: http://oaa-anaes.ac.uk/content.asp?contentid=367

The Royal College of Anaesthetists, 2004. Good practice in the management of continuous epidural analgesia in the hospital setting. Online. Available at: www.rcoa.ac.uk/docs/Epid.Analg.pdf.

MCQs

In the following lists, which of the statements (a) to (e) are true?

1. Epidural catheters and filters:
   a) A minimum of 10 cm of the catheter should be inserted into the epidural space.
   b) The catheter should not be withdrawn through the Tuohy needle once it has been threaded beyond the bevel.
   c) Catheters with a single port at the distal tip reduce the incidence of vascular or dural puncture.
   d) The filter should be changed every 8 hours.
   e) Catheters can be radio-opaque.

2. Regional anaesthesia using a nerve stimulator:
   a) The needles used have sharp tips to aid in localizing the nerves/plexuses.
   b) AC current is used to locate the nerve.
   c) A current of 1 A is usually used to locate a nerve.
   d) Paraesthesia is not required for successful blocks.
   e) 50-Hz frequency stimuli are used.

3. Nerve stimulators in regional anaesthesia:
   a) They enable the block to be performed even without full knowledge of the anatomy.
   b) In the insulated nerve block needle, the current passes through the tip only.
   c) In the non-insulated nerve block needle, the current passes through the tip and the shaft.
   d) A catheter can be used for continuous nerve/plexus blockade.
   e) The immobile needle technique improves the success rate of the block.

4. Incidence of spinal headache:
   a) Yale and Quincke needle design have lower incidence of spinal headache.
   b) It is inversely proportional to the size of the needle used.
   c) It is similar in young and elderly patients.
   d) It is proportional to the number of dural punctures.
   e) It is reduced using a pencil-shaped needle tip.

5. Which of the following is/are true:
   a) Using ultrasound guidance in regional anaesthesia, a frequency range of 10–14 kHz is adequate.
   b) It is important to prevent free flow from the syringe pump.
   c) There is no need to use anti-reflux valves in other infusion lines.
   d) Sector transducers can achieve better images when in regional anaesthesia.
   e) Syringe pumps should be positioned at the same level as the patient.

SINGLE BEST ANSWER (SBA)

6. Spinal needles:
   a) Can be used to perform epidural block.
   b) Have an opaque hub to allow identification of CSF fluid.
   c) Dural puncture headache is eliminated with the cutting bevels.
   d) New guidelines make it impossible to administer drugs.
   e) Can be used as part of a combined spinal/epidural procedure.

Answers

1. Epidural catheters and filters:
   a) False. 3–5 cm of the catheter is left in the epidural space. This reduces the incidence of vascular or dural puncture, segmental or unilateral block (as the catheter can pass through an intervertebral foramina) and knotting.
   b) True. The withdrawal of the catheter through the Tuohy needle after it has been threaded beyond the bevel can lead to the transection of the catheter. This usually happens when the catheter punctures a vessel during insertion. The needle and the catheter should be removed together and another attempt should be made to reinsert the needle and catheter.
   c) False. Catheters with a single port at the distal tip increase the incidence of vascular or dural puncture. This is due to the 'sharp' point at the end of the catheter. In contrast, catheters with side ports have a closed and rounded end thus reducing the incidence of vascular or dural puncture.
   d) False. The filter can be used for up to 24 h.
   e) True. Some catheters are designed to be radio-opaque. They are more rigid than the standard design. They are mainly used in patients with chronic pain to ensure the correct placement of the catheter.

2. Regional anaesthesia using a nerve stimulator:
   a) False. There is a need for feedback from the needle as it goes through the different layers of tissue. A sharp needle will pass the different layers of tissues easily with minimal feedback. A blunt needle will provide much better feedback.
   b) False. DC current from a battery is used to operate nerve stimulators. By avoiding AC current, patient safety is improved.
   c) False. This is a very high current. A current range of up to 5 mA is needed in locating the nerve. A current of 0.25–0.5 mA is used to stimulate the nerve fibres. Using a very high current, the tip of the needle might be far away from the nerve but might still lead to stimulation of the nerve fibres or the muscle fibres directly leading to the failure of the block.
   d) True. There is no need for paraesthesia in order to achieve a successful block using a nerve stimulator. Paraesthesia implies that the needle is touching the nerve. With a nerve stimulator, the nerve can be stimulated electrically without being touched.
   e) False. Stimuli with a frequency of 1–2 Hz are used. Tetanic stimuli (e.g. 50-Hz frequency) are not used because of the discomfort caused.

3. Nerve stimulators in regional anaesthesia:
   a) False. Full knowledge of the anatomical structure is essential for a successful block.
   b) True. As the tip is the only non-insulated part of the needle, the current passes only through it. Using a small current, the tip of the needle has to be very close to the nerve before stimulation is visible.
   c) True. In a non-insulated needle, the current passes through both the tip and shaft. This might lead to nerve stimulation by current from the shaft even when the tip is far away from the nerve. This obviously leads to a failed block.
   d) True. After successful nerve stimulation, a catheter can be inserted. This allows a prolonged and continuous block using an infusion or boluses.
   e) True. The immobile needle technique allows one operator to maintain the needle in the correct position while the second operator injects the local anaesthetic. This also reduces the risk of accidental intravascular injection.

4. Incidence of spinal headache:
   a) False. Yale and Quincke have a higher incidence of spinal headache. This is due to the traumatic bevel cutting the dural fibres producing a ragged tear which allows CSF leakage.
   b) False. The incidence is directly proportional to the size of the needle used. Using a 20-G spinal needle causes a 30% incidence of spinal headache whereas a 26-G needle has a 1% incidence of headache.
   c) False. The incidence of spinal headache is much higher in the young than in elderly patients.
   d) True. The incidence of spinal headache is increased with multiple dural punctures.

e) *True.* The pencil-shaped needle tip separates rather than cuts the longitudinal dural fibres. After removal of the needle, the dura has a higher chance of sealing, reducing the incidence of spinal headache.

5. Which of the following is/are true:
a) *False.* The frequencies needed for nerve blocks are in the range of 10–14 MHz. Most modern ultrasound devices can generate these frequencies.
b) *True.* Anti-siphon valves are used to prevent free flow from the syringe pump. In addition, the syringe should be securely clamped to the pump. Siphoning can also occur if there is a crack in the syringe allowing air entry.
c) *False.* An anti-reflux valve should be inserted in any other line that is connected to the infusion line. Anti-reflux valves prevent backflow up the secondary (usually with lower pressure) should a distal occlusion occur and avoid a subsequent inadvertent bolus.
d) *False.* Sector transducers emit diverging sound waves, such that the echotexture of the nerves will only be displayed in the centre of the image.

The true echogenicity of a nerve is only captured if the sound beam is oriented perpendicularly to the nerve axis. This can best be achieved with linear array transducers with parallel sound beam emission.
e) *True.* Gravitational pressure can be generated to overcome the friction between a non-secured plunger and barrel especially if the pump is positioned more than 100 cm above the patient.

6. e)

Chapter 13

Additional equipment used in anaesthesia and intensive care

Continuous positive airway pressure (CPAP)

CPAP is a spontaneous breathing mode used in the intensive care unit, during anaesthesia and for patients requiring respiratory support at home. It increases the functional residual capacity (FRC) and improves oxygenation. CPAP prevents alveolar collapse and possibly recruits already collapsed alveoli.

Components

1. A flow generator producing high flows of gas (Fig. 13.1), or a large reservoir bag may be needed.
2. Connecting tubing from the flow generator to the inspiratory port of the mask. An oxygen analyser is fitted along the tubing to determine the inspired oxygen concentration.

3. A tight-fitting mask or a hood. The mask or hood has both inspiratory and expiratory ports. A CPAP valve is fitted to the expiratory port.
4. If the patient is intubated and spontaneously breathing, a T-piece with a CPAP valve fitted to the expiratory limb can be used.

Mechanism of action

1. Positive pressure within the lungs (and breathing system) is maintained throughout the whole of the breathing cycle.
2. The patient's peak inspiratory flow rate can be met.
3. The level of CPAP varies depending on the patient's requirements. It is usually 5–15 cm H_2O.
4. CPAP is useful in weaning patients off ventilators especially when positive end expiratory pressure (PEEP) is used. It is also useful in improving oxygentaion in type 1 respiratory failure,

where CO_2 elemination is not a problem.
5. Two levels of airway pressure support can be provided using *inspiratory positive airway pressure* (IPAP) and *expiratory positive airway pressure* (EPAP). IPAP is the pressure set to support the patient during inspiration. EPAP is the pressure set for the period of expiration This is commonly used in reference to bilevel positive airway pressure (BiPAP©). Using this mode, the airway pressure during inspiration is independent from expiratory airway pressure. This mode is useful in managing patients with type 2 respiratory failure as the work of breathing is reduced with improvements in tidal volume and CO_2 removal.

Problems in practice and safety features

1. CPAP has cardiovascular effects similar to PEEP but to a lesser extent. Although the arterial oxygenation may be improved, the cardiac output can be reduced. This may reduce the oxygen delivery to the tissues.
2. Barotrauma can occur.
3. A loose-fitting mask allows leakage of gas and loss of pressure.
4. A nasogastric tube is inserted in patients with depressed consciousness level to prevent gastric distension.
5. Skin erosion caused by the tight-fitting mask. This is minimized by the use of soft silicone masks or protective dressings or by using a CPAP hood. Rhinorrhoea and nasal dryness can also occur.
6. Nasal masks are better tolerated but mouth breathing reduces the effects of CPAP.

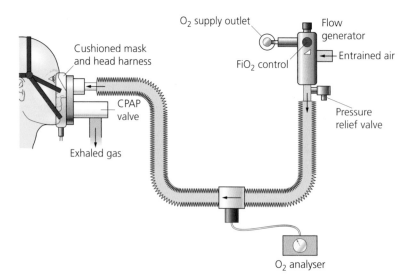

Fig. 13.1 A CPAP breathing system set-up.

Haemofiltration

Haemofiltration is a process of acute renal support used for critically ill patients. It is the ultrafiltration of blood.

Ultrafiltration is the passage of fluid under pressure across a semipermeable membrane where low molecular weight solutes (up to 20 000 Da) are carried along with the fluid by solvent drag (convection) rather than diffusion. This allows the larger molecules such as plasma proteins, albumin (62 000 Da) and cellular elements to be preserved.

The widespread use of haemofiltration has revolutionized the management of critically ill patients with acute renal failure within the intensive therapy environment (Fig. 13.2). Haemofiltration is popular because of its relative ease of use and higher tolerability in the cardiovascularly unstable patient.

In the critical care setting, haemofiltration can be delivered by:

1. *Continuous low flow therapy*, which is typically run 24 h per day for more than 1 day, but may be stopped for procedures and filter or circuit changes. Continuous treatments are said

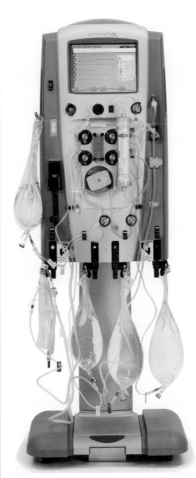

Fig. 13.2 The Prismaflex 1 haemofiltration system. (Courtesy of Gambro Lundia AB.)

to offer better cardiovascular stability and more efficient solute removal because of the steady biochemical correction and gradual fluid removal. Continuous therapy is also better suited to the frequently changing fluid balance situation in patients with multiorgan dysfunction in critical care.

2. *Intermittent high flow systems*, often 4-hour sessions with a new filter and circuit for each session.

Components

1. Intravascular access lines. These can either be arteriovenous lines (such as femoral artery and vein or brachial artery and femoral vein) or venovenous lines (such as the femoral vein or the subclavian vein using a single double-lumen catheter). The extracorporeal circuit is connected to the intravascular lines. The lines should be as short as possible to minimize resistance.

2. Filter or membrane (Fig. 13.3). Synthetic membranes are ideal for this process. They are made of polyacrylonitrile (PAN), polysulphone or polymethyl methacrylate. They have a large pore size to allow efficient diffusion (in contrast to the smaller size of dialysis filters).

3. Two roller pumps, one on each side of the circuit. Each pump peristaltically propels about 10 mL of blood per revolution and is positioned slightly below the level of the patient's heart.

4. The collection vessel for the ultrafiltrate is positioned below the level of the pump.

Mechanism of action

1. At its most basic form, the haemofiltration system consists of a circuit linking an artery to a vein with a filter positioned between the two.

2. The patient's blood pressure provides the hydrostatic pressure necessary for ultrafiltration of the plasma. This technique is suitable for fluid-overloaded patients who have a stable, normal blood pressure.

3. Blood pressure of less than a mean of 60 or 70 mmHg reduces the flow and the volume of filtrate and leads to clotting despite heparin.

4. In the venovenous system, a pump is added making the cannulation of a large artery

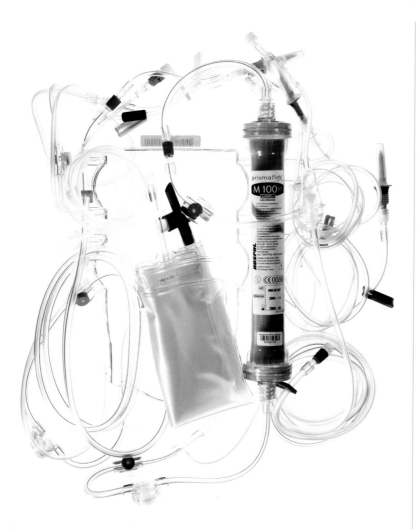

Fig. 13.3 The M100 Haemofilter set showing the filter, tubes and collecting bag. (Courtesy of Gambro Lundia AB.)

low post-pump pressures can happen in line occlusion or disconnection respectively.

7. Some designs have the facility to weigh the filtrate and automatically supply the appropriate amount of reinfusion fluid.

8. Heparin is added as the anticoagulant with a typical loading dose of 3000 IU followed by an infusion of 10 IU per kg body weight. Heparin activity is monitored by activated partial thromboplastin time or activated clotting time. Prostacyclin or low molecular weight heparin can be used as alternatives to heparin.

9. The filters are supplied either in a cylinder or flat box casing. The packing of the filter material ensures a high surface area to volume ratio. The filter is usually manufactured as a parallel collection of hollow fibres packed within a plastic canister. Blood is passed, or pumped, from one end to the other through these tubules. One or more ports provided in the outer casing are used to collect the filtrate and/or pass dialysate fluid across the effluent side of the membrane tubules.
   a) They are highly biocompatible causing minimal complement or leucocyte activation.
   b) They are also highly wettable achieving high ultrafiltration rates.
   c) They have large pore size allowing efficient diffusion.
   d) The optimal surface area of the membrane is 0.3–1.9 m².
   e) Both small molecules (e.g. urea, creatinine and potassium) and large molecules (e.g. myoglobin and some antibiotics) are cleared efficiently. Proteins do not pass through the membrane because of their larger molecular size.

unnecessary (Fig. 13.4). The speed of the blood pump controls the maintenance of the transmembrane pressure. The risk of clotting is also reduced. This is the most common method used. Blood flows of 30–750 mL/min can be achieved, although flow rates of 150–300 mL/min are generally used. This gives an ultrafiltration rate of 25–40 mL/min.

5. The fluid balance is maintained by the simultaneous reinfusion of a sterile crystalloid fluid. The fluid contains most of the plasma electrolytes present in their normal values (sodium, potassium, calcium, magnesium, chloride, lactate and glucose) with an osmolality of 285–335 mosmol/kg. Large amounts of fluid are needed such as 2–3 L/h.

6. Pressure transducers monitor the blood pressure in access and return lines. Air bubble detection facilities are also incorporated. Low inflow pressures can happen during line occlusion. High and

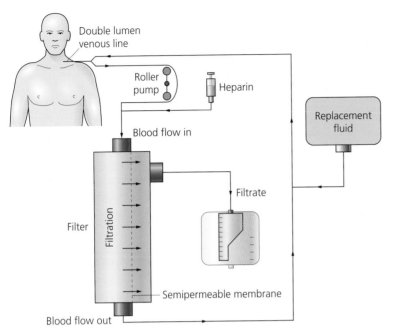

Fig. 13.4 Diagrammatic representation of venovenous haemofiltration.

Problems in practice and safety features

1. The extracorporeal circuit must be primed with 2 L of normal saline prior to use. This removes all the toxic ethylene oxide gas still present in the filter. (Ethylene oxide is used to sterilize the equipment after manufacture.)
2. Haemolysis of blood components by the roller pump.
3. The risk of cracks to the tubing after long-term use.
4. The risk of bleeding must be controlled by optimizing the dose of anticoagulant.

Haemofiltration

- An effective method of renal support in critically ill patients using ultrafiltration of the blood.
- Arteriovenous or venovenous lines are connected to the extracorporeal circuit (filter and a pump).
- Synthetic filters with a surface area of 0.5–1.5 m^2 are used.

Arterial blood gas analyser (Fig. 13.5)

In order to measure arterial blood gases, a sample of heparinized, anaerobic and fresh arterial blood is needed.

1. Heparin should be added to the sample to prevent clotting during the analysis. The heparin should only fill the dead space of the syringe and form a thin film on its interior. Excess heparin, which is acidic, lowers the pH of the sample.
2. The presence of air bubbles in the sample increases the oxygen partial pressure and decreases carbon dioxide partial pressure.
3. An old blood sample has a lower pH and oxygen partial pressure and a higher carbon dioxide partial pressure. If there is a need to delay the analysis (e.g. machine self-calibration), the sample should be kept on ice.

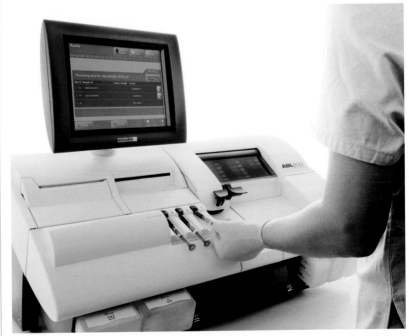

Fig. 13.5 The ABL800FLEX blood gas analyser. (Courtesy of Radiometer Medical ApS.)

The measured parameters are:

1. arterial blood oxygen partial pressure
2. arterial carbon dioxide partial pressure
3. the pH of the arterial blood.

From these measurements, other parameters can be calculated, e.g. actual bicarbonate, standard bicarbonate, base excess and oxygen saturation.

Polarographic (Clark) oxygen electrode

This measures the oxygen partial pressure in a blood (or gas) sample (Fig. 13.6).

Components

1. A platinum cathode sealed in a glass body.
2. A silver/silver chloride anode.
3. A sodium chloride electrolyte solution.
4. An oxygen-permeable Teflon membrane separating the solution from the sample.
5. Power source of 700 mV.

Mechanism of action

1. Oxygen molecules cross the membrane into the electrolyte solution at a rate proportional to their partial pressure in the sample.
2. A very small electric current flows when the polarization potential is applied across the electrode in the presence of oxygen molecules in the electrolyte solution. Electrons are donated by the *anode* and accepted by the *cathode*, producing an electric current within the solution. The circuit is completed by the input terminal of the amplifier.

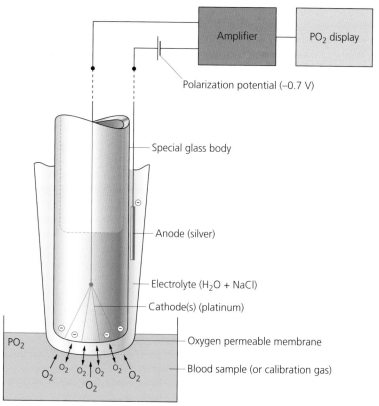

Fig. 13.6 Mechanism of action of the oxygen electrode. (Reproduced with permission from AVL Medical Instruments UK Ltd.)

Cathode reaction:

$$O_2 + 2H_2O + 4e^- = 4OH^-$$

Electrolyte reaction:

$$NaCl + OH^- = NaOH + Cl^-$$

Anode reaction:

$$Ag + Cl^- = AgCl + e^-$$

3. The oxygen partial pressure in the sample can be measured since the amount of current is linearly proportional to the oxygen partial pressure in the sample.
4. The electrode is kept at a constant temperature of 37°C.

Problems in practice and safety features

1. The membrane can deteriorate and perforate, affecting the performance of the electrode. Regular maintenance is essential.
2. Protein particles can precipitate on the membrane affecting the performance.

> **Polarographic oxygen electrode**
> - Consists of a platinum cathode, silver/silver chloride anode, electrolyte solution, membrane and polarization potential of 700 mV.
> - The flow of the electrical current is proportional to the oxygen partial pressure in the sample.
> - Requires regular maintenance.

pH electrode

This measures the activity of the hydrogen ions in a sample. Described mathematically, it is:

$$pH = -\log[H^+]$$

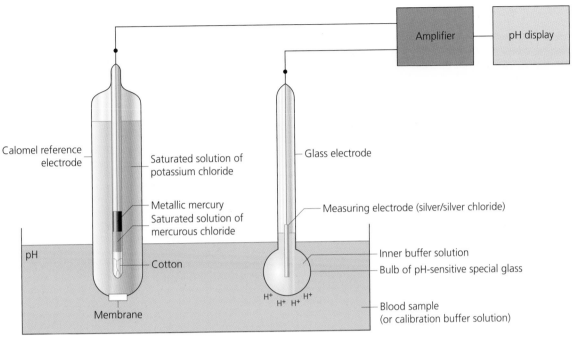

Fig. 13.7 Mechanism of action of the pH electrode.

It is a versatile electrode which can measure samples of blood, urine or CSF (Fig. 13.7).

Components

1. A glass electrode (silver/silver chloride) incorporating a bulb made of pH-sensitive glass holding a buffer solution.
2. A calomel reference electrode (mercury/mercury chloride) which is in contact with a potassium chloride solution via a cotton plug. The arterial blood sample is in contact with the potassium chloride solution via a membrane.
3. A meter to display the potential difference across the two electrodes.

Mechanism of action

1. The reference electrode maintains a constant potential.
2. The pH within the glass remains constant due to the action of the buffer solution. However, a pH gradient exists between the sample and the buffer solution. This gradient results in an electrical potential.
3. Using the two electrodes to create an electrical circuit, the potential can be measured. One electrode is in contact with the buffer and the other is in contact with the blood sample.
4. A linear electrical output of about 60 mV per unit pH is produced.
5. The two electrodes are kept at a constant temperature of 37°C.

Problems in practice and safety features

1. It should be calibrated before use with two buffer solutions.
2. The electrodes must be kept clean.

> **pH electrode**
> - Two half cells linked via the sample.
> - The electrical potential produced is proportional to the pH of the sample.

Carbon dioxide electrode (Severinghaus electrode)

A modified pH electrode is used to measure carbon dioxide partial pressure, as a result of change in the pH of an electrolyte solution (Fig. 13.8).

Components

1. A pH-sensitive glass electrode with a silver/silver chloride reference electrode forming its outer part.
2. The electrodes are surrounded by a thin film of an electrolyte solution (sodium bicarbonate).
3. A carbon dioxide permeable rubber or Teflon membrane.

Mechanism of action

1. Carbon dioxide (not hydrogen ions) diffuses in both directions

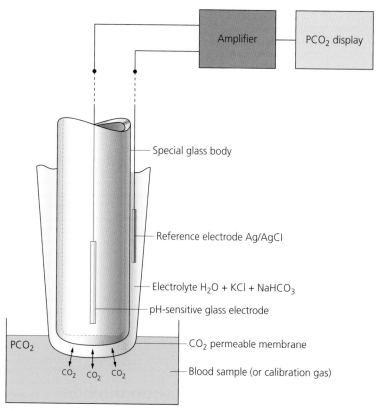

Fig. 13.8 Mechanism of action of the carbon dioxide electrode.

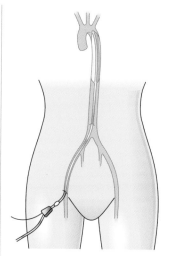

Fig. 13.9 The intra-aortic balloon pump in situ.

until equilibrium exists across the membrane between the sample and the electrolyte solution.

2. Carbon dioxide reacts with the water present in the electrolyte solution producing hydrogen ions resulting in a change in pH:

$$CO_2 + H_2O \rightarrow H^+ + HCO_3^-$$

3. The change in pH is measured by the glass electrode.
4. The electrode should be maintained at a temperature of 37°C. Regular calibration is required.

Problems in practice and safety features

1. The integrity of the membrane is vital for accuracy.

2. Slow response time because diffusion of carbon dioxide takes up to 2–3 min.

Carbon dioxide electrode

- A modified pH electrode measures changes in pH due to carbon dioxide diffusion across a membrane.
- Maintained at 37°C.
- Slow response time.

Intra-aortic balloon pump (IABP)

This is a catheter incorporating a balloon which is inserted into the aorta to support patients with severe cardiac failure. Its core principle

is synchronized counterpulsation. It is usually inserted using a percutaneous femoral approach, over a guidewire, under fluoroscopic or transoesophageal echo guidance. The correct position of the pump is in the descending aorta, just distal to the left subclavian artery (Fig 13.9).

Components

1. A 7- up to 8-FG catheter with a balloon.
2. The catheter has two lumens, an outer lumen for helium gas exchange to and from the balloon and a fluid-filled central lumen for continuous aortic pressure monitoring via a transducer. The most modern versions use fibre-optics instead to monitor aortic pressure, which is faster and more sensitive, generating faster response times.
3. The usual volume of the balloon is 40 mL. A 34-mL balloon is available for small individuals. The size of the balloon should be 80–90% of the diameter of the aorta. The pump is attached to a console (Fig. 13.10) which

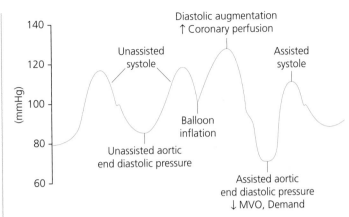

Fig. 13.11 The changes that intra-aortic balloon pump therapy causes to the arterial waveform and their consequences.

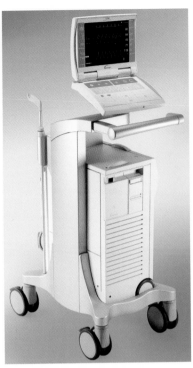

Fig. 13.10 Intra-aortic ballon pump console. (Courtesy of MAQUET Ltd.)

controls the flow of helium in and out of the balloon and monitors the patient's blood pressure and ECG. The console allows the adjustment of the various parameters in order to optimize counterpulsation.

Mechanism of action

1. The balloon is inflated in early diastole, immediately after the closure of the aortic valve. This leads to an increase in peak diastolic blood pressure (diastolic augmentation) and an increase in coronary artery perfusion pressure. This increases myocardial oxygen supply. Inflation should be at the dicrotic notch on the arterial pressure waveform (Fig. 13.11).
2. The balloon is deflated at the end of diastole just before the aortic

valve opens and remains deflated during systole. This leads to a decrease in aortic end-diastolic pressure causing a decrease in left ventricular afterload and decreased myocardial oxygen demand. This will lead to an increase in left ventricular performance, stroke work and ejection fraction. Deflation should be at the lowest point of the arterial diastolic pressure.
3. During myocardial ischaemia, the main benefits of the IABP are the reduction of myocardial oxygen demand (by lowering of the left ventricular pressure) and the increase in myocardial oxygen supply (by increasing the coronary artery perfusion).
4. The effectiveness of the balloon depends on the ratio of the balloon to aorta size, heart rate and rhythm, compliance of the aorta and peripheral vessels and the precise timing of the counterpulsation. Correctly timed IABP should be able to increase the augmented diastolic pressure to higher then the systolic pressure. IABP is expected to increase diastolic pressure by 30%, decrease the systolic pressure by 20% and improve cardiac output by 20%.

Indications for use of IABP

- Refractory ventricular failure.
- Acute myocardial infarction complicated with cardiogenic shock, mitral regurgitation, ventricular septal defect.
- Impending myocardial infarction.
- Unstable angina refractory to medical treatment.
- High risk angioplasty.
- Ischaemia-related ventricular arrythmias.
- Pre- and post-coronary bypass surgery, including weaning from cardiopulmonary bypass.

Contraindications for use of IABP

- Severe aortic regurgitation.
- Aortic dissection.
- Major coagulopathy.
- Severe bilateral peripheral arterial disease.
- Bilateral femoral–popliteal bypass graft.
- Sepsis.

Problems in practice and safety features

1. If the balloon is too large, it may damage the aorta. If it is

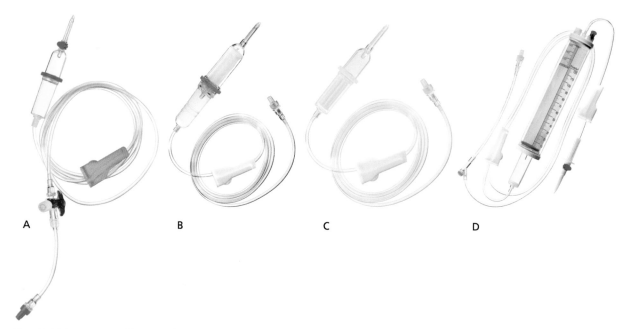

Fig. 13.12 Intravenous giving sets: (A) Intrafix Safe Set adult fluid set; (B) SangofixB blood adult giving set with a 200-μm filter; (C) Sangopur adult blood set with a 40-μm filter; (D) Dosifix paediatric fluid set with burette. (Courtesy of B Braun Medical.)

too small, counterpulsation will be ineffective.
2. Limb ischaemia.
3. Thrombosis and embolism. Low-dose heparinization is often used to counteract this.
4. Arterial dissection or perforation.
5. Bleeding.
6. Infection.

Intra-aortic balloon pump
- 7- up to 8-FG catheter with a balloon positioned in the descending aorta.
- Two lumens: a central one to monitor blood pressure and an outer one for inflation and deflation of the balloon with helium.
- Balloon inflation occurs at the dicrotic notch of the arterial pressure waveform.
- Balloon deflation occurs at the lowest point of the arterial diastolic pressure.

Intravenous giving sets

These are designed to administer intravenous fluids, blood and blood products (Fig. 13.12).

Components

1. Adult giving set:
   a) A clear plastic tube of about 175 cm in length and 4 mm in internal diameter. One end is designed for insertion into the fluid bag whereas the other end is attached to an intravascular cannula with a Luer-lock connection.
   b) Blood giving sets have a filter with a mesh of about 150–200 μm and a fluid chamber (Fig. 13.12B). Giving sets with finer mesh filter of about 40 μm are available (Fig. 13.12C).

   c) Some designs have a one-way valve and a three-way tap attachment or a rubber injection site at the patient's end. The maximum size needle used for injection should be 23 G.
   d) A flow controller determines the drip rate (20 drops of clear fluid is 1 mL and 15 drops of blood is 1 mL).
2. Paediatric set (Fig. 13.12D):
   a) In order to attain accuracy, a burette (30–200 mL) in 1 mL divisions is used to measure the volume of fluid to be infused. The burette has a filter, air inlet and an injection site on its top. At the bottom, there is a flap/ball valve to prevent air entry when the burette is empty.
   b) There are two flow controllers: one is between the fluid bag and the burette and is used to fill the burette; the second is between the burette

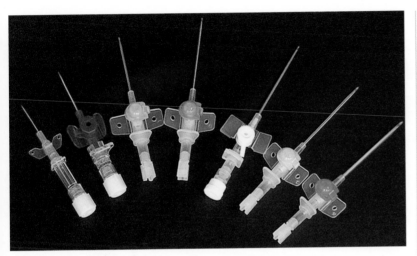

Fig. 13.13 A range of intravenous cannulae.

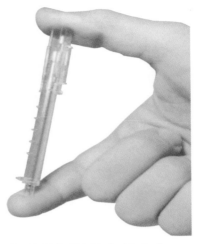

Fig. 13.14 Smith's Medical Protective Acuvance cannula designed to reduce the risk of needle stick injury.

and the patient and controls the drip rate. An injection site should be close to the patient to reduce the dead space.

c) Drop size is 60 drops per 1 mL of clear fluid. A burette with a drop size similar to the adult's version (15 drops per mL) is used for blood transfusion.

d) 0.2-micron filters can be added in line to filter out air and foreign bodies, e.g. glass or plastic particles. Infusion-related thrombophlebitis can be reduced by the use of these filters.

More recent designs are the 'closed and integrated' cannulae (Fig. 13.15). A 'closed' system may offer better protection against bacterial exposure than conventional 'open' ports. As the blood does not naturally escape from the catheter hub, these devices further minimize the risk of exposing the clinician to blood during the insertion procedure.

Using distilled water at a temperature of 22°C and under a pressure of 10 kPa, the flow through a 110-cm tubing with an internal diameter of 4 mm is as follows:

20 G: 40–80 mL/min.
18 G: 75–120 mL/min.
16 G: 130–220 mL/min.
14 G: 250–360 mL/min.

Blood warmers

These are used to warm blood (and other fluids) before administering them to the patient. The aim is to

Intravenous cannulae

Intravenous cannulae are made of plastic. They are made by different manufacturers with different characteristics (Fig. 13.13).

Intravenous cannulae can be either with or without a port. Some designs offer protection against the risk of needle stick injuries (Fig. 13.14), covering the sharp needle tip with a blunt end.

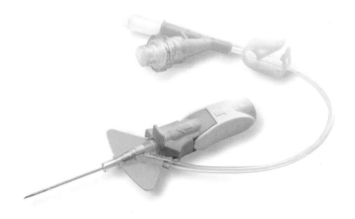

Fig. 13.15 The BD Nexiva IV closed and integrated cannula. (Courtesy of BD Medical.)

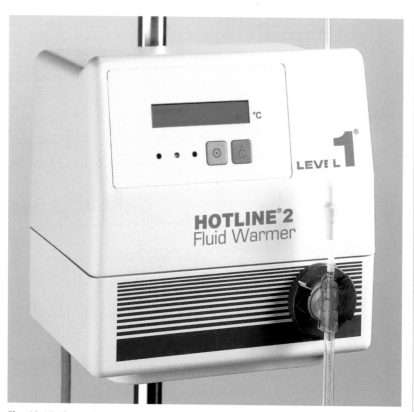

Fig. 13.16 The Hotline 2 Fluid Warmer. (Courtesy of Smiths Medical.)

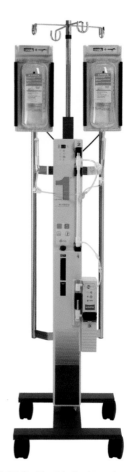

Fig. 13.17 Smiths Medical Level 1 H 1200 fast fluid warmer with an integrated air detector.

deliver blood/fluids to the patient at 37°C. At this temperature, there is no significant haemolysis or increase in osmotic fragility of the red blood cells. There are various designs with the coaxial fluid/blood warmer devices are most popular (Fig. 13.16). A coaxial tubing is used to heat and deliver the fluids to the patient. The outside tubing carries heated sterile water. The inside tubing carries the intravenous fluid. The sterile water is heated to 40°C and stored by the heating case. The water is circulated through the outside tubing. The intravenous fluid does not come in contact with the circulating water. The coaxial tubing extends to the intravenous cannula reducing the loss of heat as fluid is exposed to room temperature.

For patients requiring large and rapid intravenous therapy, special devices are used to deliver warm fluids (Fig. 13.17). Fluids are pressurized to 300 mmHg and warmed with a countercurrent recirculation fluid at a temperature of 42°C.

Forced-air warmers (Fig. 13.18)

These devices are used to maintain the temperature of patients during surgery. They have been found to be effective even when applied to a limited surface body area. They consist of a case where warm ambient air is pumped at variable temperatures between 32 and 37°C. The warm air is delivered via a hose to a thin-walled channelled bag positioned on the patient's body.

There are different bags available depending on which part of the body is covered (e.g. upper or lower body). A thermostat to prevent overheating controls the temperature of the warm air. Cooling versions also exist for surgery where body temperature >37°C is desirable, e.g. neurosurgery.

Defibrillator

This is a device that delivers electrical energy to the heart causing simultaneous depolarization of an adequate number of myocardial

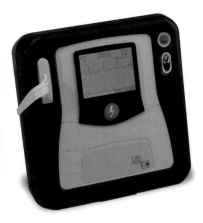

Fig. 13.18 Level 1 forced-air warmer.

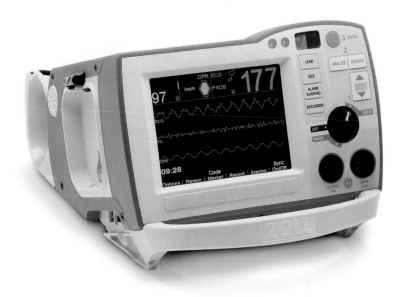

Fig. 13.20 The Zoll R manual defibrillator. (Courtesy of Zoll Medical.)

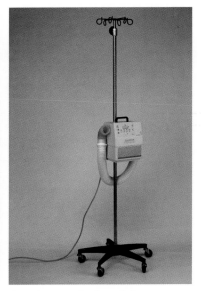

Fig. 13.19 The Zoll Pro AED. (Courtesy of Zoll Medical.)

cells to allow a stable rhythm to be established. Defibrillators can be divided into the automated external defibrillators (AEDs) (Fig. 13.19) and manual defibrillators (Fig. 13.20). AEDs offer interaction with the rescuer through voice and visual prompts.

Components

1. The device has an on/off switch, Joules setting control, charge and discharge buttons.

2. Paddles can be either external (applied to the chest wall) or internal (applied directly to the heart). The external paddles/pads are usually 8–8.5 cm in size.

Mechanism of action

1. DC energy rather than AC energy is used. DC energy is more effective causing less myocardial damage and being less arrhythmogenic than AC energy. The lower the energy used, the less the damage to the heart.

2. Transformers are used to step up mains voltage from 240 V AC to 5000–9000 V AC. A rectifier converts it to 5000 V DC. A variable voltage step-up transformer is used so that different amounts of charge may be selected. Most defibrillators have internal rechargeable batteries that supply DC in the absence of mains supply. This is then converted to AC by means of an inverter, and then amplified to 5000 V DC by a

step-up transformer and rectifier (Fig. 13.21).

3. The DC shock is of brief duration and produced by discharge from a capacitor. The capacitor stores energy in the form of an electrical charge, and then releases it over a short period of time. The current delivered is maintained for several milliseconds in order to achieve successful defibrillation. As the current and charge delivered by a discharging capacitor decay rapidly and exponentially, inductors are used to prolong the duration of current flow.

4. The external paddles/pads are positioned on the sternum and on the left midaxillary line (fifth–sixth rib). An alternative placement is one paddle positioned anteriorly over the left precordium and the other positioned posteriorly behind the heart. Firm pressure on the paddles is required in order to reduce the transthoracic impedance and achieve a higher

Charging circuit

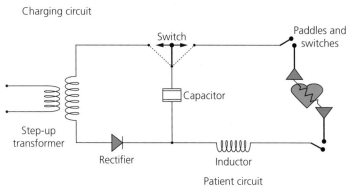

Fig. 13.21 Defibrillator electric circuit.

peak current flow. Using conductive gel pads helps in reducing the transthoracic impedance. Disposable adhesive defibrillator electrode pads are currently used instead of paddles, offering hands-free defibrillation.

5. Most of the current is dissipated through the resistance of the skin and the rest of the tissues and only a small part of the total current (about 35 A) flows through the heart. The impedance to the flow of current is about 50–150 Ohms; however, repeated administration of shocks in quick succession reduces impedance.

6. Waveform:
   a) *Monophasic defibrillators* deliver current that is unipolar (i.e. one direction of current flow) (Fig. 13.22A). They are not used in modern practice as they were likely to have waveform modification depending on transthoracic impedance (e.g. larger patients with high transthoracic impedance received considerably less transmyocardial current than smaller patients).
   b) *Biphasic defibrillators* deliver a two-phased current flow in which electrical current flows in one direction for a specified duration, then

reverses and flows in the opposite direction for the remaining milliseconds of the electrical discharge. Biphasic defibrillators can either be *biphasic truncated exponential* (BTE) (Fig. 13.22B) or *rectilinear biphasic* (RLB) (Fig. 13.22C). Biphasic defibrillators compensate for the wide variations in transthoracic impedance by

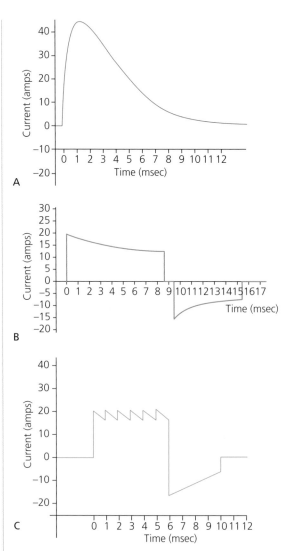

Fig. 13.22 Defibrillator waveforms. (A) Monophasic defibrillator waveform. (B) Biphasic truncated exponential defibrillator waveform. (C) Biphasic rectilinear defibrillator waveform.

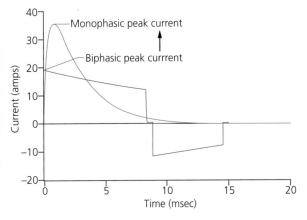

Fig. 13.23 Performance of monophasic versus biphasic defibrillator current.

— Monophasic waveform — Biphasic waveform

electronically adjusting the waveform magnitude and duration to ensure optimal current delivery to the myocardium, irrespective of the patient's size.

c) *Monophasic vs biphasic performance*: as can be seen in Figure 13.23 the highest part of the current waveform is known as the 'peak current' when the most current is flowing. Note the difference in height (amps) between the monophasic peak current and the biphasic peak current. Too much peak current during the shock can injure the heart. It's the peak current, not energy, that can injure the heart. The goal of defibrillation is to deliver enough current to the heart to stop the lethal rhythm but with a low peak current to decrease risk of injury to the heart muscle.

7. For internal defibrillation, the shock delivered to the heart depends on the size of the heart and the paddles.

8. Some designs have an ECG oscilloscope and paper recording facilities. DC defibrillation can be synchronized with the top of the R-wave in the treatment of certain arrhythmias such as atrial fibrillation.

9. The implantable automatic internal defibrillator (Fig. 13.24) is a self-contained diagnostic and therapeutic device placed next to the heart. It consists of a battery and electrical circuitry (pulse generator) connected to one or more insulated wires. The pulse generator and batteries are sealed together and implanted under the skin, usually near the shoulder. The wires are threaded through blood vessels from the implantable cardiac defibrillator (ICD) to the heart muscle. It continuously monitors the rhythm, and when malignant tachyarrhythmias are detected, a defibrillation shock is automatically delivered. ICDs are subject to malfunction due to internal short circuit when attempting to deliver an electrical shock to the heart or due to a memory error. Newer devices also provide overdrive pacing to electrically convert a sustained ventricular tachycardia, and 'back-up' pacing if bradycardia occurs. They also offer a host of other sophisticated functions (such as storage of detected arrhythmic events and the ability to do 'non-invasive' electrophysiologic testing).

Problems in practice and safety features

1. Skin burns.
2. Further arrythmias.

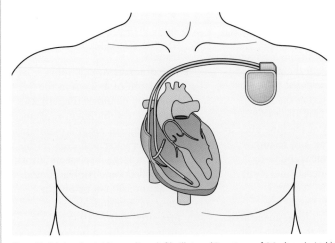

Fig. 13.24 Implantable cardiac defibrillator. (Courtesy of Medtronic Ltd.)

Defibrillators
- AED and manual versions are available.
- A step-up transformer increases mains voltage then a rectifier converts it to direct current. DC energy is discharged from a capacitor.
- Modern defibrillators use a biphasic current flow.
- Implanted automatic internal defibrillators are becoming more popular with pacemaker capabilities.

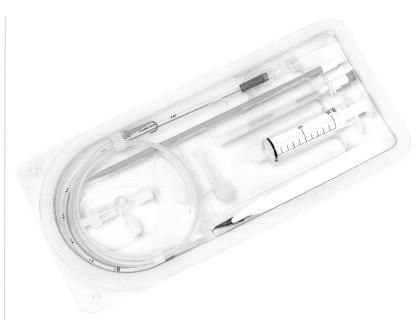

Fig. 13.25 Seldinger chest drainage kit. (Courtesy of Smiths Medical.)

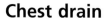

Chest drain

Used for the drainage of air, blood and fluids from the pleural space.

Components

1. A drainage tubing with distal ports (Fig. 13.25).
2. An underwater seal and a collection chamber of approximately 20-cm diameter.

Mechanism of action

1. An air-tight system is required to maintain a subatmospheric intrapleural pressure. The underwater seal acts as a one-way valve through which air is expelled from the pleural space and prevented from re-entering during the next inspiration. This allows re-expansion of the lung after a pneumothorax and restores haemodynamic stability by minimizing mediastinal shift.
2. Under asepsis, skin and subcutaneous tissues are infiltrated with local anaesthetic at the level of the fourth–fifth intercostal space in the midaxillary line. The chest wall is incised and blunt dissection using artery forceps through to the pleural cavity is performed. Using the tip of the finger, adherent lung is swept away from the insertion site.
3. The drain is inserted into the pleural cavity and slid into position (usually towards the apex). The drain is then connected to an underwater seal device.
4. Some designs have a flexible trocar to reduce the risk of trauma.
5. The drainage tube is submerged to a depth of 1–2 cm in the collection chamber (Fig. 13.26). This ensures minimum resistance to drainage of air and maintains the underwater seal even in the face of a large inspiratory effort.
6. The collection chamber should be about 100 cm below the chest as subatmospheric pressures up to −80 cm H_2O may be produced during obstructed inspiration.

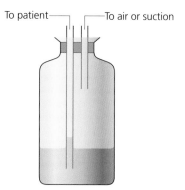

Fig. 13.26 Chest drain underwater seal.

7. A Heimlich flutter one-way valve can be used instead of an underwater seal, allowing better patient mobility.
8. Drainage can be allowed to occur under gravity or suction of about −15–20 mmHg may be applied.

Problems in practice and safety features

1. Retrograde flow of fluid may occur if the collection chamber

is raised above the level of the patient. The collection chamber should be kept below the level of the patient at all times to prevent fluid being siphoned into the pleural space.

2. Absence of oscillations may indicate obstruction of the drainage system by clots or kinks, loss of subatmospheric pressure or complete re-expansion of the lung.
3. Persistent bubbling indicates a continuing bronchopleural air leak.
4. Clamping a pleural drain in the presence of a continuing air leak may result in a tension pneumothorax.

Chest drain

- An air-tight system to drain the pleural cavity usually inserted at the fourth–fifth intercostal space in the midaxillary line.
- The underwater seal chamber should be about 100 cm below the level of the patient.
- Absence of oscillation is seen with complete lung expansion, obstruction of the system or loss of negative pressure.
- Persistent bubbling is seen with a continuing bronchopleural air leak.

The ultrasound machine (Fig. 13.27)

Ultrasound is a longitudinal high-frequency wave. It travels through a medium by causing local displacement of particles. This particle movement causes changes in pressures with no overall movement of the medium. An ultrasound machine consists of a probe

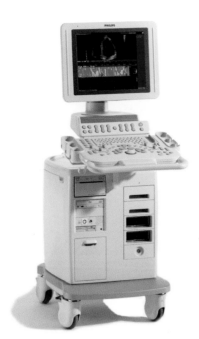

Fig. 13.27 The XD11XE Philips ultrasound machine. (Courtesy of Philips Health Care.)

connected to a control unit that displays the ultrasound image.

Components

1. Beamformer: applies high-amplitude voltage to energize the crystals.
2. Transducer: converts electrical energy to mechanical (US) energy and vice versa.
3. Receiver: detects and amplifies weak signals.
4. Memory: stores video display.

Mechanism of action

1. The probe transmits and receives the ultrasound beam once placed in contact with the skin via 'acoustic coupling' jelly.
2. Ultrasound is created by converting electrical energy into mechanical vibration utilizing the piezoelectric (PE) effect. The PE materials vibrate when a varying voltage is applied. The frequency of the voltage applied determines the frequency of the sound waves produced. The thickness of the PE element determines the frequency at which the element will vibrate most efficiently, i.e. its resonant frequency (RF). RF occurs when the thickness of element is half the wavelength of the sound wave generated.
3. An image is generated when the pulse wave emitted from the transducer is transmitted into the body, reflected off the tissue interface and returned to the transducer. Returning US waves cause PE crystals (elements) within the transducer to vibrate. This causes the generation of a voltage. Therefore, the same crystals can be used to send and receive sound waves.
4. Two-dimensional images of structures are displayed. Procedures requiring precise needle placement such as venous cannulation or nerve blocks can be performed under direct ultrasound control. This helps to minimize the possible risks of the procedure.
5. The image can be displayed in a number of modes:
   a) A-mode (amplitude); not used any more
   b) B-mode (brightness); most commonly used for regional anaesthesia
   c) M-mode (motion); most commonly for cardiac and foetal imaging
   d) 2D-real time.
6. Structures can then be identified via their ultrasound characteristics and anatomical relationships.
7. Increasing the depth allows visualization of deeper structures. The depth of the image should be optimized so

that the target is centred in the display image.

8. Transducer probes come in many shapes and sizes (Fig. 13.28). The shape of the probe determines its field of view, and the frequency of emitted sound waves determines how deep the sound waves penetrate and the resolution of the image.

Problems in practice and safety features

1. One of the commonest mistakes in ultrasound imaging is the use of incorrect gain settings. Insufficient gain can result in missed structures of low reflectivity, such as thrombus. Excessive gain can result in artifacts.

2. The characteristics differentiating vein from artery are listed below.

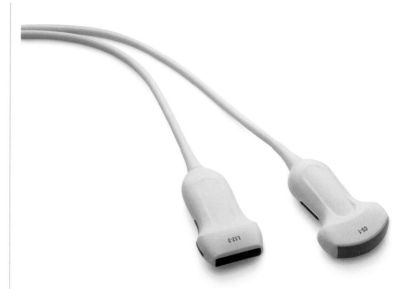

Fig. 13.28 Different ultrasound probes. The probe on the left can be used for superficial nerve blocks whereas the curved probe on the right can be used for deeper nerve blocks. (Courtesy of Philips Health Care.)

	Vein	Artery
Appearance	Black	Black
Movement	None	Pulsatile
Compressible	Yes	No
Colour flow	Constant flow	Pulsatile

Ultrasound machine

- Ultrasound is longitudinal high-frequency waves.
- Created by converting electrical energy into mechanical vibration using piezoelectric effect.
- Same crystals can be used to send and receive sound wave.
- Shape of probe determines its field of view whereas frequency of emitted sounds determines the depth of penetration and resolution of image.

FURTHER READING

Alaour, B., English, W., 2011. Intra-aortic balloon pump counterpulsation. World Anaesthesia Society. Online. Available at: http://www.anaesthesiauk.com/Documents/220%20Intra-aortic%20Balloon%20Pump%20Counterpulsation.pdf.

MHRA, 2010. Infusion systems DB 2003(02) v2.0. Online. Available at: http://www.mhra.gov.uk/Publications/Safetyguidance/DeviceBulletins/CON007321.

MHRA, 2010. Medical device alert: all chest drains when used with high-flow, low-vacuum suction systems (wall mounted) (MDA/2010/040). Online. Available at: http://www.mhra.gov.uk/Publications/Safetywarnings/MedicalDeviceAlerts/CON081890.

MHRA, 2010. Medical device alert: intravenous (IV) extension sets with multiple ports: all brands (MDA/2010/073). Online. Available at: http://www.mhra.gov.uk/Publications/Safetywarnings/MedicalDeviceAlerts/CON093966.

MHRA, 2010. Medical device alert: IV extension sets with multiple ports and vented caps. Various manufacturers (MDA/2010/068). Online. Available at: http://www.mhra.gov.uk/Publications/Safetywarnings/MedicalDeviceAlerts/CON093757.

MHRA, 2010. Medical device alert: SleepStyle CPAP devices manufactured by Fisher & Paykel Healthcare (MDA/2010/076). Online. Available at: http://www.mhra.gov.uk/Publications/Safetywarnings/MedicalDeviceAlerts/CON094175.

NHS, 2009. Chest drains: risks associated with the insertion of chest drains. Online. Available at: http://www.nrls.npsa.nhs.uk/resources/?entryid45=59887&p=10.

NHS, 2010. Non-invasive ventilation. Online. Available at: http://www.nrls.npsa.nhs.uk/resources/?entryid45=83759&p=2.

MCQs

In the following lists, which of the statements (a) to (e) are true?

1. Concerning defibrillators:
   a) Alternating current is commonly used instead of direct current.
   b) The electric current released is measured in watts.
   c) Consists of an inductor which releases the electric current.
   d) Can cause skin burns.
   e) The same amount of electrical energy is used for external and internal defibrillation.

2. Concerning arterial blood gases analysis:
   a) Excess heparin in the sample increases the hydrogen ion concentration.
   b) Blood samples with air bubbles have a lower oxygen partial pressure.
   c) If there is delay in the analysis, the blood sample can be kept at room temperature.
   d) Normal H^+ ion concentration is 40 mmol/L.
   e) CO_2 partial pressure can be measured by measuring the pH.

3. Concerning the CO_2 electrode:
   a) KCl and $NaHCO_3$ are used as electrolyte solutions.
   b) A carbon dioxide-sensitive glass electrode is used.
   c) The electrical signal generated is directly proportional to the log of CO_2 tension in the sample.
   d) It has a response time of 10 s.
   e) It should be kept at room temperature.

4. CPAP:
   a) CPAP is a controlled ventilation mode.
   b) It can improve oxygenation by increasing the FRC.
   c) Pressures of up to 15 kPa are commonly used.
   d) It has no effect on the cardiovascular system.
   e) A nasogastric tube can be used during CPAP.

5. Haemofiltration:
   a) Solutes of molecular weight up to 20 000 Da can pass through the filter.
   b) It should not be used in the cardiovascularly unstable patient.
   c) Blood flows of 150–300 mL/min are generally used.
   d) Warfarin is routinely used to prevent the filter clotting.
   e) The optimal membrane surface area is 0.5–1.5 cm^2.

6. Intra-aortic balloons:
   a) The usual volume of the balloon is 40 mL.
   b) The inflation of the balloon occurs at the upstroke of the arterial waveform.
   c) The deflation of the balloon occurs at the end of diastole just before the aortic valve opens.
   d) It is safe to use in aortic dissection.
   e) Helium is used to inflate the balloon.

7. Chest drains:
   a) The underwater seal chamber can be positioned at any level convenient to the patient.
   b) Persistent air bubbling may be a sign of a continuing bronchopleural air leak.
   c) They function by expelling intrapleural fluids during deep inspiration.
   d) Negative pressure of about −15–20 mmHg may be applied to help in the drainage.
   e) Clamping a pleural drain in the presence of a continuing air leak may result in a tension pneumothorax.

SINGLE BEST ANSWERS (SBA)

8. CPAP repiratory support:
   a) Should be administered by a loose-fitting mask.
   b) Can only be used in type 2 respiratory failure.
   c) Can be used with high inspired oxygen concentrations.
   d) Typically uses an expiratory valve between 20–30 cm H_2O
   e) Has no effects on the cardiovascular system.

9. The blood gas analyser:
   a) Can use either heparinized or unheparinized samples.
   b) All the results are individually measured by the machine.
   c) The pH is related to the $[H^+]$.
   d) Its results are unaffected by temperature.
   e) Only blood samples can be analysed.

Answers

1. Concerning defibrillators:

a) *False. DC current is used as the energy generated is more effective and causes less myocardial damage. Also DC energy is less arrhythmogenic than AC energy.*

b) *False. Joules, not watts, are used to measure the electric energy released.*

c) *False. The defibrillator consists of a capacitor that stores then discharges the electric energy in a controlled manner. Step-up transformers are used to change mains voltage to a much higher AC voltage. A rectifier converts that to a DC voltage. Inductors are used to prolong the duration of current flow as the current and charge delivered by a discharging capacitor decay rapidly and exponentially.*

d) *True. Because of the high energy release, skin burns can be caused by defibrillators especially if gel pads are not used.*

e) *False. The amount of electrical energy used in internal defibrillation is a very small fraction of that used in external defibrillation. In internal defibrillation, the energy is delivered directly to the heart. In external defibrillation, a large proportion of the energy is lost in the tissues before reaching the heart.*

2. Concerning arterial blood gases analysis:

a) *True. Heparin is added to the blood sample to prevent clotting during the analysis. Heparin should only fill the dead space of the syringe and form a thin layer on its interior. Heparin is acidic and in excess will increase the hydrogen ion concentration (lowering the pH) of the sample.*

b) *False. As air consists of about 21% oxygen in nitrogen, the addition of an air bubble(s) to the blood sample will increase the oxygen partial pressure in the sample.*

c) *False. At room temperature, the metabolism of the cells in the blood sample will continue. This leads to a low oxygen partial pressure and a high H^+ concentration and CO_2 partial pressure. If there is a delay in the analysis, the sample should be kept on ice.*

d) *False. The normal H^+ concentration is 40 nanomol/L, which is equivalent to a pH of 7.4.*

e) *True. CO_2 partial pressure in a sample can be measured by measuring the changes in pH of an electrolyte solution using a modified pH electrode. The CO_2 diffuses across a membrane separating the sample and the electrolyte solution. The CO_2 reacts with the water present producing H^+ ions resulting in changes in pH.*

3. Concerning the carbon dioxide electrode:

a) *True. KCl, $NaHCO_3$ and water are the electrolyte solutions used. The CO_2 reacts with the water producing hydrogen ions.*

b) *False. A pH-sensitive glass electrode is used to measure the changes in pH caused by the formation of H^+ ions resulting from the reaction between water and CO_2.*

c) *True. The electrical signal generated at the electrode is directly proportional to the pH of the sample or the –log of H^+ concentration. The latter is related to the CO_2 tension in the sample.*

d) *False. The CO_2 electrode has a slow response time as the CO_2 takes 2–3 min to diffuse across the membrane.*

e) *False. The CO_2 electrode, like the pH electrode, should be kept at 37°C. Dissociation of acids or bases changes when temperature changes.*

4. CPAP:

a) *False. CPAP is continuous positive airway pressure used in spontaneously breathing patients via a face mask or a tracheal tube.*

b) *True. Oxygenation can be improved by CPAP as the alveoli are held open throughout the ventilatory cycle preventing airway closure thus increasing the FRC.*

c) *False. Pressures of up to 15 cm H_2O are commonly used during CPAP.*

d) *False. CPAP reduces the cardiac output (similar to PEEP, although to a lesser extent). The arterial oxygenation might improve with the application of CPAP, but oxygen delivery might be reduced because of the reduced cardiac output.*

e) *True. A nasogastric tube is inserted in patients with depressed consciousness level to prevent gastric distension.*

5. Haemofiltration:
   a) *True.* Solutes of up to 20 000 Da molecular weight are carried along the semipermeable membrane with the fluid by solvent drag (convection).
   b) *False.* One of the reasons for the popularity of haemofiltration in the intensive care unit setup is that it has a higher tolerability in cardiovascularly unstable patients.
   c) *True.* Although blood flows of 30–750 mL/min can be achieved during haemofiltration, blood flows of 150–300 mL/min are commonly used. This gives a filtration rate of 25–40 mL/min.
   d) *False.* Heparin is the anticoagulant of choice during haemofiltration. If there is a contraindication for its use, prostacyclin can be used instead.
   e) *False.* The filters have a large surface area with large pore size and are packed in such a way as to ensure a high surface area to volume ratio. The optimal surface area is 0.5–1.5 m².

6. Intra-aortic balloons:
   a) *True.* The usual volume of the balloon is 40 mL. A smaller version, 34 mL, can be used in small patients. The size of the balloon should be 80–90% of the diameter of the aorta.
   b) *False.* The balloon should be inflated in early diastole immediately after the closure of the aortic valve at the dicrotic notch of the arterial waveform. This leads to an increase in coronary artery perfusion pressure.
   c) *True.* This leads to a decrease in aortic end-diastolic pressure so reducing the left ventricular afterload and myocardial oxygen demand.
   d) *False.* Aortic dissection is one of the absolute contraindications to intra-aortic balloon pump.
   e) *True.* Helium is used to inflate the balloon. Because of its physical properties (low density) it allows rapid and complete balloon inflation and deflation.

7. Chest drains:
   a) *False.* The collection chamber should be about 100 cm below the chest as subatmospheric pressures up to –80 cm H_2O may be produced during obstructed inspiration. Retrograde flow of fluid may occur if the collection chamber is raised above the level of the patient.
   b) *True*
   c) *False.* Deep inspiration helps in expanding the lung whereas deep expiration helps in the drainage of fluids from the pleural space.
   d) *True.* Drainage can be allowed to occur under gravity, or suction of about –15–20 mmHg may be applied.
   e) *True.*

8. c)

9. c)

Chapter 14

Electrical safety

The electrical equipment used in the operating theatre and intensive care unit is designed to improve patient care and safety. At the same time, however, there is the potential of exposing both the patient and staff to an increased risk of electric shock. It is essential for the anaesthetist to have a thorough understanding of the basic principles of electricity, even though these devices include specific safety features.

In the UK, mains electricity is supplied as an alternating current with a frequency of 50 Hz. The current travels from the power station to the substation where it is converted to mains voltage by a transformer. From the substation, the current travels in two conductors, the live and neutral wires. The live wire is at a potential of 240 V (or more accurately 240 RMS (root mean square)). The neutral is connected to the earth at the substation so keeping its potential approximately the same as earth. The live wire carries the potential to the equipment whereas the neutral wire returns the current back to the source, so completing the circuit.

Principles of electricity (Fig. 14.1)

Electric current (I)

An electric current is the flow of electrons through a conductor past a given point per unit of time, propelled by the driving force, i.e. the voltage (potential difference). The current is measured in amperes (A). One ampere represents a flow of 6.24×10^{18} electrons (one coulomb of charge) past a specific point in 1 second.

1. *Direct current (DC)*: the current flows in one direction (e.g. flow from a battery).
2. *Alternating current (AC)*: the flow of electrons reverses direction at regular intervals (e.g. mains supply); in the UK, the frequency of AC is 50 cycles per second (Hz).

Potential difference or voltage (V)

It is the electrical force that drives the electric current. When a current of 1 A is carried along a conductor, such that 1 watt (W) of power is dissipated between two points, the potential difference between those points is 1 volt (V).

Electrical resistance (R)

Electrical resistance is the resistance along a conductor to the flow of electrical current. It is not dependent on the frequency of the current. Electrical resistance is measured in ohms (Ω).

Impedance (Z)

Impedance is the sum of the forces that oppose the movement of electrons in an AC circuit. The unit for impedance is the ohm (Ω). The term impedance covers resistors, capacitors and inductors and is dependent on the frequency of the current. Substances with high impedance are known as insulators. Substances with low impedance are known as conductors. The impedance through capacitors and inductors is related to the frequency (Hz) at which AC reverses direction. Such an impedance, i.e. frequency related, is known as reactance (X).

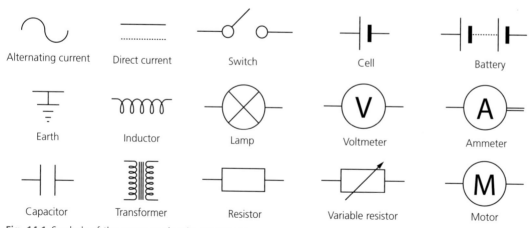

Fig. 14.1 Symbols of the common electric components.

1. Capacitor: impedance $\propto 1/$ frequency
2. Inductor: impedance $\propto$ frequency.

Ohm's law

Electric potential (volts) = current (amperes) × resistance (ohms)
$[E = I \times R]$

Capacitance

Capacitance is a measure of the ability of a conductor or system to store an electrical charge. A capacitor consists of two parallel conducting plates separated by an insulator (dielectric). The unit for capacitance is the farad.

With AC, the plates change polarity at the same current frequency (e.g. 50/s). This will cause the electrons to move back and forth between the plates so allowing the current to flow.

The impedance of a capacitor = distance between the plates/current frequency × plate area.

Inductance

Inductance occurs when electrons flow in a wire resulting in a magnetic field being induced around the wire. If the wire is coiled repeatedly around an iron core, as in a transformer, the magnetic field can be very powerful.

Identification of medical electrical equipment

A *single-fault condition* is a condition when a single means for protection against hazard in equipment is defective or a single external abnormal condition is present, e.g. short circuit between the live parts and the applied part.

The following classes of equipment describe the method used to protect against electrocution according to an International Standard (IEC 60601).

Class I Equipment

This type of equipment offers basic protection whereby the live, neutral and earth wires do not come into contact with each other. There is a secondary protection whereby parts that can be touched by the user, such as the metal case, are insulated from the live electricity and connected to an earth wire via the plug to the mains supply. There are fuses positioned on the live and neutral supply in the equipment. In addition, in the UK, a third fuse is positioned on the live wire in the mains plug. This fuse melts and disconnects the electrical circuit in the event of a fault, protecting the user from electrical shock. The fault can be due to deteriorating insulation, or a short circuit, making the metal case 'live'. Current will pass to earth causing the fuse to blow (this current is called 'leakage current'). Some tiny non-fault leakage currents are always present as insulation is never 100% perfect. A faultless earth connection is required for this protection to function.

Class II Equipment

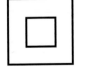

This type of equipment, also called double-insulated equipment, has double or reinforced insulation protecting the accessible parts. There is no need to earth this type of equipment. The power cable has only 'live' and 'neutral' conductors with only one fuse.

Class III Equipment

This type of equipment does not need electrical supply exceeding 24 V AC or 50 V DC. The voltage used is called *safety extra low voltage* (SELV). Although this does not cause an electrical shock, there is still a risk of a microshock. This equipment may contain an internal power source or be connected to the mains supply by an adaptor or a SELV transformer. The power input port is designed to prevent accidental connection with another cable.

The following types of equipment define the degree of protection according to the maximum permissible leakage current.

Type B Equipment

This may be class I, II or III mains-powered equipment or equipment with an internal power source. This equipment is designed to have low leakage currents, even in fault conditions, such as 0.5 mA for class I and 0.1 mA for class II. It may be connected to the patient externally or internally but is not considered safe for direct connection to the heart.

The equipment may be provided with defibrillator protection.

Type BF Equipment

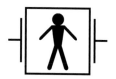

This is similar to type B equipment, but the part applied to the patient is isolated from all other parts of the equipment using an isolated (or floating) circuit. This isolation means that allowable leakage current under single fault conditions is not exceeded even when 1.1 times the rated mains voltage is applied between the attachment to the patient and the earth. The maximum AC leakage current is 0.1 mA under normal conditions and under a single fault condition is 0.5 mA. It is safer than type B but still not safe enough for direct connection to the heart.

The equipment may be provided with defibrillator protection.

Type CF Equipment

This can be class I or II equipment powered by mains with an internal electrical power source, but considered safe for direct connection to the heart. Isolated circuits are used. There is no risk of electrocution by leakage currents (allows 0.05 mA per electrode for class I and 0.01 mA per electrode for class II). This provides a high degree of protection against electrical shock. This is used in ECG leads, pressure transducers and thermodilution computers.

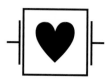

The equipment may be provided with defibrillator protection.

Attention!

The user must consult the accompanying documents for any equipment. A black triangle on a yellow background with an exclamation mark means that there is no standardized symbol for the hazard:

High voltage and risk of electrocution!

Protective Earth

The equipment itself has its own earth connection via the green-and-yellow lead in the conventional three-pin plug. The earth lead is connected to the external case of the equipment so reducing it to zero potential. Although this provides some protection, it does not guarantee it.

Functional Earth

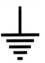

This is part of the main circuit. The current is returned via the neutral wire back to the substation and so to earth. In effect, all conventional electrical circuits have functional earth. It is necessary for proper functioning of electrical equipment and is not a safety feature. On older equipment, the same symbol may have been used to denote protective earth.

Additional Protective Earth

This equipment carries an additional protective earth. This protects against electric shock in cases of a single fault condition.

Equipotentiality

This is used to ensure that all metalwork is normally at or near zero voltage. Therefore, under fault conditions, all the metalwork will increase to the same potential. Simultaneous contact between two such metal appliances would not cause a flow of current because they are both at the same potential, therefore no shock results. This provides some protection against electric shock by joining together all the metal appliances and connecting to earth.

Drip Proof, Splash Proof, Water Tight

Depending on the nature and use of the equipment, some are drip proof, splash proof or water proof.

Anaesthetic-proof equipment

AP equipment standards are based on the ignition energy required to ignite the most flammable mixture of ether and air. They can be used within 5–25 cm of gas escaping from a breathing system. The temperature should not exceed 200°C. It is a less stringent requirement.

Anaesthetic-proof equipment category G

APG standards are based on the ignition energy required to ignite the most flammable mixture of ether and oxygen. Can be used within 5 cm of gas escaping from a breathing system. The temperature should not exceed 90°C. This is a more stringent requirement as the energy level should be less than 1 mJ.

CE

This is one of the most important symbols. It means conformity according to the Council of Europe Directive 93/42/EEC concerning medical devices.

Isolated or Floating Circuit

This is a safety feature whereby current is not allowed to flow between the electrical source and earth. These circuits are used to isolate individual equipment. An isolating transformer is used with two coils insulated from each other. The mains circuit is earthed whereas the patient's circuit is not earthed, so floating. As current flows through the mains coil (producing an electromagnetic field), a current is induced in the patient's coil. To complete the patient's circuit, the wires A and B should be connected. Contact with wire A or B alone will not complete a circuit, even if the subject is earthed.

Current-Operated Earth Leakage Circuit Breakers (COELCB)

These safety features are also known as an *earth trip* or *residual circuit breakers*. They consist of a transformer with a core that has an equal number of windings of a live and neutral wire around it. These are connected via a third winding to the coil of a relay that operates the circuit breaker. Under normal conditions, the magnetic fluxes cancel themselves out, as the current in the live and neutral wires is the same. In the case of a fault (e.g. excessive leakage current), the current in the live and neutral wires will be different so resulting in a magnetic field. This induces a current in the third winding causing the relay to break circuit. The COELCB are designed to be very sensitive. A very small current is needed to trip the COELCB (e.g. 30 mA) for a very short period of time reducing the risk of electrocution.

Maintenance of equipment

Two factors should be checked during the maintenance of equipment (details of the tests are beyond the scope of this book):

1. *Earth leakage*: the maximum current allowed is less than 0.5 mA. Devices that are connected directly to the patient's heart should have a leakage current of less than 10 mA.
2. *Earth continuity*: the maximum resistance allowed is less than 0.1 Ω.

Hazards of electrical shock

An electric shock can occur whenever an individual becomes part of the electric circuit. The person has to be in contact with the circuit at two points with a potential difference between them for the electrons to flow. This can happen either with a faulty high-leakage current or by a direct connection to the mains. Mains frequency is very dangerous as it can cause muscle spasm or tetany. As the frequency increases, the stimulation effect decreases but with an increase in heating effect. With a frequency of over 100 kHz, heating is the only effect. Electric shock can happen with both AC and DC. The DC required to cause ventricular fibrillation is very much higher than the AC.

If a connection is made between the live wire and earth, electricity will flow through that connection to earth. This connection can be a patient or member of staff. Mains supplies are maintained at a constant voltage (240 V in the UK). According to Ohm's law, current flow is ∝1/impedance. A high impedance will reduce the current flow and vice versa. The main impedance is the skin resistance which can vary from a few hundred thousand ohms to one million ohms. Skin impedance can be reduced in inflamed areas or when skin is covered with sweat.

Current density is the amount of current per unit area of tissues. In the body, the current diffusion tends to be in all directions. The larger the current or the smaller the area over which it is applied, the higher the current density.

Regarding the heart, a current of 100 mA (100 000 µA) is required to cause ventricular fibrillation when the current is applied to the surface of the body. However, only 0.05–0.1 mA (50–100 µA) is required to cause ventricular fibrillation when the current is applied directly to the myocardium. This is known as *microshock*.

Methods to reduce the risk of electrocution

- General measures: adequate maintenance and testing of electrical equipment at regular intervals, wearing anti-static shoes and having anti-static flooring in theatres.
- Ensuring that the patient is not in contact with earthed objects.
- Equipment design: all medical equipment used in theatres must comply with British Standard 5724 and *International Electro-technical Committee* (IEC) 60601–1 describing the various methods used for protection and the degree of protection (see above).
- Equipotentiality (see above).
- Isolated circuits (see above).
- Circuit breakers (COELCB) (see above).

Electricity can cause electrocution, burns or ignition of a flammable material so causing fire or explosion. Burns can be caused as heat is generated due to the flow of the current. This is typically seen in the skin. Fires and explosions can occur through sparks caused by switches or plugs being removed from wall sockets and igniting inflammable vapours.

Damage caused by electrical shock can occur in two ways:

1. Disruption of the normal electrical function of cells. This can cause contraction of muscles, alteration of the cerebral function, paralysis of respiration and disruption of normal cardiac function resulting in ventricular fibrillation.
2. Dissipation of electrical energy throughout all the tissues of the body. This leads to a rise in temperature due to the flow of electrons, and can result in burns.

The severity of the shock depends on:

1. The size of current (number of amperes) per unit of area.
2. Current pathway (where it flows). A current passing through the chest may cause ventricular fibrillation or tetany of the respiratory muscles leading to asphyxia. A current passing vertically through the body may cause loss of consciousness and spinal cord damage.
3. The duration of contact. The shorter the contact, the less damage caused.
4. The type of current (AC or DC) and its frequency. The higher the frequency, the less risk to the patient. A 50-Hz current is almost the most lethal frequency. The myocardium is most susceptible to the arrthymogenic effects of electric currents at this frequency and muscle spasm prevents the victim letting go of the source. As the frequencies increase to >1 kHz, the risks decrease dramatically.

THE EFFECTS OF ELECTROCUTION

As a general guide to the effects of electrocution, the following might occur:

1. 1 mA: tingling pain.
2. 5 mA: pain.
3. 15 mA: tonic muscle contraction and pain.
4. 50 mA: tonic contraction of respiratory muscles and respiratory arrest.

5. 75–100 mA: ventricular fibrillation.
6. 1000 mA: extensive burns and charring.

The body can form part of an electrical circuit either by acting as the plate of a capacitor (capacitance coupling) without being in direct contact with a conductor or as an electrical resistance (resistive coupling).

Resistive coupling

This can be caused by:

1. faulty equipment allowing a contact with a live wire if it touches the casing of the equipment
2. leakage current. As there is no perfect insulation or infinite resistance, some small currents will flow to earth because the equipment is at a higher potential than earth.

Diathermy

Diathermy is frequently used to coagulate a bleeding vessel or to cut tissues. Unipolar diathermy is commonly used. As the current frequency increases above 100 kHz (i.e. radiofrequency), the entire effect is heat generating.

Components

1. Diathermy active or live electrode.
2. Patient's neutral or passive plate.
3. Diathermy case where the frequency and voltage of the current used can be adjusted. An isolating capacitor is situated between the patient's plate and earth.

Mechanism of action

1. Heat is generated when a current passes through a resistor depending on the current density (current per unit area). The amount of heat generated (H) is proportional to the square of current (I^2) divided by the area (A) ($H = I^2/A$). So the smaller the area, the greater the heat generated. The current density around the active electrode can be as much as 10 A/cm^2 generating a heating power of about 200 W.
2. A large amount of heat is produced at the tip of the diathermy forceps because of its small size (high current density). Whereas at the site of the patient's plate, because of its large surface area, no heat or burning is produced (low current density).
3. A high-frequency current (in the radiofrequency range) of 500 000 to more than 1 000 000 Hz is used. This high-frequency current behaves differently from the standard 50-Hz current. It passes directly across the precordium without causing ventricular fibrillation. This is because high-frequency currents have a low tissue penetration without exciting the contractile cells.
4. The isolating capacitor has low impedance to a high-frequency current, i.e. diathermy current. The capacitor has a high impedance to 50-Hz current thus protecting the patient against electrical shock.
5. Earth-free circuit diathermy can be used. The patient, the tip of the diathermy forceps and the patient plate are not connected to earth. This reduces the risk of burns to the patient. This type of circuit is known as a floating patient circuit.
6. Cutting diathermy uses a continuous sine waveform at a voltage of 250–3000 V. Coagulation diathermy uses a modulated waveform.

Coagulation can be achieved by fulguration or desiccation. Blended modes (cutting and coagulation) can be used with a variable mixture of both cutting and coagulation.

7. Bipolar diathermy does not require a patient plate. The current flows through one side of the forceps, through the patient and then back through the other side of the forceps. The current density and heating effect are the same at both electrodes. Usually low power can be achieved from a bipolar diathermy with good coagulation effect but less cutting ability. Bipolar diathermy is frequently used during neurosurgery or ophthalmic surgery.

Problems in practice and safety features

1. If the area of contact between the plate and patient is reduced, the patient is at risk of being burned at the site of the plate. If the plate is completely detached, current might flow through any point of contact between patient and earth, for example earthed ECG electrodes or temperature probes. Modern diathermy machines do not function with any of the above.
2. Electrical interference with other electrical monitoring devices. The use of electrical filters can solve this problem.
3. Interference with the function of cardiac pacemakers. Damage to the electrical circuits or changes in the programming can occur. This is more of a hazard with cutting diathermy than with coagulation diathermy. Modern pacemakers are protected against diathermy.
4. Fires and explosions may be caused by sparks igniting

flammable material such as skin cleansing solutions or bowel gas.

Diathermy
- High-frequency current is used.
- An isolating capacitor is used to protect the patient against mains frequency current.
- Floating patient circuit (earth-free circuit) is used.
- There is a high current density at the tip of the diathermy forceps generating heat.

Static electricity

Measures to stop the build-up of static electricity in the operating theatre are necessary to prevent the risk of sparks, fire and explosions. The electrical impedance of equipment should allow the leakage of charge to earth, but should not be so low that there is a risk of electrocution and electrical burns.

Some of the measures used to prevent the build-up of static electricity are:

1. Tubings, reservoir bags and face masks are made of carbon-containing rubber; they are black in colour with yellow labels.
2. Staff wear anti-static footwear.
3. Trolleys have conducting wheels.
4. The relative humidity in the operating theatre is kept at more than 50% with a room temperature of more than 20°C.

With modern anaesthesia, the significance of these measures is questionable as the flammable inhalational agents (e.g. ether and cyclopropane) are not used any more.

Lasers

Lasers are being used more frequently, both in and outside the operating theatre. Lasers have the ability to cut tissue with precision with almost perfect haemostasis. They are used in thoracic surgery (excision of central airway tumours such as bronchial carcinoma), ENT (e.g. excision of vocal cord tumours), gynaecology (excision of endometriosis), urology (benign prostatic hyperplasia), skin lesion and myopia. Basic knowledge of laser principles is essential for both patient and staff safety.

Laser stands for *l*ight *a*mplification by the *s*timulated *e*mission of *r*adiation. Laser produces a non-divergent light beam of a single colour or frequency (monochromatic) with a high-energy intensity and has a very small cross-sectional area. The energy of the beam depends on the frequency.

Types of laser

- Solid-state laser such as the Nd–YAG laser that emits light at 1064 nm (infrared).
- Semiconductor laser such as the gallium arsenide (GaAs) laser. The power output tends to be low.
- Liquid laser.
- Gas laser such as the helium–neon laser (emits red light), carbon dioxide laser (emits infrared light) and argon lasers (emits green light).

Problems in practice and safety features

Increasing the distance from the laser offers little increase in safety as the laser is a high-energy non-divergent beam.

1. Permanent damage to the eye retina or the head of the optic nerve can be caused by laser beams in the visible portion. Infrared light can cause damage to cornea, lens and aqueous and vitreous humours. All staff should wear eye protection appropriate for the type of laser and within the laser-controlled area. This should offer adequate protection against accidental exposure to the main beam. Spectacles do not give reliable peripheral visual field protection.
2. Burning can be caused if the laser hits the skin.
3. A non-water-based fire extinguisher should be used immediately.
4. All doors should be locked and all windows covered in order to protect those outside the operating theatre.

Table 14.1 shows the different classes of laser products.

AIRWAY LASER SURGERY

There is a high risk of fire due to the combination of an oxygen-enriched environment and the very high thermal energy generated by the laser. The risk can be reduced by avoiding the use of nitrous oxide, the use of lower oxygen concentrations (25% or less), the use of the laser-resistant tracheal tubes, protecting other tissues with wet swabs and using non-reflective matt-black surgical instruments so reducing reflection of the main laser beam.

If fire occurs, the laser should be switched off and the site of surgery flooded with saline. The breathing system should be disconnected and the tracheal tube removed. The patient can then be ventilated with air using a bag–valve–mask system.

Table 14.1 Classification of laser products

Class 1	Power not to exceed maximum permissible exposure for the eye, or safe because of engineering design
Class 2	Visible laser beam only (400–700 nm), powers up to 1 mW, eye protected by blink-reflex time of 0.25 s
Class 2m	As class 2, but not safe when viewed with visual aids such as eye loupes
Class 3a	Relaxation of class 2 to 5 mW for radiation in the visible spectrum (400–700 nm) provided the beam is expanded so that the eye is still protected by the blink reflex Maximum irradiance must not exceed 25 W/m for intrabeam viewing For other wavelengths, hazard is no greater than class 1
Class 3b	Powers up to 0.5 W Direct viewing hazardous Can be of any wavelength from 180 nm to 1 mm
Class 4	Powers over 0.5 W Any wavelength from 180 nm to 1 mm Capable of igniting inflammable materials. Extremely hazardous

FURTHER READING

Boumphrey, S., Langton, J.A., 2003. Electrical safety in the operating theatre. BJA CPED Reviews 3, 10–14.

ebme.co.uk, no date. Safety testing of medical and electrical equipment.

Online. Available at: http://www.ebme.co.uk/arts/safety/index.htm.

Kitching, A.J., Edge, C.E., 2003. Laser and surgery. BJA CPED Reviews 8, 143–146.

MHRA, 2008. DB 2008(03): guidance on the safe use of lasers, IPL systems and LEDs. Online. Available at: http://www.mhra.gov.uk/Publications/Safetyguidance/DeviceBulletins/CON014775.

MHRA, 2012. Electrosurgery. Online. Available at: http://mhra.gov.uk/learningcentre/ESUGenericModuleCertificate/player.html.

MCQs

In the following lists, which of the statements (a) to (e) are true?

1. Concerning electric current:
   a) Inductance is a measure of the ability to store a charge.
   b) Mains current in the UK is at a frequency of 50 Hz.
   c) The leakage current of a central venous pressure monitoring device should be less than 10 mA.
   d) Current density is the current flow per unit of area.
   e) In alternating current, the flow of electrons is in one direction.

2. Electrical impedance:
   a) When current flow depends on the frequency, impedance is used in preference to resistance.
   b) The impedance of an inductor to low-frequency current is high.
   c) Isolating capacitors in surgical diathermy are used because of their low impedance to high-frequency current.
   d) With ECG, skin electrodes need a good contact to reduce impedance.
   e) Ohms are the units used to measure impedance.

3. Which of the following statements are correct?
   a) With equipotentiality, all metal work is normally at or near zero voltage.
   b) Functional earth found on medical devices acts as a safety feature.
   c) Ohm's law states that electric resistance = current × potential difference.
   d) Type CF equipment can be safely used with direct connection to the heart.
   e) Defibrillators can not be used with type B equipment.

4. Electrical shock:
   a) It does not happen with direct current.
   b) The main impedance is in the muscles.
   c) A current of 50 Hz is lethal.
   d) A current of 100 mA applied to the surface of the body can cause ventricular fibrillation.
   e) It can result in burns.

5. Diathermy:
   a) The current density at the patient's plate should be high to protect the patient.
   b) An isolating capacitor is incorporated to protect the patient against low-frequency electrical shock.
   c) A floating patient circuit can be used.
   d) Filters can reduce interference with ECG.
   e) A current of 50 Hz is used to cut tissues.

Answers

1. Concerning electric current:
   a) *False. Inductance occurs when a magnetic field is induced as electrons flow in a wire. The ability to store a charge is known as capacitance. In an inductor, the impedance is proportional to the frequency of the current. In a capacitor, impedance is inversely proportional to the current frequency.*
   b) *True. The frequency of the mains supply in the UK is 50 Hz. At this relatively low frequency, the danger of electric shock is high.*
   c) *True. A central venous pressure monitoring device can be in direct contact with the heart. Ventricular fibrillation can occur with very small current, between 50 and 100 mA, as the current is applied directly to the myocardium (microshock). Such devices should have a leakage current of less than 10 mA to prevent microshock.*
   d) *True. The amount of current flow per unit of area is known as the current density. This is important in the function of diathermy. At the tip of the diathermy forceps, the current density is high so heat is generated. At the patient plate, the current density is low and no heat is generated.*
   e) *False. In alternating current, the flow of electrons reverses direction at regular intervals. In the UK, the AC is 50 cycles per second (Hz). In direct current, the flow of electrons is in one direction only.*

2. Electrical impedance:
   a) *True. Impedance is the sum of the forces that oppose the movement of electrons in an AC circuit. In capacitors, the impedance is low to high-frequency current and vice versa. The opposite is correct in inductors.*
   b) *False. Inductors have low impedance to low-frequency current and vice versa.*
   c) *True. Capacitors have low impedance to high-frequency current and high impedance to low-frequency current. The latter is of most importance in protecting the patient from low-frequency current. High-frequency currents have low tissue penetration without exciting the contractile cells, allowing the current to pass directly across the heart without causing ventricular fibrillation.*
   d) *True. The skin forms the main impedance against the conduction of the ECG signal. In order to reduce the skin impedance, there should be good contact between the skin and the electrodes.*
   e) *True. Ohms are used to measure both impedance and electrical resistance. Ohm = volt/ampere.*

3. Which of the following statements are correct?
   a) *True. Equipotentiality is a safety feature when, under fault conditions, all metalwork increases to the same potential. Current will not flow during simultaneous contact between two such*

metal appliances as they are both at the same potential and no shock results.
   b) *False. Functional earth is not a safety feature. It is necessary for the proper functioning of the device. It is part of the main circuit where the current, via the neutral wire, is returned to the substation and so to earth.*
   c) *False. Ohm's law states that the potential difference (volts) = current (ampere) × resistance (ohms).*
   d) *True. Type CF equipment can be used safely in direct contact with the heart. The leakage current is less than 50 µA in class I and less than 10 µA in class II, providing a high degree of protection against electrical shock.*
   e) *False. Type B equipment can be provided with defibrillator protection. The same applies to type BF and type CF equipment.*

4. Electrical shock:
   a) *False. Electric shock can happen with direct current although the amount of current required to cause ventricular fibrillation is much higher than that of alternating current.*
   b) *False. The main impedance is in the skin and not the muscles. Skin impedance is variable and can be from 100 000 to 1 000 000 Ω depending on the area of contact and whether or not the skin is wet.*
   c) *True. The severity of the electric shock depends on the*

frequency of the current. The lower the frequency, the higher the risk. A current of 50 Hz is almost the most lethal frequency.

d) *True.* A current of 100 mA, when applied to the surface of the body, can cause ventricular fibrillation. Most of the current is lost as the current travels through the body and only 50–100 µA are required to cause ventricular fibrillation.

e) *True.* The electrical energy is dissipated throughout the tissues of the body leading to a rise in temperature and resulting in burns.

---

5. Diathermy:

a) *False.* In order to protect the patient from burns, the current density at the plate should be low. The same current is passed through the tip of the diathermy forceps where the current density is high, thus producing heat. The current density at the plate is low because of its large surface area.

b) *True.* The isolating capacitor protects the patient from low-frequency current (50 Hz) shock because of its high impedance to low-frequency currents. It has low impedance to high-frequency (diathermy) currents.

c) *True.* A floating patient circuit can be used to reduce the risk of burns. The diathermy circuit is earth free. The patient, the tip of the diathermy forceps and the patient's plate are not connected to earth.

d) *True.* Diathermy can cause electrical interference with ECG and other monitoring devices. The use of electrical filters can solve this.

e) *False.* Very-high-frequency current (in the radiofrequency range) of 500 000 to 1 000 000 Hz is used. This high-frequency current behaves differently from the standard 50-Hz current; because of its low tissue penetration, it passes directly through the heart without causing ventricular fibrillation.

Appendices

Appendix A

Checking anaesthetic equipment

(Reproduced with the permission of The Association of Anaesthetists of Great Britain and Ireland (AAGBI).)

Summary

A pre-use check to ensure the correct functioning of anaesthetic equipment is essential to patient safety. The anaesthetist has a primary responsibility to understand the function of the anaesthetic equipment and to check it before use. Anaesthetists must not use equipment unless they have been trained to use it and are competent to do so. A self-inflating bag must be immediately available in any location where anaesthesia may be given. A two-bag test should be performed after the breathing system, vaporizers and ventilator have been checked individually. A record should be kept with the anaesthetic machine that these checks have been done. The 'first user' check after servicing is especially important and must be recorded.

Checklist for anaesthetic equipment
(AAGBI safety guideline 2012)

Checks at the start of every operating session
Do not use this equipment unless you have been trained

Check self-inflating bag available

Perform manufacturer's (automatic) machine check

Power supply	Plugged in Switched on Back-up battery charged
Gas supplies and suction	Gas and vacuum pipelines – 'tug test' Cylinders filled and turned off Flowmeters working (if applicable) Hypoxic guard working Oxygen flush working Suction clean and working
Breathing system	Whole system patent and leak-free using 'two-bag' test Vapourizers – fitted correctly, filled, leak free, plugged in (if necessary) Soda lime – colour checked Alternative systems (Bain, T-piece) – checked Correct gas outlet selected
Ventilator	Working and configured correctly
Scavenging	Working and configured correctly
Monitors	Working and configured correctly Alarms limits and volumes set
Airway equipment	Full range required, working, with spares

Record this check in the patient record

Don't forget!	Self-inflating bag Common gas outlet Difficult airway equipment Resuscitation equipment TIVA and/or other infusion equipment

This guideline is not a standard of medical care. The ultimate judgement with regard to a particular clinical procedure or treatment plan must be made by the clinician in the light of the clinical data presented and the diagnostic treatment options available
©The Association of Anaesthetists of Great Britain and Ireland 2012

Checks before each case

Breathing system	Whole system patent and leak free using 'two-bag' test Vapourizers – fitted correctly, filled, leak free, plugged in (if necessary) Alternative systems (Bain, T-piece) – checked Correct gas outlet selected
Ventilator	Working and configured correctly
Airway equipment	Full range required, working, with spares
Suction	Clean and working

The two-bag test

A two-bag test should be performed after the breathing system, vapourizers and ventilator have been checked individually:

a) Attach the patient end of the breathing system (including angle piece and filter) to a test lung or bag.
b) Set the fresh gas flow to 5 L/min and ventilate manually. Check the whole breathing system is patent and unidirectional valves are moving. Check the function of the APL valve by squeezing both bags.
c) Turn on the ventilator to ventilate the test lung. Turn off the fresh gas flow, or reduce to a minimum. Open and close each vapourizer in turn. There should be no loss of volume in the system.

This checklist is an abbreviated version of the publication by the Association of Anaesthesia of Great Britain and Ireland 'Checking Anaesthesia Equipment 2012' (endorsed by the Chief Medical Officers)

Appendix B

Recommendations for standards of monitoring during anaesthesia and recovery

Summary

The Association of Anaesthetists of Great Britain and Ireland (AAGBI) regards it as essential that certain core standards of monitoring must be used whenever a patient is anaesthetized. These minimum standards should be uniform irrespective of duration, location or mode of anaesthesia.

1. The anaesthetist must be present and care for the patient throughout the conduct of an anaesthetic.
2. Monitoring devices must be attached before induction of anaesthesia and their use continued until the patient has recovered from the effects of anaesthesia.
3. The same standards of monitoring apply when the anaesthetist is responsible for a local/regional anaesthetic or sedative technique for an operative procedure.
4. A summary of information provided by monitoring devices should be recorded on the anaesthetic record. Electronic record keeping systems are now recommended.
5. The anaesthetist must ensure that all equipment has been checked before use. Alarm limits for all equipment must be set appropriately before use. Audible alarms must be enabled during anaesthesia.
6. These recommendations state the monitoring devices which are essential and those which must be immediately available during anaesthesia. If it is necessary to continue anaesthesia without a device categorized as 'essential', the anaesthetist must clearly note the reasons for this in the anaesthetic record. In hospitals employing anaesthetic practitioners (APs), this responsibility may be delegated to an AP supervised by a consultant anaesthetist in accordance with guidelines published by the Royal College of Anaesthetists.
7. Additional monitoring may be necessary as deemed appropriate by the anaesthetist.
8. A brief interruption of monitoring is only acceptable if the recovery area is immediately adjacent to the operating theatre. Otherwise, monitoring should be continued during transfer to the same degree as any other intra- or interhospital transfer.
9. Provision, maintenance, calibration and renewal of equipment are institutional responsibilities.

Introduction

The presence of an appropriately trained and experienced anaesthetist is the main determinant of patient safety during anaesthesia. However, human error is inevitable, and many studies of critical incidents and mortality associated with anaesthesia have shown that adverse incidents and accidents are frequently attributable, at least in part, to error by anaesthetists. Monitoring will not prevent all adverse incidents or accidents in the perioperative period. However, there is substantial evidence that it reduces the risks of incidents and accidents both by detecting the consequences of errors and by giving early warning that the condition of a patient is deteriorating for some other reason.

The introduction of routine monitoring in anaesthesia coincided with numerous improvements in clinical facilities, training and other factors likely to affect patient outcomes. The progressive reduction in anaesthesia-related morbidity and mortality is therefore linked to instrumental monitoring by association rather than proof from prospective randomized trials. The overwhelming view is that such studies would today be unethical and the circumstantial evidence that is already available indicates clearly that the use of such monitoring improves the safety of patients. Consequently, it is appropriate that the AAGBI should make clear recommendations about the standards of monitoring which anaesthetists in the United Kingdom and Ireland must use. New monitoring modalities such as those describing depth of anaesthesia have not yet become established as 'routine' and the opportunity exists to critically evaluate their utility before general introduction. A clear distinction may reasonably be made between consensus-based recommendations for 'core' monitoring and requiring that new monitoring techniques be shown by clinical trials to improve patient outcomes.

The anaesthetist's presence during anaesthesia

An anaesthetist of appropriate experience must be present throughout general anaesthesia, including any period of cardiopulmonary bypass. Using clinical skills and monitoring equipment, the anaesthetist must care for the patient continuously.

The same standards must apply when an anaesthetist is responsible for a local/regional anaesthetic or sedative technique for an operative procedure. When there is a known potential hazard to the anaesthetist, for example during imaging procedures, facilities for remotely observing and monitoring the patient must be available.

Accurate records of the measurements provided by monitors must be kept. It has become accepted that core data (heart rate, blood pressure and peripheral oxygen saturation) should be recorded at intervals no longer than every 5 min, and more frequently if the patient is clinically unstable. It is recognized that contemporaneous records may be difficult to keep in emergency circumstances. Electronic record keeping systems are now available, and the Association recommends that departments consider their procurement. It is likely that their use will become routine.

Local circumstances may dictate that handing over of responsibility for patient care under anaesthetic may be necessary. If so, hand-over time must be sufficient to apprise the incoming anaesthetist of all information concerning the patient's anaesthesia and the time and details must be noted in the anaesthetic record.

Very occasionally, an anaesthetist working single-handedly may be called upon to perform a brief life-saving procedure nearby. Leaving an anaesthetized patient in these circumstances is a matter for individual judgement. If this should prove necessary, the surgeon must stop operating until the anaesthetist returns. Observation of the patient and monitoring devices must be continued by a trained anaesthetic assistant. Any problems should be reported to available medical staff.

Monitoring the anaesthetic equipment

It is the responsibility of the anaesthetist to check all equipment before use as recommended in 'Checking Anaesthetic Equipment' (see Appendix A).

Anaesthetists must ensure that they are familiar with all equipment that they intend to use and that they have followed any specific checking procedure recommended by individual manufacturers. More complex equipment will require more formal induction and training in its use.

Oxygen supply

The use of an oxygen analyser with an audible alarm is essential during anaesthesia. It must be placed in such a position that the composition of the gas mixture delivered to the patient is monitored continuously. The positioning of the sampling port will depend on the breathing system in use.

Breathing systems

During spontaneous ventilation, observation of the reservoir bag may reveal a leak, disconnection, high pressure or abnormalities of ventilation. Carbon dioxide concentration monitoring will detect most of these problems. Capnography is therefore an essential part of routine monitoring during anaesthesia.

Vapour analyser

The use of a vapour analyser is essential during anaesthesia whenever a volatile anaesthetic agent is in use.

Infusion devices

When any component of anaesthesia (hypnotic, analgesic, muscle relaxant) is administered by infusion, the infusion device unit must be checked before use. Alarm settings and infusion limits must be verified and set to appropriate levels before commencing anaesthesia. It is essential to verify that these drugs are delivered to the patient. The infusion site should be secure and preferably visible.

Alarms

Anaesthetists must ensure that all alarms are set at appropriate values. The default alarm settings incorporated by the manufacturer are often inappropriate and during the checking procedure the anaesthetist must review and reset the upper and lower limits as necessary. Audible alarms must be enabled when anaesthesia commences.

When intermittent positive pressure ventilation is used during anaesthesia, airway pressure alarms must also be used to detect excessive pressure within the airway and also to give warning of disconnection or leaks. The upper and lower alarm limits must be reviewed and set appropriately before anaesthesia commences.

Provision, maintenance, calibration and renewal of equipment are institutional responsibilities.

Monitoring the patient

During anaesthesia, the patient's physiological state and depth of anaesthesia need continual assessment. Monitoring devices supplement clinical observation in order to achieve this. Appropriate clinical observations may include mucosal colour, pupil size, response to surgical stimuli and movements of the chest wall and/or the reservoir bag. The anaesthetist should undertake palpation of the pulse, auscultation of breath sounds and, where appropriate, measurement of urine output and blood loss. A stethoscope must always be available.

MONITORING DEVICES

The following monitoring devices are essential to the safe conduct of anaesthesia. If it is necessary to continue anaesthesia without a particular device, the anaesthetist must clearly record the reasons for this in the anaesthetic record.

The AAGBI recommends that any monitor providing continuous values, such as SpO_2 and ECG, should only display a static non-invasive blood pressure value for a maximum of 5 min, after which the value should blink or disappear altogether. The value should remain stored.

A: Induction and maintenance of anaesthesia

1. Pulse oximeter.
2. Non-invasive blood pressure monitor.
3. Electrocardiograph.
4. Airway gases: oxygen, carbon dioxide and vapour.
5. Airway pressure.

The following must also be available:

1. A nerve stimulator whenever a muscle relaxant is used.
2. A means of measuring the patient's temperature.

During induction of anaesthesia in children and in unco-operative adults it may not be possible to attach all monitoring before induction. In these circumstances, monitoring must be attached as soon as possible and the reasons for delay recorded in the patient's notes.

B: Recovery from anaesthesia

A high standard of monitoring should be maintained until the patient is fully recovered from anaesthesia. Clinical observations must be supplemented by the following monitoring devices:

1. Pulse oximeter.
2. Non-invasive blood pressure monitor.

The following must also be immediately available:

1. Electrocardiograph.
2. Nerve stimulator.
3. Means of measuring temperature.
4. Capnograph.

If the recovery area is not immediately adjacent to the operating theatre, or if the patient's general condition is poor, adequate mobile monitoring of the above parameters will be needed during transfer. The anaesthetist is responsible for ensuring that this transfer is accomplished safely.

Facilities and staff needed for the recovery area are detailed in the Association booklets, 'The Anaesthesia Team' and 'Immediate Post Anaesthetic Recovery'.

C: Additional monitoring

Some patients will require additional, mainly invasive, monitoring, e.g. vascular or intracranial pressures, cardiac output or biochemical variables. Specific devices designed to monitor loss of consciousness using adaptations of either surface EEG monitoring or auditory evoked potentials have become available.

However, their routine use has yet to be fully considered as part of our recommended minimum monitoring standards. The American Society of Anaesthesiologists (ASA) recently published a report from a task force set up to assess the use of brain function monitoring to prevent intraoperative awareness. This report summarized the state of the literature and reported the opinions derived from task force members, expert consultants, open forums and public commentary. It concluded that 'brain function monitoring is not routinely indicated for patients undergoing general anaesthesia, either to reduce the frequency of intraoperative awareness or to monitor depth of anaesthesia'. It was the consensus of the task force that the decision to use a brain function monitor should be made on a case-by-case basis by the individual practitioner for selected patients. The task force reported that patients have experienced intraoperative awareness in spite of monitored values which would imply an adequate depth of anaesthesia. The AAGBI endorses the views of the ASA taskforce.

D: Regional techniques and sedation for operative procedures

Patients must have appropriate monitoring, including a minimum of the following devices:

1. Pulse oximeter.
2. Non-invasive blood pressure monitor.
3. Electrocardiograph.

MONITORING DURING TRANSFER WITHIN THE HOSPITAL

It is essential that the standard of care and monitoring during transfer is as high as that applied in the controlled operating theatre environment and that personnel with adequate knowledge and experience accompany the patient.

The patient should be physiologically as stable as possible on departure. Prior to transfer, appropriate monitoring must be commenced. Oxygen saturation and arterial pressure should be monitored in all patients and an ECG must be attached. Intravascular or intracranial pressure monitoring may be necessary in special cases. A monitored oxygen supply of known content sufficient to last the maximum duration of the transfer is essential for all patients. If the patient's lungs are ventilated, expired carbon dioxide should be monitored continuously. Airway pressure, tidal volume and respiratory rate must also be monitored when the lungs are mechanically ventilated.

Anaesthesia outside hospital

The Association's view is that the standards of monitoring used during general and regional analgesia and sedation should be exactly the same in all locations.

AAGBI safety statement

CAPNOGRAPHY OUTSIDE THE OPERATING THEATRE

A statement from the Association of Anaesthetists of Great Britain and Ireland (AAGBI), January 2009

In 2007, the AAGBI published the fourth edition of its guidance document 'Recommendations for standards of monitoring during anaesthesia and recovery'. This document noted that continuous capnography must be used during induction and maintenance of general anaesthesia. It also recommended that continuous expired carbon dioxide monitoring be used for patients whose tracheas are intubated and who are undergoing transfer from one clinical area to another.

Because of the recognized safety advantages of using capnography in these situations, it is difficult to justify not using it when caring for patients in similar circumstances throughout the hospital. Following serious untoward incidents arising from patients being treated outside the operating theatre in intensive care units, high-dependency units and recovery rooms, the AAGBI has decided to update its guidance on the use of capnography. The AAGBI now makes the following recommendation.

Continuous capnography should be used in the following patients, regardless of location within the hospital:

1. Those whose tracheas are intubated.
2. Those whose airways are being maintained with supraglottic or other similar airway devices.

Capnographs should be available for use wherever it is possible that a patient's trachea will be intubated, such as anaesthetic rooms, operating theatres, recovery rooms, other treatment rooms in which general anaesthesia is given, intensive care units, high-dependency units and accident and emergency departments. It is also recommended that a capnograph be immediately available during the treatment of cardiac arrests in hospital.

To enhance patient safety, the AAGBI recommends that gas monitoring is normally set up directly from the breathing circuit just proximal to the patient breathing filter so that safer breathing filters without monitoring ports can be used routinely. This will decrease the number of breathing circuit connections and reconnections, and will minimize the potential for disconnections, leaks and the need for extra plastic caps, the use of which has been associated with the obstruction of airway equipment.

It is also recommended that continuous capnography should be considered during sedation:

1. For all patients receiving deep sedation.
2. For all patients receiving moderate sedation whose ventilation cannot be directly observed.

Notes

Detection of expired carbon dioxide requires the following four processes to be intact:

1. Metabolism to generate carbon dioxide.
2. Adequate circulation to deliver carbon dioxide to the lungs.
3. Ventilation of the lungs through a patent airway to expel carbon dioxide.
4. A functioning carbon dioxide analyser to quantify the gas.

Failure at any of the steps of this pathway can lead to a failure to detect expired carbon dioxide. Because the first three processes are indicators of patient wellbeing, detection of expired carbon dioxide has become a standard of safety monitoring. Also expired carbon dioxide monitoring has become a standard for assessing correct endotracheal tube placement.

Minimal sedation: a minimally depressed level of consciousness, produced by a pharmacological method, that retains the patient's ability to independently and continuously maintain an airway and respond normally to tactile stimulation and verbal command.

Moderate sedation: a drug-induced depression of consciousness during which patients respond purposefully to verbal commands, either alone or accompanied by light tactile stimulation. No interventions are required to maintain a patent airway, and spontaneous ventilation is adequate.

Deep sedation: a drug-induced depression of consciousness during which patients cannot easily be aroused but respond purposefully following repeated or painful stimulation. The ability to independently maintain ventilatory function may be impaired.

Addendum to 'Standards of Monitoring During Anaesthesia and Recovery (4) 2007' regarding the non-invasive blood pressure monitors, 18 April 2011

The AAGBI Council has approved the following as an addendum to this guideline.

The AAGBI recommends that any monitor providing continuous values, such as $SpO2$ and ECG, should only display a static non-invasive blood pressure value for a maximum of 5 minutes, after which the value should blink or disappear altogether. The value should remain stored.

Appendix C

Graphical symbols for use in labelling medical devices

LOT

Batch code

134°C

Can be autoclaved

Cannot be autoclaved

REF

Catalogue number

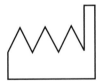

Certified to British Standards

Date of manufacture

Expiry date

SN

Serial number

Do not reuse (single use only)

STERILE

Sterile

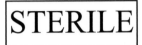

Method of sterilization using ethylene oxide

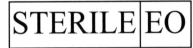

Method of sterilization using irradiation

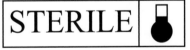

Method of sterilization using dry heat or steam

Do not use if package is opened or damaged. Do not use if the product sterilization barrier or its packaging is compromised

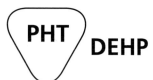

Contains phthalate – DEHP – The potential effects of phthalates on pregnant/nursing women or children have not been fully characterized and there may be concern for reproductive and developmental effects.

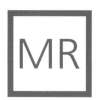

MR safe. This means the item poses no known hazards in *all* magnetic resonance imaging (MRI) environments

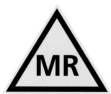

MR conditional. This means an item has been demonstrated to pose no known hazards in a *specified* MRI environment with *specified* conditions of use

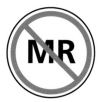

MR unsafe. This means an item is known to pose hazards in all MRI environments

Manufacturer. This symbol is accompanied by the name and address of the manufacturer

Order Number = Reference Number = Catalogue Number

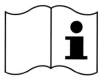

Consult instructions for use

Appendix D

Decontamination of medical equipment

Healthcare-associated infections are the leading cause of preventable disease. In the UK, they are responsible for more than 5000 deaths per year and cost the NHS over £1 billion every year. Failure to adequately decontaminate equipment carries not only the risk associated with breach of the host barriers but the additional risk of person-to-person transmission (e.g. hepatitis B virus) and transmission of environmental pathogens. Decontamination is a term encompassing all the processes necessary to enable a reusable device to be reused. This includes cleaning, disinfection, inspection, packaging, sterilization, transport, storage and use (Table AppD.1). The decontamination process is required to make medical devices:

1. safe for users to handle
2. safe for use on the patient.

Clean, disinfect or sterilize instruments?

As there is no need to sterilize all clinical items and some items can't be sterilized, healthcare policies must identify whether cleaning, disinfection or sterilization is indicated based primarily on the items' intended use.

Earle H Spaulding devised a classification system where instruments and items used for patient care are divided into three categories based on the degree of risk of infection involved in the use of the items (Table AppD.2).

Table AppD.1 Cleaning, disinfection and sterilization

Cleaning	Disinfection	Sterilization
Cleaning is the removal of visible soil (e.g. organic and inorganic material) from objects and surfaces It is normally accomplished by manual or mechanical means using water with detergents or enzymatic products Cleaning does much to reduce risk of vCJD	Disinfection describes a process that eliminates many or all pathogenic micro-organisms on inanimate objects with the exception of bacterial spores It is usually accomplished by the use of liquid chemical and heat (washer disinfector)	Sterilization is the complete elimination or destruction of all forms of microbial life This is accomplished in healthcare facilities by either physical or chemical processes

Table AppD.2 Spaulding classification

Critical	Semi-critical	Non-critical
Items which enter normally sterile tissue or the vascular system or through which blood flows They have a high risk of infection These items should be sterile Examples: surgical instruments and needles	Items that touch the mucous membranes or skin that is not intact They require a high-level disinfection process; i.e. mycobactericidal As intact mucous membranes are generally resistant to infection, such items pose an intermediate risk Such devices should ideally be sterilized but chemical disinfection is usually reserved for those that are intolerant of heat sterilization Example: laryngoscopes	Items that touch only intact skin require low-level disinfection As skin is an effective barrier to micro-organisms, such items pose a low risk of infection Examples: bedpans and blood pressure cuffs.

This classification has been successfully used by infection control professionals and others when planning methods for disinfection or sterilization.

The ease of inactivation differs according to the micro-organisms involved (see Fig. AppD.1).

Cleaning

Involves physical removal of the infectious material or organic matter on which micro-organisms thrive. The critical parameters for cleaning are the following:

1. Temperature: initial wash temperatures must be below 45°C to prevent coagulation of tissue/blood residues.

2. Chemicals: detergents used are a complex formulation of chemicals designed to remove soil (proteins, carbohydrates, lipids, etc.) from instruments. Detergents have an optimal concentration and pH to work effectively.

3. Energy: may take the form of manual washing, ultrasonic energy or water jets/sprays in automated washer disinfectors.

4. Time: cleaning cycle requires a suitable time period to achieve its desired effect.

Cleaning can be achieved either by:

Manual cleaning

1. Immersion in a diluted detergent at 35°C:

Non-immersion techniques involve a cloth soaked in cleaning solution and used

???? Prions ????
• Bacterial Spores
• Mycobacteria
• Non-lipid or Small Viruses
• Fungi
• Vegetative Bacteria
• Lipid or Medium-Size Viruses

Fig. AppD.1 Descending order of resistance of micro-organisms against inactivation.

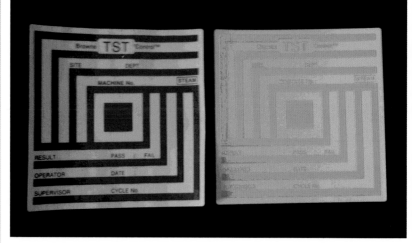

Fig. AppD.3 Bowie Dick test. This is a daily test to ensure that the steam sterilizer is functioning appropriately. Paper patches with heat-sensitive inks are used. The blue patch (left) is a PASS, the yellow patch (right) is FAILED.

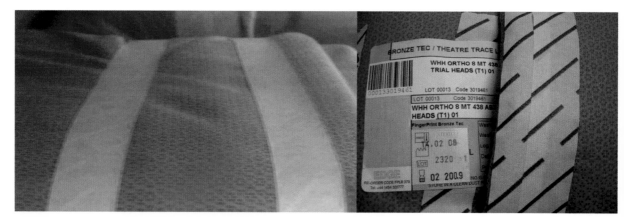

Fig. AppD.2 Heat- or chemical-sensitive inks that change colour. Right: presterilization. Left: poststerilization with the sterilization trace label. Note the date of sterilization that is valid for 1 year and details to track any object.

to wipe the items. This can be used for electrical equipment.
2. Mechanical cleaning: uses thermal disinfection, chemical disinfection (see later) or ultrasonic cleaners.

Ultrasonic cleaning is used in areas that are difficult to access. The ultrasonic waves create small bubbles on the surfaces of the instruments. These bubbles expand until they cavitate and collapse, producing areas of vacuum that dislodge the contaminants.

Disinfection

Involves reduction of micro-organisms on devices.

1. Thermal washer disinfectors combine cleaning and disinfection. Powerful water and detergent jets heated to about 80°C are used. Most organisms are inactivated except for bacterial spores, some heat-resistant viruses and cryptosporidia.
2. Chemical disinfection is the destruction of micro-organisms by chemical or physiochemical means. This process is difficult to control and validate. It is frequently used for devices that are heat sensitive in the semicritical category such as endoscopes. Examples are

glutaraldehyde 2% for 20 min, hydrogen peroxide 6–7.5% for 20–30 min, peracetic acid 0.2–0.35% for 5 min and orthophthalaldehyde (OPA) for 5–12 min.
3. Pasteurization (heat disinfection): heating to 60–100°C for approximately 30 min to reduce the number of pathogens by killing a significant number of them. The higher the temperature, the shorter the time needed.

Sterilization

The complete destruction of all micro-organisms. Sterility is the probability of complete sterilization. This probability is known as the *sterility assurance level* (SAL). A sterile device has a SAL of 10^{-6}, which means that the probability of an organism surviving on that device is one in a million using a validated process.

The methods used to achieve sterility include the following:

1. *Steam sterilization* is currently the gold standard method (Table AppD.3). It is reliable, easy to monitor, non-toxic, inexpensive, sporicidal and has high lethality, rapid heating and good penetration of fabrics. The temperature and pressure reached determine the time

to sterilization. Usually a temperature of 134°C maintained for a period of 3 min under a pressure of 2.25 bars is used.
2. *Ionizing radiation* using γ rays to produce sterility. It is ideal for prepacked heat-labile single-use items such as IV cannulae and syringes. This technique of sterilization is widely used in industry.
3. *Dry heat sterilization* (hot air oven): a constant supply of electricity is needed. Used for reusable glass, metal instruments, oil, ointments and powders.
4. *Ethylene oxide* can effectively sterilize most equipment that can withstand temperatures of 50–60°C. However, it is used under carefully controlled conditions because it is extremely toxic, carcinogenic, flammable and an explosion risk. Although it is very versatile and can be used for heat-sensitive equipment, fluids and rubber, a long period of aeration is necessary to remove all traces of gas before the equipment can be distributed. The processing time ranges from 2 to 24 h and is a very costly process.

Sterilization monitoring

The sterilization process should demonstrate a spore kill to achieve a SAL of 1×10^{-6}. To ensure that sterilization has been successful, indicators are used (Table AppD.4). For steam sterilization, for example, this requires the direct contact of saturated steam with the device in question in the absence of air at the required pressure/temperature and time.

Table AppD.3 Steam sterilization

Advantages	Disadvantages
Highly effective	Items must be heat and moisture resistant
Rapid heating and penetration of instruments	Does not sterilize powders, ointments or oils
Non-toxic	Needs good maintenance
Inexpensive	
Can be used to sterilize liquids	

Table AppD.4 Indicators used to monitor sterilization

Physical indicators	Chemical indicators	Biological indicators
These indicators are part of the steam sterilizer itself They record and allow the observation of time, temperature and pressure readings during the sterilization cycle	There are different chemical indicators There are tapes with heat- or chemical-sensitive inks that change colour when the intended temperature, time and pressure are reached (Fig. AppD.2) Such a tape does not assure sterility It merely states that the pack has been through a heating process Bowie Dick test uses heat-sensitive inks to ensure that the steam sterilizer is functioning appropriately (Fig. AppD.3)	These are rarely used in UK hospitals *Bacillus* spores that are heat sensitive can directly measure sterilization They are inherently unreliable but can be used as an additional method of validation for some forms of sterilization such as ethylene oxide

SINGLE-USE ITEMS

The use of single-use items should be encouraged when possible. This practice ensures the sterility of the equipment and prevents cross-infection. The quality of such devices must be the same as the reusable ones. As a large proportion of these devices are made from PVC plastic materials, a balance should be struck between the reduction in infection risk and effect on the environment. Incinerating PVC has no or very small effect on the levels of dioxin produced. The operating conditions of an incineration plant are the key factor in determining dioxin production and emissions, rather than the quantity or source of the chlorine entering the incinerator. It must be emphasized that any equipment that is designated 'single-use' must be used for one patient only and for a single treatment episode, and not reused even for the same patient during subsequent visits.

FURTHER READING

Association of Anaesthetists in Great Britain and Ireland, 2008. Infection control in anaesthesia. AAGBI, London. Online. Available at: http://www.aagbi.org/sites/default/files/infection_control_08.pdf

MHRA, 2010. Sterilization, disinfection and cleaning of medical equipment: guidance on decontamination from the Microbiology Advisory Committee (the MAC manual). Online. Available at: http://www.mhra.gov.uk/Publications/Safetyguidance/Otherdevicesafetyguidance/CON007438

TSE Working Group, 2008. Transmissible spongiform encephalopathy agents: safe working and the prevention of infection. Guidance from the Advisory Committee on Dangerous Pathogens. Online. Available at: http://www.advisorybodies.doh.gov.uk/acdp/tseguidance/Index.htm

Appendix E

Latex allergy

Allergy to natural rubber latex has become a major source of concern for patient safety in clinical practice and a potentially serious occupational hazard to operating theatre staff. It is estimated that 8% of the general population in the United States are allergic to products containing latex and thus subject to severe intraoperative allergic reactions. In France, it is estimated that 16.6% of anaphylactoid reactions during anaesthesia are due to latex allergy, second only to reactions due to muscle relaxants.

Latex is a milky liquid derived from the *Hevea brasiliensis* rubber tree. It contains a mixture of lipids, sugars and proteins. In addition, several chemicals are added to this liquid during its transportation, processing and manufacturing. Allergic reactions seem to be against proteins naturally present, which constitute about 1% of liquid latex sap. A protein of a molecular weight of 14 000 Da seems to be the major allergen. The use of latex in medical equipment has increased dramatically since the 1980s following health legislation introduced recommending the use of latex gloves to prevent transmission of blood-borne pathogens, such as HIV and hepatitis B, during medical procedures. This resulted in a global demand for latex medical gloves resulting in changes in quality during manufacture.

Clinical manifestations

1. Irritant contact dermatitis is the most common reaction. It is a non-allergic condition following chronic exposure to latex gloves. Dry, crusty and itchy skin predominantly affects the hands. The symptoms resolve when contact with latex ceases.
2. Delayed type IV hypersensitivity (allergic contact dermatitis) is a chemical reaction resulting from exposure to substances incorporated in the harvesting, processing and manufacturing of latex. It is a cell-mediated allergic reaction. Rash, dryness and itching occur within 24–48 h after exposure to latex. This may progress to skin blistering and spread to surround areas of contact.
3. Immediate type I hypersensitivity is the most serious reaction but the least common. It is an IgE-mediated response triggering the release of inflammatory mediators with a massive release of histamine at a local or whole body level. This results from binding of the latex allergen to sensitized receptors on mast cells. The symptoms may begin within minutes or a few hours following exposure to latex equipment. They can vary from skin redness and itching (local or generalized), rhinitis, conjunctivitis, bronchospasm and laryngeal oedema, to life-threatening anaphylactic shock.

Exposure to latex can be via cutaneous (gloves), inhalation of air-borne particles, intravascular (cannulae, giving sets, syringes), internal tissue (surgical equipment), mucous membrane (mouth, rectum, vagina, urethra, eyes and ears) and intrauterine routes. Anaesthetists must have a high index of suspicion as allergy to latex is an important cause of unexplained perioperative collapse.

High risk individuals are the following:

1. Healthcare workers such as theatre staff. It is estimated that this allergy affects 5–15% of healthcare workers.
2. Children and young adults with cerebral palsy and spina bifida. This is due to the increased early exposure to latex with repeated bladder catheterization and multiple surgical procedures. About 40% of spina bifida patients have IgE antibodies specific for latex.
3. Atopic individuals. Approximately 50% of people with latex allergy have a history of another type of allergy.
4. Those with allergy to certain foods such as avocado, banana, chestnut, kiwi, potato, tomato and nectarines.

Diagnosis can be made clinically, by skin prick testing, skin patch testing and radio-immunoassay test (RAST).

Management

The American Academy of Allergy and Immunology and the American Society of Anesthesiologists recommend:

1. Patients in high-risk groups should be identified with careful history.
2. All patients, regardless of risk status, should be questioned about history of latex allergy. High-risk patients should be offered testing for latex allergy.
3. Patients who have suggestive history and/or confirmatory laboratory findings must be managed with complete latex avoidance.
4. Procedures on all patients with spina bifida, regardless of history, should be performed in a latex-free environment.
5. When possible, patients should be scheduled for elective surgery as the first case of the day with induction done in theatre with

minimal staff present. 'Latex Allergy' signs should be posted on all operating theatre doors.

6. Anaphylactic reactions can occur 20–60 min after exposure. Patients should remain in the recovery area for a minimum of 1 h.

7. Preview all equipment to be used. A cart containing latex-free equipment should accompany the patient throughout their hospital stay.

8. Patients identified as latex allergic (by history or testing) should be advised to obtain a Medic Alert bracelet and self-injectable adrenaline (epinephrine) with medical records appropriately labelled.

Contact dermatitis and type IV reactions are treated by avoiding irritating skin cleansers and the use of topical corticosteroids application. Type I latex reactions are managed according to their severity. This can include anti-histamines, topical nasal and systemic steroids, H_2 blockers, oxygen, bronchodilators, tracheal intubation and adrenaline (epinephrine). However, routine preoperative H_1 and H_2 blockers and steroids are no longer recommended. Filters used in anaesthesia have been shown to prevent the spread of air-borne latex particles thus protecting patients against inhalation exposure.

A special 'latex allergy trolley' should be made with suggested items

- Glass syringes unless latex-free plastic syringes are available.
- Drugs in latex-free vials; stoppers can be removed and drugs drawn up.
- IV giving sets without latex injection ports. Use three-way stopcocks or tape all injection ports and do not use them.
- Cotton wool or similar as a barrier between skin and latex-containing items.
- Silicone resuscitation bags.
- Neoprene/latex-free sterile gloves.
- Plastic face masks.
- Teflon cannulae.

Appendix F

Directory of manufacturers

ANAEQUIP UK

2 Millstream Bank
Worthen
Shrewsbury SY5 9EY
UK
Tel: 01743 891140
www.anaequip.com

ARGON MEDICAL DEVICES UK

Unit 85C Centurion Court
Milton Park
Abington
Oxon OX14 4RY
UK
Tel: 01865 601270
www.argonmedical.com

BD

The Danby Building
Edmund Halley Road
Oxford Science Park
Oxford OX4 4DQ
UK
Tel: 01865 74884
www.bd.com

BLEASE MEDICAL EQUIPMENT LTD

Unit 3
Chiltern Court
Asheridge Rd Industrial Estate
Asheridge Road
Chesham
Buckinghamshire HP5 2PX
UK
Tel: 01494 784422
www.spacelabshealthcare.com

BLUE BOX MEDICAL LTD

Unit 29 New Forest Enterprise
    Centre
Chapel Lane
Totton
Southampton
Hants SO40 9LA
UK
Tel: 0238 066 9000
www.blueboxmedical.co.uk

B BRAUN MEDICAL LTD

Thorncliffe Park
Sheffield S35 2PW
UK
Tel: 0114 225 9000
www.bbraun.co.uk

CHART BIOMEDICAL LIMITED

Unit 2
The Maxdata Centre
Downmill Rd
Bracknell,
Berkshire RG12 1QS
UK
Tel: 01344 403100
www.sequal.com

COOK MEDICAL

O'Halloran Road
National Technology Park
Limerick
Ireland
Tel: 00353 61 334440
www.cookmedical.com

COVIDIEN PLC

20 Lower Hatch Street
Dublin 2
Ireland
Tel: +353 1 438 1700
www.covidien.com

DRAEGER MEDICAL UK LTD

The Willows
Mark Road
Hemel Hempstead
Hertfordshire HP2 7BW
UK
Tel: 01442 213542
www.draeger.com

GAMBRO LUNDIA AB

Lundia House
Unit 3
The Forum
Minerva Business Park
Peterborough PE2 6FT
UK
Tel: 01733 396100
www.gambro.com

GE DATEX-OHMEDA MEDICAL
EQUIPMENT SUPPLIES LTD

71 Great North Road,
Hatfield
Herts AL9 5EN
UK
Tel: 01707 263570
www.gehealthcare.com

INTAVENT DIRECT

14 Cordwallis Park,
Clivemont Road,
Maidenhead,
Berkshire SL6 7BU
UK
Tel: 01628 560020
www.intavent.co.uk

INTERSURGICAL

Crane House
Molly Millars Lane
Wokingham
Berkshire RG41 2RZ
UK
Tel: 0118 965 6300
www.intersurgical.com

KIMBERLY-CLARK HEALTH CARE

I-Flow Corporation
20202 Windrow Drive
Lake Forest
CA 92630
USA
www.iflo.com

MAQUET LTD

14–15 Burford Way
Boldon Business Park
Sunderland
Tyne & Wear NE35 9PZ
UK
Tel: 0191 519 6200
www.maquet.com

OLYMPUS KEYMED (MEDICAL &
INDUSTRIAL EQUIPMENT) LTD

Keymed House
Stock Road
Southend-on-Sea SS2 5QH
UK
Tel: 01702 616333
www.keymed.co.uk

PENLON LTD

Abingdon Science Park
Barton Lane
Abingdon
Oxon OX14 3PH
UK
Tel: 01235 547000
www.penlon.com

PHILIPS HEALTH CARE

Philips Centre
Guildford Business Park
Guildford
Surrey GU2 8XH
Tel: 01483 792004
www.healthcare.philips.com

RADIOMETER LTD

Manor Court
Manor Royal
Crawley
West Sussex RH10 9FY
Tel: 01293 531597
www.radiometer.co.uk

RIMER ALCO LTD

4–8 Kelvin Place
Stephenson Way
Thetford
Norfolk IP24 3RR
UK
Tel: 01842 766557
www.i4innovation.co.uk

SIEMENS HEALTHCARE

Newton House
Sir William Siemens Square
Frimley
Camberley
Surrey GU16 8QD
UK
Tel: 01276 696000
www.medical.siemens.com

SMITHS MEDICAL

1500 Eureka Park
Lower Pemberton
Ashford
Kent TN25 4BF
UK
Tel: 01233 722351
www.smiths-medical.com

TELEFLEX

St Mary's Court
The Broadway
Old Amersham
Buckinghamshire HP7 0UT
UK
Tel: 01494 53 27 61
www.teleflex.com

VERATHON MEDICAL UNITED KINGDOM LTD.

Stokenchurch House
First Foor
Oxford Road
Stokenchurch
High Wycombe
Buckinghamshire HP14 3SX
UK
Tel: 01494 682650
www.verathon.com

VYGON (UK) LTD

The Pierre Simonet Building
V Park
Gateway North
Latham Road
Swindon
Wiltshire SN25 4DL
UK
Tel: 01793 748800
www.vygon.co.uk

UAM GLOBAL

OES Global
Unit 10
Area D
Radley Road Industrial Estate
Abingdon
Oxfordshire OX14 3RY
UK
Tel: 01235 539618
www.uamglobal.org

ZOLL MEDICAL UK

16 Seymour Court
Tudor Road
Manor Park
Runcorn
Cheshire WA7 1SY
Tel: 01928 595160
www.zollaed.co.uk

Glossary

Absolute pressure This is the total pressure exerted on a system; i.e. the gauge pressure plus atmospheric pressure.

Absolute pressure = gauge pressure + atmospheric pressure.

Absolute temperature This is the temperature measured in relation to the absolute zero using the Kelvin temperature scale with the absolute zero, or 0K, that corresponds to $-273.15°C$.

Absolute zero The temperature at which molecular energy is minimum and below which temperatures do not exist.

Cardiac index The cardiac output divided by the body surface area. Normally, it is about 3.2 L/min/m².

Dead space That volume of inspired air that does not take part in gas exchange. It is divided into:

1. *Anatomical dead space*: that part of the patient's respiratory tract into which fresh gases enter without undergoing gas exchange. Gases are warmed and humidified in the anatomical dead space.
2. *Alveolar dead space*: that part of the lungs where perfusion is impaired resulting in ventilation/perfusion mismatch.

End-tidal gas concentration This is an estimation of the alveolar gas composition. In cases of severe ventilation/perfusion mismatch, it is an inaccurate estimation of the alveolar gas composition.

FGF Fresh gas flow from the anaesthetic machine or other source supplied to the patient.

Flow The amount of fluid (gas or liquid) moving per unit of time.

1. *Laminar flow*: flow (through a smooth tube with no sharp edges or bends) is even with no eddies. Laminar flow can be described by the Hagen–Poiseuille equation.

$$Q = \frac{\pi P r4}{8 \eta l}$$

where:
Q = flow
P = pressure across tube
r = radius of tube
η = viscosity
l = length of tube

2. *Turbulent flow*: flow through a tube with a constriction (an orifice) is uneven and eddies occur.
   In this situation, flow (Q) is:
   proportional to the square of the radius of the tube $\propto r^2$
   proportional to the square root of the pressure gradient (P) $\propto \sqrt{P}$
   inversely proportional to the length of the tube (l) $\propto \frac{1}{l}$
   inversely proportional to the density of the fluid (ρ) $\propto \frac{1}{\rho}$

FRC The functional residual capacity. It is the sum of the expiratory reserve volume and the residual volume. In an adult male, it is normally about 2.5–3 litres.

Gas laws
Dalton's law of partial pressures: in a mixture of gases, each gas exerts the same pressure which it would if it alone occupied the container.
Boyle's law: at a constant temperature, the volume of a given mass of gas varies inversely with the absolute pressure.

$$Volume = constant \times \frac{1}{pressure}$$

Charles' law: at a constant pressure, the volume of a given mass of gas varies directly with the absolute temperature.

$$Volume = constant \times temperature$$

Gay-Lussac's law: at a constant volume, the absolute pressure of a given mass of gas varies directly with the absolute temperature.

$$Pressure = constant \times temperature$$

Humidity

1. *Absolute humidity*: the mass of water vapour present in a given volume of air. The unit is mg/L.
2. *Relative humidity*: the ratio of the mass of water vapour in a given volume of air to that required to saturate the same volume at the same temperature. The unit is %.

I/E ratio The ratio of the length of inspiration to the length of expiration, including the expiratory pause. The commonly used ratio is 1:2.

Implantation testing (IT) In order to ensure that tracheal tubes are safe for use in the human body, tube material is cut into strips and inserted usually into rabbit muscle. After a period of time the effect of the implant on the tissue is compared to controls.

IPPV Intermittent positive pressure ventilation includes both controlled and assisted ventilation. The pressure within the lung increases during inspiration (e.g. 15–20 cm H_2O) and decreases during expiration to atmospheric pressure. This reverses the pressures found during spontaneous ventilation.

Latent heat of vaporization The energy needed to change a substance from liquid to gas, without changing its temperature.

Minute volume The sum of the tidal volumes in 1 min. It is the tidal volume × respiratory rate.

Oscilloscope A device capable of displaying recorded electrical signals. It is particularly useful in displaying high-frequency signals and allowing analysis of their shapes.

Partial pressure The pressure exerted by each gas in a gas mixture.

PCWP Pulmonary capillary wedge pressure is a reflection of the pressure in the left atrium. It is obtained by using a balloon-tipped flow-guided pulmonary artery catheter.

PEEP Positive end-expiratory pressure where the pressure during expiration is prevented from reaching atmospheric pressure (zero). It prevents the closure of airways during expiration thus improving oxygenation.

Plenum A chamber where the pressure inside is greater than the pressure outside. Most modern vaporizers are plenum vaporizers

where compressed gases are driven under pressure over or through a liquid anaesthetic.

Pulmonary vascular resistance (PVR) The resistance against which the right heart pumps. The unit is dyne/s/cm^{-5}. Normally, PVR = 80–120 dyne/s/cm^{-5}.

Pulse pressure The difference between the arterial systolic and diastolic pressures.

SI units

Length	Metre, m
Mass	Kilogram, kg
Time	Second, s
Electric current	Ampere, A
Thermodynamic temperature	Kelvin, K
Luminous intensity	Candela, cd
Amount of substance	Mole, mol
Other units are derived, e.g.:	
pressure (force + area)	Pascal, P
Force	Newton, N
Volume	cubic metre, m^3

SIMV Synchronized intermittent mandatory ventilation where the patient is allowed to breathe spontaneously between the preset mechanical breaths delivered by the ventilator. The ventilator synchronizes the patient's spontaneous breaths if they coincide.

Stroke volume The amount of blood expelled from a ventricle at each beat. In an adult it is about 70–125 mL.

$$\text{Stroke volume} = \frac{\text{cardiac output}}{\text{heart rate}}$$

Systemic vascular resistance (SVR) The resistance against which the left heart pumps. The unit is dyne/s/cm^{-5}. Normally, SVR = 1000–1500 dyne/s/cm^{-5}.

Tidal volume This is the volume of a single breath. It is about 10 mL/kg body weight.

Transducer A device which changes one form of energy to another. An example is the pressure transducer used to measure pressures in the body. Mechanical energy is converted to electrical energy.

Venturi principle A constriction in a tube causing an area of low pressure leading to the entrainment of a fluid (gas or liquid) via a side arm.

$$\text{PVR} = \frac{\text{mean pulmonary artery pressure} - \text{left atrial pressure}}{\text{cardiac output}} \times 80 \text{ (correction factor)}$$

$$\text{SVR} = \frac{\text{mean arterial pressure} - \text{right atrial pressure}}{\text{cardiac output}} \times 80 \text{ (correction factor)}$$

Index

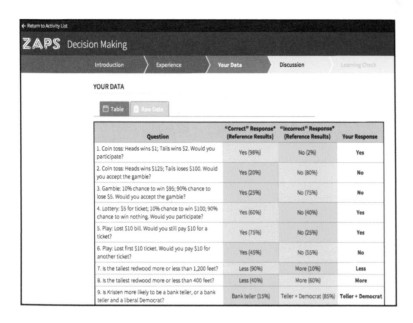

Instructor support in this completely revised ZAPS for the cognitive psychology course includes the following:

- **Summaries of students' performance** for each ZAPS lab assigned, so credit can be given for the lab.

- **Access to all the data students generate** in ZAPS, which can be shared with the class to help students see how psychological concepts influence their lives.

- **Instructor-only notes** and **activity ideas** for each ZAPS lab, available through the *Cognition* Interactive Instructor's Guide.

Visit **http://digital.wwnorton.com/cognition6**

Cognition

sixth edition

Cognition 6e

exploring the science of the mind

Daniel Reisberg

REED COLLEGE

W. W. Norton & Company
New York • London

W. W. Norton & Company has been independent since its founding in 1923, when William Warder Norton and Mary D. Herter Norton first published lectures delivered at the People's Institute, the adult education division of New York City's Cooper Union. The firm soon expanded its program beyond the Institute, publishing books by celebrated academics from America and abroad. By midcentury, the two major pillars of Norton's publishing program—trade books and college texts—were firmly established. In the 1950s, the Norton family transferred control of the company to its employees, and today—with a staff of four hundred and a comparable number of trade, college, and professional titles published each year—W. W. Norton & Company stands as the largest and oldest publishing house owned wholly by its employees.

Editor: Ken Barton
Project Editor: Sujin Hong
Assistant Editor: Scott Sugarman
Manuscript Editor: Alice Vigliani
Managing Editor, College: Marian Johnson
Managing Editor, College Digital Media: Kim Yi
Production Manager: Ashley Horna
Media Editor: Patrick Shriner
Associate Media Editor: Stefani Wallace
Assistant Media Editor: George Phipps
Marketing Manager: Lauren Winkler
Design Director: Rubina Yeh
Art Director: Jillian Burr
Designer: Lisa Buckley
Photo Editor: Kathryn Bryan
Photo Researcher: Elyse Rieder
Permissions Manager: Megan Jackson
Permissions Clearer: Elizabeth Trammell
Composition/Illustrations: Cenveo® Publisher Services
Manufacturing: Transcontinental

Library of Congress Cataloging-in-Publication Data.

Reisberg, Daniel.
  Cognition : exploring the science of the mind / Daniel Reisberg, Reed College.—Sixth edition.
    pages cm
  Includes bibliographical references and index.
  ISBN 978-0-393-93867-8 (hardcover)
  1. Cognitive psychology.   I. Title.
  BF201.R45   2013
  153—dc23   2015017228

W. W. Norton & Company, Inc., 500 Fifth Avenue, New York, NY 10110-0017
wwnorton.com
W. W. Norton & Company Ltd., Castle House, 75/76 Wells Street, London
W1T 3QT

1 2 3 4 5 6 7 8 9 0

For all my teachers,
and all they've taught me,
and for all my students,
and all they've taught me.

Brief Contents

Contents

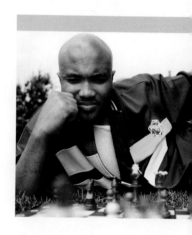
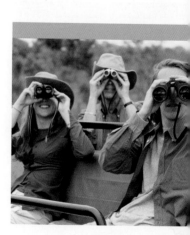

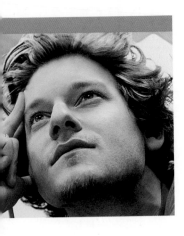
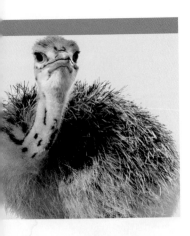

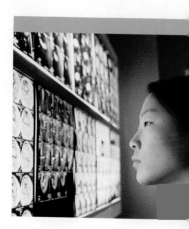

Preface

I was a college sophomore when I took my first course in cognitive psychology. I was excited about the material then, and now, many years later, the excitement hasn't faded. Part of the reason is that cognitive psychologists are pursuing profound questions that have intrigued humanity for thousands of years: Why do we think the things we think? Why do we believe the things we believe? What is "knowledge," and how *secure* (complete, accurate) is our knowledge of the world around us?

Other questions cognitive psychologists ask, though, are more immediate and personal: How can I help myself to remember more of the material that I'm studying in my classes? Is there some better way to solve the problems I encounter? Why is it that my roommate can study with the radio on but I can't?

And sometimes the questions have important consequences for our social and political institutions: If an eyewitness reports what he or she saw at a crime scene, should we trust the witness's recollection? If a newspaper raises questions about a candidate's integrity, how will voters react?

Of course we want more than interesting questions—we want *answers* to these questions, and this is another reason I find cognitive psychology so exciting. In the last half-century or so, the field has made extraordinary progress on many fronts, providing us with a rich understanding of the nature of memory, the processes of thought, and the content of knowledge. There are still many things to be discovered, and that's part of the fun. Even so, we already have something to say about all of the questions just posed, and many more. We can speak to the specific questions and the general, to the theoretical issues and the practical. Our research has uncovered principles useful for improving the process of education and we have made discoveries of considerable importance for the courts. What I've learned as a cognitive psychologist has changed how I think about my own memory, how I make decisions, and how I draw conclusions when I'm thinking about events in my life.

On top of all this, I'm also excited about the connections that cognitive psychology makes possible. In the academic world, intellectual disciplines are often isolated from each other, sometimes working on closely related problems without even realizing it. In the last decades, though, cognitive psychology has forged rich connections with its neighboring disciplines, and in this book, we'll touch on topics in philosophy, neuroscience, economics, linguistics, politics, computer science, and medicine. These connections bring obvious benefits, since insights and information can be traded back and forth between the domains. In addition, these connections highlight the importance of the material we'll be examining, since they make it clear that the issues before us are of interest to a wide range of scholars. This is a strong signal that we're working on questions of considerable power and scope.

I've tried to convey all this excitement in this text. I've done my best to describe the questions being asked within my field and the substantial answers we can provide, and finally, given some indications of how cognitive psychology is (and must be) interwoven with other intellectual endeavors.

I've also had other goals in writing this text. In my own teaching, I try to maintain a balance among many different elements—the nuts and bolts of how our science proceeds, the data provided by the science, the practical implications of our findings, and the theoretical framework that holds all of these pieces together. I've tried to find the same balance in this text. Perhaps most important, though, both in my teaching and throughout this book, I try to "tell a good story," one that conveys how the various pieces of our field fit together into a coherent package. I certainly want the specific evidence for our claims to be in view, so that readers can see how our field tests its hypotheses. And I want readers to see that our hypotheses *have been* tested, so that our claims must be taken seriously. But I also put a strong emphasis on the flow of ideas—how theories lead to new experiments, and how those experiments can lead to new theory. I also emphasize the ways in which different forms of evidence weave together, so that, for example, the coverage of neuroscience is not just presented as an adjunct to the discussion, but instead is used to address psychological questions that have long been of interest to the field.

The notion of telling a "good story" also emerges in another way. I've always been impressed with the ways in which the different parts of cognitive psychology are interlocked. Our claims about attention, for example, have immediate implications for how we can theorize about memory; and our theories about object recognition are linked to our proposals for how knowledge is stored in the mind. Linkages like these are intellectually satisfying, because they ensure that the pieces of the puzzle really do fit together. But, in addition, these linkages make the material within cognitive psychology easier to learn and remember. Indeed, if I were to emphasize one crucial fact about memory, it would be that memory is best when the memorizer perceives the organization and interconnections within the material being learned. (We'll discuss this point in Chapter 6.) With an eye on this point, I've made sure to highlight the interconnections among various topics so that readers can appreciate the beauty of our field, and can also be helped in their learning by the orderly nature of our theorizing.

I've also worked hard to help readers in other ways. First, I've tried throughout the book to make the prose approachable. I want my readers to gain a sophisticated understanding of the material in this text, but I certainly don't want them to struggle with the ideas. Therefore, I've kept the presentation as straightforward and focused as possible by highlighting the themes that bind the field together. This edition also includes many more illustrations—including many new data figures—to facilitate readers' understanding.

Second, I've taken steps that I hope will foster an "alliance" with readers. My strategy here grows out of the fact that, like most teachers, I value the questions I receive from students and the discussions I have with them. In a classroom, this two-way flow of information unmistakably improves the educational process. Of course, a two-way flow is not possible in a book, but I've offered what I hope is a good approximation: Often, the questions I hear from students, and the discussions I have with them, focus on the relevance of the material we're covering to their own lives, or the relevance of the material to the world outside of academics. I've tried to capture this dynamic, and to present my answers to these student questions in the Applying Cognitive Psychology essays at the end of each chapter (and I'll say more about these essays in a moment). Roughly half of these essays appear under the banner "Cognitive Psychology and Education," and as the label suggests, these essays will help readers understand how the materials covered in that chapter matter for (and might change!) the reader's own learning. The other essays appear under the banner "Cognitive Psychology and the Law," and explore how that chapter's materials matter in another arena: the enormously important domain of the justice system. I hope that both types of essays—Education and Law—will help readers see that all of this material is indeed relevant to their lives and, perhaps, is as exciting for them as it is for me.

Have I met all of these goals? You, the readers, will need to be the judges of this. I would love to hear from you about what I've done well and what I could have done better; and what I've covered (but perhaps should have omitted) and what I've left out. I'll do my best to respond to every comment. You can reach me via email (reisberg@reed.edu). I've been delighted to get comments from readers of the previous editions and look forward to more with this edition.

Organization of the Book

The fourteen chapters in this book are designed to cover the major topics within cognitive psychology. The first section lays the foundation. Chapter 1 provides the conceptual and historical background for the subsequent chapters. In addition, this chapter seeks to convey the extraordinary scope of this field and why research on cognition is so important. This chapter also highlights the relationship between theory and evidence in cognitive psychology, and discusses the logic on which this field is built.

Chapter 2 then offers a brief introduction to the study of the brain. Most of cognitive psychology is concerned with the functions that our brains make possible, and not the brain itself. Nonetheless, our understanding of cognition has been enhanced by the study of the brain, and throughout this book, we'll use biological evidence as one means of evaluating our theories. Chapter 2 is designed to make this evidence fully accessible to readers by providing a quick survey of the research tools used in studying the brain, an overview of the brain's anatomy, and also an example of how we can use brain evidence as a source of insight into cognitive phenomena.

In the next section of the book, we consider the problems of perception, object recognition, and attention. Chapter 3 is new to this edition and covers visual perception. At the outset, the chapter links to the previous (neuroscience) chapter with a description of the eyeball and basic mechanisms within early visual processing. In this context, the chapter introduces the crucial concept of parallel processing and the prospect of mutual influence among separate neural mechanisms. From this base, the chapter builds toward a discussion of the perceiver's *activity* in shaping and organizing the visual world, and explores this point by discussing the rich topics of perceptual constancy and perceptual illusions.

Chapter 4 discusses how we recognize the objects that surround us. This seems a straightforward matter—what could be easier than recognizing a telephone, or a coffee cup, or the letter *Q*? As we will see, however, recognition is surprisingly complex, and discussion of this complexity allows me to amplify key themes introduced in earlier chapters: how *active* people are in organizing and interpreting the information they receive from the world, the degree to which people *supplement* the information by relying on prior experience, and the ways in which this knowledge can be built into a *network*.

Chapter 5 then considers what it means to "pay attention." The first half of the chapter is concerned largely with selective attention (cases in which a person tries to focus on a target while ignoring distractors), while the second half is concerned with divided attention (cases in which a person tries to focus on more than one target or task at the same time). Here, too, we will see that seemingly simple processes turn out to be more complicated than one might suppose.

The third section turns to the broad problem of memory. Chapters 6, 7, and 8 start with a discussion of how information is "entered" into long-term storage, but then turn to the complex interdependence between how information is first learned and how that same information is subsequently retrieved. A recurrent theme in this section is that learning that is effective for one sort of task, or one sort of use, may be quite ineffective for other uses. This theme is examined in several contexts and leads to a discussion of unconscious memories—so-called "memory without awareness." These chapters also offer a broad assessment of human memory: How accurate are our memories? How complete or long-lasting are they? These issues are pursued with regard to theoretical treatments of memory, as well as the practical consequences of memory research, including the application of this research to the assessment in the courtroom of eyewitness testimony. These chapters—like the entire book—have expanded coverage in three major domains: fuller discussion of the relevant neuroscience; a broader exploration of theory, including working memory's role in making someone *intelligent*; and a greater emphasis on key applied issues, such as eyewitness memory.

The book's fourth section is about knowledge. Earlier chapters show over and over that humans are, in many ways, guided in their thinking and experiences by what they already know—that is, the broad pattern of knowledge they bring into each new experience. This invites the questions posed in Chapters 9, 10, and 11: What is knowledge? How is it represented in the mind? Chapter 9 tackles the question of how "concepts"—the building blocks of our knowledge—are represented in the mind. Chapters 10 and 11 focus on two special types of knowledge. Chapter 10 examines our knowledge about language, with discussion of both *linguistic competence* and *linguistic performance*. Chapter 11 considers *visual knowledge*, and examines what is known about mental imagery.

The chapters in the fifth section are concerned with the topic of thinking. Chapter 12 examines how each of us draws conclusions from evidence, including cases in which we are trying to be careful and deliberate in our judgments, and also cases of informal judgments of the sort we make in our everyday lives. The chapter then turns to the question of how we reason from our beliefs—that is, how we check on whether our beliefs are correct, and how we draw conclusions based on things we already believe. The chapter also considers the pragmatic issue of how errors in thinking can be diminished through education. This chapter has updated coverage of theorizing from Nobel Laureate Daniel Kahneman and expanded discussion of the role of *emotion* within decision making.

Chapter 13 is also about thinking, but with a different perspective. This chapter considers some of the ways people differ from each other in their ability to solve problems, in their creativity, and in their intelligence. The chapter also addresses the often heated, often misunderstood debate about how different groups—specifically Whites and African Americans—might (or might not) differ in their intellectual capacities.

Chapter 14, the final chapter in the book, does double service. First, it pulls together many of the strands of contemporary research relevant to the topic of consciousness: what consciousness is and what it is for. In addition, most readers will reach this chapter at the end of a full semester—a point at which they are well-served by a review of the topics already covered and ill-served by the introduction of much new material. Therefore, this chapter draws many of its themes and evidence from previous chapters, and so it can be used as a review of points that appear earlier in the book. Chapter 14 also highlights the fact that we are using these materials to approach some of the greatest questions ever asked about the mind, and in that way, should help convey the power of the material we have been discussing.

New to this Edition

What's new in this edition? I've already noted that the perception chapter is new (Chapter 3), and fills what I believe was a conspicuous gap in the previous edition. And, of course, material has been updated throughout the book to make the coverage as current as possible. I've also updated the art program for the entire book with several goals: I wanted to make the book as attractive as possible. I wanted the art to deepen and supplement readers' understanding. And, in addition, I've used the art to showcase the many points of contact between cognitive psychology and cognitive neuroscience—and so the new art will help readers grasp both the relevant brain anatomy and the nature of cognitive neuroscience research.

This edition also contains a number of entirely new elements. At the start of each chapter, the "What if…" section serves several aims. The mental capacities described in each chapter (the ability to recognize objects, the ability to pay attention, and so on) are crucial for our day-to-day functioning, and to help readers understand this point, most of the "What if…" sections explore what someone's life is like if they *lack* the relevant capacity. The "What if…" sections are rooted in concrete, human stories, and I hope these stories will be inviting and thought-provoking for readers, motivating them to engage the material in a richer way. Moreover, most of the "What if…" sections involve people who have lost the relevant capacity through some sort of brain damage. These sections therefore provide another avenue through which to highlight the linkage between cognitive psychology and cognitive neuroscience.

The sixth edition also includes explicit coverage of Research Methods. Much of this material was in the *Cognitive Workbook* for the previous edition, but I've updated and reorganized the material, and more importantly, moved the material into the text itself to make it easily accessible to all readers. At the same time, I've set the Methods coverage as an appendix to accommodate readers (or instructors) who prefer to focus on the book's substantive content. The appendix is divided into "modules" for each chapter, so that it can be used in a chapter-by-chapter basis. This organization will help readers see, for each chapter, how the research described in the chapter unfolds, and will simultaneously provide a context for each of the modules, so that readers can see why the methods are so important.

The appendix is surely no substitute for a research methods course, but nonetheless, is sequenced in a fashion that builds toward a broad understanding of how the scientific method plays out in our field. An early module, for example, works through the question of what a "testable hypothesis" is and why this is so important. Another module works through the power of random assignment, and another discusses how we deal with confounds. In all cases, my hope is that the appendix will guide readers toward a sophisticated understanding of why our research is as it is, and why, therefore, our research is so persuasive.

I've already mentioned another new element: the end-of-chapter essays. As I've discussed, these essays illustrate for readers why the chapter's materials are so important, and also how the materials are *useful*. In addition, I hope these end-of-chapter essays are inviting and maybe even *fun*, and so some readers may want to see more of them. For that reason, a fuller set of end-of-chapter essays is contained in the text's ebook, available to all readers at no additional cost.

As I flagged before, the end-of-chapter essays (both in the text and in the ebook) are of two types. For some, I draw on my own experience working with law enforcement and the criminal justice system. In this work, I'm called on to help juries understand how an eyewitness might be certain in his or her recollection, yet *mistaken*. I also work with police officers to help them draw as much information from a witness as possible without leading the witness in any way. Based on this experience, many of the essays discuss how the material in the chapter might be useful for the legal system. These essays, I hope, will be interesting for readers and persuade them that the material they're studying has important real-world consequences. In turn, it's my hope that this will make it obvious to readers why it's crucial that the science be done carefully and well, so that we bring only high-quality information into the legal system.

In addition, my students often seek take-home messages from the material that will, in a direct way, benefit them. We are, after all, talking about memory, and students obviously are engaged in an endeavor of putting a lot of new information—information they're learning in their courses—into their memories! We're also talking about attention, and students often struggle with the chore of keeping themselves "on task" and "on target." In light of these points of contact, the other end-of-chapter essays build a bridge between the course materials and the real-life concerns of students. This will, I hope, make the material more useful for students, and make it clear just how important an enterprise cognitive psychology really is.

As in the previous editions, I've also included in the ebook various Demonstrations to accompany the book's description of research. Many of these demonstrations are miniature versions of experimental procedures, allowing students to see for themselves what these experiments involve and just how powerful many of our effects are. Margin icons in the text signal points for which demonstrations are available, but it's of course up to instructors (or readers) to decide how best to use the demonstrations. Readers who want to run the demonstrations for themselves as they read along certainly can, and instructors who want to run the demonstrations in their classrooms (as I sometimes do) are certainly encouraged to do so. Instructors who want to use the demonstrations in discussion sections, aside from the main course, can do that as well. In truth, I suspect that some demonstrations will work better in one of these venues, and some will work better in others. But in all cases, I hope the demonstrations help bring the material to life—putting students directly in contact with both our experimental methods and our experimental results.

Finally, I'm excited about another element I've added for this edition in the *Instructors' Manual*. Students love videos, and they probably spend more time than they should surfing the Internet (YouTube in particular) for fun clips. As it turns out, though, YouTube contains far more than cute-pet videos. It also contains intriguing, powerful material directly relevant to the topics in this text. The *Instructors' Manual* therefore provides a list of carefully selected online videos to accompany each chapter. In many cases, these videos introduce students to the individuals briefly described in the "What if…" sections, making these sections even more compelling. I'll leave it to instructors to decide how best to use these videos in their courses, but I also want to issue an invitation: I'm sure there are other videos available that I haven't seen yet, and I would be grateful to any readers who can help me broaden this list, so we can make this resource even better.

For Students

As in previous editions, this edition of *Cognition* comes with various supplementary materials, some for students and some for instructors.

ZAPS 2.0 Cognition Labs. Every copy of the text comes packaged with free access to ZAPS 2.0 Cognition Labs—a completely updated revision of Norton's popular online psychology labs. Crafted specifically to support cognitive psychology courses, this version helps students learn about core psychological phenomena. Each lab (1 or 2 per chapter) is introduced in a brief video that relates the topic to students' lives. Students then engage in a hands-on experience that, for most labs, produces data based on their individual responses. The theories behind the concepts are then explained alongside the data the student has generated. A new assessment component lets students confirm that they understand the concept. By illustrating how research is conducted in the field, these ZAPS labs underscore that psychology is indeed a science.

Interactive Ebook. Every print copy of the text comes packaged with free access to the Interactive Ebook. This ebook can also be purchased separately at a fraction of the price of the print version. The ebook has several advantages over the printed text. First, the ZAPS 2.0 Cognition Labs are linked to the relevant topics in the ebook. Second, the ebook includes Demonstrations (mentioned earlier) designed to show students what key experiments described in the text actually involve. Third, the ebook has additional Applying Cognitive Psychology essays. While the printed text includes one of these essays at the end of each chapter, the ebook includes more. In addition, the ebook can be viewed on any device—laptop, tablet, phone, even a public computer—and will stay synced between devices. The ebook is therefore a perfect solution for students who want to learn more in more convenient settings, and pay far less doing so.

For Instructors

Interactive Instructor's Guide. This online repository of teaching assets offers materials for every chapter that both veteran and novice instructors of the course will find helpful. Searchable by chapter or asset class, the Interactive Instructor's Guide provides multiple ideas for teaching: links to YouTube-style video clips (selected and annotated by the author), teaching suggestions, and other class activities and exercises. This continually updated repository of lecture and teaching materials functions both as a course prep tool and as a means of tracking the latest ideas in teaching the cognitive psychology course.

Test Bank. The Test Bank features 980 questions, including 60 multiple-choice and 10 short-answer questions for each chapter. All questions have been updated according to Norton's assessment guidelines to make it easy for instructors to construct quizzes and exams that are meaningful and diagnostic. All questions are classified according to educational objective, student text section, difficulty, and question type. This Norton Test Bank is available with ExamView Test Generator software, allowing instructors to create, administer, and manage assessments. The convenient and intuitive test-making wizard makes it easy to create customized exams. Other key features include the ability to create paper exams with algorithmically generated variables and export files directly to your LMS.

Lecture PowerPoints. These text-focused PowerPoints follow the chapter outlines and include figures from the text and feature instructor-only notes.

Art Slides. All the figures, photos, and tables from the text are offered as JPEGs, both separately and embedded in a PowerPoint set for each chapter. All text art is enhanced for optimal viewing when projected in large classrooms.

Coursepack (Blackboard, Canvas, Angel, Moodle, and other LMS systems). Available at no cost to professors or students, Norton Coursepacks for online, hybrid, or lecture courses are available in a variety of formats. With a simple download from the instructor's website, adopters can bring high-quality Norton digital media into new or existing online courses (no extra student passwords required), and it's theirs to keep. Instructors can edit assignments at the question level and set up custom grading policies to assess student understanding. In addition to the instructor resources listed above, the Norton Coursepack includes additional chapter quizzes, flashcards, chapter outlines, chapter summaries, and questions to follow up on the essays that appear in the printed text (as end-of-chapter essays) and in the ebook.

Acknowledgements

Finally, let me turn to the happiest of chores—thanking all of those who have contributed to this book. I begin with those who helped with the previous editions: Bob Crowder (Yale University) and Bob Logie (University of Aberdeen) both read the entire text of the first edition, and the book was unmistakably improved by their insights. Other colleagues who read, and helped enormously with, specific chapters: Enriqueta Canseco-Gonzalez (Reed College); Rich Carlson (Pennsylvania State University); Henry Gleitman (University of Pennsylvania); Lila Gleitman (University of Pennsylvania); Peter Graf (University of British Columbia); John Henderson (Michigan State University); Jim Hoffman (University of Delaware); Frank Keil (Cornell University); Mike McCloskey (Johns Hopkins University); Hal Pashler (UCSD); Steve Pinker (MIT); and Paul Rozin (University of Pennsylvania).

The second edition was markedly strengthened by the input and commentary provided by: Martin Conway (University of Bristol); Kathleen Eberhard (Notre Dame University); Howard Egeth (Johns Hopkins University); Bill Gehring (University of Michigan); Steve Palmer (University of California,

Berkeley); Henry Roediger (Washington University); and Eldar Shafir (Princeton University).

In the third edition, I was again fortunate to have the advice, criticism, and insights provided by a number of colleagues who, together, made the book better than it otherwise would have been. I'd like to thank: Rich Carlson (Penn State); Richard Catrambone (Georgia Tech); Randall Engle (Georgia Tech); Bill Gehring and Ellen Hamilton (University of Michigan); Nancy Kim (Rochester Institute of Technology); Steve Luck (University of Iowa); Michael Miller (University of California, Santa Barbara); Evan Palmer, Melinda Kunar, and Jeremy Wolfe (Harvard University); Chris Shunn (University of Pittsburgh); and Daniel Simons (University of Illinois).

A number of colleagues also provided their insights and counsel for the fourth edition—for either the textbook or *The Cognition Workbook*. I'm therefore delighted to thank: Ed Awh (University of Oregon); Glen Bodner (University of Calgary); William Gehring (University of Michigan); Katherine Gibbs (University of California, Davis); Eliot Hazeltine (University of Iowa); William Hockley (Wilfrid Laurier University); James Hoffman (University of Delaware); Helene Intraub (University of Delaware); Vikram Jaswal (University of Virginia); Karsten Loepelmann (University of Alberta); Penny Pexman (University of Calgary); and Christy Porter (College of William and Mary).

And even more people to thank for their help with the fifth edition: Karin M. Butler (University of New Mexico); Mark A. Casteel (Penn State University, York); Alan Castel (University of California, Los Angeles); Robert Crutcher (University of Dayton); Kara D. Federmeier (University of Illinois, Urbana-Champaign); Jonathan Flombaum (Johns Hopkins University); Katherine Gibbs (University of California, Davis); Arturo E. Hernandez (University of Houston); James Hoeffner (University of Michigan); Timothy Jay (Massachusetts College of Liberal Arts); Timothy Justus (Pitzer College); Janet Nicol (University of Arizona); Robyn T. Oliver (Roosevelt University); Raymond Phinney (Wheaton College, and his comments were especially thoughtful!); Brad Postle (University of Wisconsin, Madison); Erik D. Reichle (University of Pittsburgh); Eric Ruthruff (University of New Mexico); Dave Sobel (Brown University); Martin van den Berg (California State University, Chico); and Daniel R. VanHorn (North Central College).

And now, happily, for the current edition: Michael Dodd (University of Nebraska—Lincoln); James Enns (University of British Columbia); E. Christina Ford (Penn State University); Danielle Gagne (Alfred University); Marc Howard (Boston University); B. Brian Kuhlman (Boise State University); Guy Lacroix (Carleton University); Ken Manktelow (University of Wolverhampton); Aidan Moran (University College Dublin, Ireland); Joshua New (Barnard College); Janet Nicol (University of Arizona); Mohammed K. Shakeel (Kent State University); David Somers (Boston University); and Stefan Van der Stigchel (Utrecht University).

I also want to thank the people at Norton. I've had a succession of terrific editors, and I'm grateful to Jon Durbin, Sheri Snavely, Aaron Javsicas, and Ken Barton for their support and fabulous guidance over the years. There's simply no question that the book is stronger, clearer, and *better* because of their input and advice.

I also want to thank Scott Sugarman for doing a fabulous job of keeping this project on track, and also Sujin Hong, Patrick Shriner, Kathryn Bryan, and Elyse Rieder for their extraordinary work in helping me bring out a book of the highest quality. Thanks in advance to Lauren Winkler and the Norton sales team—I am, of course, deeply grateful for all you do. Thanks also to Patrick Shriner, George Phipps, and Pepper Williams for developing the new ZAPS labs, and Stefani Wallace for her skilled management of the supplements package. Thanks, finally, to Ben Morris, who did a fabulous job of helping find the "neuro-art." Last—but FAR from least—may Alice Vigliani's peonies always flourish. I assume she tends her flowers with the same care that she devotes to her editing and, if so, her garden must be marvelous indeed.

Finally, I lovingly reiterate the words I said in the previous edition: In dozens of ways, Friderike makes all of this possible and worthwhile. She forgives me the endless hours at the computer, tolerates the tension when I'm feeling overwhelmed by deadlines, and is always ready to read my pages and offer thoughtful, careful, instructive insights. My gratitude to, and love for, her are boundless.

Daniel Reisberg
Portland, Oregon

The Foundations of Cognitive Psychology

What is cognitive psychology? In Chapter 1, we'll define this discipline and offer a sketch of what this field can teach us—through its theories and practical applications. We'll also provide a brief history to explain why cognitive psychology has taken the form that it does.

Chapter 2 has a different focus. In the last decade or two, cognitive psychology has formed a productive partnership with the field of *cognitive neuroscience*—the effort toward understanding our mental functioning by close study of the brain and nervous system. In this book, our emphasis will be on psychology, not neuroscience, but even so, we'll rely on evidence from neuroscience at many points. To make sure this evidence is useful, we need to provide some background, and that's the main purpose of Chapter 2. In that chapter, we'll offer a rough mapping of what's where in the brain, and we'll describe the functioning of many of the brain's parts. We'll also discuss the broad issue of *what it means* to describe the functioning of this or that brain region, because, as we will see, each of the brain's parts is enormously specialized in what it does. As a result, mental achievements such as reading or remembering or deciding depend on the coordinated functioning of many different brain regions, with each contributing its own small bit to the overall achievement.

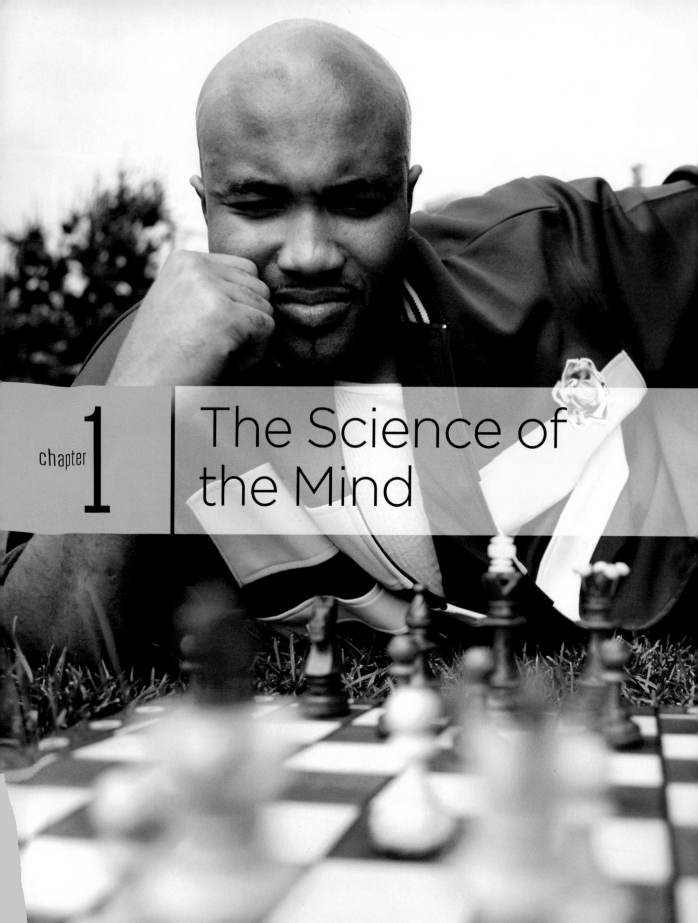

chapter **1** | The Science of
the Mind

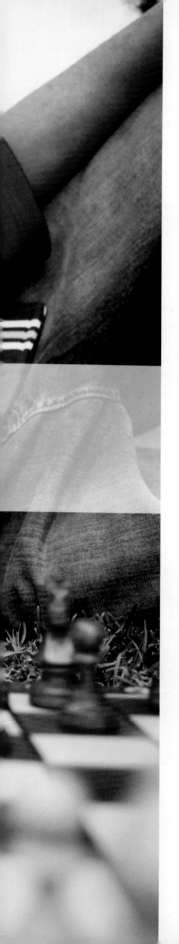

Almost everything you do, and everything you feel or say, depends on your *cognition*—what you know, what you remember, and what you think. As a result, the book you're now reading—a textbook on cognition—describes the foundation for virtually every aspect of who you are.

As illustrations of this theme, in a few pages we'll consider the way in which your ability to cope with grief depends on how your memory functions. We'll also discuss the role that memory plays in shaping your self-image—and, hence, your self-esteem. As a more mundane example, we'll also discuss a case in which your understanding of a simple story depends on the background knowledge that you supply. Examples like these make it clear that cognition matters in an extraordinary range of circumstances, and it is on this basis that our focus in this book is, in a real sense, on the intellectual foundation of almost every aspect of human experience.

The Scope of Cognitive Psychology

When the field of cognitive psychology was first launched, it was broadly focused on the *scientific study of knowledge*, and this focus led immediately to a series of questions: How is knowledge acquired? How is knowledge retained so that it's available when needed? How is knowledge used—whether as a basis for making decisions or as a means of solving problems?

These are great questions, and it's easy to see that answering them might be quite useful. For example, imagine that you're studying for next Wednesday's exam, but for some reason the material just won't "stick" in your memory. You find yourself wishing, therefore, for a better strategy to use in studying and memorizing. What would that strategy be? Is it possible to have a "better memory"?

As a different case, let's say that while you're studying, your friend is moving around in the room, and you find this to be quite distracting. Why can't you just shut out your friend's motion? Why don't you have better control over your attention and your ability to concentrate?

Here's one more example: You pick up the morning newspaper, and you're horrified to learn how many people have decided to vote for candidate X. How do people decide whom to vote for? For that matter, how do people decide what college to attend, or which car to buy, or even what to have for dinner? And how can we help people make *better* decisions—so that, for example, they choose healthier foods, or vote for the candidate who (in your view) is obviously preferable?

- The chapter begins with a description of the *scope* of cognitive psychology. The domain of this field includes activities that are obviously "intellectual" (such as remembering, or attending, or making judgments) but also a much broader range of activities that depend on these intellectual achievements.

- What form should a "science of the mind" take? We discuss the difficulties in trying to study the mind by means of direct observation. But we also explore why we *must* study the mental world if we are to understand behavior; the

reason, in brief, is that our behavior depends, in crucial ways, on how we *perceive* and *understand* the world around us.

- Combining these themes, we are led to the view that we must study the mental world *indirectly*, but as we will see, the (inferential) method for doing this is the same method used by most sciences.

- Finally, we consider examples of research in cognitive psychology to illustrate the types of data that psychologists consider and the logic they use in testing their theories.

Before we're through, we'll consider evidence pertinent to all of these questions. Let's note, though, that in these examples, things aren't going as you might have wished: You remember less than you want to; you're unable to ignore a distraction; the voters make a choice you don't like. But what about the other side of the picture? What about the remarkable intellectual feats that humans achieve—brilliant deductions or creative solutions to complex problems? In this text, we'll also discuss these cases and explore how it is that people accomplish the great things they do.

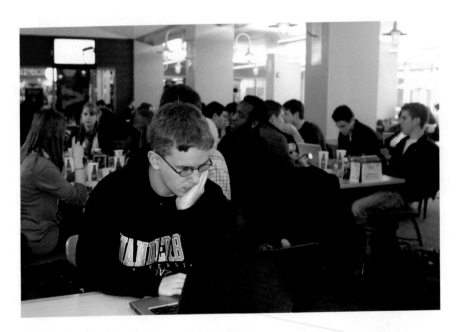

TRYING TO FOCUS

Often, you want to focus your attention on just one thing, and you want to shut out the other sights and sounds that are making it hard for you to concentrate. What steps should you take to promote this focus and to avoid distraction?

The Broad Role for Memory

Clearly there is an important set of issues in play here, but even so, the various questions just catalogued risk a misunderstanding, because they make it sound like cognitive psychology is concerned only with our functioning as intellectuals—our ability to remember, or to pay attention, or to think through options when making a choice. As we said at the start, though, the relevance of cognitive psychology is far broader—thanks to the fact that a huge range of our actions, thoughts, and feelings *depend on knowledge*. As one illustration of this point, let's look at the study of *memory* and ask: When we investigate how memory functions, what exactly is it that we're investigating? Or, to turn this around, what aspects of your life depend on memory?

You obviously rely on memory when you're taking an exam—memory for what you have learned during the term. Likewise, you rely on memory when you're at the supermarket and trying to remember the cheesecake recipe so that you can buy the right ingredients. You also rely on memory when you're reminiscing about childhood. But what else draws on memory?

Consider this simple story (adapted from Charniak, 1972):

> Betsy wanted to bring Jacob a present. She shook her piggy bank. It made no sound. She went to look for her mother.

This four-sentence tale is easy to understand, but *only because you provided some important bits of background yourself*. For example, you weren't at all puzzled about why Betsy was interested in her piggy bank; you weren't puzzled, specifically, about why the story's first sentence led naturally to the second. This is because you already knew (a) that the things one gives as presents are often things bought for the occasion (rather than things already owned), (b) that buying things requires money, and (c) that money is stored in piggy banks. Without these facts, you would have been bewildered as to why a desire to give a gift would lead someone to her piggy bank. (Surely you did not think she intended to give the piggy bank itself as the present!) Likewise, you immediately understood why Betsy *shook* her piggy bank. You didn't suppose that she was shaking it in frustration or trying to find out if it would make a good percussion instrument. Instead, you understood that she was trying to determine its contents. But you knew this fact only because you already knew (d) that children don't keep track of how much money is in their bank, and (e) that one cannot simply look into the bank to learn its contents. Without these facts, Betsy's shaking of the bank would make no sense. Similarly, you understood what it meant that the bank made no sound. That's because you know (f) that it's usually coins (not bills) that are kept in piggy banks, and (g) that coins make noise when they are shaken. If you didn't know these facts, you might have interpreted the bank's silence, when it was shaken, as good news, indicating perhaps that the bank was jammed full of $20 bills—an inference that would have led you to a very different expectation for how the story would unfold from there.

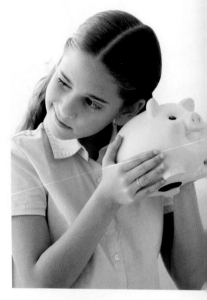

A SIMPLE STORY

What is involved in your understanding of this simple story? Betsy wanted to bring Jacob a present. She shook her piggy bank. It made no sound. She went to look for her mother.

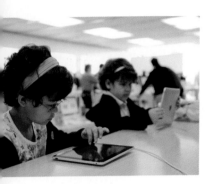

CELEBRATING HUMAN ACHIEVEMENTS

Many of the text's examples involve *failures* or *limitations* in our cognition. But we also need to explain our species' incredible intellectual achievements—the complex problems we've solved or the extraordinary devices we've invented.

Of course, there's nothing special about the "Betsy and Jacob" story, and it seems likely that we'd uncover a similar reliance on background knowledge if we explored how you understand some other narrative, or how you follow a conversation, or comprehend a TV show. Our suggestion, in other words, is that many (and perhaps all) of your encounters with the world depend on your supplementing your experience with knowledge that you bring to the situation. And perhaps this *has* to be true. After all, if you didn't supply the relevant bits of background, then anyone telling the "Betsy and Jacob" story would need to spell out all the connections and all the assumptions. That is, the story would have to include all the facts that, *with* memory, are supplied by you. As a result, the story would have to be many times longer, and the telling of it much slower. The same would be true for every story you hear, every conversation you participate in. Memory is thus crucial for each of these activities.

Amnesia and Memory Loss

Here is a different sort of example: In Chapter 7, we will consider various cases of clinical *amnesia*—cases in which someone, because of brain damage, has lost the ability to remember certain materials. These cases are fascinating at many levels, including the fact that they provide us with key insights into what memory is *for*: Without memory, what is disrupted?

H.M. was in his mid-20's when he had brain surgery intended to control his severe epilepsy. He survived for more than 50 years after the operation, and for all of those years, he had little trouble remembering events *prior to* the surgery. However, H.M. seemed completely unable to recall any event that occurred *after* his operation. If asked who the president is, or about recent events, he reported facts and events that were current at the time of the surgery. If asked questions about last week, or even an hour ago, he recalled nothing.

This memory loss had massive consequences for H.M.'s life, and some of the consequences are perhaps surprising. For example, H.M. had an uncle he was very fond of, and he occasionally asked his hospital visitors how his uncle was doing. Unfortunately, the uncle died sometime after H.M.'s surgery, and H.M. was told this sad news. The information came as a horrible shock, but because of his amnesia, he soon forgot about it.

Sometime later, though, because he'd *forgotten* about his uncle's death, H.M. again asked how his uncle was doing and was again told of the death. However, with no memory of having heard this news before, he was once more hearing it "for the first time," with the shock and grief every bit as strong as it was initially. Indeed, each time he heard this news, he was hearing it "for the first time." With no memory, he had no opportunity to live with the news, to adjust to it. Hence, his grief could not subside. Without memory, H.M. had no way to come to terms with his uncle's death.

A different glimpse of memory function comes from H.M.'s poignant comments about his state and about "who he is." Each of us has a conception

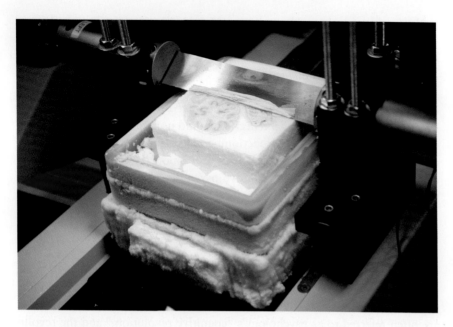

H.M.'S BRAIN

H.M. died in 2008, and the world then learned his full name, Henry Molaison. Throughout his life, H.M. had cooperated with researchers in many studies of his memory loss. Even after his death, H.M. is contributing to science: His brain (shown here) was frozen and has now been sliced into sections for detailed anatomical study.

of who we are, and that conception is supported by numerous memories: We know whether we're deserving of praise for our good deeds or blame for our transgressions because we remember our good deeds and our transgressions. We know whether we've kept our promises or achieved our goals because, again, we have the relevant memories. None of this is true for people who suffer from amnesia, and H.M. sometimes commented on the fact that in important ways, he didn't know who he was. He didn't know if he should be proud of his accomplishments or ashamed of his crimes; he didn't know if he'd been clever or stupid, honorable or dishonest, industrious or lazy. In a sense, then, without a memory, there is no self. (For broader discussion, see Conway & Pleydell-Pearce, 2000; Hilts, 1995.)

What, then, is the scope of cognitive psychology? As we mentioned earlier, this field is sometimes defined as the scientific study of the acquisition, retention, and use of knowledge. We've now seen, though, that "knowledge" (and, hence, the study of how we gain and use knowledge) is relevant to a huge range of concerns. Our self-concept, it seems, depends on our knowledge (and, in particular, on our episodic knowledge). Our emotional adjustments to the world, as we have seen, rely on our memories. Or, to take a much more ordinary case, our ability to understand a story we've read, or a conversation, or, presumably, any of our experiences, depends on our supplementing that experience with some knowledge.

The suggestion, then, is that cognitive psychology can help us understand capacities relevant to virtually every moment of our lives. Activities that don't, on the surface, appear intellectual would nonetheless collapse without the support of our cognitive functioning. The same is true whether we're considering our actions, our social lives, our emotions, or almost any other domain. This is the scope of cognitive psychology and, in a real sense, the scope of this book.

The Cognitive Revolution

The enterprise that we now call "cognitive psychology" is roughly 50 years old, and the emergence of this field was in some ways dramatic. Indeed, the science of psychology went through changes in the 1950s and 1960s that are often referred to as psychology's "cognitive revolution," and the revolution brought a huge shift in the style of research used by most psychologists. The new style was intended initially for studying problems we've already met: problems of memory, decision making, and so on. But this new type of research, and its new approach to theorizing, was soon exported to other domains, with the consequence that in important ways the cognitive revolution changed the intellectual map of our field.

The Limits of Introspection

The cognitive revolution centered on a small number of key ideas. One idea is that the science of psychology cannot study the mental world directly. A second idea is that the science of psychology *must* study the mental world if we are going to understand behavior.

As a path toward understanding each of these ideas, let's look at a pair of earlier traditions in psychology that offered a rather different perspective. We'll start with a research framework, prominent more than a century ago, that assumed we *could* study the mental world directly. Note, though, that our purpose here is not to describe the full history of modern cognitive psychology. That history is rich and interesting, but our goal is a narrow one—to explain why the cognitive revolution's themes were as they were. (For readers interested in the history, though, see Bartlett, 1932; Benjamin, 2008; Broadbent, 1958; Malone, 2009; Mandler, 2011.)

In the late 19th century, Wilhelm Wundt (1832–1920) and his student Edward Bradford Titchener (1867–1927) launched a new research enterprise, and according to many scholars, it was their work that eventually led to the modern field of experimental psychology. In Wundt's and Titchener's view, psychology needed to focus largely on the study of conscious mental events—feelings, thoughts, perceptions, and recollections. But how should

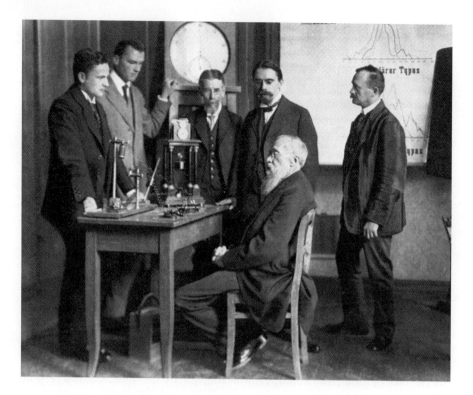

these events be studied? These early researchers started with the obvious fact that there is no way for you to experience my thoughts, or I yours. The only person who can experience or observe your thoughts is you. Wundt, Titchener, and their colleagues concluded, therefore, that the only way to study thoughts is for each of us to **introspect**, or "look within," to observe and record the content of our own mental lives and the sequence of our own experiences.

Wundt and Titchener insisted, though, that this introspection could not be casual. Instead, introspectors had to be meticulously trained: They were given a vocabulary to describe what they observed; they were taught to be as careful and as complete as possible; and above all, they were trained simply to report on their experiences, with a minimum of interpretation.

This style of research was enormously influential for several years, but psychologists gradually became disenchanted with it, and it's easy to see why. As one concern, these investigators were soon forced to acknowledge that some thoughts are *un*conscious, and this meant that introspection was inevitably limited as a research tool. After all, by its very nature introspection is the study of conscious experiences, and so of course it can tell us nothing about unconscious events.

Indeed, we now know that unconscious thought plays a huge part in our mental lives. For example, what is your phone number? It's likely that the moment you read this question, the number "popped" into your thoughts without any effort, noticeable steps, or strategies on your part. But, in fact, there's good reason to think that this simple bit of remembering requires a complex series of steps. These steps take place outside of awareness; and so, if we rely on introspection as our means of studying mental events, we have no way of examining these processes.

But there is also another and deeper problem with introspection: In order for any science to proceed, there must be some way to test its claims; otherwise, we have no means of separating correct assertions from false ones, accurate descriptions of the world from fictions. Hand in hand with this requirement, science needs some way of resolving disagreements: If you claim that Earth has one moon and I insist that it has two, we need some way of determining who is right. Otherwise, we cannot locate the facts of the matter, and so our "science" will become a matter of opinion, not fact.

With introspection, this testability of claims is often unattainable. To see why, imagine that I insist my headaches are worse than yours. How could we ever test my claim? It might be true that I describe my headaches in extreme terms: I talk about my "agonizing, excruciating" headaches. But that might mean only that I'm inclined toward extravagant descriptions; it might reflect my verbal style, not my headaches. Similarly, it might be true that I need bed rest whenever one of my headaches strikes. Does that mean my headaches are truly intolerable? It might mean instead that I'm self-indulgent and rest even in the face of mild pain. Perhaps our headaches are identical, but you're stoic about yours and I'm not.

How, therefore, should we test my claim about my headaches? What we need is some means of directly comparing my headaches to yours, and that would require transplanting one of my headaches into your experience, or vice versa. Then one of us could make the appropriate comparison. But (setting aside the science fiction notion of telepathy) there's no way to do this, leaving us, in the end, unable to determine whether my headache reports are exaggerated, distorted, or accurate. We're left, in other words, with the brute fact that our only information about my headaches is what comes to us through the filter of my description, and we have no way to know how (or whether) that filter is coloring the evidence.

For purposes of science, this is unacceptable. Ultimately, we do want to understand conscious experience, and so, in later chapters, we will consider introspective reports. For example, we'll talk about the subjective feeling of "familiarity" and the conscious experience of mental imagery; in Chapter 14, we'll talk about consciousness itself. In these settings, though, we'll rely on introspection as a source of observations that need to be explained; we won't rely on introspective data as a means of evaluating our hypotheses—because, usually, *we can't*. To test hypotheses, we need data we can rely on, and, among other requirements, this means we need data that aren't dependent on a particular point of view or a particular descriptive style. Scientists generally achieve this objectivity by making sure the raw data are out in plain view, so that you can inspect my evidence, and I yours. In that way, we can be certain that neither of us is distorting or misreporting or exaggerating the facts. And that is precisely what we cannot do with introspection.

The Years of Behaviorism

Historically, the concerns just described led many psychologists to abandon introspection as a research tool. Psychology could not be a science, they argued, if it relied on this method. Instead, psychology needed objective data, and that meant data that were out in the open for all to observe.

What sorts of data does this allow? First, an organism's *behaviors* are obviously observable in the right way: You can watch my actions, and so can anyone else who is appropriately positioned. Therefore, data concerned with behavior are objective data and, thus, grist for the scientific mill. Likewise, *stimuli* in the world are in the same "objective" category: These are measurable, recordable, physical events.

In addition, you can arrange to record the stimuli I experience day after day after day and also the behaviors I produce each day. This means that you can record how the pattern of behaviors changes with the passage of time and with the accumulation of experience. Thus, my *learning history* can also be objectively recorded and scientifically studied.

In contrast, my *beliefs*, *wishes*, *goals*, and *expectations* are all things that cannot be directly observed, cannot be objectively recorded. These "mentalistic" notions can be observed only via introspection; and introspection, we have suggested, has little value as a scientific tool. Hence, a scientific psychology needs to avoid these invisible internal entities.

It was this perspective that led researchers to the **behaviorist theory** movement, a movement that dominated psychology in America for the first half of the 20th century. This movement was a success in many ways and uncovered a range of principles concerned with how behavior changes in response to

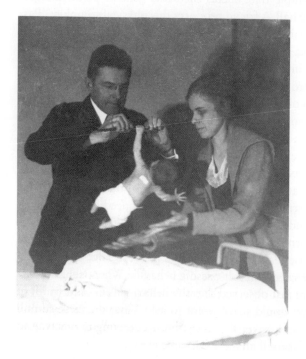

JOHN B. WATSON

John B. Watson (1878–1958) was a prominent and persuasive advocate for the behaviorist movement. Given his focus on learning and learning histories, it is unsurprising that Watson was intrigued by babies' behavior and learning. Here, he tests the grasp reflex displayed by all human neonates.

various stimuli (including the stimuli we call "rewards" and "punishments"). By the late 1950s, however, psychologists were convinced that a lot of our behavior could not be explained in these terms. The reason, in brief, is that the ways people act, and the ways that they feel, are guided by how they *understand* or *interpret* the situation, and not by the objective situation itself. Therefore, if we follow the behaviorists' instruction and focus only on the objective situation, we will regularly misunderstand why people are doing what they're doing and make the wrong predictions about how they'll behave in the future. To put this point another way, the behaviorist perspective demands that we not talk about mental entities such as beliefs, memories, and so on, because these things cannot be studied directly and therefore cannot be studied scientifically. Yet it seems that these subjective entities play a pivotal role in guiding behavior, and so we *must* consider these entities if we want to understand behavior.

Evidence pertinent to these assertions is threaded throughout the chapters of this book. Over and over, we'll find it necessary to mention people's perceptions and strategies and understanding, as we strive to explain why (and how) they perform various tasks and accomplish various goals. Indeed, we've already seen an example of this pattern. Imagine that we present the "Betsy and Jacob" story to people and then ask them various questions: Why did Betsy shake her piggy bank? Why did she go to look for her mother? People's responses will surely reflect their understanding of the story, which in turn depends on far more than the physical stimulus—that is, the 29 syllables of the story itself. If we want to predict someone's responses to these questions, therefore, we'll need to refer to the stimulus (the story itself) *and also* to the person's knowledge and understanding of this stimulus.

Here's a different example that makes the same general point. Imagine you're sitting in the dining hall. A friend produces this physical stimulus: "Pass the salt, please," and you immediately produce a bit of salt-passing behavior. In this exchange, there is a physical stimulus (the words that your friend uttered) and an easily defined response (your passing of the salt), and so this simple event seems fine from the behaviorists' perspective: The elements are out in the open, for all to observe, and can easily be objectively recorded. But let's note that the event would have unfolded in the same way if your friend had offered a different stimulus. "Could I have the salt?" would have done the trick. Ditto for "Salt, please!" or "Hmm, this sure needs salt!" If your friend is both loquacious and obnoxious, the utterance might have been, "Excuse me, but after briefly contemplating the gustatory qualities of these comestibles, I have discerned that their sensory qualities would be enhanced by the addition of a number of sodium and chloride ions, delivered in roughly equal proportions and in crystalline form; could you aid me in this endeavor?" You might giggle (or snarl) at your friend, but you would still pass the salt.

Now let's work on the science of salt-passing behavior. When is this behavior produced? Since we've just observed that the behavior is evoked by all of these different stimuli, we would surely want to ask: What do these stimuli have in common? If we can answer that question, we're well on our way to understanding why these stimuli all have the same effect.

If we focus entirely on the observable, objective aspects of these stimuli, they actually have little in common. After all, the actual sounds being produced are rather different in that long utterance about sodium and chloride ions and the utterance, "Salt, please!" And in many circumstances, *similar* sounds would not lead to salt-passing behavior. Imagine that your friend says, "Salt the pass" or "Sass the palt." These are acoustically similar to "Pass the salt" but wouldn't have the same impact. Or imagine that your friend says, "She has only a small part in the play. All she gets to say is, 'Pass the salt, please.'" In this case, exactly the right syllables were uttered, but you wouldn't pass the salt in response.

It seems, then, that our science of salt passing won't get very far if we insist on talking only about the physical stimulus. Stimuli that are physically different from each other ("Salt, please" and the bit about ions) have similar effects. Stimuli that are physically similar to each other ("Pass the salt" and "Sass the palt") have different effects. Physical similarity, therefore, is plainly not what unites the various stimuli that evoke salt passing.

It is clear, though, that the various stimuli that evoke salt passing do have something in common with each other: *They all mean the same thing.* Sometimes this meaning derives easily from the words themselves ("Please pass the salt"). In other cases, the meaning depends on certain pragmatic rules. (For example, we pragmatically understand that the question "Could you pass the salt?" is not a question about arm strength, although, interpreted literally, it might be understood that way.) In all cases, though, it seems plain that to predict your behavior in the dining hall, we need to ask what these stimuli *mean to you.* This seems an extraordinarily simple point, but it is a point, echoed over and over by countless other examples, that indicates the impossibility of a complete behaviorist psychology.[1]

The Roots of the Cognitive Revolution

It seems, then, that we're caught in a trap: We need to talk about the mental world if we hope to explain behavior. This is because how people act is shaped by how they *perceive* the situation, how they *understand* the stimuli, and so on. The only direct means of studying the mental world, however, is introspection, and introspection is scientifically unworkable. Thus, in brief: We need to study the mental world, but we can't.

There is, however, a solution to this impasse, and it was actually suggested many years ago by philosopher Immanuel Kant (1724–1804). To use Kant's **transcendental method**, you begin with the observable facts and then work backward from these observations. In essence, you ask: How could these observations have come about? What must the underlying *causes* be that led to these *effects*?

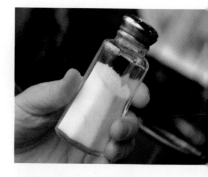

PASSING THE SALT

If a friend requests the salt, your response will depend on how you understand your friend's words. This is a simple point, echoed in example after example, but it is the reason why a rigid behaviorist perspective will not allow us to explain your behavior.

---

1. We should note that the behaviorists themselves quickly realized this point. Hence, modern behaviorism has abandoned the radical rejection of mentalistic terms; indeed, it's hard to draw a line between modern behaviorism and a field called "animal cognition," a field that often employs mentalistic language! The behaviorism being criticized here is a historically defined behaviorism, and it's this perspective that, in large measure, gave birth to modern cognitive psychology.

This method, sometimes called "inference to best explanation," is at the heart of most modern science. Physicists, for example, routinely use this method to study objects or events that cannot be observed directly. To take just one case, no physicist has ever observed an electron, but this has not stopped physicists from learning a great deal about electrons. How do the physicists proceed? Even though electrons themselves are not observable, their presence often leads to observable results—in essence, *visible effects* from an *invisible cause*. Thus, among other things, electrons leave observable tracks in cloud chambers, and they produce momentary fluctuations in a magnetic field. Physicists can then use these observations the same way a police detective uses clues—asking what the "crime" must have been like if it left this and that clue. (A size 11 footprint? That probably tells us what size feet the criminal has, even though no one observed his feet. A smell of tobacco smoke? That suggests the criminal was a smoker. And so on.) In the same fashion, physicists observe the clues that electrons leave behind, and from this information they form hypotheses about what electrons must be like in order to have produced these specific effects.

Of course, physicists (and other scientists) have a huge advantage over a police detective: If the detective has insufficient evidence, she can't arrange for the crime to happen again in order to produce more evidence. (She can't say to the robber, "Please visit the bank again, but this time don't wear a mask.") Scientists, in contrast, can arrange for a repeat of the "crime" they're seeking to explain. More precisely, they can arrange for new experiments, with new measures. Better still, they can set the stage in advance, to maximize the likelihood that the "culprit" (in our example, the electron) will leave useful clues behind. They can, for example, add new recording devices to the situation, or they can place various obstacles in the electron's path. In this way, scientists can gather more and more data, including data that are crucial for testing the specific predictions of a particular theory. This prospect—of reproducing experiments and varying the experiments to test hypotheses—is what gives science its power. It's what enables scientists to assert that their hypotheses have been rigorously tested, and it's what gives scientists assurance that their theories are correct.

Psychologists work in the same fashion—and the notion that we *could* work in this fashion was one of the great contributions of the cognitive revolution. The idea, in essence, is simply this: We know that we need to study mental processes; that's what we learned from the limitations of behaviorism. But we also know that mental processes cannot be observed directly; we learned that from the downfall of introspection. Our path forward, therefore, is to study mental processes *indirectly*, relying on the fact that these processes, themselves invisible, have visible consequences: measurable delays in producing a response, performances that can be assessed for accuracy, errors that can be scrutinized and categorized. By examining these (and other) effects produced by mental processes, we can develop—and then *test*—hypotheses about what the mental processes must have been. In this fashion, we use Kant's method, just as physicists (or biologists or chemists or astronomers) do, to develop a science that does not rest on direct observation.

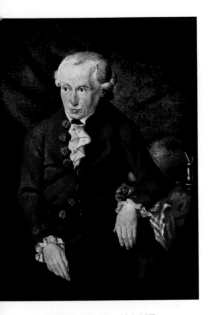

IMMANUEL KANT

Philosopher Immanuel Kant (1724–1804) made major contributions to many fields, and his transcendental method enabled him to ask what qualities of the mind make experience possible.

Research in Cognitive Psychology: The Diversity of Methods

In setting after setting, cognitive psychologists have applied the Kantian logic to explain how people remember, make decisions, pay attention, or solve problems. In each case, we begin with a particular performance—say, a memory task—and then hypothesize a series of unseen mental events that made the performance possible. But, crucially, we don't stop there. We also ask whether some other, perhaps simpler, sequence of events might explain the data or whether a different sequence might explain both these data and some other findings. In this fashion, we do more than ask how the data came about; we also seek the *best* way to think about the data.

For some data, the sequence of events we hypothesize resembles the processing steps that a computer might use. (For classic examples of this approach, see Broadbent, 1958; Miller, Galanter, & Pribram, 1960.) For other data, we might cast our hypotheses in terms of the strategies a person is using or the inferences she is making. No matter what the form of the hypothesis, though, the next step is crucial: The hypothesis is tested by collecting more data. Specifically, we seek to derive new predictions based on our hypothesis: "If this is the mechanism behind the original findings, then things should work differently in *this* circumstance or *that* one." If these predictions are tested and confirmed, this outcome suggests that the proposed hypothesis was correct. If the predictions are not confirmed, then a new hypothesis is needed.

But what methods do we use, and what sorts of data do we collect? The answer, in brief, is that we use *diverse* methods and collect many types of data. In other words, what unites cognitive psychology is not an allegiance to any particular procedure in the laboratory. Instead, what unites the field is the logic that underlies our research, no matter what method is in use. (We discuss this logic more fully in the appendix for this textbook; the appendix contains a series of modules, "keyed" to individual chapters. Each module explores an aspect of research methodology directly related to its associated chapter.)

Let's explore this point with a concrete example. We'll return to this example in Chapter 6, where we'll put it into a richer context. For now, though, you shouldn't worry too much about the theory involved in this example; our focus here is on how the research unfolds.

Working Memory: Some Initial Observations

Many of the sentences in this book—including the one you are reading right now, which consists of 23 words—are rather long. In these sentences, words that must be understood together (such as "sentences . . . are . . . long") are often widely separated (note the 16 words interposed between "sentences" and "are"). Yet you have no trouble understanding these sentences.

We begin, therefore, with a simple fact—that you are able to read, even though ordinary reading requires you to integrate words that are widely separated on the page. How should we explain this fact? What is the (unseen) cause that leads to this (easily observed) fact? The obvious suggestion is that you're relying on some form of *memory* that enables you to remember the early words in the sentence as you forge ahead. Then, once you've read enough, you can integrate what you have decoded so far. In this section's very first sentence, for example, you needed to hang on to the first seven words ("Many of the sentences in this book") while you read the interposed phrase ("including the one . . . 23 words"). Then, you had to bring those first seven words back into play, to integrate them with the sentence's end ("are rather long").

The form of memory proposed here is called **working memory**, to emphasize that this is the memory you use for information that you are actively working on. Working memory holds information in an easily accessible form, so that the information is, so to speak, at your fingertips, instantly available when you need it. This instant availability is promoted by several factors, including, quite simply, working memory's *size*: Working memory is hypothesized to have a small capacity, and so, with only a few items held in this store, you will never have a problem locating just the item you want. (If you have only two keys on your key ring, it's easy to find the one that unlocks your door. If you had a hundred keys on the ring, the situation would be rather different.)

Can we test this proposal? One way to measure working memory's capacity is via a **span test**. In this test, we read to someone a list of, say, four items, perhaps four letters ("A D G W"). The person has to report these back, immediately, in sequence. If she succeeds, we try it again with five letters ("Q D W U F"). If she can repeat these back correctly, we try six letters, and so on, until we find a list that the person cannot report back accurately. Generally, people start making errors with sequences of seven or eight letters. Most people's letter span, therefore, is about seven or eight. This finding confirms our hypothesis that working memory is limited in size; but more important for our purposes here, it also provides a simple example of how we can learn about this memory's properties by seeing how this (unseen) memory influences observable performance.

Working Memory: A Proposal

As it turns out, the span test also puts another observation into view— another "effect" for which we need to seek a "cause." Specifically, when we measure memory span, we find that people often make errors—they report letters that they hadn't heard at all—and these errors follow a simple pattern: When people make mistakes in this task, they generally substitute one letter for another with a similar *sound*. Having heard "S," they'll report back "F"; or having heard "D," they'll report back "T." The problem is not in hearing the letters in the first place: We get similar sound-alike confusions if the letters are presented visually. Thus, having *seen* "F," people are likely to report back "S"; they are not likely, in this situation, to report back the similar-looking "E."

This finding provides another clue about working memory's nature, and two British researchers—Alan Baddeley and Graham Hitch—proposed a model to explain both this finding and many other results as well (e.g., Baddeley & Hitch, 1974, or, for a more recent treatment, see Baddeley, 2000). We'll have more to say about their model later; but for now, the key idea is that working memory actually has several different parts, and so it's more accurate to speak of the **working-memory system**. At the heart of the system is the **central executive**; this is the part that runs the show and does the real work. The executive is helped out, though, by low-level "assistants." These assistants are not sophisticated; and so, if you need to analyze or interpret some information, the assistants can't do it—the executive is needed for that. What the assistants can do, however, is provide storage, and this function, simple though it is, makes the assistants extremely useful.

Specifically, information that will soon be needed, but isn't needed right now, can be sent off to the assistants for temporary storage. As a result, the executive isn't burdened by the mere storage of this information and so is freed up to do other tasks. In effect, therefore, the assistants serve the same function as a piece of scratch paper on your desk. When you're going to need some bit of information soon (a phone number, perhaps), you write it down on the scratch paper. Of course, the scratch paper has no mind of its own, and so it can't do anything with the "stored" information; all it does is hold on to the information. But that's helpful enough: With the scratch paper "preserving" this information, you can cease thinking about it with no risk that the information will be lost. This enables you to focus your attention more productively on other, more complex chores. Then, when you're ready for the stored information (perhaps just a moment later), you glance at your note, and there the information will be.

Working memory's assistants provide the same benefit, and one of the most important assistants is the **articulatory rehearsal loop**. To see how it works, try reading the next few sentences while holding on to this list of numbers: "1, 4, 6, 4, 9." Got them? Now read on. You are probably repeating the numbers over and over to yourself, rehearsing them with your inner voice. But this turns out to require very little effort, so you can continue reading while doing this rehearsal. Nonetheless, the moment you need to recall the numbers (what were they?), they are available to you. How did you do this? The numbers were maintained by working memory's rehearsal loop, and with the numbers thus out of the way, the central executive was free to continue reading. And that is the advantage of this system: With storage handled by the helpers, the executive is available for other, more demanding tasks.

To launch the rehearsal loop, you rely on the process of **subvocalization**—silent speech. In other words, you quietly say the numbers to yourself. This "inner voice," in turn, produces a representation of these numbers in the **phonological buffer**. In other words, an auditory image is created in the "inner ear" (see **Figure 1.1**). This image will fade away after a second or two, but before it does, subvocalization can be used once again to create a new image, sustaining the material in this buffer.

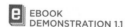 EBOOK
DEMONSTRATION 1.1

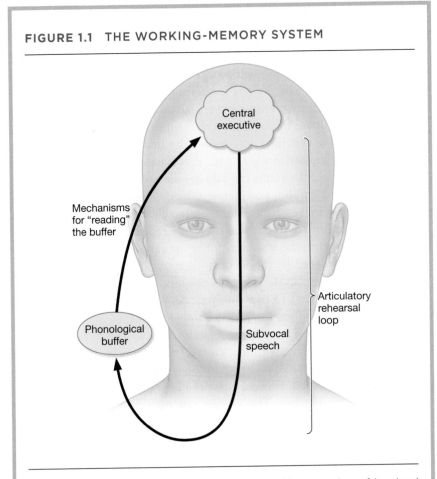

FIGURE 1.1   THE WORKING-MEMORY SYSTEM

Central
executive

Mechanisms
for "reading"
the buffer

Articulatory
rehearsal
loop

Phonological
buffer

Subvocal
speech

Working memory's central executive is supported by a number of low-level assistants. One assistant, the articulatory rehearsal loop, involves two components: subvocal speech (the "inner voice") and a phonological buffer (the "inner ear"). Items are rehearsed by using subvocalization to "load" the buffer. While this is going on, the executive is free to work on other matters.

Evidence for the Working-Memory System

Baddeley and Hitch proposed their model as an explanation for the available evidence; it was, in their view, the best way to explain the facts collected so far. For example, why do people make "sound-alike" errors in a span task? It's because they're relying on the rehearsal loop, which involves a mechanism (the "inner ear") that stores the memory items as (internal representations of) sounds, and so it's no surprise that errors, when they occur, are shaped by this mode of storage.

Notice, then, that we're using the Kantian logic described earlier: generating a hypothesis about unseen mechanisms (e.g., the operation of the rehearsal loop) in order to explain visible data (e.g., the pattern of the errors).

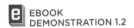 EBOOK
DEMONSTRATION 1.2

FIGURE 1.2   THE EFFECTS OF CONCURRENT ARTICULATION

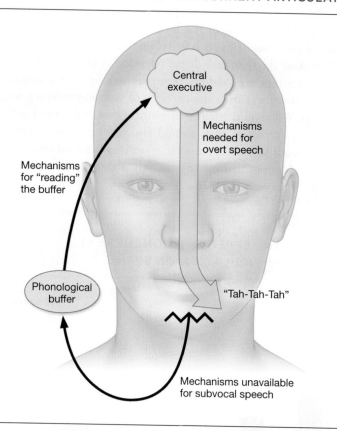

The mechanisms needed to control subvocal speech (the "inner voice") overlap significantly with those needed for the control and production of overt speech. Therefore, if these mechanisms are in use for actual speech, they are not available for subvocal rehearsal. Hence, many experiments block rehearsal by requiring participants to say "Tah-Tah-Tah" out loud.

Crucially, though, this hypothesis also leads to many new predictions, and this enables us to test the hypothesis—by asking whether its predictions are accurate. It is this step that turns a "mere" hypothesis into solid scientific knowledge.

For example, imagine that we ask people to take the span test while simultaneously saying "Tah-Tah-Tah" over and over, out loud. This **concurrent articulation task** obviously requires the mechanisms for speech production. Therefore, these mechanisms are not available for other use, including subvocalization. (If you're directing your lips and tongue to produce the "Tah-Tah-Tah" sequence, you can't at the same time direct them to produce the sequence needed for the subvocalized materials; see **Figure 1.2**.)

According to the model, how will this constraint matter? First, note that our original span test measured the combined capacities of the central executive and the loop. That is, when people take a span test, they store some of the to-be-remembered items in the loop and others via the central executive. (This is a poor use of the executive, underutilizing its talents, but that's okay here, because the span task doesn't demand anything beyond mere storage.) With concurrent articulation, though, the loop isn't available for use, and so we are now measuring the capacity of working memory without the rehearsal loop. We should predict, therefore, that concurrent articulation, even though it's extremely easy, should cut memory span drastically. This prediction turns out to be correct. Span is ordinarily about seven items; with concurrent articulation, it drops by roughly a third—to four or five items (Chincotta & Underwood, 1997; see **Figure 1.3**).

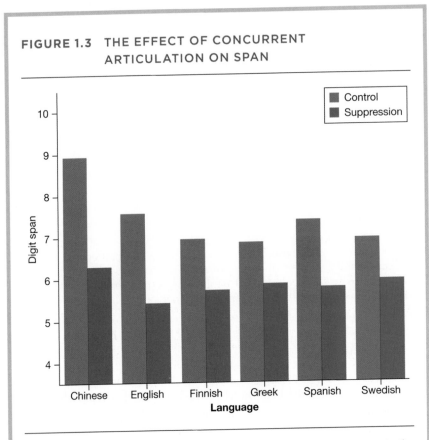

FIGURE 1.3   THE EFFECT OF CONCURRENT ARTICULATION ON SPAN

In the Control condition, people were given a normal digit-span test. In the Suppression condition, people were required to do concurrent articulation while taking the test. Concurrent articulation is easy, but it blocks use of the articulatory loop and consistently decreases memory span, from roughly seven items to five or so. And plainly this use of the articulatory loop is not an occasional strategy; instead, it can be found in a wide range of countries and languages.   AFTER CHINCOTTA & UNDERWOOD, 1997.

Second, with visually presented items, concurrent articulation should eliminate the sound-alike errors. Repeatedly saying "Tah-Tah-Tah" blocks use of the articulatory loop, and it is in this loop, we've proposed, that the sound-alike errors arise. This prediction, too, is correct: With concurrent articulation and visual presentation of the items, sound-alike errors are largely eliminated.

Third, we can also test people's memory spans by using complex visual shapes. People are shown these shapes and then must echo the sequence back by drawing what they have just seen. If we choose shapes that are not easily named, then the shapes cannot be rehearsed via the inner-voice/inner-ear combination. (What would you subvocalize to rehearse them?) With these stimuli, therefore, there should be no effect of concurrent articulation: If people aren't using the rehearsal loop, there should be no cost attached to denying them use of the loop. This prediction is also correct.

Finally, here is a different sort of prediction. We have claimed that the rehearsal loop is required only for storage; this loop (like all of working memory's assistants) is incapable of any more sophisticated operations. Therefore, these other operations should not be compromised if the loop is unavailable. This, too, turns out to be correct: Concurrent articulation blocks use of the loop but has no effect on someone's ability to read brief sentences, to do simple logic problems, and so on. (Blocking use of the loop *does* have an effect when you're reading more complex sentences or doing harder problems; that's because these harder tasks require analysis *and* the storage of interim steps, and so require the entire working-memory system—the executive *and* the assistants.)

The Nature of the Working-Memory Evidence

No one has ever seen the "inner voice" or the "inner ear" directly. Nonetheless, we're confident that these entities exist, because they are essential parts of our explanation for the data and—crucially—there seems to be no other way to explain the data. Moreover, our claims about the inner voice and the inner ear have consistently led us to new predictions that have been confirmed by further testing. In this way, our claims have been *useful* (leading to new observations) as well as *accurate* (leading to correct predictions).

Let's note also that in supporting our account, there are many forms of data available to us. We can manipulate research participants' activities, as we did with concurrent articulation, and then we can look at how this manipulation changes their performance (e.g., the size of the measured memory span). We can also manipulate the stimuli themselves, as we did in testing memory for visual shapes, and see how this changes things. We can also look in detail at the nature of the performance, asking not just about someone's overall level of success in our tasks but also about his or her specific errors (sound-alike vs. look-alike). We can also measure the speed of participants' performance and ask how it is influenced by various manipulations. We do this, for example, when we ask whether problem solving is compromised by concurrent articulation. The assumption here is that mental processes are very fast but nonetheless do take a measurable amount of time. By timing how quickly participants answer various questions or perform various tasks, we can ask what factors speed up mental processes and what factors slow them down.

We can also gather data from another source. So far, we've been concerned with people's *performance* on our tasks—for example, how much or how well they remember. There's much to learn, though, by considering the biological mechanisms that make this performance possible. That is, we can draw evidence from the realm of **cognitive neuroscience**—the study of the biological basis for cognitive functioning.

For example, what exactly is the nature of subvocalization? Is it just like actual speech, but silent? If so, does it involve movements (perhaps tiny movements) of the tongue, the vocal cords, and so on? One way to find out would be to paralyze the relevant muscles. Would this action disrupt use of the rehearsal loop? As it turns out, we don't have to perform this experiment; nature has performed it for us. Because of specific forms of neurological damage, some individuals have no ability to move these various muscles and so suffer from **anarthria**—an inability to produce overt speech. Data indicate, however, that these individuals show sound-alike confusions in their span data, just as ordinary participants do; they also show other results (e.g., something called "the word-length effect") associated with the use of the rehearsal loop (e.g., Vallar & Cappa, 1987). These observations suggest that actual muscle movements aren't needed for subvocalization, because the results are the same *without* these movements. It seems likely, therefore, that "inner speech" relies on the brain areas responsible for *planning* and *controlling* the muscle movements of speech and not on the movements themselves. This is by itself an interesting fact, but for present purposes, let's note the use of yet another type of data: observations from **neuropsychology**, concerned with how various forms of brain dysfunction influence observed performance.

We can pursue related questions by examining the brain activity of people with fully intact (undamaged) brains. Recent developments in brain-imaging technology tell us that when a participant is engaged in working-memory rehearsal, considerable activity is observed in brain areas that we know (from other evidence) are crucially involved in the production of spoken language, as well as in areas that play an important role in the perception of spoken language. These findings suggest that claims about the "inner voice" and "inner ear" are more than casual metaphors; instead, the "inner voice" uses brain mechanisms that are ordinarily used for overt speech, and the "inner ear" uses mechanisms ordinarily used for actual hearing (cf. Jonides, Lacey, & Nee, 2005; for more on the neuroscience of working memory, see Jonides et al., 2008).

We can also gain insights by comparing diverse populations—for example, by comparing people who speak different languages (see Figure 1.3), or comparing people with normal hearing to people who have been deaf since

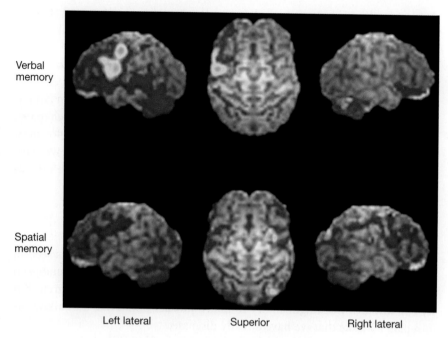

Verbal memory

Spatial memory

Left lateral   Superior   Right lateral

BRAIN ACTIVITY AND WORKING-MEMORY REHEARSAL

Color is used here as an indication of increased brain activity (measured in this case by positron emission tomography). When people are engaged in a verbal memory task (and so using the articulatory loop), activation increases in areas ordinarily used for language production and perception. A very different pattern is observed when people are engaged in a task requiring memory for spatial position.

birth and who communicate via sign language. It turns out, for example, that the deaf rely on a different assistant for working memory: They use an "inner hand" (and covert sign language) rather than an "inner voice" (and covert speech). As a result, they are disrupted if they are asked to wiggle their fingers during a memory task (akin to a hearing person saying "Tah-Tah-Tah"), and they also tend to make "same-hand-shape" errors in working memory (analogous to the sound-alike errors made by the hearing population). These results speak not only to the generality of the claims made here but also to the need to fine-tune these claims when we consider other groups of people.

Finally, let's emphasize the importance of building our argument with *multiple lines* of evidence. That's because, in most cases, no single line of evidence is decisive by itself. There are, after all, probably other ways to explain our initial observations about span, if those results were all we had to go on. There are also other ways to explain the other individual findings we have mentioned, if these likewise were considered in isolation. It's only when we take the results as a package that we can make headway, and if we have done our work well, there will be just one theoretical account that fits with the entire data pattern. At that point, with no other way to explain the

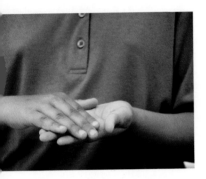

THE INNER HAND, RATHER THAN THE INNER VOICE

People who can speak and hear rely on the articulatory rehearsal loop as part of the working-memory system; as a result, errors in working memory are often "sound-alike errors." Members of the deaf community, in contrast, rely on a "signing rehearsal loop," using an "inner hand" rather than an "inner voice." Their errors often involve confusions between different words that happen to have similar hand shapes when expressed in sign language.

data, we will conclude that we have understood the evidence and that we have correctly reconstructed what is going on in the mind, invisibly, never directly observed.

Let's be clear, though, that there's no reason for you, as a reader, to memorize this catalogue of different types of evidence. That's because we'll encounter each of these forms of data again and again in this text. In addition (and as we said earlier), we'll return to the working memory system in later chapters, and there we'll say more about the theory just sketched. Our point for now, therefore, is to highlight—and, indeed, to celebrate—the fact that we have multiple tools with which we can test, and eventually confirm, our various claims.

Working Memory in a Broader Context

Having made all of these methodological points, let's round out this section with one final comment. We introduced the example of working memory in order to showcase the diversity of methods used in cognition research. But we can also use working memory to make another point, one that allows us to replay an issue that we have already discussed.

Why should you care about the structure of working memory? The memory-span task itself seems quite unnatural: How often do you need to memorize a set of unrelated letters? For that matter, how often do you need to work on a problem while simultaneously saying "Tah-Tah-Tah" over and over? In short, what does this task, or this procedure, have to do with things you care about?

The answer to these questions lies in the fact that you rely on working memory in a vast number of circumstances; and so, if we understand working memory, we move toward an understanding of this far broader set of problems and issues. For example, bear in mind our initial comments about the role of working memory in reading or in any other task in which you must store early "products," keeping them ready for integration with later "products." One might imagine that many tasks have this character; reading, reasoning, and problem solving are a few. If you make effective use of working memory, therefore, you will have an advantage in all of these domains. Indeed, some scholars have suggested that "intelligence" in many domains amounts to nothing more than having a larger capacity in working memory. (We'll return to this point in Chapter 13.)

In a similar vein, the use of articulatory rehearsal seems a simple trick— one you use spontaneously, a trick in which you take no special pride. But it is a trick you had to learn, and young children, for example, often seem not to know it. There is some indication that this lack can be a problem for these children in learning to read: Without the option of relying on articulatory rehearsal, reading becomes much more difficult. It also appears that the rehearsal loop plays an important role when someone is learning new vocabulary, including vocabulary in a new language (Baddeley, Gathercole, & Papagno, 1998; Gathercole, Service, Hitch, Adams, & Martin, 1999;

Majerus, Poncelet, Elsen, & van der Linden, 2006). So here, too, is an important function of the working-memory system.

These examples can easily be multiplied, but by now the point should be clear: Working memory and articulatory rehearsal are relevant to a wide range of mental activities in adults and in children. Understanding working memory, therefore, may give us insight into a broad range of tasks. Similar claims can be made about many other cognitive resources: By understanding what it means to pay attention, we move toward an understanding of all the contexts in which attention plays a role. By understanding how we comprehend text, or how we use our knowledge to supplement our perceptions, we move toward an understanding of all the contexts in which these abilities play a part. And in each case, the number of such contexts is vast.

We end this chapter, therefore, by echoing a comment we have already made: The machinery of cognition is essential to virtually all of our waking activities (and perhaps some of our sleeping activities as well). The scope of cognitive psychology is broad indeed, and the relevance of our research is wide.

APPLYING COGNITIVE PSYCHOLOGY

Research in cognitive psychology helps us understand deep theoretical issues, such as what it means to be rational or what the function of consciousness might be. But our research also has practical implications, and studies often provide lessons for how we should conduct many aspects of our day-to-day lives.

To help you see these implications—and so to help you understand just how important our research is—each chapter in this text ends with an essay on one of the applications of cognitive psychology. In all cases, the essay explores how the material in that chapter can be applied to a real-world concern.

Some of the pragmatic lessons from cognitive psychology are obvious. For example, research on memory can help students who are trying to learn new materials in the classroom; studies of how people draw conclusions can help people to draw smarter, more defensible conclusions. Following these leads, many of the end-of-chapter essays are aimed at educational issues. The essay at the end of Chapter 4, for example, will teach you how to speed-read (but will also explain the limitations of speed-reading). The essay at the end of Chapter 6 offers concrete suggestions for how you should study the material you're hoping to learn.

Other implications of our work, though, are more surprising. Consider, for example, the implications of cognitive psychology for the criminal justice system. More specifically, think about what happens in a criminal investigation. Eyewitnesses provide evidence, based on what they paid attention to during a crime and what they remember. Police officers question the witnesses, trying to maximize what each witness recalls—but without leading the witness in any way. Then the police try to deduce, from the evidence, who the perpetrator was. Then later, during the trial, jurors listen to evidence and make a judgment about the defendant's innocence or guilt.

Cast in these terms, it should be obvious that an understanding of *attention*, *memory*, *reasoning*, and *judgment* (to name just a few processes) is directly relevant to what happens in the legal system. It's on this basis, therefore, that some of the end-of-chapter essays focus on the interplay between cognitive psychology and the law. The essay at the end of Chapter 3, for example, uses what we know about visual perception to ask what we can expect witnesses to see. The essay for Chapter 7 explores a research-based procedure for helping witnesses to recall more of what they've observed.

Of course, cognitive psychology also has implications for other domains— the practice of medicine, for example, or the training of businesspeople. One reason I focus on the justice system, though, is my own involvement with these issues: As a psychologist specializing in memory, I consult with police, lawyers, and the courts on questions about eyewitness evidence. This work has made it clear for me just how important our science is, and it also provides a constant reminder that we need to be careful in our work—so that we don't mislead the courts with unfounded advice. I hope these essays will persuade you of the same crucial points.

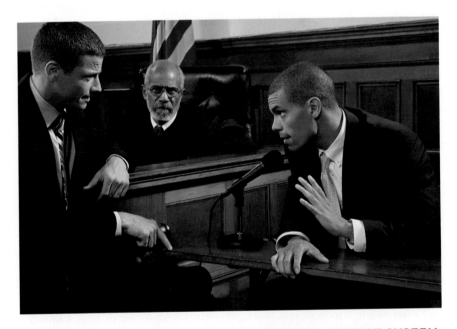

COGNITIVE PSYCHOLOGY AND THE CRIMINAL JUSTICE SYSTEM

Eyewitnesses in the courtroom are relying on what they *remember* about the key events, and what they remember depends crucially on what they *perceived* and *paid attention to*. Therefore, our understanding of memory, perception, and attention can help the justice system in its evaluation of witness evidence.

chapter summary

- Cognitive psychology is concerned with how people remember, pay attention, and think. The importance of all these issues arises in part from the fact that most of what we do, think, and feel is guided by things we already know. One example is the comprehension of a simple story, which turns out to be heavily influenced by the knowledge we supply.

- Cognitive psychology emerged as a separate discipline in the late 1950s, and its powerful impact on the wider field of psychology has led many academics to speak of this emergence as the cognitive revolution. One predecessor of cognitive psychology was the 19th-century movement that emphasized introspection as the main research tool for psychology. Psychologists soon became disenchanted with this movement, however, for several reasons: Introspection cannot inform us about unconscious mental events; even with conscious events, claims rooted in introspection are often untestable because there is no way for an independent observer to check on the accuracy or completeness of an introspective report.

- The behaviorist movement rejected introspection as a method, insisting instead that psychology speak only of mechanisms and processes that were objective and out in the open for all to observe. However, evidence suggests that our thinking, behavior, and feelings are often shaped by our perception or understanding of the events we experience. This is problematic for the behaviorists: Perception and understanding are exactly the sorts of mental processes that the behaviorists regarded as subjective and not open to scientific study.

- In order to study mental events, psychologists have turned to a method in which one focuses on observable events but then asks what (invisible) events must have taken place in order to make these (visible) effects possible.

- Research in working memory provides an example of how cognitive psychologists use evidence. One theory of working memory proposes that this memory consists of a central executive and a small number of low-level assistants, including the articulatory rehearsal loop, which stores material by means of covert speech. Many forms of evidence are used in supporting this account: measures of working memory's holding capacity in various circumstances, the nature of errors people make when using working memory, the speed of performance in working-memory tasks, evidence drawn from the study of people with brain damage, and evidence drawn from brain-imaging technology.

eBook Demonstrations & Essays

Online Demonstrations:
- Demonstration 1.1: The Articulatory Rehearsal Loop
- Demonstration 1.2: Sound-Based Coding

Online Applying Cognitive Psychology Essays:
- Cognitive Psychology and Education: Enhancing Classroom Learning

ZAPS 2.0 Cognition Labs

- Go to **http://digital.wwnorton.com/cognition6** for the online labs relevant to this chapter.

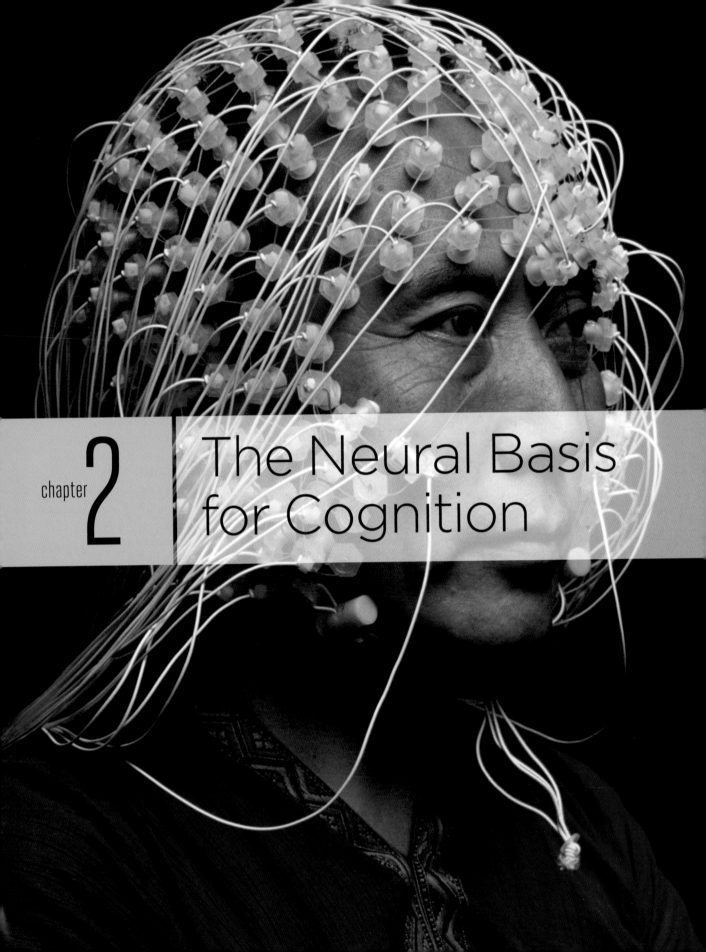

chapter **2**

The Neural Basis for Cognition

what if... Throughout this text, we'll be examining ordinary achievements. A friend asks: "Where'd you grow up?" and you immediately answer. You're meeting a friend at the airport, and you instantly recognize her the moment she steps into view. An instructor says, "Examine this picture carefully," and you have no trouble focusing your attention on the image.

Ordinary or not, achievements like these are crucial for you, and your life would be massively disrupted if you couldn't draw information from your own memory, or recognize the objects that you encounter, or choose where you'll point your attention. As a way of dramatizing this point, we'll begin each chapter by asking: What would happen to someone if one of these fundamental capacities *didn't work* as it normally does? What if...?

The disorder known as Capgras syndrome (Capgras & Reboul-Lachaux, 1923) is relatively rare, but it can result from various injuries to the brain (Ellis & De Pauw 1994) and is sometimes one of the accompaniments to Alzheimer's syndrome (Harwood, Barker, Ownby, & Duara, 1999). Someone with this syndrome is fully able to recognize the people in her world—her husband, her parents, her friends—but is utterly convinced that these people are not who they appear to be. The real husband or the real son, the afflicted person insists, has been kidnapped (or worse). The person now on the scene, therefore, isn't the genuine article; instead, he or she must be a well-trained impostor—a fraud of some sort, impersonating the (allegedly) absent person.

Imagine what it is like to have this disorder. You turn, let's say, to your father—and exclaim, "You look like my father, sound like him, and act like him. But I can tell that you're not my father. *Who are you?*"

Often, a person with Capgras syndrome insists that there are slight differences between the "impostor" and the person he has supposedly replaced—subtle changes in personality or tiny changes in appearance. Of course, no one else detects these (nonexistent) differences, and this can lead to all sorts of paranoid suspicions about why a loved one has been replaced and why no one is willing to acknowledge this replacement. In the extreme, these suspicions can lead a Capgras sufferer to desperate steps. In a few cases, patients suffering from this syndrome have murdered

* We begin by exploring the example of *Capgras syndrome* to illustrate how seemingly simple achievements actually depend on many parts of the brain; we also highlight the ways that the study of the brain, and of brain damage, can illuminate questions about the mind.

* We then survey the brain's anatomy, emphasizing the function carried out by each region. The identification of these functions is supported by neuroimaging data, which can assess the activity levels in different areas, and also by studies of the effects of brain damage.

* We then take a closer look at the various parts of the cerebral cortex—arguably the most important part of the brain for our cognitive functioning. These parts include the motor areas, the sensory areas, and the so-called association cortex.

* Finally, we turn to the individual cells that make up the brain—the *neurons* and *glia*—and discuss the basic principles of how these cells function.

the supposed impostor in an attempt to end the charade and relocate the "genuine" character. Indeed, in one case, a Capgras patient was convinced his father had been replaced by a robot and so decapitated him in order to look for the batteries and microfilm in his head (Blount, 1986).

What is going on here? The answer likely lies in the fact that facial recognition involves two separate systems in the brain, one of which leads to a cognitive appraisal ("I know what my father looks like, and I can perceive that you closely resemble him"), and the other to a more global, emotional appraisal ("You look familiar to me and also trigger a warm response in me"). The concordance of these two appraisals then leads to the certainty of recognition ("You obviously are my father"). In Capgras syndrome, though, the emotional processing is disrupted, leading to an intellectual identification without a familiarity response (Ellis & Lewis, 2001; Ellis & Young, 1990; Ramachandran & Blakeslee, 1998): "You resemble my father but trigger no sense of familiarity, so you must be someone else." The result? Confusion, and sometimes bizarre speculation about why a loved one has been kidnapped and replaced—and, as we have seen, a level of paranoia that even can lead to homicide.

Explaining Capgras Syndrome

We began this chapter with a description of Capgras syndrome, and we've offered an account of the mental processes that cause this disorder. Specifically, we've suggested that someone with this syndrome is able to recognize a loved one's face, but with no feeling of familiarity. Is this the right way to think about Capgras syndrome?

One line of evidence comes from **neuroimaging techniques**, developed in the last few decades, that enable researchers to take high-quality, three-dimensional "pictures" of living brains without in any way disturbing the brains' owners. We'll have more to say about neuroimaging later; but first, what do these techniques tell us about Capgras syndrome?

The Neural Basis for Capgras Syndrome

Some types of neuroimaging data provide portraits of the physical makeup of the brain: What's where? How are structures shaped or connected to each other? Are there structures present (such as tumors) that shouldn't be there, or structures that are missing (perhaps because of disease or birth defects)? These facts about structure were gained in older studies from PET scans; current studies usually rely on MRI scans (see **Figure 2.1**). These scans suggest a link between Capgras syndrome and abnormalities in several brain areas, indicating that our

FIGURE 2.1 NEUROIMAGING

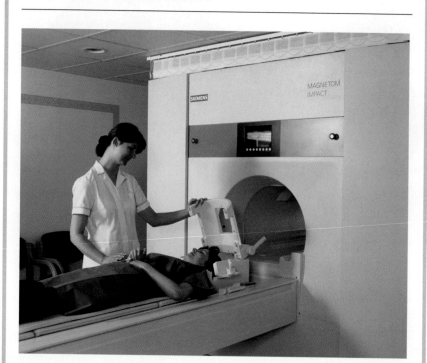

Scanners like this one are used for both MRI and fMRI scans. MRI scans tell us about the structure of the brain; fMRI scans tell us which portions of the brain are especially active during the scan. An fMRI scan usually results in color images, with each hue indicating a particular activity level.

account of the syndrome will need to consider several elements (Edelstyn & Oyebode, 1999; also see O'Connor, Walbridge, Sandson, & Alexander, 1996).

One site of damage in Capgras patients is in the temporal lobe (see **Figure 2.2**), particularly on the right side of the head. This damage probably disrupts circuits involving the **amygdala**, an almond-shaped structure that—in the intact brain—seems to serve as an "emotional evaluator," helping an organism to detect stimuli associated with threat or danger (see **Figure 2.3**). The amygdala is also important for detecting positive stimuli—indicators of safety or indicators of available rewards. With *damaged* amygdalae, therefore, people with Capgras syndrome won't experience the warm sense

FIGURE 2.2   THE LOBES OF THE HUMAN BRAIN

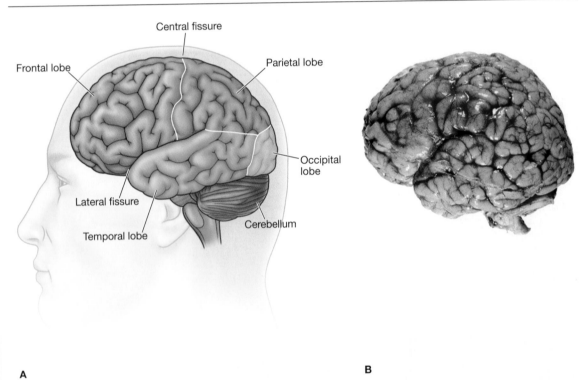

A   **B**

Panel A identifies the various lobes and some of the brain's prominent features. Actual brains, however, are uniformly colored, as shown in the photograph in Panel B. The four lobes of the forebrain surround (and hide from view) the midbrain and most of the hindbrain. (The cerebellum is the only part of the hindbrain that is visible, and, in fact, the temporal lobe has been pushed upward a bit in the left panel to make the cerebellum more visible.) This side view shows the left cerebral hemisphere; the structures on the right side of the brain are similar. However, the two halves of the brain have somewhat different functions, and so the results of brain injury depend on which half is damaged. The symptoms of Capgras syndrome, for example, result from damage to specific sites on the right side of the frontal and temporal lobes.

of feeling good (and safe and secure) when looking at a loved one's familiar face. This lack of an emotional response is probably why these faces don't feel familiar to them, and it is, of course, fully in line with the two-systems hypothesis we've already sketched.

Patients with Capgras syndrome also have brain abnormalities in the frontal lobe, specifically in the right **prefrontal cortex**. What is this area's normal function? To find out, we turn to a different neuroimaging technique, fMRI, which enables us to track moment-by-moment *activity levels* in different sites in a living brain. (We'll say more about fMRI in a later section.) This technique allows us to answer such questions as: When a person is reading, which brain regions

---

FIGURE 2.3   THE AMYGDALA AS AN "EMOTION EVALUATOR"

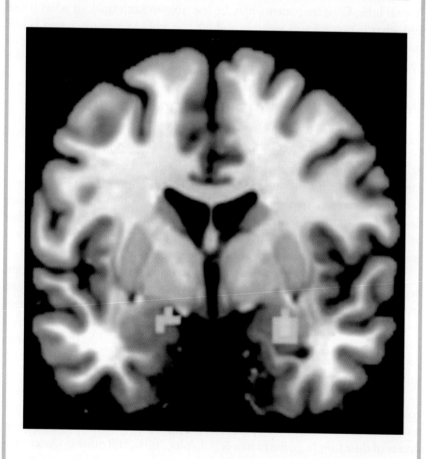

The area shown in yellow marks the location of the amygdala. In this image, the yellow is a reflection of increased activity created by a fear memory—the memory of receiving an electric shock.

are particularly active? How about when a person is listening to music? With data like these, we can ask which tasks make heavy use of a brain area, and from that base we can draw conclusions about what the brain area's function is.

Studies make it clear that the prefrontal cortex is especially active when a person is engaged in tasks that require planning or careful analysis. Conversely, this area is less active when someone is *dreaming*. Plausibly, this latter pattern reflects the *absence* of careful analysis of the dream material, which in turn helps us understand why dreams are often illogical or bizarre.

Related, consider fMRI scans of patients suffering from schizophrenia (e.g., Silbersweig et al., 1995). Neuroimaging reveals diminished activity in the frontal lobes whenever these patients are experiencing hallucinations. One interpretation is that the diminished activity reflects a decreased ability to distinguish internal events (thoughts) from external ones (voices) or to distinguish imagined events from real ones (cf. Glisky, Polster, & Routhieaux, 1995).

How is all of this relevant to Capgras syndrome? With damage to the frontal lobe, Capgras patients may be less able to keep track of what is real and what is not, what is sensible and what is not. As a result, weird beliefs can emerge unchecked, including delusions (about robots and the like) that you or I would find utterly bizarre.

What Do We Learn from Capgras Syndrome?

As it turns out, we have other lines of evidence that help us understand the symptoms of Capgras syndrome (e.g., Ellis & Lewis, 2001; Ramachandran & Blakeslee, 1998). Some of the evidence comes from the psychology laboratory and confirms the suggestion that recognition of all stimuli (and not just faces) involves two separate mechanisms—one that hinges on factual knowledge, and one that's more "emotional" and tied to the warm sense of familiarity (see Chapter 7). These findings join the neuroscience evidence we've just described, providing further support for our account so far.

Let's emphasize, though, that our understanding of Capgras syndrome depends on a combination of evidence drawn from cognitive psychology and from cognitive neuroscience. We use both perspectives to test (and, ultimately, to confirm) the hypothesis we've offered. In addition, just as both perspectives can illuminate Capgras syndrome, both can be *illuminated by* the syndrome. That is, we can use Capgras syndrome (and other biological evidence) to illuminate broader issues about the nature of the brain and of the mind.

For example, Capgras syndrome suggests that the amygdala plays a crucial role in supporting the feeling of familiarity. Other evidence suggests that the amygdala also plays a central part in helping people remember the emotional events of their lives (e.g., Buchanan & Adolphs, 2004). Still other evidence indicates that the amygdala plays a role in decision making (e.g., Bechara, Damasio, & Damasio, 2003), especially for decisions that rest on emotional evaluations of one's options. Facts like these tell us a lot about the various functions that make cognition possible and, more specifically, tell us that our theorizing needs to include a broadly useful "emotional evaluator," involved in many cognitive processes. Moreover, Capgras syndrome tells us that this emotional evaluator works in a fashion separate from the evaluation of factual information, providing us a way to think about the occasions in which someone's evaluation of the facts points toward one conclusion, while an emotional evaluation points toward a different conclusion. These are clues of great value as we seek to understand the processes that support ordinary remembering or decision making. (For more on the role of the emotion evaluator, see Chapter 12.)

What does Capgras syndrome teach us about the brain itself? One lesson focuses on the fact that many different parts of the brain are needed for even the simplest achievement. In order to recognize your father, for example, one part of your brain needs to store the factual memory of what your father looks like. Another part of the brain is responsible for analyzing the visual input you receive when looking at a face. Yet another brain area has the job of comparing this now-analyzed input to the factual information provided from memory, to determine whether there's a match. Another site provides the emotional evaluation of the input. A different site presumably assembles the data from all these other sites, and so registers the fact that the face being inspected does match the factual recollection of your father's face, and also produces a warm sense of familiarity.

Ordinarily, all of these brain areas work together, allowing the recognition of your father's face to go smoothly forward. If they don't work together—that is, if the coordination among these areas is disrupted—yet another area works to make sure you offer plausible hypotheses about this, and not zany ones. (Thus, if your father looks less familiar to you on some occasion, you're likely to explain this by saying, "I guess he must have gotten new glasses" rather than "I bet he's been replaced by a robot.")

Unmistakably, then, this apparently easy task—seeing your father and recognizing who he is—requires multiple brain areas. The same is true of most tasks, and in this way Capgras syndrome illustrates this crucial aspect of brain function.

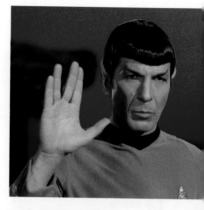

HUMANS AREN'T VULCANS

The TV show *Star Trek* (and its various offshoots) provided a prominent role for Vulcans—people who were entirely logical and felt no emotion, and so were not influenced by emotion. As the show made clear, though, humans are different—and emotional evaluations are an important aspect of many cognitive processes.

The Study of the Brain

In order to discuss Capgras syndrome, we needed to refer to different brain areas; we also had to rely on several different research techniques. Thus, the syndrome also illustrates another point—namely, that this is a domain in which we need some technical foundations before we can develop our theories. Let's start building those foundations.

The human brain weighs between 3 and 4 pounds; it's roughly the size of a small melon. Yet this structure has been estimated to contain a trillion nerve cells (that's 10^{12}), each of which is connected to 10,000 or so others—for a total of roughly 10 million billion connections. The brain also contains a huge number of *glial* cells (and, by some estimates, the glia outnumber the nerve cells by roughly 10 to 1, so there are roughly 10 trillion of these). We'll have much more to say about nerve cells and glial cells later; but more immediately, how should we begin our study of this densely packed, incredibly complex organ?

One place to start is with a simple fact we've already met: that different parts of the brain perform different jobs. We've known this fact about the brain for many years, thanks to clinical evidence showing that the symptoms produced by brain damage depend heavily on the location of the damage. In 1848, for example, a horrible construction accident caused Phineas Gage to suffer damage in the frontmost part of his brain (see **Figure 2.4**); this damage led to severe personality and emotional problems. In 1861, physician Paul Broca noted that damage in a different location, on the left side of the brain, led to a disruption of language skills. In 1911, Édouard Claparède (1911/1951) reported his observations with patients who suffered from profound memory loss, a loss produced by damage in still another part of the brain.

Clearly, therefore, we need to understand brain functioning with reference to brain anatomy. Where was the damage that Gage suffered? Where exactly was the damage in Broca's patients or Claparède's? In this section, we fill in some basics of brain anatomy.

EBOOK
DEMONSTRATION 2.1

FIGURE 2.4 PHINEAS GAGE

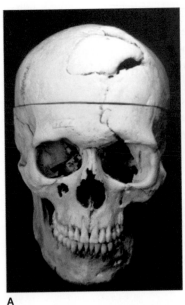
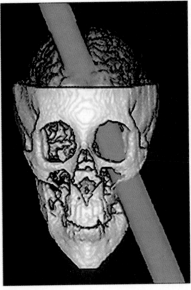
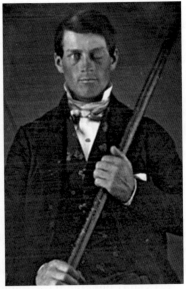

A   B   C

Phineas Gage was working as a construction foreman when some blasting powder misfired and launched a piece of iron into his cheek and through the front part of his brain. Remarkably, Gage survived and continued to live a more-or-less normal life, but his pattern of intellectual and emotional impairments provide valuable cues about the function of the brain's frontal lobes. Panel A is a photo of Gage's skull; the drawing in Panel B depicts the iron bar's path as it blasted through his head. Panel C is an actual photograph of Gage, and he's holding the bar that went through his brain!

Hindbrain, Midbrain, Forebrain

The human brain is divided into three main structures: the hindbrain, the midbrain, and the forebrain. The **hindbrain** sits directly atop the spinal cord and includes structures crucial for controlling key life functions. It's here, for example, that the rhythm of heartbeats and the rhythm of breathing are regulated. The hindbrain also plays an essential role in maintaining the body's overall tone: specifically, the hindbrain helps maintain the body's posture and balance; it also helps control the brain's level of alertness.

The largest area of the hindbrain is the **cerebellum**. For many years, investigators believed this structure's main role was in the coordination of bodily movements and balance. Some studies suggest, however, that the cerebellum plays a diverse set of further roles and that damage to this organ can cause problems in spatial reasoning, in discriminating sounds, and in integrating the input received from various sensory systems (Bower & Parsons, 2003).

The **midbrain** has several functions. It plays an important part in coordinating your movements, including the skilled, precise movements of your eyes as you explore the visual world. Also in the midbrain are circuits that relay auditory information from the ears to the areas in the forebrain where this information is processed and interpreted. Still other structures in the midbrain help to regulate the experience of pain.

For our purposes, though, the most interesting brain region (and, in humans, the largest region) is the **forebrain**. Drawings of the brain (like the one shown in Figure 2.2) show little other than the forebrain, because this structure surrounds (and so hides from view) the entire midbrain and most of the hindbrain. Of course, it is only the outer surface of the forebrain—the **cortex**—that is visible in such pictures. In general, the word "cortex" (from the Latin word for "tree bark") refers to an organ's outer surface, and many organs each have their own cortex; what's visible in the drawing, then, is the *cerebral* cortex.

The cortex is just a thin covering on the outer surface of the forebrain; on average, it is a mere 3 mm thick. Nonetheless, there's a great deal of cortical tissue; by some estimates, the cortex constitutes 80% of the human brain. This considerable volume is made possible by the fact that the cerebral cortex, thin as it is, consists of a large sheet of tissue; if stretched out flat, it would cover more than 2 square feet. (For comparison, an extra-large, 18-inch pizza covers roughly 1.4 square feet.) But the cortex isn't stretched flat; instead, it is all crumpled up and jammed into the limited space inside the skull. It's this crumpling that produces the brain's most obvious visual feature—the wrinkles, or **convolutions**, that cover the brain's outer surface.

Some of the "valleys" between the wrinkles are actually deep grooves that divide the brain into different sections. The deepest groove is the **longitudinal fissure**, running from the front of the brain to the back, which separates the left **cerebral hemisphere** from the right. Other fissures divide the cortex in each hemisphere into four lobes (again, look back at Figure 2.2), and these are named after the bones that cover them—bones that, as a group, make up the skull. The **frontal lobes** form the front of the brain—right behind the forehead. The **central fissure** divides the frontal lobes on each side of the brain from the **parietal lobes,** the brain's topmost part. The bottom edge of the frontal lobes is marked by the **lateral fissure,** and below it are the **temporal lobes.** Finally, at the very back of the brain, connected to the parietal and temporal lobes, are the **occipital lobes.**

Subcortical Structures

Hidden from view, underneath the cortex, are the **subcortical** parts of the forebrain. One of these parts, the **thalamus,** acts as a relay station for nearly all the sensory information going to the cortex. Directly underneath the thalamus is the **hypothalamus,** a structure that plays a crucial role in controlling motivated behaviors such as eating, drinking, and sexual activity.

Surrounding the thalamus and hypothalamus is another set of interconnected structures that together form the **limbic system.** Included here is the amygdala, and close by is the **hippocampus,** both located underneath the cortex in the temporal lobe (plurals: amygdalae and hippocampi; see **Figure 2.5**). These structures are essential for learning and memory, and the

FIGURE 2.5   THE LIMBIC SYSTEM AND THE HIPPOCAMPUS

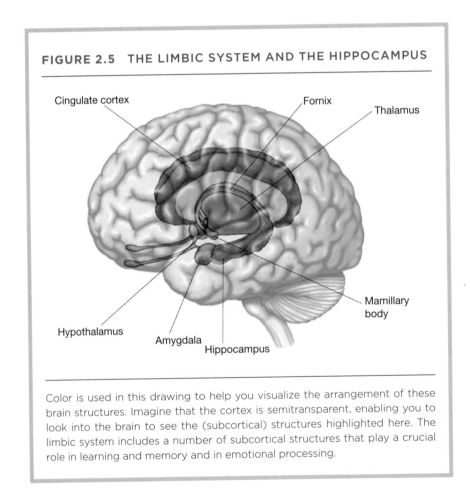

Color is used in this drawing to help you visualize the arrangement of these brain structures. Imagine that the cortex is semitransparent, enabling you to look into the brain to see the (subcortical) structures highlighted here. The limbic system includes a number of subcortical structures that play a crucial role in learning and memory and in emotional processing.

patient H.M., discussed in Chapter 1, developed his profound amnesia after surgeons removed these structures—a strong confirmation of their role in the formation of new memories.

We mentioned earlier that the amygdala plays a key role in emotional processing, and this role is reflected in many findings. For example, presentation of frightful faces causes high levels of activity in the amygdala (Williams et al., 2006). Likewise, people ordinarily show more complete, longer-lasting memories for emotional events, compared to similar but emotionally flat events. This memory advantage for emotional events is especially pronounced in people who showed greater activation in the amygdala while they were witnessing the event in the first place. Conversely, the memory advantage for emotional events is diminished (and may not be observed at all) in people who (through sickness or injury) have suffered damage to the amygdala.

Lateralization

Virtually all parts of the brain come in pairs, and so there is a hippocampus on the left side of the brain and another on the right, a left-side amygdala and a right-side one. Of course, the same is true for the cerebral cortex itself: There is a temporal cortex (i.e., a cortex of the temporal lobe) in the left hemisphere and another in the right, a left occipital cortex and a right one, and so on. In all cases, cortical and subcortical, the left and right structures in each pair have roughly the same shape and the same pattern of connections to other brain areas. Even so, there are differences in function between the left-side and right-side structures, with the left-hemisphere structure playing a somewhat different role from the corresponding right-hemisphere structure.

Let's bear in mind, though, that the two halves of the brain work together; the functioning of one side is closely integrated with that of the other side. This integration is made possible by the **commissures**, thick bundles of fibers that carry information back and forth between the two hemispheres. The largest commissure is the **corpus callosum**, but several other structures also ensure that the two brain halves work as partners in nearly all mental tasks.

In some cases, though, there are medical reasons to sever the corpus callosum and some of the other commissures. (For many years, this surgery was a last resort for extreme cases of epilepsy.) The person is then said to be a "split-brain patient"—still having both brain halves, but with communication between the halves severely limited. Research with these patients has taught us a great deal about the specialized function of the brain's two hemispheres and has provided evidence, for example, that language capacities are generally lodged in the left hemisphere, while the right hemisphere seems crucial for a number of tasks involving spatial judgment (see **Figure 2.6**).

However, it is important not to overstate the contrast between the two brain halves, and it's misleading to claim (as some people do) that we need

FIGURE 2.6 STUDYING SPLIT-BRAIN PATIENTS

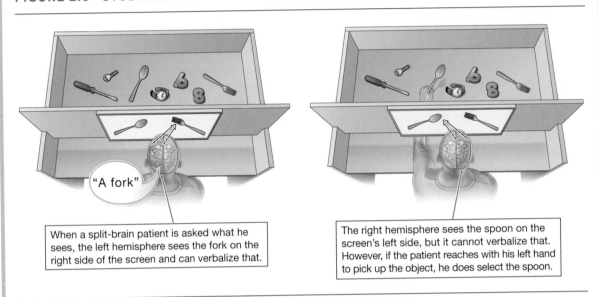

"A fork"

When a split-brain patient is asked what he sees, the left hemisphere sees the fork on the right side of the screen and can verbalize that.

The right hemisphere sees the spoon on the screen's left side, but it cannot verbalize that. However, if the patient reaches with his left hand to pick up the object, he does select the spoon.

In this experiment, the patient is shown two pictures, one of a spoon and one of a fork. If asked what he sees, his verbal response is controlled by the left hemisphere, which has seen only the fork (because it's in the right visual field). If asked to pick up the object shown in the picture, however, the patient—reaching with his left hand—picks up the spoon. That happens because the left hand is controlled by the right hemisphere, and this hemisphere receives visual information from the left-hand side of the visual world.

to silence our "left-brain thinking" in order to be more creative, or that intuitions grow out of "right-brain thinking." Instead, in people with intact commissures, the two hemispheres work together, with each hemisphere providing its own specialized skills that contribute to overall performance. Put differently, the complex, sophisticated skills we each display (including creativity, intuition, and more) depend on the whole brain. Our hemispheres are not cerebral competitors, each trying to impose its style of thinking on the other. Instead, the hemispheres pool their specialized capacities to produce a seamlessly integrated single mental self.

Data from Neuropsychology

How can we learn about these various structures—and many others that we have not named? Just as cognitive psychology relies on many types of evidence in order to study the mind, cognitive neuroscience relies on many types of evidence to study the brain and nervous system.

We've already encountered one form of evidence—the study of individuals who (tragically) have suffered brain damage, whether through accident, disease, or in some cases birth defect. The study of these cases generally falls within the domain of *neuropsychology*: the study of the brain's structures and how they relate to brain function. Within neuropsychology, the specialty of *clinical neuropsychology* seeks (among other goals) to understand the functioning of intact, undamaged brains by careful scrutiny of cases involving brain damage.

Data drawn from clinical neuropsychology will be important for us throughout this text. For now, though, let's note once again that the symptoms resulting from brain damage depend significantly on the site of the damage. A **lesion** (a specific area of damage) in the hippocampus produces memory problems but not language disorders; a lesion in the occipital cortex produces problems in vision but spares the other sensory modalities. Likewise, the consequences of brain lesions depend on which hemisphere is damaged: Damage to the left side of the frontal lobe, for example, is likely to produce a disruption of language use; damage to the right side of the frontal lobe generally doesn't have this effect. In obvious ways, all of these patterns confirm that different brain areas perform different functions and provide a rich source of data that help us develop and test hypotheses about those functions.

Data from Neuroimaging

We can also learn a great deal from neuroimaging data. As we mentioned earlier, neuroimaging allows us to take precise three-dimensional pictures of the brain. For many years, researchers used **computerized axial tomography (CT scans)** to study the brain's structure and **positron emission tomography (PET scans)** to study the brain's activity. CT scans rely on X-rays and thus—in essence—provide a three-dimensional X-ray picture of the brain. PET scans, in contrast, start by introducing a tracer substance such as glucose into the body; the molecules of this tracer have been tagged with a low dose of radioactivity, and the scan keeps track of this radioactivity, allowing us to tell which tissues are using more of the glucose (the body's main fuel) and which are using less. For both types of scan, though, the primary data (X-rays or radioactive emissions) are collected by a bank of detectors surrounding the head; a computer then compares the signals received by each of the detectors and uses this information to pinpoint the source of each signal. In this way, the computer reconstructs a three-dimensional map of the brain. For CT scans, the map tells us the shape, size, and position of structures within the brain. For PET scans, the map tells us what regions are particularly active at any point in time.

More recent studies have turned to two newer techniques, introduced earlier in the chapter. **Magnetic resonance imaging (MRI)** relies on the magnetic properties of the atoms that make up the brain tissue, and it yields fabulously detailed pictures of the brain. A closely related technique, **functional magnetic resonance imaging (fMRI)**, measures the oxygen content in the blood flowing through each region of the brain; this turns out to be an accurate index of the level of neural activity in that region.

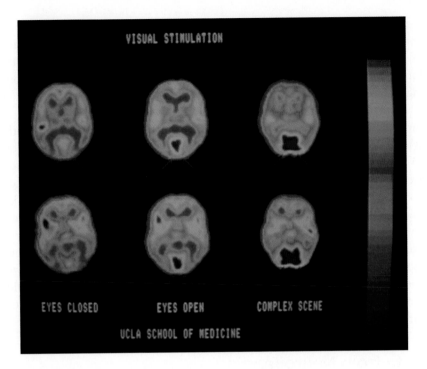

PET SCANS

PET scans can measure how much glucose (the brain's fuel) is being used at specific locations within the brain; this provides a measurement of each location's activity level at a certain moment in time. In the figure, the brain is viewed from above, with the front of the head at the top and the back at the bottom. The various colors indicate relative activity levels (the brain itself is not colored!), using the ordered palette shown on the right side of the figure. As the figure shows, visual processing involves increased activity in the occipital lobe.

In this way, fMRI scans provide an incredibly precise picture of the brain's moment-by-moment activities.

The results of a CT or MRI scan are relatively stable, changing only if the person's brain structure changes (because of an injury, perhaps, or the growth of a tumor). The results of PET or fMRI scans, in contrast, are highly variable, because the results depend on what task the person is performing. This linkage between the scan data and mental activity once again confirms a fundamental point: Different brain areas perform different functions and are involved in different tasks.

More ambitiously, though, we can use the neuroimaging procedures as a means of exploring brain function—using fMRI scans, for example, to ask which brain sites are especially activated when someone is listening to Mozart or when someone is engaged in memory rehearsal. In this fashion, the neuroimaging data can provide crucial information about how these complex activities are made possible by specific brain functioning.

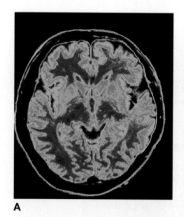
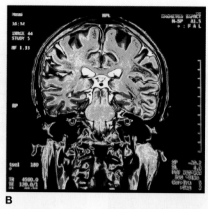
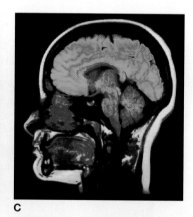

A   B   C

MAGNETIC RESONANCE IMAGING

Magnetic resonance imaging produces magnificently detailed pictures of the brain. Panel A shows a "slice" of the brain viewed from the top of the head (the front of the head is at the top of the image); clearly visible is the longitudinal fissure, which divides the left cerebral hemisphere from the right. Panel B shows a slice of the brain viewed from the front; again, the separation of the two hemispheres is clearly visible, and so are some of the commissures linking the two brain halves. Panel C shows a slice of the brain viewed from the side; many of the structures in the limbic system (see Figure 2.5) are easily seen.

Data from Electrical Recording

Neuroscientists have another technique in their toolkit: electrical recording of the brain's activity. To explain this point, though, we need to say a bit about how the brain functions. As we mentioned earlier, the brain contains a trillion nerve cells—more properly called "neurons"—and it is the neurons that do the brain's main work. (We'll say more about these cells later in the chapter.) Neurons vary in their shape, size, and functioning, but for the most part they communicate with one another via chemical signals called "neurotransmitters." Once a neuron is "activated," it releases the transmitter, and this chemical can then activate (or, in some cases, *de*-activate) other, immediately adjacent neurons. The adjacent neurons, in other words, "receive" this chemical signal, and they, in turn, can send their own signal onward to other neurons.

Let's be clear, though, that the process we just described is communication *between* neurons: One neuron releases the transmitter substance and this activates (or de-activates) another neuron. But, in addition, there's also communication *within* each neuron. The reason—to put it roughly—is that neurons have an "input" end and an "output" end. The "input" end is the portion of the neuron that's most sensitive to neurotransmitters; this is where the signal from other neurons is received. The "output" end is the portion of the neuron that releases neurotransmitters, sending the signal on to other neurons. These two ends can sometimes be far apart. (For example, some neurons in your body run from the base of your spine down to your

FIGURE 2.7   RECORDING THE BRAIN'S ELECTRICAL ACTIVITY

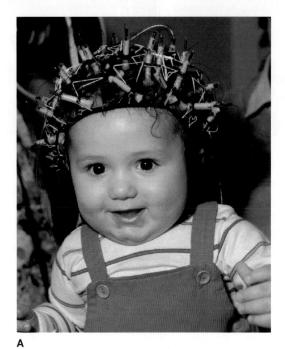

A

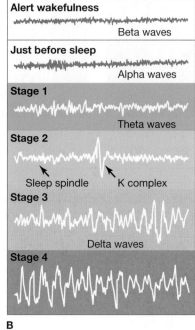

B

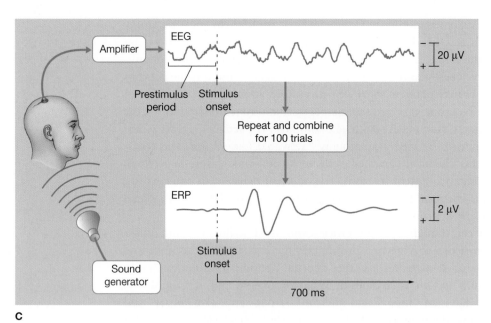

C

To record the brain's electrical signals, researchers generally use a cap that has electrodes attached to it. The procedure is easy and entirely safe—it can even be used to measure brain signals in a baby (Panel A). In some procedures, researchers measure recurrent rhythms in the brain's activity, including the rhythms that distinguish the stages of sleep (Panel B). In other procedures, they measure the brain activity produced in response to a single event—such as the presentation of a well-defined stimulus (Panel C).

toes; for these cells, the input and output ends are likely to be almost a meter apart.) The question, then, is how neurons get a signal from one end of the cell to the other.

The answer involves an electrical pulse, made possible by a flow of charged atoms (ions) in and out of the neuron (again, we will say more about this process later in the chapter). The amount of electrical current involved in this ion flow is minute; but, of course, many millions of neurons are active at the same time, and the current generated by all of them together is strong enough to be detected by sensitive electrodes placed on the surface of the scalp. This is the basis for **electroencephalography**—a recording of voltage changes occurring at the scalp that reflect activity in the brain underneath. The result of this procedure is an *electroencephalogram,* or EEG—a recording of the brain's electrical activity.

Often, EEGs are used to study broad rhythms in the brain's activities. Thus, for example, an *alpha rhythm* (with the activity level rising and falling seven to ten times per second) can usually be detected in the brain of someone who is awake but calm and relaxed; a *delta rhythm* (with the activity rising and falling roughly one to four times per second) is observed when someone is deeply asleep.

Sometimes, though, we want to know about the brain's electrical activity over a shorter period of time—for example, when the brain is responding to a specific input or a particular stimulus. In this case, we measure the changes in EEG in the brief period just before, during, and after the event; these changes are referred to as an **event-related potential** (see **Figure 2.7**).

The Power of Combining Techniques

Each of the research tools we have described has its own strengths and weaknesses. CT scans and MRI data tell us about the shape and size of brain structures, but they tell us nothing about the activity levels within these structures. PET scans and fMRI studies do tell us about brain activity, and they can locate the activity rather precisely (within a millimeter or two). However, these techniques are less precise about *when* the activity took place. For example, fMRI data summarize the brain's activity over a period of several seconds and cannot tell us when exactly, within this time window, the activity took place. EEG data give us much more precise information about timing but are much weaker in telling us *where* the activity took place.

Researchers deal with these limitations by means of a strategy commonly used in science: We seek data from multiple sources, so that we can use the strengths of one technique to make up for the shortcomings of another. Thus, some studies combine EEG recordings with fMRI scans, with the EEGs telling us when certain events took place in the brain, and the scans telling us where the activity took place. Likewise, some studies combine fMRI scans with CT data, so that we can link our findings about brain activation to a detailed portrait of the person's brain anatomy.

Researchers also need to deal with another limitation on their findings: the fact that many of the techniques described so far provide only *correlational data*. To understand this point, consider the finding that a brain area often called the **fusiform face area (FFA)** seems especially active whenever a face is being perceived (see **Figure 2.8**). Does this mean the FFA is needed for face perception? A different possibility is that the FFA activation may just be

FIGURE 2.8   BRAIN ACTIVITY AND AWARENESS

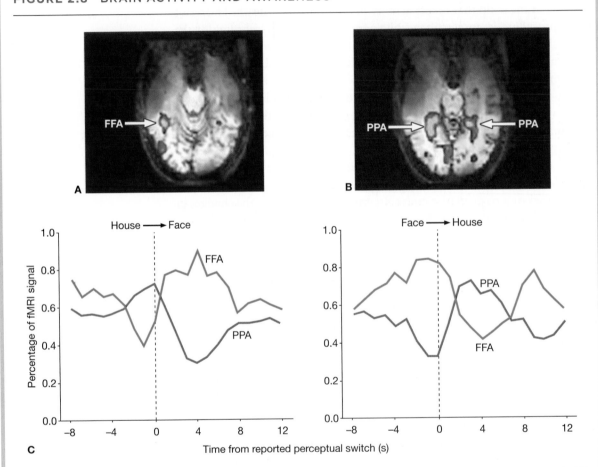

Panel A shows an fMRI scan of a subject looking at faces. Activation levels are high in the fusiform face area (FFA), an area that is apparently more responsive to faces than to other visual stimuli. Panel B shows a scan of the same subject looking at pictures of places; now activity levels are high in the parahippocampal place area (PPA). Panel C compares the activity in these two areas when the subject has a picture of a face in front of one eye, and a picture of a house in front of the other eye. When the viewer's attention shifts from the house to the face, activation increases in the FFA. When the viewer's attention shifts from the face to the house, PPA activation increases. Thus, the activation level reflects what the subject is aware of, and not just the pattern of incoming stimulation.   AFTER TONG, NAKAYAMA, VAUGHAN, & KANWISHER, 1998.

a by-product of face perception and does not play a crucial role. As an analogy, think about the fact that a car's speedometer becomes "more activated" (i.e., shows a higher value) whenever the car goes faster. That doesn't mean that the speedometer *causes* the speed or *is necessary* for the speed. Indeed, the car would go just as fast and would, for many purposes, perform just as well if the speedometer were removed. The speedometer's state, in other words, is *correlated* with the car's speed but in no sense causes (or promotes, or is needed for) the car's speed.

In the same way, neuroimaging data can tell us that a brain area's activity is correlated with a particular function, but we need other data to ask whether the brain site plays a role in *causing* (or supporting, or allowing) that function. In many cases, those other data come from the study of brain lesions: If damage to a brain site disrupts a function, that's an indication that the site does play some role in supporting that function. (And, in fact, the FFA does play an important role in face recognition.)

Also helpful here is a technique called **transcranial magnetic stimulation (TMS)**. This technique creates a series of strong magnetic pulses at a specific location on the scalp, causing a (temporary!) disruption in the brain region directly underneath this scalp area (Helmuth, 2001). This allows us to ask, in an otherwise normal brain, what functions are compromised when a particular bit of brain tissue is temporarily "turned off." The results of a TMS procedure can therefore provide crucial information about the functional role of that brain area.

Localization of Function

Overall, then, the data make it clear that different portions of the brain each have their own jobs to do. Indeed, drawing on the techniques we have described, neuroscientists have learned a great deal about the function of specific brain structures—a research effort broadly referred to as the **localization of function**, an effort (to put it crudely) aimed at figuring out what's happening where within the brain.

Localization data are useful in many ways. For example, think back to the discussion of Capgras syndrome earlier in this chapter. Brain scans told us that people with this syndrome have damaged amygdalae. To interpret this observation, though, we needed to ask about the function of the amygdalae: Yes, we can locate the brain damage in these patients, but how does the brain damage affect them? To tackle this question, we relied on localization of function—and, in particular, on data telling us that the amygdala is involved in many tasks involving emotional appraisal. This combination of points, then, helped us to build (and test) our claims about this syndrome and, more broadly, claims about the role of emotional processing within the ordinary experience of "familiarity."

As a different illustration, consider the experience of calling up a "mental picture" before the "mind's eye." We'll have more to say about this experience in Chapter 11, but we can already ask: How much does this experience

FIGURE 2.9 A PORTRAIT OF THE BRAIN AT WORK

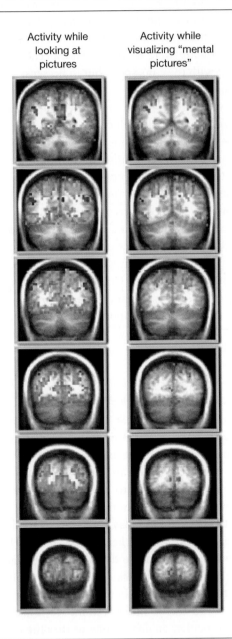

These fMRI images show different "slices" through the living brain, revealing levels of activity in different brain sites. More-active regions are shown in yellow, orange, and red. The first column shows brain activity while a person is making judgments about simple pictures. The second column shows brain activity while the person is making the same sorts of judgments about "mental pictures," visualized before the "mind's eye."

have in common with ordinary seeing—that is, placing a real picture before the actual eyes? As it turns out, localization data reveal enormous overlap between the brain structures needed for these two activities (visualizing and actual vision), telling us immediately that these activities do have a great deal in common (see **Figure 2.9**). Thus, again, we build on localization—this time to ask how exactly two mental activities are related to each other.

The Cerebral Cortex

As we've already noted, the largest portion of the human brain is the cerebral cortex—the thin layer of tissue covering the cerebrum. This is the region in which an enormous amount of information processing takes place, and so, for many topics, it is the brain region of greatest interest for cognitive psychologists. The cortex includes many distinct regions, each with its own function, but these regions are traditionally divided into three categories: *motor areas*, which contain brain tissue crucial for organizing and controlling bodily movements; *sensory areas*, which contain tissue essential for organizing and analyzing the information we receive from the senses; and *association areas*. These latter areas support many functions, including the essential (but not well defined) human activity we call "thinking."

Motor Areas

Certain regions of the cerebral cortex serve as the "departure points" for signals leaving the cortex and controlling muscle movement. Other areas are the "arrival points" for information coming from the eyes, ears, and other sense organs. In both cases, these areas are called "primary projection areas," with the departure points known as the **primary motor projection areas** and the arrival points contained in regions known as the **primary sensory projection areas**.

Evidence for the motor projection area comes from studies in which investigators apply mild electrical current to this area in anesthetized animals. This stimulation often produces specific movements, so that current applied to one site causes a movement of the left front leg, while current applied to a different site causes the ears to prick up. These movements show a pattern of **contralateral control**, with stimulation to the left hemisphere leading to movements on the right side of the body, and vice versa.

Why are these areas called "projection areas"? The term is borrowed from mathematics and from the discipline of map making, because these areas seem to form "maps" of the external world, with particular positions on the cortex corresponding to particular parts of the body or particular locations in space. In the human brain, the map that constitutes the motor projection area is located on a strip of tissue toward the rear of the frontal lobe, and the pattern of mapping is illustrated in **Figure 2.10**; in this illustration, a drawing of a person has been overlaid on a depiction of the brain, with each part of the little person positioned on top of the brain area that controls its movement. The figure makes clear that areas of the body that we can move

FIGURE 2.10   THE PRIMARY PROJECTION AREAS

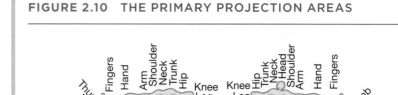

The primary motor projection area is located at the rearmost edge of the frontal lobe, and each region within this projection area controls the motion of a specific body part, as illustrated on the top left. The primary somatosensory projection area, receiving information from the skin, is at the forward edge of the parietal lobe; each region within this area receives input from a specific body part. The primary projection areas for vision and hearing are located in the occipital and temporal lobes, respectively. These two areas are also organized systematically. For example, in the visual projection area, adjacent areas of the brain receive visual inputs that come from adjacent areas in visual space.

with great precision (e.g., fingers and lips) have a lot of cortical area devoted to them; areas of the body over which we have less control (e.g., the shoulder and the back) receive less cortical coverage.

Sensory Areas

Information arriving from the skin senses (your sense of touch or your sense of temperature) is projected to a region in the parietal lobe, just behind the motor projection area; this is labeled the "somatosensory" area in Figure 2.10. If a patient's brain is stimulated in this region (with electrical current or touch), the patient will typically report a tingling sensation in a specific part of the body. Figure 2.10 also shows the region (in the temporal lobes) that functions as the primary projection area for hearing (the "auditory" area). If the brain is directly stimulated here, the patient will hear clicks, buzzes, and hums. An area in the occipital lobes is the primary projection area for vision; stimulation here produces the experience of seeing flashes of light or visual patterns.

The sensory projection areas differ from each other in important ways, but they also have features in common, and they're features that parallel the attributes of the motor projection area. First, each of these areas provides a "map" of the sensory environment. In the somatosensory area, each part of the body's surface is represented by its own region on the cortex; areas of the body that are near to each other are typically represented by similarly nearby areas in the brain. In the visual area, each region of visual space has its own cortical representation, and again, adjacent areas of space are usually represented by adjacent brain sites. In the auditory projection area, different

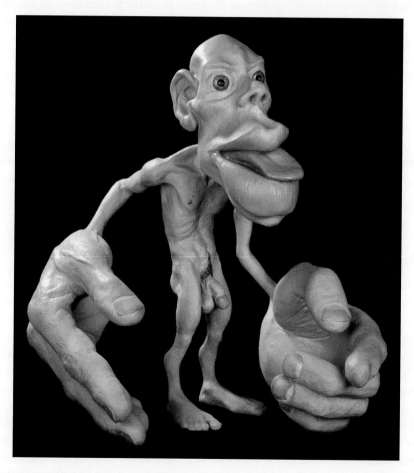

THE SENSORY HOMUNCULUS

An artist's rendition of what a man would look like if his appearance were proportional to the area allotted by the somatosensory cortex to his various body parts.

EBOOK
DEMONSTRATION 2.2

frequencies of sound have their own cortical sites, and adjacent brain sites are responsive to adjacent frequencies.

Second, in each of these sensory maps the assignment of cortical space is governed by function, not by anatomical proportions. In the parietal lobes, parts of the body that are not very discriminating with regard to touch, even if they're physically large, get relatively little cortical area. Other, more sensitive areas of the body (the lips, tongue, and fingers) get far more space. In the occipital lobes, more cortical surface is devoted to the fovea, the part of the eyeball that is most sensitive to detail. And in the auditory areas, some frequencies of sound get more cerebral coverage than others; it's surely no coincidence that these "advantaged" frequencies are those essential for the perception of speech.

Finally, we also find evidence here of contralateral connections. The somatosensory area in the left hemisphere, for example, receives its main input from the right side of the body; the corresponding area in the right hemisphere receives its input from the left side of the body. Likewise for the visual projection areas, although here the projection is not contralateral with regard to body parts; instead, it's contralateral with regard to physical space. Specifically, the visual projection area in the right hemisphere receives information from both the left eye and the right, but the information it receives corresponds to the left half of visual space (i.e., all of the things visible to your left when you're looking straight ahead). The reverse is true for the visual area in the left hemisphere: It receives information from both eyes, but from only the right half of visual space. The pattern of contralateral organization is also evident—although not as clear-cut—for the auditory cortex, with roughly 60% of the nerve fibers from each ear sending their information to the opposite side of the brain.

Association Areas

The areas described so far, both motor and sensory, make up only a small part of the human cerebral cortex—roughly 25%. The remaining cortical areas are traditionally referred to as the **association cortex**. This terminology is falling out of use, however, in part because this large volume of brain tissue can be subdivided further on both functional and anatomical grounds. These subdivisions are perhaps best revealed by the diversity of symptoms that result if the cortex is damaged in one or another specific location. For example, some lesions in the frontal lobe produce **apraxias**, disturbances in the initiation or organization of voluntary action. Other lesions (generally in the occipital cortex, or in the rearmost part of the parietal lobe) lead to **agnosias**, disruptions in the ability to identify familiar objects. Agnosias usually affect one modality only, so a patient with visual agnosia, for example, can recognize a fork by touching it but not by looking at it. A patient with auditory agnosia, by contrast, might be unable to identify familiar voices but might still recognize the face of the person speaking.

Still other lesions (usually in the parietal lobe) produce **neglect syndrome**, in which the individual seems to ignore half of the visual world. A patient afflicted with this syndrome will shave only half of his face and eat food from only half of his plate. If asked to read the word "parties," he will read "ties," and so on.

Damage in other areas causes still other symptoms. We mentioned earlier that lesions in areas near the lateral fissure (again, the deep groove that separates the frontal and temporal lobes) can result in disruption to language capacities, a problem referred to as **aphasia**.

Finally, damage to the frontmost part of the frontal lobe, the **prefrontal** area, causes problems in problems of planning and implementing strategies. In other cases, patients with damage here show problems in inhibiting their own behaviors, relying on habit even in situations for which habit is inappropriate. Frontal lobe damage can also (as we mentioned in our discussion of Capgras syndrome) lead to a variety of confusions, such as whether a remembered episode actually happened or was simply imagined.

We will have much more to say about these diagnostic categories—aphasia, agnosia, neglect, and more—in upcoming chapters, where we'll consider these disorders in the context of other things we know about object recognition, attention, and so on. Our point for the moment, though, is a simple one: These clinical patterns make it clear that the so-called association cortex contains many subregions, each specialized for a particular function, but with all of the subregions working together in virtually all aspects of our daily lives.

Brain Cells

The brief tour presented above has described only the large-scale structures in the brain. For many purposes, though, we need to zoom in for a closer look, in order to see how the brain's functions are actually carried out.

Neurons and Glia

We've already mentioned that the human brain contains roughly a trillion **neurons** and a much greater number of **glia**. The glia perform many functions: They help to guide the development of the nervous system in the fetus and young infant; they support repairs if the nervous system is damaged; they also control the flow of nutrients to the neurons. Specialized glial cells also provide a layer of electrical insulation surrounding parts of some neurons; this insulation dramatically increases the speed with which neurons can send their signals. Finally, some research suggests the glia may also constitute their own signaling system within the brain, separate from the information flow provided by the neurons (e.g., Bullock et al, 2005; Gallo & Chitajullu, 2001).

There is no question, though, that the main flow of information through the brain—from the sense organs inward, from one part of the brain to the others, and then from the brain outward—is made possible by the neurons. As we noted earlier, neurons come in many shapes and sizes; but, in general,

FIGURE 2.11   NEURONS

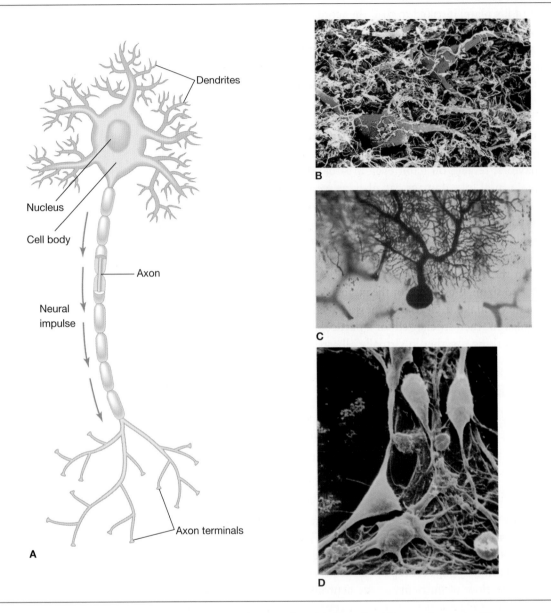

A

Dendrites

Nucleus

Cell body

Axon

Neural impulse

Axon terminals

B

C

D

Most neurons have three identifiable regions, as shown in Panel A: The *dendrites* are the part of the neuron that usually detects incoming signals. The *cell body* contains the metabolic machinery that sustains the cell. The *axon* is the part of the neuron that transmits a signal to another location. When the cell fires, neurotransmitters are released from the terminal endings at the tip of the axon. We should note, though, that neurons actually come in many shapes and sizes. Panel B shows neurons from the spinal cord (stained in red); Panel C shows neurons from the cerebellum; Panel D shows neurons from the cerebral cortex. Neurons usually have the same basic parts (dendrites, a cell body, and at least one axon), but the dimensions and configuration of these parts can vary widely.

neurons have three major parts (see **Figure 2.11**). The **cell body** is the portion of the cell that contains the neuron's nucleus and all the elements needed for the normal metabolic activities of the cell. The **dendrites** are usually the "input" side of the neuron, receiving signals from many other neurons. In most neurons, the dendrites are heavily branched, like a thick and tangled bush. The **axon**, finally, is the "output" side of the neuron; it sends neural impulses to other neurons. Axons can vary enormously in length; the giraffe, for example, has neurons with axons that run the full length of its neck.

The Synapse

We've already noted that communication from one neuron to the next is generally made possible by a chemical signal: When a neuron has been sufficiently stimulated, it releases a minute quantity of a **neurotransmitter**. The molecules of this substance drift across the tiny gap between neurons and latch on to the dendrites of the adjacent cell. If the dendrites receive enough of this substance, the next neuron will "fire," and so the signal will be sent along to other neurons.

EBOOK
DEMONSTRATION 2.3

Notice, then, that neurons usually don't touch each other directly. Instead, at the end of the axon there is a gap separating each neuron from the next. This entire site—the end of the axon, plus the gap, plus the receiving membrane of the next neuron—is called a **synapse**. The space between the neurons is the *synaptic gap*; the bit of the neuron that releases the transmitter into this gap is the **presynaptic membrane**, and the bit of the neuron on the other side of the gap, affected by the transmitters, is the **postsynaptic membrane**.

When the neurotransmitters arrive at the postsynaptic membrane, they cause changes in this membrane that enable certain ions to flow into and out of the postsynaptic cell (see **Figure 2.12**). If these ionic flows are relatively small, then the postsynaptic cell quickly recovers and the ions are transported back to where they were initially. But if the ionic flows are large enough, they trigger a response in the postsynaptic cell. In formal terms, if the incoming signal reaches the postsynaptic cell's **threshold**, then the cell **fires**; that is, it produces an **action potential**—a signal that moves down its axon, which in turn causes the release of neurotransmitters at the next synapse, potentially causing the next cell to fire.

Let's emphasize several points about this sequence of events. First, note once again that neurons depend on two different forms of information flow. Communication from one neuron to the next is (for most neurons) mediated by a chemical signal. In contrast, communication from one end of the neuron to the other (usually from the dendrites down the length of the axon) is made possible by an electrical signal, created by the flow of ions in and out of the cell.

Second, note that the postsynaptic neuron's initial response can vary in size; the incoming signal can cause a small ionic flow or a large one. Crucially, though, once these inputs reach the postsynaptic neuron's firing threshold,

FIGURE 2.12   SCHEMATIC VIEW OF SYNAPTIC TRANSMISSION

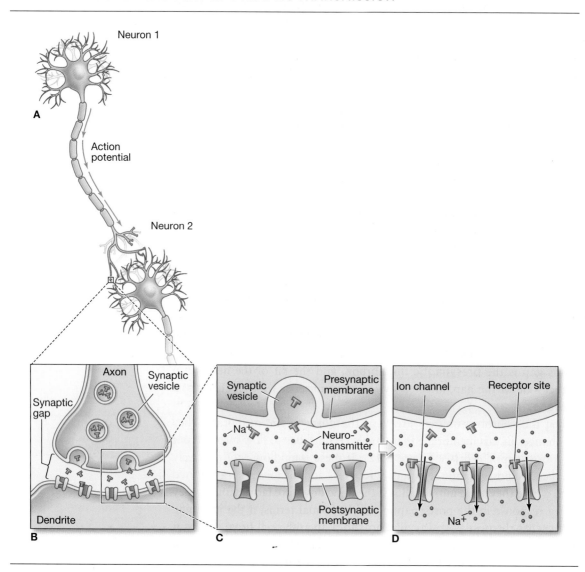

(Panel A) Neuron 1 transmits a message across the synaptic gap to Neuron 2. The neurotransmitters are initially stored in structures called *synaptic vesicles* (Panel B). When a signal travels down the axon, the vesicles are stimulated and some of them burst (Panel C), ejecting neurotransmitter molecules into the synaptic gap, and thus toward the postsynaptic membrane. (Panel D) Neurotransmitter molecules settle on receptor sites, ion channels open, and sodium (Na+) floods in.

there's no variability in the response: Either a signal is sent down the axon or it is not; if the signal is sent, it is always of the same magnitude, a fact referred to as the **all-or-none law**. Just as pounding on a car horn won't make the horn any louder, a stronger stimulus won't produce a stronger action potential. A neuron either fires or it doesn't; there's no in-between.

This does not mean, however, that neurons always send exactly the same information. A neuron can fire many times per second or only occasionally. A neuron can fire just once and then stop, or it can keep firing for an extended span. But, even so, each individual response by the neuron is always the same size.

Third, we should note also that the brain relies on many different neurotransmitters. Roughly a hundred transmitters have been catalogued so far, and this diversity enables the brain to send a variety of different messages. Some transmitters have the effect of stimulating subsequent neurons; some do the opposite and *inhibit* other neurons. Some transmitters play an essential role in learning and memory; others play a key role in regulating the level of arousal in the brain; still others influence motivation and emotion.

Finally, let's be clear about the central role of the synapse. The synaptic gap is actually quite small—roughly 20 to 30 nanometers across. (For contrast's sake, the diameter of a human hair is roughly 80,000 nanometers.) Even so, transmission across this gap slows down the neuronal signal, but this is a tiny price to pay for the *advantages* created by this mode of signaling: Each neuron receives information from (i.e., has synapses with) many other neurons, and this allows the "receiving" neuron to integrate information from many sources. This pattern of many neurons feeding into one also makes it possible for a neuron to "compare" signals and to adjust its response to one input according to the signal arriving from a different input. In addition, communication at the synapse is *adjustable*: The strength of a synaptic connection can be altered by experience, and this adjustment is crucial for the process of *learning*—the storage of new knowledge and new skills within the nervous system.

Moving On

We've now described the brain's basic anatomy and have also zoomed in for a brief look at the brain's microscopic parts—the individual neurons. But how do all of these elements, large and small, function in ways that enable us to think, remember, learn, speak, or feel? As a step toward tackling this issue, the next chapter takes a closer look at the portions of the nervous system that allow us to *see*. We'll use the visual system as our example for two important reasons. First, vision is the modality through which we humans acquire a huge amount of information, whether by reading or simply by viewing the world around us. If we understand vision, therefore, we understand the processes that bring us much of our knowledge. Second, investigators have made enormous progress in mapping out the neural "wiring" of the visual system, providing us with a detailed and sophisticated portrait of how this system operates. As a result, the study of vision provides an excellent illustration of how the study of the brain can proceed and what it can teach us.

Food Supplements and Cognition

Various businesses try to sell you food supplements that (they claim) will improve your memory, help you think more clearly, and so on. Unfortunately, most of these supplements have not been tested in any systematic way, and so there's little (and often no) solid evidence to support these promotional claims.

One supplement, though, has been rigorously tested: *Ginkgo biloba* is an extract derived from a tree of the same name and advertised as capable of enhancing memory. Is *Ginkgo biloba* effective? The answer begins with the fact that for its normal functioning, the brain requires an excellent blood flow and, with that, a lot of oxygen and a lot of nutrients. Indeed, it's estimated that the brain, constituting just 2% of your body weight, consumes 15% percent of your body's energy supply.

It's not surprising, therefore, that the brain's operations are impaired if some change in your health interferes with the flow of oxygen or nutrients. If (for example) you're ill, or not eating enough, or not getting enough sleep, these conditions affect virtually all aspects of your biological functioning. However, since the brain is so demanding of nutrients and oxygen, it's one of the first organs to suffer if the supply of these necessities is compromised. This is why poor nutrition or poor health almost inevitably undermines your ability to think, to remember, or to pay attention.

Within this context, it's important that *Ginkgo* extract can improve blood circulation and reduce some sorts of bodily inflammation. Because of these effects, *Ginkgo* can be helpful for people who have circulatory problems or who are at risk for nerve damage, and, in fact, evidence suggests a benefit from this food supplement for patients with Alzheimer's disease and several other conditions. *Ginkgo* helps these patients to remember more and to think more clearly, but let's be clear that *Ginkgo* is not making these patients "smarter" in any direct fashion. Instead, the *Ginkgo* is broadly improving the patients' blood circulation and the health status of their nerve cells, allowing these cells to do their work.

What about healthy people—people not suffering from bodily inflammations or damage to their brain cells? Here, the evidence is mixed, but most studies have failed to observe any benefit from this food supplement. Apparently, *Ginkgo*'s effects, if they exist at all in healthy adults, are so small that they are difficult to detect.

Are there other steps that *will* improve the mental functioning of healthy young adults? Answers here have to be tentative, because new "smart pills" and "smart foods" are being proposed all the time, and, of course, each one has to be tested before we can know its effects. For now, though, we've already indicated part of a positive answer: Good nutrition, plenty of sleep, and adequate exercise will keep your blood supply in good condition, and this will help your brain to do its job. In addition, there may be something

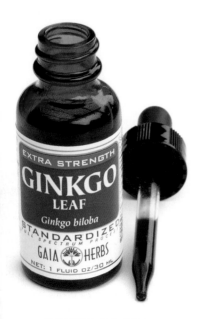

GINKGO BILOBA

A variety of food supplements have been derived from the *Ginkgo* tree, and are alleged to improve cognitive functioning. Current understanding, though, suggests that the benefits of *Ginkgo* are indirect: This supplement improves functioning because it can improve blood circulation and can help the body to fight some forms of inflammation.

else you can do: The brain needs "fuel" to do its work, and the body's fuel comes from the sugar *glucose*. You can protect yourself, therefore, by making sure that your brain has all the glucose it needs. This is not, however, a recommendation to jettison all other aspects of your diet and eat nothing but chocolate bars. In fact, most of the glucose your body needs doesn't come from sugary foods; most comes from the breakdown of carbohydrates, and so you get it from the grains, dairy products, fruits, and vegetables you eat. Thus, it might be a good idea to have a slice of bread and a glass of milk just before you take an exam or just before you walk into a particularly challenging class. These steps will help ensure that you're not caught by a glucose shortfall that could interfere with your brain's functioning.

In addition, be careful not to ingest *too much* sugar. If you eat a big candy bar just before your exam, you might produce an upward spike in your blood glucose followed by a sudden drop, and these abrupt changes can produce problems of their own.

Overall, though, it seems that food supplements tested so far offer no "fast track" toward better cognition. *Ginkgo* is helpful, but mostly for special populations. A high-carb snack may help, but it will be of little value if you're already adequately nourished. Thus, on all these grounds, the best path toward better cognition seems for now to be the one that common sense would already recommend—eating a balanced diet, getting a good night's sleep, and paying careful attention during your studies.

chapter summary

● The brain is divided into several different structures, but of particular importance for cognitive psychology is the forebrain. In the forebrain, each cerebral hemisphere is divided into the frontal lobe, parietal lobe, temporal lobe, and occipital lobe. In understanding these brain areas, one important source of evidence comes from studies of brain damage, enabling us to examine what sorts of symptoms result from lesions in specific brain locations. This has allowed a localization of function, an effort that is also supported by neuroimaging research, which shows that the pattern of activation in the brain depends on the particular task being performed.

● Different parts of the brain perform different jobs; but for virtually any mental process, different brain areas must work together in a closely integrated fashion. When this integration is lost (as it is, for example, in Capgras syndrome), bizarre symptoms can result.

● The primary motor projection areas are the departure points in the brain for nerve cells that initiate muscle movement. The primary sensory projection areas are the main points of arrival in the brain for information from the eyes, ears, and other sense organs. These projection areas generally show a pattern of contralateral control, with tissue in the left hemisphere sending or receiving its main signals from the right side of the body, and vice versa. Each projection area provides a map of the environment or the relevant body part, but the assignment of space in this map is governed by function, not by anatomical proportions.

● Most of the forebrain's cortex has traditionally been referred to as the association cortex, but this area is itself subdivided into specialized regions. This subdivision is reflected in the varying consequences of brain damage, with lesions in the occipital lobes leading to visual agnosia, damage in the temporal lobes leading to aphasia, and so on. Damage to the prefrontal area causes many different problems, but these are generally problems in the forming and implementing of strategies.

● The brain's functioning depends on neurons and glia. The glia perform many functions, but the main flow of information is carried by the neurons. Communication from one end of the neuron to the other is electrical and is governed by the flow of ions in and out of the cell. Communication from one neuron to the next is generally chemical, with a neuron releasing neurotransmitters that affect neurons on the other side of the synapse.

Online Demonstrations & Essays

Online Demonstrations:
● Demonstration 2.1: Brain Anatomy
● Demonstration 2.2: "Acuity" in the Somatosensory System
● Demonstration 2.3: The Speed of Neural Transmission

Online Applying Cognitive Psychology Essays:
● Cognitive Psychology and Education: The So-Called "Smart Pills"
● Cognitive Psychology and the Law: Detecting Lies

ZAPS 2.0 Cognition Labs

● Go to **http://digital.wwnorton.com/cognition6** for the online labs relevant to this chapter.

Learning about the World around Us

I n setting after setting, you rely on your knowledge and beliefs, but where does this knowledge come from? The answer, usually, is *experience*, but this point simply demands a further question: What is it that makes experience possible? Tackling this issue will force us to examine mental processes that turn out to be surprisingly complex.

In Chapter 3, we'll ask how visual perception operates—and thus how you manage to perceive the world around you. We'll start with events in the eye and then move to how you organize and interpret the visual information you receive. We'll also consider the ways in which you can *mis*interpret this information, so that you're vulnerable to illusions.

Chapter 4 takes a further step and asks how you manage to recognize and categorize the objects that you see. We'll start with a simple case: how you recognize printed letters. We'll then turn to the recognition of more complex (three-dimensional) objects.

In these chapters, we'll discuss the active role that you play in shaping your experience. We'll see, for example, that your perceptual apparatus doesn't just "pick up" the information that's available to you. You don't, in other words, just open your eyes and let the information "flow in." Instead, we'll discuss the ways in which you supplement and interpret the information you receive. In Chapter 3, we'll see that this activity begins very early in the sequence of biological events that support visual perception. In Chapter 4, these ideas will lead us to a mechanism made up of very simple components, but nonetheless shaped by a broad pattern of knowledge.

Chapter 5 then turns to the study of attention. As we'll see, paying attention is a complex achievement involving many elements. We'll discuss how the mechanisms of attention can sometimes limit what people achieve, and so part of what's at stake in Chapter 5 is the question of what people ultimately can or cannot accomplish, and whether there may be ways to escape these apparent limits on human performance.

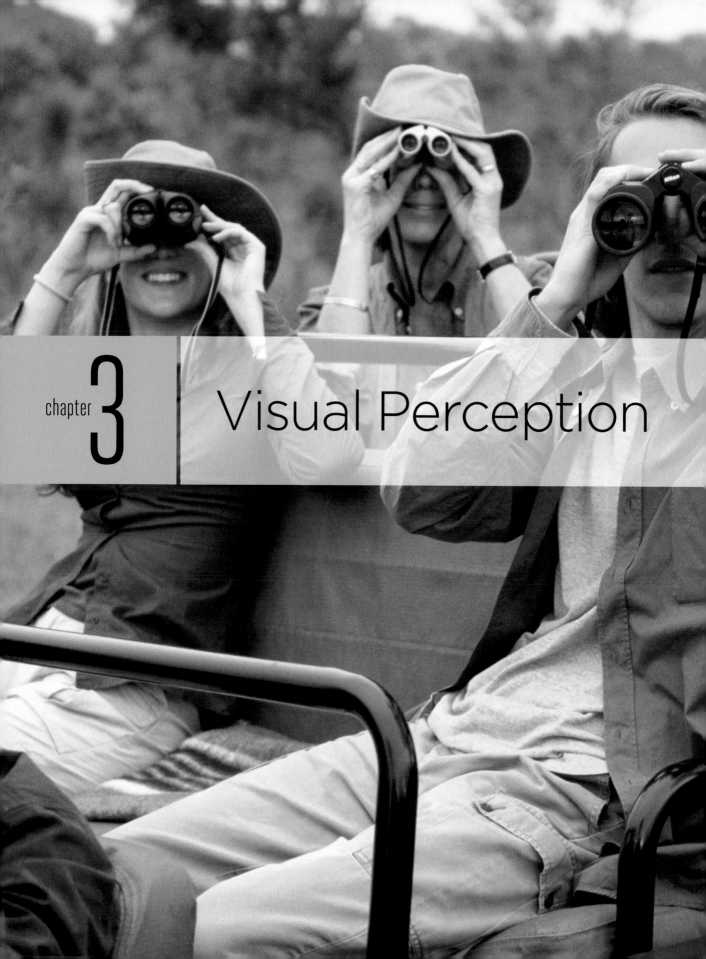

chapter **3** | Visual Perception

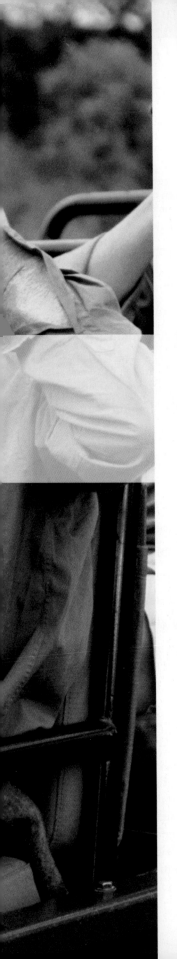

what if... You look around the world and you instantly, effortlessly, recognize the objects that surround you—words on this page, objects in the room in which you're sitting, things you can view out the window. Perception, in other words, seems fast, easy, and automatic. But even so, there is complexity here, and your ability to perceive the world depends on many separate and individually complicated processes.

Consider, for example, the case of *akinetopsia* (Zeki, 1991). This condition is rare, and much of what we know comes from a single patient—L.M.—who developed this disorder (because of a blood clot in her brain) at age 43. L.M. was completely unable to perceive motion—even though other aspects of her vision (e.g., her ability to recognize objects, to see color, or to discern detail in a visual pattern) seemed normal.

Because of her akinetopsia, L.M. can detect that an object *now* is in a position different from its position a moment ago, but she reports seeing "nothing in between." As a way of capturing this experience, consider a rough analogy in which you're looking at really slow movement. If, for example, you stare at the hour hand on a clock as it creeps around the clock face, you cannot discern its motion. But you can easily see the hand is now pointing, say, at the 4, and if you come back a while later, you can see that it's now at a position closer to the 5. Thus, you can *infer* motion from the change in position, but you cannot at all *perceive* the motion. This is your experience with very slow movement; someone with akinetopsia has the same experience with *all* movement.

What's it like to have this disorder? L.M. complained, as one concern, that it was hard to cross the street because she couldn't tell which of the cars in view were moving and which were parked. (She eventually learned to estimate the position and movement of traffic by listening to cars' *sounds* as they approached, even though she couldn't see their movement.)

Other problems caused by akinetopsia are more surprising. For example, L.M. complained about difficulties in following conversations, because she was essentially blind to the speaker's lip movement

* We explore vision—humans' dominant sensory modality. We discuss the mechanisms through which the visual system detects patterns in the incoming light, but we also showcase the *activity* of the visual system, in interpreting and shaping the incoming information, so that, in many ways, the visual system goes "beyond the information given" in the input itself.

* We also highlight the ways in which perception of one aspect of the input is shaped by perception of other aspects—so that the detection of simple features depends on how the overall form is organized, and the perception of size is shaped by the perceived distance of the target object.

* We emphasize that the interpretation of the visual input is usually accurate—but the same mechanisms can lead to illusions, and the study of those illusions can often illuminate the processes through which perception functions.

or changing facial expressions. She also felt insecure in some social settings: If more than two people were moving around in a room, she felt anxious because "people were suddenly here or there, but [she had] not seen them moving" (Zihl, von Cramon, & Mai, 1983, p. 315). Or, as a different example: She had trouble in everyday activities like pouring a cup of coffee; she couldn't see the fluid level's gradual rise as she poured, and so she didn't know when to stop pouring. For her, "the fluid appeared to be frozen, like a glacier" (Zihl et al., 1983, p. 315; also Schenk, Ellison, Rice, & Milner, 2005).

We will have more to say about cases of disordered perception later in the chapter. For now, though, let's note the specificity of this disorder—a disruption of movement perception, with other aspects of perception still intact. Let's also highlight the perhaps obvious but deeply important point that each of us is, in countless ways, dependent on our perceptual contact with the world. That point demands that we ask: What makes this perception possible?

The Visual System

You receive information about the world through various sensory modalities: You hear the sound of the approaching train, you smell the chocolate cake almost ready to come out of the oven, you feel the tap on your shoulder. There's no question, though, that for humans vision is the dominant sense. This is reflected in how much brain area is devoted to *vision* compared to any of the other senses. It's also reflected in many aspects of our behavior. For example, if visual information conflicts with information received from other senses, you usually place your trust in vision. This is the basis for ventriloquism, in which you see the dummy's mouth moving while the sounds themselves are coming from the dummy's master. Vision wins out in this contest, and so you experience the illusion that the voice is coming from the dummy.

The Photoreceptors

How does vision operate? The process begins, of course, with light. Light is produced by many objects in our surroundings—the sun, lamps, candles—and this light then reflects off most other objects. In most cases, it's this reflected light—reflected from this book page or from a friend's face—that launches the processes of visual perception. Some of this light hits the front surface of the eyeball, passes through the **cornea** and the **lens**, and then hits the **retina**, the light-sensitive tissue that lines the back of the eyeball (see **Figure 3.1**).

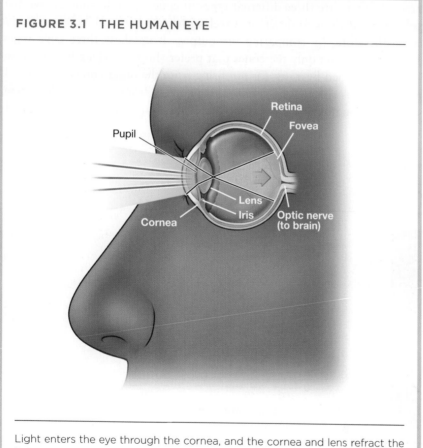

FIGURE 3.1 THE HUMAN EYE

Light enters the eye through the cornea, and the cornea and lens refract the light rays to produce a sharply focused image on the retina. The iris can open or close to control the amount of light that reaches the retina. The retina is made up of three main layers: the rods and cones, which are the photoreceptors; the bipolar cells; and the ganglion cells, whose axons make up the optic nerve.

The cornea and lens focus the incoming light, just as a camera lens might, so that a sharp image is cast onto the retina. Adjustments in this process are made possible by the fact that the lens is surrounded by a band of muscle. When the muscle tightens, the lens bulges somewhat, creating the proper shape for focusing images cast by nearby objects; when the muscle relaxes, the lens returns to a flatter shape, allowing the proper focus for objects farther away.

On the retina, there are two types of **photoreceptors**—specialized neural cells that respond directly to the incoming light (see **Figure 3.2**). One type, the **rods**, are sensitive to very low levels of light and so play an essential role whenever you're moving around in semidarkness or trying to view a fairly dim stimulus. But the rods are also color-blind: They can distinguish different intensities of light (and so contribute to your perception of brightness), but they provide no means of discriminating one hue from another.

Cones, in contrast, are less sensitive than rods and so need more incoming light to operate at all. But cones are sensitive to color differences. More precisely, there are three different types of cones, each having its own pattern of sensitivities to different wavelengths (see **Figure 3.3**). You perceive color, therefore, by comparing the outputs from these three cone types. Strong firing from only the cones that prefer short wavelengths, for example, accompanied by weak (or no) firing from the other cone types, signals purple. Blue is signaled by equally strong firing from the cones that prefer short wavelengths and those that prefer medium wavelengths, with only

FIGURE 3.2 RODS AND CONES

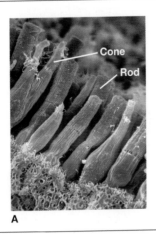

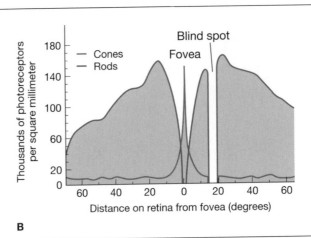

A   B

(Panel A) Rods and cones are the light-sensitive cells at the back of the retina that launch the neural process of vision. In this (colorized) photo, cones appear green; rods appear brown. (Panel B) Distribution of photoreceptors. Cones are most frequent at the fovea, and the number of cones drops off sharply as we move away from the fovea. In contrast, there are no rods at all on the fovea. There are neither rods nor cones at the retina's blind spot.

modest firing by cones that prefer long wavelengths. And so on, with other patterns of firing, across the three cone types, corresponding to different perceived hues.

Cones have another crucial function: They enable you to discern fine detail. The ability to see detail is referred to as **acuity,** and acuity is much higher for the cones than it is for the rods. This explains why you point our eyes toward a target whenever you wish to perceive it in detail. What you are

FIGURE 3.3   WAVELENGTHS OF LIGHT

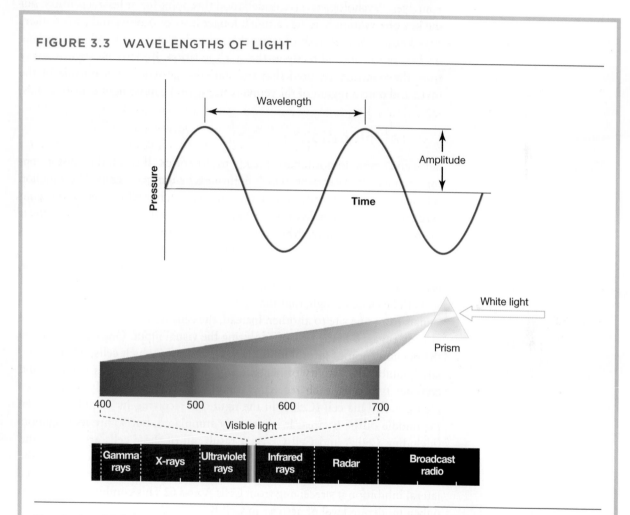

The physics of light are complex, but for many purposes light can be thought of as a wave, and the shape of the wave can be described in terms of its amplitude and its wavelength (i.e., the distance from "crest" to "crest"). The wavelengths our visual system can sense are only a tiny part of the broader electromagnetic spectrum. Light with a wavelength longer than 750 nanometers is invisible to us, although we do feel these longer infrared waves as heat. Ultraviolet light, which has a wavelength shorter than 360 nanometers, is also invisible to us. That leaves the narrow band of wavelengths between 750 and 360 nanometers—the so-called visible spectrum. Within this spectrum, we usually see wavelengths close to 400 nanometers as violet, those close to 700 nanometers as red, and those in between as the rest of the colors in the rainbow.

actually doing is positioning your eyes so that the image of the target falls onto the **fovea**, the very center of the retina. Here, cones far outnumber rods (and, in fact, the center of the fovea has no rods at all). As a result, this is the region of the retina with the greatest acuity.

In portions of the retina more distant from the fovea (i.e., portions of the retina in the so-called visual periphery), the rods predominate; well out into the periphery, there are no cones at all. This distribution of photoreceptors explains why you're better able to see very dim lights out of the corner of your eyes. Psychologists have understood this point for at least a century, but the key observation here has a much longer history: Sailors and astronomers have known for hundreds of years that when looking at a barely visible star, it's best not to look directly at the star's location. By looking slightly away from the star, they ensured that the star's image would fall outside of the fovea and onto a region of the retina dense with the more light-sensitive rods.

Lateral Inhibition

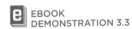
EBOOK
DEMONSTRATIONS
3.1 AND 3.2

EBOOK
DEMONSTRATION 3.3

Rods and cones do not report directly to the cortex. Instead, the photoreceptors stimulate **bipolar cells**, which in turn excite **ganglion cells**. The ganglion cells are spread uniformly across the entire retina, but all of their axons converge to form the bundle of nerve fibers that we call the **optic nerve**; this is the nerve tract that leaves the eyeball and carries information to various sites in the brain. This information is sent first to an important way station in the thalamus called the **lateral geniculate nucleus (LGN)**; from there, information is transmitted to the primary projection area for vision, in the occipital lobe.

Let's be clear, though, that the optic nerve is not just a cable that conducts signals from one site to another. Instead, the cells that link retina to brain are already engaged in the task of analyzing the visual input. One example lies in the phenomenon of **lateral inhibition**, a pattern in which cells, when stimulated, inhibit the activity of neighboring cells. To see why this is important, consider two cells, each receiving stimulation from a brightly lit area (see **Figure 3.4**). One cell (Cell B in the figure) is receiving its stimulation from the middle of the lit area. It is intensely stimulated, but so are its neighbors (including Cell A and Cell C). As a result, all of these cells are active, and therefore each one is trying to inhibit its neighbors. The upshot is that the activity level of Cell B is *increased* by the stimulation but *decreased* by the lateral inhibition it's receiving from Cells A and C. This combination leads to only a moderate level of activity in Cell B.

In contrast, another cell (Cell C in the figure) is receiving its stimulation from the edge of the lit area. It is intensely stimulated, and so are its neighbors *on one side*. Therefore, this cell will receive inhibition from one side but not from the other (in the figure: inhibition from Cell B but *not* from Cell D), and so it will be less inhibited than Cell B (which, you'll remember, is receiving inhibition from both sides). Thus, Cells B and C initially receive the same input, but C is less inhibited than B and so will end up firing more strongly than B.

FIGURE 3.4 LATERAL INHIBITION

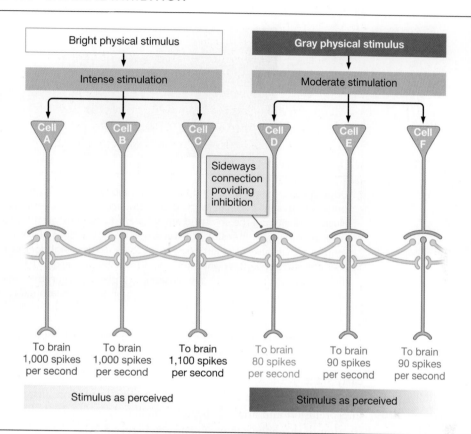

Cell B receives strong inhibition from all its neighbors, because its neighbors are intensely stimulated. Cell C, in contrast, receives inhibition only from one side (because its neighbor on the other side, Cell D, is only moderately stimulated). As a result, Cells B and C start with the same input, but Cell C, receiving less inhibition, sends a stronger signal to the brain, emphasizing the edge in the stimulus. The same logic applies to Cells D and E, and it explains why Cell D sends a weaker signal to the brain. Note, by the way, that the spikes per second numbers are hypothetical and are intended only to illustrate lateral inhibition's effects.

Notice, then, that the pattern of lateral inhibition highlights a surface's edges, because the response of cells detecting the edge of the surface (such as Cell C) will be stronger than that of cells detecting the middle of the surface (such as Cell B). For that matter, by *increasing* the response by Cell C and *decreasing* the response by Cell D, lateral inhibition actually exaggerates the contrast at the edge—a process called **edge enhancement**. This process is of enormous importance, because it's obviously highlighting the information that defines an object's shape—information crucial for figuring out what the object *is*. And let's emphasize that this edge enhancement occurs at a very

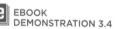
EBOOK
DEMONSTRATION 3.4

FIGURE 3.5 MACH BANDS

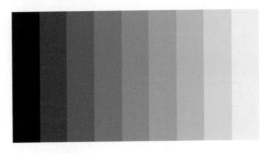

Edge enhancement, produced by lateral inhibition, helps us to perceive the outline that defines an object's shape. But the same process can produce illusions—including the so-called Mach bands. Each vertical strip in this figure is of uniform light intensity, but the strips do not appear uniform. For each strip, contrast makes the left edge (next to its darker neighbor) look brighter than the rest, while the right edge (next to its lighter neighbor) looks darker. To see that the differences are illusions, try placing some thin object (such as a toothpick or a straightened paper clip) on top of the boundary between strips. With the strips separated in this manner, the illusion disappears.

early stage of the visual processing. In other words, the information sent to the brain isn't a mere copy of the incoming stimulation; instead, the steps of interpretation and analysis begin immediately, in the eyeball. (For a demonstration of this edge enhancement, see **Figure 3.5**.)

Single Neurons and Single-Cell Recording

Part of what we know about the visual system—indeed, part of what we know about the entire brain—comes from a technique called **single-cell recording**. As the name implies, this is a procedure through which investigators can record, moment by moment, the pattern of electrical changes within a single neuron.

We mentioned in Chapter 2 that when a neuron fires, each response is the same size; this is, again, the *all-or-none law*. However, neurons can, we've said, vary in *how often* they fire, and when investigators record the activity of a single neuron, what they're usually interested in is the cell's firing rate, measured in "spikes per second." The investigator can then vary the circumstances (either in the external world or elsewhere in the nervous system) in order to learn what makes the cell fire more and what makes it fire less. In this way, we can figure out what job the neuron does within the broad context of the entire nervous system.

The technique of single-cell recording has been used with enormous success in the study of vision. In a typical procedure, the animal being studied is first immobilized. Then, electrodes are placed just outside a neuron in the animal's optic nerve or brain. Next, a computer screen is placed in front of the animal's eyes, and various patterns are flashed on the screen: circles, lines at various angles, or squares of various sizes at various positions. Researchers can then ask: Which patterns cause that neuron to fire? To what visual inputs does that cell respond?

By analogy, we know that a smoke detector is a smoke detector because it "fires" (makes noise) when smoke is on the scene. We know that a motion detector is a motion detector because it "fires" when something moves nearby. But what kind of detector is a given neuron? Is it responsive to any light in any position within the field of view? In that case, we might call it a "light detector." Or is it perhaps responsive only to certain shapes at certain positions (and therefore is a "shape detector")? With this logic, we can map out precisely what it is that the cell responds to—what kind of detector it is. More formally, this procedure allows us to define the cell's **receptive field**—that is, the size and shape of the area in the visual world to which that cell responds.

Multiple Types of Receptive Fields

The neurophysiologists David Hubel and Torsten Wiesel were awarded the Nobel Prize for their exploration of the mammalian visual system (e.g., Hubel & Wiesel, 1959, 1968). They documented the existence of specialized neurons within the brain, each of which has a different type of receptive field, a different kind of visual trigger. For example, some neurons seem to function as "dot detectors." These cells fire at their maximum rate when light is presented in a small, roughly circular area, in a specific position within the field of view. Presentations of light just outside of this area cause the cell to fire at *less* than its usual "resting" rate, so the input must be precisely positioned to make this cell fire. **Figure 3.6** depicts such a receptive field.

These cells are often called **center-surround cells**, to mark the fact that light presented to the central region of the receptive field has one influence, while light presented to the surrounding ring has the opposite influence. If both the center and the surround are strongly stimulated, the cell will fire neither more nor less than usual; for this cell, a strong uniform stimulus is equivalent to no stimulus at all.

Other cells fire at their maximum only when a stimulus containing an edge of just the right orientation appears within their receptive fields. These cells, therefore, can be thought of as "edge detectors." Some of these cells fire at their maximum rate when a horizontal edge is presented; others, when a vertical edge is in view; still others fire at their maximum to orientations in between horizontal and vertical. Note, though, that in each case, these orientations merely define the cells' "preference," because these cells are not oblivious to edges of other orientations. If a cell's preference is for, say, horizontal edges, then the cell will still respond to other orientations but will respond less strongly than it does for horizontals. Specifically, the further the edge is

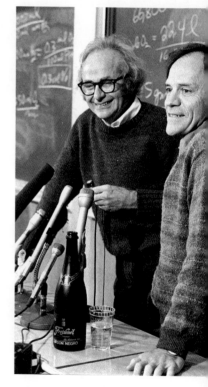

TORSTEN WIESEL AND DAVID HUBEL

Much of what we know about the visual system derives from the pioneering work done by David Hubel and Torsten Wiesel. This pair of researchers won the 1981 Nobel Prize for their discoveries. (The Nobel Prize was shared with Roger Sperry for his independent research on the cerebral hemispheres.)

FIGURE 3.6   CENTER-SURROUND CELLS

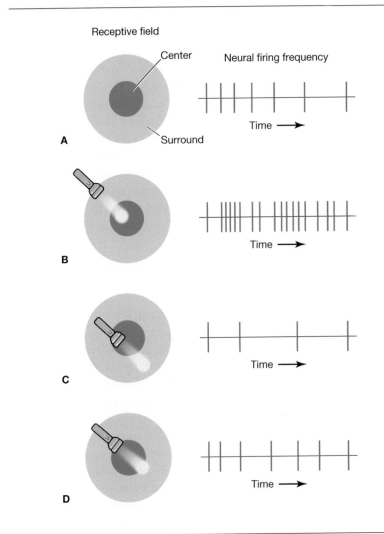

Stimuli are presented to various regions of the retina. The data show that different cells have different patterns of responding. For example, Panels A through D show the firing frequency of a particular ganglion cell. (A) This graph shows the baseline firing rate when no stimulus is presented. (B) The cell's firing rate goes up when a stimulus is presented in the middle of the cell's receptive field. (C) In contrast, the cell's firing rate goes down if a stimulus is presented at the edge of the cell's receptive field. (D) If a stimulus is presented both to the center of the receptive field and to the edge, the cell's firing rate does not change from its baseline level. Cells with this pattern of responding are called "center-surround" cells, to highlight their opposite responses to stimulation in the center of the receptive field and the surrounding region.

FIGURE 3.7 ORIENTATION-SPECIFIC VISUAL FIELDS

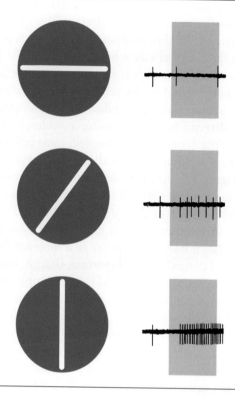

Some cells in the visual system fire only when the input contains a line segment at the proper orientation. For example, one cell might fire very little in response to a horizontal line, fire only occasionally in response to a diagonal, and fire at its maximum rate only when a vertical line is present. In this figure, the circles show the stimulus that was presented. The right side shows records of neural firing. Each vertical stroke represents a firing by the cell; the left–right position reflects the passage of time.   AFTER HUBEL, 1963.

from the cell's preferred orientation, the weaker the firing will be, and edges sharply different from the cell's preferred orientation (say, a vertical edge for a cell that prefers horizontal) will elicit virtually no response (see **Figure 3.7**).

Other cells, elsewhere in the visual cortex, have receptive fields that are more specific. Some cells fire maximally only if an angle of a particular size appears in their receptive fields; others fire maximally in response to corners and notches. Still other cells appear to be "movement detectors" and fire strongly if a stimulus moves, say, from right to left across the cell's receptive field. Other cells favor left-to-right movement, and so on through the various possible directions of movement.

Parallel Processing in the Visual System

This proliferation of cell types highlights another important principle for us—namely, that the visual system relies on a "divide and conquer" strategy, with different types of cells, located in different areas of the cortex, each specializing in a particular kind of analysis. This pattern is plainly evident in **Area V1**, the site on the occipital lobe where axons from the LGN first reach the cortex (see **Figure 3.8**). In this brain area, some cells fire to (say) horizontals in *this* position in the visual world, others to horizontals in *that* position, others to verticals in specific positions, and so on. The full ensemble of cells in this area provides a detector for every possible stimulus, making certain that no matter what the input is or where it's located, some cell will respond to it.

The pattern of specialization becomes all the more evident as we consider other brain areas. **Figure 3.9**, for example, reflects one summary of the brain areas known to be involved in vision. The details of the figure aren't crucial, but it is noteworthy that some of these areas (V1, V2, V3, V4, PO, and MT) are in the occipital cortex; other areas are in the parietal cortex; others are in the temporal cortex (we'll have more to say in a moment about these areas outside of the occipital cortex). Most important, though, each area seems to have its own function. Neurons in Area MT, for example, are acutely sensitive to direction and speed of movement. (This area is the brain region that has suffered damage in cases involving akinetopsia.) Cells in Area V4 fire most strongly when the input is of a certain color and a certain shape.

Let's also emphasize that all of these specialized areas are active at the same time, so that (for example) cells in Area MT are detecting movement in the visual input at the same time that cells in Area V4 are detecting shapes. In other words, the visual system relies on **parallel processing**—a system in which many different steps (in this case, different kinds of analysis) are going on simultaneously. (Parallel processing is usually contrasted with **serial processing**, in which steps are carried out one at a time—i.e., in a series.)

One advantage of this simultaneous processing is speed: Brain areas trying to discern the shape of the incoming stimulus don't need to wait until the motion analysis or the color analysis is complete. Instead, all of the analyses go forward immediately when the input appears before your eyes, with no waiting time.

Another advantage of parallel processing is the possibility of mutual influence among multiple systems. To see why this is important, consider the fact that sometimes your interpretation of an object's motion depends on your understanding of the object's three-dimensional shape. This suggests that it might be best if the perception of shape happened first. That way, you could use the results of this processing step as a guide to later analyses. In other cases, though, it turns out that the relationship between shape and motion is reversed: In these cases, your interpretation of an object's three-dimensional shape depends on your understanding of its motion. To allow for this possibility, it might be best if the perception of motion happened first, so that it could guide the subsequent analysis of shape.

FIGURE 3.8   AREA V1 IN THE HUMAN BRAIN

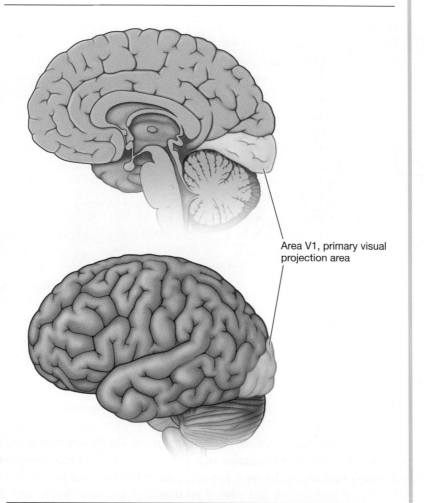

Area V1, primary visual
projection area

Area V1 is the site on the occipital lobe where axons from the LGN first reach
the cortex. The top panel shows the brain as if sliced vertically down the middle, revealing the "inside" surface of the brain's right hemisphere; the bottom
panel shows the left hemisphere of the brain viewed from the side. As the two
panels show, most of Area V1 is located on the cortical surface *between* the
two cerebral hemispheres.

How does the brain deal with these contradictory demands? Parallel
processing provides the answer: Since both sorts of analysis go on simultaneously,
each type of analysis can be informed by the other. Put differently, neither
the shape-analyzing system nor the motion-analyzing system gets priority.
Instead, the two systems work concurrently and "negotiate" a solution that
satisfies both systems (Van Essen & DeYoe, 1995).

FIGURE 3.9 THE VISUAL PROCESSING PATHWAYS

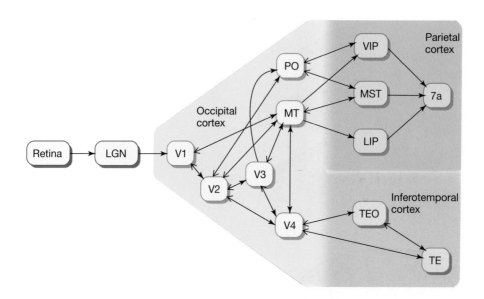

Each box in this figure refers to a specific location within the visual system. Notice that vision depends on many brain sites, each performing a specialized type of analysis. Note also that the flow of information is complex, so there's no strict sequence of "this step" of analysis followed by "that step." Instead, everything happens at once, with a great deal of back-and-forth communication among the various elements.

Parallel processing is easy to document throughout the visual system. As we have seen, the retina contains two types of specialized receptors (rods and cones) each doing its own job (e.g., the rods detecting stimuli in the periphery of your vision and stimuli presented at low light levels, and the cones detecting hues and detail at the center of your vision). Both types of receptors function at the same time—another case of parallel processing.

Likewise, within the optic nerve itself, there are two types of cells, **P cells** and **M cells.** The P cells provide the main input for the LGN's **parvocellular cells** and appear to be specialized for spatial analysis and the detailed analysis of form. M cells provide the input for the LGN's **magnocellular cells** and are specialized for the detection of motion and the perception of depth.[1] And, again, both of these systems are functioning at the same time—more parallel processing.

1. A quick note on terminology: The names here refer to the relative sizes of the relevant cells: *parvo* derives from the Latin word for "small," and *magno* from the word for "large." To remember the function of these two types of cells, many students find it useful to think of the P cells as specialized roughly for the perception of *pattern* and M cells as specialized for the perception of *motion.* These descriptions are crude, but they're easy to remember.

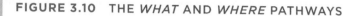

FIGURE 3.10   THE *WHAT* AND *WHERE* PATHWAYS

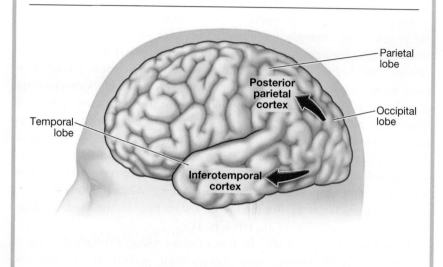

Information from the primary visual cortex at the back of the head is transmitted to the inferotemporal cortex (the so-called *what* system) and to the posterior parietal cortex (the *where* system). The term "inferotemporal" refers to the lower part of the temporal lobe. The term "posterior parietal cortex" refers to the rearmost portion of this cortex.

Parallel processing remains in evidence when we move beyond the occipital cortex. As **Figure 3.10** indicates, some of the activation from the occipital lobe is passed along to the cortex of the temporal lobe. This pathway, often called the **what system**, plays a major role in the identification of visual objects, telling you whether the object is a cat, an apple, or whatever. At the same time, activation from the occipital lobe is also passed along a second pathway, leading to the parietal cortex, in what is often called the **where system**. This system seems to perform the function of guiding your action, based on your perception of where an object is located—above or below you, to your right or to your left (Goodale & Milner, 2004; Humphreys & Riddoch, 2014; Ungerleider & Haxby, 1994; Ungerleider & Mishkin, 1982; for some complications, though, see Borst, Thompson, & Kosslyn, 2011; de Haan & Cowey, 2011).

The contrasting roles of these two systems can be revealed in many ways, including studies of brain damage. Patients with lesions in the *what* system show visual agnosia—an inability to recognize visually presented objects, including such common things as a cup or a pencil. However, these patients show little disorder in recognizing visual orientation or in reaching. The reverse pattern is observed with patients who have suffered lesions in the *where* system: They have difficulty in reaching, but no problem in object identification (Damasio, Tranel, & Damasio, 1989; Farah, 1990; Goodale, 1995; Newcombe, Ratcliff, & Damasio, 1987).

Still other data echo this broad theme of parallel processing among separate systems. For example, we noted earlier that different brain areas are critical for the perception of color, motion, and form. If this is right, then someone who has suffered damage in just one of these areas should show problems in the perception of color but not the perception of motion or form, or problems in the perception of motion but not the perception of form or color. These predictions are correct: As we mentioned at the chapter's start, some patients suffer damage to the motion system and so develop akinetopsia (Zihl, Von Cramon, & Mai, 1983). For such patients, the world is described as a succession of static photographs. They're unable to report the speed or direction of a moving object; as one patient put it, "When I'm looking at the car first, it seems far away. But then when I want to cross the road, suddenly the car is very near" (Zihl et al., 1983, p. 315).

Other patients suffer a specific loss of color vision through damage to the central nervous system, even though their perception of form and motion remains normal (Damasio, 1985; Gazzaniga, Ivry, & Mangun, 2014; Meadows, 1974). To them, the entire world is clothed only in "dirty shades of gray."[2]

Cases like these provide dramatic confirmation of the separateness of our visual system's various elements and the ways in which the visual system is vulnerable to very specific forms of damage. (For further evidence with neurologically intact participants, see Bundesen, Kyllingsbaek, & Larsen, 2003.)

Putting the Pieces Back Together

Let's emphasize once again, therefore, that even the simplest of our intellectual achievements depends on an array of different, highly specialized brain areas all working together in parallel. This was evident in Chapter 2, in our consideration of Capgras syndrome, and the same pattern has emerged in our description of the visual system. Here, too, many brain areas must work together: the *what* system and the *where* system, areas specialized for the detection of movement and areas specialized for the identification of simple forms.

We have identified certain advantages that derive from this division of labor and the parallel processing it allows. But the division of labor also creates a problem: If multiple brain areas contribute to an overall task, how is their functioning coordinated? When you see a ballet dancer in a graceful leap, the leap itself is registered by motion-sensitive neurons, but the recognition of the ballet dancer depends on shape-sensitive neurons. How are the

---

2. This is different from ordinary color blindness, which is usually present from birth and results from abnormalities that are outside the brain itself—for example, abnormalities in the photoreceptors.

pieces put back together? When you reach for a coffee cup but stop midway because you see that the cup is empty, the reach itself is guided by the *where* system; the fact that the cup is empty is registered by the *what* system. How are these two streams of processing coordinated?

Investigators refer to this broad issue as the **binding problem**—the task of reuniting the various elements of a scene, elements that are initially addressed by different systems in different parts of the brain. And obviously this problem is solved: What you perceive is not an unordered catalogue of sensory elements. Instead, you perceive a coherent, integrated perceptual world. Apparently, then, this is a case in which the various pieces of Humpty Dumpty are reassembled to form an organized whole.

Visual Maps and Firing Synchrony

Look around you. Your visual system registers whiteness and blueness and brownness; it also registers a small cylindrical shape (your coffee cup), a medium-sized rectangle (this book page), and a much larger rectangle (your desk). How do you put these pieces together so that you see that it's the coffee cup, and not the book page, that's blue; the desktop, and not the cup, that's brown?

There is still debate about how the visual system solves this problem, but we can identify three elements that contribute to the solution. One element is *spatial position*. The part of the brain registering the cup's shape is separate from the parts registering its color or its motion; nonetheless, these various brain areas all have something in common: They each keep track of where the target is—where the cylindrical shape was located, and where the blueness was; where the motion was detected, and where things were still. Thus, the reassembling of these pieces can be done with reference to position. In essence, you can overlay the map of *which forms are where* on top of the map of *which colors are where* to get the right colors with the right forms, and likewise for the map showing *which motion patterns are where*.

Information about spatial position is of course important for its own sake: You have a compelling reason to care whether the tiger is close to you or far away, or whether the bus is on your side of the street or the other. But in addition, location information apparently provides a frame of reference used to solve the binding problem. Given this double function, we shouldn't be surprised that spatial position is a major organizing theme within all the various brain areas concerned with vision, with each area seeming to provide its own map of the visual world.

Spatial position, however, is not the whole story. Evidence also suggests that the brain uses a special *rhythm* to identify which sensory elements belong with which. Imagine two groups of neurons in the visual cortex. One group of neurons fires maximally whenever a vertical line is in view; another group fires maximally whenever a stimulus is in view moving from a high position to a low one. Let's also imagine that right now a vertical line is presented and it is moving downward; as a result, both groups of neurons are firing strongly.

How does the brain encode the fact that these attributes are bound together, different aspects of a single object? There is evidence that the visual system marks this fact by means of **neural synchrony:** If the neurons detecting a vertical line are firing in synchrony with those signaling movement, then these attributes are registered as belonging to the same object. If they are not in synchrony, the features are not bound together (Buzsáki & Draguhn, 2004; Csibra, Davis, Spratling, & Johnson, 2000; Elliott & Müller, 2000; Fries, Reynolds, Rorie, & Desimone, 2001).

What causes this synchrony? How do the neurons become synchronized in the first place? Here, another factor appears to be crucial: *attention.* We will have more to say about attention in Chapter 5, but for now let's just note that attention plays a key role in binding together the separate features of a stimulus. (For a classic statement of this argument, see Treisman & Gelade, 1980; Treisman, Sykes, & Gelade, 1977. For a more recent and more complex view, see Quinlan, 2003; Rensink, 2012; and also Chapter 5.)

Evidence for attention's role comes from many sources, including the fact that when we overload someone's attention, she is likely to make **conjunction errors**—correctly detecting the features present in a visual display, but making mistakes about how the features are bound together (or *conjoined*). Thus, someone shown a blue *H* and a red *T* might report seeing a blue *T* and a red *H*—an error in binding. Similarly, individuals who suffer from severe attention deficits (because of brain damage in the parietal cortex) are particularly impaired in tasks that require them to judge how features are conjoined to form complex objects (e.g., Robertson, Treisman, Friedman-Hill, & Grabowecky, 1997). Finally, studies suggest that synchronized neural firing is observed in an animal's brain when the animal is attending to a specific stimulus but is not observed in neurons activated by an unattended stimulus (e.g., Buschman & Miller, 2007; Saalman, Pigarev, & Vidyasagar, 2007; Womelsdorf et al., 2007). All of these results point toward the claim that attention is indeed crucial for the binding problem and, moreover, that attention is linked to the neural synchrony that seems to unite a stimulus's features.

Notice, then, that there are several ways in which information is represented in the brain. In Chapter 2, we noted that the brain uses different chemical signals (i.e., different types of neurotransmitters) to transmit different types of information. We now see that there is information reflected in *which* cells are firing, *how often* they are firing, whether the cells are firing in *synchrony* with other cells, and also, it turns out, the *rhythm* in which they are firing. Plainly, then, this is a system of considerable complexity!

Form Perception

So far in this chapter, we've been discussing how visual perception begins: with the detection of simple attributes in the stimulus—its color, its motion, and its catalogue of simple features. But this detection is just the *start* of

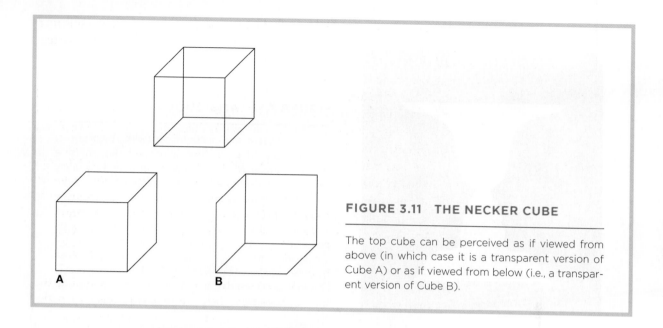

FIGURE 3.11 THE NECKER CUBE

The top cube can be perceived as if viewed from above (in which case it is a transparent version of Cube A) or as if viewed from below (i.e., a transparent version of Cube B).

the process. As one indication of further complexities, it turns out that our perception of the visual world is organized in ways that the stimulus input is not—a point documented early in the 20th century by a group called the "Gestalt psychologists."[3] The Gestaltists argued, therefore, that the organization must be contributed by the perceiver; this is why, they claimed, the perceptual whole is often different from the sum of its parts. Some years later, Jerome Bruner (1973) voiced related claims and coined the phrase "beyond the information given" to describe some of the ways that our perception of a stimulus differs from (and goes beyond) the stimulus itself.

For example, consider the form shown in the top of **Figure 3.11**: the **Necker cube**. This drawing is an example of a *reversible figure*—so-called because people routinely perceive it first one way and then another. Specifically, this form can be perceived as a drawing of a cube viewed from above (in which case it's similar to the cube marked "A" in the figure); it can also be perceived as a cube viewed from below (in which case it's similar to the cube marked "B"). Both perceptions fit perfectly well with the information received by your eyes, and so the drawing itself is fully compatible with either of these perceptions. Put differently, the lines on the page are entirely neutral with regard to the shape's configuration in depth; the lines on the page don't specify which is the "proper" interpretation. Your perception of the cube, however, is not neutral. Instead, you perceive the cube as having one configuration or the other—similar either to Cube A or to Cube B. Your perception,

---

3. *Gestalt* is the German word for "shape" or "form." The Gestalt psychology movement was, overall, committed to the view that our theories need to emphasize the organization of the entire shape, not just focus on the shape's parts.

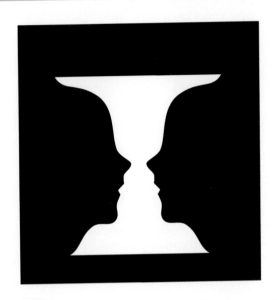

FIGURE 3.12   AMBIGUOUS FIGURES

Many stimuli that you encounter can (with a bit of effort) be reinterpreted. Little effort is needed, though, for a smaller number of stimuli, which easily and naturally lend themselves to reinterpretation. These figures are often called "reversible" or "bistable," because there are two prominent and stable interpretations of the figure. The vase/profiles figure, for example, is spontaneously perceived by many people to be a white vase (or candlestick) on a black background, but it is perceived by other people to be two black faces, shown in profile and looking at each other. (A similar bistable form, by the way, is visible in the Canadian flag!)

in other words, goes beyond the information given in the drawing, by specifying an arrangement in depth.

The same point can be made for many other stimuli. **Figure 3.12** (after Rubin, 1915, 1921) can be perceived either as a vase centered in the picture or as two profiles facing each other. The drawing by itself, it seems, is fully compatible with either of these perceptions, and so, once again, the drawing is neutral with regard to perceptual organization. In particular, it is neutral with regard to **figure/ground organization**, the determination of what is the figure (the depicted object, displayed against a background) and what is the ground. Your perception of this figure, however, isn't neutral about this point. Instead, your perception somehow specifies that you're looking at the vase and not at the profiles, or that you're looking at the profiles and not at the vase.

In these examples, then, your perception contains information—about how the form is arranged in depth, or about which part of the form is figure and which is ground—that is not contained within the stimulus itself. Apparently, then, this is information contributed by you, the perceiver.

The Gestalt Principles

With figures like the Necker cube or the vase-profiles, your role in shaping the perception seems obvious and undeniable. If you stare at either of these figures, your perception flips back and forth: First you see the figure one way, then another, then back to the first way. With these figures, though, the information that's actually reaching your eyes is constant; the exact geometry of the figure is the same, no matter how you perceive it. Any changes in perception, therefore, are caused by *you* and not by some change in the stimulus.

One might argue, though, that reversible figures are special—carefully designed to support multiple interpretations. On this basis, perhaps you play a smaller role when perceiving other, more "natural" stimuli.

This position is plausible—but wrong, because many stimuli (and not just the reversible figures) are ambiguous and in need of interpretation. We often don't detect this ambiguity, but that's because the interpretation is done so quickly that we don't notice it. Consider, for example, the scene shown in **Figure 3.13**. It's almost certain that you perceive segments B and E as being united, forming a complete apple, but notice that this information isn't provided by the stimulus; instead, it's your interpretation. (If we simply go with the information in the figure, it's possible that segments B and E are parts of entirely different fruits, with the "gap" between the two fruits hidden from view by the banana.) It's also likely that you perceive the banana as entirely banana-shaped and, thus, continuing downward out of your view into the bowl, where it eventually terminates with the sort of point that's normal for a banana. Similarly, surely

---

FIGURE 3.13 THE ROLE OF INTERPRETATION IN PERCEIVING AN ORDINARY SCENE

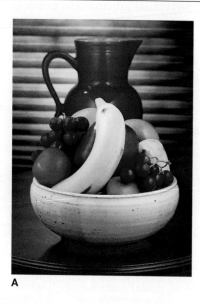

A

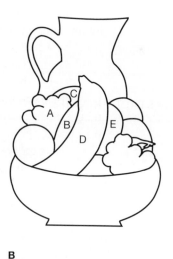

B

(A) The text emphasizes that perception must go "beyond the information given" in important ways. Most of the examples in the text involve simple line drawings, but the same points apply to real-life scenes. For example, consider the still life (B) and an overlay designating five different segments of the scene. For this picture to be perceived correctly, the perceptual system must first decide what goes with what—for example, that Segment B and Segment E are different bits of the same object (even though they are separated by Segment D) and that Segment B and Segment A are different objects (even though they are adjacent and the same color).

you perceive the horizontal stripes in the background as continuous and merely hidden from view by the pitcher. (You'd likely be surprised if we removed the pitcher and revealed a pitcher-shaped gap in the stripes.) But, of course, the stimulus doesn't in any way "guarantee" the banana's shape or the continuity of the stripes; these points are, again, just your interpretation.

Even with this ordinary scene, therefore, your perception goes "beyond the information given," and so the unity of the two apple slices and the continuity of the stripes is "in the eye of the beholder," not in the stimulus itself. Of course, you don't feel like you're "interpreting" this picture or extrapolating beyond what's on the page. But your role becomes clear the moment we start cataloguing the differences between your perception and the information that's truly present in the photograph.

Let's emphasize, though, that your interpretation of the stimulus isn't careless or capricious. Instead, you're guided by a few straightforward principles, and these were catalogued by the Gestalt psychologists many years ago. For example, your perception is guided by principles of *proximity* and *similarity*: If, within the visual scene, you see elements that are close to each other, or elements that resemble each other, you assume these elements are parts of the same object (**Figure 3.14**). You also tend to assume that contours are smooth, not jagged, and you avoid interpretations that involve coincidences.

These perceptual principles are—as we said—quite straightforward, but they're essential if your perceptual apparatus is going to make sense of the often ambiguous, often incomplete information provided by your senses. In addition, it's worth mentioning that everyone's perceptions are guided by the same principles, and that's why you generally perceive the world the

---

FIGURE 3.14   GESTALT PRINCIPLES OF ORGANIZATION

    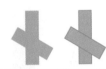

Similarity
We tend to group these dots into columns rather than rows, grouping dots of similar colors.

Proximity
We tend to perceive groups, linking dots that are close together.

Good continuation
We tend to see a continuous green bar rather than two smaller rectangles.

Closure
We tend to perceive an intact triangle, reflecting our bias toward perceiving closed figures rather than incomplete ones.

Simplicity
We tend to interpret a form in the simplest way possible. We would see the form on the left as two intersecting rectangles (as shown on the right) rather than as a single 12-sided irregular polygon.

As Figure 3.13 illustrated, your ordinary perception of the world requires that you make decisions about what goes with what—which elements are part of the same object, and which elements belong to different objects. Your decisions are guided by a few simple principles, catalogued many years ago by the Gestalt psychologists.

same way that other people do. Each of us imposes our own interpretation on the perceptual input, but we all tend to impose the *same* interpretation, because we're all governed by the same rules.

Organization and "Features"

We've now considered two broad topics—the detection of simple attributes in the stimulus, and then the ways in which you *organize* those attributes. In thinking about these topics, you might want to think about them as separate steps: First, you collect information about the stimulus, so that you know (for example) what corners or angle or curves are contained in the input. Then, once you've gathered the "raw data," you interpret this information, and that's when you "go beyond the information given"—deciding how the form is laid out in depth (as in Figure 3.11), deciding what is figure and what is ground (Figure 3.12), and so on.

The notion we're considering, then, is that perception can be divided (roughly) into an "information gathering" step followed by an "interpretation" step. Once again, though, this view is plausible, but certainly wrong. In fact, it's easy to show that in many settings, your interpretation of the input happens *before* you start cataloguing the input's basic features, not after. Consider, for example, **Figure 3.15**. Initially, these shapes seem to have no meaning, but after a moment most people discover the word hidden in the figure. That is, people find a way to reorganize the figure so that the familiar letters come into view. But let's be clear about what this means. At the start, the form seems not to contain the features needed to identify the *L*, the *I*, and

FIGURE 3.15   A HIDDEN FIGURE

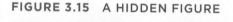

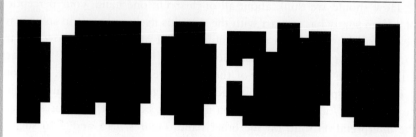

Initially, these dark shapes have no meaning, but after a moment the hidden figure becomes clearly visible. Notice, therefore, that at the start the figure seems not to contain the features needed to identify the various letters. Once the figure is reorganized, with the white parts (not the dark parts) making up the figure, the features are easily detected. Apparently, therefore, the analysis of features depends on a prior step, one in which the figure is first organized by the viewer.

FIGURE 3.16 MISSING FEATURES

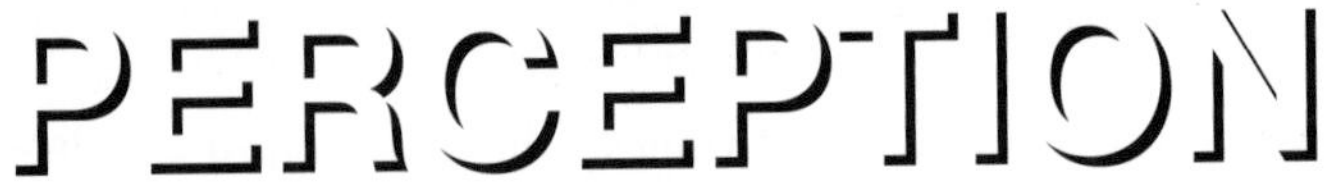

PERCEPTION

People have no trouble reading this word, despite the fact that most of the features needed for recognition are absent from the stimulus. People easily "supply" the missing features, emphasizing once again that the analysis of features depends on how the overall figure has been interpreted and organized.

so on. Once the form is reorganized, though, it does contain these features, and the letters are immediately recognized. In other words, with one organization, the features are absent; with another, they're plainly present. It would seem, then, that the features themselves depend on how the form is organized by the viewer, and so the features are as much "in the eye of the beholder" as they are in the figure itself.

As a different example, you have no difficulty reading the word printed in **Figure 3.16**, although most of the features needed for this recognition are absent from the figure. You easily "provide" the missing features, though, thanks to the fact that you interpret the black marks in the figure as shadows cast by solid letters. Given this interpretation and the extrapolation it entails, you can, with no trouble, "fill in" the missing features and in this way read the word.

How should we think about all of this? On one hand, your perception of a form surely has to start with the stimulus itself and must in some ways be governed by what's in that stimulus. (After all, no matter how you try to interpret Figure 3.16, it won't look to you like a photograph of Queen Elizabeth—the basic features of the queen are just not present, and your perception respects this obvious fact.) This suggests that the features must be in place *before* an interpretation is offered, because the features govern the interpretation. But, on the other hand, Figures 3.15 and 3.16 suggest that the opposite is the case: that the features you find in an input depend on how the figure is interpreted. Therefore, it's the interpretation, not the features, that must be first.

The solution to this puzzle, however, is easy, and it hinges on points we've already met: Many aspects of the brain's functioning depend on parallel processing, with different brain areas all doing their work at the same time. In addition, the various brain areas all influence one another, so that what's going on in one brain region is shaped by what's going on elsewhere. Thus, the brain areas that analyze a pattern's basic features do their work at the same time as the brain areas that analyze the pattern's large-scale configuration, and these brain areas interact, so that the perception of the features is guided by the configuration, and analysis of the configuration is guided by the features. In other words, neither type of processing "goes first." Neither has priority. Instead, they work together, with the result that the perception that is achieved makes sense at both the large-scale and fine-grained levels.

Constancy

We've now seen many indications of the perceiver's active role in "going beyond the information given" in the stimulus itself. This theme is also evident in another—and crucial—aspect of perception: namely, the achievement of **perceptual constancy**. This term refers to the fact that we perceive the constant properties of objects in the world (their sizes, shapes, and so on) even though the sensory information we receive about these attributes changes whenever our viewing circumstances change.

To illustrate this point, consider the perception of size. If you happen to be far away from the object you're viewing, then the image cast onto your retinas by that object will be relatively small. If you approach the object, then the image size will increase. This change in image size is a simple consequence of physics, but of course you're not fooled by this variation. Instead, you manage to achieve **size constancy**—correctly perceiving the sizes of objects in the world despite the changes in retinal-image size created by changes in viewing distance (see **Figure 3.17**).

Similarly, if you view a door straight on, the retinal image will be rectangular; but if you view the same door from an angle, the retinal image will have a different shape (see **Figure 3.18**). Still, you achieve **shape constancy**—that is, you correctly perceive the shapes of objects despite changes in the retinal image created by shifts in your viewing angle. You also achieve **brightness constancy**—you correctly perceive the brightness of objects whether they're illuminated by dim light or strong sun.

Unconscious Inference

How do you achieve each of these forms of constancy? One hypothesis focuses on relationships within the retinal image. In judging size, for example, you might be helped by the fact that you generally see objects against some background, providing a basis for comparison with the target object. Thus, the dog sitting nearby on the kitchen floor is half as tall as the chair and hides eight of the kitchen's floor tiles from view. If you take several steps back from the dog, none of these relationships changes, even though the sizes of all the retinal images are reduced (see **Figure 3.19** on p. 90). Size constancy, therefore, might be achieved by focusing not on the images themselves but on these unchanging relationships.

FIGURE 3.17 THE RELATIONSHIP BETWEEN IMAGE SIZE AND DISTANCE

Closer objects cast larger retinal images

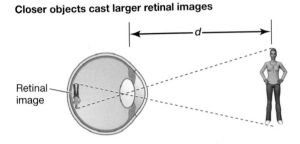

Retinal image

Farther objects cast smaller retinal images

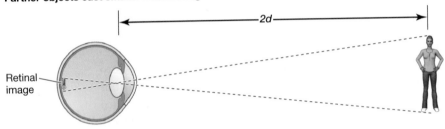

Retinal image

If you view an object from a greater distance, the object casts a smaller image on your retina. Nonetheless, you generally achieve size constancy—perceiving the object's actual size.

Relationships do contribute to size constancy, and that's why you are better able to judge size when comparison objects are in view or when the target you're judging sits on a surface that has a uniform visual texture (like the floor tiles in the example). But these relationships don't tell the whole story. Size constancy is found even when the visual scene offers no basis for comparison—if, for example, the object to be judged is the only object in view—provided that other cues signal the distance of the target object (Harvey & Leibowitz, 1967; Holway & Boring, 1947).

How does your visual system use this distance information? More than a century ago, the German physicist Hermann von Helmholtz developed an influential hypothesis regarding this question. Helmholtz started with the fact that there's a simple inverse relationship between distance and retinal image size: If an object doubles its distance from the viewer, the size of its image is reduced by half. If an object triples its distance, the size of its image is reduced to a third of its initial size (see Figure 3.17). This relationship is guaranteed to hold true because of the principles of optics, and the relationship makes it possible for perceivers to achieve size constancy by means of a

FIGURE 3.18 SHAPE CONSTANCY

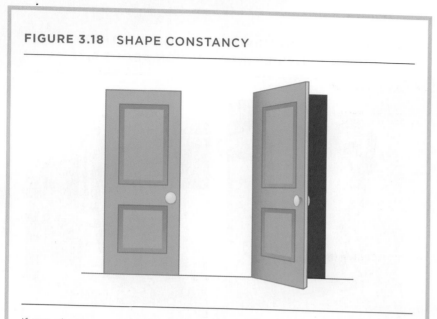

If you change your viewing angle, the shape of the retinal image cast by a target changes—and so the door viewed straight on casts a rectangular image on your retina; the door viewed from an angle casts a trapezoidal image. Nonetheless, you generally achieve shape constancy.

simple calculation. Of course, Helmholtz knew that we don't run through a conscious calculation every time we perceive an object's size; but he believed we were calculating nonetheless—and so he referred to the process as an **unconscious inference** (Helmholtz, 1909).

What is the calculation that enables someone to perceive size correctly? It's simply multiplication: the size of the image on the retina, multiplied by the distance between you and the object. (We'll have more to say about how you know this distance in a later section.) Thus, imagine an object that, at a distance of 10 feet, casts an image on the retina that's 4 millimeters across. Because of straightforward principles of optics, the same object, at a distance of 20 feet, casts an image of 2 millimeters. In both cases, the product—10×4 or 20×2—is the same. If, therefore, your size estimate depends on that product, your size estimate won't be thrown off by viewing distance—and of course, that's exactly what we want.

What's the evidence that size constancy does depend on this sort of inference? In many experiments, researchers have shown participants an object and, without changing the object's retinal image, have changed the apparent distance of the object. (There are many ways to do this—lenses that change how the eye has to focus to bring the object into sharp view, or mirrors that change how the two eyes have to angle inward so that the object's image is centered on both foveas.) If people are—as Helmholtz proposed—using

FIGURE 3.19 AN INVARIANT RELATIONSHIP THAT PROVIDES INFORMATION ABOUT SIZE

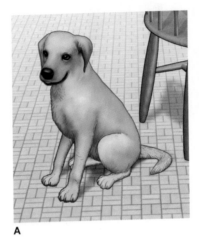
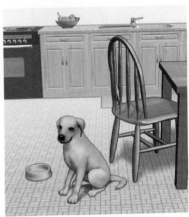

A

B

One proposal is that you achieve size constancy by focusing on *relationships* in the visual scene. Thus, the dog sitting nearby on the kitchen floor (Panel A) is half as tall as the chair and hides eight of the kitchen's floor tiles from view. If you take several steps back from the dog (Panel B), none of these relationships changes, even though the sizes of all the retinal images are reduced.

distance information to judge size, then these manipulations should affect size perception. Any manipulation that makes an object seem farther away (without changing retinal image size) should make that object seem bigger (because, in essence, the perceiver would be "multiplying" by a larger number). Any manipulation that makes the object seem closer should make it look smaller. And, in fact, these predictions are correct—a powerful confirmation that people do use distance to judge size.

A similar proposal explains how people achieve shape constancy. Here, you take the slant of the surface into account and make appropriate adjustments—again, an unconscious inference—in your interpretation of the retinal image's shape. Likewise for brightness constancy: Perceivers are sensitive to how a surface is oriented relative to the available light sources, and they take this information into account in estimating how much light is reaching the surface. Then, they use this assessment of lighting to judge the surface's brightness (e.g., whether it's black or gray or white). In all these cases, therefore, it appears that the perceptual system does draw some sort of unconscious inference, taking viewing circumstances into account in a way that enables you to perceive the constant properties of the visual world.

Illusions

This process of taking information into account—whether it's distance (in order to judge size), viewing angle (to judge shape), or illumination (to judge brightness)—is crucial for achieving constancy. More than that, it's another indication that you don't just "receive" visual information; instead, you *interpret* it. The interpretation is an essential part of your perception and generally helps you perceive the world correctly.

The role of the interpretation becomes especially clear, however, in circumstances in which you *misinterpret* the information available to you and end up misperceiving the world. Consider the two tabletops shown in **Figure 3.20**. The table on the left looks appreciably longer and thinner than the one on the right; a tablecloth that fits one table surely won't fit the other. Objectively, though, the parallelogram depicting the left tabletop is exactly the same shape as the one depicting the right tabletop. If you were to cut out the left tabletop, rotate it, and slide it onto the right tabletop, they'd be an exact match. (Not convinced? Just lay another piece of paper on top of the page, trace the left tabletop, and then move your tracing onto the right tabletop.)

Why do people misperceive these shapes? The answer involves the normal mechanisms of shape constancy. Cues to depth in this figure cause

FIGURE 3.20   TWO TABLETOPS

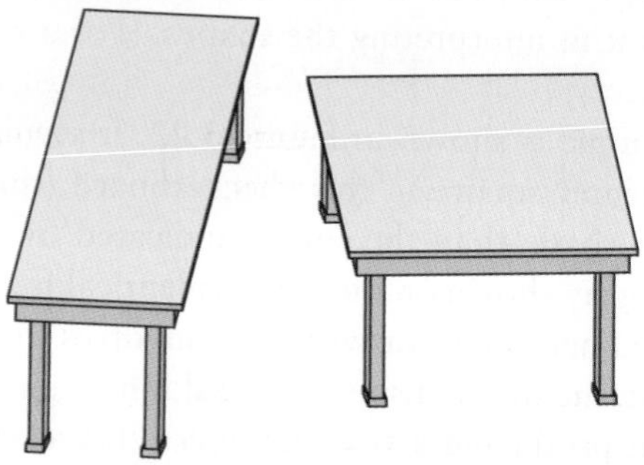

These two tabletops seem to have markedly different shapes and sizes. However, this contrast is an illusion—and the shapes drawn on the page (the two parallelograms depicting the tabletops) are identical in shape and size. The illusion is caused by the same mechanisms that, in most circumstances, allow you to achieve constancy.

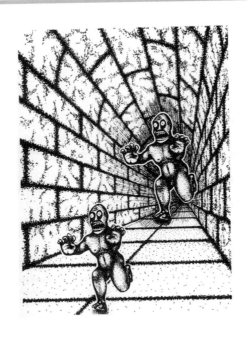

FIGURE 3.21 THE MONSTER ILLUSION

The two monsters appear rather different in size. But, again, this is an illusion, and the two drawings are exactly the same size. The illusion is created by the distance cues in the picture, which make the monster on the right appear to be farther away. This (mis)perception of distance leads to a (mis)perception of size.

you to perceive the figure as a drawing of three-dimensional objects, each viewed from a particular angle. This leads you—quite automatically—to adjust for the (apparent) viewing angles in order to perceive the two table-tops, and it's this adjustment that causes the illusion. Notice then, that this illusion about shape is caused by a misperception of depth: You misperceive the depth relationships in the drawing and then take this faulty information into account in interpreting the shapes. (For a related illusion, see **Figure 3.21**.)

A different example is shown in **Figure 3.22**. It seems obvious to most viewers that the center square in this checkerboard (third row, third column) is a brighter shade than the square indicated by the arrow. But, in truth, the shade of gray shown on the page is identical for these two squares. What has happened here? The answer again involves the normal processes of perception. First, the mechanisms of lateral inhibition (described earlier) play a role here in producing a *contrast effect*: The central square in this figure is surrounded by dark squares, and the contrast makes the central square look brighter. The square marked at the edge of the checkerboard, however, is surrounded by white squares; here, contrast makes the marked square look darker.

But, in addition, the visual system also detects that the central square is in the shadow cast by the cylinder. Your vision compensates for this fact—again, an example of unconscious inference that takes the shadow into account in judging brightness—and therefore powerfully magnifies the illusion.

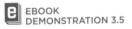
EBOOK
DEMONSTRATION 3.5

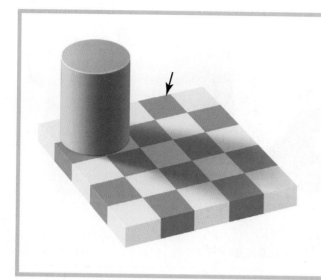

FIGURE 3.22 A BRIGHTNESS ILLUSION

The central square (third row, third column) appears much brighter than the square marked by the arrow. Once again, though, this is an illusion. If you don't believe it, use your fingers or pieces of paper to cover everything in the figure except for these two squares.

The Perception of Depth

In discussing constancy, we said that perceivers take distance, slant, and illumination into account in judging size, shape, and brightness. But to do this, they obviously need to know what the distance is (how far away is the target object?), what the viewing angle is ("Am I looking at the shape straight on or at an angle?"), and what the illumination is. Otherwise, they'd have no way to take these factors into account and, thus, no way to achieve constancy.

Let's pursue this issue by asking how people judge *distance*. We've just said that distance perception is crucial for size constancy, but, of course, information about where things are in your world is also valuable for its own sake. If you want to walk down a hallway without bumping into obstacles, you need to know which obstacles are close to you and which are far off. If you wish to caress a loved one, you need to know where he or she is; otherwise, you're likely to swat empty space when you reach out with your caress or (worse) poke him or her in the eye. Plainly, then, you need to know where objects in your world are located.

Binocular Cues

The perception of distance depends on various **distance cues**—features of the stimulus that indicate an object's position. For example, one important cue comes from the fact that your two eyes look out on the world from slightly different positions; as a result, each eye has a slightly different view. This difference between the two eyes' views is called **binocular disparity**, and it provides important information about distance relationships in the world (see **Figure 3.23**).

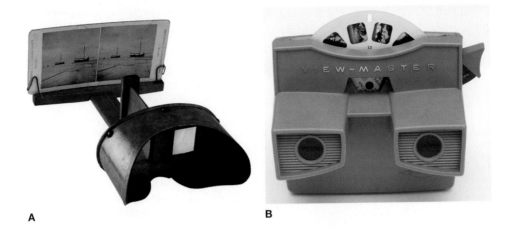

A

B

POPULAR USES OF BINOCULAR DISPARITY

Binocular disparity was the principle behind the stereoscope (Panel A), a device popular in the 19th century that presented a slightly different photograph to each eye, creating a vivid sense of depth. The ViewMaster (Panel B), a popular children's toy, works exactly the same way. The photos on the wheel are actually in pairs—and so, at any rotation, the left eye views one photo in the pair (the one at 9 o'clock on the wheel) and the right eye views a slightly different photo (the one at 3 o'clock), one that shows the same scene from a slightly different angle. Again, the result is a powerful sense of depth.

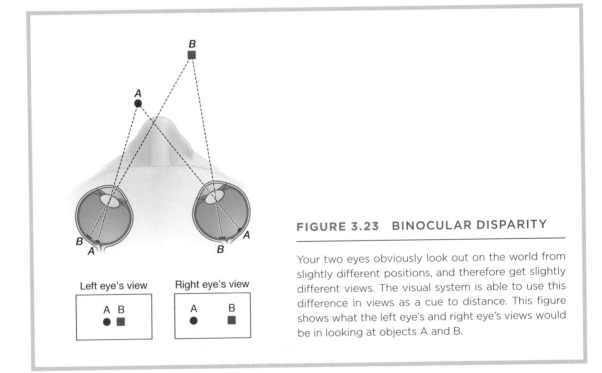

Left eye's view

Right eye's view

FIGURE 3.23 BINOCULAR DISPARITY

Your two eyes obviously look out on the world from slightly different positions, and therefore get slightly different views. The visual system is able to use this difference in views as a cue to distance. This figure shows what the left eye's and right eye's views would be in looking at objects A and B.

Binocular disparity can induce the perception of depth even when no other distance cues are present. For example, the bottom panels of Figure 3.23 show the views that each eye would receive while looking at a pair of nearby objects. If we present each of these views to the appropriate eye (e.g., by drawing the views on two cards and placing one card in front of each eye), we can obtain a striking impression of depth.

Monocular Cues

Binocular disparity is a powerful determinant of perceived depth. But we can also perceive depth with one eye closed; plainly, then, there are also depth cues that depend only on what each eye sees by itself. These are the **monocular distance cues.**

One of the monocular cues depends on the adjustment that the eye must make to see the world clearly. We've already mentioned that in each eye, muscles adjust the shape of the lens to produce a sharply focused image on the retina. The amount of adjustment depends on how far away the viewed object is—there's a lot of adjustment for nearby objects, less for those a few steps away, and virtually no adjustment at all for objects more than a few meters away. It turns out that perceivers are sensitive to the amount of adjustment and use it as a cue indicating how far away the object is.

Other monocular cues have been exploited for centuries by artists to create an impression of depth on a flat surface—that is, within a picture—and that's why these cues are often called **pictorial cues.** In each case, these cues rely on straightforward principles of physics. For example, imagine a situation in which a man is trying to admire a sports car, but a mailbox is in the way (see **Figure 3.24A**). In this case, the mailbox will inevitably block the

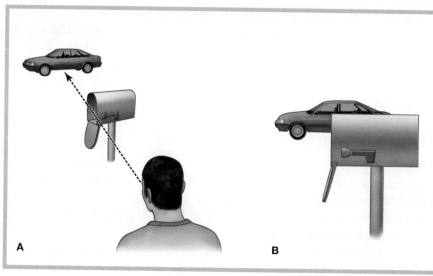

**FIGURE 3.24
INTERPOSITION AS
A DEPTH CUE**

This man is looking at the sports car, but the mailbox blocks part of his view (Panel A). Here's how the scene looks from the man's point of view (Panel B). Because the mailbox blocks the view, the man gets a simple but powerful cue that the mailbox must be closer to him than the sports car is.

A

B

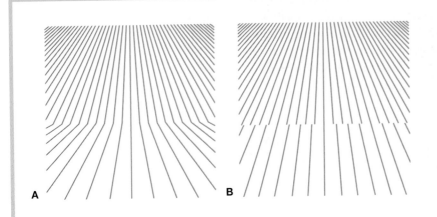

view simply because light can't travel through an opaque object. This fact about the physical world provides a cue you can use in judging distance. The cue is known as **interposition**—the blocking of your view of one object by some other object. In Figure 3.24B, interposition tells the man that the mailbox is closer than the car.

In the same way, distant objects necessarily produce a smaller retinal image than do nearby objects of the same size; this is a fact about optics. But this physical fact again gives you perceptual information you can use. In particular, it's the basis for the cue of **linear perspective**, the name for the pattern in which parallel lines seem to converge as they get farther and farther from the viewer.

A related pictorial cue is provided by texture gradients. Consider what meets your eye when you look at cobblestones on a street or patterns of sand on a beach. The retinal projection of the sand or cobblestones shows a pattern of continuous change in which the elements of the texture grow smaller and smaller as they become more distant. This pattern of change by itself can reveal the spatial layout of the relevant surfaces. If, in addition, there are discontinuities in these textures, they can tell you even more about how the surfaces are laid out (see **Figure 3.25**; Gibson, 1950, 1966).

The Perception of Depth through Motion

Whenever you move your head, the images projected by the objects in your view necessarily move across your retinas. For reasons of geometry, the projected images of nearby objects move more than those of distant ones; this pattern of motion in the retinal images gives you another distance cue, called **motion parallax** (Helmholtz, 1909).

A different motion cue is produced when you move toward or away from objects. As you approach an object, its image gets larger and larger; as you

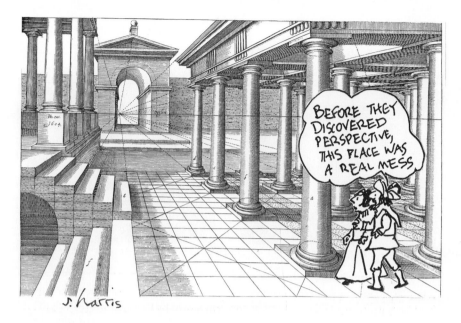

move away, it gets smaller. The pattern of stimulation across the entire visual field also changes as you move toward an object, resulting in a pattern of change in the retinal stimulation that's called **optic flow**. This flow gives you another type of information about depth and plays a large role in the coordination of your movements (Gibson, 1950, 1979).

The Role of Redundancy

One might think that the various distance cues all end up providing the same information—each one tells you which objects are close by and which ones are distant. On that basis, it might be efficient for the visual system to focus on just one or two cues and ignore the others. The fact is, however, that you make use of all these cues, as well as several others we haven't described (e.g., see **Figure 3.26**).

Why do we have a visual system influenced by so many cues, especially since these cues do, in fact, often provide redundant information? It's because different distance cues become important in different circumstances. For example, binocular disparity is a powerful cue, but it's informative only when objects are relatively close by. (For targets farther than 30 feet away, the two eyes receive virtually the same image.) Likewise, motion parallax tells you a great deal about the spatial layout of your world, but only if you're moving. Texture gradients are informative only if there's a suitably uniform texture in view. So while these various cues are often redundant, each type of cue can provide information when the others cannot. By being sensitive to them all, you're able to judge distance in nearly any situation

FIGURE 3.26 MONOCULAR CLUES TO DEPTH: LIGHT AND SHADOW

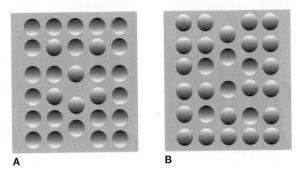

In this chapter, we've covered only a subset of the cues to distance that are used by our visual system. Another cue is provided by the shadows "attached" to an object. In Panel A, most viewers will say that the figure contains six "bulges" in a smiley-face configuration (two eyes, a nose, a mouth). In Panel B, the same figure has simply been turned upside-down. Now the bulges appear to be "dents," and the other circles that had appeared concave, now look like bulges. The reason is the location of the shadows: When the shadow is at the bottom, the object looks convex, a point that makes sense because in our day-to-day lives light almost always comes from above us, not below.

you encounter. This turns out to be a consistent theme of perception—with multiple cues to distance, multiple cues to illumination, multiple paths through which you can detect motion, and so on. The result is a system that sometimes seems inelegant and inefficient, but it's one that guarantees flexibility and versatility.

COGNITIVE PSYCHOLOGY AND THE LAW

Viewing Opportunity

Eyewitness testimony provides a crucial source of evidence for the justice system: "That's the guy I saw in the park that night; I'm sure!" Common sense, however, tells us that eyewitnesses can't report on things they didn't see in the first place—and so can't report on an event if they were too far away from it or if the lighting was too dim. Careful science, however, allows us to go considerably beyond common sense. For example, how far is "too far"?

One study addressed this issue by exploring the "best case scenario" (Loftus & Harley, 2004). Participants were trying to recognize highly familiar faces and were cued in advance whose face they might see. (Roughly, the procedure is one in which research participants are told: "In the next block of trials, you will be seeing faces drawn from the following list of 16 celebrities…") Prior to the test trials, participants were also shown photos of these celebrities, to remind them of the celebrities' appearance. In addition, the participants were all calm and focused on their task; the illumination was fine and the air was clear.

In this procedure, participants recognized at least 80% of the celebrities at a viewing distance of approximately 30 feet. At greater distances, recognition accuracy fell off, and (for example) at a distance of 64 feet (about 20 meters), the error rate was greater than 40%. By 128 feet (about 40 meters), more than 80% of the identifications were mistaken.

It's also valuable here to contrast these results, obtained from careful research, with the "results" obtained with a commonsense "experiment." Loftus and Harley describe a criminal trial that hinged on an identification at a distance of roughly 450 feet. After the verdict was in, some of the jurors "confirmed that they did their own experiment in broad daylight during a break. They had one or more jurors pace off a given distance and then they all stood and decided if they could recognize them [*sic*]" (pg. 23). Of course, this "experiment" was problematic at many levels: The crime took place in the evening, when light levels were low. The jurors, in contrast, did their experiment with good illumination. The crime was fast-paced and involved four assailants carrying out complex actions. The jurors' experiment was slow-paced and involved people standing still while they were being viewed. Most important, the witness to the actual crime was trying, at this distance, to perceive and perhaps memorize never-seen-before faces for a subsequent I.D. The jurors, in contrast, were viewing a face they knew well (one of the other jurors) and asking one another some version of "You can still see it's Fred, can't you?" These are massively different conditions, and performance is certain to be vastly better under the latter conditions than in the former.

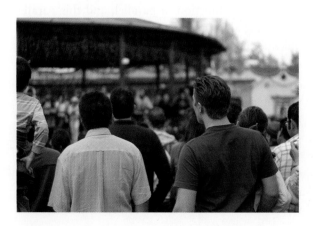

VIEWING OPPORTUNITY

Eyewitness identifications are dramatic and persuasive. But these identifications are only informative if the witness got an adequate view of the perpetrator—and we can use psychological science to evaluate that view.

In addition, we need to consider how the justice system finds out about a witness's view. Often, a police officer asks the witness, an hour after the crime, "How far away was he?" Sometimes an attorney might ask the same question months after the crime. In either case, it's important to realize that people are quite poor at estimating distances. In one study, viewers were asked to use ranges to describe their estimates ("I was at least ___ feet away, but no more than ___ feet away"), and the actual distance was outside of the reported range in more than half the cases, with viewers often underestimating near distances and overestimating longer distances (Lindsay et al., 2008).

Accuracy is even lower if we rely on a witness's *memory* for viewing distance, and one reason is the distorting effect of feedback. Often, witnesses make an identification and then are given some confirmation of their choice. ("Good; that was our suspect," or "Another witness made the same choice.") This feedback seems to trigger an (entirely unconscious) inference, along the lines of "Apparently, I made a good choice, so I must have gotten a good view after all." Guided by this inference, witnesses who receive feedback remember their viewing distance as closer than it actually was, remember the event duration as longer than it actually was, remember the lighting as better than it actually was, and so on.

There is no denial that a witness's viewing opportunity is a crucial determinant of the witness's accuracy; indeed, this factor is emphasized in many court rulings. In ways that should be clear, though, our assessment of viewing opportunity needs to be guided by an understanding of both perception (e.g., how far is "too far") and memory. Otherwise, we'll be unable to interpret this crucial aspect of witness evidence.

chapter summary

• One brain area that has been mapped in considerable detail is the visual system. This system takes its main input from the rods and cones on the retina. Then, information is sent via the optic nerve to the brain. An important point is that cells in the optic nerve do much more than transmit information; they also begin the analysis of the visual input. This is reflected in the phenomenon of lateral inhibition, which leads to edge enhancement.

• Part of what we know about the brain comes from single-cell recording, which can record the electrical activity of an individual neuron. In the visual system, this recording has allowed researchers to map the receptive fields for many cells. The mapping has provided evidence for a high degree of specialization among the various parts of the visual system, with some parts specialized for the perception of motion, others for the perception of color, and so on. These various areas function in parallel, and this parallel processing allows great speed; it also allows mutual influence among multiple systems.

• Parallel processing begins in the optic nerve and continues throughout the visual system. For example, the *what* system (in the temporal lobe) appears to be specialized for the identification of visual objects; the *where* system (in the parietal lobe) seems to tell us where an object is located.

• The reliance on parallel processing creates a problem of reuniting the various elements of a scene so that these elements are perceived in an integrated fashion. This is the binding problem. One key in solving this problem, though, lies in the fact that different brain systems are organized in terms of maps, so that spatial position can be used as a framework for reuniting the separately analyzed aspects of the visual scene.

● Visual perception requires more than the "pickup" of features. Those features must be organized into wholes—a process apparently governed by the so-called Gestalt principles. The visual system also must interpret the input, a point that is especially evident with reversible figures. Crucially, though, these interpretive steps aren't separate from, and occurring after, the pickup of elementary features, because the features themselves are shaped by the perceiver's organization of the input.

● The active nature of perception is also evident in perceptual constancy. We achieve constancy through a process of unconscious inference, taking one aspect of the input (e.g., the distance to the target) into account in interpreting another aspect (e.g., the target's size). This process is usually quite accurate, but it can produce illusions.

● The perception of distance relies on many cues—some dependent on binocular vision, and some on monocular vision. The diversity of cues enables us to perceive distance in a wide range of circumstances.

eBook Demonstrations & Essays

Online Demonstrations:
● Demonstration 3.1: Foveation
● Demonstration 3.2: Eye Movements
● Demonstration 3.3: The Blind Spot and the Active Nature of Vision
● Demonstration 3.4: A Brightness Illusion
● Demonstration 3.5: A Motion Illusion

Online Applying Cognitive Psychology Essays:
● Cognitive Psychology and Education: Memorable "Slogans"

ZAPS 2.0 Cognition Labs

● Go to **http://digital.wwnorton.com/cognition6** for the online labs relevant to this chapter.

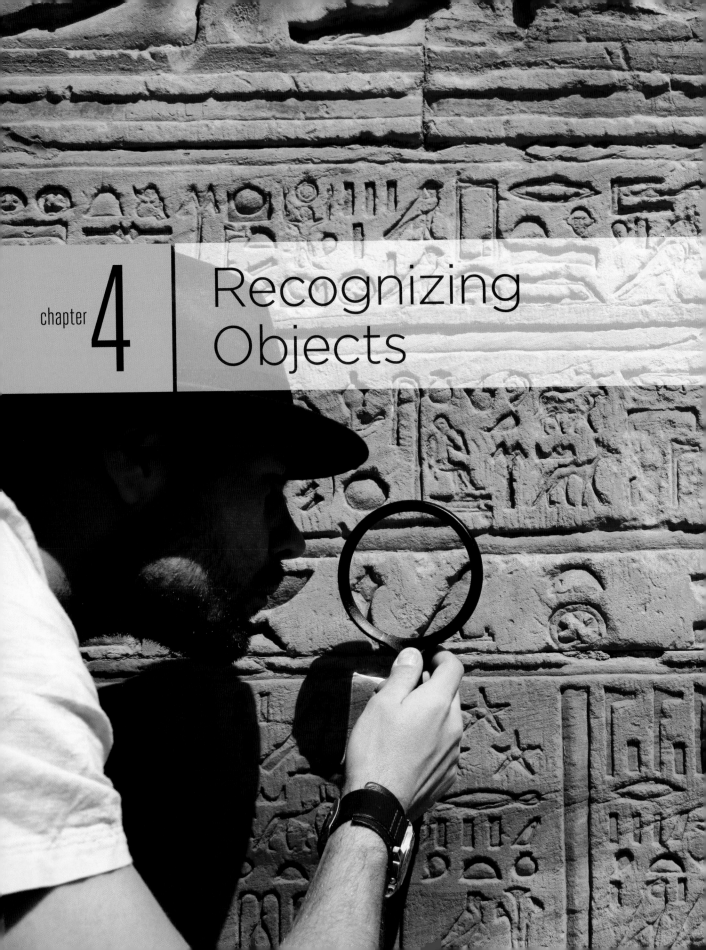

chapter **4** | Recognizing
Objects

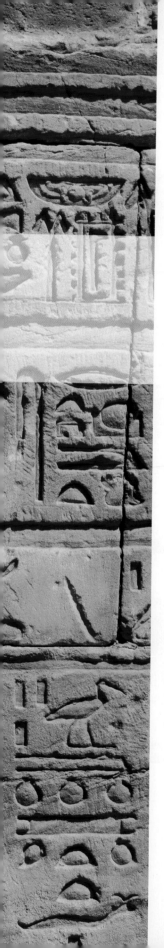

what if... In Chapter 3, we discussed some of the steps involved in visual perception. But, of course, you don't just perceive objects; you also *recognize* them and can identify what they are. This recognition is usually very easy for you, and so you have no difficulty at all in recognizing a vast array of objects in your world—whether the object is a squirrel or a shoe or a frying pan or a pickup truck. But, easy or not, recognition relies on processes that are surprisingly sophisticated, and your life would be massively disrupted if you couldn't manage this (seemingly simple) achievement.

We mentioned in Chapter 2 that certain types of brain damage produce a disorder called "agnosia." In some cases, patients suffer from **apperceptive agnosia**. These patients seem able to see an object's shape and color and position, but they cannot put these elements together to perceive the intact object. For example, one patient—identified only as D.F.—suffered from brain damage in the sites shown in **Figure 4.1.** D.F. was asked to copy drawings that were in plain view (**Figure 4.2A**). The resulting attempts are shown in Figure 4.2B. The limit here is not some problem in drawing ability, and Figure 4.2C shows what happened when D.F. was asked to draw various forms *from memory*. Plainly D.F. can draw; the problem instead is in her ability to see and to assemble the various elements that she sees.

Other patients suffer from **associative agnosia**. They see but cannot link what they see to their basic visual knowledge. One remarkable example comes from a case described by neurologist Oliver Sacks:

> "What is this?" I asked, holding up a glove.
>
> "May I examine it?" he asked, and, taking it from me, he proceeded to examine it. "A continuous surface," he announced at last, "infolded in itself. It appears to have"—he hesitated—"five outpouchings, if this is the word."
>
> "Yes," I said cautiously. ". . .Now tell me what it is."
>
> "A container of some sort?"
>
> "Yes," I said, "and what would it contain?"
>
> "It would contain its contents!" said Dr. P., with a laugh. "There are many possibilities. It could be a change purse, for example, for coins of five sizes. It could . . ." (Sacks, 1985, p. 14)

preview of chapter themes

- Recognition of visual inputs begins with features, but it's not just the features that matter. How easily we recognize a pattern also depends on how frequently or recently we have viewed the pattern and on whether the pattern is well formed (such as letter sequences with "normal" spelling patterns).

- We explain these findings in terms of a feature net—a network of detectors, each of which is "primed" according to how often or how recently it has fired. The network relies on distributed knowledge to make inferences, and this process gives up some accuracy in order to gain efficiency.

- The feature net can be extended to other domains, including the recognition of three-dimensional objects. However, the recognition of faces requires a different sort of model, sensitive to configurations rather than to parts.

- Finally, we consider top-down influences on recognition. The existence of these influences tells us that object recognition is not a self-contained process; instead, knowledge external to object recognition is imported into and clearly shapes the process.

FIGURE 4.1   D.F.'S LESIONS

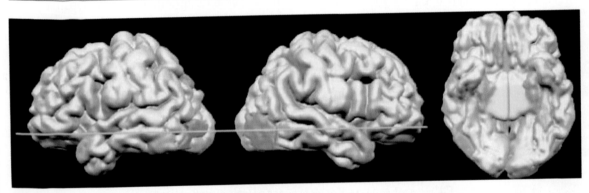

A Lesions in subject D.F.

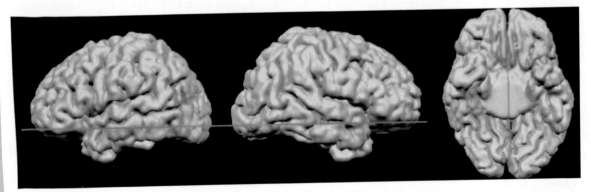

B Location of LOC in neurologically intact subjects

Panel A shows the location of the brain damage in D.F. Panel B shows the areas in the "lateral occipital complex" that are especially activated when neurologically healthy people are recognizing objects.

FIGURE 4.2 DRAWINGS FROM PATIENT D.F.

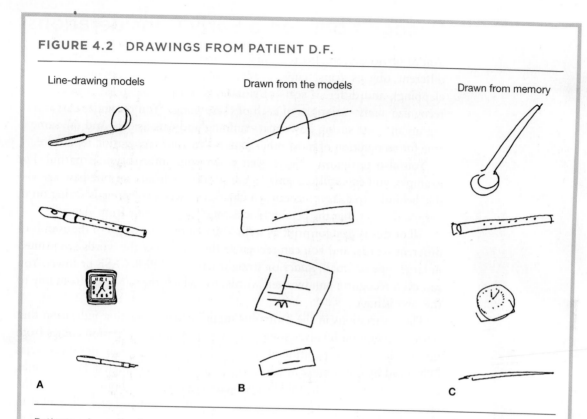

Line-drawing models	Drawn from the models	Drawn from memory

A   B   C

Patients who suffer from *apperceptive agnosia* can see, but cannot organize the elements they see to perceive an intact object. This deficit was evident when patient D.F. was asked to copy the drawings shown in Panel A. His attempts are shown in Panel B. The problem is in D.F.'s perception, not in his drawing ability, because his performance was much better (as shown in Panel C), when he was asked to draw the same forms from memory, rather than from a model.

Dr. P. obviously can see, and he uses his (considerable) intelligence to figure out what he is seeing. Nonetheless, his agnosia profoundly disrupts his life. Sacks describes one incident in which Dr. P. failed to put on his shoe, because he did not recognize it as a shoe. (In fact, Sacks notes that at one point Dr. P. was confused about which object was his shoe and which was his foot.) Then, at the end of their time together, Sacks reports that Dr. P. "reached out his hand and took hold of his wife's head, tried to lift it off, to put it on. He had apparently mistaken his wife for a hat!" (p. 11).

Thus, object recognition may not be a glamorous skill, but it is nonetheless a skill that we all rely on for even our most ordinary commerce with the world.

Recognition: Some Early Considerations

You're obviously able to recognize a huge number of different patterns—different objects (cats, cups, coats), various actions (crawling, climbing, clapping), and different sorts of situations (crises, comedies). You can also recognize many variations of each of these things. You recognize cats standing up and cats sitting down, cats running and cats asleep. And the same is true for recognition of most other patterns in your recognition repertoire.

You also recognize objects even when your information is partial. For example, you can still recognize a cat if only its head and one paw are visible behind a tree. You recognize a chair even when someone is sitting on it, despite the fact that the person blocks much of the chair from view.

All of this is true for print as well: You can recognize tens of thousands of different words, and you can recognize them whether the words are printed in large type or small, *italics* or straight letters, UPPER CASE or lower. You can even recognize handwritten words, for which the variation from one to the next is huge.

These variations in the "stimulus input" provide our first indication that object recognition involves some complexity. Another indication comes from the fact that your recognition of various objects, whether print or otherwise, is influenced by the *context* in which the objects are encountered. For example, consider **Figure 4.3**. The middle character is the same in both words, but the character looks more like an *H* in the word on the left and more like an *A* in the word on the right. With this, you unhesitatingly read the word on the left as "THE" and not "TAE" and the word on the right as "CAT" and not "CHT."

Of course, object recognition is powerfully influenced by the stimulus itself—that is, by the features that are in view. Processes that are directly shaped by the stimulus are sometimes called "data driven" but are more commonly termed **bottom-up processes**. The effect of context, however, reminds us that recognition is also influenced by your knowledge and expectations. Thus, your reading of Figure 4.3 is guided by your knowledge that "THE" and "CAT" are common words but that "TAE" and "CHT" are not. This sort of influence—relying on

---

FIGURE 4.3 CONTEXT INFLUENCES PERCEPTION

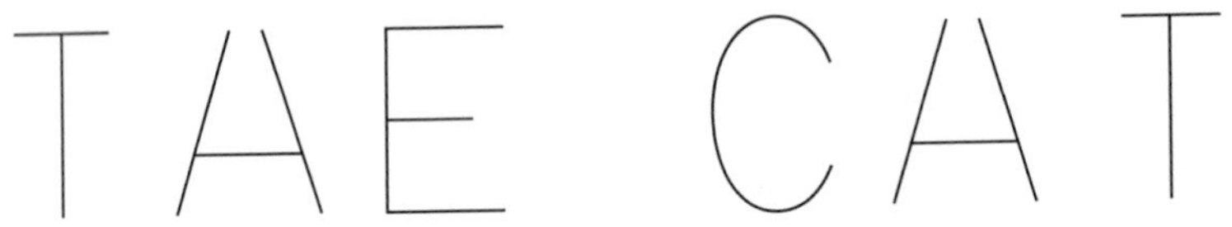

You are likely to read this sequence as "THE CAT," reading the middle symbol as an *H* in one case and as an *A* in the other.   AFTER SELFRIDGE, 1955.

your knowledge—is sometimes called "concept-driven," and processes shaped by knowledge are commonly called **top-down processes.**

How should we think about all this? What mechanism underlies both the top-down and bottom-up influences? In the next section, we'll consider a classic proposal for what the mechanism might be. We'll then build on this base, as we discuss more recent elaborations of this proposal.

The Importance of Features

Common sense suggests that many objects are recognized by virtue of their parts. You recognize an elephant because you see the trunk, the thick legs, the large body. You know a lollipop is a lollipop because you can see the circle shape on top of the straight stick. These notions, though, invite a further question: How do you recognize the parts themselves? How, for example, do you recognize the trunk on the elephant or the circle in the lollipop? The answer may be simple: Perhaps you recognize the parts by looking at *their* parts—the arcs, for example, that make up the circle, or the (roughly) parallel lines that identify the elephant's trunk.

To put this more generally, recognition might begin with the identification of **visual features** in the input pattern—the vertical lines, curves, diagonals, and so on. With these features appropriately catalogued, you can then start assembling the larger units: If you detect a horizontal together with a vertical, you know you're looking at a right angle; if you've detected four right angles, you know you're looking at a square.

This broad proposal lines up well with the neuroscience evidence we discussed in Chapter 3. There, we saw that specialized cells in the visual system do seem to act as "feature detectors," firing whenever the relevant input (i.e., the appropriate feature) is in view. In addition, we've already noted that people can recognize many variations on the objects they encounter—cats in different positions, *A*'s in different fonts or different handwritings. An emphasis on features, though, might help with this point: The various *A*'s, for example, differ from one another in overall shape, but they do have certain things in common: two inwardly sloping lines and a horizontal crossbar. Thus, focusing on features might allow us to concentrate on elements shared by the various *A*'s and so might allow us to recognize *A*'s despite their apparent diversity.

The importance of features is also evident in the fact that people are remarkably efficient when searching for a target defined by a simple feature—for example, finding a vertical segment in a field of horizontals or a green shape in a field of red shapes. People are much slower, in contrast, in searching for a target defined as a *combination* of features (see **Figure 4.4**). This is just what we would expect if feature analysis is an early step in your analysis of the visual world—and separate from the step in which you combine the features you've detected. (For more on this point, see Chapter 5.)

Further support for these claims comes from studies of brain damage. At the start of the chapter, we mentioned *apperceptive agnosia*—a disorder, it seems, that involves an inability to assemble the various aspects of an input

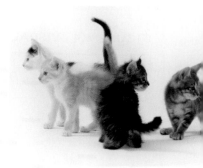

THE VARIABILITY OF STIMULI WE RECOGNIZE

We recognize cats from the side or the front, whether we see them close up or far away.

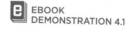
EBOOK
DEMONSTRATION 4.1

FIGURE 4.4 VISUAL SEARCH

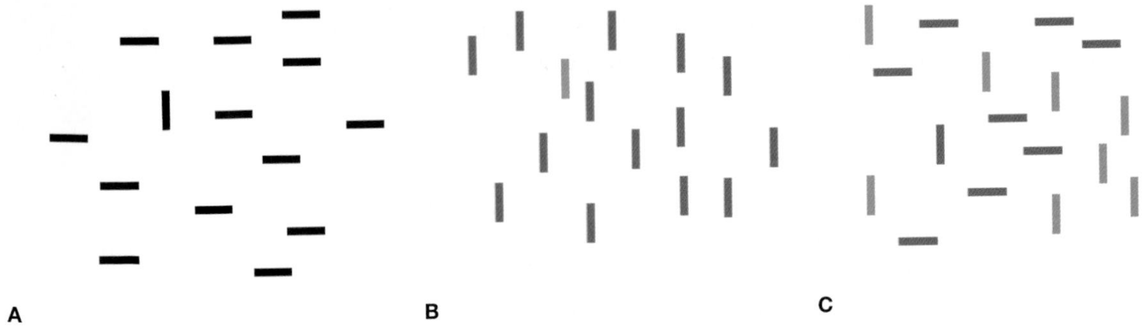

A   B   C

In Panel A, you can immediately spot the vertical, distinguished from the other shapes by just one feature. Likewise, in Panel B, you can immediately spot the lone green bar in the field of reds. In Panel C, it takes much longer to find the one red vertical, because now you need to search for a combination of features—not just for red or vertical, but for the one form that has both of these attributes.

into an organized whole. A related disorder derives from damage to the parietal cortex: Patients who suffer from **integrative agnosia** appear relatively normal in tasks requiring them simply to detect features in a display. However, these people are markedly impaired in tasks that require them to judge how the features are bound together to form complex objects (e.g., Behrmann, Peterson, Moscovitch, & Suzuki, 2006; Humphreys & Riddoch, 2014; Robertson, Treisman, Friedman-Hill, & Grabowecky, 1997; for related results, in which *transcranial magnetic stimulation* was used to disrupt portions of the brain in healthy individuals, see Ashbridge, Walsh, & Cowey, 1997).

Word Recognition

Several lines of evidence, therefore, indicate that object recognition does begin with the detection of simple features. Then, once this detection has occurred, separate mechanisms are needed to put the features together, assembling them into complete objects. But how does this assembly proceed, so that we end up seeing not just the features but whole words, for example, or Chihuahuas, or fire hydrants? In tackling this question, it will be helpful to fill in some more facts that we can then use as a guide to our theory building.

Factors Influencing Recognition

In many studies, participants have been shown stimuli for just a brief duration—perhaps 20 or 30 ms (milliseconds). Older research did this by means of a **tachistoscope,** a device specifically designed to present stimuli for precisely controlled amounts of time. More modern research uses computers for this purpose, but the brief displays are still called "tachistoscopic presentations."

Each stimulus is followed by a poststimulus **mask**—often, just a random jumble of letters, such as "XJDKEL." The mask serves to interrupt any continued processing that participants might try to do for the stimulus just presented. This way, researchers can be certain that a stimulus presented for (say) 20 ms is visible for exactly 20 ms and no longer.

Can people recognize these briefly visible stimuli? The answer depends on many factors, including how *familiar* a stimulus is. If the stimulus is a word, for example, we can measure familiarity by literally counting how often that word appears in print, and these counts are an excellent predictor of tachistoscopic recognition. In one early experiment, Jacoby and Dallas (1981) showed participants words that were either very frequent (appearing at least 50 times in every million printed words) or infrequent (occurring only 1 to 5 times per million words of print). Participants viewed these words for 35 ms, followed by a mask; under these circumstances, they recognized twice as many of the frequent words (see **Figure 4.5A**).

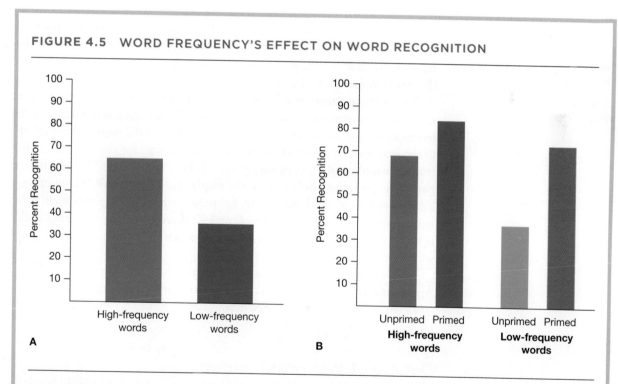

FIGURE 4.5 WORD FREQUENCY'S EFFECT ON WORD RECOGNITION

In one study, recognition was much more likely for words appearing often in print, in comparison to words appearing only rarely—an effect of frequency. Similarly, words that had been viewed recently were more often recognized, an effect of recency that in this case creates a benefit termed "repetition priming." AFTER JACOBY & DALLAS, 1981.

Another factor influencing recognition is recency of view. If participants view a word and then, a little later, view it again, they will recognize the word much more readily the second time around. The first exposure **primes** the participant for the second exposure; more specifically, this is a case of **repetition priming.**

As an example, participants in one study read a list of words aloud. The participants were then shown a series of words in a tachistoscope. Some of these words were from the earlier list and so had been primed; others were unprimed. For words that were high in frequency, 68% of the unprimed words were recognized, compared to 84% of the primed words. For words low in frequency, 37% of the unprimed words were recognized, compared to 73% of the primed words (see Figure 4.5B; Jacoby & Dallas, 1981).

The Word-Superiority Effect

Words that are viewed frequently are, it seems, easier to perceive, as are words that have been viewed recently. It also turns out that words themselves are easier to perceive than isolated letters. This finding is referred to as the **word-superiority effect.**

This effect is usually demonstrated with a "two-alternative, forced-choice" procedure. Thus, in some trials, we might present a single letter—let's say *K*—followed by a poststimulus mask, and follow that with a question: "Which of these was in the display: an *E* or a *K*?" In other trials, we present a word—let's say "DARK"—followed by a mask, followed by a question: "Which of these was in the display: an *E* or a *K*?"

Notice that a participant has a 50-50 chance of guessing correctly in either of these situations, and so any contribution from guessing is the same for the letters as it is for the words. Note in addition that for the word stimulus, both of the letters we've asked about are plausible endings for the stimulus; either ending would create a common word ("DARE" or "DARK"). Therefore, a participant who saw only part of the display (perhaps "DAR") couldn't use his knowledge of the language to figure out what the display's final letter was. In order to choose between *E* and *K*, therefore, the participant really needs to have seen the relevant letter—and that, of course, is exactly what we want.

In this procedure, accuracy rates are reliably higher in the word condition. Apparently, then, recognizing words is easier than recognizing isolated letters (see **Figure 4.6**; Johnston & McClelland, 1973; Reicher, 1969; Rumelhart & Siple, 1974; Wheeler, 1970).

Degree of Well-Formedness

The data are telling us, then, that it's easier to recognize an *E*, say, if the letter appears in context than it is if the letter appears on its own (and likewise for any other letter). But this benefit emerges only if the context is of the right sort. There's no context effect if we present a string like "HZYE"

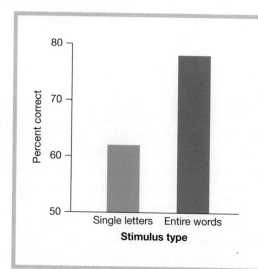

FIGURE 4.6 THE WORD-SUPERIORITY EFFECT

The word-superiority effect is usually demonstrated with a two-alternative forced-choice procedure (and so a participant can get a score of 50% just by guessing randomly). Performance is much better if the target letter is shown in context (within an intact word) than if the target letter is shown on its own. AFTER JOHNSTON & MCCLELLAND, 1973.

or "SBNE." An *E* presented within these strings will *not* show the word-superiority effect—that is, it will not be recognized more readily than an *E* presented in isolation.

What about a context like "FIKE" or "LAFE"? These letter strings are not English words and are not familiar, but they nonetheless look like English strings and (related) are easy to pronounce. Strings like these *do* produce a context effect, and so letters in these contexts are easier to identify than letters alone (or letters in random strings).

The pattern is similar if we ask participants to report all of what they have seen, not just to detect specific letters. Thus, a letter string like "JPSRW" is extremely difficult to recognize if presented briefly. With a stimulus like this and, say, a 30-ms exposure, participants may report that they only saw a flash and no letters at all; at best, they may report a letter or two. But with the same 30-ms exposure, participants will generally recognize (and be able to report) strings like "FIKE" or "LAFE," although they do better still if the stimuli presented are actual, familiar words.

How should we think about these facts? One approach emphasizes the statistically defined regularities in English spelling. Specifically, we can work through a dictionary, counting how often (for example) the letter combination "FI" occurs, or the combination "LA," or "HZ." We can do the same for three-letter sequences ("FIK," "LAF," "HZY," and so on). All of these counts will leave us with a tally that reveals which letter combinations are more probable in English spelling and which are less. We can then use this tally to evaluate new strings—asking, for any string, whether its letter sequences are high-probability ones (occurring often) or low-probability (occurring rarely).

These statistical measures enable us to evaluate how "well formed" a letter string is—that is, how well the letter sequence conforms to the usual spelling patterns of English. Well-formedness, in turn, is a good predictor of word recognition: The more English-like the string is (measured statistically), the easier it will be to recognize that string, and the greater the context benefit the string will produce. This well-documented pattern has been known for more than a century (see, for example, Cattell, 1885) and has been replicated in many studies (Gibson, Bishop, Schiff, & Smith, 1964; Miller, Bruner, & Postman, 1954).

Making Errors

Let's recap some important points. First, it seems that a letter will be easier to recognize if it appears in a well-formed sequence, but not if it appears in a random sequence. Second, well-formed strings are, overall, easier to perceive than ill-formed strings; this advantage remains in place even if the well-formed strings are made-up ones that you've never seen before (strings like "HAKE" or "COTER"). All of these facts suggest that you somehow are using your knowledge of spelling patterns when you look at, and recognize, the words you encounter—and so you have an easier time with letter strings that conform to these patterns.

The influence of spelling patterns also emerges in another way: in the mistakes you make. With brief exposures, word recognition is good but not perfect, and the errors that occur are quite systematic: There is a strong tendency to misread less-common letter sequences as if they were more-common patterns. Thus, for example, "TPUM" is likely to be misread as "TRUM" or even "DRUM." But the reverse errors are rare: "DRUM" is unlikely to be misread as "TRUM" or "TPUM."

These errors can sometimes be quite large—so that someone shown "TPUM" might instead perceive "TRUMPET." But, large or small, the errors show the pattern described: Misspelled words, partial words, or nonwords are read in a way that brings them into line with normal spelling. In effect, people perceive the input as being more regular than it actually is. Once again, therefore, our recognition seems to be guided by (or, in this case, misguided by) some knowledge of spelling patterns.

Feature Nets and Word Recognition

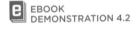
EBOOK
DEMONSTRATION 4.2

What lies behind this broad pattern of evidence? What are the processes inside of us that lead to the various findings we've described? Psychology's understanding of these points grows out of a theory published more than 50 years ago (Selfridge, 1959). Let's start with that theory and then build on that base as we look at more modern work. (For a glimpse of some of the modern research, including work that links theorizing to neuroscience, see Carreiras, Armstrong, Perea, & Frost, 2014.)

The Design of a Feature Net

Imagine that we want to design a system that will recognize the word "CLOCK" whenever it is in view. How might our "CLOCK" detector work? One option is to "wire" this detector to a C-detector, an L-detector, an

O-detector, and so on. Then, whenever these letter detectors are activated, this would activate the word detector. But what activates the letter detectors? Perhaps the *L*-detector is "wired" to a horizontal-line detector, and also a vertical-line detector, and maybe also a corner detector, as shown in **Figure 4.7**. When all of these feature detectors are activated as a group, this activates the letter detector.

The idea, then, is that there could be a network of detectors, organized in layers. The "bottom" layer is concerned with features, and that is why networks of this sort are often referred to as **feature nets**. As we move "upward" in the network, each subsequent layer is concerned with larger-scale objects; and using the term we introduced earlier, the flow of information would be *bottom-up*—from the lower levels toward the upper levels.

But what does it mean to "activate" a detector? At any point in time, each detector in the network has a particular **activation level**, which reflects the status of the detector at just that moment—roughly, how energized the detector is. When a detector receives some input, its activation level increases. A strong input will increase the activation level by a lot, and so will a series of weaker inputs. In either case, the activation level will eventually reach the detector's **response threshold**, and at that point the detector will *fire*—that is, send its signal to the other detectors to which it is connected.

These points parallel our description of neurons in Chapter 2, and that's no accident. If the feature net is to be a serious candidate for how humans recognize patterns, then it has to use the same sorts of building blocks that the brain does. However, let's be careful not to overstate this point: No one

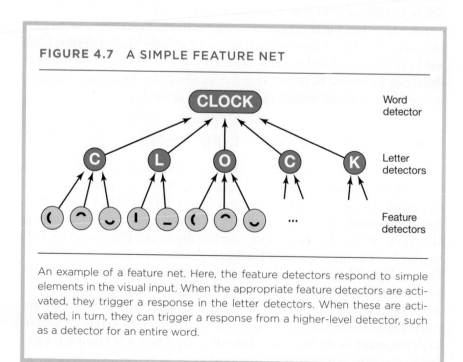

FIGURE 4.7   A SIMPLE FEATURE NET

An example of a feature net. Here, the feature detectors respond to simple elements in the visual input. When the appropriate feature detectors are activated, they trigger a response in the letter detectors. When these are activated, in turn, they can trigger a response from a higher-level detector, such as a detector for an entire word.

is suggesting that detectors are neurons or even large groups of neurons. Instead, detectors likely involve complex assemblies of neural tissue. Nonetheless, it's plainly attractive that the hypothesized detectors in the feature net function in a way that's biologically sensible.

Within the net, some detectors will be easier to activate than others—that is, some detectors will require a strong input to make them fire, while others will fire even with a weak input. This difference is created in part by how activated each detector is to begin with. If the detector is moderately activated at the start, then only a little input is needed to raise the activation level to threshold, and so it will be easy to make this detector fire. If a detector is not at all activated at the start, then a strong input is needed to bring the detector to threshold, and so it will be more difficult to make this detector fire.

What determines a detector's starting activation level? As one factor, detectors that have fired recently will have a higher activation level (think of it as a "warm-up" effect). In addition, detectors that have fired frequently in the past will also have a higher activation level (think of it as an "exercise" effect). Thus, in simple terms, activation level is dependent on principles of *recency* and *frequency*.

We now can put these mechanisms to work. Why are frequent words in the language easier to recognize than rare words? Frequent words, by definition, appear often in the things you read. Therefore, the detectors needed for recognizing these words have been frequently used, and so they have relatively high levels of activation. Thus, even a weak signal (e.g., a brief or dim presentation of the word) will bring these detectors to their response threshold and so will be enough to make these detectors fire. Hence, the word will be recognized even with a degraded input.

Repetition priming is explained in similar terms. Presenting a word once will cause the relevant detectors to fire. Once they have fired, activation levels will be temporarily lifted (because of recency of use). Therefore, only a weak signal will be needed to make the detectors fire again. As a result, the word will be more easily recognized the second time around.

The Feature Net and Well-Formedness

The net we've described so far cannot, however, explain all of the data. Consider, for example, the effects of well-formedness—for instance, the fact that people are able to read letter strings like "PIRT" or "HICE" even when they're presented very briefly (or dimly or in low contrast), but not strings like "ITPR" or "HCEI." How can we explain this result? One option is to add another layer to the net, a layer filled with detectors for *letter combinations*. Thus, in **Figure 4.8**, we've added a layer of **bigram detectors**—detectors of letter pairs. These detectors, like all the rest, will be triggered by lower-level detectors and send their output to higher-level detectors. And just like any other detector, each bigram detector will start out with a certain activation level, influenced by the frequency with which the detector has fired in the past and by the recency with which it has fired.

FIGURE 4.8 BIGRAM DETECTORS

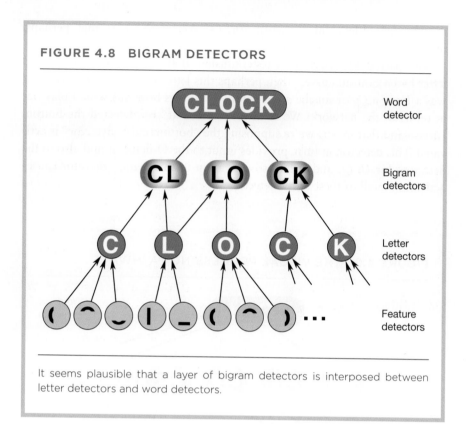

It seems plausible that a layer of bigram detectors is interposed between letter detectors and word detectors.

This turns out to be all the theory we need. You have never seen the sequence "HICE" before, but you have seen the letter pair *HI* (in "HIT," "HIGH," or "HILL") and the pair *CE* ("FACE," "MICE," "JUICE"). The detectors for these letter pairs, therefore, have high activation levels at the start, and so they don't need much additional input to reach their threshold. As a result, these detectors will fire with only weak input. That will make the corresponding letter combinations easy to recognize, facilitating the recognition of strings like "HICE." None of this is true for "IJPV" or "RSFK." Because none of these letter combinations is familiar, these strings will receive no benefits from priming. A strong input will therefore be needed to bring the relevant detectors to threshold, and so these strings will be recognized only with difficulty. (For more on bigram detectors and how they work, see Grainger, Rey, & Dufau, 2008; Grainger & Whitney, 2004; Whitney, 2001; for some complications, though, see Rayner & Pollatsek, 2011.)

Recovery from Confusion

Imagine that we present the word "CORN" for just 20 ms. In this setting, the visual system has only a limited opportunity to analyze the input, so it's possible that you'll miss some of the input's features. For example, let's imagine that the second letter in this word—the *O*—is hard to see, so that, perhaps, only the bottom curve is detected.

This partial information invites confusion: If all you know is "the second letter had a bottom curve," then perhaps this letter was an *O*, or perhaps it was a *U*, or a *Q*, or maybe an *S*. **Figure 4.9** shows how this would play out in terms of the network: We've already said that you detected the bottom curve—and that means we're supposing the "bottom-curve detector" is activated. This detector, in turn, provides input to the *O*-detector and also to the detectors for *U*, *Q*, and *S*, and so activation in this *feature* detector causes activation in all of these *letter* detectors.

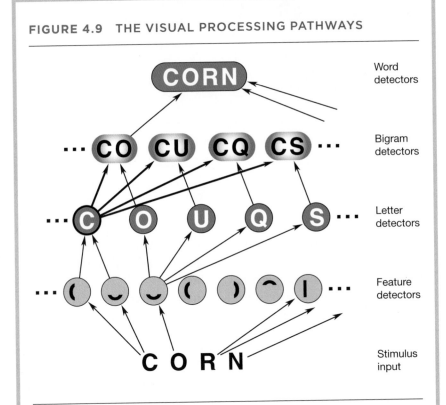

FIGURE 4.9   THE VISUAL PROCESSING PATHWAYS

If "CORN" is presented briefly, not all of its features will be detected. Imagine, for example, that only the bottom curve of the *O* is detected, and not the *O*'s top or sides. This will (weakly) activate the *O*-detector, but it will also activate the detectors of various other letters having a bottom curve, including *U*, *Q*, and *S*. This will, in turn, send weak activation to the appropriate bigram detectors. The *CO*-detector, however, is well primed and so is likely to respond even though it is receiving only a weak input. The other bigram detectors (for *CQ* or *CS*) are less well primed and so will not respond to this weak input. Therefore, "CORN" will be correctly perceived, despite the confusion at the letter level caused by the weak signal.

Of course, each of these letter detectors is wired so that it can also receive input from other feature detectors. (And so usually the O-detector also gets input from detectors for left curves and right curves and top curves.) We've already said, though, that with this brief input these other features weren't detected this time around. As a result, the O-detector will only be weakly activated (because it's not getting its customary full input), and the same is true for the detectors for *U*, *Q*, and *S*.

In this situation, therefore, the network has partial information at the feature level (because only one of the O's features was detected), and this leads to confusion at the letter level: Too many letter detectors are firing (because, again, the now-activated bottom-curve detector is wired to all of them). And, roughly speaking, all of these letter detectors are firing in a fashion that signals uncertainty, because they're each receiving input from only *one* of their usual feature detectors.

The confusion continues in the information sent upward from the letter level to the bigram level. The detector for the CO bigram will receive a strong signal from the C detector (because the C was clearly visible) but only a weak signal from the O detector (because the O wasn't clearly visible). The *CU* detector will get roughly the same input—a strong signal from the C-detector and a weak signal from the *U*-detector. Likewise for the *CQ* and *CS* detectors. Thus, to put this state-of-affairs crudely, the signal being sent from the letter-detectors is, "maybe *CO* or maybe *CU* or maybe *CQ* or maybe *CS*."

The confusion is, however, sorted out at the bigram level. All four bigram detectors in this situation are receiving the same input—a strong signal from one of their letters and a weak signal from the other. However, the four detectors don't all respond in the same way. The CO-detector is well primed (because this is a frequent pattern), and so the activation this detector is receiving will probably be enough to fire this (primed) detector. The CU-detector is less primed (because this is a less frequent pattern); the CQ- and CS-detectors, if they even exist, are not primed at all. The input to these latter detectors is therefore unlikely to activate them—because, again, they're less-well primed and so won't respond to this weak input.

What will be the result of all this? The network was "understimulated" at the feature level (with only a subset of the input's features detected) and therefore confused at the letter level (with too many detectors firing). But then, at the bigram level, it's only the CO-detector that fires, because, at this level, this is the detector (because of priming) most likely to respond to the weak input. Thus, in a totally automatic fashion, the network recovers from its own confusion and, in this case, avoids an error.

Ambiguous Inputs

Look again at Figure 4.3. The second character is exactly the same as the fifth, but the left-hand string is perceived as "THE" (and the character is identified as an *H*) and the right-hand string is perceived as "CAT" (and the character as an *A*).

What's going on here? In the string on the left, the initial *T* is clearly in view, and so presumably the T-detector will fire strongly in response. The next character in the display will likely trigger some of the features normally associated with an *A* and some normally associated with an *H*. This will cause the *A*-detector to fire, but only weakly (because only some of the *A*'s features are present), and likewise for the *H*-detector. At the letter level, then, there will be uncertainty about what this character is.

What happens next, though, follows a by-now familiar logic: With only weak activation of the *A*- and *H*-detectors, only a moderate signal will be sent upward to the *TH*- and *TA*-detectors. Likewise, it seems plausible that only a moderate signal will be sent to the *THE*- and *TAE*-detectors at the word level. But, of course, the *THE*-detector is enormously well primed; if there is a *TAE*-detector, it would be barely primed, since this is a string rarely encountered. Thus, the *THE*- and *TAE*-detectors might be receiving similar input, but this input is sufficient only for the (well-primed) *THE*-detector, and so only it will respond. In this way, the net will recognize the ambiguous pattern as "THE," not "TAE." (And the same is true, with appropriate adjustment, for the ambiguous pattern on the right, perceived as "CAT," not "CHT.")

A similar explanation will handle the word-superiority effect (see, e.g., Rumelhart & Siple, 1974). To take a simple case, imagine that we present the letter *A* in the context "AT." If the presentation is brief enough, participants may see very little of the *A*, perhaps just the horizontal crossbar. This would not be enough to distinguish among *A*, *F*, or *H*, and so all these letter detectors would fire weakly. If this were all the information the participants had, they'd be stuck. But let's imagine that the participants did perceive the second letter in the display, the *T*. It seems likely that the *AT* bigram is far better primed than the *FT* or *HT* bigrams. (That is because you often encounter words like "CAT" or "BOAT"; words like "SOFT" or "HEFT" are used less frequently.) Thus, the weak firing of the *A*-detector would be enough to fire the *AT* bigram detector, while the weak firing for the *F* and *H* might not trigger their bigram detectors. In this way, a "choice" would be made at the bigram level that the input was "AT" and not something else. Once this bigram has been detected, answering the question "Was there an *A* or an *F* in the display?" is easy. In this manner, the letter will be better detected in context than in isolation. This is not because context enables you to see more; instead, context allows you to make better use of what you see.

Recognition Errors

There is, however, a downside to all this. Imagine that we present the string "CQRN" to participants. If the presentation is brief enough, study participants will register only a subset of the string's features. Let's imagine, in line with an earlier example, that they register only the bottom bit of the string's second letter. This detection of the bottom curve will weakly activate the

FIGURE 4.10   RECOGNITION ERRORS

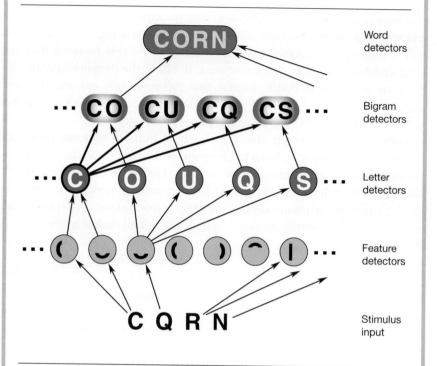

If "CQRN" is presented briefly, not all of its features will be detected. Perhaps only the bottom curve of the *Q* is detected, and this will (weakly) activate various other letters having a bottom curve, including *O*, *U*, and *S*. However, this is the same situation that would result from a brief presentation of "CORN" (as shown in Figure 4.9); therefore, by the logic we have already discussed, this stimulus is likely to be misperceived as "CORN."

Q-detector and also the *U*-detector and the *O*-detector. The resulting pattern of network activation is shown in **Figure 4.10**.

Of course, the pattern of activation in this case is exactly the same as it was in Figure 4.9. In both cases, perceivers have seen the features for the *C*, *R*, and *N* and have only seen the second letter's bottom curve. And we've already walked through the network's response to this feature pattern: This configuration will lead to confusion at the letter level, but this confusion will get sorted out at the bigram level, with the (primed) *CO*-detector responding to this input and other (less well primed) detectors *not* responding. Thus, the stimulus will be identified as "CORN." In the situation we described in Figure 4.9, the stimulus actually was "CORN," and so the dynamic built in to the net aids performance, allowing the network to recover from its initial confusion. In the case we're considering now (with "CQRN" as the stimulus), the exact same dynamic causes the network to misread the stimulus.

This example helps us understand how recognition errors come about and why those errors tend to make the input look more regular than it really is. The basic idea is that the network is biased, inevitably favoring frequent letter combinations over infrequent ones. In effect, the network operates on the basis of "when in doubt, assume that the input falls into the frequent pattern." The reason, of course, is simply that the detectors for the frequent pattern are well primed—and therefore easier to trigger.

Let's emphasize, though, that the bias built into the network *facilitates* perception if the input is, in fact, a frequent word, and these (by definition) are the words you encounter most of the time. The bias will pull the network toward errors if the input happens to have an unusual spelling pattern, but (by definition) these inputs are less common in your experience. Hence, the network's bias necessarily helps perception more often than it hurts.

Distributed Knowledge

We've now seen many indications that the network's functioning is guided by knowledge of spelling patterns. This point is evident in the fact that letter strings are easier to recognize if they conform to normal spelling. The same point is shown by the fact that letter strings provide a context benefit only if they conform to normal spelling. Still more evidence comes from the fact that errors, when they occur, "shift" the perception toward the patterns of normal spelling.

To explain these results, we've suggested that the network "knows" (for example) that *CO* is a common bigram in English, while *CF* is not, and likewise "knows" that *THE* is a common sequence but *TAE* is not. The network seems to rely on this "knowledge" in "choosing" its "interpretation" of unclear or ambiguous inputs. Similarly, the network seems to "expect" certain patterns and not others, and is more efficient when the input lines up with those "expectations."

Obviously, though, we've wrapped quotations around several of these words in order to emphasize that the sense in which the net "knows" facts about spelling, or the sense in which it "expects" things or makes "interpretations," is a bit peculiar. Knowledge about spelling patterns is not explicitly stored anywhere in the network. Nowhere within the net is there a sentence like "*CO* is a common bigram in English; *CF* is not." Instead, this memory (if we even want to call it that) is manifest only in the fact that the *CO*-detector happens to be more primed than the *CF*-detector. The *CO*-detector doesn't "know" anything about this advantage, nor does the *CF*-detector know anything about its disadvantage. Each simply does its job, and in the course of doing their jobs, occasions will arise that involve a "competition" between these detectors. (This sort of competition was illustrated in Figures 4.9 and 4.10.) When these competitions occur, they'll be "decided," in a straightforward way, by activation levels: The better-primed detector will be more likely to respond, and so that detector will be more likely to influence subsequent events. That's the entire mechanism through which these "knowledge effects" arise. That's how "expectations" or "inferences" emerge—as a direct consequence of the activation levels.

To put this into technical terms, the network's "knowledge" is not **locally represented** anywhere; it is not stored in a particular location or built into a specific process. Thus, we cannot look just at the level of priming in the CO-detector and conclude that this detector represents a frequent bigram, nor can we look at the CF-detector to conclude that it represents a rare bigram. Instead, we need to look at the *relationship* between their levels of priming, and we also need to look at how this relationship will lead to one detector being more influential than the other. The knowledge about bigram frequencies, in other words, is **distributed knowledge**—that is, it is represented in a fashion that's distributed across the network and detectable only if we consider how the entire network functions.

What is perhaps most remarkable about the feature net, then, lies in how much can be accomplished with a distributed representation, and thus with simple, mechanical elements correctly connected to one another. The net appears to make inferences and to know the rules of English spelling. But the actual mechanics of the net involve neither inferences nor knowledge (at least, not in any conventional sense). You and I can see how the inferences unfold by taking a bird's-eye view and considering how all the detectors work together as a system. But nothing in the net's functioning depends on the bird's-eye view. Instead, the activity of each detector is locally determined—influenced by just those detectors feeding into it. When all of these detectors work together, though, the result is a process that acts as if it knows the rules. But the rules themselves play no role in guiding the network's moment-by-moment activities.

Efficiency versus Accuracy

One other point about the network also needs emphasis: The network does make mistakes, misreading some inputs and misinterpreting some patterns. As we've seen, though, these errors are produced by exactly the same mechanisms that are responsible for the network's main advantages—its ability to deal with ambiguous inputs, for example, or to recover from confusion. Perhaps, therefore, we should view the errors as the price you pay in order to gain the benefits associated with the net: If you want a mechanism that's able to deal with unclear or partial inputs, you simply have to live with the fact that sometimes the mechanism will make mistakes.

This framing of things, however, invites a question: Do you really need to pay this price? After all, outside of the lab you're unlikely to encounter fast-paced tachistoscopic inputs. Instead, you see stimuli that are out in view for long periods of time, stimuli that you can inspect at your leisure. Why, therefore, don't you take the moment to scrutinize these inputs so that you can rely on fewer inferences and assumptions, and in that fashion gain a higher level of accuracy in recognizing the objects you encounter?

The answer to this question is straightforward. To maximize accuracy, you could, in principle, scrutinize every character on the page. That way, if a character were missing or misprinted, you would be sure to detect it. But the cost associated with this strategy would be insufferable: Reading would be unspeakably slow (in part because the speed with which you move your eyes is relatively slow—no more than four or five eye movements per second). In contrast, it's possible to make inferences about a page with remarkable speed, and this leads readers to adopt the obvious strategy: They read some of the letters and make inferences about the rest. And for the most part, those inferences are safe—thanks to the simple fact that our language (like most aspects of our world) contains some redundncies, so that one doesn't need every lettr to identify what a wrd is; oftn the missng letter is perfctly predctable from the contxt, virtually guaranteeing that inferences will be correct.

Thus, the efficient reader is not being careless, or hasty, or lazy. Given the redundancy of text, and given the slowness of letter-by-letter reading, the inferential strategy is the only strategy that makes sense.

EBOOK
DEMONSTRATION 4.3

Descendants of the Feature Net

As we mentioned early on, we've been focusing on the "classic" version of the feature net. This has enabled us to bring a number of important themes into view—including the trade-off between efficiency and accuracy and the notion of distributed knowledge built into a network's functioning.

Over the years, though, researchers have offered improvements on this basic conceptualization, and in the next sections we'll consider three of their proposals. All three preserve the basic idea of a network of interconnected detectors, but all three extend this idea in important ways. We'll look first at a proposal that highlights the role of *inhibitory* connections among detectors. Then we'll turn to a proposal that applies the network idea to the recognition of complex three-dimensional objects. Finally, we'll consider a proposal that rests on the idea that your ability to recognize objects may depend on your viewing perspective when you encounter those objects.

The McClelland and Rumelhart Model

In the network proposal we've considered so far, activation of one detector serves to *activate* other detectors. Other models involve a mechanism through which detectors can *inhibit* one another, so that activation of one detector can *decrease* the activation in other detectors.

One highly influential model of this sort was proposed by McClelland and Rumelhart (1981); a portion of their model is illustrated in **Figure 4.11**. This network, like the one we've been discussing, is better able to identify well-formed strings than irregular strings; this net is also more efficient in

FIGURE 4.11   AN ALTERNATIVE CONCEPTION OF
THE FEATURE NETWORK

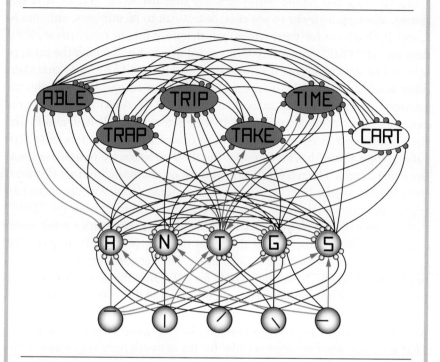

The McClelland and Rumelhart (1981) pattern-recognition model includes both excitatory connections (indicated by red arrows) and inhibitory connections (indicated by connections with dots). Connections within a specific level are also possible—so that, for example, activation of the "TRIP" detector will inhibit the detectors for "TRAP," "TAKE," or "TIME."

identifying characters in context as opposed to characters in isolation. However, several attributes of this net make it possible to accomplish all this without bigram detectors.

In Figure 4.11, **excitatory connections**—connections that allow one detector to activate its neighbors—are shown as arrows; for example, detection of a *T* serves to "excite" the "TRIP" detector. Other connections are *inhibitory*, and so (for example) detection of a *G* deactivates, or inhibits, the "TRIP" detector. These **inhibitory connections** are shown in the figure with dots. In addition, this model also allows for more complicated signaling than we've used so far. In our discussion, we have assumed that lower-level detectors trigger upper-level detectors, but not the reverse. The flow of information, it seemed, was a one-way street. In the McClelland and Rumelhart model, higher-level detectors (word detectors) can influence lower-level detectors, and detectors at any level can also influence other detectors at the same level (e.g., letter detectors inhibit other letter detectors; word detectors inhibit other word detectors).

To see how this would work, let's say that the word "TRIP" is briefly shown, allowing a viewer to see enough features to identify, say, only the *R*, *I*, and *P*. Detectors for these letters will therefore fire, in turn activating the detector for "TRIP." Activation of this word detector will inhibit the firing of other word detectors (e.g., detectors for "TRAP" or "TAKE"), so that these other words are less likely to arise as distractions or competitors with the target word. At the same time, activation of the "TRIP" detector will excite the detectors for its component letters—that is, detectors for *T*, *R*, *I*, and *P*. The *R*-, *I*-, and *P*-detectors, we've assumed, were already firing, so this extra activation "from above" has little impact. But the *T*-detector, we've supposed, was not firing before. The relevant features were on the scene but in a degraded form (thanks to the brief presentation); this weak input was insufficient to trigger an unprimed detector. However, once the excitation from the "TRIP" detector primes the *T*-detector, it's more likely to fire, even with a weak input.

In effect, then, activation of the word detector for "TRIP" implies that this is a context in which a *T* is quite likely. The network therefore responds to this suggestion by "preparing itself" for a *T*. Once the network is suitably prepared (by the appropriate priming), detection of this letter is facilitated. In this way, the detection of a letter sequence (the word "TRIP") makes the network more sensitive to elements that are likely to occur within that sequence. That is exactly what we need in order for the network to be responsive to the regularities of spelling patterns.

Let's also note that the two-way communication being showcased here is ubiquitous in the nervous system. Thus, in the model, letters can activate words, and words can activate letters. In the nervous system, neurons in the eyeballs send activation to the brain but also *receive* activation from the brain; neurons in the lateral geniculate nucleus (LGN) send activation to the visual cortex but also receive activation from the cortex. Facts like these make it clear that visual processing is not a one-way process, with information flowing simply from the eyes toward the brain. Instead, signaling occurs in both an ascending (toward the brain) and a descending (away from the brain) direction, just as the McClelland and Rumelhart model claims.

Recognition by Components

The McClelland and Rumelhart model—like the feature net we started with—was designed initially as an account of how people recognize *printed language*. But, of course, we recognize many objects other than print, including the three-dimensional objects that fill our world—chairs and lamps and cars and trees. Can these objects also be recognized by a feature network? The answer turns out to be yes.

Conside a network theory known as the **recognition by components (RBC) model** (Hummel & Biederman, 1992; Hummel, 2013). This model includes several important innovations, one of which is the inclusion of an intermediate level of detectors, sensitive to **geons** (short for "geometric ions"). The idea is that geons might serve as the basic building blocks of all the objects we recognize; geons are, in essence, the alphabet from which all objects are constructed.

Geons are simple shapes, such as cylinders, cones, and blocks (see **Figure 4.12A**) And only a small set of these shapes is needed: According to Biederman (1987, 1990), we need (at most) three dozen different geons to describe every object in the world, just as 26 letters are all we need to spell all the words of English. These geons can be combined in various ways—in a top-of relation, or a side-connected relation, and so on—to create all the objects we perceive (see Figure 4.12B).

The RBC model, like the other networks we've been discussing, uses a hierarchy of detectors. The lowest-level detectors are feature detectors, which respond to edges, curves, vertices, and so on. These detectors in turn activate the geon detectors. Higher levels of detectors are then sensitive to combinations of geons. More precisely, geons are assembled into complex

FIGURE 4.12   GEONS

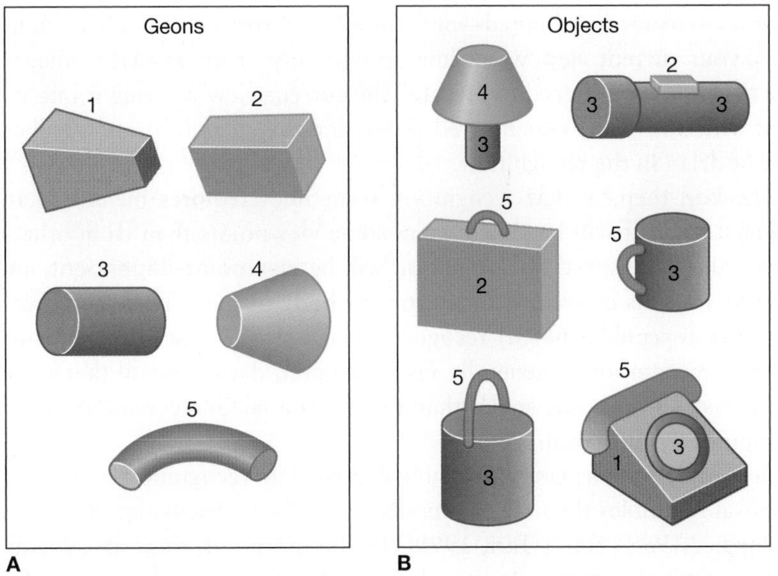

Panel A shows five different geons; Panel B shows how these geons can be assembled into objects. The numbers in Panel B identify the specific geons; for example, a bucket contains Geon 5 top-connected to Geon 3.

arrangements called "geon assemblies," which explicitly represent the relations between geons (e.g., top-of or side-connected). These assemblies, finally, activate the *object model*, a representation of the complete, recognized object.

The presence of the geon and geon-assembly levels within this hierarchy buys us several advantages. For one, geons can be identified from virtually any angle of view, and so recognition based on geons is **viewpoint-independent**. Thus, no matter what your position is relative to a cat, you'll be able to identify its geons and thus identify the cat. Moreover, it seems that most objects can be recognized from just a few geons. As a consequence, geon-based models like RBC can recognize an object even if many of the object's geons are hidden from view.

Recognition via Multiple Views

A number of researchers (Hayward & Williams, 2000; Tarr, 1995; Tarr & Bülthoff, 1998; Vuong & Tarr, 2004; Wallis & Bülthoff, 1999) have offered a different approach to object recognition. They propose that people have stored in memory a number of different views of each object they can recognize: an image of what a cat looks like when viewed head-on, an image of what it looks like from the left, and so on. According to this perspective, then, you'll recognize Felix (let's say) as a cat only if you can match your current view of Felix with one of these views in memory. However, the number of views in memory is limited—perhaps a half dozen or so—and so, in many cases, your current view won't line up with any of the available images. In that situation, you'll need to "rotate" the current view to bring it into alignment with one of the remembered views, and this mental rotation will cause a slight delay in the recognition.

The key, then, is that recognition sometimes requires mental rotation, and as a result it will be slower from some viewpoints than from others. In other words, the speed of recognition will be **viewpoint-dependent**, and in fact this claim is confirmed by a growing body of data. To be sure, we can (as we've repeatedly noted) recognize objects from many different angles, and our recognition is generally fast. However, data indicate that recognition is faster from some angles than others, in a fashion consistent with this multiple-views proposal.

According to this perspective, how exactly does recognition proceed? One proposal resembles the network models we've been discussing (Riesenhuber & Poggio, 1999, 2002; Tarr, 1999). In this proposal, there is a hierarchy of detectors, with each successive layer within the network concerned with more complex aspects of the whole. Thus, low-level detectors respond to lines at certain orientations; higher-level detectors respond to corners and notches. At the top of the hierarchy are detectors that respond to the sight of whole objects. It is important, though, that these detectors each represent what the object looks like from a particular vantage point, and so the detectors fire when there is a match to one of these view-tuned representations.

These representations are probably supported by tissue in the inferotemporal cortex, near the terminus of the *what* pathway. Recording from cells in this area has shown that many neurons here seem object-specific—that is, they fire preferentially when a certain type of object is on the scene. (For an example of just how specific these cells can be in their "preferred" target, see **Figure 4.13**.) Crucially, though, many of these neurons are view-tuned: They fire most strongly to a particular view of the target object. This is just what one might expect with the multiple-views proposal (Peissig & Tarr, 2007).

Let's emphasize, though, that there has been energetic debate between advocates of the RBC approach (with its claim that recognition is largely viewpoint-independent) and the multiple-views approach (with its argument that recognition is viewpoint-dependent). And this may be a case in which both sides are right—with some brain tissue sensitive to viewpoint, and some brain tissue not sensitive (see **Figure 4.14**). In addition, still other approaches to object recognition are also being explored (e.g., Hummel, 2013; Peissig & Tarr, 2007; Ullman, 2007). Plainly, then, there is disagreement in this domain. Even so, let's be clear that all of the available proposals involve the sort of hierarchical network we've been discussing. In other words, no matter how the debate about object recognition turns out, it looks like we're going to need a network model along the lines we've considered.

FIGURE 4.13 THE JENNIFER ANISTON CELL

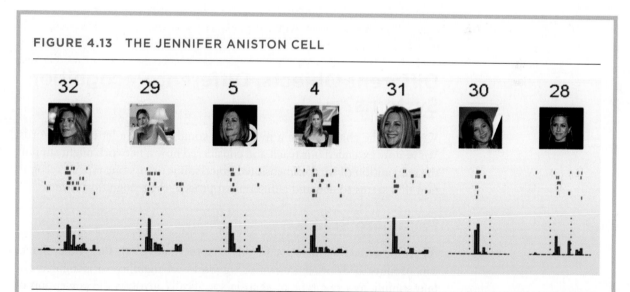

Researchers in one study were able to do single-cell recording within the brains of people who were undergoing surgical treatment for epilepsy. The researchers located cells that fired strongly whenever a picture of Jennifer Aniston was in view—whether the picture showed her close up (picture 32) or far away (picture 29), with long hair (picture 32) or shorter (picture 5). These cells are to a large extent viewpoint-independent; other cells, though, are viewpoint-dependent.

FIGURE 4.14 VIEWPOINT INVARIANCE

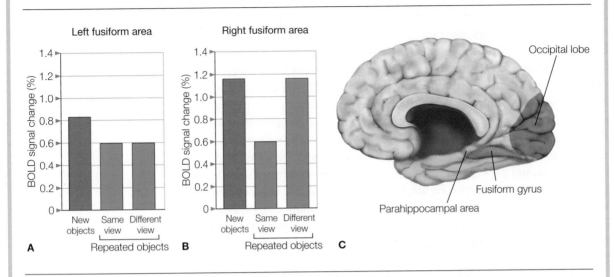

Is object recognition viewpoint-dependent? Some aspects of object recognition may be viewpoint-dependent while other aspects are not. Here, researchers documented viewpoint independence in the left occipital cortex (and so the activity in the fusiform area was the same, even when an object was viewed from a novel perspective). However, the data show viewpoint dependence in the right occipital cortex.

Different Objects, Different Recognition Systems?

We began the chapter with a model that could recognize letters and words. We've now extended our reach and considered how a network might support the recognition of three-dimensional objects. But there's one type of recognition that seems to demand a different approach: the recognition of *faces*.

Faces Are Special

As we described at the start of this chapter, damage to the visual system can produce a disorder known as *agnosia*—an inability to recognize certain stimuli, and one type of agnosia specifically involves the perception of faces. People who suffer from **prosopagnosia** generally have normal vision. Indeed, they can look at a photograph and correctly tell you whether the photo shows a face or something else; they can generally tell you whether a face is a man's or a woman's, and whether it belongs to someone young or someone old. But they cannot recognize individual faces—and so they cannot recognize their own parents or children, whether from photographs or "live."

They cannot recognize the faces of famous performers or politicians. In fact, they cannot recognize *themselves* (and so they sometimes believe they are looking through a window at some stranger when, in truth, they're looking at themselves in a mirror).

Often, this condition is the result of brain damage, but in some people it appears to be present from birth, without any detectable brain damage (e.g., Duchaine & Nakayama, 2006). Whatever its origin, prosopagnosia seems to imply the existence of special neural structures involved almost exclusively in the recognition and discrimination of faces. Presumably, prosopagnosia results from some damage to (or malfunction in) this brain tissue (Behrman & Avidan, 2005; Burton, Young, Bruce, Johnston, & Ellis, 1991; Damasio, Tranel, & Damasio, 1990; De Renzi, Faglioni, Grossi, & Nichelli, 1991).

Face recognition is also distinctive in another way—in its strong dependence on orientation. We've mentioned that there is debate about whether the recognition of houses, or teacups, or automobiles is viewpoint-dependent, but there can be no question about this issue when we're considering faces. In one study, four categories of stimuli were considered—right-side-up faces, upside-down faces, right-side-up pictures of common objects other than faces, and upside-down pictures of common objects. As can be seen in **Figure 4.15**, performance suffered for all of the upside-down stimuli. However, this effect was much larger for faces than for other kinds of stimuli (Yin, 1969).

The same point can be made informally. **Figure 4.16** shows two upside-down photographs of former British prime minister Margaret Thatcher (from Thompson, 1980). You can probably detect that something is odd about them, but now try turning the book upside down so that the faces are right side up. As you can see, the difference between these faces is immense, and yet this fiendish contrast is largely lost when the faces are upside down.

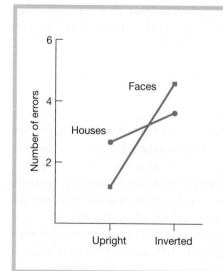

FIGURE 4.15 FACES AND THE INVERSION EFFECT

People's memory for faces is quite good, when compared with memory for other pictures (in this case, pictures of houses). However, performance is very much disrupted when the pictures of faces are inverted. Performance with houses is also worse with inverted pictures, but the effect of inversion is far smaller.   AFTER YIN, 1969.

FIGURE 4.16 PERCEPTION OF UPSIDE-DOWN FACES

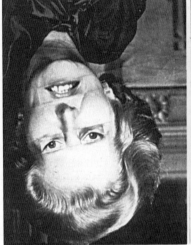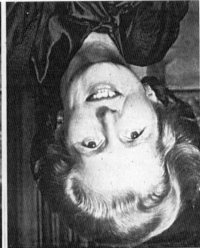

The left-hand picture looks somewhat odd, but the two pictures still look relatively similar to each other. Now, try turning the book upside down (so that the faces are upright). In this position, the left-hand face (now on the right) looks ghoulish, and the two pictures look very different from each other. Perception of upside-down faces is apparently quite different from our perception of upright faces.   FROM THOMPSON, 1980.

Once again, it seems that the perception of faces is strikingly different from other forms of perception, with face perception being more strongly dependent on orientation. (Also see Rhodes, Brake, & Atkinson, 1993; Valentine, 1988.)

Let's pause, though, to acknowledge an ongoing debate. According to some authors, the recognition of faces really is in a category by itself, distinct from all other forms of recognition (e.g., Kanwisher, McDermott & Chun, 1997). Other authors, though, offer a different perspective: They agree that face recognition is special, but they argue that certain other types of recognition, in addition to faces, are special in the same way. As one line of evidence, they argue that prosopagnosia is not just a disorder of *face* recognition. In one case, for example, a prosopagnosic bird-watcher has lost not only the ability to recognize faces but also the ability to distinguish the different types of warblers (Bornstein, 1963; Bornstein, Sroka, & Munitz, 1969). Another patient with prosopagnosia lost the ability to tell cars apart; she is able to locate her car in a parking lot only by reading all the license plates until she finds her own (Damasio, Damasio, & Van Hoesen, 1982).

Likewise, in Chapter 2, we mentioned neuroimaging data showing that a particular brain site—the fusiform face area (FFA)—is specifically responsive to faces. One study, however, suggests that tasks requiring subtle distinctions among birds, or among cars, can also produce high levels of activation in this area (Gauthier, Skudlarski, Gore, & Anderson, 2000; also Bukach, Gauthier, & Tarr, 2006). Thus, the neural tissue "specialized" for faces isn't used *only* for faces. (But, for a response to these findings, see Grill-Spector, Knouf, & Kanwisher, 2004; Weiner & Grill-Spector, 2013).

What should we make of all this? There's no debate that humans do have a specialized recognition system that's crucial for face recognition. This system certainly involves the FFA brain area, and damage to this system causes prosopagnosia. What's controversial is how exactly we should describe this system. According to some authors, this system is truly a *face* recognition system and will be used for other stimuli only if those stimuli happen to be "face-like" (cf. Kanwisher & Yovel, 2006). According to other authors, this specialized system needs to be defined more broadly: The system is used whenever you are trying to recognize specific individuals within a highly familiar category (e.g., Gauthier et al., 2000). The recognition of faces certainly has these traits (and so you are trying to distinguish Fred from George from Jacob within the familiar category of "faces"), but other forms of recognition may have the same traits (e.g., if a bird-watcher is distinguishing different types within the familiar category of "warblers").

The available data do not provide a clear resolution of this debate; both sides of the argument have powerful evidence supporting their view. But, amid these disagreements, let's focus on the key point of agreement: Face recognition is achieved by a process that's different from the process described earlier in this chapter. We need to ask, therefore, how face recognition proceeds.

Holistic Recognition

The networks we have been considering so far all begin with an analysis of a pattern's *parts* (features, geons); the networks then assemble those parts into larger wholes. Face recognition, in contrast, seems not to depend on an inventory of a face's parts; instead, this recognition seems to depend on *holistic perception* of the face. In other words, the recognition depends on complex relationships created by the face's overall configuration—the spacing of the eyes relative to the length of the nose, the height of the forehead relative to the width of the face, and so forth. (For a detailed model of face recognition, see Bruce & Young, 1986, also Duchaine & Nakayama, 2006.)

Of course, a face's features still matter in this holistic process. The key, however, is that the features can't be considered one by one, apart from the context of the face. Instead, the features matter by virtue of the relationships and configurations they create. It's these relationships, and not the features

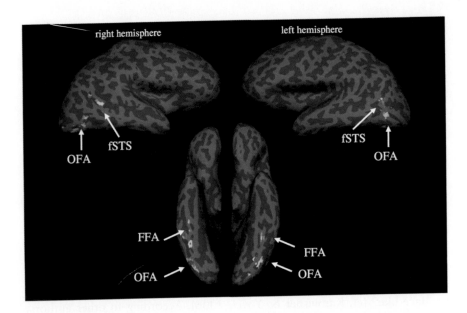

BRAIN AREAS CRUCIAL FOR FACE PERCEPTION

Several brain sites seem to be especially activated when people are looking at faces. These sites include the fusiform face area (FFA), the occipital face area (OFA), and also the superior temporal sulcus (fSTS).

on their own, that guide face recognition (cf. Fitousi, 2013; Rakover, 2013; Rhodes, 2012; Wang, Li, Fang, Tian, & Liu, 2012, but also see Richler & Gauthier, 2014).

Some of the evidence for this holistic processing comes from the *composite effect* in face recognition. In an early demonstration of this effect, Young, Hellawell, and Hay (1987) combined the top half of one face with the bottom half of another, and participants were asked to identify just the top half. This task is difficult if the two halves are properly aligned. In this setting, participants seemed unable to focus only on the top half; instead, they saw the top of the face as part of the whole (see **Figure 4.17A**). Thus, in the figure, it's difficult to see that the top half of the face is Harrison Ford's (shown in normal view in Figure 4.17C). This task is relatively easy, though, if the halves are misaligned (as in Figure 4.17B). Now, the stimulus itself breaks up the configuration, making it possible to view the top half on its own. (For related results, see Amishav & Kimchi, 2010.)

Further work is needed to specify exactly how the configurational system functions. In addition, there are some complications involved in facial recognition—including the fact that processes used for *familiar* faces (ones you've seen over and over) may be different from the processes for faces you've just seen once or twice (Burton, Jenkins, & Schweinberg, 2011). Likewise, people seem to differ in their ability to recognize faces: Some

FIGURE 4.17 THE COMPOSITE EFFECT IN FACE RECOGNITION

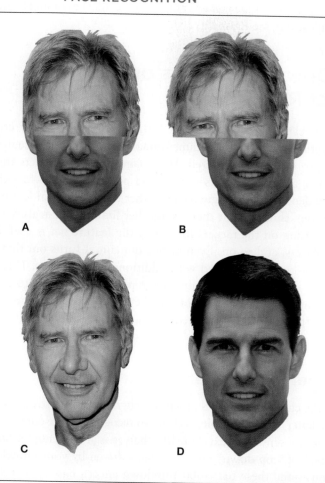

Participants were asked to identify the top half of composite faces like those in Panels A and B. This task was much harder if the halves were properly aligned (as in Panel A), easier if the halves weren't aligned (as in Panel B). With the aligned faces, participants have a difficult time focusing on just the face's top (and so have a hard time recognizing Harrison Ford—shown in Panel C). Instead, they view the face as a whole, and this context changes their perception of Ford's features, making it harder to recognize him. (The bottom of the composite face belongs to Tom Cruise, shown in Panel D.)

people seem to be "super-recognizers," while others edge on prosopagnosia (Bindemann, Brown, Koyas, & Russ, 2012; DeGutis, Wilmer, Mercado, & Cohan, 2013; Russell, Duchaine, & Nakayama, 2009). Plainly, therefore, we have work to do in explaining how we recognize our friends, our family, and our foes—not to mention how we manage to remember and recognize someone we've seen only once before. (For examples of other research on memory for faces, see Jones & Bartlett, 2009; Kanwisher, 2006; Michel, Rossion, Han, Chung, & Caldara, 2006; Rhodes, 2012; for discussion of how these issues play out in the *justice system*, with evidence coming from eyewitness identifications, see Reisberg, 2014.)

Top-Down Influences on Object Recognition

Feature nets can accomplish a great deal, and they are plainly crucial for the recognition of print, three-dimensional objects in our visual environment, and probably sounds as well. At the same time, feature nets are limited, because there are some targets—faces, and perhaps others—for which our recognition depends on configurations, rather than individual features.

It turns out, though, that there is another limit on the feature net, even if we're focusing on the targets for which the feature net *is* useful—print, common objects, and so on. Even in this domain, it turns out that the feature net must be supplemented with additional mechanisms. This requirement doesn't in any way undermine the importance of the feature net idea; the net is plainly needed as part of our theoretical account. The key word, however, is "part," because we need to place the feature net within a larger theoretical frame.

The Benefits of Larger Contexts

Earlier in the chapter, we saw that letter recognition is improved by context, so that the letter *V*, for example, is easier to recognize in the context "VASE," or even the nonsense context "VIMP," than it is if presented alone. These are examples of "top-down" effects—effects driven by your knowledge and expectations—and these particular top-down effects, based on spelling patterns, are easily accommodated by the network: As we have discussed, priming (from recency and frequency of use) guarantees that detectors that have often been used in the past will be easier to activate in the future. In this way, the network "learns" which patterns are common and which are not, and it is more receptive to inputs that follow the usual patterns.

Other top-down effects, however, require a different type of explanation. Consider, for example, the fact that words are easier to recognize if you see them as part of a sentence than they are if you see them in isolation. There are many formal demonstrations of this effect (e.g., Rueckl & Oden, 1986; Spellman, Holyoak, & Morrison, 2001; Tulving & Gold, 1963; Tulving, Mandler, & Baumal, 1964), but for our purposes, an informal example will be sufficient. Imagine that we tell research participants, "I am about to show you a word very briefly on a computer screen; the word is the name of something that you can eat." If we forced the participants to guess the word at this point, they would be unlikely to name the target word. (There are, after all, many things you can eat, and so the chances are slim of guessing just the right one.) But if we now briefly show the word "CELERY," we're likely to observe a large priming effect; that is, participants are more likely to recognize "CELERY" with this cue than they would have been without the cue.

Think about what this priming involves. First, the person needs to understand each of the words in the instruction. If she did not understand the word "eat" (if, for example, she mistakenly thought we had said, "something that you can beat"), we would not get the priming. Second, the person must understand the syntax of the instruction and thus the relations among the words in the instruction. Again, if she mistakenly thought we said "something that can eat you," we would expect a very different sort of priming. Third, the person has to know some facts about the world—namely, the kinds of things that can be eaten; without this knowledge, we would expect no priming.

Obviously, then, this instance of priming relies on a broad range of knowledge, and there is nothing special about this example. We could, after all, observe similar priming effects if we tell someone that the word about to be shown is the name of a historical figure or that the word is related to the Harry Potter books. In each case, this instruction would facilitate perception, with the implication that in explaining these various priming effects we'll need to hook up our object-recognition system to a much broader library of information.

Notice, though, where all of this brings us: Examples like we have just considered tell us that we cannot view object recognition as a self-contained process. Instead, knowledge that is external to object recognition (e.g., knowledge about what is edible) is imported into and clearly influences the process. Put differently, the "CELERY" example (and others as well) does not depend just on the specific stimuli you've encountered recently or frequently. Instead, what is crucial for this sort of priming is what you know coming into the experiment—knowledge derived from a wide range of life experiences.

We have, therefore, reached an important juncture. We have tried in this chapter to examine object recognition in isolation from other cognitive processes, considering how a separate object-recognition module might function, with the module then handing its product (the object it had recognized) on to subsequent processes. We have made good progress in this attempt and have described how a significant piece of object recognition might proceed. But in the end we have run up against a problem—namely, top-down priming that draws on knowledge from outside of object recognition per se. (For neuroscience evidence that word and object recognition interacts with other sorts of information, see Carreiras et al., 2014; also **Figure 4.18**.) This sort of priming depends on what is in memory and on how that knowledge is accessed and used, and so we cannot tackle this sort of priming until we have said a great deal more about memory, knowledge, and thought. We therefore must leave object recognition for now in order to fill in some other pieces of the puzzle. We will have more to say about object recognition in later chapters, once we have some more theoretical machinery in place.

FIGURE 4.18   THE FLOW OF TOP-DOWN PROCESSING

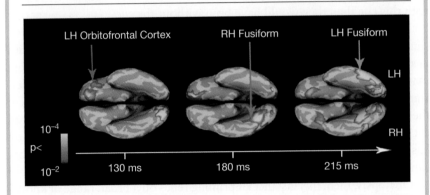

When viewers had only a very brief glimpse of a target object, brain activity indicating top-down processing was evident in the prefrontal cortex 50 ms before activity further back in the brain, indicating successful recognition. This pattern was not evident when object recognition was easy (because of a longer presentation of the target). Sensibly, top-down processing plays a larger role when bottom-up processing is somehow limited or inadequate.

COGNITIVE PSYCHOLOGY AND EDUCATION

Speed-Reading

Students often wish they could read more quickly, and, in fact, it's easy to teach people how to speed-read. It's important to understand, however, how speed-reading works, because this will help you see when speed-reading is a good idea—and when it's a terrible strategy.

In normal reading, there's no need to look at every word on the page. Printed material (like language in general) follows predictable patterns, and so, having read a few words, you're often able to guess what the next words will be. And without realizing you're doing it, you routinely exploit this predictability: you ordinarily skip over many of the words on the page, relying on rapid inference to fill in what you've skipped.

The same process is central for speed-reading. Courses that teach you how to speed-read actually rely on simple strategies that help you to *skip more*, as you move down the page, and, with this, to increase your use of inference. As a result, speed-reading is not really "reading faster"; it is instead "reading *less* and inferring more."

How does this process work? First, before you speed-read some text, you need to lay the groundwork for the inference process—so that you'll make the inferences efficiently and accurately. Specifically, before you speed-read a text, you should flip through it quickly. Look at the figures and the figure captions. If there's a summary at the end or a preview at the beginning, read these. These steps will give you a broad sense of what the material is about, preparing you to make rapid—and sensible—inferences about the material.

Second, you need to make sure you do rely on inference, rather than word-by-word scrutiny of the page. To achieve this, read for a while holding an index card just under the line you're reading, or perhaps using your finger to slide along the line of print to indicate what you are reading at that moment. These procedures establish a physical marker that helps you keep track of where you are as you move from word to word. This use of a pointer will become easy and automatic after a bit of practice, and once it does, you're ready for the key step.

Rather than using the marker to *follow* your eye-position, use the marker to *lead* your eyes. Specifically, try moving the index card or your finger a bit more quickly than you have so far, and try to move your eyes to "keep up" with this marker.

Of course, if you suddenly realize that you don't have a clue what's on the page, then you're trying to go too fast. Just move quickly enough so that you have to hustle along to keep up with your pointer. Don't move so quickly that you lose track of what you're reading.

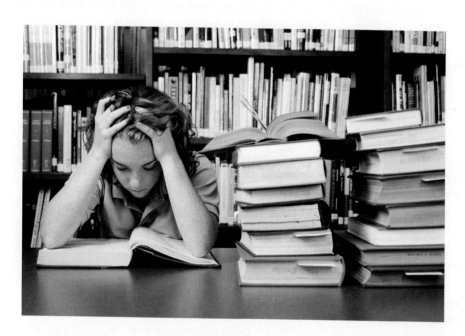

WHEN SHOULD YOU SPEED-READ?

Students are often assigned an enormous amount of reading, and so strategies for speed-reading can be extremely helpful. It is crucial, though, to understand *why* speed-reading works as it does; knowing this will help you decide when speed-reading is appropriate and when it is unwise.

This procedure will feel awkward at first, but it will become easier with some practice, and you'll gradually learn to move the pointer faster and faster. As a result, you'll increase your reading speed by 30%, 40%, or more. But let's be clear about what's going on here: You're simply shifting the balance between how much input you're taking in and how much you're filling in the gaps with sophisticated guesswork. Often, though, this is a fine strategy. Many of the things you read are highly predictable, and so your inferences about the skipped words are likely to be correct. In this setting, you might as well use the faster process of making inferences, rather than the slower process of looking at individual words.

Of course, speed-reading is a bad bet if the material is hard to understand; in that case, you won't be able to figure out the skipped words via inference, and so speed-reading will hurt you. Speed-reading is also a poor choice if you're trying to appreciate an author's style. If, for example, you speed-read Shakespeare's *Romeo and Juliet*, you probably will be able to make inferences about the plot, but you won't be able to make inferences about the specific words you're skipping over, and so you won't be able to make inferences about the *language* that Shakespeare actually used. And, of course, if you miss the language of Shakespeare and miss the poetry, you've missed the point.

Speed-reading will enable you to zoom through many assignments. But do not speed-read material that is technical, filled with details that you'll need, or beautiful for its language. In those cases, what you want is to pay attention to the words on the page and not rely on your own inferences.

chapter summary

- We easily recognize a wide range of objects in a wide range of circumstances. Our recognition is significantly influenced by context, which can determine how or whether we recognize an object. To study these achievements, investigators have often focused on the recognition of printed language, using this case as a microcosm within which to study how object recognition in general might proceed.

- Many investigators have proposed that recognition begins with the identification of features in the input pattern. Crucial evidence for this claim comes from neuroscience studies showing that the detection of features is separate from the processes needed to assemble these features into more complex wholes.

- To study word recognition, investigators often use tachistoscopic presentations. In these studies, words that appear frequently in the language are easier to identify, and so are words that have been recently viewed—an effect known as repetition priming. The data also show a pattern known as the "word-superiority effect"; this refers to the fact that words are more readily perceived than isolated letters. In addition, well-formed nonwords are more readily perceived than letter strings that do not conform to the rules of normal spelling. Another reliable pattern is that recognition errors, when they occur, are quite systematic, with the input typically perceived as being more regular than it actually is. These findings together indicate that recognition is influenced by the regularities that exist in our environment (e.g., the regularities of spelling patterns).

- These results can be understood in terms of a network of detectors. Each detector collects input and fires when the input reaches a threshold level. A network of these detectors can accomplish a great deal; for example, it can interpret ambiguous inputs, recover from its own errors, and make inferences about barely viewed stimuli.

- The feature net seems to "know" the rules of spelling and "expects" the input to conform to these rules. However, this knowledge is distributed across the entire network and emerges only through the network's parallel processing. This setup leads to enormous efficiency in our commerce with the world because it enables us to recognize patterns and objects with relatively little input and under highly diverse circumstances. But these gains come at the cost of occasional error. This trade-off may be necessary, though, if we are to cope with the informational complexity of our world.

- A feature net can be implemented in different ways—with or without inhibitory connections, for example. With some adjustments (e.g., the addition of geon detectors), the net can also recognize three-dimensional objects. However, some stimuli—for example, faces—probably are not recognized through a feature net but instead require a different sort of recognition system, one that is sensitive to relationships and configurations within the stimulus input.

- The feature net also needs to be supplemented to accommodate top-down influences on object recognition. These influences can be detected in the benefits of larger contexts in facilitating recognition and in forms of priming that are plainly concept-driven rather than data-driven. These other forms of priming demand an interactive model that merges bottom-up and top-down processes.

eBook Demonstrations & Essays

Online Demonstrations:
- Demonstration 4.1: Features and Feature Combination
- Demonstration 4.2: The Broad Influence of the Rules of Spelling
- Demonstration 4.3: Inferences in Reading

Online Applying Cognitive Psychology Essays:
- Cognitive Psychology and the Law: Cross-Race Identification

ZAPS 2.0 Cognition Labs

- Go to **http://digital.wwnorton.com/cognition6** for the online labs relevant to this chapter.

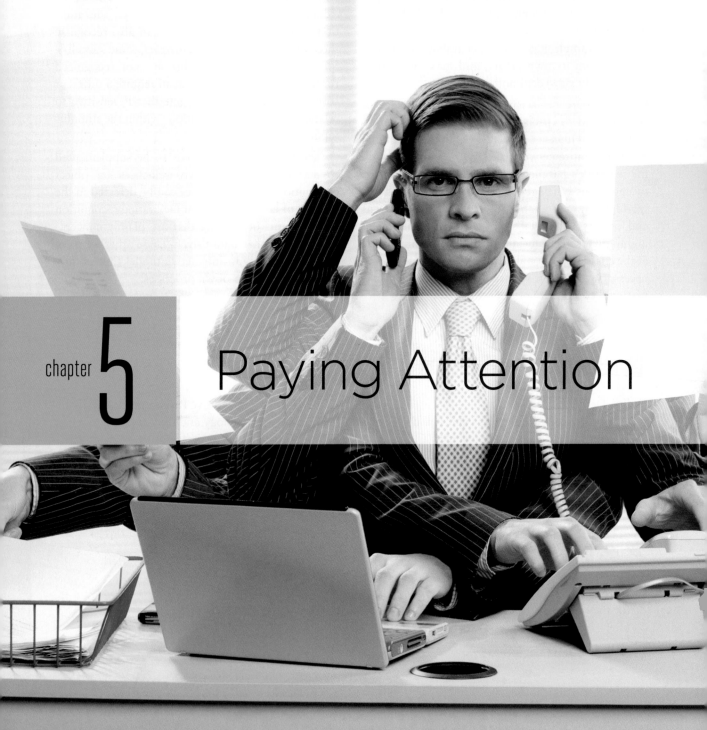

chapter **5** Paying Attention

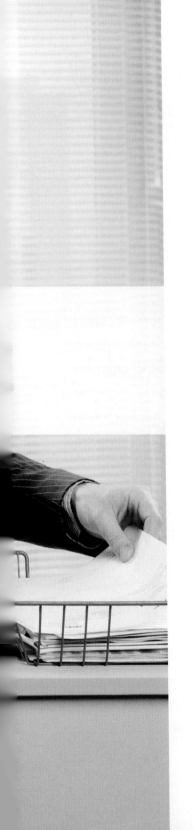

what if...

Right now, you're paying attention to this page, reading these words. But you could, if you chose, pay attention to the other people in the room, or your plans for the weekend, or even, if you wished, the feel of the floor under your feet.

What would your life be like if you couldn't control your attention in this way? Every one of us has, at one point or another, suffered through the maddening experience of being distracted when we're trying to concentrate. For example, there you are on the bus, trying to read your book. You have no interest in the conversation going on in the seats behind you, but you seem unable to shut it out, and so you make no progress at all in your book.

The frustration in this experience is surely fueled, though, by the fact that usually you *can* control your own attention, so that it's especially irritating when you can't focus in the way you want to. The life challenge is much worse, therefore, for people who suffer from *attention deficit disorder*. These individuals are often overwhelmed by the flood of information available to them, and they're unable to focus on just their chosen target. They can have trouble following a conversation and are easily distracted by an unimportant sight or sound in the environment. Even their own thoughts can distract them—and so they can be pulled off track by their own daydreams.

In many cases, people with attention deficit also have problems with hyperactivity and impulsivity—and so they suffer from *attention deficit hyperactivity disorder (ADHD)*. They hop from activity to activity; they're unable to sit still. They're likely to reach out toward (and touch and play with) anything that's in sight. In powerful ways, ADHD reminds us just how important the ability to control your own focus, and to resist distraction, is in everyday life.

The term "ADHD" covers a spectrum of problems, ranging from relatively mild to rather serious. Nothing in this range, however, approaches a far more extreme disruption in attention, termed **unilateral neglect syndrome**. This pattern is generally the result of damage to the parietal

• In this chapter, we argue that multiple mechanisms are involved in the seemingly simple act of paying attention. In other words, people must take many different steps to facilitate the processing of desired inputs; in the absence of these steps, their ability to pick up information from the world is dramatically reduced.

• Many of the steps you take in order to perceive have a "cost" attached to them: They require the commitment of mental resources. These resources are limited in availability, and this is part of the reason you usually cannot pay attention to two inputs at once: Doing so would require more resources than you have.

• Divided attention (the attempt to do two things at once) can also be understood in terms of resources: You can perform two activities at the same time only if the activities do not require more resources than you have available.

• Some of the mental resources you use are specialized, and so they are required only for tasks of a certain sort. Other resources are more general, needed for a wide range of tasks. The resource demand of a task can, however, be diminished through practice.

• We emphasize that attention is best understood not as a process or mechanism but as an *achievement*. Like most achievements, paying attention involves many different elements, all of which help you to be aware of the stimuli you're interested in and not be pulled off track by irrelevant distractors.

cortex, and patients with this syndrome generally ignore all inputs coming from one side of the body. A patient with neglect syndrome will eat food from only one side of the plate, will wash only half of his or her face, and will fail to locate sought-for objects if they're on the neglected side (see Logie, 2012; Sieroff, Pollatsek, & Posner, 1988). Someone with this disorder surely cannot drive a car and, as a pedestrian, is likely to trip over unnoticed obstacles.

This syndrome typically results from damage to the *right* parietal lobe, and so the neglect is for the *left* side of space. (Remember the brain's contralateral organization; see Chapter 2.) Neglect patients will therefore read only the right half of words shown to them: they'll read "threat" as "eat," "parties" as "ties." If asked to draw a clock, they'll likely remember that the numbers from 1 to 12 need to be included, but jam all the numbers into the clock's right side.

All of these observations, then, remind us just how crucial the ability to pay attention is—so that you can focus on the things you want to focus on and not be pulled off track by distraction. But what is "attention"? As we'll see in this chapter, the ability to pay attention involves many independent elements.

Selective Attention

William James is one of the historical giants of our field, and his writing, late in the 19th century, set out many of the key issues that psychology continues to pursue today. James is often quoted in the modern literature, and one of his most famous quotes provides a starting point in this chapter. Roughly 125 years ago, James wrote:

> Everyone knows what attention is. It is the taking possession by the mind, in clear and vivid form, of one out of what seem several simultaneously possible objects or trains of thought. Focalization, concentration, of consciousness are of its essence. It implies withdrawal from some things in order to deal effectively with others, and is a condition which has a real opposite in the confused, dazed, scatterbrained state which in French is called distraction. . . . (James, 1890, pp. 403–404)

In this quote, James describes what attention *achieves,* but what processes or mechanisms produce these effects? What steps do you need to take in order to achieve this "focus," and why is it that the focus "implies withdrawal from some things in order to deal effectively with others"?

Dichotic Listening

Early studies of attention often used a setup called **dichotic listening**: Participants wore headphones and heard one input in the left ear and a different input in the right ear. The participants were instructed to pay attention to one of these inputs—the **attended channel**—and told simply to ignore the message in the other ear—the **unattended channel**.

To make sure participants were paying attention, they were usually given a task called **shadowing**. The attended channel contained a recording of someone speaking, and as participants listened to this speech, they were required to repeat it back, word for word, so that they were, in essence, simply echoing what they heard. Shadowing is initially challenging, but it becomes relatively easy after a minute of practice. (You might try it, shadowing a voice on the radio or TV.)

Participants' shadowing performance is generally close to perfect: They repeat almost 100% of the words they hear. At the same time, however, they hear remarkably little from the unattended channel. If we ask them, after a minute or so of shadowing, to report what the unattended message was about, they indicate that they have no idea at all (see Cherry, 1953, for an early study documenting this point). They can't even tell if the unattended channel contained a coherent message or just random words. In fact, in one study, participants shadowed coherent prose in the attended channel, while in the unattended channel they heard a text in Czech, read with English pronunciation. The individual sounds, therefore (the vowels, the consonants), resembled English, but the message itself was (for an English speaker) gibberish. After a minute of shadowing, only 4 of 30 participants detected the peculiar character of the unattended message (Treisman, 1964).

FIGURE 5.1 THE INVISIBLE GORILLA

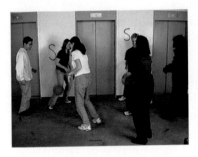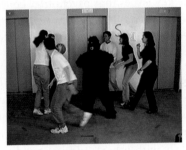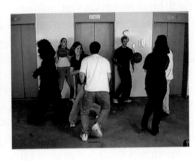

In this experiment, participants were instructed to keep track of the ballplayers in the white shirts. Intent on their task, they were oblivious to what the black-shirted players were doing. They also failed to see the person in the (black) gorilla suit strolling through the scene.   FIGURE PROVIDED BY DANIEL J. SIMONS.

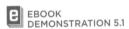 EBOOK
DEMONSTRATION 5.1

More-recent studies have documented a similar pattern with *visual* inputs. Participants in one study watched a TV screen that showed a team of players in white shirts passing a ball back and forth; the participants had to signal each time the ball changed hands. Interwoven with these players (and visible on the same TV screen) was another team, wearing black shirts, also passing a ball back and forth; participants were instructed to ignore these players. Participants easily did this selective task, but they were so intent on the white team that they didn't see other, rather salient, events that also appeared on the screen, right in front of their eyes. For example, they failed to notice when someone wearing a gorilla costume walked through the middle of the game, pausing briefly to thump his chest before exiting. (See **Figure 5.1**; Neisser & Becklen, 1975; Simons & Chabris, 1999; also see Jenkins, Lavie, & Driver, 2005.)

However, people are not altogether oblivious to the unattended channel. In selective listening experiments, they easily and accurately report whether the unattended channel contained human speech, musical instruments, or silence. If the unattended channel actually did contain human speech, they can report whether the speaker was male or female, had a high or low voice, or was speaking loudly or softly. (For reviews of this early work, see Broadbent, 1958; Kahneman, 1973.) Apparently, then, *physical attributes* of the unattended channel are heard, even though participants seem oblivious to the unattended channel's semantic content.

Some Unattended Inputs Are Detected

Some results, however, don't fit this pattern, because some bits of the unattended input do get noticed. In one study, participants were asked to shadow one passage while ignoring a second passage. Embedded within the unattended channel was a series of names, and roughly one third of the participants did hear their own name when it was spoken—even though (just like in other studies) they heard almost nothing else from the unattended input (Moray, 1959).

And it's not just names that can "catch" your attention. Mention of a movie you just saw, or mention of your favorite restaurant, will often be noticed in the unattended channel. More generally, words with some personal importance are often (but not always) noticed, even though the rest of the unattended channel is perceived only as an undifferentiated blur (Conway, Cowan, & Bunting, 2001; Wood & Cowan, 1995).

How can we put all these results together? How can we explain both your general insensitivity to the unattended channel and also the cases in which the unattended channel "leaks through"?

Perceiving and the Limits on Cognitive Capacity

One option for explaining these results focuses on what you do with the *unattended* input. Specifically, the proposal is that you somehow block processing of the inputs you're not interested in, much as a sentry blocks the path of unwanted guests but stands back and does nothing when legitimate guests are in view, allowing them to pass through the gate unimpeded.

This sort of proposal was central for early theories of attention; these theories suggested that you erect a **filter** that shields you from potential distractors. Desired information (the attended channel) is not filtered out and so goes on to receive further processing (Broadbent, 1958). Recent evidence confirms this notion, but also suggests that this filtering is rather specific and occurs on a distractor-by-distractor basis—as if the sentry lacked the broad ability to separate desirable guests in general from undesirable ones. Instead, the sentry seems to have the assignment of blocking specific, already identified gate-crashers. Thus, you seem able to inhibit your response to *this* distractor and do the same for *that* distractor, but these efforts are of little value if some new, unexpected distractor comes along. In that case, you need to develop a new skill aimed specifically at blocking the new intruder (Fenske, Raymond, Kessler, Westoby, & Tipper, 2005; Jacoby, Lindsay, & Hessels, 2003; Tsushima, Sasaki, & Watanabe, 2006; Frings & Wühr, 2014; for a glimpse of some of the brain mechanisms that make ignoring possible, see Payne & Sekuler, 2014).

It seems, then, that the ability to ignore certain distractors—to shut them out—needs to be part of our theory. Other evidence, though, indicates that this is not the whole story. That's because you not only block the processing of distractors, but you are also able to *promote* the processing of *desired* stimuli.

Inattentional Blindness

We saw in Chapters 3 and 4 that perception involves a lot of activity, as you organize and interpret the incoming stimulus information. It seems plausible that this activity would require some initiative and some resources from you—and the evidence suggests that it does.

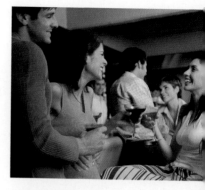

THE COCKTAIL PARTY EFFECT

We have all experienced some version of the so-called cocktail party effect. There you are at a party, engaged in conversation. Other conversations are taking place in the room, but somehow you're able to "tune them out." All you hear is the single conversation you're attending to, plus a buzz of background noise. But now imagine that someone a few steps away from you mentions the name of a close friend of yours. Your attention is immediately caught, and you find yourself listening to that other conversation and (momentarily) oblivious to the conversation you had been engaged in. This experience, easily observed outside the laboratory, is parallel to the pattern of experimental data.

In one experiment, participants were told that they would see large "+" shapes on a computer screen, presented for 200 milliseconds, followed by a pattern mask. (The "mask" is just a meaningless jumble on the screen, designed to interrupt any further processing.) If the horizontal bar of the "+" was longer than the vertical, participants were supposed to press one button; if the vertical bar was longer, they had to press a different button. As a complication, participants weren't allowed to look directly at the "+." Instead, they fixated (pointed their eyes at) a mark in the center of the computer screen—a **fixation target**—and the "+" shapes were shown just off to one side (see **Figure 5.2**).

For the first three trials of the procedure, events proceeded just as the participants expected, and the task was relatively easy. On Trial 3, for example, participants made the correct response 78% of the time. On Trial 4, though, things were slightly different: While the target "+" was on the screen, the fixation target disappeared and was replaced by one of three shapes—a triangle, a rectangle, or a cross. Then, the entire configuration (the "+" target and this new shape) was replaced by the mask.

Immediately after the trial, participants were asked: Was there anything different on this trial? Was anything present, or anything changed, that wasn't there on previous trials? Remarkably, 89% of the participants reported that

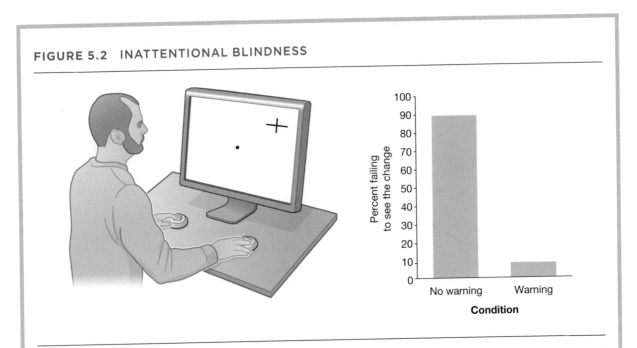

FIGURE 5.2   INATTENTIONAL BLINDNESS

Participants were instructed to point their eyes at the dot and to make judgments about the cross shown just off to the side. However, the dot itself briefly changed to another shape. If participants were not warned about this (and so were not paying attention to the dot), they routinely failed to detect this change—even though they had been pointing their eyes right at the dot the whole time. If participants were warned, though, and therefore alert to possible changes, then virtually all participants detected the change.   AFTER MACK & ROCK, 1998.

there was no change; they had apparently failed to see anything other than the (attended) "+." To probe the participants further, the researchers told them (correctly) that during the previous trial the fixation target had momentarily disappeared and had been replaced by a shape. The participants were then asked what that shape had been and were explicitly given the choices of a triangle, a rectangle, or a cross. The responses to this question were essentially random. Even when probed in this fashion, participants seemed not to have seen the shape that had been directly in front of their eyes (Mack & Rock, 1998; also see Mack, 2003).

What's going on here? Some researchers have proposed that the participants in this experiment did see the target shapes but, a moment later, couldn't *remember* what they'd just seen (e.g., Wolfe, 1999). However, Mack and Rock, the researchers who conducted the study, offer a stronger claim— namely, that the participants literally failed to see the shapes, even though they were staring straight at them. This failure to see, Mack and Rock argue, was caused by the fact that the participants were not expecting any shapes to appear and were not in any way prepared for them. The researchers dubbed this pattern inattentional blindness (Mack & Rock, 1998; also see Mack, 2003; for a similar effect in *hearing*, see Dalton & Fraenkel, 2012).

Which of these accounts is correct? Did participants fail to see the input? Or did they see it but then, just a few milliseconds later, forget what they'd seen? For purposes of theory, this distinction is crucial, but for the moment let's emphasize what the two proposals have in common: By either account, our normal ability to see what's around us, and to make use of what we see, is dramatically diminished in the absence of attention.

There's more to be said about these issues, but before we press on, let's note the important "real-world" implications of these findings. Chabris and Simons (2010) call attention to the reports of traffic accidents in which (for example) a driver says, "I never saw the bicyclist! He came out of nowhere! But then— suddenly—there he was, right in front of me." Drew, Võ, and Wolfe (2013) showed that experienced radiologists often miss obvious anomalies in a patient's CT scan, even though they're looking right at the anomaly. Or, as a much more mundane case, you go to the refrigerator to find the mayonnaise (or the ketchup or the juice), and fail to find it, even though it is directly in front of you.

In these cases, we lament the neglectful driver and the careless radiologist. Your inability to find the mayonnaise may cause you to worry that you're losing your mind as well as your condiments. The response to all this, though, is to realize that these cases of failing-to-see are entirely normal. Perception requires more than "merely" having a stimulus in front of your eyes. Perception requires some work.

Change Blindness

The active nature of perception is also evident in studies of change blindness— observers' inability to detect changes in scenes they're looking directly at. In some experiments, participants are shown pairs of pictures separated by a brief blank interval (e.g., Rensink, O'Regan, & Clark, 1997). The pictures

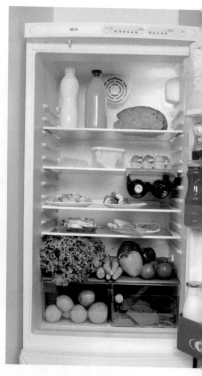

INATTENTIONAL BLINDNESS OUTSIDE THE LAB

Inattentional blindness is usually demonstrated in the laboratory, but it has a number of real-world counterparts. Most people, for example, have experienced the peculiar situation in which they are unable to find the mayonnaise in the refrigerator (or the ketchup or the salad dressing) even though they are staring right at the bottle. This is a situation in which the person is so absorbed in thoughts about other matters that he or she becomes blind to an otherwise salient stimulus.

FIGURE 5.3 CHANGE BLINDNESS

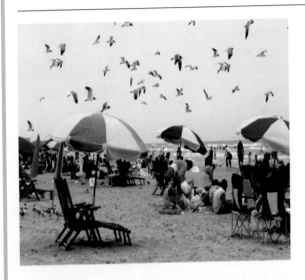
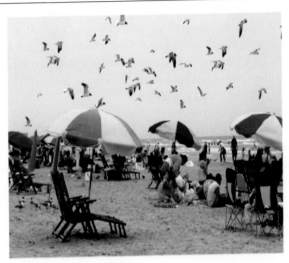
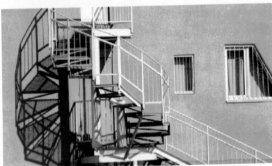
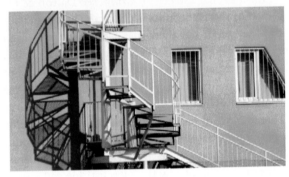

In some change-blindness demonstrations, participants see one picture, then a second, then the first again, then the second, and must spot the difference between the two pictures. Here, we've displayed the pictures side by side, rather than putting them in alternation. Can you find the differences? For most people, it takes a surprising amount of time and effort to locate the differences—even though some of the differences are quite large. Apparently, therefore, having a stimulus directly in front of your eyes is no guarantee that you will perceive the stimulus.

in each pair are identical except for some single aspect: an "extra" engine shown on the airplane in one picture and not in the other; a man not wearing a hat in one picture but wearing one in the other; and so on (see **Figure 5.3**). Participants know from the start that their task is to detect these changes, but even so, the task is difficult. If the change involves something central to the scene, observers may need as many as a dozen alternations between the pictures before they detect the change. If the change involves some peripheral aspect of the scene, as many as 25 alternations may be required.

A related pattern emerges when participants watch videos. In one study, observers watched a movie of two women having a conversation. The camera

EBOOK
DEMONSTRATION 5.2

FIGURE 5.4   CHANGE BLINDNESS

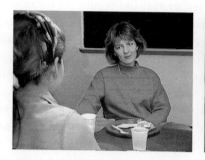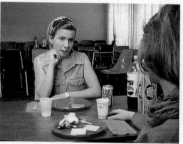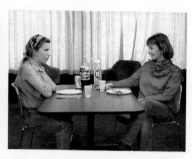

In this video, every time there was a shift in camera angle, there was a change in the scene—so that the woman in the red sweater abruptly gained a scarf, the plates that had been red were suddenly white, and so on. When viewers watched the video, though, they noticed none of these changes.

first focused on one woman, then on the other, just as it would in an ordinary TV show or movie. The crucial element of this experiment, though, was that aspects of the scene changed every time the camera angle changed. For example, when the camera was pointing at Woman A, you could plainly see the red plates on the table between the women. When the camera was shifted to point at Woman B just a fraction of a second later, Woman A inexplicably has a scarf (see **Figure 5.4**). Most observers, however, noticed none of these changes (D. T. Levin & Simons, 1997; Shore & Klein, 2000; Simons & Rensink, 2005).

Incredibly, the same pattern can be documented with live (i.e., not filmed) events. In a remarkable study, an investigator (let's call him "Leon") approached pedestrians on a college campus and asked for directions to a certain building. During the conversation, two men carrying a door approached and deliberately walked *between* Leon and the research participant. As a result, Leon was momentarily hidden (by the door) from the participant's view, and in that moment Leon traded places with one of the men carrying the door. A second later, therefore, Leon was able to walk away, unseen, while the new fellow (who had been carrying the door) stayed behind and continued the conversation with the participant.

Roughly half of the participants failed to notice this switch. They continued the conversation as though nothing had happened—despite the fact that Leon and his replacement were wearing different clothes and had easily distinguishable voices. When asked directly whether anything odd had happened in this event, many participants commented only that it was rude that the guys carrying the door had walked right through their conversation (Simons & Ambinder, 2005; Chabris & Simons, 2010). (For other studies of change blindness, see Most et al., 2001; Rensink, 2002; Seegmiller, Watson, & Strayer, 2011. For similar effects with auditory stimuli, see Gregg & Samuel, 2008; Vitevitch, 2003.)

Early versus Late Selection

In several paradigms, then, it's clear that people are oblivious to stimuli directly in front of their eyes—whether the stimuli are simple displays on a computer screen, photographs, movies, or real-life events. As we've said, though, there are two ways we might think about these results: These studies may reveal genuine limits on *perception*, so that participants literally don't see these stimuli; or these studies may reveal limits on *memory*, so that people do see the stimuli but immediately forget what they've just seen.

Which proposal is correct? One approach to this question hinges on *when* the perceiver selects the desired input and (correspondingly) when the perceiver ceases the processing of the unattended input. According to the **early selection** hypothesis, the attended input is privileged from the start, so that the unattended input receives little (maybe even zero?) analysis (and so is never perceived). According to the **late selection** hypothesis, all inputs receive relatively complete analysis, and the selection occurs after the analysis is finished. Perhaps the selection occurs just before the stimuli reach consciousness, and so we become aware only of the attended input.

FIGURE 5.5   UNCONSCIOUS PERCEPTION

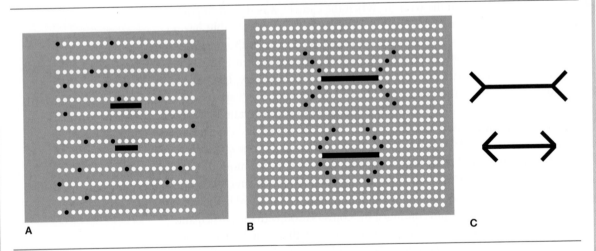

One study, apparently showing "late selection," indicated that participants perceived (and were influenced) by background material, even though the participants had not consciously perceived this material. Specifically, participants in this study were shown a series of images, each containing a pair of horizontal lines; their task was to decide which of the two lines was longer. For the first three trials, the background dots in the display were arranged randomly (Panel A). For the fourth trial, the dots were arranged as shown in Panel B, roughly reproducing the configuration of the Müller-Lyer illusion; Panel C shows the standard form of this illusion. The participants in this study did not perceive the "fins" consciously, but they were nonetheless influenced by the fins—judging the top horizontal line in Panel B to be longer, fully in accord with the usual misperception of this illusion.

Or perhaps the selection occurs later still—so that all inputs make it (briefly) into consciousness, but then the selection occurs, so that only the attended input is remembered.

It turns out that each hypothesis captures part of the truth. On the one side, there are cases in which people seem unaware of distractors but are nevertheless influenced by them—so that the (apparently unnoticed) distractors guide the interpretation of the attended stimuli (e.g., Moore & Egeth, 1997; see **Figure 5.5**). This seems a case of *late selection*: The distractors are perceived (so that they do have an influence) but are selected out before they make it to consciousness. On the other side, though, we can also find evidence for *early selection*, with distractor stimuli falling out of the stream of processing at a very early stage. Relevant evidence comes, for example, from studies that record the electrical activity of the brain in the milliseconds (ms) after a stimulus has arrived. These studies confirm that the brain activity for attended inputs is distinguishable from that for unattended inputs just 80 ms or so after the stimulus presentation—a time interval in which early sensory processing is still under way (Hillyard, Vogel, & Luck, 1998). Apparently, in these cases, the attended input is privileged from the start (see **Figure 5.6**).

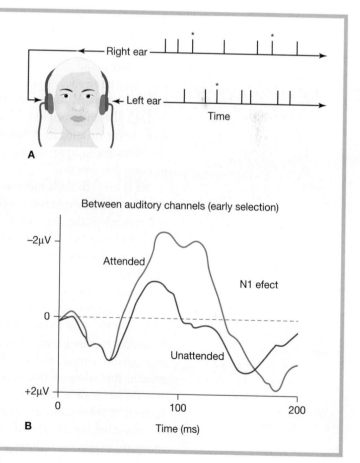

FIGURE 5.6 EVIDENCE FOR EARLY SELECTION

Participants were instructed to pay attention to the signals arriving in one ear, but to ignore signals in the other ear (Panel A). During this task, researchers monitored the electrical activity in the participants' brains, with a special focus on a brain wave termed the N1 (so called because the wave reflects a negative voltage roughly 100 ms after the target). As can be seen in Panel B, the N1 effect is different for the attended and unattended inputs within 80 ms of the target's arrival—indicating that the attended and unattended inputs are processed differently from a very early stage.

Other data also provide evidence for early selection. For example, recordings from neurons in Area V4 of the visual cortex show that these neurons are more responsive to attended inputs than to unattended ones (Carrasco, Ling, & Read, 2004; Carrasco, Penpeci-Talgar, & Eckstein, 2000; McAdams & Reid, 2005; Reynolds, Pasternak, & Desimone, 2000; also see O'Connor, Fukui, Pinsk, & Kastner, 2002; Yantis, 2008). These results suggest that attention doesn't just change what we remember or what we're aware of. Attention can literally change what we perceive.

Selective Priming

Whether selection is early or late, though, it's clear that people often fail to see stimuli that are directly in front of them, in plain view. But what exactly is the obstacle here? Why *don't* people perceive these stimuli?

In Chapter 4, we proposed that recognition requires a network of detectors, and we argued that these detectors fire most readily, and most quickly, if they're suitably primed. In some cases, the priming is produced by your visual experience—specifically, whether each detector has been used recently or frequently in the past. But we suggested at the end of Chapter 4 that priming can also come from another source: your expectations about what the stimulus will be.

The proposal, then, is that you can literally prepare yourself for perceiving by priming the relevant detectors. In other words, you somehow "reach into" the network and deliberately activate just those detectors that, you believe, will soon be needed. Then, once primed in this fashion, those detectors will be on "high alert" and ready to fire.

Let's also suppose that this priming isn't "free." Instead, you need to spend some effort or allocate some resources in order to do the priming, and these resources are in limited supply. As a result, there is a limit on just how much priming you can do.

We'll need to flesh out this proposal in several ways, but even so, we can already use it to explain some of the findings we've already met. Why don't participants notice the shapes in the inattentional blindness studies? The answer lies in the fact that they don't expect any stimulus to appear, so they have no reason to prepare for any stimulus. As a result, the stimulus, when it's presented, falls on unprepared (thus, unprimed, unresponsive) detectors. The detectors therefore don't respond to the stimulus, so participants end up not perceiving the stimulus.

What about selective listening? In this case, you've been instructed to *ignore* the unattended input, and so you have no reason to devote any resources to this input. Hence, the detectors needed for the distractor message are unprimed, and this literally makes it more difficult to hear the distractor. But why, on this account, does attention sometimes "leak," so that you do hear some aspects of the unattended input? Think about what will happen if your name is uttered on the unattended channel. The detectors for this stimulus are already primed, but this is not because you are, at that moment, expecting to hear your name. Instead, the detectors for your name are primed simply because this is a stimulus you've often encountered in the past. Thanks to this prior exposure, the activation level of these detectors is already high; you don't need to prime them further. So these detectors will fire even if your attention is elsewhere.

Two Types of Priming

The idea before us, in short, has three elements. First, perception is vastly facilitated by the *priming* of relevant detectors. Second, the priming is sometimes stimulus-driven—that is, produced by the stimuli you've encountered (recently or frequently) in the past. This type of priming takes no effort on your part and requires no resources. This is the sort of priming that enables you to hear your name on the unattended channel. But third, a different sort of priming is also possible. This priming is expectation-driven and is under your control: Specifically, you can deliberately prime detectors for inputs you think are upcoming, so that you're ready for those inputs when they arrive. You don't do this priming for inputs you have no interest in, and you *can't* do this priming for inputs you can't anticipate.

Can we test these claims? In a classic series of studies, Posner and Snyder (1975) gave people a straightforward task: A pair of letters was shown on a computer screen, and participants had to decide, as swiftly as they could, whether the letters were the same or different. So someone might see "AA" and answer "same" or might see "AB" and answer "different."

Before each pair, participants saw a warning signal. In the neutral condition, the warning signal was a plus sign ("+"). This signal notified participants that the stimuli were about to arrive but provided no other information. In a different condition, the warning signal was itself a letter and actually matched the stimuli to come. So someone might see the warning signal "G" followed by the pair "GG." In this case, the warning signal served to prime the participants for the stimuli. In a third condition, though, the warning signal was misleading. The warning signal was again a letter, but it was a letter different from the stimuli to come. Participants might see "H" followed by the pair "GG." Let's consider these three conditions *neutral*, *primed*, and *misled*.

In this simple task, accuracy rates are very high, but in addition Posner and Snyder recorded how *quickly* people responded. By comparing these **response times (RTs)** in the *primed* and *neutral* conditions, we can ask what benefit there is from the prime. Likewise, by comparing RTs in the *misled* and *neutral* conditions, we can ask what cost there is, if any, from being misled.

Before we turn to the results, though, we need one further complication: Posner and Snyder ran this procedure in two different versions. In one version, the warning signal was an excellent predictor of the upcoming stimuli: For example, if the warning signal was an *A*, there was an 80% chance that the upcoming stimulus pair would contain *A*'s. In Posner and Snyder's terms, the warning signal provided a "high validity" prime. In a different version of the procedure, the warning signal was a poor predictor of the upcoming stimuli: If the warning signal was an *A*, there was only a 20% chance that the upcoming pair would contain *A*'s. This is the "low validity" condition (see **Table 5.1**).

TABLE 5.1 DESIGN OF POSNER AND SNYDER'S EXPERIMENT

		TYPICAL SEQUENCE		Provides Repetition Priming?	Provides Basis for Expectation?
	Type of Trial	Warning Signal	Test Stimuli		
Low-validity Condition	Neutral	+	AA	No	No
	Primed	G	GG	Yes	No
	Misled	H	GG	No	No
High-validity Condition	Neutral	+	AA	No	No
	Primed	G	GG	Yes	Prime leads to correct expectation
	Misled	H	GG	No	Prime leads to incorrect expectation

In the low-validity condition, misled trials occurred four times as often as primed trials (80% versus 20%). Therefore, participants had no reason to trust the primes and, correspondingly, no reason to generate an expectation based on the primes. In the high-validity condition, things were reversed: Now, *primed* trials occurred four times as often as *misled* trials. Therefore, participants had good reason to trust the primes and good reason to generate an expectation based on the prime.

Let's consider the low-validity condition first, and let's focus on those rare occasions in which the prime did match the subsequent stimuli. That is, we're focusing on 20% of the trials and ignoring the other 80% for the moment. In this condition, the participant can't use the prime as a basis for predicting the stimuli because, after all, the prime is a poor indicator of things to come. Therefore, the prime should not lead to any specific expectations. Nonetheless, we do expect faster RTs in the *primed* condition than in the *neutral* condition. Why? Thanks to the prime, the relevant detectors have just fired, and so the detectors should still be warmed up. When the target stimuli arrive, therefore, the detectors should fire more readily, allowing a faster response.

The results bear this out. RTs were reliably faster (by roughly 30 ms) in the *primed* condition than in the *neutral* condition (see **Figure 5.7**, left side). Apparently, then, detectors can be primed by mere exposure to a stimulus. Or, put differently, priming is observed even in the absence of expectations. This priming, therefore, seems truly stimulus-based.

What about the *misled* condition? With a low-validity prime, misleading the participants had no effect: Performance in the *misled* condition was the same as performance in the *neutral* condition. Priming the "wrong" detector, it seems, takes nothing away from the other detectors—including the detectors actually needed for that trial. This fits with our discussion in Chapter 4: Each of the various detectors works independently of the others, and so priming one detector obviously influences the functioning of that specific detector but neither helps nor hinders the other detectors.

Let's look next at the high-validity primes. In this condition, people might see, for example, a "J" as the warning signal and then the stimulus pair "JJ."

FIGURE 5.7 THE EFFECTS OF PRIMING ON
STIMULUS PROCESSING

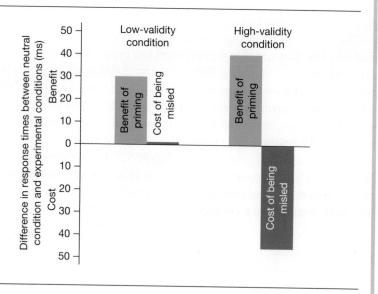

As one way of assessing the Posner and Snyder (1975) results, we can subtract the response times for the neutral condition from those for the primed
condition; in this way, we measure the benefits of priming. Likewise, we can
subtract the response times for the neutral condition from those for the misled
condition; in this way, we measure the costs of being misled. In these terms,
the low-validity condition shows a small benefit (from repetition priming) but
zero cost from being misled. The high-validity condition, in contrast, shows a
larger benefit—but also a substantial cost. The results shown here reflect trials
with a 300 ms interval between the warning signal and the test stimuli; the
results were somewhat different at other intervals.

Presentation of the prime itself will fire the *J*-detectors, and this should, once
again, "warm up" these detectors, just as the low-validity primes did. Thus, we
expect a stimulus-driven benefit from the prime. However, the high-validity
primes may also have another influence: High-validity primes are excellent
predictors of the stimulus to come. Participants are told this at the outset, and
they have lots of opportunity to see that it is true. High-validity primes will
therefore produce a warm-up effect *and also* an expectation effect, whereas
low-validity primes produce only the warm-up. We should therefore expect
the high-validity primes to help participants more than low-validity primes—
and that's exactly what the data show (Figure 5.7, right side). The combination of warm-up and expectations, in other words, leads to faster responses
than warm-up alone. From the participants' point of view, it pays to know
what the upcoming stimulus might be.

Explaining the Costs and Benefits

Thus, we need to distinguish two types of primes. One type is stimulus-based—produced merely by presentation of the priming stimulus, with no role for expectations. The other type is expectation-based and is created only when the participant believes the prime allows a prediction of what's to come.

These types of primes can be distinguished in various ways, including the biological mechanisms that support them (see **Figure 5.8**; Corbetta & Shulman, 2002; Hahn, Ross, & Stein, 2006) and also a difference in what they "cost." Stimulus-based priming appears to be "free," and so we can prime one detector without taking anything away from other detectors. (We saw this in the low-validity condition, in the fact that the *misled* trials lead to responses just as fast as those in the *neutral* trials.) Expectation-based priming, in contrast, does have a cost, and we see this in an aspect of Figure 5.7 that we've not yet mentioned: With high-validity primes, responses in the *misled* condition were slower than responses in the *neutral* condition. That is, misleading the participants actually hurt performance. As a concrete example, *F*-detection was slower if *G* was

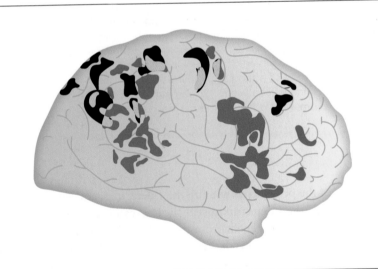

FIGURE 5.8   BIOLOGICAL MECHANISMS FOR THE TWO TYPES OF PRIMING

The text argues that there are two types of priming—one that is stimulus-based and one that is expectation-based. Evidence suggests that these two types depend on activity in distinct brain areas. Sites shown in black have been identified in various studies as involved in expectation-based (sometimes called "goal directed") attention; sites shown in blue have been implicated in "stimulus-driven" attention; and sites shown in gray have been identified as involved in both types of attention.

primed, compared to *F*-detection when the prime was simply the neutral warning signal ("+"). Put more broadly, it seems that priming the "wrong" detector takes something away from the other detectors, and so participants are worse off when they're misled than when they received no prime at all.

What produces this cost? As an analogy, let's say that you have just $50 to spend on groceries. You can spend more on ice cream if you wish, but if you do, you'll have that much less to spend on other foods. Any increase in the ice cream allotment must be covered by a decrease somewhere else. This trade-off arises, though, only because of the limited budget. If you had unlimited funds, you could spend more on ice cream and still have enough money for everything else.

Expectation-based priming shows the same pattern. If the *Q*-detector is primed, this takes something away from the other detectors. Getting prepared for one target seems to make people less prepared for other targets. But we just said that this sort of pattern implies a limited "budget." If an unlimited supply of activation were available, you could prime the *Q*-detector and leave the other detectors just as they were. And that is the point: Expectation-based priming, by virtue of revealing costs when misled, reveals the presence of a **limited-capacity system**.

We can now put the pieces together. Ultimately, we need to explain the facts of selective attention, including the fact that while listening to one message you hear little content from other messages. To explain this, we've proposed that perceiving involves some work, and this work requires some limited mental resources. That is why you can't listen to two messages at the same time; doing so would require more resources than you have. And now, finally, we're seeing evidence for those limited resources: The Posner and Snyder research (and many other results) reveals the workings of a limited-capacity system, just as our hypothesis demands.

Chronometric Studies and Spatial Attention

The Posner and Snyder study shows us that your expectations about an upcoming stimulus can influence the processing of that stimulus. But what exactly is the nature of these expectations? How precise or vague are they?

As one way of entering this issue, imagine that participants in a study are told, "The next stimulus will be a *T*." In this case, they know exactly what to get ready for. But now imagine that participants are told, "The next stimulus will be a letter" or "The next stimulus will be on the left side of the screen." Will these cues allow people to prepare themselves?

These issues have been examined in studies of **spatial attention**—that is, the ability to focus on a particular position in space and, thus, to be better prepared for any stimulus that appears in that position. In an early study, Posner, Snyder, and Davidson (1980) required their participants simply to detect letter presentations; the task was just to press a button as soon as a letter appeared. Participants kept their eyes pointed at a central fixation mark, and letters could appear either to the left or to the right of this mark.

For some trials, a neutral warning signal was presented, so that participants knew a trial was about to start but had no information about stimulus location. For other trials, an arrow was used as the warning signal. Sometimes the arrow pointed left, sometimes right; and the arrow was generally an accurate predictor of the location of the stimulus-to-come: If the arrow pointed right, the stimulus would be on the right side of the computer screen. (In the terms we used earlier, this is a high-validity cue.) On 20% of the trials, however, the arrow misled participants about location.

The results show a familiar pattern (Posner et al., 1980). With high-validity priming, the data show a benefit from cues that correctly signal where the upcoming target will appear. The differences between conditions aren't large (a few hundredths of a second), but keep the task in mind: All participants had to do was detect the input. Even with the simplest of tasks, it pays to be prepared (see **Figure 5.9**).

What about the trials in which participants were misled? RTs in this condition were about 12% slower than those in the neutral condition. Once again, therefore, we're seeing evidence of a limited-capacity system: In order to devote more attention to (say) the left position, you have to devote *less*

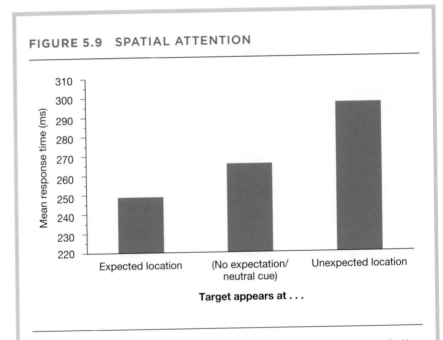

FIGURE 5.9 SPATIAL ATTENTION

In the Posner et al. (1980) study, participants simply had to press a button as soon as they saw the target. If participants knew where the target would appear, they were slightly faster (although the procedure prevented them from moving their eyes to this target location). If, however, participants were misled about the target's position (so that the target appeared in an unexpected location), their responses were slower than they were when the participants had no expectations at all.

attention to the right. If the stimulus then shows up on the right, you're less prepared for it—hence, the cost of being misled.

Attention as a Spotlight

Studies of spatial attention suggest to some psychologists that visual attention can be compared to a spotlight beam that can "shine" anywhere in the visual field. The "beam" marks the region of space for which you are prepared, so inputs within the beam are processed more efficiently. The beam can be wide or narrowly focused (see **Figure 5.10**), and it can be moved about at will as you explore (attend to) one aspect of the visual field or another.

FIGURE 5.10 ADJUSTING THE "BEAM" OF ATTENTION

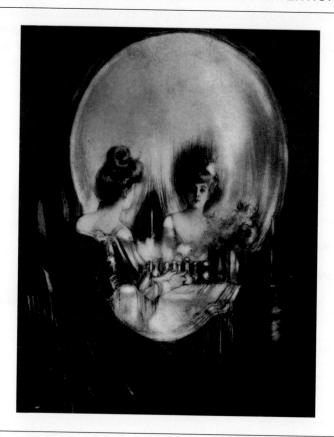

Charles Allan Gilbert's painting *All Is Vanity* can be perceived either as a woman at her dressing table or as a human skull. As you shift from one of these perceptions to the other, you need to adjust the spotlight beam of attention—to a narrow beam to see details (e.g., to see the woman) or to a wider beam to see the whole scene (e.g., to see the skull).

Let's emphasize, though, that the spotlight idea is referring to movements of *attention*, not movements of the eyes. Of course, eye movements do play an important role in your selection of information from the world: If you want to learn more about something, you generally look at it. (For more on how you move your eyes to explore a scene, see Henderson, 2013.) Even so, movements of the eyes can be separated from movements of attention, and it's attention, not the eyes, that's moving around in the Posner et al. study. We know this because of the timing of the effects: Eye movements are surprisingly slow, requiring 180 to 200 ms. But the benefits of primes can be detected within the first 150 ms after the priming stimulus is presented. Thus, the benefits of attention occur *prior to* any eye movement, so they cannot be a consequence of eye movements.

But what does it mean to "move attention?" Obviously, the spotlight beam is just a metaphor, and so we need to ask what's really going on in the brain to produce these effects. Evidence suggests that the control of attention actually depends on a network of brain sites in the frontal cortex and parietal cortex. According to one proposal (Posner & Rothbart, 2007; see **Figure 5.11**), one cluster of sites (the *orienting* system) is needed to disengage attention

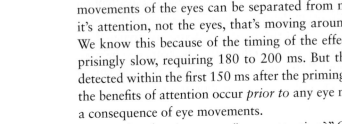

EBOOK
DEMONSTRATION 5.3

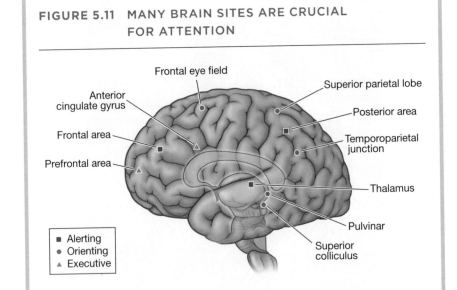

FIGURE 5.11   MANY BRAIN SITES ARE CRUCIAL
FOR ATTENTION

Frontal eye field
Anterior cingulate gyrus
Superior parietal lobe
Posterior area
Frontal area
Temporoparietal junction
Prefrontal area
Thalamus
Pulvinar
Superior colliculus

■ Alerting
● Orienting
▲ Executive

Many brain sites are important for controlling attention. Some brain sites play a pivotal role in "alerting" the brain, so that it is ready for an upcoming event. Other sites play a key role in "orienting" attention, so that you're focused on this position or that, on one target or another. Still other sites are crucial for controlling the brain's "executive" function—a function we'll discuss further, later in the chapter.   AFTER POSNER & ROTHBART, 2007.

from one target, shift attention to a new target, and then engage attention on the new target. A second set of sites (the *alerting* system) is responsible for achieving and maintaining an alert state in the brain. A third set of sites (the *executive* system) controls voluntary actions.

Notice that these points echo a theme we first met in Chapter 2. There, we argued that most of our cognitive capacities depend on the coordinated activity of multiple brain regions, with each region providing a specialized process necessary for the overall achievement. As a result, a problem in *any* of these regions can disrupt the overall capacity, and if there are problems in *several* regions, the disruption can be substantial.

As an illustration of this interplay between brain sites and symptoms, consider a disorder we mentioned at the start of this chapter—ADHD. **Table 5.2** summarizes a recent proposal about ADHD. Symptoms of this disorder are listed in the left column, grouped according to the cognitive processes leading to that symptom. The right column then identifies brain areas that may be the main source of each problem. Let's be clear, though, that the proposal shown in the table is not the only way to think about ADHD; nonetheless,

TABLE 5.2 ATTENTION-DEFICIT/HYPERACTIVITY DISORDER SYMPTOMS, COGNITIVE PROCESSES, AND NEURAL NETWORKS

Symptom Domains	Neural Networks
Problems in the "Alerting" system	
Has difficulty sustaining attention	Right frontal cortex
Fails to finish	Right posterior parietal
Avoids sustained efforts	Locus ceruleus
Problems in the "Orienting" system	
Is distracted by stimuli	Bilateral parietal
Does not appear to listen	Superior colliculus
Fails to pay close attention	Thalamus
Problems in the "Executive" system	
Blurts out answers	Anterior cingulate
Interrupts or intrudes	Left lateral frontal
Cannot wait	Basal ganglia

Earlier in the chapter, we mentioned the problem known as ADHD. The table summarizes a recent proposal about this disorder, linking the symptoms of ADHD to the three broad processes described in the text (Swanson, Posner, Cantwell, Wigal, Crinella, Filipek, Emerson, Tuckiker, & Nalcioglu, 2000; for a somewhat different proposal, though, see Barkley, Murphy, & Fischer, 2008). ZILLMER ET AL., p. 328.

FIGURE 5.12 SELECTIVE ATTENTION ACTIVATES THE VISUAL CORTEX

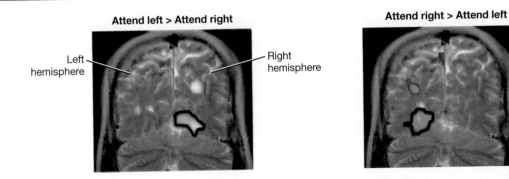

The brain sites that *control* attention are separate from the brain sites that do the actual analysis of the input. Thus, the intention to attend to, say, stimuli on the left is implemented through the many brain sites shown in Figure 5.11. However, these sites collectively activate a different set of sites—in the visual cortex—to promote the actual processing of the incoming stimulus. Shown here are activity levels in a single participant (measured through fMRI scans) overlaid on a structural image of the brain (obtained through MRI scans). Bear in mind that, because of the brain's contralateral organization, the intention to pay attention to the left side of space requires activation in the right hemisphere; the intention to pay attention to the right requires activation in the left.

the proposal illustrates the complex, many-part relationship between overall function (in this case: the ability to pay attention) and brain anatomy.

In all cases, though, these sites should be understood as forming the control systems for attention. To implement these controls, neural connections from all of these areas send activity to other brain regions (like the visual areas in the occipital cortex) that do the actual analysis of the incoming information (see **Figure 5.12**). In this way, expectations (based on your goals and the information you've received so far) are supported by one group of brain areas and are used to modulate activity in other areas directly responsible for handling the input (Corbetta & Shulman, 2002; Hampshire, Duncan, & Owen, 2007; Hon, Epstein, Owen, & Duncan, 2006; Hung, Driver, & Walsh, 2005; Miller & Cohen, 2001; for parallel arguments for how you pay attention to your own *memories*, see Cabeza, Ciaramelli, Olson, & Moscovitch, 2008).

Thus, there is no spotlight beam. Instead, neural mechanisms are in place that enable you to adjust your sensitivity to certain inputs. This is, of course, entirely in line with the proposal we're developing—namely, that a large part of "paying attention" involves priming: For stimuli you don't care about, you don't bother to prime yourself, and so those stimuli fall on unprepared (and unresponsive) detectors. For stimuli you do care about, you do your best to anticipate the input, and then you use these anticipations to prime the relevant processing channel. This increases your sensitivity to the desired input, which is of course just what you want.

Attending to Objects or Attending to Positions

Although it's just a metaphor, the spotlight beam is a useful way to think about attention. (For further discussion of the spotlight notion, see Cave, 2013; Rensink, 2012; Wright & Ward, 2008; but also Awh & Pashler, 2000; Morawetz, Holz, Baudewig, Treue, & Dechent, 2007.) But the comparison to a spotlight raises a new question. Think about how an actual spotlight works. If, for example, a spotlight shines on a donut, then part of the beam will fall on the donut's hole and so illuminate the plate underneath the donut. Similarly, if the beam isn't aimed quite accurately, it may also illuminate the plate just to the left of the donut. The region illuminated by the beam, in other words, is defined purely in spatial terms: a circle of light at a particular position. That circle may or may not line up with the boundaries of the object you're shining the beam on.

Is this how attention works—so that you pay attention to whatever it is that falls in a certain region of space? In this case, you might on some occasions end up paying attention to part of this object, part of that. An alternative is that you pay attention to *objects* rather than to *positions in space*. To continue the example, the target of your attention might be the donut itself rather than the donut's location. In that case, the plate just to the left and the bit of plate visible through the donut's hole might be close to your focus, but they aren't part of the attended object and so aren't attended.

Which is the correct view of attention? Do you pay attention to regions in space, whatever the objects (or parts of objects) are that fall in that region? Or do you pay attention to objects? It turns out that each view captures part of the truth.

One line of evidence comes from the study of people we mentioned at the chapter's start—people who suffer from unilateral neglect syndrome (see **Figure 5.13**). Taken at face value, the symptoms shown by these patients

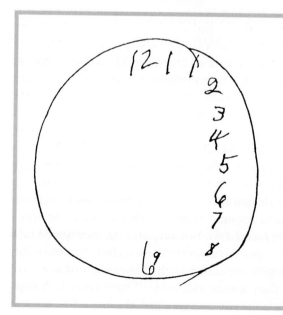

FIGURE 5.13   NEGLECT SYNDROME

A patient with damage to the right parietal cortex was asked to draw a typical clock face. In his drawing, the patient seemed unaware of the left side, but he still recalled that all 12 numbers had to be displayed. The drawing shows how he resolved this dilemma.

FIGURE 5.14 SPACE-BASED OR OBJECT-BASED ATTENTION

Patient initially sees:

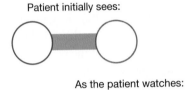

As the patient watches:

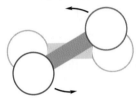

Patient now sees:

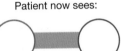

Patients with unilateral neglect syndrome were much more sensitive to targets appearing within the red circle (on the right) and missed many of the targets appearing within the blue circle (on the left); this observation simply confirms their clinical diagnosis. Then, as the patients watched, the "barbell" frame rotated, so that now the red circle was on the left and the blue circle was on the right. After this rotation, participants were still more sensitive to targets in the red circle (now on the left), apparently focusing on this attended object even though it had moved into their "neglected" side.

seem to support a space-based account of attention: The afflicted patient seems insensitive to all objects within a spatially defined region—namely, everything to the left of his current focus. If an object falls half within the region and half outside of it, then the spatially defined region is what matters, not the object's boundaries. This is clear, for example, in how these patients read words (likely to read "BOTHER" as "HER" or "CARROT" as "ROT")—responding only to the word's right half, apparently oblivious to the word's overall boundaries.

Other evidence, however, demands further theory. In one study, patients with neglect syndrome had to respond to targets that appeared within a barbell-shaped frame (see **Figure 5.14**). Not surprisingly, they were much more sensitive to the targets appearing within the red circle (on the right) and missed many of the targets appearing in the blue circle (on the left); this result simply confirms the patients' diagnosis. What's crucial, though, is what happened next: While the patients watched, the barbell frame was slowly spun around, so that the red circle, previously on the right, was now on the left and the blue circle, previously on the left, was now on the right.

What should we expect in this situation? If the patients consistently neglect a region of space, they should now be more sensitive to the (right-side) blue circle. A different possibility is more complicated: Perhaps these patients have a powerful bias to attend to the right side, and so initially they attend to the red circle. Once they have "locked in" to this circle, however, it's the object, and not the position in space, that defines their focus of attention. According to this view, if the barbell form rotates, they will continue attending to the red circle (this is, after all, the focus of their attention), even though it now appears on their "neglected" side. This prediction turns out to be correct: When the barbell rotates, the patients' focus of attention seems to rotate with it (Behrmann & Tipper, 1999).

To describe these patients, therefore, we need a two-part account. First, the symptoms of neglect syndrome plainly reveal a spatially defined bias: These patients neglect half of space. But, second, once attention is directed toward a target, it's the target itself that defines the focus of attention; if the target moves, the focus moves with it. In this way, the focus of attention is object-based, not space-based. (For more on these issues, see Chen & Cave, 2006; Logie & Della Salla, 2005; Richard, Lee, & Vecera, 2008.)

And it's not just people with brain damage who show this complex pattern; people with intact brains also show a mix of space-based and object-based attention. We've already seen evidence for the spatial base: The Posner et al. (1980) study and many results like it show that participants can focus on a particular region of space in preparation for a stimulus. In this situation, the stimulus has not yet appeared; there is no object to focus on. Therefore, the attention must be spatially defined.

In other cases, though, your attention is heavily influenced by object boundaries. For example, in some studies, participants have been shown displays with visually superimposed stimuli, as if a single television set were showing two channels at the same time (Neisser & Becklen, 1975; Simons & Chabris, 1999). Participants can easily pay attention to one of these stimuli and ignore the other. This selection cannot be space-based (because both stimuli are in the same place) and so must be object-based.

This two-part account is also demanded by neuroscience evidence. For example, various studies have examined the pattern of brain activation when participants are attending to a particular position in space, and the pattern of activation when participants are attending to a particular object or when they are searching for a target having specific features. These data suggest that the tasks involve different brain circuits—with one set of circuits, near the top of the head, primarily concerned with spatial attention, and a different set of circuits crucial for nonspatial tasks (e.g., Cave, 2013; Cohen, 2012; Corbetta & Shulman, 2011). Once again, therefore, our description of attention needs to include a mix of object-based and space-based mechanisms.

Feature Binding

We're almost finished with our discussion of selective attention, but there's one more topic to consider. Earlier, we argued that expectation-based priming draws on a limited-capacity system. Therefore, priming the detectors for a specific target or a particular location will inevitably take resources away from other detectors, and so you'll be less prepared if the input that arrives is not the one you expected.

One might think, therefore, that you'd be better off if you had *un*limited capacity, so that you could prime all of your detectors and thus be ready for anything. However, this suggestion is wrong. If in some fashion you tried to handle *all* of the inputs available to you, you'd likely be overwhelmed by input overload, buried in an avalanche of information. In an obvious fashion, therefore, your limited capacity *helps you*, by allowing you only a manageable flow of stimulation.

But there's another regard in which your limited capacity helps you. In Chapters 2 and 3, we emphasized that different analyses of the input all go on in the brain *in parallel*. In other words, you figure out the color of the object in front of you at the same time that you figure out its shape and its position. A separate step is then needed to put these elements together, so that you perceive a single, unified object. In other words, you need to solve the *binding problem,* so that you don't just perceive orange + round + close by + moving, but instead see the basketball in its trajectory toward you.

Attention plays a key role in solving this problem. That's evident in the fact (which we mentioned in Chapter 3) that if we overload attention (by giving participants some other task to perform while they're perceiving our displays), participants often make *errors* in binding. Thus, we might show them a red triangle and blue circle, and yet the participants report seeing a blue triangle and a red circle. In other words, these distracted participants correctly catalogue the features that are in view, but with attention diverted to another task, they fail to bundle the features the right way.

Further evidence comes from *visual search tasks*. We discussed these tasks in Chapter 4, when we mentioned that it's easy to search through a set of stimuli looking for a red object, for example, in a crowd of greens, or finding a round shape in a group of triangles. This was part of the evidence that *features* really do have priority in your perception.

In fact, we probably shouldn't use the term "search" when we're talking about a target defined by a single feature. That's because this sort of target seems to "pop out" from the display, with no effort (and little time) spent in hunting for it. Things are different, though, if you're searching for a target defined by a *combination* of features. Imagine, for example, that you're looking at a computer screen, and some of the lines in view are red and some are green. Some of the lines in view are horizontal and some are vertical. But there's just one line that's red *and* horizontal, and it's your job to find it. In this case, the time you'll need depends on how many items (in total) are in view; to put the matter simply, the larger the crowd to be searched through, the longer it takes.

To understand these results, imagine two hypothetical participants, both hunting for the combination red + horizontal. One participant (shown in **Figure 5.15A**) is trying to take in the whole display. He'll be able to catalogue quickly all the features that are in view (because he's looking at all the inputs simultaneously), but he'll also fail in his search for the red + horizontal combination: His catalogue of features tells him that both redness and horizontality are present, but the catalogue doesn't help him in figuring out if these features are linked or not. The observer in Figure 5.15B, in contrast, has focused his mental spotlight, so he's looking at just one stimulus at a time. This process is slower, because he'll have to examine the stimuli one by one, but this focusing gives the participant the information he needs: If, at any moment, he's only analyzing one item, he can be sure that the features he's detecting are all coming from that item. That tells him directly which features are linked to each other, and for this task (and for many other purposes as well), that's the key. (For the "classic" statement of these ideas, see Treisman & Gelade, 1980; for a more modern take and some complications, see Rensink, 2012.)

FIGURE 5.15   THE COSTS AND BENEFITS OF SELECTION

With attention aimed . . .

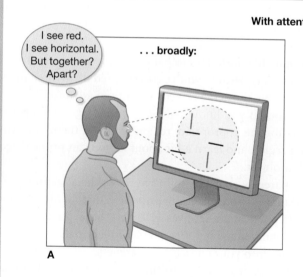

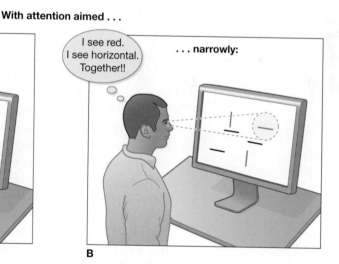

A

B

Focusing your attention involves a trade-off: If you focus your attention broadly, you can take in many inputs at once, and this is faster (because you don't have to search through the items one by one). But, since you're taking in multiple inputs simultaneously, you may not know which feature belongs with which (Panel A). In contrast, if you focus your attention narrowly, you'll be slower in your search (because now you do have to search item by item), but with information coming from just one input, you'll know how the features are combined (Panel B).

Now, let's put these pieces together. Expectation-based priming is selective: You prime the detectors for just one location or one type of feature, and this creates a processing advantage for stimuli in that location or stimuli with that feature. Of course, by shining the spotlight of attention on just one stimulus, your "pickup" of information from the display will be slower (because with this focus you won't pick up information from other stimuli, and so you'll need to turn to them later). But this selectivity gives you a substantial benefit: You've primed just one stimulus, so you're receiving information from just one stimulus. Thus, there's no risk of confusion about where the information is coming from, and you can be sure that all the information you're picking up at a particular moment (the redness, the orientation, and the size) is linked. In this way, the selectivity that's built into priming helps you solve the binding problem.

Perceiving and the Limits on Cognitive Capacity: An Interim Summary

At the broadest level, then, we've suggested that two different mechanisms are involved in selective attention. One mechanism serves to *inhibit*, or block out, the processing of *unwanted* inputs; this mechanism is especially important for intrusive distractors—distractors likely to seize your attention whether you like it or not. A second mechanism, though, is the one you more commonly rely on, and this is a mechanism that *facilitates* the processing of *desired* inputs.

We've also seen, though, that the latter mechanism has several parts. You're primed for some stimuli simply because you've encountered them often in the past. For other stimuli, if you know the target's identity in advance, you can prime the relevant detectors. If you know only *where* the target will appear, you can prime detectors for the appropriate region of space; then, once you locate the object in that region and learn a bit about it, you can prime detectors appropriate for that object.

Moreover, there's apparently some flexibility in *when* the selection takes place. In some circumstances, you make an early selection of the desired input, so that the unattended input receives relatively little processing. In other circumstances, the unattended input receives a fuller analysis—even if that input never penetrates into your conscious awareness.

In light of all these points, it's best not to think of the term "attention" as referring to a particular process or a particular mechanism. Instead, we need to think of paying attention as an *achievement*, something that you're able to do. Like many other achievements (e.g., doing well in school, staying healthy, earning a good salary), paying attention involves many elements, and the exact set of elements needed will vary from one occasion to the next. In all cases, though, multiple steps are needed to ensure that you end up aware of the stimuli you're interested in, and not pulled off track by irrelevant inputs.

Divided Attention

So far in this chapter, we've emphasized situations in which you're trying to focus on a single input. If other tasks and other stimuli are on the scene, they are mere distractors.

There are surely circumstances, however, in which you want to do multiple things at once—that is, settings in which you want to divide your attention among various tasks or various inputs. In the last decade or so, people have referred to this as "multitasking," but psychologists use the term **divided attention**—the effort to divide your focus between multiple tasks or multiple inputs.

Sometimes divided attention is easy. For example, almost anyone can walk and sing simultaneously; many people like to knit while they're holding a conversation or listening to a lecture. It's far harder, though, to do your calculus homework while listening to the lecture; and trying to get your reading done while watching TV is surely a bad bet. What lies behind this pattern? Why are some combinations difficult while others are easy?

Our first step toward answering these questions is already in view. We've proposed that perceiving requires resources that are in short supply; the same is presumably true for other tasks—remembering, reasoning, problem solving. They, too, require resources, and without these resources these processes cannot go forward. What are these resources? The answer includes a mix of things: certain mechanisms that do specific jobs, certain types of memory that hold on to information while you're working on it, energy supplies to keep the mental machinery going, and more. No matter what the resources are, though, a task will be possible only if you have the needed resources—just as a dressmaker can produce a dress only if he has the raw materials, the tools, the time needed, the energy to run the sewing machine, and so on.

All of this leads to a straightforward proposal: You can perform concurrent tasks only if you have the resources needed for both. If the two tasks, when combined, require more resources than you've got, divided attention will fail.

The Specificity of Resources

We need to be more specific, though, about how this competition for "mental resources" unfolds. Imagine two relatively similar tasks—say, reading a book and listening to a lecture. Both of these tasks involve the use of language, and so it seems plausible that these tasks will have similar resource requirements. As a result, if you try to do these tasks at the same time, they're likely to *compete* for resources, and therefore this sort of multitasking will be difficult.

Now, think about two very different tasks, such as the example we mentioned earlier: *knitting* and listening to a lecture. These tasks are unlikely to interfere with each other: Even if all of your language-related resources are in use for the lecture, this won't matter for knitting, because it's not a language-based task.

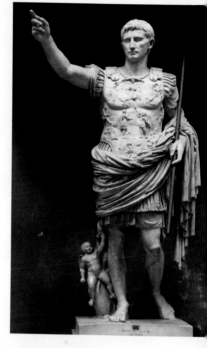

CAESAR THE MULTITASKER

Some writers lament the hectic pace at which we live and view this as a sad fact about the pressured reality of the modern world. But were things that different in earlier times? More than 2,000 years ago, Julius Caesar was praised for his ability to multitask. (That term is new, but the capacity is not.) According to the Roman historian Suetonius, Caesar could write, dictate letters, and read at the same time. Even on the most important subjects, he could dictate four letters at once— and if he had nothing else to do, as many as seven letters at once.

More broadly, the prediction here is that divided attention will be easier if the simultaneous tasks are very different from each other, because, again, different tasks are likely to have distinct resource requirements. Thus, resources consumed by Task 1 won't be needed for Task 2, so it doesn't matter for Task 2 that these resources are tied up in another endeavor.

Is this the pattern of the research data? In an early study by Allport, Antonis, and Reynolds (1972), participants heard a list of words presented through headphones into one ear, and their task was to shadow these words. At the same time, they were also presented with a second list. No immediate response was required to this second list, but later on, memory was tested for these items. In one condition, the second list (the memory items) consisted of words presented into the other ear, so the participants were hearing (and shadowing) a list of words in one ear while simultaneously hearing the memory list in the other. In a second condition, the memory items were presented visually. That is, while the participants were shadowing one list of words, they were also seeing, on a screen before them, a different list of words. Finally, in a third condition, the memory items consisted of pictures, also presented on a screen.

These three conditions have the same requirements—namely, shadowing one list while memorizing another. But the first condition (hear words + hear words) involves very similar tasks; the second condition (hear words + see words) involves less similar tasks; the third condition (hear words + see pictures), even less similar tasks. On the logic we've discussed, we should expect the most interference in the first condition, the least in the third. And that is what the data show (see **Figure 5.16**).

FIGURE 5.16 DIVIDED ATTENTION AMONG DISTINCT TASKS

Participants perform poorly if they are trying to shadow one list of words while hearing other words. They do somewhat better if shadowing while seeing other words. They do better still if shadowing while seeing pictures. In general, the greater the difference between two tasks, the easier it will be to combine the tasks. AFTER ALLPORT, ANTONIS, & REYNOLDS, 1972.

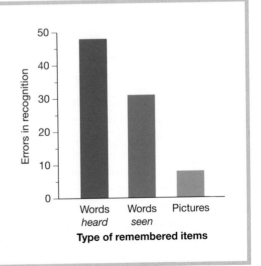

The Generality of Resources

Thus, task similarity matters for divided attention—but is not the whole story. If it were, then we'd observe less and less interference as we consider tasks further and further apart. Eventually, we'd find tasks that were so different from each other that we'd observe *no* interference at all between them. But that's not the pattern of the evidence.

Consider a situation that touches many of our lives: talking on a cell phone while driving. When you're on the phone, the main stimulus information comes into your ear, and your primary response is by talking. When you're driving, the main stimulation comes into your eyes, and your primary response involves control of your hands on the steering wheel and your feet on the pedals. For the phone conversation, you're relying on language skills. For driving, you need spatial skills. Overall, it looks like there's little overlap in the specific demands of these two tasks, and so little chance that the tasks will compete for resources.

It turns out, however, that driving and cell-phone use do interfere with each other; this is reflected, for example, in the fact that phone use has been implicated in many automobile accidents (Lamble, Kauranen, Laakso, & Summala, 1999). Even with a hands-free phone, drivers engaged in cell-phone conversations are more likely to be involved in accidents, more likely to overlook traffic signals, and slower to hit the brakes when they need to (Kunar, Carter, Cohen, & Horowitz, 2008; Levy & Pashler, 2008; Strayer & Drews, 2007; Strayer, Drews, & Johnston, 2003; for some *encouraging* data, though, on why these problems don't occur even more often, see Garrison & Williams, 2013; for a potential complication, see Bergen, Medeiros-Ward, Wheeler, Drews & Strayer, 2013).

We should mention, though, that the data pattern is different if the driver is instead talking to a *passenger* in the car rather than using the phone. Conversations with passengers seem to cause little interference with driving (Drews, Pasupathi, & Strayer, 2008; see **Figure 5.17**), and the reason is simple: If the traffic becomes complicated or the driver has to perform some tricky maneuver, the passenger can see this—either by looking out of the car's window or by detecting the driver's tension and focus. In these cases, passengers helpfully slow down their side of the conversation, which takes the load off of the driver, enabling the driver to focus on the road (Hyman, Boss, Wise, McKenzie, & Caggiano, 2010; Gaspar, Street, Windsor, Carbonari, Kaczmarski, Kramer, & Mathewson, 2014; Nasar, Hecht & Wener, 2008).

Identifying General Resources

Apparently, tasks as different as driving and talking compete with each other for some mental resource. But what is this resource—evidently needed for verbal tasks and spatial ones, tasks with visual inputs and tasks with auditory inputs?

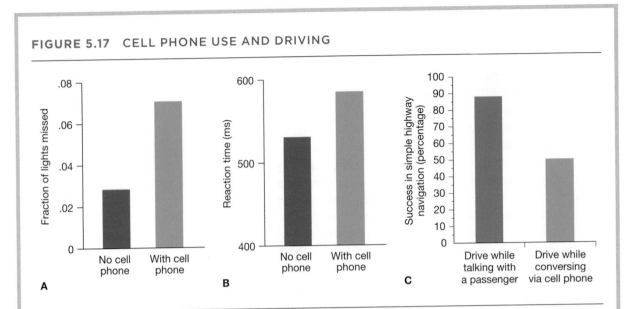

FIGURE 5.17 CELL PHONE USE AND DRIVING

Many studies show that driving performance is impaired when the driver is on the phone (whether it's a hand-held or hands-free phone). (Panel A) On the phone, drivers are more likely to miss a red light, and (Panel B) are certainly slower in responding to a red light. (Panel C) Disruption is not observed, however, if the driver is conversing with a passenger rather than on the phone. That's because the passenger is likely to adjust her conversation to accommodate changes in driving—such as not speaking while the driver is navigating an obstruction.
AFTER STRAYER & JOHNSTON, 2001.

The answer to this question has several parts, because *multiple* resources contribute to the limits on how (or whether) you can divide attention between tasks. Some authors, for example, describe resources that serve (roughly) as an energy supply, drawn on by all tasks (Eysenck, 1982; Kahneman, 1973; Lavie, 2001; 2005; Lavie, Lin, Zokaei, & Thoma, 2009; Macdonald & Lavie, 2008). Other authors describe resources best thought of as "mental tools" rather than as some sort of mental "energy supply" (Allport, 1989; Baddeley, 1986; Bourke & Duncan, 2005; Dehaene, Sergent, & Changeux, 2003; Johnson-Laird, 1988; Just, Carpenter, & Hemphill, 1996; Norman & Shallice, 1986; Ruthruff, Johnston, & Remington, 2009; Vergaujwe, Barrouillet, & Camos, 2010; for an alternative perspective on these resources, though, see Franconeri, 2013; Franconeri, Alvarez, & Cavanagh, 2013). One of these tools, for example, is a mechanism that seems to be required for *selecting* and *initiating* responses, including both physical responses and mental ones (such as the beginning of a memory search or the making of a decision; McCann & Johnston, 1992; Pashler, 1991, 1992, 1996; Pashler & Johnston, 1989; but also see Tombu & Jolicoeur, 2003). This **response selector** presumably plays a key role in coordinating the timing of your various activities and thus serves as a mental traffic cop, controlling which processes go forward at any moment in time.

Executive Control

A different mental resource is needed for many tasks: namely, the mind's **executive control**. This is the mechanism that sets goals and priorities, chooses strategies, and controls the sequence of cognitive processes.

Researchers have offered a variety of proposals for how exactly the executive operates and how the brain tissue enables executive function (Baddeley, 1986, 1996; Brown, Reynolds & Braver, 2007; Duncan et al., 2008; Engle & Kane, 2004; Gilbert & Shallice, 2002; Kane, Conway, Hambrick, & Engle, 2007; Miller & Cohen, 2001; Miyake & Friedman, 2012; Stuss & Alexander, 2007; Unsworth & Engle, 2007; Vandierendonck, Liefooghe, & Verbruggen, 2010). Across these various proposals, though, theorists agree about several key points. Let's start with the observation that much of your day-to-day functioning is guided by habit and prior associations. After all, many of the situations you find yourself in resemble those you've encountered in the past, so you don't need to start from scratch in figuring out how to behave. Instead, you can rely on responses or strategies you've used previously.

In some cases, though, you want to behave in a fashion that's different from how you've behaved in the past—because your goals have changed or because the situation itself has changed in some way. In such cases, you need to overrule the action or strategy supplied by memory. As a related problem, some circumstances contain triggers that powerfully evoke certain responses. If you wish to make some *other* response, you need to take steps to avoid the obvious trap.

With this context, the proposal is that executive control is needed whenever you want to avoid interference either from habits supplied by memory or from habits triggered by situational cues. This control provides several functions. First, it works to maintain the desired goal in mind, so that this goal (and not habit) will guide your actions. Second, the executive ensures that your mental steps are organized into the right sequence—one that will in fact move you toward your goal. This sequencing, in turn, requires that the executive have some means of monitoring the progress of your mental operations, so that the executive knows when to launch the next step in your plan. The monitoring will also allow the executive to shift plans, or change strategy, if your current operations aren't moving you toward your goal. Finally, executive control also serves to *inhibit* automatic responses, helping to ensure that these responses won't occur.

We can see how important these functions are when we consider people who have *diminished* executive control. Evidence comes, for example, from studies of people who have suffered damage to the prefrontal cortex (or PFC); this is (roughly) the brain area right behind your eyes. People with this damage (including Phineas Gage, whom we met in Chapter 2) can lead relatively normal lives, because in their day-to-day behavior they can often rely on habit or routine or can simply respond to prominent cues in their environment. With appropriate tests, though, we can reveal the disruption

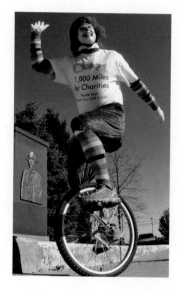

CELL-PHONE DANGERS FOR PEDESTRIANS

It's not just driving that's disrupted by cell-phone use. Pedestrians engaged in phone conversations tend to walk more slowly and more erratically, change directions more often, and are less likely to check traffic carefully before they cross a street. They're also less likely to notice things along their path. In one study, researchers observed pedestrians walking across a public square. If the pedestrian was walking with a friend (and so engaged in a "live" conversation), there was a 71% chance the pedestrian would notice the unicycling clown, just off the pedestrian's path. If the pedestrian was instead on the phone (and thus engaged in a telephonic conversation), the person had only a 25% chance of detecting the clown. HYMAN, BOSS, WISE, MCKENZIE, & CAGGIANO, 2010.

that results from frontal lobe damage. For example, in one commonly used task, patients with frontal lesions are asked to sort a deck of cards into two piles. At the start, the patients have to sort the cards according to color; later, they need to switch strategies and sort according to the shapes shown on the cards. The patients have enormous difficulty in making this shift and continue to sort by color, even though the experimenter tells them again and again that they're placing the cards on the wrong piles (Goldman-Rakic, 1998). This is referred to as a **perseveration error**, a tendency to produce the same response over and over even when it's plain that the task requires a change in the response.

These patients also show a pattern of **goal neglect**—failing to organize their behavior in a way that moves them toward their goals. For example, one patient was asked to copy **Figure 5.18A**; the patient produced the drawing shown in Figure 5.18B. The copy preserves features of the original, but close inspection reveals that the patient drew the copy with no particular plan in mind. The large rectangle that defines the shape was never drawn; the diagonal lines that organize the figure were drawn in a piecemeal fashion. Many details are correctly reproduced but were not drawn in any sort of order; instead, these details were added whenever they happened to catch the patient's attention (Kimberg, D'Esposito, & Farah, 1998). Another patient, asked to copy the same figure, produced the drawing shown in Figure 5.18C.

FIGURE 5.18 GOAL NEGLECT

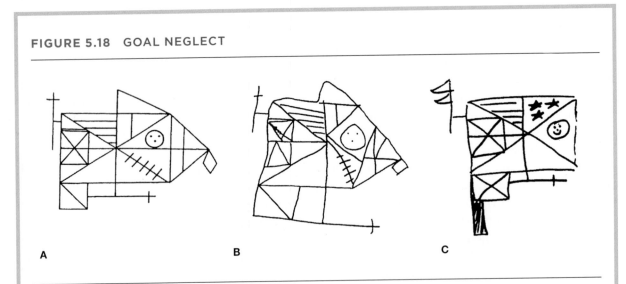

A   B   C

Patients who had suffered damage to the prefrontal cortex were asked to copy the drawing in Panel A. One patient's attempt is shown in Panel B; the drawing is reasonably accurate but seems to have been drawn with no overall plan (and so, for example, the large rectangle in the original, and the main diagonals, were created piecemeal rather than being used to organize the drawing). Another patient's attempt is shown in Panel C; this patient started to re-create the drawing but then got swept up in her own artistic impulses.

This patient started to draw the figure in a normal way, but then she got swept up in her own artistic impulses, adding stars and a smiley face (Kimberg et al., 1998). (For more on executive control, see Aron, 2008; Courtney, Petit, Maisog, Ungerleider, & Haxby, 1998; Duncan et al., 2008; Gilbert & Shallice, 2002; Huey, Krueger, & Grafman, 2006; Kane & Engle, 2003; Kimberg et al., 1998; Logie & Della Salla, 2005; Ranganath & Blumenfeld, 2005; Stuss & Levine, 2002.)

Divided Attention: An Interim Summary

Let's pause once again to take stock. Our consideration of *selective* attention drove us toward a several-part account, with one mechanism apparently serving to block out unwanted distractors and a number of other mechanisms serving to promote the processing of interesting stimuli. Now, in our discussion of *divided* attention, we again seem to require several elements in our theory. Interference between tasks is plainly increased if the tasks are similar to each other, presumably because similar tasks overlap in their processing requirements and so make competing demands on mental resources that are specialized for that sort of task.

But interference can also be demonstrated with tasks that are entirely different from each other—such as driving and talking on a cell phone. Thus, our account needs to include resources that are general enough in their use that they're drawn on by almost any task. We've noted that there are, in fact, several of these general resources: an energy supply needed for mental tasks; a response selector needed whenever a task involves the launching of successive steps; executive control, needed whenever a task requires "rising above" prior habits and tendencies; and probably others as well. No matter what the resource, though, the key principle will be the same: Tasks will interfere with each other if their combined demand for a resource is greater than the amount available—that is, if the demand exceeds the supply.

Practice

Let's return once again to the example of talking on a cell phone while driving. For a skilled driver, this task combination is easy if the driving is straightforward and the conversation is simple. Things fall apart, though, the moment the conversation becomes complex or the driving becomes challenging; that's when these two tasks interfere with each other. Engaged in deep conversation, the driver misses a turn; while maneuvering through the intersection, the driver suddenly stops talking.

The situation is different, though, for a *novice* driver. For the novice, driving is difficult all by itself, even on a straight road with no traffic. If, therefore, we ask the novice to do anything else at the same time—whether it's talking on a cell phone or even listening to the radio—we put the driver (and other cars) at substantial risk. Why is this? Why are things so different after practice?

Practice Diminishes Resource Demand

We've already said that mental tasks require resources, with the particular resources required—and the *amount* of resources required—dependent on the nature of the task. Let's now add a further claim: As a task becomes more practiced, it requires *fewer* resources, or perhaps it requires *less frequent* use of these resources.

In fact, this decrease in a task's resource demand may be inevitable, given the function of some resources. Recall, for example, that executive control is needed whenever you want to rise above habit and do things in a new way. Conversely, executive control *isn't* needed when your available habits are sufficient for your needs. (This is, remember, why patients with PFC damage can live nearly normal lives—often, our habits do serve us well.) But, of course, the option of relying on habits is only possible if you *have* habits, and early in practice, when a task is brand new, you haven't formed any relevant habits yet, so you have no habits to fall back on. As a result, executive control is needed all the time. Once you've done the task over and over, though, you can acquire a repertoire of suitable habits, and as you rely on them more and more, the demand for executive control decreases.

Roughly the same logic applies to other mental resources, on the broad notion that these resources are in various ways involved in the *control* of mental performance—making plans for what to do, launching each step, and so on. Once a routine is established, there's less need for this control and, with that, less need for the resources.

Of course, we've already argued that tasks will interfere with each other if their *combined resource demand* is greater than the amount of resources available. Interference is less likely, therefore, if the "cognitive cost" of a task is low; in that case, you'll have an easier time accommodating the task within your "resource budget." And we've now added the idea that the resource demand (the "cost") will be lower after practice than before. Thus, it's no surprise that practice makes divided attention easier—enabling the skilled driver to continue chatting with her passenger as they cruise down the highway, even though this combination is hopelessly difficult for the novice driver.

Automaticity

These points about practice have an important implication: With practice, we've said, you develop habits and routines, and so you have less need for executive control. We've described some of the ways this is helpful—since (among other benefits) this diminished reliance on control mechanisms makes it easier for you to "multitask." But this gain comes at a significant price: Once a task is well practiced, you can lose the option of controlling your own mental operations. Said differently, practice enables many mental processes to go forward untouched by control mechanisms, with the result that these processes are now uncontrollable.

To capture this idea, psychologists say that tasks that have been frequently practiced can achieve a state of **automaticity**. With this, many psychologists distinguish between **controlled tasks** and **automatic tasks** (Shiffrin & Schneider, 1977; also Moors & De Houwer, 2006). Controlled tasks are typically novel (i.e., not yet practiced) or are tasks that continually vary in their demands (so that it's not possible for you to develop standardized "routines"). Automatic tasks, in contrast, are typically highly familiar and do not require great flexibility. With some practice, then, you can approach these tasks with a well-rehearsed procedure—a sequence of responses (often triggered by specific stimuli) that have gotten the job done in the past. Of course, this procedure is usually established through practice, but it can also be learned from some good advice or a skilled teacher (cf. Yamaguchi & Proctor, 2011). In any case, once the routine is acquired, the automatic task doesn't need to be supervised or controlled, and so it requires few resources.

Automaticity can be beneficial, because (as we've discussed) if resources are not needed for a task, then those resources are available for other chores. But automaticity also has a downside: Automatic tasks are not governed by the mind's control mechanisms, with the result that they are not controlled and, thus, can act as if they were "mental reflexes."

A striking example of this lack of control involves an effect known as **Stroop interference**. In the classic demonstration of this effect, study participants were shown a series of words and asked to name aloud the color of the ink used for each word. The trick, though, was that the words themselves were color names. So people might see the word "BLUE" printed in green ink and would have to say "green" out loud, and so on (see **Figure 5.19**; Stroop, 1935).

EBOOK DEMONSTRATION 5.4

This task turns out to be extremely difficult. There is a strong tendency to read the printed words themselves rather than name the ink color, and people make many mistakes in this task. Presumably, this reflects the fact that word recognition, especially for college-age adults, is enormously well practiced and, as a consequence, can proceed automatically. This is a condition, therefore, in which mental control should be minimal, and that is certainly consistent with the errors that we observe. (For discussion of the specific mechanisms that produce this interference, see Besner & Stolz, 1999a, 1999b; Durgin, 2000; Engle & Kane, 2004; Jacoby et al., 2003; Kane & Engle, 2003.)

Where Are the Limits?

We are nearing the end of our discussion of attention, and so it again may be useful to summarize where we are. Two simple ideas lie at the heart of our account: First, tasks require resources, and second, you cannot "spend" more resources than you have. These claims are central for almost everything we have said about selective and divided attention.

As we have seen, though, we need to add some complexity to this account. There seem to be different types of resources, and the exact resource demand

FIGURE 5.19 STROOP INTERFERENCE

Column A	Column B
ZYP	RED
QLEKF	BLACK
SUWRG	YELLOW
XCIDB	BLUE
WOPR	RED
ZYP	GREEN
QLEKF	YELLOW
XCIDB	BLACK
SUWRG	BLUE
WOPR	BLACK

As rapidly as you can, name out loud the colors of the *ink* in Column A. (And so you'll say, "black, green" and so on.) Next, do the same for Column B—again, naming out loud the colors of the ink. You will probably find it much easier to do this for Column A, because in Column B, you experience interference from the automatic habit of reading the words.

of a task depends on several factors. The nature of the task matters, of course, so that the resources required by a verbal task (e.g., reading) are different from those required by a spatial task (e.g., remembering a shape). The novelty of the task and the amount of flexibility the task requires also matter. Connected to this, *practice* matters, with well-practiced tasks requiring fewer resources.

What, then, sets the limits on divided attention? When can you do two tasks at the same time, and when not? The answer varies, case by case. If two tasks make competing demands on task-specific resources, the result will be interference. If two tasks make competing demands on task-general resources (the response selector or executive control), again the result will be interference. In addition, it will be especially difficult to combine tasks that involve similar stimuli—combining two tasks that both involve printed text, for example, or that both involve speech. The problem here is that these stimuli can "blur together," with a danger that you'll lose track of which elements belong in which input ("Was it the man who said 'yes,' or was it the woman?"; "Was the red dog in the top picture or the bottom one?"). This sort of "crosstalk" (leakage of bits of one input into the other input) can itself compromise performance.

In short, it seems again like we need a multipart theory of attention, with performance limited by different factors on different occasions. This perspective draws us back to a claim we made earlier in the chapter: Attention cannot be thought of as a skill or a mechanism or a capacity. Instead, attention is an achievement—an achievement of performing multiple activities simultaneously or an achievement of successfully avoiding distraction when you wish to focus on a single task. And, as we have seen, this achievement rests on an intricate base, so that many skills, mechanisms, and capacities contribute to our ability to attend.

Finally, one last point. We have discussed various limits on human performance—that is, limits on how much you can do at any one time. How rigid are these limits? We have discussed the improvements in divided attention that are made possible by practice, but are there boundaries on what practice can accomplish? Can you perhaps gain new mental resources or, more plausibly, find new ways to accomplish a task in order to avoid the bottleneck created by some limited resource? At least some evidence indicates that the answer to these questions may be yes; if so, many of the claims made in this chapter must be understood as claims about what is *usual*, not as claims about what is *possible* (Hirst, Spelke, Reaves, Caharack, & Neisser, 1980; Spelke, Hirst, & Neisser, 1976). With this, many traditions in the world—Buddhist meditation traditions, for example—claim it is possible to *train* attention so that one has better control over one's mental life; how do these claims fit into the framework we have developed in this chapter? These are issues in need of further exploration, and in truth, what is at stake here is a question about the boundaries on human potential, making these issues of deep interest for future researchers to pursue.

COGNITIVE PSYCHOLOGY AND THE LAW

What Do Witnesses Pay Attention To?

Throughout Chapter 5, we have emphasized how little information people seem to gain about stimuli that are plainly visible (or plainly audible) *if they are not paying attention to these stimuli*. Thus, people fail to see a gorilla that's directly in front of their eyes, a large-scale color change that's plainly in view, and more.

Think about what this means for law enforcement. Imagine, for example, a customer in a bank during a robbery. Perhaps the customer waited in line directly behind the robber. Will the customer remember what the robber looked like? Will the customer remember the robber's clothing? There's no way to tell unless we have some indications of what the customer was paying attention to—even though the robber's appearance and clothing were salient stimuli in the customer's environment.

Of course, the factors governing a witness's attention will vary from witness to witness and from crime to crime. One factor, though, is often important: the presence of a *weapon* during the crime. If a gun (for example) is in view, then of course witnesses will want to know whether the gun is pointed at them and whether the criminal's finger is on the trigger. After all, what else in the scene could be more important to the witness? But with this focus on the weapon, other things in the scene will be unattended, so that the witness will fail to notice—and later on fail to remember—many bits of information crucial for law enforcement.

Consistent with these suggestions, witnesses to crimes involving weapons are said to show a pattern called "weapon focus." They are able to report to the police many details about the weapon (its size, its color) and, often, details about the hand that was holding the weapon (e.g., whether the person was wearing any rings or a bracelet). However, because of this focus, the witness may have a relatively poor memory for other aspects of the scene—including the crucial information of what the perpetrator looked like. Indeed, studies suggest that eyewitness identifications of the perpetrator may be systematically *less accurate* in crimes involving weapons—presumably because the witness's attention was focused on the weapon, not on the perpetrator's face.

The weapon-focus pattern has been demonstrated in many studies, including those that literally track where participants are pointing their eyes during the event. Scientists have also used a statistical technique called "meta-analysis" to provide an overall summary of these data. Meta-analysis confirms the overall pattern and, importantly, shows that the weapon-focus effect is stronger and more reliable in studies that are closer to actual forensic settings. Thus, the weapon-focus effect is not a peculiar by-product of the artificial situations created in the lab; indeed, the effect may be *underestimated* in laboratory studies.

Surprisingly, though, the weapon-focus pattern is less consistent in actual crimes. In some cases, witnesses tell us directly that they experienced weapon focus: "All I remember is that huge knife." "I couldn't take my eyes off of that gun." But this pattern is not reliable, and several studies, examining the memories of real victims of real crimes, have found little indication of weapon focus: In these studies, the accuracy of witness I.D.'s is the same whether the crime involves a weapon or does not—with the implication that the weapon just doesn't matter for the witness's attention.

What's going on here? The answer probably has several parts, including whether violence is overtly threatened during the crime (this will make weapon focus more likely) and whether the perpetrator happens to be distinctive in his or her appearance (this will make weapon focus *less* likely). In addition, the *duration* of the crime is important. A witness may focus initially

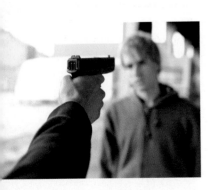

WEAPON FOCUS

Witnesses to crimes involving a weapon are likely to focus their attention on the weapon. After all, they surely want to know if the weapon is pointed at them or not! But, with their focus on the weapon, they are less likely to notice—and later remember—other aspects of the scene.

on the weapon (and so *will* show the pattern of weapon focus), but then, if the crime lasts long enough, the witness has time to look around and observe other aspects of the scene as well. This would, of course, decrease the overall impact of the weapon-focus effect.

Even with these complications, consideration of weapon focus is important for the justice system. Among other considerations, police officers and attorneys often ask whether a witness was "attentive" or not, and they use this point in deciding how much weight to give the witness's testimony. Weapon focus reminds us, however, that it's not enough to ask, in a general way, whether someone was attentive. Instead, we need to ask a more fine-grained question: What, within the crime scene, was the witness paying attention to? Research is clear that attention will always be selective and that unattended aspects of an event won't be perceived and won't be remembered later. We should therefore welcome any clue—including the weapon-focus pattern—that helps us figure out what the witness paid attention to, as part of an overall effort toward deciding when we can rely on a witness's report and when we cannot.

chapter summary

● People are often oblivious to unattended inputs; they are unable to tell if an unattended auditory input was coherent prose or random words, and they often fail altogether to detect unattended visual inputs, even though such inputs are right in front of the viewers' eyes. However, some aspects of the unattended inputs are detected. For example, people can report on the pitch of the unattended sound and whether it contained human speech or some other sort of noise. Sometimes they can also detect stimuli that are especially meaningful; some people, for example, hear their own name if it is spoken on the unattended channel.

● These results suggest that perception may require the commitment of mental resources, with some of these resources helping to prime the detectors needed for perception. This proposal is supported by studies of inattentional blindness—that is, studies showing that perception is markedly impaired if the perceiver commits no resources to the incoming stimulus information. The proposal is also supported by results showing that you perceive more efficiently when you can anticipate the upcoming stimulus (and so can prime the relevant detectors). In many cases, this anticipation is spatial—if, for example, you know that a stimulus is about to arrive at a particular location. This priming, however, seems to draw on a limited-capacity system, and so priming one stimulus or one position takes away resources that might be spent on priming some other stimulus.

● The ability to pay attention to certain regions of space has encouraged many researchers to compare attention to a spotlight beam, with the idea that stimuli falling "within the beam" are processed more efficiently than stimuli that fall "outside the beam." However, this spotlight analogy is potentially misleading. In many circumstances, you do seem to devote attention to identifiable regions of space, no matter what falls within those regions. In other circumstances, though, attention seems to be object-based, not space-based, and so you pay attention to specific objects, not specific positions.

- Perceiving, it seems, requires the commitment of resources, and so do most other mental activities. This provides a ready account of divided attention: It is possible to perform two tasks simultaneously only if the two tasks do not in combination demand more resources than are available. Some of the relevant mental resources are task-general and so are called on by a wide variety of mental activities. These include the response selector and executive control. Other mental resources are task-specific, required only for tasks of a certain type.

- Divided attention is clearly influenced by practice, with the result that it is often easier to divide attention between familiar tasks than between unfamiliar tasks. In the extreme, practice may produce automaticity, in which a task seems to require virtually no mental resources but is also difficult to control. One proposal is that automaticity results from the fact that decisions are no longer needed for a well-practiced routine; instead, one can simply run off the entire routine, doing on this occasion just what one did on prior occasions.

e eBook Demonstrations & Essays

Online Demonstrations:
- Demonstration 5.1: Shadowing
- Demonstration 5.2: Color-Changing Card Trick
- Demonstration 5.3: The Control of Eye Movements
- Demonstration 5.4: Automaticity and the Stroop Effect

Online Applying Cognitive Psychology Essays:
- Cognitive Psychology and Education: ADHD
- Cognitive Psychology and the Law: Guiding the Formulation of New Laws

ZAPS 2.0 Cognition Labs

- Go to **http://digital.wwnorton.com/cognition6** for the online labs relevant to this chapter.

Memory

As we move through our lives, we encounter new facts, gain new skills, and have new experiences. And we are often *changed* by all of this, and so, later on, we know things and can do things that we couldn't know or do before. How do these changes happen? How do we get new information into our memories, and then how do we retrieve this information when we need it? And how much trust can we put in this process? Why is it, for example, that we sometimes fail to remember things (including important things)? And why is it that our memories are sometimes *wrong*—so that, in some cases, you remember an event one way, but your friend who was present at the same event remembers things differently?

We'll tackle all these issues in this section, and they will lead us to both theoretical claims and practical applications. We'll offer suggestions, for example, about how students should study their class materials to maximize retention. We'll also discuss how police should question crime witnesses to maximize the quality of information the witnesses provide.

In our discussion, several themes will emerge again and again. One theme concerns the active nature of learning, and we'll discuss the fact that passive exposure to information, with no intellectual engagement, leads to poor memory. From this base, we'll consider why some forms of engagement with to-be-learned material lead to especially good memory but other forms do not.

A second theme will be equally prominent: the role of memory connections. In Chapter 6 we'll see that at its essence, learning involves the creation of connections, and the more connections formed, the better the learning. In Chapter 7 we'll argue that these connections serve as "retrieval paths" later on—paths that, you hope, will lead you from your memory search's starting point to the information you're trying to recall. As we'll see, this notion has clear implications for when you will remember a previous event and when you won't.

Chapter 8 then explores a different ramification of the connections idea: Memory connections can actually be a source of memory errors. We'll ask what this means for memory accuracy overall, and we'll discuss what you can do to minimize error and to improve the completeness and accuracy of your memory.

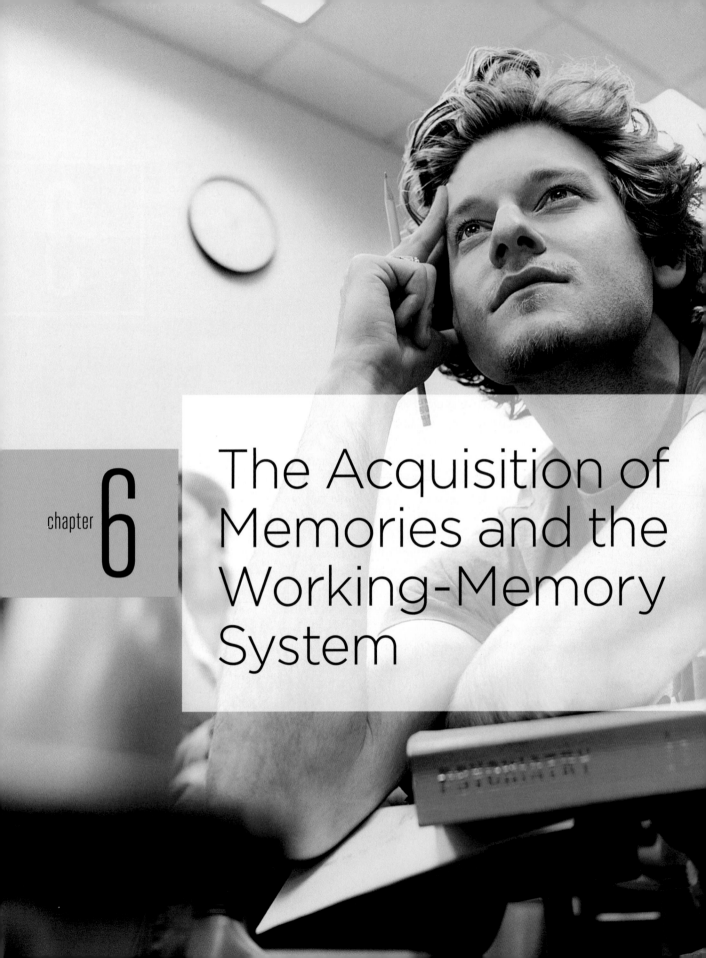

chapter 6

The Acquisition of Memories and the Working-Memory System

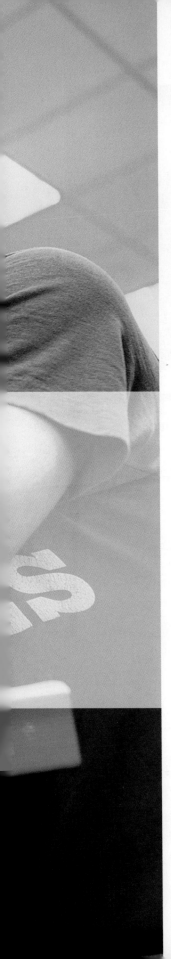

what if...

Clive Wearing is an accomplished musician and a scholar of Renaissance music. When he was 47 years old, however, his brain was invaded and horribly damaged by a Herpes virus, and he now has profound amnesia. He is still articulate and intelligent, able to participate in an ongoing conversation, and he is still able to play music (beautifully) and conduct. But Wearing has no episodic memories. Every few minutes, he realizes he can't remember anything from just a few seconds back, and so he concludes that he must have just woken up. He grabs his diary and writes "8:31 a.m. Now I am really, completely awake." A short while later, though, he again realizes he can't recall the last seconds, and so he decides that *now* he has just woken up. He picks up his diary to record this event and immediately sees his previous entry. Puzzled by the entry, he crosses it out and replaces it with "9:06 a.m. Now I am perfectly, overwhelmingly awake." But then the process repeats, and so this entry, too, gets scribbled out and a new entry reads "9:34 a.m.: Now I am superlatively, actually awake."

Wearing is deeply in love with his wife, Deborah, and his love is in no way diminished by his amnesia. Each time Deborah enters his room—even if she's been away just a few minutes—he races to embrace her as though it's been countless lonely months since they last met. If asked directly, he has no recollection of her previous visits—even if she'd been there just an hour earlier.

We met a different case of amnesia in Chapter 1—the famous patient H.M. He, too, was unable to recall his immediate past—and the many, deep problems this produced included an odd sort of disorientation: If you were smiling at him, was it because you'd just said something funny? Or because he'd said something embarrassing? Or had you been smiling all along? As H.M. put it, "Right now, I'm wondering. Have I done or said anything amiss? You see, at this moment, everything looks clear to me, but what happened just before? That's what worries me" (Milner, 1970, p. 37; also see Corkin, 2013).

Cases like these remind us of how profoundly our memories shape our everyday lives. But these cases also raise many questions: Why is it that Wearing still remembers who his wife is? How is it possible that

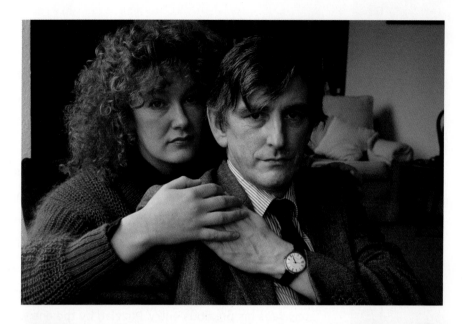

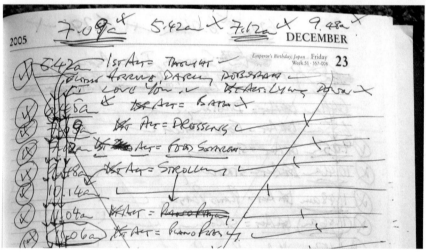

CLIVE WEARING

Clive Wearing (shown here with his wife) developed profound amnesia as a result of viral encephalitis, and now he seems to have only a moment-to-moment consciousness. With no memory at all of what he was doing just moments ago, he is often convinced he just woke up, and he repeatedly writes in his diary "Now perfectly awake (1st time)." On the diary page shown here, he has recorded his bath as his "1st act" because he has no memory of any prior activity. A few minutes later, though, he seems to realize again that he has no memory of any earlier events, and so he scribbles out the 6:45 entry and now records that dressing is his "1st act." The sequence repeats over and over, with Wearing never recalling what he did before his current activity, and so he records act after act as his "first."

● We begin the chapter with a discussion of the broad architecture of memory. We then turn to a closer examination of one component of this architecture: working memory.

● We emphasize the active nature of working memory—activity that is especially evident when we discuss working memory's "central executive," a mental resource that serves to order, organize, and control our mental lives.

● The active nature of memory is also evident in the process of *rehearsal*. Rehearsal is effective only if the person engages the materials in some way; this is reflected, for example,

in the contrast between deep processing (which leads to excellent memory) and mere maintenance rehearsal (which produces virtually no memory benefit).

● Activity during learning appears to establish *memory connections*, which can serve as retrieval routes when it comes time to remember the target material. For complex material, the best way to establish these connections is to seek to understand the material; the better the understanding, the better the memory will be.

even with his amnesia, Wearing remains such a talented musician? Why does H.M. still remember his young adult years, even though he cannot remember what he said just five minutes earlier? We'll tackle questions like these in this chapter and the next two.

Acquisition, Storage, and Retrieval

How does new information—whether it's a friend's phone number or a fact you hope to memorize for the bio exam—become established in memory? Are there ways to learn that are particularly effective? And then, once information is in storage, how do you locate it and "reactivate" it later? And why does search through memory sometimes fail—so that (for example) you forget the name of that great restaurant downtown (but then, to your chagrin, remember the name when you're midway through a mediocre dinner someplace else)?

In tackling these questions, there is an obvious way to organize our inquiry. Before there can be a memory, you need to gain, or "acquire," some new information. On this basis, **acquisition**—the process of gaining information and placing it into memory—should be our first topic. Then, once you've acquired this information, you need to hold it in memory until the information is needed. We refer to this as the **storage** phase. Finally, you *remember*. In other words, you somehow locate the information in the vast warehouse that is memory and you bring it into active use; this is called **retrieval.**

This organization seems sensible; it fits, for example, with the way most "electronic memories" (e.g., computers) work. Information ("input") is provided to a computer (the acquisition phase). The information then resides in some dormant form, generally on the hard drive (the storage phase). Finally, the information can be brought back from this dormant form, often via a search process that hunts through the disk (the retrieval phase). And, of course, there's nothing special about a computer here; "low-tech" information storage works the same way. Think about a file drawer: Information is acquired (i.e., filed), rests in this or that folder, and then is retrieved.

Guided by this framework, we'll begin our inquiry by focusing on the acquisition of new memories, leaving discussion of storage and retrieval for later. As it turns out, though, we'll soon find reasons for challenging this overall approach to memory. In discussing acquisition, for example, we might wish to ask: What is good learning? What guarantees that material is firmly recorded in memory? As we will see, evidence indicates that what is good learning depends on how the memory is to be used later on, so that good preparation for one kind of use may be poor preparation for a different kind of use. Claims about acquisition, therefore, must be interwoven with claims about retrieval. These interconnections between acquisition and retrieval will be the central theme of Chapter 7.

In the same way, we cannot separate claims about memory acquisition from claims about memory storage. This is because *how you learn* (acquisition) depends *on what you already know* (information in storage). This relationship needs to be explored and explained, and it will provide a recurrent theme in both this chapter and Chapter 8.

With these caveats in view, we'll nonetheless begin by describing the acquisition process. Our approach will be roughly historical. We'll start with a simple model, emphasizing data collected largely in the 1970s. We'll then use this as the framework for examining more recent research, adding refinements to the model as we proceed.

The Route into Memory

For many years, theorizing in cognitive psychology focused on the process through which information was perceived and then moved into memory storage—that is, on the process of information acquisition. There was disagreement about the details but reasonable consensus on the bold outline of events. An early version of this model was described by Waugh and Norman (1965); later refinements were added by Atkinson and Shiffrin (1968). The consensus model came to be known as the **modal model**, and **Figure 6.1** provides a (somewhat simplified) depiction of this model.

Updating the Modal Model

According to the modal model, when information first arrives, it is stored briefly in *sensory memory*, which holds on to the input in "raw" sensory form—an *iconic memory* for visual inputs and an *echoic memory* for auditory inputs. A process of selection and interpretation then moves the information into *short-term memory*—the place where you hold information while you're working on it. Some of the information is then transferred into *long-term memory*, a much larger and more permanent storage place.

This early conception of memory captures some important truths, but it needs to be updated in several ways. As one concern, the idea of "sensory

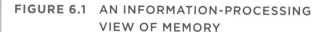

FIGURE 6.1   AN INFORMATION-PROCESSING VIEW OF MEMORY

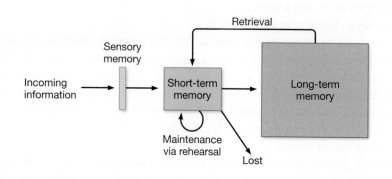

Diagrams like this one depict the flow of information hypothesized by the "modal model." The model captures many important truths, but it must be updated in important ways. Current theorizing, for example, emphasizes that short-term memory (now called "working memory") is not a place serving as a "loading dock" outside of long-term memory. Instead, working memory is best understood as an activity, in ways described in the chapter.

memory" plays a much smaller role in modern theorizing, and so modern discussions of perception (like our discussion in Chapters 2 and 3) often make no mention of this memory. In addition, modern proposals use the term "working memory" rather than "short-term memory," to emphasize the function of this memory: Ideas or thoughts in this memory are currently activated, currently being thought about, and so they're the ideas you are currently *working on*. **Long-term memory (LTM)**, in contrast, is the vast repository that contains all of your knowledge and all of your beliefs—most of which you happen not to be thinking about (i.e., not working on) at this moment.

The modal model also needs updating in another way. Pictures like the one in Figure 6.1 suggest that working memory is a *storage place*, sometimes described as the "loading dock" just outside of the long-term memory "ware-house." The idea, roughly, is that information has to "pass through" working memory on the way into longer-term storage. Likewise, the picture implies that memory retrieval involves the "movement" of information out of storage and back into working memory.

In contrast, contemporary theorists do not conceive of working memory as a "place" at all. Instead, working memory is (as we will see) simply the name we give to a *status*. Thus, when we say that ideas are "in working memory," this simply means that these ideas are currently activated and being worked on by a specific set of operations.

We'll have much more to say about this modern perspective before we're through. It's important to emphasize, though, that the modern perspective also preserves some key ideas in the modal model. Specifically, modern theorizing continues to build on several of the modal model's claims about how working memory and long-term memory differ from each other, so let's start by counting through those differences.

First, working memory is limited in size; long-term memory is enormous. Indeed, long-term memory has to be enormous, because it contains all of your knowledge—including specific knowledge (e.g., how many siblings you have) and more general themes (e.g., you know that water is wet, that Dublin is in Ireland, that unicorns don't exist). Long-term memory also contains all your knowledge about events, including events early in your life as well as your more recent experiences.

Second, getting information into working memory is easy. If you think about some idea or some content, then you are, in effect, "working on" that idea or content, and so this information—by definition—is now in your working memory. In contrast, we'll see later in the chapter that getting information into long-term memory often involves some work.

Third, getting information out of working memory is also easy. Since (by definition) this memory holds the ideas you are thinking about right now, this information is already available to you. Finding information in long-term memory, in contrast, can sometimes be effortful and slow—and in some settings can fail altogether.

Finally, the contents of working memory are quite fragile. Working memory, we emphasize, contains the ideas you're thinking about right now. If you shift your thoughts to a new topic, these new ideas will now occupy working memory, pushing out what was there a moment ago. Long-term memory, in contrast, is not linked to the current focus of your thoughts, and so it is far less fragile: Information remains in storage whether or not you're thinking about it right now.

We can make all these claims more concrete by looking at some classic findings. These findings come from a task that's quite artificial (i.e., not the sort of memorizing you do every day) but also quite informative.

Working Memory and Long-Term Memory: One Memory or Two?

In many studies, researchers have asked study participants to listen to a series of words, like "bicycle, artichoke, radio, chair, palace." In a typical experiment, the list contains 30 words and is presented at a rate of one word per second. Immediately after the last word is read, participants are asked to repeat back as many words as they can. They are free to report the words in any order they choose, which is why this is referred to as a **free recall** procedure.

People usually remember 12 to 15 words in this test, in a consistent pattern. They are very likely to remember the first few words on the list,

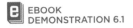
EBOOK
DEMONSTRATION 6.1

FIGURE 6.2 PRIMACY AND RECENCY EFFECTS IN FREE RECALL

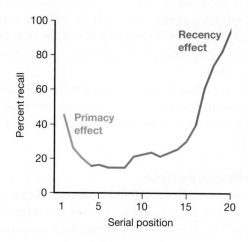

Research participants heard a list of 20 common words presented at a rate of 1 word per second. Immediately after hearing the list, participants were asked to write down as many of the words on the list as they could recall. The results show that position in the series strongly affected recall—participants had better recall for words at the beginning of the list (the primacy effect) and for words at the end of the list (the recency effect).

something known as the **primacy effect**, and they're also likely to remember the last few words on the list, a **recency effect**. The resulting pattern is a U-shaped curve describing the relation between position within the series—or **serial position**—and likelihood of recall (see **Figure 6.2**; Baddeley & Hitch, 1977; Deese & Kaufman, 1957; Glanzer & Cunitz, 1966; Murdock, 1962; Postman & Phillips, 1965).

Explaining the Recency Effect

What produces this pattern? We've already said that working memory contains the material someone is *working on* at just that moment. In other words, this memory contains whatever the person is currently thinking about; and of course, during the list presentation, the participants are thinking about the words they're hearing. Therefore, it's these words that are in working memory. This memory, however, is limited in its size, capable of holding only five or six words. Consequently, as participants try to keep up with the list presentation, they will be placing the words *just heard* into working memory, and this will bump the previous words out of this memory. Thus, as participants proceed through the list, their working memories will, at each moment, contain only the half dozen words that arrived most recently. Any words earlier than these will have been pushed out by later arrivals.

Of course, the last few words on the list don't get bumped out of working memory, because no further input arrives to displace these words. Therefore, when the list presentation ends, those last few words stay in place. Moreover, our hypothesis is that materials in working memory are readily available—easily and quickly retrieved. When the time comes for recall, then, working memory's contents (the list's last few words) are accurately and completely recalled.

The key idea, then, is that the list's ending is still in working memory when the list ends (because nothing has arrived to push out these items), and we know that working memory's contents are easy to retrieve. This is the source of the recency effect.

Explaining the Primacy Effect

The primacy effect comes from a different source. We've suggested that it takes some work to get information into long-term memory (LTM), and it seems likely that this work requires some time and attention. Let's examine, then, how participants allocate their attention to the list items. As participants hear the list, they do their best to be good memorizers, and so when they hear the first word, they typically repeat it over and over to themselves ("bicycle, bicycle, bicycle")—a process referred to as memory rehearsal. When the second word arrives, they rehearse it, too ("bicycle, artichoke, bicycle, artichoke"). Likewise for the third ("bicycle, artichoke, radio, bicycle, artichoke, radio"), and so on through the list. Note, though, that the first few items on the list are privileged: For a brief moment, "bicycle" is the only word participants have to worry about, and so it has 100% of their attention; no other word receives this privilege. When "artichoke" arrives a moment later, participants divide their attention between the list's first two words, and so "artichoke" gets only 50% of the participants' attention—less than "bicycle" got, but still a large share of the participants' efforts. When "radio" arrives, it has to compete with "bicycle" and "artichoke" for the participants' time, and so it receives only 33% of their attention.

Words arriving later in the list receive even less attention. Once six or seven words have been presented, the participants need to divide their attention among all of these words, which means that each one receives only a small fraction of the participants' focus. As a result, words later in the list are rehearsed fewer times than words early in the list—a fact we can confirm simply by asking participants to rehearse out loud (Rundus, 1971).

This view of things leads immediately to our explanation of the primacy effect—that is, the observed memory advantage for the early list items. These early words didn't have to share attention with other words (because the other words hadn't arrived yet), and so more time and more rehearsal were devoted to them than to any others. This means that the early words have a greater chance of being transferred into LTM—and so a greater chance of being recalled after a delay. That's what shows up in our data as the primacy effect.

Testing Claims about Primacy and Recency

This account of the serial-position curve leads to many further predictions. First, note that we're claiming the recency portion of the curve is coming from working memory, while the other items on the list are being recalled from LTM. Therefore, any manipulation of working memory should affect recall of the recency items but should have little impact on the other items on the list. To see how this works, consider a modification of our procedure. In the standard setup, we allow participants to recite what they remember immediately after the list's end. In place of this, we can delay recall by asking participants to perform some other task prior to their report of the list items. For example, we can ask them, immediately after hearing the list, to count backward by threes, starting from 201. They do this for just 30 seconds, and then they try to recall the list.

We've hypothesized that at the end of the list working memory still contains the last few items heard from the list. But the chore of counting backward will itself require working memory (e.g., to keep track of where you are in the counting sequence). Therefore, this chore will *displace* working memory's current contents; that is, it will bump the last few list items out of working memory. As a result, these items won't benefit from the swift and easy retrieval that working memory allows, and, of course, that retrieval was the presumed source of the recency effect. On this basis, the simple chore of counting backward, even if only for a few seconds, will eliminate the recency effect. In contrast, the counting backward should have no impact on recall of the items earlier in the list: These items are (by hypothesis) being recalled from long-term memory, not working memory, and there's no reason to think the counting task will interfere with LTM. (That's because LTM, unlike working memory, is not dependent on current activity.)

Figure 6.3 shows that these predictions are correct. An activity interpolated between the list and recall essentially eliminates the recency effect, but it has no influence elsewhere in the list (Baddeley & Hitch, 1977; Glanzer & Cunitz, 1966; Postman & Phillips, 1965). In contrast, merely delaying the recall for a few seconds after the list's end, with no interpolated activity, has no impact. In this case, participants can continue rehearsing the last few items during the delay and so can maintain them in working memory. With no new materials coming in, nothing pushes the recency items out of working memory, and so, even with a delay, a normal recency effect is observed.

The outcome should be different, though, if we manipulate long-term memory rather than working memory. In this case, the manipulation should affect all performance *except* for recency (which, again, is dependent on working memory, not LTM). For example, what happens if we slow down the presentation of the list? Now, participants will have more time to spend on all of the list items, increasing the likelihood of transfer into more permanent storage. This should improve recall for all items coming from LTM. Working memory, in contrast, is limited by its size, not by ease of entry or ease of access. Therefore, the slower list presentation should have no influence on working-memory performance. The results confirm these claims:

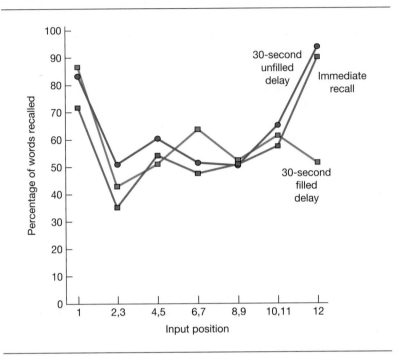

FIGURE 6.3   THE IMPACT OF INTERPOLATED ACTIVITY ON THE RECENCY EFFECT

With immediate recall, or if recall is delayed by 30 seconds with no activity during this delay, a strong recency effect is detected. In contrast, if participants spend 30 seconds on some other activity between hearing the list and the subsequent memory test, the recency effect is eliminated. This interpolated activity has no impact on the pre-recency portion of the curve.

Slowing the list presentation improves retention of all the pre-recency items but does not improve the recency effect (see **Figure 6.4**).

Other variables that influence long-term memory have similar effects. Using more familiar or more common words, for example, would be expected to ease entry into long-term memory and does improve pre-recency retention, but it has no effect on recency (Sumby, 1963).

Over and over, therefore, the recency and pre-recency portions of the curve are open to separate sets of influences and obey different principles. This strongly indicates that these portions of the curve are the products of different mechanisms, just as our theorizing proposes. In addition, fMRI scans suggest that memory for early items on a list depends on brain areas (in and around the hippocampus) that are associated with long-term memory; memory for later items on the list do not show this pattern (Talmi, Grady, Goshen-Gottstein, & Moscovitch, 2005; see **Figure 6.5**). This provides further (and powerful) confirmation for our memory model.

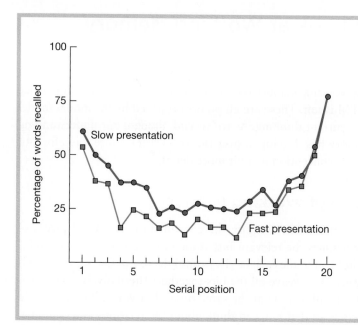

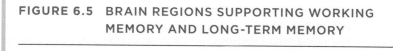

FIGURE 6.4 RATE OF LIST PRESENTATION AND THE SERIAL-POSITION EFFECT

Presenting the to-be-remembered materials at a slower rate improves pre-recency performance but has no effect on recency. The slow rate in this case was 9 seconds per item; the fast rate was 3 seconds per item.

FIGURE 6.5 BRAIN REGIONS SUPPORTING WORKING MEMORY AND LONG-TERM MEMORY

Retrieval from long-term memory specifically activates the hippocampus.

Retrieval from working memory specifically activates the perirhinal cortex.

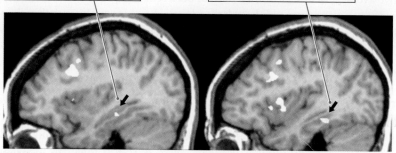

We can confirm the distinction between working memory and long-term memory with fMRI scans. These scans suggest that memory for early items on a list depends on brain areas (in and around the hippocampus) that are associated with long-term memory; memory for later items on the list do not show this pattern. TALMI, GRADY, GOSHEN-GOTTSTEIN, & MOSCOVITCH, 2005.

A Closer Look at Working Memory

We earlier counted four fundamental differences between working memory and LTM—the *size* of these two stores, the *ease of entry*, the ease of *retrieval*, and the fact that working memory is dependent on current activity (and hence *fragile*) while LTM is not. These are all points proposed by the modal model and preserved in current thinking. As we've said, though, our understanding of working memory has developed over the years. Let's pause, therefore, to examine the newer conception in a bit more detail.

The Function of Working Memory

Virtually all mental activities require the coordination of several pieces of information. Sometimes the relevant bits come into view one by one, and if so, you need to hold on to the early-arrivers until the rest of the information is available, and only then weave all the bits together. Alternatively, sometimes the relevant bits are all in view at the same time—but you still need to hold on to them together, so that you can think about the relations and combinations. In either case, you'll end up with multiple ideas in your thoughts, all activated simultaneously, and thus several bits of information in the status we describe as "in working memory." (For more on how you manage to focus on these various bits, see Oberauer & Hein, 2012.)

Framing things in this way makes it clear how important working memory is: You use working memory whenever you have multiple ideas in your mind, multiple elements that you're seeking to combine or compare. Let's now add that people differ in the "holding capacity" of their working memories. Some people are able to hold on to (and work with) more elements, and some with fewer. How exactly does this matter? To find out, we first need a means of *measuring* working memory's capacity, to find out if your memory capacity is above average, below, or somewhere in between. The procedure for obtaining this measurement, however, has changed over the years; looking at this change will help clarify what working memory *is*, and what working memory *is for*.

Digit Span

For many years, the holding capacity of working memory was measured with a digit-span task. In this task, people are read a series of digits (e.g., "8, 3, 4") and must immediately repeat them back. If they do so successfully, they're given a slightly longer list (e.g., "9, 2, 4, 0"). If they can repeat this one without error, they're given a still longer list ("3, 1, 2, 8, 5"), and so on. This procedure continues until the person starts to make errors—something that usually happens when the list contains more than seven or eight items. The number of digits the person can echo back without errors is referred to as that person's digit span.

Procedures such as this imply that working memory's capacity is typically around seven items or, more cautiously, at least five items and probably not more than nine items. These estimates are often summarized by the statement that this memory holds **"7 plus-or-minus 2"** items (Chi, 1976; Dempster, 1981; Miller, 1956; Watkins, 1977).

However, we immediately need a refinement of these measurements. If working memory can hold 7 plus-or-minus 2 items, what exactly is an "item"? Can we remember seven sentences as easily as seven words? Seven letters as easily as seven equations? In a classic paper, George Miller (one of the founders of the field of cognitive psychology) proposed that working memory holds 7 plus-or-minus 2 **chunks** (Miller, 1956). The term "chunk" is deliberately unscientific-sounding in order to remind us that a chunk does not hold a fixed quantity of information. Instead, Miller proposed, working memory holds 7 plus-or-minus 2 packages, and what those packages contain is largely up to the individual person.

The flexibility in how people "chunk" input can easily be seen in the span test. Imagine that we test someone's "letter span" rather than their "digit span," using the procedure we've already described. Thus, the person might hear "R, L" and have to repeat this sequence back, and then "F, J, S," and so on. Eventually, let's imagine that the person hears a much longer list, perhaps one starting "H, O, P, T, R, A, S, L, U. . . ." If the person thinks of these as individual letters, she'll only remember 7 of them, more or less. But the same person might reorganize the list into "chunks" and, in particular, think of the letters as forming syllables ("HOP, TRA, SLU, . . ."). In this case, she'll still remember 7 plus-or-minus 2 items, but the items are the *syllables*, and by remembering them she'll be able to report back at least a dozen letters and probably more.

How far can this process be extended? Chase and Ericsson (1982; Ericsson, 2003) studied a remarkable individual who happens to be a fan of track events. When he hears numbers, he thinks of them as finishing times for races. The sequence "3, 4, 9, 2," for example, becomes "3 minutes and 49.2 seconds, near world-record mile time." In this fashion, four digits become one chunk of information. This person can then retain 7 finishing times (7 chunks) in memory, and this can involve 20 or 30 digits! Better still, these chunks can be grouped into larger chunks, and these into even larger chunks. For example, finishing times for individual racers can be chunked together into heats within a track meet, so that, now, 4 or 5 finishing times (more than a dozen digits) become one chunk. With strategies like this and with a considerable amount of practice, this person has increased his apparent memory span from the "normal" 7 digits to 79 digits.

However, let's be clear that what has changed through practice is merely this person's chunking strategy, not the capacity of working memory itself. This is evident in the fact that when tested with sequences of letters, rather than numbers, so that he can't use his chunking strategy, this individual's memory span is a normal size—just 6 consonants. Thus, the 7-chunk limit is still in place for this man, even though (with numbers) he is able to make extraordinary use of these 7 slots.

EBOOK
DEMONSTRATION 6.2

Operation Span

Chunking provides one complication in our measurement of working memory's capacity. Another—and deeper—complication grows out of the very nature of working memory. Early theorizing about working memory, we've said, was guided by the modal model, and this model implies that working memory is something like a box in which information is stored, or perhaps a location in which information can be displayed. The traditional digit-span test fits well with this conception. If working memory is like a "box," then it's sensible to ask how much "space" there is in the box: How many slots, or spaces, are there in it? This is precisely what the digit span measures, on the notion that each digit (or each chunk) is placed in its own slot.

We've suggested, though, that the modern conception of working memory is more dynamic—so that working memory is best thought of as a *status* (something like "currently activated") rather than a *place* (see **Figure 6.6**). On this basis, perhaps we need to rethink how we measure this memory's capacity—seeking a measure that reflects working memory's active operation.

Modern researchers therefore measure this memory's capacity in terms of **operation span,** a procedure explicitly designed to measure working memory when it is "working." There are several ways to measure operation span, with the types differing in what "operation" they use (Conway et al., 2005; but also see Cowan, 2010). One type, for example, is *reading span*; to

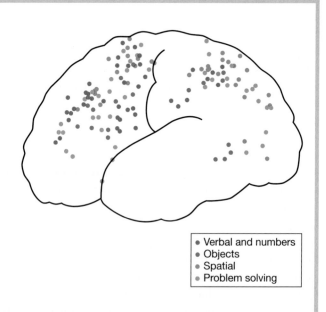

FIGURE 6.6   IS WORKING MEMORY A "PLACE"?

Modern theorists argue that working memory is not a place at all, but is instead the name we give for a certain set of mental activities. Consistent with this modern view, there's no specific location within the brain that serves as working memory. Instead, working memory is associated with a wide range of brain sites, as shown here.
AFTER CABEZA & NYBERG, 2000.

- Verbal and numbers
- Objects
- Spatial
- Problem solving

measure this span, research participants might be asked to read aloud a series of sentences, like these:

Due to his gross inadequacies, his position as director was terminated abruptly.

It is possible, of course, that life did not arise on Earth at all.

Immediately after reading the sentences, the participant is asked to recall each sentence's final word—in this case, "abruptly" and "all." If the participant can do this with these two sentences, she's asked to do the same task with a group of three sentences, and then with four, and so on, until the limit on her performance is located. This limit defines the person's working-memory capacity, typically abbreviated WMC.

Think about what this task involves: storing materials (the ending words) for later use in the recall test, while simultaneously working with other materials (the full sentences). This juggling of processes, as you move from one part of the task to the next, is exactly what working memory must do in its functioning in day-to-day life. Therefore, performance in this test is likely to reflect the efficiency with which working memory will operate in more natural settings.

Is the operation span a valid measure—that is, does it measure what it's supposed to? Our hypothesis, of course, is that someone with a higher span has a larger working memory, and if this is right, then someone with a higher span should have an advantage in tasks that make heavy use of this memory. Which tasks are these? They're tasks that require you to keep multiple ideas active at the same time, so that you can coordinate and integrate various bits of information. Thus, here's our prediction: People with a larger span (i.e., a greater WMC) should do better in tasks that require the coordination of different pieces of information.

Consistent with this claim, people with a greater WMC do have an advantage in many settings—in tests of reasoning, assessments of reading comprehension, standardized academic tests (including the verbal SAT), and more (e.g., Ackerman, Beier, & Boyle, 2002; Butler, Arrington & Weywadt, 2011; Daneman & Hannon, 2001; Engle & Kane, 2004; Gathercole & Pickering, 2000; Gray, Chabris, & Braver, 2003; Salthouse & Pink, 2008).

These results actually convey several messages. First, these correlations provide indications about when it's helpful to have a larger working memory, which in turn helps us understand when and how working memory is used. Second, the link between WMC and measures of intellectual performance provides an intriguing hint about what we're measuring with tests (like the SAT) that seek to measure "intelligence." We'll return to this issue in Chapter 13 when we discuss the nature of intelligence. Third, it's important that these various correlations are obtained with the more active measure of working memory (operation span) but not with the more traditional (and more static) span measure. (We note, however, that there

FIGURE 6.7 DYNAMIC MEASURES OF WORKING MEMORY

$(7 \times 7) + 1 = 50$; dog
$(10/2) + 6 = 10$; gas
$(4 \times 2) + 1 = 9$; nose
$(3/1) + 1 = 5$; beat
$(5/5) + 1 = 2$; tree

Operation span can be measured in several different ways. In one procedure, participants must announce whether each of these "equations" is true or false, and then recall the words that were appended to each equation. If participants can do this with two equations, we ask them to do three; if they can do that, we ask them to try four. By finding out how far they can go, we measure their working-memory capacity.

are several ways to measure operation span—see **Figure 6.7**.) This point confirms the advantage of the more dynamic measures and, more broadly, strengthens the idea that we're now thinking about working memory in the right way: not as a passive storage box but instead as a highly active information processor.

The Working-Memory System

Working memory's active nature is also evident in another way: in the actual structure of this memory. In Chapter 1, we introduced the idea that working memory is not a single entity but is instead a *system* built out of several components (Baddeley, 1986, 1992, 2002, 2012; Baddeley & Hitch, 1974). At the center of the system is a set of processes we discussed in Chapter 5: the executive control processes that govern the selection and sequence of our thoughts. In discussions of working memory, these processes have been playfully dubbed the *central executive*, as if there were a tiny agent somehow embedded in your mind, running your mental operations. Of course, there is no agent, and the central executive is merely a name we give to the set of mechanisms and processes that do run the show.

The central executive is needed for the "work" in working memory; thus, if you have to plan a response or make a decision, these steps require the executive. But there are many settings in which you need less than this from working memory. Specifically, there are settings in which you need to keep ideas in mind, not because you're analyzing or integrating them but because you're likely to need them *soon*. In this case, you don't need the executive.

Instead, you can rely on the executive's "helpers," leaving the executive itself free to work on more difficult matters.

In Chapter 1, we discussed the fact that the executive has several helpers, including the *articulatory rehearsal loop*, used for storing verbal material. Another helper is the *visuospatial buffer*, used for storing visual materials, such as mental images (see Chapter 11). Both of these helpers function in much the same way a piece of scratch paper on your desk does: Imagine that a friend tells you a phone number and that you'll need to dial the number in a few minutes. Odds are that you'll jot the number down on whatever piece of paper is nearby. That way, the number is "stored" so that you don't have to keep it in your thoughts, allowing you to turn your attention to other chores. Then, a few minutes later, when you're ready to dial the number, you can glance at the paper and see the digits, ready for use. Working memory's helpers function in roughly the same way—providing brief interim storage for information you'll need soon, but doing so in a way that does not burden the executive.

The Central Executive

In Chapter 1, we described the functioning of working memory's rehearsal loop and discussed some of the evidence confirming this loop's existence. But what can we say about the main player within working memory—the central executive? Here, too, we can rely on earlier chapters, because (as we've already flagged) the central executive (a crucial concept for theorizing about working memory) is really the same thing as the *executive control processes* we described in Chapter 5 (where we introduced the executive as a key concept in our theorizing about attention; also see Repovš & Baddeley, 2006).

In Chapter 5, we argued that executive control processes are needed to govern the sequence of your thoughts and actions; these processes enable you to set goals, to make plans for reaching those goals, and to select the steps needed for implementing those plans. Executive control also helps you whenever you want to rise above habit or routine, in order to "tune" your words or deeds to the current circumstances.

For purposes of the current chapter, though, let's emphasize that the same processes control the selection of ideas that are active at any moment in time. And, of course, these active ideas constitute the contents of working memory. It's inevitable, then, that we would link executive control with this type of memory.

With all these points in view, we're ready to move on. We've now updated the modal model (Figure 6.1) in important ways, and in particular we've abandoned the notion of a relatively passive *short-term memory* serving largely as storage container. We've shifted instead to a dynamic conception of *working memory*, with the proposal that this term is merely the name we give to an organized set of activities—especially the complex activities of the central executive. (For more on this updated view of working memory, see Jonides et al., 2008; Nee, Berman, Moore, & Jonides, 2008.)

But let's also emphasize that in this modern conception, just as in the modal model, working memory is quite fragile: Each shift in attention brings new information into working memory, and this newly arriving material displaces earlier items. Storage in this memory, therefore, is temporary. Obviously, then, we also need some sort of enduring memory storage, so that we can remember things that happened an hour, or a day, or even years ago. Let's turn, therefore, to the functioning of long-term memory.

Entering Long-Term Storage: The Need for Engagement

We've already seen an important clue regarding how information gets established in long-term storage: In discussing the primacy effect, we suggested that the more an item is rehearsed, the more likely it is that you'll remember that item later. In order to pursue this point, though, we need to ask what exactly rehearsal is and how it might work to promote memory.

Two Types of Rehearsal

The term "rehearsal" really means little beyond "thinking about." In other words, when a research participant rehearses an item on a memory list, she's simply thinking about that item—perhaps once, perhaps over and over; perhaps mechanically, or perhaps with close attention to what the item means. Clearly, therefore, there's considerable variety within the activities that count as rehearsal, and, in fact, psychologists find it useful to sort this variety into two broad types.

As one option, people can engage in **maintenance rehearsal**, in which they simply focus on the to-be-remembered items themselves, with little thought about what the items mean or how they are related to each other. This is a rote, mechanical process, recycling items in working memory simply by repeating them over and over. In contrast, **relational**, or **elaborative**, **rehearsal** involves thinking about what the to-be-remembered items mean and how they're related to each other and to other things you already know.

In general, relational rehearsal is vastly superior to maintenance rehearsal for establishing information in memory. Indeed, in many settings maintenance rehearsal provides no long-term benefit whatsoever. As an informal demonstration of this point, consider the following experience (although, for a more formal demonstration of this point, see Craik & Watkins, 1973). You're watching your favorite reality show on TV. The announcer says, "To vote for Contestant #4, dial 800-233-4830!" You reach into your pocket for your phone but realize you left it in the other room. You therefore recite the number to yourself while scurrying for your phone, but then, just before you dial, you see that you've got a text message. You pause, read the message, and then you're ready to dial, but . . . you realize at that moment that you don't have a clue what the number was.

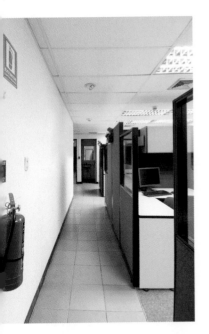

WE DON'T REMEMBER THINGS WE DON'T PAY ATTENTION TO

To promote public safety, many buildings have fire extinguishers and automatic defibrillators positioned in obvious and easily accessible locations. But in a moment of need, will people in the building remember where this safety equipment is located? Will they even remember that the safety equipment is conveniently available? Research suggests they may not. Occupants of the building have passed by the safety equipment again and again— but have had no reason to take notice of the equipment. As a result, they are unlikely to remember where the equipment is located. AFTER CASTEL, VENDETTI, & HOLYOAK, 2012.

What went wrong? You certainly heard the number, and you rehearsed it a couple of times while you were moving to fetch your phone. But despite these rehearsals, the brief interruption (from reading the text) seems to have erased the number from your memory. But this isn't ultra-rapid forgetting. Instead, you never established the number in memory in the first place, because in this setting you relied only on maintenance rehearsal. This kept the number in your thoughts while you were moving across the room, but it did nothing to establish the number in long-term storage. And when you try to dial the number (again: after reading the text), it's long-term storage that you need.

The idea, then, is that if you think about something only in a mindless and mechanical fashion, the item will not be established in your memory. In the same way, long-lasting memories are not created simply by repeated exposures to the items to be remembered. If you encounter an item over and over but, on each encounter, barely think about it (or think about it only in a mechanical fashion), then this, too, will not produce a long-term memory. As a demonstration, consider the ordinary penny. Adults in the United States have probably seen pennies tens of thousands of times. Adults in other countries have seen their own coins just as often. If sheer exposure is what counts for memory, people should remember perfectly what these coins look like.

But, of course, most people have little reason to pay attention to the penny. Pennies are a different color from the other coins, so they can be identified at a glance with no need for further scrutiny. If it's scrutiny that matters for memory, or, more broadly, *if we remember what we pay attention to and think about*, then memory for the coin should be quite poor.

The evidence on this point is clear: People's memory for the penny is remarkably bad. For example, most people know that Lincoln's head is on the "heads" side, but which way is he facing? Is it his right cheek that's visible or his left? What other markings are on the coin? Most people do very badly with these questions; their answers to the "Which way is he facing?" question are close to random (see **Figure 6.8**; Nickerson & Adams, 1979); performance is similar for people in other countries remembering their own coins. (Also see Bekerian & Baddeley, 1980; Rinck, 1999, for a much more consequential example.)

The Need for Active Encoding

Apparently, it takes some work to get information into long-term memory. Merely having an item in front of your eyes is not enough—even if the item is there over and over and over. Likewise, having an item in your thoughts doesn't, by itself, establish a memory. That's evident in the fact that maintenance rehearsal seems ineffective at promoting memory.

Further support for these claims comes from studies of brain activity during learning. In several procedures, researchers have used fMRI recording to keep track of the moment-by-moment brain activity in people who were studying a list of words (Brewer, Zhao, Desmond, Glover, & Gabrieli, 1998; Wagner, Koutstaal, & Schacter, 1999; Wagner et al., 1998; also see Levy,

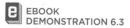

EBOOK
DEMONSTRATION 6.3

FIGURE 6.8 MEMORY FOR PENNIES

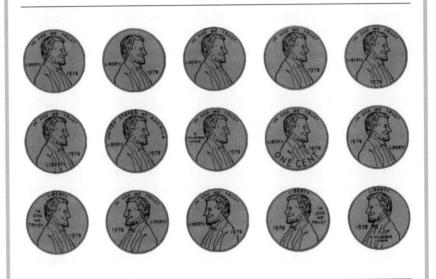

Despite having seen the U.S. penny thousands and thousands of times, people seem to have little recollection of its layout. Test yourself. Which of these versions is most accurate?

Kuhl & Wagner, 2010). Later, the participants were able to remember some of the words they had learned, but not others, which allowed the investigators to return to their initial recordings and compare brain activity *during the learning process* for words that were later remembered and words that were later forgotten. **Figure 6.9** shows the results, with a clear difference, during the initial encoding, between these two types of words. Specifically, greater levels of brain activity (especially in the hippocampus and regions of the prefrontal cortex) were reliably associated with greater probabilities of retention later on.

These fMRI results are telling us, once again, that learning is not a passive process. Instead, activity is needed to lodge information into long-term memory, and, apparently, higher levels of this activity lead to better memory. But this raises some new questions: What is this activity? What does it accomplish? And if—as it seems—*maintenance* rehearsal is a poor way to memorize, what type of rehearsal is more effective?

Incidental Learning, Intentional Learning, and Depth of Processing

Consider a student taking a course in college. The student knows that her memory for the course materials will be tested later (e.g., in the course's final exam). And presumably the student will take various steps to help

FIGURE 6.9 BRAIN ACTIVITY DURING LEARNING

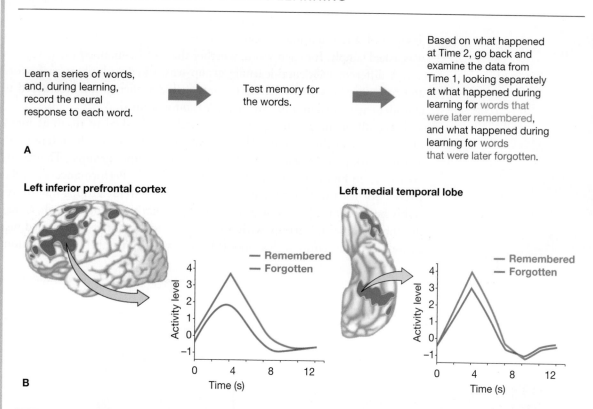

(Panel A) Participants in this study were given a succession of words to memorize, and their brain activity was recorded during this initial presentation. These brain scans were then divided into two types: those showing brain activity during the encoding of words that were remembered later on in a subsequent test, and those showing activity during encoding of words that were forgotten in the test. (Panel B) As the figure shows, activity levels during encoding were higher for the later-remembered words than they were for the later-forgotten words. This confirms that whether a word is forgotten or not depends on participants' mental activity when they encountered the word in the first place.

herself remember: She may read through her notes again and again; she may discuss the material with friends; she may try outlining the material. Will these various techniques work—so that the student will have a complete and accurate memory when the exam takes place? And notice that the student is taking these steps in the context of wanting to memorize, hoping to memorize. How do these elements influence performance? Or, put another way, how does the intention to memorize influence how or how well material is learned?

In an early experiment, participants in one condition heard a list of 24 words; their task was to remember as many of these words as they could.

This is **intentional learning**—learning that is deliberate, with an expectation that memory will be tested later. Other groups of participants heard the same 24 words but had no idea that their memories would be tested. This allows us to examine the impact of **incidental learning**—that is, learning in the absence of any intention to learn. One of these incidental-learning groups was asked simply, for each word, whether the word contained the letter *e* or not. A different incidental-learning group was asked to look at each word and to report how many letters it contained. Another group was asked to consider each word and to rate how *pleasant* it seemed.

Later, all of the participants were tested—and asked to recall as many of the words as they could. (The test was as expected for the intentional-learning group, but it was a surprise for all of the other groups.) The results are shown in **Figure 6.10A** (Hyde & Jenkins, 1969). Performance was relatively poor for the "Find the *e*" and "Count the letters" groups but appreciably better for the "How pleasant?" group. What's striking, though, is that the "how pleasant?" group, with no intention to memorize, performed just as well as the intentional-learning ("Learn these!") group. The suggestion,

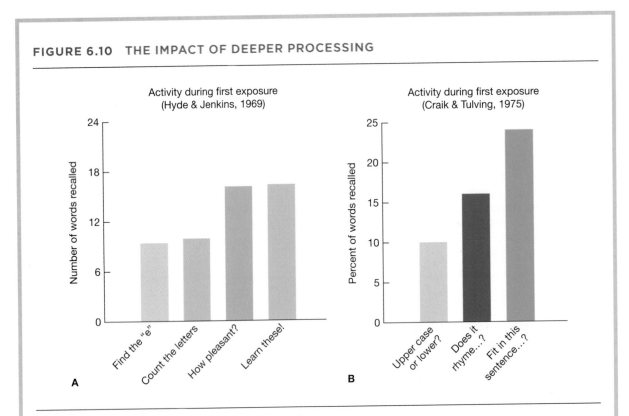

FIGURE 6.10   THE IMPACT OF DEEPER PROCESSING

The two sets of results here derive from studies described in the text, but are just part of an avalanche of data confirming the broad pattern: Shallow processing leads to poor memory. Deeper processing (paying attention to meaning) leads to much better memory. And what matters seems to be the level of engagement; the specific intention to learn (because someone knows their memory will be tested later on) contributes little.

then, is that the intention to learn doesn't add very much; memory can be just as good without this intention, provided that you approach the materials in the right way.

This broad pattern has been reproduced in countless other experiments (to name just a few: Bobrow & Bower, 1969; Craik & Lockhart, 1972; Hyde & Jenkins, 1973; Jacoby, 1978; Lockhart, Craik, & Jacoby, 1976; Parkin, 1984; Slamecka & Graf, 1978). As one example, consider a study by Craik and Tulving (1975). Their participants were again led to do incidental learning (i.e., the participants did not know their memories would be tested). For some of the words shown, the participants did **shallow processing**—that is, they engaged the material in a superficial fashion. Specifically, they had to say whether the word was printed in CAPITAL letters or not. (Other examples of shallow processing would be decisions about whether the words are printed in red or in green, high or low on the screen, and so on.) For other words, the participants had to do a moderate level of processing: They had to judge whether each word shown *rhymed* with a particular cue word. Then, finally, for other words, participants had to do **deep processing**. This is processing that requires some thought about what the words *mean*; specifically, Craik and Tulving asked whether each word shown would fit into a particular sentence.

The results are shown in Figure 6.10B. Plainly, there is a huge effect here of **level of processing**, with deeper processing (i.e., more attention to meaning) leading to better memory. In addition, Craik and Tulving (and many other researchers) have confirmed the Hyde and Jenkins finding that the intention to learn adds little. That is, memory performance is roughly the same in conditions in which participants do shallow processing *with* an intention to memorize, and in conditions in which they do shallow processing *without* this intention. Likewise, the outcome is the same whether people do deep processing *with* the intention to memorize or *without*. In study after study, what matters is how people approach the material they're seeing or hearing. It's that approach, that manner of engagement, that determines whether memory will be excellent or poor later on. The intention to learn seems, by itself, not to matter.

The Role of Meaning and Memory Connections

The message so far seems clear: If you want to remember the sentences you're reading in this text, or the materials you're learning in the training sessions at your job, you should pay attention to what these materials mean. That is, you should try to do deep processing. And, in fact, if you do deep processing, it won't matter if you're trying hard to memorize the materials (intentional learning) or merely paying attention to the meaning because you find the material interesting, with no plan for memorizing (incidental learning).

But what lies behind these effects? Why does attention to meaning lead to such good recall? Let's start with a broad proposal; we'll then fill in the evidence for this proposal.

EBOOK
DEMONSTRATION 6.4

Connections Promote Retrieval

Perhaps surprisingly, the benefits of deep processing may not lie in the learning process itself. Instead, deep processing may influence subsequent events. More precisely, attention to meaning may help you by virtue of facilitating *retrieval* of the memory later on. To understand this point, consider what happens whenever a library acquires a new book. On its way into the collection, the new book must be catalogued and shelved appropriately. These steps happen when the book arrives, but the cataloguing doesn't literally influence the arrival of the book into the building. The moment the book is delivered, it's physically in the library, catalogued or not, and the book doesn't become "more firmly" or "more strongly" in the library because of the cataloguing.

But the cataloguing is crucial. If the book were merely tossed on a random shelf somewhere, with no entry in the catalogue, users might never be able to find it. Indeed, without a catalogue entry, users of the library might not even realize that the book was in the building. Notice, then, that cataloguing happens at the time of arrival, but the benefit of cataloguing isn't for the arrival itself. (If the librarians all went on strike, so that no books were being catalogued, books would continue to arrive, magazines would still be delivered, and so on. Again: The *arrival* doesn't depend on cataloguing.) Instead, the benefit of cataloguing is for events subsequent to the book's arrival: Cataloguing makes it possible (and maybe makes it *easy*) to find the book later on.

The same is true for the vast library that is your memory. The task of learning is not merely a matter of placing information into long-term storage. Learning also needs to establish some appropriate indexing; it must, in effect, pave a path to the newly acquired information, so that this information can

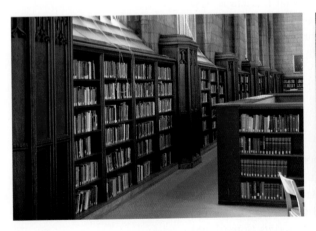 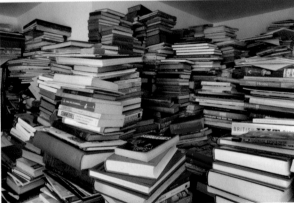

WHY DO MEMORY CONNECTIONS HELP?

When books arrive in a library, the librarians must catalog them. This doesn't facilitate the "entry" of books into the library—the books are in the building whether they are catalogued or not. But cataloguing makes the books vastly easier to find later on. Memory connections may serve the same function: The connections don't "bring" material into memory, but they do make the material "findable" in long-term storage later.

be retrieved at some future point. Thus, one of the main chores of memory acquisition is to lay the groundwork for memory retrieval.

But what is it that facilitates memory retrieval? There are, in fact, several ways to search through memory, but a great deal depends on memory *connections*. Connections allow one memory to trigger another, and then that memory to trigger another, so that you are "led," connection by connection, to the sought-after information. In some cases, the connections link one of the items you're trying to remember to some of the other items; if so, finding the first will lead you to the others. In other settings, the connections might link some aspect of the context-of-learning to the target information, so that when you think again about the context ("I recognize this room—this is where I was last week"), you'll be led to other ideas ("Oh, yeah, I read that sad story in this room"). In all cases, though, this triggering will happen only if the relevant connections are in place—and establishing those connections is a large part of what happens during learning.

This line of reasoning has many implications, and we can use those implications as a basis for testing whether this proposal is correct. But, right at the start, it should be clear why, according to this account, deep processing (i.e., attention to meaning) promotes memory. The key here is that attention to meaning involves thinking about relationships: "What words are related in meaning to the word I'm now considering? What words have *contrasting* meaning? What is the relationship between the start of this story and the way the story turned out?" Points like these are likely to be prominent when you're thinking about what some word (or sentence or event) means, and these points will help you to find (or, perhaps, to *create*) connections among your various ideas. It's these connections, we're proposing, that really matter for memory.

Elaborate Encoding Promotes Retrieval

We need to be clear, though, that, on this account, attention to meaning is not the only way to improve memory. Other strategies should also be helpful, provided that they help you to establish memory connections. As an example, consider another study by Craik and Tulving (1975). Participants were shown a word and then shown a sentence with one word left out. Their task was to decide whether the word fit into the sentence. For example, they might see the word "chicken," then the sentence "She cooked the _____." The appropriate response would be yes, since the word does fit in this sentence. After a series of these trials, there was a surprise memory test, with participants asked to remember all the words they had seen.

There was, however, an additional element in this experiment: Some of the sentences shown to participants were simple, while others were more elaborate. For example, a more complex sentence might be "The great bird swooped down and carried off the struggling _____." Sentences like this one produced a large memory benefit. More precisely, words were much more likely to be remembered if they appeared with these rich, elaborate sentences than if they had appeared in the simpler sentences (see **Figure 6.11**).

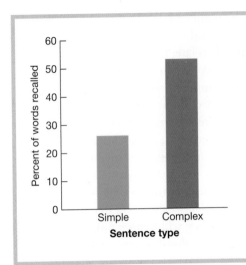

FIGURE 6.11 DEEP AND ELABORATE ENCODING

Deep processing (paying attention to meaning) promotes memory, but it is not the only factor that has this benefit. More elaborate processing (e.g., by thinking about the word in the context of a complex sentence, rich with relationships) also has a powerful effect on memory. AFTER CRAIK & TULVING, 1975.

Apparently, then, deep *and elaborate* processing leads to better recall than deep processing on its own. Why is this? The answer hinges on memory connections. Perhaps the "great bird swooped" sentence calls to mind a barnyard scene with the hawk carrying a chicken away. Or perhaps it calls to mind thoughts about predator-prey relationships. One way or another, the richness of this sentence offers the potential for many connections as it calls other thoughts to mind, each of which can be connected, in your thinking, to the target sentence. These connections, in turn, provide potential **retrieval paths**—paths that can, in effect, guide your thoughts toward the content to be remembered. All of this seems less likely for the impoverished sentences, which will evoke fewer connections and so establish a narrower set of retrieval paths. Consequently, words associated with these sentences are less likely to be recalled later on.

Organizing and Memorizing

Sometimes, we've said, memory connections link the to-be-remembered material to other information already in memory. In other cases, the connections link one aspect of the to-be-remembered material to another aspect of the same material. Such a connection ensures that if any part of the material is recalled, then all will be recalled.

In all settings, though, the connections are important, and that leads us to ask how people go about discovering (or creating) these connections. More than 60 years ago, a psychologist named George Katona argued that the key lies in *organization* (Katona, 1940). Katona's argument, in fact, was that the processes of organization and memorization are inseparable: You memorize well when you discover the order within the material. Conversely, if you find (or impose) an organization on the material, you will easily remember it. These suggestions are fully compatible with the conception we're developing here, since what organization provides is, once again, memory connections.

Mnemonics

For thousands of years, people have longed for "better" memories; guided by this wish, people in the ancient world devised various techniques to improve memory—techniques known as **mnemonic strategies**. In fact, many of the mnemonics still in use date back to ancient Greece. (It is therefore appropriate that these techniques are named in honor of Mnemosyne, the goddess of memory in Greek mythology.)

How do mnemonics work? In general, these strategies simply provide some means of organizing the to-be-remembered material. For example, one broad class of mnemonic, often used for memorizing sequences of words, links the *first letters* of the words into some meaningful structure. Thus, children rely on ROY G. BIV to memorize the sequence of colors in the rainbow (*red, orange, yellow* . . .) and learn the lines in music's treble clef via "Every Good Boy Deserves Fudge" or ". . . Does Fine" (the lines indicate the musical notes *E, G, B, D,* and *F*). Biology students use a sentence like "King Philip Crossed the Ocean to Find Gold and Silver" (or: ". . . to Find Good Spaghetti") to memorize the sequence of taxonomic categories: *kingdom, phylum, class, order, family, genus,* and *species.*

Other mnemonics involve the use of mental imagery, relying on "mental pictures" to link the to-be-remembered items to each other. (We'll have much more to say about "mental pictures" in Chapter 11.) For example, imagine a student trying to memorize a list of word pairs. For the pair *eagle-train*, the student might imagine the eagle winging back to its nest with a locomotive in its beak. Evidence indicates that images of this sort can be enormously helpful. It's important, though, that the images show the objects in some sort of relationship or interaction—again highlighting the role of organization. It doesn't help just to form a picture of an eagle and a train sitting side-by-side (Wollen, Weber, & Lowry, 1972; for an example of the *wrong* sort of mnemonic use, *not* providing the linkage, see **Figure 6.12**).

A different type of mnemonic provides an external "skeleton" for the to-be-remembered materials, and here too mental imagery can be useful. Imagine, for example, that you want to remember a list of largely unrelated items, perhaps the entries on your shopping list or a list of questions you want to ask when you next see your adviser. For this purpose, you might rely on one of the so-called **peg-word systems**. These systems begin with a well-organized structure, such as this one:

One is a bun.

Two is a shoe.

Three is a tree.

Four is a door.

Five is a hive.

Six are sticks.

Seven is heaven.

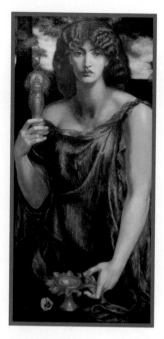

MNEMOSYNE

Strategies used to improve memory are known as mnemonic strategies; the term derives from the name of the goddess of memory in Greek mythology—Mnemosyne.

FIGURE 6.12   MNEMONIC STRATEGIES

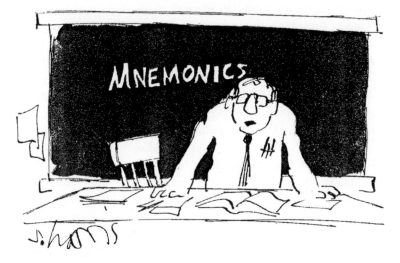

"YOU SIMPLY ASSOCIATE EACH NUMBER WITH A WORD, SUCH AS 'TABLE' AND 3,476,029."

To be effective, a mnemonic must provide some rich linkage among the items being memorized. Merely putting the items side-by-side is not enough.

Eight is a gate.

Nine is a line.

Ten is a hen.

This rhyme provides ten "peg words" ("bun," "shoe," and so on), and in memorizing something you can "hang" the materials to be remembered on these "pegs." Let's imagine, therefore, that you want to remember the list of topics you need to discuss with your adviser. If you want to discuss your unhappiness with your chemistry class, you might form an association between chemistry and the first peg, "bun." You might, for example, form a mental image of a hamburger bun floating in an Erlenmeyer flask. If you also want to discuss your after-graduation plans, you might form an association between some aspect of those plans and the next peg, "shoe." (Perhaps you might think about how you plan to pay your way after college by selling shoes.) Then, when the time comes to meet with your adviser, all you have to do is think through that silly rhyme again. When you think of "one is a bun," it is highly likely that the image of the flask (and therefore of chemistry lab) will come to mind. When you think of "two is a shoe," you'll be reminded of your job plans. And so on.

Hundreds of variations on these techniques—the first-letter mnemonics, visualization strategies, peg-word systems—are available. Some of the variations are taught in self-help books (you've probably seen the ads—"How to Improve Your Memory!"); some are presented by corporations as part of management training. All the variations, though, use the same basic scheme. To remember a list with no apparent organization, you impose an organization on it by using a skeleton or scaffold that is itself tightly organized. And, crucially, these systems all work: They help you remember individual items, and they also help you remember those items in a specific sequence. **Figure 6.13** shows some of the data from one early study; many other studies confirm this pattern (e.g., Bower, 1970, 1972; Bower & Reitman, 1972; Christen & Bjork, 1976; Higbee, 1977; Roediger, 1980;

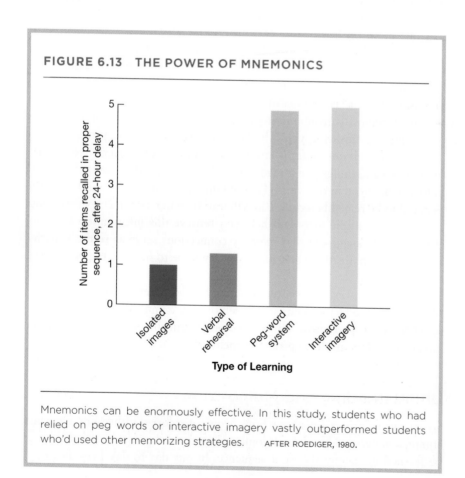

FIGURE 6.13   THE POWER OF MNEMONICS

Mnemonics can be enormously effective. In this study, students who had relied on peg words or interactive imagery vastly outperformed students who'd used other memorizing strategies.   AFTER ROEDIGER, 1980.

Ross & Lawrence, 1968; Yates, 1966). All of this strengthens our central claim: Mnemonics work because they impose an organization on the materials you're trying to memorize, and, consistently and powerfully, organizing improves recall.

Given the power of mnemonics, it's unsurprising that students often use these strategies to help them in their studies. Indeed, for many topics there are online databases containing thousands of useful mnemonics—helping medical students to memorize symptom lists, chemistry students to memorize the periodic table, neuroscientists to remember the brain's anatomy, and more.

Use of these mnemonics is sensible. We've already said that mnemonics can improve memory. But there's also a downside to mnemonics in educational settings: When you're using a mnemonic, you typically focus on just one aspect of the material you're trying to memorize—for example, just the first letter of the word to be remembered—and this focus usually means that you don't pay much attention to *other* aspects of the material. As a result, you may cut short your effort toward understanding this material, and likewise your effort toward finding multiple connections between the material and other things you know.

To put this point differently, mnemonic use involves a trade-off: If you focus your attention on just one or two memory connections, you'll spend little time thinking about *other* possible connections, including other connections that might help you understand the material. This trade-off will be fine if you don't care very much about the meaning of the material. (Do you care why, in taxonomy, "order" is a subset of "class," rather than the other way around?) But this trade-off is troubling if you're trying to memorize material that is meaningful. In this case, you'd be better served by a memory strategy that leads you to seek out *multiple* connections between the material you're trying to learn and things you already know. Indeed, this effort toward multiple links will help you in two ways. First, it will foster your understanding of the material to be remembered, and so will lead to better, richer, deeper learning. Second, the multiple links will help you retrieve this information later on: We've already suggested that memory connections serve as retrieval paths, and the more paths there are, the easier it will be to find the target material later.

For these reasons, mnemonic use may be ill-advised in many situations. Nonetheless, the fact remains that mnemonics are immensely useful in some settings (What were those rainbow colors?), and this in turn confirms our initial point: Organization promotes memory.

Understanding and Memorizing

So far, we've said a lot about how people memorize rather impoverished stimulus materials—lists of randomly selected words, or colors that have to be learned in exactly the right sequence. In our day-to-day lives, however, we typically want to remember more meaningful, and more complicated, material. We want to remember the episodes we experience, the details of rich scenes we have observed, or the many-step arguments we have read in a book. Do the same memory principles apply to these cases?

The answer is clearly yes (although we'll have more to say about this broad issue in Chapter 8). In other words, your memory for events, or pictures, or complex bodies of knowledge is enormously dependent on your being able to organize the material to be remembered. With these more complicated materials, though, we've already suggested that your best bet for organization is not some arbitrary skeleton like those used in the various mnemonics. Instead, the optimal organization of these complex materials is generally dependent on understanding. That is, you remember best what you understand best.

There are many ways to show that this is true. For example, we can give people a sentence or paragraph to read and test their comprehension by asking questions about the material. Sometime later, we can test their memory. The results are straightforward: The better the participants' understanding of a sentence or a paragraph, if questioned immediately after viewing the material, the greater the likelihood that they will remember the material after a delay (e.g., Bransford, 1979).

Likewise, consider the material you are learning right now in the courses you are taking. Will you remember this material 5 years from now, or 10, or 20? The answer depends on how well you understand the material, and one measure of understanding is the grade you earn in a course: With full and rich understanding, you're likely to earn an A; with poor understanding, your grade is likely to be lower. This leads to an obvious prediction: If understanding is (as we've proposed) important for memory, then the higher someone's grade in a course, the more likely that person is to remember the course contents, even years later. This is exactly what the data show, with A students remembering the material quite well, and C students remembering much less (Conway, Cohen, & Stanhope, 1992).

The relationship between understanding and memory can also be demonstrated in another way: by *manipulating* whether people understand the material or not. For example, in an experiment by Bransford and Johnson (1972, p. 722), participants read this passage:

The procedure is actually quite simple. First you arrange items into different groups. Of course one pile may be sufficient depending on how much there is to do. If you have to go somewhere else due to lack of facilities that is the next step; otherwise you are pretty well set. It is important not to overdo things. That is, it is better to do too few things at once than too many. In the short run, this may not seem important but complications can easily arise. A mistake can be expensive as well. At first, the whole procedure will seem complicated. Soon, however, it will become just another facet of life. It is difficult to foresee any end to the necessity for this task in the immediate future, but then, one never

FIGURE 6.14   MEMORY FOR DIGITS

1 4 9 1 6 2 5 3 6 4 9 6 4 8 1

Examine this series of digits for a moment, and then turn away from the page and try to recall all 15 in their proper sequence. The chances are good that you will fail in this task—perhaps remembering the first few and the last few digits, but not the entire list. Things will go differently, though, if you discover the pattern within the list. Now, you'll easily be able to remember the full sequence. What is the pattern? Try thinking of the series this way: 1, 4, 9, 16, 25, 36. . . . Here, as always, organizing and understanding aid memory.

can tell. After the procedure is completed one arranges the materials into different groups again. Then they can be put into their appropriate places. Eventually they will be used once more and the whole cycle will then have to be repeated. However, that is part of life.

You are probably puzzled by this passage; so are most research participants. The story is easy to understand, though, if we give it a title: "Doing the Laundry." In the experiment, some participants were given the title before reading the passage; others were not. Participants in the first group easily understood the passage and were able to remember it after a delay. The second group, reading the same words, were not confronting a meaningful passage and did poorly on the memory test. (For related data, see Bransford & Franks, 1971; Sulin & Dooling, 1974; for another example, see **Figure 6.14**.)

Similar effects can be documented with nonverbal materials. Consider the picture shown in **Figure 6.15**. At first it looks like a bunch of meaningless blotches; with some study, though, you may discover that a familiar object is depicted. Wiseman and Neisser (1974) tested people's memory for this picture. Consistent with what we have seen so far, their memory was good if they understood the picture—and bad otherwise. (Also see Bower, Karlin, & Dueck, 1975; Mandler & Ritchey, 1977; Rubin & Kontis, 1983.)

The Study of Memory Acquisition

This chapter has largely been about memory acquisition. How do we acquire new memories? How is new information, new knowledge, established in long-term memory? Or, in more pragmatic terms, what is the best, most

FIGURE 6.15 COMPREHENSION ALSO AIDS MEMORY FOR PICTURES

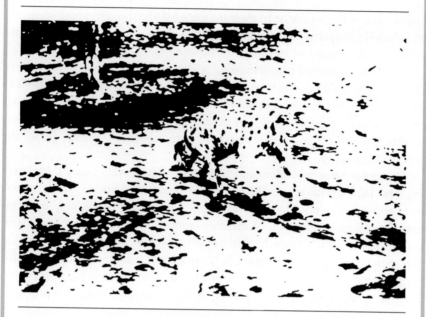

People who perceive this picture as a pattern of meaningless blotches are unlikely to remember the picture. People who perceive the "hidden" form do remember the picture. AFTER WISEMAN & NEISSER, 1974.

effective way to learn? We now have answers to these questions, but our discussion has also indicated that we need to place these questions into a broader context—with attention to the substantial contribution from the memorizer, and also a consideration of the interconnections among acquisition, retrieval, and storage.

The Contribution of the Memorizer

Over and over, we've seen that memory depends on *connections* among ideas. These connections, in turn, are fostered by the steps you take in your effort toward organizing and understanding the materials you encounter. Hand in hand with this, it appears that memories are not established by sheer contact with the items you're hoping to remember. If you are merely exposed to the items without giving them any thought, then subsequent recall of those items will be poor.

These points draw our attention to the huge role played by the memorizer. If, for example, we wish to predict whether this or that event will be recalled, it isn't enough to know that someone was exposed to the event. Instead, we need to ask what the person was *doing* during the event. Did she do mere maintenance rehearsal, or did she engage the material in some other way? If the latter, how did she think about the material? Did she pay attention to the appearance of the words or to their meaning? If she thought about meaning, was she able to understand the material? These considerations are crucial for predicting the success of memory.

The contribution of the memorizer is also evident in another way. We've argued that learning depends on your making connections, but connections to what? If you want to connect the to-be-remembered material to other knowledge, to other memories, then you need to have that other knowledge—you need to have other (potentially relevant) memories that you can "hook" the new material on to.

This point helps us understand why sports fans have an easy time learning new facts about sports, and why car mechanics can easily learn new facts about cars, and why memory experts easily memorize new information about memory. In each of these situations, the person enters the learning situation with a considerable advantage—a rich framework that the new materials can be woven into. But, conversely, if someone enters a learning situation with little relevant background, then there is no framework, nothing to connect to, and learning will be correspondingly more difficult. Plainly, then, if we want to predict someone's success in memorizing, we need to consider what other knowledge the individual brings into the situation.

The Links among Acquisition, Retrieval, and Storage

These points lead us to another theme of considerable importance. Our emphasis in this chapter has been on memory acquisition, but we've now seen that claims about acquisition cannot be separated from claims about storage and retrieval. For example, why is memory acquisition improved by organization? We've suggested that organization provides retrieval paths, making the memories "findable" later on, and this is, of course, a claim about retrieval. Plainly, therefore, our claims about acquisition are intertwined with claims about retrieval.

Likewise, we just noted that your ability to learn new material depends, in part, on your having a framework of prior knowledge to which the new materials can be tied. In this way, claims about memory acquisition need to be coordinated with claims about the nature of what is already in storage.

These interactions among acquisition, knowledge, and retrieval are crucial for our theorizing. But these interactions also have important implications for learning, for forgetting, and for memory accuracy. The next two chapters explore some of those implications.

How Should I Study?

Throughout your life, you encounter information that you hope to remember later. This point is particularly salient, though, for students in college courses or workers getting trained for a new job. These groups spend hours trying to master new information and new skills. If you're in one of these groups, what helpful lessons might you draw from memory research?

For a start, bear in mind that the *intention to memorize*, on its own, has no effect. Therefore, you don't need any special "memorizing steps." Instead, you should focus your efforts on making sure you *understand* the material, because if you do, you're likely to remember it.

As a specific strategy, it's often useful to quiz yourself with questions like these: "Does this new fact fit with other things I know?" or "Do I know why this fact is as it is?" or "Do I see why this conclusion is justified?" Answering these questions will help you find meaningful connections within the material you're learning, and also between this material and other information already in your memory—and all of these connections powerfully promote memory. In the same spirit, it's useful to rephrase material you encounter, putting it into your own words; this will force you to think about what the words mean—again a good thing for memory.

We should also note that students sometimes rely on study strategies that are far too passive. They simply read their notes or re-read an assignment over and over. In some cases, they listen again to an audio recording of an instructor's lecture. The students' idea here seems to be that the materials studied in this fashion will somehow "soak in" to their memories. But the flaw in this logic is obvious: As the chapter explains, memories are produced by active engagement with materials, not by passive exposure. Once again, therefore, we're led to the idea that your goal in studying should be an active search for understanding and connections—connections that will both enrich your comprehension and also serve as retrieval paths later.

As a related point, it's often useful to study with a friend—so that he or she can explain topics to you, and you can do the same in return. This step has several advantages. In explaining things, you're obviously forced into a more active role, in contrast to the passive stance you might take in reading or listening. Working with a friend is also likely to enhance your understanding, because each of you can help the other to understand bits you're having trouble with. You'll also benefit from hearing your friend's insights and perspective on the materials being learned. This additional perspective offers the possibility of creating new connections among ideas, making the information easier to recall later on.

Memory will also be best if you spread your studying out across multiple occasions—using *spaced learning* (essentially, taking breaks between study sessions) rather than *massed learning* (essentially, "cramming" all at once).

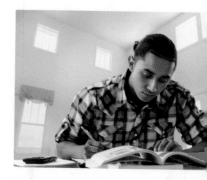

MEANINGFUL CONNECTIONS

What sort of connections will help you to remember? The answer, in truth, is that almost any connection can be helpful. Here's a silly—but useful!—example. Students learning about the nervous system have to learn that *efferent* fibers carry information away from the brain and central nervous system, while *afferent* fibers carry information inward. How to keep these terms straight? It may be helpful to notice that efferent fibers carry information *exiting* the nervous system, while afferent fibers provide *access* to the nervous system. And, as a bonus, the same connections will help you remember that you can have an *effect* on the world (an influence outward, from you), but that the world can also *affect* you (an influence coming in, toward you).

There are several reasons for this, including the fact that spaced learning makes it likely that you'll bring a slightly different perspective to the material each time you turn to it. This new perspective will enable you to see connections you didn't see before; and—again—the new connections create new links among ideas, which will provide retrieval paths that promote recall.

What about mnemonic strategies, such as a peg-word system? These are enormously helpful—but often at a cost. As the chapter mentions, focusing on the mnemonic may divert your time and attention away from efforts at understanding the material, and so you'll end up understanding the material less well. You will also be left with only the one or two retrieval paths that the mnemonic provides, not the multiple paths created by comprehension. There are surely circumstances in which these drawbacks are not serious, and so mnemonics are often useful for remembering specific dates or place names or particular bits of terminology. But for richer, more meaningful material, mnemonics may hurt you more than they help.

Finally, let's emphasize that there's more to say about these issues because our discussion here (like Chapter 6 itself) focuses on the "input" side of memory—getting information into storage, so that it's available for use later on. There are also steps you can take that will help you locate information in the vast warehouse of your memory, and still other steps that you can take to avoid forgetting materials you've already learned. Discussion of those steps, however, depends on materials we'll cover in Chapters 7 and 8.

chapter summary

● It is convenient to think of memorizing as having separate stages. First, one acquires new information (acquisition). Next, the information remains in storage until it is needed. Finally, the information is retrieved. However, this separation among the stages may be misleading. For example, in order to memorize new information, you form connections between this information and things you already know. In this fashion, the acquisition stage is intertwined with the retrieval of information already in storage.

● Information that is currently being considered is held in working memory; information that is not currently active but is nonetheless in storage is in long-term memory. The distinction between these two forms of memory has traditionally been described in terms of the modal model and has been examined in many studies of the serial-position curve. The primacy portion of this curve reflects those items that have had extra opportunity to reach long-term

memory; the recency portion of this curve reflects the accurate retrieval of items currently in working memory.

● Our conception of working memory has evolved in important ways in the last few decades. Crucially, psychologists no longer think of working memory as a "storage container" or even as a "place." Instead, working memory is a status—and so we say items are "in working memory" when they are being actively thought about, actively contemplated. This activity is governed by working memory's central executive. For mere storage, the executive often relies on a number of low-level assistants, including the articulatory rehearsal loop and the visuospatial buffer, which work as mental scratch pads. The activity inherent in this overall system is reflected in the flexible way material can be chunked in working memory; the activity is also reflected in current measures of working memory, via operation span.

Maintenance rehearsal serves to keep information in working memory and requires little effort, but it has little impact on subsequent recall. To maximize your chances of recall, elaborative rehearsal is needed, in which you seek connections within the material to be remembered or connections between the material to be remembered and things you already know.

In many cases, elaborative processing takes the form of attention to meaning. This attention to meaning is called "deep processing," in contrast to attention to sounds or visual form, which is considered "shallow processing." Many studies have shown that deep processing leads to good memory performance later on, even if the deep processing occurred with no intention of memorizing the target material. In fact, the intention to learn has no direct effect on performance; what matters instead is how someone engages or thinks about the material to be remembered.

Deep processing has beneficial effects by creating effective retrieval paths that can be used later on. Retrieval paths depend on connections linking one memory to another; each connection provides a path potentially leading to a target memory. Mnemonic strategies build on this idea and focus on the creation of specific memory connections, often tying the to-be-remembered material to a frame (e.g., a strongly structured poem).

Perhaps the best way to form memory connections is to understand the material to be remembered. In understanding, you form many connections within the material to be remembered, as well as between this material and other knowledge. With all of these retrieval paths, it becomes easy to locate this material in memory. Consistent with these suggestions, studies have shown a close correspondence between the ability to understand some material and the ability to recall that material later on; this pattern has been demonstrated with stories, visual patterns, number series, and many other sorts of stimuli.

e eBook Demonstrations & Essays

Online Demonstrations:
- Demonstration 6.1: Primacy and Recency Effects
- Demonstration 6.2: Chunking
- Demonstration 6.3: The Effects of Unattended Exposure
- Demonstration 6.4: Depth of Processing

Online Applying Cognitive Psychology Essays:
- Cognitive Psychology and the Law: The Video-Recorder View

ZAPS 2.0 Cognition Labs

- Go to **http://digital.wwnorton.com/cognition6** for the online labs relevant to this chapter.

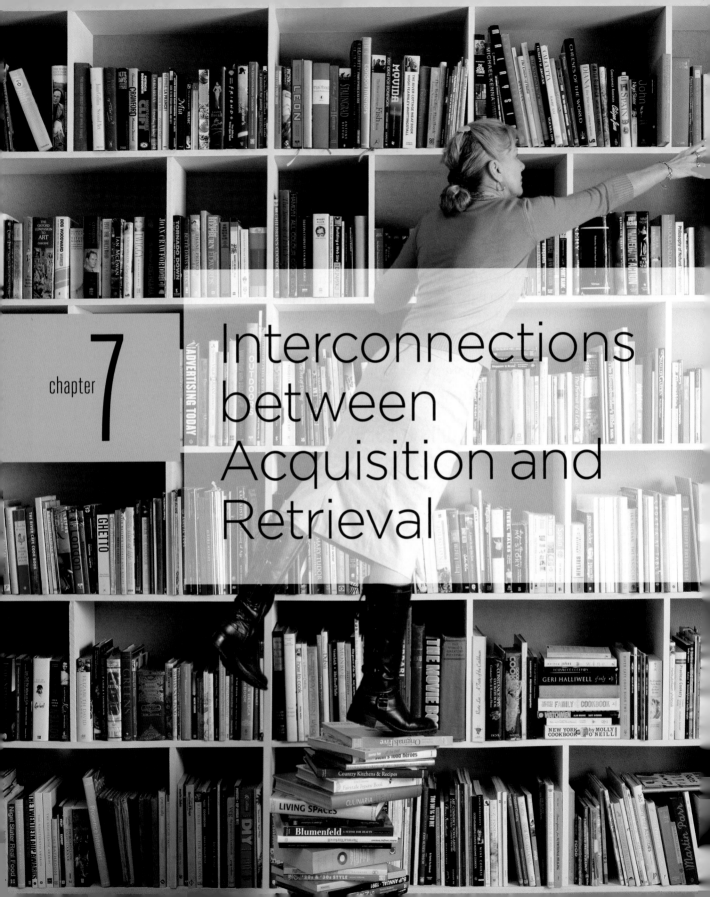

chapter **7**

Interconnections between Acquisition and Retrieval

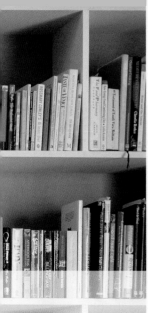
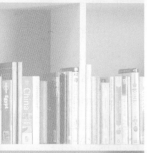
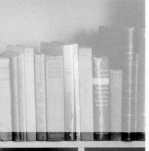
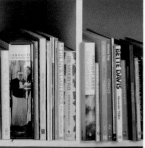
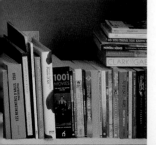

what if...

In Chapter 1, we introduced the case of H.M. (We also mentioned H.M. briefly in Chapters 2 and 6.) H.M., you'll recall, was in his mid-20's when he had brain surgery intended to control his epilepsy. The surgery was, in one regard, a success, and H.M.'s seizures were curtailed. But the surgery also had an unexpected and horrible consequence: H.M. lost the ability to form new, specific, episodic memories. If asked what he did last week, or yesterday, or even an hour ago, H.M. had no idea. He could not recognize the faces of medical staff he'd seen day after day. He could read and reread a book yet never realize that he'd read the same book many times before.

H.M.'s case is unique, but a related pattern of memory loss is observed among patients who suffer from Korsakoff's syndrome. We'll have more to say about this syndrome later in the chapter, but for now let's highlight a paradox. These patients, like H.M., are profoundly amnesic; they're completely unable to recall the events of their own lives. But these patients (again, like H.M.) seem to have "unconscious" memories— memories that they do not know they have.

We can reveal these unconscious memories if we test Korsakoff's patients *indirectly*. Thus, if we ask them, "Which of these melodies did you hear an hour ago?" they will answer randomly—confirming their amnesia. But if we ask them, "Which of these melodies do you prefer?" they're likely to choose the ones that, in fact, they heard an hour ago— indicating that they do somehow remember (and are influenced by) the earlier experience. If we ask them, "Have you ever seen a puzzle like this one before?" they'll say no. But if we ask them to solve the puzzle, their speed will be much faster the second time—even though they insist it's the *first* time they've seen the puzzle. They'll be faster still the third time they solve the puzzle and the fourth, although again and again they'll tell us that they're seeing the puzzle for the very first time. Likewise, they'll fail if we ask them, "I showed you some words a few minutes ago; can you tell me which of those words began 'CHE . . .'?" But, alternatively, we can ask them, "What's the first word that comes to mind that starts 'CHE . . .'?"

preview of chapter themes

● Learning does not simply place information in memory; instead, learning prepares you to retrieve the information in a particular way. As a result, learning that is good preparation for one sort of memory retrieval may be inadequate for other sorts of retrieval.

● In general, retrieval seems to be most likely if your mental perspective is the same during learning and during retrieval, just as we would expect if learning establishes retrieval paths that help you later when you "travel" the same path in your effort toward locating the target material.

● Some experiences seem to produce unconscious memories. Consideration of these "implicit memory" effects will help us understand the broad set of ways in which memory influences you and will also help us see where the feeling of familiarity comes from.

● Finally, an examination of amnesia confirms a central theme of the chapter—namely, that we cannot speak of "good" or "bad" memory in general; instead, we need to evaluate memory by considering how, and for what purposes, the memory will be used.

With this question, they're likely to respond with the word they'd seen earlier—a word that ostensibly they could not remember.

We get similar results if we teach these patients a new skill. For example, we can ask them to trace a figure—but with a setup in which they can only observe the figure (and their hand holding a stylus) through a mirror (see **Figure 7.1**). This task is challenging, but performance improves if we give the person an opportunity to practice this sort of "mirror-writing." Patients with amnesia—just like everyone else—get better and better in this task with practice, although each time they try the task they insist they're doing it for the first time.

All of these observations powerfully suggest that there must be different types of memory—including a type that is massively disrupted in these amnesic patients, but one that is apparently intact. But, of course, this raises several questions: How many types of memory are there? How does each one function? Is it possible that processes or strategies that create one type of memory might be less useful for some other type? These questions will be central for us in this chapter.

Learning as Preparation for Retrieval

Putting information into long-term memory helps you only if you can retrieve that information later on. Otherwise, it would be like putting money into a savings account without the option of ever making withdrawals, or writing books that could never be read. But let's emphasize that there are different ways to retrieve information from memory. You can try to *recall* the information ("What was the name of your tenth-grade homeroom teacher?") or to *recognize* it ("Was the name perhaps Miller?"). If you try to recall the

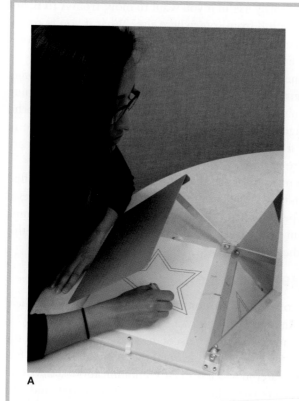

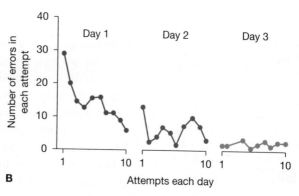

FIGURE 7.1 MIRROR DRAWING

In a mirror-drawing task, participants must draw a precisely defined shape—and so might be asked, for example, to trace a line between the inner and outer star. The trick, though, is that the participants can see the figure (and their own hand) only in the mirror. Performance is usually poor at first but gradually gets better. Remarkably, the same pattern of improvement is observed with amnesic patients, even though on each attempt they insist that they are performing this task for the very first time.

information, a variety of cues may or may not be available (you might be told, as a hint, that the name began with an *M* or rhymed with "tiller").

In Chapter 6, we largely ignored these variations in retrieval. We talked as if material was well established in memory or was not, with no regard for how the material would be retrieved from memory. There's every reason to believe, however, that we cannot ignore these variations in retrieval, and in this chapter we'll examine the interactions between how exactly a bit of information was learned and how it is retrieved later on.

Crucial Role of Retrieval Paths

In Chapter 6, we argued that when you are learning, you're making connections between the newly acquired material and other information already in your memory. These connections help you because they make the new knowledge "findable" later on. Specifically, the connections serve as *retrieval paths*: When you want to locate information in memory, you travel on those paths, moving from one memory to the next until you reach the target material.

These claims seem simple enough, but they have an important implication. To see this, bear in mind that retrieval paths—like any paths—have a starting point and an ending point: The path leads you from a certain Point A to a certain Point B. That's obviously useful if you want to move from A to B, but what if you're trying to reach B from somewhere else? What if you're trying to reach Point B, but at the moment you happen to be nowhere close to Point A? In that case, the path linking A and B may not help you.

As an analogy, imagine that you're trying to reach Chicago from somewhere to the west. For this purpose, what you need is some highway coming in from the west. It won't be helpful that you've constructed a wonderful road coming into Chicago from the *east*. That road might be valuable in other circumstances, but it's not the path you need to get from where you are right now to where you're heading.

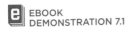
EBOOK
DEMONSTRATION 7.1

Do retrieval paths in memory work the same way? If so, we might find cases in which your learning is excellent preparation for one sort of retrieval but useless for other types of retrieval—as if you've built a road coming in from one direction but now need a road from another direction. Is this indeed the pattern that the data show?

Context-Dependent Learning

Consider a broad class of studies on **context-dependent learning** (Eich, 1980; Overton, 1985). In one such study, Godden and Baddeley (1975) asked scuba divers to learn various materials. Some of the divers learned the material while sitting on dry land; others learned the material while 20 feet underwater, hearing the material via a special communication set. Within each group, half of the divers were then tested while above water, and half were tested below (see **Figure 7.2**).

Underwater, the world has a different look, feel, and sound, and this could easily influence what thoughts come to mind for the divers in this situation. Imagine, for example, that a diver is feeling a bit cold while underwater. This context will probably lead the diver to think "cold-related" thoughts, so those thoughts will be in the diver's mind during the learning episode. In this setting, the diver is likely to form memory connections between these thoughts and the materials he's trying to learn.

How will all of this matter? If this diver is back underwater at the time of the memory test, it's plausible that he'll again feel cold, and this may once again lead him to "cold-related" thoughts. These thoughts, in turn, are now connected (we've proposed) to the target materials, and that gives us what we want: The cold triggers certain thoughts, and thanks to the connections formed during learning, those thoughts can trigger the target memories.

Of course, all is not lost if the diver is tested for the same memory materials *on land*. In this case, the diver might have other links, other memory connections, that will lead to the target memories. Even so, the diver will be at a disadvantage: On land, the "cold-related" thoughts are not triggered, so there will be no benefit from the connections that are now in place, linking those thoughts to the sought-after memories.

By this logic, we should expect that divers who learn material while underwater will remember the material best if they're again underwater at the time of the test. This setting will enable them to use the connections they estab-

FIGURE 7.2 THE DESIGN OF A CONTEXT-DEPENDENT LEARNING EXPERIMENT

		Test while: On land	Test while: Underwater
Learn while	On land	Learning and test circumstances match	*CHANGE* of circumstances between learning and test
	Underwater	*CHANGE* of circumstances between learning and test	Learning and test circumstances match

Half of the participants (deep-sea divers) learned the test material while underwater; half learned while sitting on land. Then, within each group, half were tested while underwater; half were tested on land. We expect a retrieval advantage if the learning and test circumstances match. Hence, we expect better performance in the top left and bottom right cells.

lished earlier. In terms of our earlier analogy: They've built certain highways, and we've put them into a situation in which they can use what they've built. And, of course, the opposite is true for divers who learned while on land; they should do best if tested on land. And that is exactly what the data show (see **Figure 7.3**).

Similar results have been obtained in many other studies, including studies designed to mimic the life situation of a college student. In one experiment, research participants read a two-page article similar to the sorts of readings they might encounter in their college courses. Half the participants read the article in a quiet setting; half read it in noisy circumstances. When later given a short-answer test, those who read the article in quiet did best if tested in quiet—67% correct answers, compared to 54% correct if tested in a noisy environment. Those who read the article in a noisy environment did better if tested in a noisy environment—62% correct, compared to 46% (Grant et al., 1998; also see Balch, Bowman, & Mohler, 1992; Cann & Ross, 1989; Schab, 1990; Smith, 1985; Smith & Vela, 2001).

Smith, Glenberg, and Bjork (1978) report the same pattern if learning and testing take place in different *rooms*—with the rooms varying in their

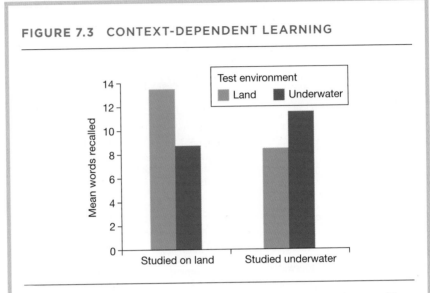

FIGURE 7.3   CONTEXT-DEPENDENT LEARNING

Scuba divers learned materials either while on land or while underwater. Then, they were tested while on land or underwater. Performance was best if the divers' circumstances at the time of test were matched to those in place during learning.   AFTER GODDEN & BADDELEY, 1975.

visual appearance, sounds, and even scent. The data showed that recall was best if done in the room in which the initial learning took place. In this study, though, there was an important twist: In one version of the procedure, the participants learned materials in one room and were tested in a different room. Just before testing, however, the participants were urged to think about the room in which they had learned—what it looked like and how it made them feel. When tested, these participants performed as well as those participants for whom there was no room change (Smith, 1979). What matters, therefore, is not the *physical* context but the *psychological* context—a result that's entirely consistent with our account of this effect. As a result, you can get the benefits of context-dependent learning through a strategy of **context reinstatement**—a strategy of re-creating the thoughts and feelings of the learning episode even if, at the time of recall, you're in a very different place. That's because, once again, what matters for memory retrieval is the mental context, not the physical environment itself.

Encoding Specificity

The results we've been describing also illuminate a further point: just what it is that's stored in memory. Let's go back to the scuba-diving experiment. The divers in this study didn't just remember the words they'd learned; apparently, they also remembered something about the context in which this learning took place. Otherwise, the data in Figure 7.3 (and related findings) make no sense: If the context left no trace in memory, there'd be no way for a *return* to the context to influence the divers later.

The suggestion, then, is that what's preserved in memory is some record of the target material (i.e., the information you're focusing on) *and also* some record of the connections you established during learning. To return to our analogy one more time: Your brain contains the target information *and* the highways you've now built, leading toward that information. These highways—the memory connections—can obviously influence your search for the target information; that's what we've been emphasizing so far. But the connections can do more: They can also change the *meaning* of what is remembered, because in many settings "memory plus *this* set of connections" has a different meaning from "memory plus *that* set of connections." That change in meaning, in turn, can have profound consequences for how you remember the past.

In one experiment, participants read target words (e.g., "piano") in either of two contexts: "The man lifted the piano" or "The man tuned the piano." In each case, the sentence led the participants to think about the target word in a particular way, and it was this thought that was encoded into memory. In other words, what was placed in memory was not just the word "piano." Instead, what was recorded in memory was the idea of "piano as something heavy" or "piano as musical instrument."

This difference in memory content became clear when participants were later asked to recall the target words. If they had earlier seen the "lifted" sentence, they were quite likely to recall the target word if given the cue "something heavy." The hint "something with a nice sound" was much less effective. But if participants had seen the "tuned" sentence, the result reversed: Now, the "nice sound" hint was effective, but the "heavy" hint was not (Barclay, Bransford, Franks, McCarrell, & Nitsch, 1974). In both cases, then, the cue was effective only if it was congruent with what was stored in memory.

Other experiments show a similar pattern, a pattern often dubbed **encoding specificity** (Tulving, 1983; also see Hunt & Ellis, 1974; Light & Carter-Sobell, 1970). This label reminds us that what you encode (i.e., place into memory) is indeed specific—not just the physical stimulus as it was encountered, but the stimulus together with its context. Then, if you're later presented with the stimulus *in some other context*, you ask yourself, "Does this match anything I learned previously?" and you *correctly* answer no. And we emphasize that this "no" response is indeed correct. It is as if you had learned the word "other" and were later asked whether you had been shown the word "the." In fact, "the" does appear as part of "other." Or, more precisely, the letters *t h e* do appear within the word "other." But it's the whole that people learn, not the parts. Therefore, if you've seen "other," it's entirely sensible to deny that you have seen "the" or, for that matter, "he" or "her," even though all these letter combinations are contained within "other."

FIGURE 7.4   REMEMBERING "RE-CREATES" AN EARLIER EXPERIENCE

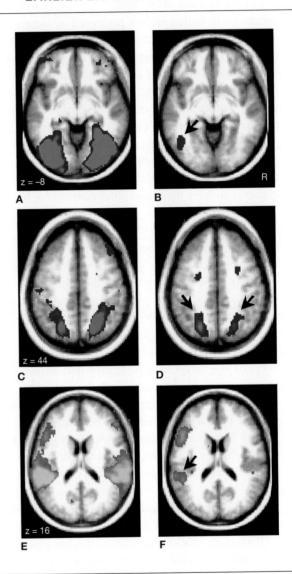

The text argues that what goes into your memory is a record of the material you've encountered *and also* a record of the connections you established during learning. On this basis, it's sensible that the brain areas activated when you're remembering a target overlap considerably with the brain areas that were activated when you first encountered the target. Here, the left panels show brain activation while viewing one picture (A) or another picture (C) or while hearing a particular sound (E). The right panels show brain activation while *remembering* the same targets.   AFTER WHEELER, PETERSON, & BUCKNER, 2000.

Learning a list of words works in the same way. The word "piano" was contained in what the research participants learned, just as "the" is contained in "other." What was learned, however, was not just this word; instead, what was learned was the broader, integrated experience: the word as the perceiver understood it. Therefore, "piano as musical instrument" *isn't* what participants learned if they saw the "lifted" sentence, and so they're correct in asserting that this item wasn't on the earlier list (also see **Figure 7.4**).

EBOOK
DEMONSTRATION 7.2

The Memory Network

In Chapter 6, we introduced the idea that memory acquisition—and, more broadly, *learning*—involves the creation (or strengthening) of memory connections. In this chapter, we've returned to the idea of memory connections, building on the notion that these connections serve as retrieval paths, guiding you toward the information you seek. But what are these connections? How do they work? And who (or what?) is traveling on these "paths"?

According to many theorists, memory is best thought of as a vast *network* of ideas. In later chapters, we'll consider how exactly these ideas are represented (as pictures? as words? in some more abstract format?). For now, though, let's just think of these representations as **nodes** within the network, just like the knots in a fisherman's net. (In fact, the word "node" is derived from the Latin word for knot, *nodus*.) These nodes are then tied to each other via connections we'll call **associations**, or **associative links**. Some people find it helpful to think of the nodes as being akin to lightbulbs that can be turned on by incoming electricity, and to imagine the associative links as wires that carry the electricity.

Spreading Activation

Theorists speak of a node becoming *activated* when it has received a strong enough input signal. Then, once a node has been activated, it can in turn activate other nodes: Energy will spread out from the just-activated node via its associations, and this will activate the nodes connected to the just-activated node.

To put all of this more precisely, nodes receive activation from their neighbors, and as more and more activation arrives at a particular node, the **activation level** for that node increases. Eventually, the activation level will reach the node's **response threshold**. Once this happens, we say that the node **fires**. This firing has several effects, including the fact that the node will now itself be a source of activation, sending energy to its neighbors and so activating them. In addition, firing of the node will summon attention to that node; this is what it means to "find" a node within the network.

Activation levels below the response threshold, so-called **subthreshold activation**, also have an important role to play: Activation is assumed to accumulate, so that two subthreshold inputs may add together, or **summate**, and bring the node to threshold. Likewise, if a node has been partially activated recently, it is in effect already "warmed up," so that even a weak input will now be sufficient to bring the node to threshold.

These claims mesh well with points we raised in Chapter 2, when we considered how neurons communicate with each other. Neurons receive activation from other neurons; once a neuron reaches its threshold, it fires, sending activation to other neurons. All of this is precisely parallel to the suggestions we're describing here.

Our current discussion also parallels the claims we offered in Chapter 4, when we described how a network of detectors might function in object recognition. Thus, the network linking *memories* to each other will resemble the networks we've described, linking *detectors* to each other (e.g., Figures 4.9 and 4.10). Detectors, like memory nodes, receive their activation from other detectors; they can accumulate activation from different inputs, and once activated to threshold levels, they fire.

Returning to long-term storage, however, the key idea here is that activation travels from node to node via the associative links. As each node becomes activated and fires, it serves as a source for further activation, spreading onward through the network. This process, known as **spreading activation**, enables us to deal with a key question: How does one navigate through the maze of associations? If you start a search at one node, how do you decide where to go from there? The answer is that, in most cases, you do not "choose" at all. Instead, activation spreads out from its starting point in all directions simultaneously, flowing through whatever connections are in place.

Retrieval Cues

This sketch of the memory network leaves a great deal unspecified, but even so it allows us to explain some well-established results. For example, why do hints help you to remember? Why is it, for example, that you draw a blank if asked, "What's the capital of South Dakota?" but then remember if given the cue, "Is it perhaps a man's name?" Here's one likely explanation. Mention of South Dakota will activate nodes in memory that represent your knowledge about this state. Activation will then spread outward from these nodes, eventually reaching nodes that represent the capital city's name. It's possible, though, that there's only a weak connection between the SOUTH DAKOTA nodes and the nodes representing PIERRE. Perhaps you're not very familiar with South Dakota, or perhaps you haven't thought about this state's capital for some time. In either case, this weak connection will do a poor job of carrying the activation, with the result that only a trickle of activation will flow into the PIERRE nodes, and so these nodes won't reach threshold and won't be "found."

Things will go differently, though, if a hint is available. If you're told, "South Dakota's capital is also a man's name," this will activate the MAN'S NAME node, with the result that activation will spread out from this source at the same time that activation is spreading out from the SOUTH DAKOTA nodes.

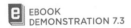
EBOOK
DEMONSTRATION 7.3

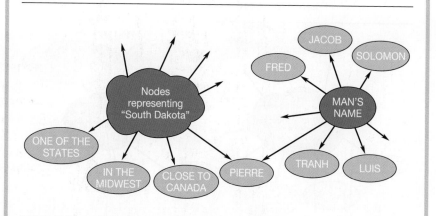

FIGURE 7.5 ACTIVATION OF A NODE FROM TWO SOURCES

A participant is asked, "What is the capital of South Dakota?" This activates the SOUTH DAKOTA nodes, and activation spreads from there to all of the associated nodes. However, it is possible that the connection between SOUTH DAKOTA and PIERRE is weak, so PIERRE may not receive enough activation to reach threshold. Things will go differently, though, if the participant is also given the hint "The capital is a man's name." Now the PIERRE node will receive activation from two sources: the SOUTH DAKOTA nodes and the man's name nodes. With this double input, it is more likely that the PIERRE node will reach threshold. This is why the hint ("man's name") makes the memory search easier.

Therefore, the nodes for PIERRE will now receive activation from two sources simultaneously, and this will probably be enough to lift the nodes' activation to threshold levels. In this way, question-plus-hint accomplishes more than the question by itself (see **Figure 7.5**).

Context Reinstatement

Likewise, why is it that memory retrieval is more likely to succeed if your state during retrieval is the same as it was during learning? Why is it that if you were underwater during learning, you'll have an easier time remembering what you learned if you're again underwater during the memory test?

We've already suggested that being underwater will bring certain thoughts to mind during your learning, and it seems likely that some of these thoughts will become associated with the materials being learned. With this base, the logic here is the same as it was in our discussion of hints. Imagine that you learn a list of words while underwater, including the words "home," "city," and "nose." If you're later asked, "What words were on the list?" activation will flow outward from the nodes representing your general thoughts

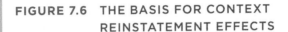

FIGURE 7.6 THE BASIS FOR CONTEXT REINSTATEMENT EFFECTS

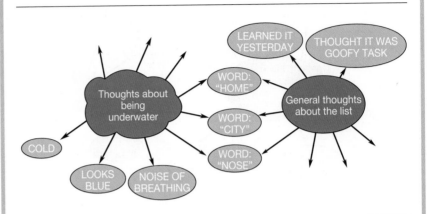

Why is it helpful, when trying to recall something, to re-create the context? The information you seek in memory is probably tied to the retrieval cue you're given (e.g., "What was on the list?"), but it's possible that the information you seek receives insufficient activation from this source. However, the information you seek may also be tied in memory to thoughts that had been triggered by the learning context (e.g., thoughts about being underwater). If you're back in that context at the time of recall, the target nodes can receive a double input (i.e., activation from two different sources), and this will help activate the target nodes.

about the list (see **Figure 7.6**). Perhaps enough of this activation will reach the HOME, CITY, and NOSE nodes to activate them, but perhaps not. If, however, you're again underwater at the time of the test, then this will trigger certain thoughts, and we just suggested that the nodes representing these thoughts may be linked to the nodes representing the learned material. As a result, the HOME, CITY, and NOSE nodes will be receiving a double input: They will receive activation not only from the nodes representing thoughts about the list, but also from the nodes representing the underwater thoughts. This double input makes it more likely that they will be activated, leading to the memory advantage that we associate with context reinstatement.

Semantic Priming

The explanations we've just offered rest on a key assumption—namely, the *summation of subthreshold activation*. In other words, we've relied on the idea that the insufficient activation received from one source can add to the insufficient activation received from another source. Either source of activation on its own would not be enough, but the two can combine to activate the target nodes.

Can we document this summation more directly? In a **lexical-decision task**, research participants are shown a series of letter sequences on a computer screen. Some of the sequences spell words; other sequences aren't words (e.g., "blar, plome"). The participants' task is to hit a "yes" button if the sequence spells a word and a "no" button otherwise. Presumably, they perform this task by "looking up" these letter strings in their "mental dictionary," and they base their response on whether they find the string in the dictionary or not. We can therefore use the participants' speed of response in this task as an index of how quickly they can locate the word in their memories.

In a series of classic studies, Meyer and Schvaneveldt (1971; Meyer, Schvaneveldt, & Ruddy, 1974) presented participants with *pairs* of letter strings, and participants had to respond "yes" if both strings were words and "no" otherwise. Thus, participants would say "yes" in response to "chair, bread" but "no" in response to "house, fime." In addition, if both strings were words, sometimes the words were semantically related in an obvious way (e.g., "nurse, doctor") and sometimes they were not ("lake, shoe"). Of central interest was how this relationship between the words would influence performance.

Consider a trial in which participants see a related pair, like "bread, butter." To choose a response, they first need to "look up" the word "bread" in memory. This means they'll search for, and presumably activate, the relevant node, and in this fashion they'll decide that, yes, this string is a legitimate word. Then, they're ready for the second word. But note that in this sequence, the node for bread (the first word in the pair) has just been activated. This will, we've hypothesized, trigger a spread of activation outward from this node, bringing activation to other, nearby nodes. These nearby nodes will surely include BUTTER, since the association between "bread" and "butter" is a strong one. Therefore, once BREAD (the first word) is activated, some activation should also spread to the BUTTER node.

Now think about what happens when the participant turns her attention to the second word in the pair. To select a response, the participant must locate "butter" in memory. If the participant finds this word (or, more precisely, finds the relevant node), then she knows that this string, too, is a word, and she can hit the "yes" button. But of course the process of activating the BUTTER node has already begun, thanks to the (subthreshold) activation this node just received from bread. This should accelerate the process of bringing this node to threshold (since it's already partway there), and so it will require less time to activate. Hence, we expect quicker responses to "butter" in this context, compared to a context in which "butter" was preceded by some unrelated word.

Our prediction, therefore, is that trials with related words will produce **semantic priming**. The term "priming" is used to indicate that a specific prior event (in this case, the presentation of the first word in the pair) will produce a state of readiness (and, hence, faster responding) later on. There are various forms of priming (in Chapter 4, we discussed *repetition* priming). In the procedure we're considering here, the priming results from the fact that the two words in the pair are related in meaning—hence, this is *semantic* priming.

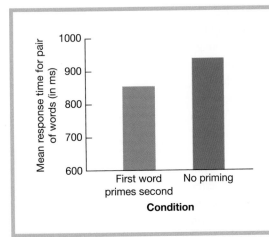

FIGURE 7.7 SEMANTIC PRIMING

Participants were given a lexical-decision task involving pairs of words. In some pairs, the words were semantically related (and so the first word in the pair primed the second); in other pairs, the words were unrelated (and so there was no priming). Responses to the second word were reliably faster if the word had been primed—providing clear evidence of the importance of subthreshold activation. AFTER MEYER & SCHVANEVELDT, 1971.

The results confirm these predictions. Participants' lexical-decision responses were faster by almost 100 ms if the stimulus words were related (see **Figure 7.7**), just as we would expect on the model we are developing. (For other relevant studies, including some alternative conceptions of priming, see Hutchison, 2003; Lucas, 2000.)

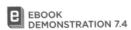
EBOOK DEMONSTRATION 7.4

Before pressing on, though, we should mention that this process of spreading activation—with one node activating nearby nodes—is not the whole story for memory search. As one complication, people have some degree of control over the *starting points* for their memory searches, relying on the processes of reasoning (Chapter 12) and the mechanisms of executive control (Chapters 5 and 6). In addition, evidence suggests that once the spreading activation has begun, people have the option of "shutting down" some of this spread if they are convinced that the wrong nodes are being activated (e.g., Anderson & Bell, 2001; Johnson & Anderson, 2004). Even so, spreading activation is a crucial mechanism: It plays a central role in retrieval, and it helps us understand why memory connections are so important and so helpful.

Different Forms of Memory Testing

Let's pause to take stock of where we are. In Chapter 6, we argued that learning involves the creation or strengthening of connections. This is why memory is promoted by understanding (because understanding consists, in large part, of seeing how new material is connected to other things you know). We also proposed that these connections later serve as retrieval paths, guiding your search through the vast warehouse that is memory. In this chapter, we've explored an important implication of this idea: that (like all paths) the paths through memory have both a starting point and an end point. Therefore, retrieval paths will be helpful only if you're at the appropriate starting point; this, we've proposed, is the basis for the advantage produced by *context reinstatement*. And, finally, we've now started to lay out what these paths really are: connections that carry activation from one memory to another.

This theoretical base also helps us with another issue: the impact of different forms of memory testing. Both in the laboratory and in day-to-day life, you often try to **recall** information from memory. This means that you're presented with a retrieval cue that broadly identifies the information you seek, but then you need to come up with the information on your own: "What was the name of that great restaurant that your parents took us to?"; "Can you remember the words to that song?"; "Where were you last Saturday?"

In other circumstances, you draw information from your memory via **recognition**. This term refers to cases in which information is presented to you, and you must decide whether it's the sought-after information or not: "Is this the man who robbed you?"; "I'm sure I'll recognize the street when we get there"; "If you let me taste that wine, I'll tell you if it's the same one we had last time."

These two modes of retrieval—recall and recognition—turn out to be fundamentally different from each other. Recall, by its very nature, requires memory search because you have to come up with the sought-after item on your own; you need to locate that item within memory. As a result, recall depends heavily on the memory connections we've been emphasizing so far. Recognition, in contrast, often depends on a sense of familiarity. Imagine, for example, that you're taking a recognition test, and the fifth word on the test is "butler." In response to this word, you might find yourself thinking, "I don't recall seeing this word on the list, but this word feels extraordinarily familiar, so I guess I must have seen it recently. Therefore, it must have been on the list." In this case you do not have what's called **source memory**; that is, you do not have any recollection of the *source* of your current knowledge. But you do have a strong sense of **familiarity**, and you're willing to make an inference about where that familiarity came from. In other words, you attribute the familiarity to the earlier encounter, and thanks to this **attribution** you'll probably respond "yes" on the recognition test.

Familiarity and Source Memory

We need no new theory to talk about *source memory*, because this type of memory depends on the connections we've been discussing all along. In other words, memory connections link the target material to thoughts about the setting in which you encountered that material, and these connections help you to recall when and where you saw that person, or heard that song, or smelled that perfume.

But what about familiarity? What does this sort of remembering involve? As a start, let's be clear that familiarity is truly distinct from source memory. This is evident, for example, in the fact that the two types of memory are independent of each other, so that it's possible for an event to be familiar without any source memory, and it's also possible for you to have source memory without any familiarity. Indeed, this independence is reflected in the common experience in which you're watching a movie and realize that one of the actors is familiar, but (with considerable frustration, and despite a lot of effort) you're unable to recall where you've seen that actor before. Or you're walking down the street, see a familiar face, and immediately find yourself asking: "Where do I know that woman from? Does she work at the grocery store I shop in? Is she the driver of the bus I often take?" You're at a loss to answer these questions; all you know is that the face is familiar.

In maddening cases like these, you cannot "place" the memory; you cannot identify the episode in which the face was last encountered. But you're certain the face is familiar, even though you don't know why—a clear example of familiarity without source memory.

The inverse case (source memory without familiarity) is less common but can also be demonstrated. For example, in Chapter 2 we discussed a disorder known as Capgras syndrome. In this syndrome, the patient has detailed, accurate memories of the past but no sense at all of familiarity, and so faces (of family members, of friends) seem hauntingly unfamiliar. (For further evidence— and, specifically, a patient who, after surgery, has intact source memory but disrupted familiarity—see Bowles et al., 2007; also see Yonelinas & Jacoby, 2012.)

We can also document the difference between source memory and familiarity in another way. In many studies, (neurologically intact) participants have been asked, during a recognition test, to make a **"remember/ know" distinction**—pressing one button (to indicate "remember") if they actually recall the episode of encountering a particular item, and pressing a different button ("know") if they don't recall the encounter but just have the broad feeling that the item must have been on the earlier list. In the latter case, participants are essentially saying, "This item seems very familiar, so I know it was on the earlier list even though I don't remember the experience of seeing it" (Gardiner, 1988; Hicks & Marsh, 1999; Jacoby, Jones, & Dolan, 1998).

We can use fMRI scans to monitor participants' brain activity while they are taking these memory tests, and the scans make it clear that "remember" and "know" judgments depend on different brain areas. The scans show heightened activity in the hippocampus when people indicate that they

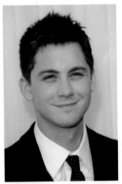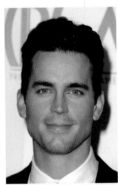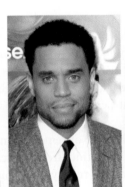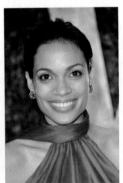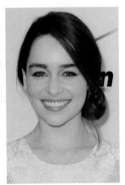

"FAMILIAR . . . BUT *WHERE DO I KNOW HIM FROM?!?*"

The photos here all show successful TV or film actors. The odds are good that for some of them you will immediately know their faces as familiar but will be uncertain why they are familiar. You know you have seen these actors in some movie, but which one? (We provide the performers' names at the chapter's end.)

"remember" a particular test item, suggesting that this brain structure is crucial for source memory. In contrast, "know" responses are associated with activity in a different area—the anterior parahippocampus, with the implication that this brain site is crucial for familiarity (Aggleton & Brown, 2006; Diana, Yonelinas, & Ranganath, 2007; Dobbins, Foley, Wagner, & Schacter, 2002; Wagner, Shannon, Kahn, & Buckner, 2005; also see Rugg & Curran, 2007; Rugg & Yonelinas, 2003).

Familiarity and source memory can also be distinguished during *learning*. Specifically, if certain brain areas (e.g., the rhinal cortex) are especially active during learning, then the stimulus is likely to seem familiar later on (thus, that stimulus is likely, later, to trigger a "know" response). Apparently, this brain site plays a key role in establishing familiarity (see **Figure 7.8**). In contrast, if

FIGURE 7.8 FAMILIARITY VERSUS SOURCE MEMORY

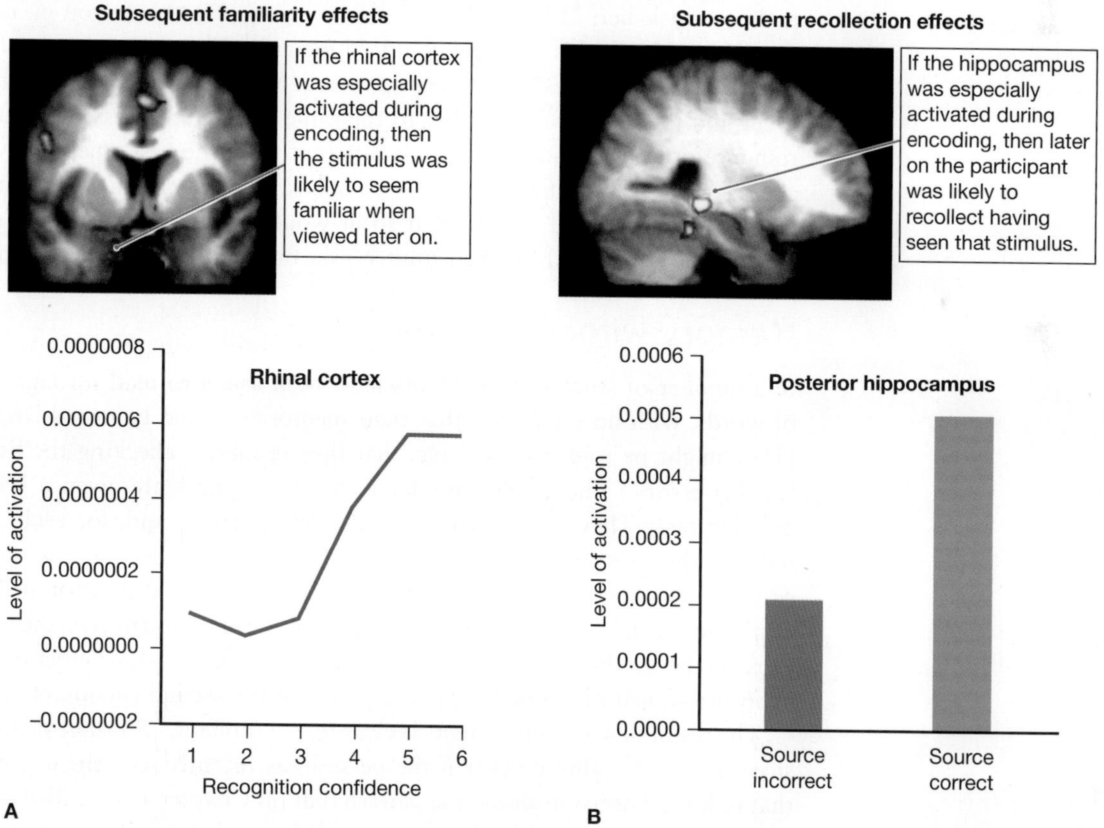

In this study, researchers tracked participants' brain activity during encoding and then analyzed the data according to what happened later, when the time came for retrieval. AFTER RANGANATH ET AL., 2003.

other brain areas (e.g., the hippocampal region) are particularly active during learning, there's a high probability that the person will offer a "remember" response to that stimulus when tested later (e.g., Davachi & Dobbins, 2008; Davachi, Mitchell, & Wagner, 2003; Ranganath et al., 2003), implying that these brain sites are crucial for establishing source memory.

We still need to ask, though, what's going on in these various brain areas to create the relevant memories. Activity in the hippocampus is presumably helping to create the memory connections we've been discussing all along, and it is these connections, we've suggested, that promote source memory: The connections link a memory item to other thoughts that help identify the episode (the source) in which that item was encountered. But what about familiarity? What "record" does it leave in memory? The answer to this question leads us to a very different sort of "memory."

Implicit Memory

How can we find out if someone remembers a previous event? The obvious path is to ask her: "How did the job interview go?"; "Have you ever seen *Casablanca*?"; "Is this the book you told me about?" But at the start of this chapter we encountered a different approach: We can expose someone to an event and then later reexpose her to the same event and assess whether her response on the second encounter is different from the first. Specifically, we can ask whether the first encounter somehow *primed* the person—got her ready—for the second exposure. If so, it would seem that the person must retain some record of the first encounter—she must have some sort of memory.

Memory without Awareness

In a number of studies, participants have been asked to read through a list of words, with no indication that their memories would be tested later on. (They might be told, for example, that they're merely checking the list for spelling errors.) Then, sometime later, the participants are given a lexical-decision task: They are shown a series of letter strings and, for each, must indicate (by pressing one button or another) whether the string is a word or not. Of course, some of the letter strings in the lexical-decision task are duplicates of the words seen in the first part of the experiment (i.e., the words were on the list they checked for spelling), enabling us to ask whether the first exposure somehow primed the participants for the second encounter.

The result of such experiments is clear (e.g., Oliphant, 1983): Lexical decisions are appreciably quicker if the person has recently seen the test word; that is, lexical decision shows the pattern that (in Chapter 4) we called *repetition priming*. Remarkably, this priming is observed even when participants have no recollection for having encountered the stimulus words before. To demonstrate this, we can show participants a list of words and then test them in two different ways. One test assesses memory directly, using a standard recognition procedure: "Which of these words were on the list I showed you earlier?" The other test is indirect and relies on lexical decision: "Which of these letter strings form real words?" In this setup, the two tests will often yield different results. At a sufficient delay, the direct memory test is likely to show that the participants have completely forgotten the words presented earlier; their recognition performance is essentially random. According to the lexical-decision results, however, the participants still remember the words— and so they show a robust priming effect. In this situation, then, participants are influenced by a specific past experience that they seem (consciously) not to remember at all—a pattern that some researchers refer to as "memory without awareness."

A different example draws on a task we alluded to earlier, a task called **word-stem completion**. In this task, participants are given three or four letters and must produce a word with this beginning. If, for example, they are given *cla-*, then "clam" or "clatter" would be acceptable responses, and the question of interest for us is which of these the participants produce. It turns out that people are more likely to offer a specific word if they've encountered it recently; once again, this priming effect is observed even if participants, when tested directly, show no conscious memory of their recent encounter with that word (Graf, Mandler, & Haden, 1982).

Results like these lead psychologists to distinguish two types of memory. **Explicit memories** are those usually revealed by **direct memory testing**— testing that specifically urges you to remember the past. Recall is a direct memory test; so is a standard recognition test. **Implicit memories**, however, are typically revealed by **indirect memory testing** and are often manifested as priming effects. In this form of testing, your current behavior is demonstrably influenced by a prior event, but you may be quite unaware of this. Lexical decision, word-stem completion, and many other tasks provide indirect means of assessing memory (see, for example, **Figure 7.9**; for a broad review, see Mulligan & Besken, 2012; for a different perspective on these data, though, see Cabeza & Moscovitch, 2012).

How exactly is implicit memory different from explicit memory? We'll have more to say about this question before we're done; first, though, we need to say more about how implicit memory *feels* from the rememberer's point of view. This will then lead us back into our discussion of familiarity and source memory.

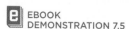 EBOOK DEMONSTRATION 7.5

False Fame

Jacoby, Kelley, Brown, and Jasechko (1989) presented participants with a list of names to read out loud. The participants were told nothing about a memory test; they thought the experiment was concerned with how they pronounced the names. Some time later, the participants were given the second step of the procedure: They were shown a new list of names and asked to rate each person on this list according to how famous each was. The list included some real, very famous people; some real but not-so-famous people; and some fictitious names (names the experimenters had invented). Crucially, the

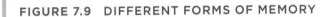

FIGURE 7.9   DIFFERENT FORMS OF MEMORY

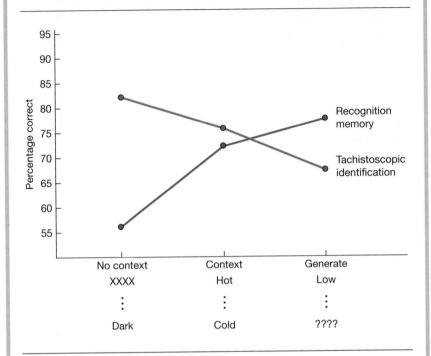

In this early study, participants were asked to read a list of words aloud and later were given a test in which words were presented very briefly ("tachistoscopically") on a computer screen; the participants' task was simply to identify each word—to say what the word was. Unbeknownst to the participants, some of the words shown had also been presented during the procedure's initial phase, while other words were novel (i.e., had not been recently viewed). The question was whether this earlier exposure would influence performance. In this task, performance was considerably improved if participants had recently viewed the test word ("No context" condition). If they'd merely thought about the word ("Generate" condition), performance was much worse. The "Context" condition produced an intermediate result because here participants had seen the word but probably only glanced at it. The results were entirely different, though, with a conventional memory test ("Recognition"). In this condition, best performance came from thinking about the word's meaning; worst performance came from passive exposure to the word.   JACOBY, 1983; ALSO JACOBY & DALLAS, 1981; WINNICK & DANIEL, 1970.

fictitious names were of two types: Some were names that had occurred on the prior ("pronunciation") list, and some were simply new names. A comparison between those two types will tell us how the prior familiarization (during the pronunciation task) influenced the participants' judgments of fame.

For some participants, the "famous" list was presented right after the "pronunciation" list; for other participants, there was a 24-hour delay between these two steps. To see how this delay matters, imagine that you're a participant in the immediate-testing condition: When you see one of the fictitious-but-familiar names, you might decide, "This name sounds familiar, but that's because I just saw it on the previous list." In this situation, you have a feeling that the (familiar) name is distinctive, but you also realize *why* it's distinctive, because you remember your earlier encounter with the name. In other words, you have both a sense of familiarity *and* a source memory, so there's nothing here to persuade you that the name belongs to someone famous, and you respond accordingly. But now imagine that you're a participant in the other condition, with the 24-hour delay. Thanks to this time span, you may not recall the earlier episode of seeing the name in the pronunciation task. Nonetheless, the broad sense of familiarity remains, so in this setting you might say, "This name rings a bell, and I have no idea why. I guess this must be a famous person." And this is indeed the pattern of the data: When the two lists are presented one day apart, the participants are likely to rate the made-up names as being famous.

Apparently, the participants in this study noted (correctly) that some of the names did "ring a bell" and so did have a certain feeling of familiarity. The false judgments of fame, however, come from the way the participants *interpreted* this feeling and what conclusions they drew from it. To put it simply, participants in the 24-hour-delay condition forgot the real source of the familiarity (appearance on a recently viewed list) and instead filled in a bogus source ("Maybe I saw this person in a movie?"). And it's not hard to see why they made this particular misattribution. After all, the experiment was described to them as being about fame, and other names on the list were indeed those of famous people. From the participants' point of view, therefore, it's a reasonable inference in this setting that any name that "rings a bell" belongs to a famous person.

Let's be clear, though, that this misattribution is possible only because the feeling of familiarity produced by these names was relatively vague, and so open to interpretation. The suggestion, then, is that implicit memories may leave people with only a broad sense that a stimulus is somehow distinctive— that it "rings a bell" or "strikes a chord." What happens after this depends on how they interpret that feeling.

Implicit Memory and the "Illusion of Truth"

How broad is this potential for *mis*interpreting an implicit memory? Participants in one study heard a series of statements and had to judge how interesting each statement was (Begg, Anas, & Farinacci, 1992). As an example, one sentence was "The average person in Switzerland eats about 25 pounds of cheese each year." (This is false; the average is closer to 18 pounds.) Another was "Henry Ford forgot to put a reverse gear in his first automobile." (This is true.) After hearing these sentences, the participants were presented with some more sentences, but now they had to judge the credibility of these sentences, rating them on a scale from *certainly true* to *certainly false*. Needless to say, some of the sentences in this "truth test" were repeats from the earlier presentation; the question of interest is how sentence credibility is influenced by sentence familiarity.

The result was a propagandist's dream: Sentences heard before were more likely to be accepted as true; that is, familiarity increased credibility (Begg, Armour, & Kerr, 1985; Brown & Halliday, 1990; Fiedler, Walther, Armbruster, Fay, & Naumann, 1996; Moons, Mackie, & Garcia-Marques, 2009; Unkelbach, 2007). To make things worse, this effect emerged even when the participants were explicitly warned in advance not to believe the sentences in the first list. In one procedure, participants were told that half of the statements had been made by men and half by women. The women's statements, they were told, were always true; the men's, always false. (Half the participants were told the reverse.) Then, participants rated how interesting the sentences were, with each sentence attributed to either a man or a woman: "Frank Foster says that house mice can run an average of 4 miles per hour" or "Gail Logan says that crocodiles sleep with their eyes open." Later, participants were presented with more sentences and had to judge their truth, with these new sentences including the earlier assertions about mice, crocodiles, and so forth.

Let's focus on the sentences initially identified as being false—in our example, Frank's claim about mice. If someone explicitly remembers this sentence ("Oh yes—Frank said such and such"), then he should judge the assertion to be false ("After all, the experimenter said that the men's statements were all lies"). But what about someone without this explicit memory? Since the person doesn't remember whether the assertion came from a man or a woman, he can't use the source as a basis for judging the sentence's veracity. Nonetheless, the person might still have an implicit memory for the sentence left over from the earlier exposure ("Gee, that statement rings a bell"), and this might increase the credibility of the statement ("I'm sure I've heard that somewhere before; I guess it must be true"). This is exactly the pattern of the data: Statements plainly identified as false when they were first heard still created the so-called **illusion of truth**; that is, these statements were subsequently judged to be more credible than sentences never heard before.

The relevance of this result to the political arena or to advertising should be clear. A newspaper headline inquires, "Is Mayor Wilson a crook?" Or perhaps the headline declares, "Known criminal claims Wilson is a crook!" In either case, the assertion that Wilson is a crook has now become familiar. The Begg et al. data indicate that this familiarity will, by itself, increase the likelihood that you'll later believe in Wilson's dishonesty. This will be true even if the paper merely raised the question; it will be true even if the allegation came from a disreputable source. Malicious innuendo does in fact work nasty effects (Wegner, Wenzlaff, Kerker, & Beattie, 1981).

Attributing Implicit Memory to the Wrong Source

Apparently, implicit memory can influence us (and, perhaps, *bias* us) in the political arena. Other evidence suggests that implicit memory can influence us in the marketplace—and can, for example, guide our choices when we're shopping (e.g., Northup & Mulligan, 2013, 2014). Yet another example involves the justice system, and it is an example with troubling implications. In a study by Brown, Deffenbacher, and Sturgill (1977), research participants witnessed a staged crime. Two or three days later, they were shown "mug shots" of individuals who supposedly had participated in the crime; but as it turns out, the people in these photos were different from the actual "criminals"—no mug shots were shown for the truly "guilty" individuals. Finally, after four or five more days, the participants were shown a lineup and asked to select the individuals seen in Step 1—namely, the original crime (see **Figure 7.10**).

FIGURE 7.10   A PHOTO LINEUP

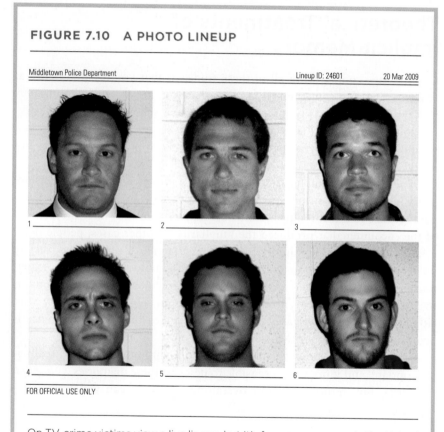

Middletown Police Department   Lineup ID: 24601   20 Mar 2009

1 _____   2 _____   3 _____

4 _____   5 _____   6 _____

FOR OFFICIAL USE ONLY

On TV, crime victims view a live lineup, but it's far more common in the United States for the victim (or witness) to see a "photo lineup" like this one. The victim (or witness) is told that the perpetrator may or may not be present and is asked to pick out the perpetrator if he's there. Unfortunately, victims sometimes pick the wrong person, and this error is more likely to occur if the suspect is familiar to the victim for some reason other than the crime. The error is unlikely, though, if the face is *very* familiar, because, in that case, your history will likely produce a feeling of familiarity and an accurate source memory. ("Number Two looks familiar, but that's because I see him at the gym all the time."

The data in this study show a pattern known as **source confusion**. The participants correctly realized that one of the people in the lineup looked familiar, but they were confused about the source of the familiarity. They falsely believed they had seen the person's face in the original "crime," when, in truth, they'd seen that face only in a subsequent photograph. In fact, the likelihood of this error was quite high, with 29% of the participants (falsely) selecting from the lineup an individual they had seen only in the mug shots. (Also see Davis, Loftus, Vanous, & Cucciare, 2008; for examples of similar errors that—sadly—interfere with a real-life criminal investigations, see Garrett, 2011; for a broader discussion of eyewitness memory and errors in identifying criminals, see Reisberg, 2014.)

Theoretical Treatments of Implicit Memory

One message coming from all of these studies is that you're often better at remembering *that* something is familiar than you are at remembering *why* it is familiar. This is why it's possible to have a sense of familiarity without source memory ("I've seen her somewhere before, but I can't figure out where!") and also why it's possible to be *correct* in judging familiarity but *mistaken* in judging source.

In addition, let's emphasize that in many of these studies participants are being influenced by memories they are not aware of. In some cases, participants realize that a stimulus is somehow familiar, but they have no memory of the encounter that produced the familiarity. In other cases, people don't even have a sense of familiarity for the target stimulus; nonetheless, they're influenced by their previous encounter with the stimulus. For example, experiments show that participants often *prefer* a previously presented stimulus over a novel stimulus, even though they have no sense of familiarity with either stimulus. In such cases, people have no idea that their preference is being guided by memory (Murphy, 2001).

It does seem, then, that the phrase "memory without awareness" really is appropriate, and it does seem sensible to describe these memories as *implicit* memories. But, returning to our overall agenda, how can we explain this form of unconscious "remembering"?

Processing Fluency

Our discussion so far—in this chapter, and in Chapters 4 and 5—has already laid the foundation for a proposal about implicit memory. Let's build the argument, though, in steps: When a stimulus arrives in front of your eyes, it triggers certain detectors, and these trigger still other detectors, and these still others, until you recognize the object ("Oh, it's my stuffed bear, Blueberry"). We can think of this sequence as involving a "flow" of activation that moves from detector to detector, and we could, if we wished, keep track of this flow and in this way identify the "path" that the activation traveled through the network. Let's refer to this path as a **processing pathway**—the sequence of detectors, and the connections *between* detectors, that the activation flows through in recognizing a specific stimulus.

In the same way, we've proposed in this chapter that *remembering* often involves the activation of a node, and this node triggers other, nearby, nodes so that they become activated; they, in turn, trigger still other nodes, leading (eventually) to the information you seek in memory. So here, too, we can speak of a processing pathway—the sequence of nodes, and connections between nodes, that the activation flows through during memory retrieval.

We've also said the use of a processing pathway *strengthens* that pathway. This is because the baseline activation level of nodes or detectors increases if the nodes or detectors have been used frequently in the past, or if they've been used recently. Likewise, connections (between detectors or nodes) grow stronger with use. Thus, by thinking about the link between, say, Jacob and Iowa, you strengthen the connection between the corresponding nodes, and this will help you remember that Jacob once lived in Iowa.

Now, let's put the pieces together. Use of a processing pathway strengthens the pathway. As a result, the pathway will be a bit more efficient, a bit faster, the next time you use it. Theorists describe this fact by saying that use of a pathway increases the **processing fluency** of that pathway—that is, the speed and ease with which the pathway will carry activation.

In many cases, this is all the theory we need to explain implicit memory effects. Consider implicit memory's effect on lexical decision. In this procedure, you first are shown a list of words, including, let's say, the word "bubble." Then, we ask you to do the lexical-decision task, and we find that you're faster for words (like "bubble") that had been included in the earlier list. It's this increase in speed that provides our evidence for implicit memory. The explanation, though, is straightforward. When we show you "bubble" early in the experiment, you read the word and this involves activation flowing through the appropriate processing pathway for this word. This warms up the pathway, and as a result, the path's functioning will be more fluent the next time you use it. Of course, when the word "bubble" shows up a bit later as part of the lexical-decision task, it's handled by the same (now more fluent) pathway, and so the word is processed more rapidly—exactly the outcome that we're trying to explain.

For other implicit-memory effects, though, we need a further assumption—namely, that people are sensitive to the *degree* of processing fluency. That is, just as people can easily tell whether they've lifted a heavy carton or a lightweight one, just as they can tell whether they've answered an easy question ("What's 2 + 2?") or a harder one ("What's 17 × 19?"), people also have a broad sense of when they have perceived easily and when they have perceived only by expending more effort. They likewise know when a sequence of thoughts was particularly fluent and when the sequence was labored. This fluency, however, is perceived in an odd way. When a stimulus is easy to perceive (for example), people do not experience something like "That stimulus sure was easy to recognize!" Instead, they merely register a vague sense of specialness. They feel that the stimulus "rings a bell." No matter how it is described, though, this sense

FIGURE 7.11   FAMILIARITY AND SPELLING

innoculate	vs.	inoculate?
embarrass	vs.	embarass?
argument	vs.	arguement?
harass	vs.	harrass?
cemetery	vs.	cemetary?
mispell	vs.	misspell?

The feeling that a stimulus somehow "rings a bell" or "strikes a chord" is rather vague, and so open to various interpretations. As a result, this feeling can influence you in a wide range of circumstances. For example, think about the strategy many people use in deciding how to spell a word. People sometimes write out the word and then ask themselves, "Does this look right?" This is often a successful strategy, and relies on processing fluency: You've encountered the correctly spelled version of the word many times, and so your processing of this version will be fluent; that's why the correct spelling "looks right." But what if you've often encountered the misspelled version of the word? These encounters can make that spelling "look right," and this will be true even if you have no recollection of those encounters—another example of the influence of implicit memory.

of specialness has a simple cause—namely, the detection of ease-in-processing, brought on by fluency, which in turn was created by practice.[1]

We need one more step in our hypothesis, but it's a step we have already introduced: When a stimulus feels special, people often want to know why. Thus, the vague, hard-to-pinpoint feeling of specialness (again, produced by fluency) can trigger an attribution process, as people seek to ask, "Why did that stimulus stand out?" In many circumstances, that question will be answered correctly, and so the specialness will be (accurately) interpreted as *familiarity* and attributed to the correct source. ("That picture seems distinctive, and I know why: It's the same picture I saw yesterday in the dentist's office.") In other situations, though, things may not go so smoothly, and so—as we have seen—people sometimes misinterpret their own processing fluency, falling prey to the errors and illusions we have been discussing. (For yet another example of how fluency can influence us, see **Figure 7.11.**)

1. Actually, what people detect, and what makes a stimulus feel "special," may not be fluency per se. Instead, what they detect may be a discrepancy between how easy (or hard) it was to carry out some mental step and how easy (or hard) they expected it to be, in light of the context and their experience. (See, e.g., Whittlesea, 2002.) A stimulus is registered as distinctive, or "rings a bell," when this discrepancy reaches too high a level. Having acknowledged this, however, we will, for simplicity's sake, ignore this complication in our discussion.

The Nature of Familiarity

All of these points provide us—at last—with a proposal for what "familiarity" is, and the proposal is surprisingly complex. One might think that familiarity is a feeling produced more or less directly when you encounter a stimulus you have met before. The findings of the last few sections, though, point toward a different proposal—namely, that "familiarity" is more like a *conclusion that you draw* rather than a *feeling triggered by a stimulus*. Specifically, the evidence suggests that a stimulus will seem familiar whenever the following list of requirements is met: First, you have encountered the stimulus before. Second, because of that prior encounter (and the "practice" it afforded), you are now faster and more efficient in your processing of that stimulus; that's what we're calling "processing fluency." Third, you detect that fluency, and this leads you to register the stimulus as somehow distinctive or special. Fourth, you try to figure out *why* the stimulus seems special, and you reach a particular conclusion—namely, that the stimulus has this distinctive quality *because* it's a stimulus you have met before in some prior episode. And then, finally, you may draw a further conclusion about when and where you encountered the stimulus—in the experimenter's list of words, or yesterday in the newspaper, and so on (see **Figure 7.12**).

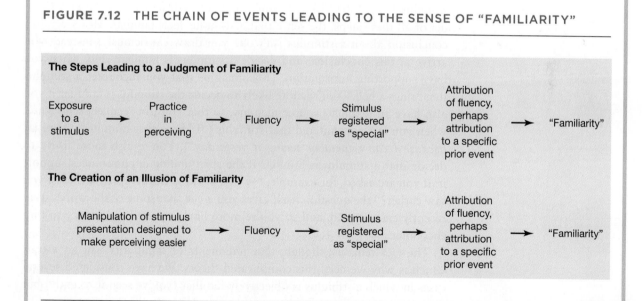

FIGURE 7.12   THE CHAIN OF EVENTS LEADING TO THE SENSE OF "FAMILIARITY"

The Steps Leading to a Judgment of Familiarity

Exposure to a stimulus → Practice in perceiving → Fluency → Stimulus registered as "special" → Attribution of fluency, perhaps attribution to a specific prior event → "Familiarity"

The Creation of an Illusion of Familiarity

Manipulation of stimulus presentation designed to make perceiving easier → Fluency → Stimulus registered as "special" → Attribution of fluency, perhaps attribution to a specific prior event → "Familiarity"

In the top line, practice in perceiving leads to fluency, and if the person attributes the fluency to some specific prior encounter, the stimulus will "feel familiar." The bottom line, however, indicates that fluency can be created in other ways: by presenting the stimulus more clearly or for a longer exposure. Once this fluency is detected, though, it can lead to steps identical to those in the top row. Hence, an "illusion of familiarity" can be created.

CHANGES IN APPEARANCE

The text emphasizes our sensitivity to increases in fluency, but we can also detect decreases. In viewing a picture of a well-known actor, for example, you might notice immediately that something is new in his appearance, but you might be unsure about what exactly the change involves. In this setting, the change in appearance disrupts your well-practiced steps of perceiving for an otherwise familiar face, and so the perception is *less* fluent than it has been in the past. This lack of fluency is what gives you the "something is new" feeling. But then the attribution step fails: You cannot identify what produced this feeling (and so you end up offering various weak hypotheses such as "Is that a new haircut?" when, in fact, it's the mustache and goatee that are new). This case therefore provides the mirror image of the cases we have been considering, in which familiarity leads to an increase in fluency, so that something "rings a bell" but you cannot say why.

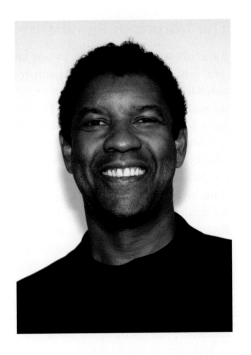

Let's be clear, though, that none of these steps happens consciously; you're not aware of seeking an interpretation or trying to explain why a stimulus feels distinctive. All you experience consciously is the end product of all these steps: the sense that a stimulus feels familiar. Moreover, this conclusion about a stimulus isn't one you draw capriciously; instead, you arrive at this conclusion, and decide a stimulus is familiar, only when you have supporting information. Thus, imagine that you encounter a stimulus that "rings a bell." You're more likely to decide the stimulus is familiar if you also have an (explicit) source memory, so that you can recollect where and when you last encountered that stimulus ("I know this stimulus is familiar *because I can remember seeing it yesterday*"). You're also more likely to decide that a stimulus is familiar if the surrounding circumstances support it: If you are asked, for example, "Which of these words were on the list you saw earlier?" the question itself gives you a cue that some of the words were recently encountered, and so you're more likely to attribute fluency to that encounter.

The fact remains, though, that judgments of familiarity can go astray, which is why we need this complicated theory. We have considered several cases in which a stimulus is objectively familiar (you've seen it recently) but does not *feel* familiar—just as our theory predicts. In these cases, you detect the fluency but attribute it to some other source ("That melody is lovely" rather than "The melody is familiar"). In other words, you go through all of the steps shown in the top of Figure 7.12 except for the last two: You do not attribute the fluency to a specific prior event, and so you do not experience a sense of familiarity.

We can also find the opposite sort of case—in which a stimulus is not familiar (i.e., you've not seen it recently) but feels familiar anyhow—and this, too, fits with the theory. This sort of *illusion of familiarity* can be produced, for example, if the processing of a completely novel stimulus is more fluent than you expected—perhaps because (without telling you) we've sharpened the focus of a computer display or presented the stimulus for a few milliseconds longer than other stimuli you're inspecting (Jacoby & Whitehouse, 1989; Whittlesea, 2002; Whittlesea, Jacoby, & Girard, 1990). In cases like these, we have the situation shown in the bottom half of Figure 7.12, and as our theory predicts, these situations do produce an illusion: Your processing of the stimulus is unexpectedly fluent; you seek an attribution for this fluency, and you are fooled into thinking the stimulus is familiar—and so you say you've seen the stimulus before when in fact you haven't. This illusion is a powerful confirmation that the sense of familiarity does rest on processes like the ones we've described. (For more on fluency, see Besken & Mulligan, 2014; Griffin, Gonzalez, Koehler, & Gilovich, 2012; Hertwig, Herzog, Schooler, & Reimer, 2008; Lanska, Old & Westerman, 2013; Oppenheimer, 2008; Tsai & Thomas, 2011. For a glimpse of what fluency amounts to in the nervous system, see Knowlton & Foerde, 2008.)

The Hierarchy of Memory Types

There's no question that we're often influenced by the past without being aware of that influence. We often respond differently to familiar stimuli than we do to novel stimuli, even if we have no subjective feeling of familiarity. Thus, our conscious recollection seriously underestimates what is in our memories, and researchers have only begun to document the ways in which unconscious memories influence what we do, think, and feel. (For examples, though, of some of the relevant research, see Coates, Butler, & Berry, 2006; Kahneman, 2011; Thomson, Milliken, & Smilek, 2010.)

In addition, the data are telling us that there are two different kinds of memory: one typically conscious and deliberate, one typically unconscious and automatic. These two broad categories can, in turn, be further subdivided, as shown in **Figure 7.13**. Explicit memories can be subdivided into episodic memories (memory for specific events) and semantic memory (more general knowledge). Implicit memory is often divided into four subcategories, as shown in the figure. Our emphasis here has been on one of the subtypes—priming—largely because of its role in producing the feeling of familiarity. However, the other subtypes of implicit memory are also important and can be distinguished from priming both in terms of their functioning (i.e., they follow somewhat different rules) and in terms of their biological underpinnings.

Some of the best evidence for these distinctions, though, comes from the clinic, not the laboratory. In other words, we can learn a great deal about these various types of memory by considering individuals who have suffered different forms of brain damage. Let's look at some of that evidence.

FIGURE 7.13   HIERARCHY OF MEMORY TYPES

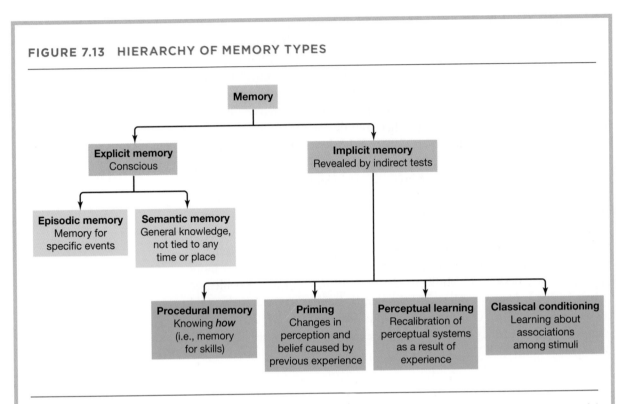

In our discussion, we've distinguished two types of memory—explicit and implicit. However, there are powerful reasons to believe that each of these categories must be subdivided further, as shown here. Evidence for these subdivisions includes functional evidence (the various types of memory follow different rules) and biological evidence (the types depend on different aspects of brain functioning).

Amnesia

As we have already mentioned, a variety of injuries or illnesses can lead to a loss of memory, or **amnesia**. Some forms of amnesia are *retrograde*, meaning that they disrupt memory for things learned *prior to* the event that initiated the amnesia (see **Figure 7.14**). **Retrograde amnesia** is often caused, for example, by blows to the head; the afflicted person is then unable to recall events that occurred just before the blow. Other forms of amnesia have the reverse effect, causing disruption of memory for experiences *after* the onset of amnesia; these are cases of **anterograde amnesia**. (We should note that many cases of amnesia involve both retrograde and anterograde memory loss.)

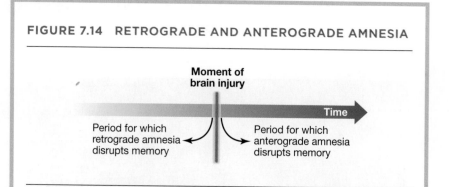

FIGURE 7.14 RETROGRADE AND ANTEROGRADE AMNESIA

Retrograde amnesia disrupts memory for experiences *before* the injury, accident, or disease that triggered the amnesia. Anterograde amnesia disrupts memory for experiences *after* the injury or disease. Some patients suffer from both retrograde and anterograde amnesia.

Disrupted Episodic Memory, but Spared Semantic Memory

Studies of amnesia can teach us many things. For example, do we need all the distinctions shown in Figure 7.13? Consider the case of Clive Wearing, whom we first met in the opening to Chapter 6. (You can find more detail about Wearing's case in an extraordinary book by his wife—see Wearing, 2011.) Wearing's episodic memory is massively disrupted, but his memory for generic information, as well as his deep love for his wife, seem to be entirely intact. Other patients show the reverse pattern—disrupted semantic memory but preserved episodic knowledge. One patient, for example suffered damage (from encephalitis) to the front portion of her temporal lobes. As a consequence, she lost her memory of many common words, important historical events, famous people, and even the fundamental traits of animate and inanimate objects. "However, when asked about her wedding and honeymoon, her father's illness and death, or other specific past episodes, she readily produced detailed and accurate recollections" (Schacter, 1996, p. 152; also see Cabeza & Nyberg, 2000). (For more on amnesia, see Brown, 2002; Conway & Fthenaki, 1999; Kopelman & Kapur, 2001; Nadel & Moscovitch, 2001; Riccio, Millin, & Gisquet-Verrier, 2003.)

These cases (and other evidence as well; see **Figure 7.15**) provide the *double dissociation* that demands a distinction between episodic and semantic memory. It is observations like these, therefore, that force us to a taxonomy like the one shown in Figure 7.13. (For evidence, though, that episodic and semantic memory are intertwined other in important ways, see McRae & Jones, 2012.)

FIGURE 7.15 SEMANTIC MEMORY WITHOUT EPISODIC MEMORY

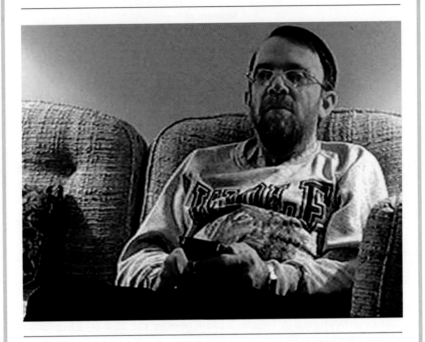

Kent Cochrane—known for years as "Patient K.C."—died in 2014. In 1981, at age 30, he skidded off the road on his motorcycle and suffered substantial brain damage. The damage caused severe disruption of Cochrane's episodic memory, but left his semantic memory intact. As a result, he could still report on the events of his life, but these reports were utterly devoid of autobiographical quality. In other words, he could remember the bare facts of, say, what happened at his brother's wedding, but the memory was totally impersonal, with no recall of context or emotion. He also knew that during his childhood his family had fled their home because a train had derailed nearby, spilling toxic chemicals. But, again, he simply knew this as factual material—the sort of information you might pick up from a reference book—and he had no recall of his own experiences during this event.

Anterograde Amnesia

We have several times mentioned the patient known as H.M. As you may recall, H.M.'s memory loss was the result of brain surgery in 1953, and over the next 55 years (until his death in 2008) H.M. participated in a vast number of studies. Some people suggest he was the most-studied individual in the entire history of psychology (and this is one of the reasons we've returned to his case several times), and the data gathering continued after his death—with careful postmortem scrutiny of his brain. (For a review of H.M.'s case, see Corkin, 2013; Milner, 1966, 1970; also O'Kane, Kensinger, & Corkin, 2004; Skotko et al., 2004; Skotko, Rubin, & Tupler, 2008.)

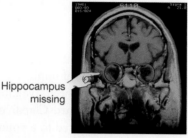
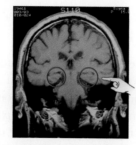

Hippocampus missing

Hippocampus intact

A Anterior   **B** Posterior

H.M.'S BRAIN

For many years, researchers thought that surgery left H.M. with no hippocampus at all. These MRI scans of H.M.'s brain show that the surgery did destroy the anterior portion of the hippocampus (the portion closer to the front of the head) but not the posterior portion (closer to the rear of the head).

H.M. was able to recall many events that had taken place *before* his surgery—and so his amnesia was anterograde, not retrograde. But the amnesia was severe: Episodes he had experienced after the surgery, people he had met, stories he had heard—all seemed to leave no enduring record, as though nothing new could get into his long-term storage. H.M. could hold a mostly normal conversation, but his deficit became instantly clear if the conversation was interrupted for some reason. If you spoke with him for a while, then (for example) left the room and came back 3 or 4 minutes later, he seemed to have totally forgotten that the earlier conversation ever took place; if the earlier conversation was your first meeting with H.M., he would, after the interruption, be certain he was now meeting you for the very first time.

H.M.'s case was unique, but a similar amnesia can be found in patients who have been longtime alcoholics. The problem is not the alcohol itself; the problem instead is that alcoholics tend to have inadequate diets, getting most of their nutrition from whatever they are drinking. It turns out, though, that most alcoholic beverages are missing several key nutrients, including vitamin B1 (thiamine). As a result, longtime alcoholics are vulnerable to a number of problems caused by thiamine deficiency, including a disorder we mentioned at the start of the chapter—the disorder known as **Korsakoff's syndrome** (Rao, Larkin, & Derr, 1986; Ritchie, 1985).

Patients suffering from Korsakoff's syndrome seem similar to H.M. in many ways. They typically have no problem remembering events that took place before the onset of alcoholism. They can also maintain current topics in mind as long as there's no interruption. New information, though, if displaced from the mind, is seemingly lost forever. Korsakoff's patients who have been in the hospital for decades will casually mention that they arrived only a week ago; if asked the name of the current president or events in the news, they unhesitatingly give answers appropriate for two or three decades earlier, whenever the disorder began (Marslen-Wilson & Teuber, 1975; Seltzer & Benson, 1974).

Anterograde Amnesia: What Kind of Memory Is Disrupted?

At the chapter's beginning, we alluded to other evidence that complicates this portrait of anterograde amnesia and returns us to issues of implicit and explicit memory. As it turns out, some of this evidence has been available for a long time. In 1911, a Swiss psychologist named Édouard Claparède (1911/1951) reported the following incident. He was introduced to a young woman suffering from Korsakoff's amnesia, and he reached out to shake her hand. However, Claparède had secretly positioned a pin in his own hand so that when they clasped hands the patient received a painful pinprick. (Respect for patients' rights would forbid any modern investigator from conducting this cruel experiment, but ethical standards were apparently different in 1911.) The next day, Claparède returned and reached out to shake hands with the patient. Not surprisingly, the patient gave no indication that she recognized Claparède or remembered anything about the prior encounter. (This simply confirms the diagnosis of amnesia.) Nevertheless, just before their hands touched, the patient abruptly withdrew her hand and refused to shake hands with Claparède. He asked her why, and after some confusion the patient simply said vaguely, "Sometimes pins are hidden in people's hands."

What's going on here? On the one side, this patient seemed to have no memory of the prior encounter with Claparède. She certainly did not mention the encounter in explaining her refusal to shake hands, and when questioned closely about the earlier encounter, she indicated no knowledge of it. On the other side, she plainly remembered something about the previous day's mishap; we see this clearly in her behavior.

A related pattern can be observed with other Korsakoff's patients. In one procedure, the researchers used a deck of cards like those used in popular trivia games. Each card contained a trivia question and some possible answers, offered in a multiple-choice format (Schacter, Tulving, & Wang, 1981). The experimenter showed each card to a Korsakoff's patient, and if the patient didn't know the answer, he was told it. Then, unbeknownst to the patient, the card was replaced in the deck, guaranteeing that the same question would come up again in a few minutes. When the question did come up again, the patient was quite likely to get it right—and so apparently had learned the answer in the previous encounter. Consistent with their diagnosis, though, the patients had no recollection of the learning: They were consistently unable to explain *why* their answers were correct. They did not say, "I know this bit of trivia because the same question came up just five minutes ago." Instead, they were likely to say things like "I read about it somewhere" or "My sister once told me about it."

Many studies show similar results, with amnesic patients showing profound memory loss on some measures but performance within the normal range on other measures (Cohen & Squire, 1980; Graf & Schacter, 1985; Moscovitch, 1982; Schacter, 1996; Schacter & Tulving, 1982; Squire & McKee, 1993). Specifically, these patients seem completely incapable of recalling episodes or events, and so, in the terms we've been using, they seem to have no explicit memory. Even so, these patients do learn and do remember and thus seem to have intact implicit memories. Indeed, in many tests of implicit memory, amnesic patients seem indistinguishable from ordinary individuals.

Can There Be Explicit Memory without Implicit?

The results with amnesic patients provide powerful evidence that explicit memory is indeed independent of implicit memory. These patients are plainly influenced (implicitly) by specific episodes in the past even though they have no conscious (explicit) recollection of those episodes.

Further data, also arguing for a separation between implicit and explicit memory, come from patients who have the reverse pattern of symptoms: implicit memory disrupted but explicit memory intact. One study involved a patient who had suffered brain damage to the hippocampus but not the amygdala and a second patient with the reverse problem—damage to the amygdala but not the hippocampus (Bechara et al., 1995). These patients were exposed to a series of trials in which a particular stimulus (a blue light) was reliably followed by a loud boat horn, while other stimuli (green, yellow, or red) were not followed by the horn. Later on, the patients were exposed to the blue light on its own and their bodily arousal was measured; would they show a fright reaction in response to this stimulus? In addition, the patients were asked directly, "Which color was followed by the horn?"

The patient with damage to the hippocampus did show a fear reaction to the blue light—assessed via the *skin conductance response* (SCR), a measure of bodily arousal—and so his data on this measure look just like results for control participants (i.e., people without brain damage; see **Figure 7.16**).

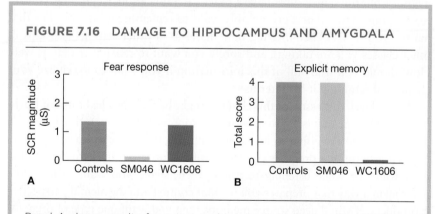

FIGURE 7.16 DAMAGE TO HIPPOCAMPUS AND AMYGDALA

Panel A shows results for a test probing implicit memory; Panel B shows results for a test probing explicit memory. Patient SM046 had suffered damage to the amygdala and shows little evidence of implicit memory (i.e., no fear response—indexed by the *skin conductance response*, or SCR) but a normal level of explicit memory. Patient WC1606 had suffered damage to the hippocampus and shows the opposite pattern: massively disrupted explicit memory but a normal fear response.   AFTER BECHARA ET AL., 1995.

However, when asked directly, this patient could not recall which of the lights had been associated with the boat horn. In contrast, the patient with damage to the amygdala showed the opposite pattern. She was able to report calmly that just one of the lights had been associated with the horn and that the light's color had been blue—demonstrating fully intact explicit memory. When presented with the blue light, however, she showed no fear response.

Optimal Learning

We're almost done with the chapter, but before closing, let's put these amnesia findings into the broader context provided by the chapter's main themes. Throughout the chapter, we've suggested that we cannot make claims about learning or memory acquisition without some reference to how the learning is going to be used later on. Thus, whether it's better to learn underwater or on land depends on where you will be tested. Whether it's better to learn while listening to jazz or while sitting in a quiet room depends on the music background of the memory test environment.

These ideas are echoed in the neuropsychology data. Specifically, it would be misleading to say that Korsakoff's amnesia disrupts someone's ability to learn or ruins their ability to create new memories. Instead, brain damage is likely to disrupt some types of learning but not others, and how this matters for the person depends on how the newly learned material will be accessed. Thus, someone who suffers hippocampal damage will likely appear normal on an indirect memory test but seem amnesic on a direct test, while someone who suffers amygdala damage will probably show the reverse pattern.

All of these points are enormously important for our theorizing about memory, but the same points have a practical implication. Right now, you are reading this material and presumably want to remember it later on. For that matter, you're also encountering new material in other settings (perhaps in other classes you are taking), and surely you want to remember that as well. How should you study all of this information if you want to maximize your chances of retaining it for later use?

At one level, the lesson of this chapter might be that the ideal form of learning would be one that is "in tune with" the approach to the material that you'll need later. If you're going to be tested explicitly, you want to learn the material in a fashion that prepares you for that form of retrieval. If you'll be tested underwater or while listening to music, then, again, you want to learn the material in a way that prepares you for that context and the mental perspective it produces. If you'll need source memory, then you want one type of preparation; if you'll need familiarity, you might want a different type of preparation.

The problem, though, is that during learning you often don't know how you'll be approaching the material later—whether your focus during retrieval will be on meaning or on sound, whether you'll need the information implicitly or explicitly, and so on. As a result, maybe the best strategy in learning would be to use *multiple perspectives*. To pick up our earlier analogy, imagine that you know that at some point in the future you'll want to reach Chicago, but you don't know yet whether you'll be approaching the city from the north, the south, or the west. In that case, your best bet might be to build multiple highways, so that you can reach your goal from any direction. Memory works the same way. If you initially think about a topic in different ways and in conjunction with many other ideas, then you'll establish many paths leading to the target material, and so you'll be able to access that material from many different perspectives. The real pragmatic message from this chapter, then, is that this multiperspective approach may, in fact, provide the optimal learning strategy.

The "Cognitive Interview"

Police investigations often depend on eyewitness reports, but what can the police do if witnesses insist they can't remember the event, and can't answer the police questions? Are there steps we can take to help witnesses remember?

A number of exotic procedures have been proposed to promote witness recollection, including hypnosis and the use of memory-enhancing medications. Evidence suggests, however, that these procedures provide little benefit (and may, in some settings, actually harm memory). Indeed, "hypnotically enhanced memory" is inadmissible as trial evidence in most jurisdictions. A much more promising approach is the *cognitive interview*, a technique developed by psychologists with the specific aim of improving eyewitness memory; a parallel procedure has been developed for interviewing *children* who have been witnesses to crimes. A related procedure is used in England (the so-called P.E.A.C.E. procedure) for questioning *suspects*.

A considerable quantity of evidence suggests that the cognitive interview is successful—and so does help people to remember more. It is gratifying, then, that the cognitive interview has been adopted by a number of police departments as their preferred interview technique.

How does the cognitive interview work? Let's start with the fact that sometimes you cannot remember things simply because you didn't notice them in the first place, and so no record of the desired information was ever placed in long-term storage. In this situation, no procedure—whether it's the cognitive interview, or hypnosis, or simply trying really hard to recall—can locate information that isn't there to be located. You cannot get water out of an empty bottle, and you cannot read words off a blank page. In the same fashion, you cannot recall information that was never placed in memory to begin with.

In other cases, though, the gaps in your recollection have a different source: The desired information is in memory, but you're unable to find it. (We'll have more to say about this point in Chapter 8, when we discuss theories of forgetting.) To overcome this problem, the cognitive interview relies on context reinstatement. The police investigator urges the witness to think back to the setting of the target event: How did the witness feel at the time of the crime? What was the physical setting? What was the weather? As

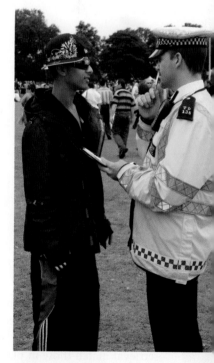

THE COGNITIVE INTERVIEW

Police in England use the Cognitive Interview both for interviewing witnesses and (in a slightly different form) for interviewing suspects.

Chapter 7 discusses, these steps are likely to put the witness back into the same mental state, the same frame of mind, that he or she had at the time of the crime—and, in many cases, these steps will promote recall.

In addition, the chapter's discussion of retrieval paths leads to the idea that sometimes you'll recall a memory only if you approach the memory from the right angle—using the proper retrieval path. But how do you choose the proper path? The cognitive interview builds on the simple notion that you don't have to choose. Instead, you can try recalling the events from lots of different angles (via lots of different paths) in order to maximize your chances of finding a path that leads to the desired information.

Thus, for example, the cognitive interview encourages witnesses first to recount the event from its start to its end, and then recount it in reverse sequence from the end back to the beginning. Sometimes witnesses are also encouraged to take a different *spatial* perspective: "You just told me what you saw; try to remember what Joe would have seen, from where he was standing."

In short, the cognitive interview builds on principles well established in research—the role of context reinstatement, for example, or the importance of retrieval paths. It's no surprise, therefore, that the cognitive interview is effective; the procedure capitalizes on mechanisms that we know to be helpful.

The cognitive interview was, as we've said, designed to help law enforcement professionals in their investigations. Note, though, that the principles involved here are general ones, and they can be useful in many other settings. Imagine, for example, a physician trying to get as complete a medical history as possible. ("When did the rash first show up? Is it worse after you have eaten certain foods?") Or think about a novice repair-person trying to recall what she learned in training. ("Did they tell me anything about this particular error code?") Or think about your own situation when you're trying to recall, say, what you read in the library last week. The ideas built into the cognitive interview are useful in these settings as well and, indeed, are useful for anyone who needs to draw as much information from memory as possible.

chapter summary

• In general, the chances that someone will remember an earlier event are greatest if the physical and mental circumstances in place during memory retrieval match those in place during learning. This is reflected, for example, in the phenomenon of context-dependent learning.

• A similar pattern is reflected in the phenomenon of "encoding specificity." This term refers to the idea that you usually learn more than the specific material to be remembered itself; you also learn that material within its associated context.

• All these results arise from the fact that learning establishes connections among memories, and these connections serve as retrieval paths. Like any path, these lead from some starting point to some target. To use a given path, therefore, you must return to the appropriate starting point. In the same way, if there is a connection between two memories, then activating the first memory is likely to call the second to mind. If the first memory is not activated, however, this connection, no matter how well established, will not help in locating the second memory—just as a large highway approaching Chicago from the south will not be helpful if you are trying to reach Chicago from the north.

- This emphasis on memory connections fits well with a conceptualization of memory as a vast "network," with individual nodes joined to each other via connections or associations. An individual node becomes activated when it receives enough of an input signal to raise its activation level to its response threshold. Once activated, the node sends activation out through its connections to all the nodes connected to it.

- Hints are effective because the target node can receive activation from two sources simultaneously—from nodes representing the main cue or question, and also from nodes representing the hint. The benefits of context reinstatement can be explained in a similar fashion.

- Activating one node does (as predicted) seem to prime nearby nodes through the process of spreading activation. This is evident (for example) in studies of semantic priming in lexical-decision tasks.

- Some learning strategies are effective as preparation for some sorts of memory tests but ineffective for other sorts of tests. Some strategies, for example, are effective at establishing source memory rather than familiarity; other strategies do the reverse. Source memory is essential for recall; recognition can often be achieved either through source memory or through familiarity.

- Different forms of learning also play a role in producing implicit and explicit memories. Implicit memories are those that influence you even when you have no awareness that you are being influenced by a specific previous event. In many cases, implicit-memory effects take the form of priming—for example, in word recognition or word-stem completion. But implicit memories can also influence you in other ways, producing a number of memory-based illusions.

- Implicit memory can be understood as the consequence of processing fluency, produced by experience in a particular task with a particular stimulus. The fluency is sometimes detected and registered as a sense of "specialness" attached to a stimulus. Often, this specialness is then attributed to some cause, but this attribution can be inaccurate.

- Implicit memory is also important in understanding the pattern of symptoms in anterograde amnesia. Amnesic patients perform badly on tests requiring explicit memory and may not even recall events that happened just minutes earlier. However, they often perform at near-normal levels on tests involving implicit memory. This disparity underscores the fact that we cannot speak in general about good and bad memories, good and poor learning. Instead, learning and memory must be matched to a particular task and a particular form of test; learning and memory that are excellent for some tasks may be poor for others.

e eBook Demonstrations & Essays

Online Demonstrations:
- Demonstration 7.1: Retrieval Paths and Connections
- Demonstration 7.2: Encoding Specificity
- Demonstration 7.3: Spreading Activation in Memory Search
- Demonstration 7.4: Semantic Priming
- Demonstration 7.5: Priming from Implicit Memory

Online Applying Cognitive Psychology Essays:
- Cognitive Psychology and Education: The Importance of Multiple Retrieval Paths
- Cognitive Psychology and Education: Familiarity Is Potentially Treacherous
- Cognitive Psychology and the Law: Unconscious Transference

ZAPS 2.0 Cognition Labs

- Go to http://digital.wwnorton.com/cognition6 for the online labs relevant to this chapter.

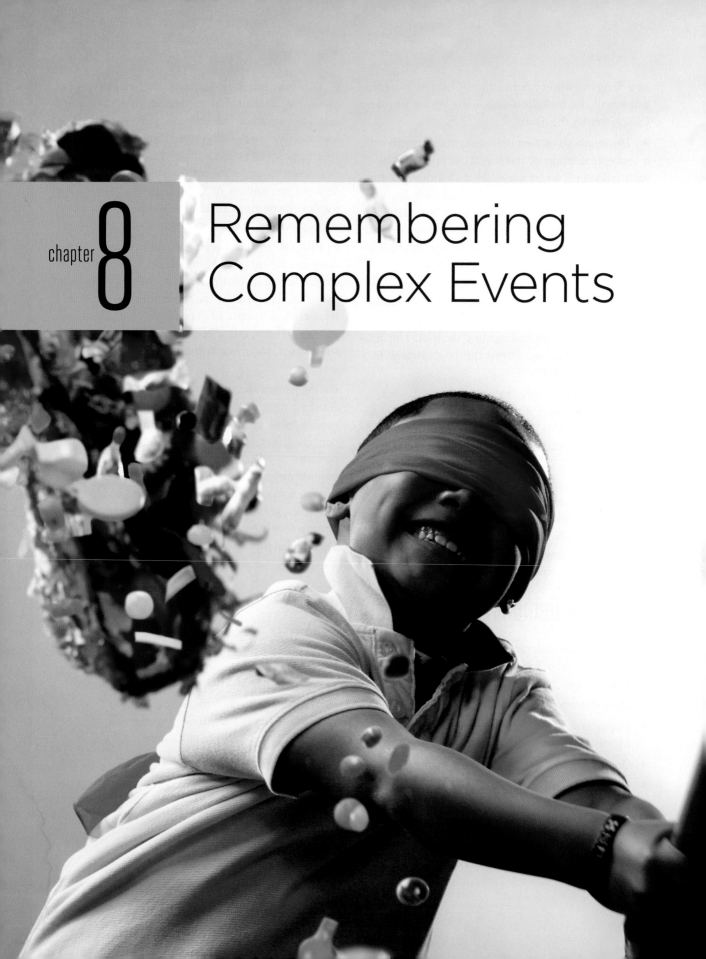

chapter 8

Remembering Complex Events

what if...

What were you doing on March 19, 2003? What did you have for lunch that day? What was the weather like? These seem like silly questions; why should you remember details of that date? But what would your life be like if you *could* remember those details—and similar details for every other day in your life? In other words, what would life be like if you had a "super memory"—so that, essentially, you never forgot anything?

Researchers have located a small number of people—just a couple of dozen—who have *hyperthymesia*, or "superior autobiographical recall." These people are able to recall every single day of their lives, over a span of many years. One of these individuals, for example, asserts that that she can recall every day of her life since she was 14. "Starting on February 5, 1980, I remember everything. That was a Tuesday."

If asked about a randomly selected date—say, February 10, 2005— these individuals can recall exactly where they were that day, what they had for lunch, what shoes they were wearing, and more. Their performance is just as good if they're asked about October 8, 2008, or March 19, 2003. And when checked, these memories turn out to be uniformly accurate, with the implication that these people can literally recall in detail every day, every episode, of their lives.

These individuals are surely remarkable in how much they remember, but it's striking that they seem quite normal in other ways. In other words, their extraordinary memory capacity hasn't made them amazing geniuses or incredible scholars. Indeed, even though these individuals have an exceptional capacity for remembering their own lives, they seem to have no advantage in remembering other sorts of content or in performing other mental tasks. This point has been documented with careful testing, but it is also evident in the fact that researchers weren't aware such people existed until just a few years ago (e.g., Parker, Cahill, & McGaugh, 2006). Apparently, these individuals, even with their incredible memory capacity, are ordinary enough in other regards so that we didn't spot them until recently.

In fact, there are at least some indications that this sort of remembering can be a *problem*, because these individuals' vivid, detailed memories

* Outside the lab, you often try to remember materials that are related in some fashion to other things you know or have experienced. Over and over, we will see that this other knowledge—the knowledge you bring to a situation—helps you to remember by promoting retrieval, but it also hurts memory by promoting error.

* The memory errors produced by your prior knowledge tend to be quite systematic, with the result that you often end up recalling the past as more "normal," more in line with your expectations, than it actually was.

* Even if we acknowledge the memory errors, our overall assessment of memory can be quite positive. This is because your memories are accurate most of the time, and the errors that do occur can be understood as the by-products of mechanisms that generally serve you well.

* Finally, we will consider three factors that play an important role in shaping memory outside of the laboratory: *involvement* with an event, *emotion*, and the *passage of time*. These factors require some additional principles as part of our overall theory, but they also confirm the power of more general principles—principles hinging (for example) on the role of memory connections.

sometimes provide uncontrollable associations, creating a disruption to their lives. Thus, A.J., the first individual confirmed with hyperthymesia, describes her recollection as "non-stop, uncontrollable and totally exhausting"; she says it is "a burden" for her. She complains that she is powerless to interrupt this flow of memories: "It's like a split screen; I'll be talking to someone and seeing something else." (We note, though, that other people with this sort of super memory offer a different report, and seem to *enjoy* having vivid access to their past; McGaugh & LePort, 2014.)

How should we think about these points? Humans have been trying for centuries to improve their own memories, but even so, a "perfect" memory may provide less of an advantage than you might think, and it may in some regards produce problems. We'll return to these points, and what they imply about memory functioning, later in the chapter.

Memory Errors, Memory Gaps

Where did you spend last summer? What country did you grow up in? Where were you five minutes ago? These are, of course, extremely easy questions, and you effortlessly retrieve this information from memory the moment you need it. If we want to understand memory, therefore, we need to understand how you locate these bits of information (and thousands of others just like them) so quickly and easily.

But we also need to account for some other observations. Sometimes, when you try to remember an episode, you simply draw a blank. On other occasions, you recall something, but with no conviction that you're correct: "I think her nickname was Dink, but I'm not sure." And sometimes, when you try to remember, things go wrong in a more serious way: You recall a past episode, but then it turns out that your memory is mistaken. Perhaps details of the event were different from the way you recall them. Or perhaps your memory is altogether wrong, misrepresenting large elements of the original episode. Worst of all, in some cases you can remember entire events that never happened at all! In this chapter, we'll consider how, and how often, these errors arise. Let's start with some examples.

Memory Errors: Some Initial Examples

In 1992, an El Al cargo plane lost power in two of its engines just after taking off from Amsterdam's Schiphol Airport. The pilot attempted to return the plane to the airport but couldn't make it; a few minutes later, the plane crashed into an 11-story apartment building in the Bijlmermeer neighborhood of Amsterdam. The building collapsed and burst into flames; 43 people were killed, including the plane's entire crew.

Ten months later, researchers questioned 193 Dutch people about the crash, asking them in particular, "Did you see the television film of the moment the plane hit the apartment building?" More than half of the participants (107 of them) reported seeing the film, even though there was no such film. No camera had recorded the crash; no film (or any reenactment) was shown on television. The participants were remembering something that never took place (Crombag, Wagenaar, & van Koppen, 1996; also see Jelicic et al., 2006; Ost, Vrij, Costall, & Bull, 2002; but for a complication, see Smeets et al., 2006).

In a follow-up study, the investigators surveyed another 93 people about the plane crash. These people were also asked whether they'd seen the (nonexistent) TV film, and then they were asked detailed questions about exactly what they had seen in the film: Was the plane burning when it crashed, or did it catch fire a moment later? In the film, did they see the plane come down vertically with no forward speed, or did it hit the building while still moving horizontally at a considerable speed?

Two thirds of these participants remembered seeing the film, and most of them confidently provided details about what they had seen. When asked about the plane's speed, for example, only 23% prudently said that they couldn't remember. The others gave various responses, presumably based on their "memory" of the (again: nonexistent) film.

This is not a case of one or two people making a mistake; instead, a large majority of the people questioned seemed to have a detailed recollection of the film. In addition, let's emphasize that this plane crash was an emotional and much-discussed event for these participants; the researchers were not asking them to recall a minor occurrence.

Perhaps these errors emerged only because the research participants were trying to remember something that had taken place almost a year earlier.

Is memory more accurate when the questions come after a shorter delay? In a study by Brewer and Treyens (1981), participants were asked to wait briefly in the experimenter's office prior to the procedure's start. After 35 seconds, participants were taken out of this office and told that there actually was no experimental procedure. Instead, the study was concerned with their memory for the room in which they'd just been sitting.

Participants' recollections of the office were powerfully influenced by their beliefs about what an academic office *typically* contains. For example, participants surely knew in advance of the study that academic offices usually contain a desk and a chair, and as it turns out, these pieces of furniture were present in this particular office. This agreement between prior knowledge and the specific experience led to accurate memory, and 29 of 30 participants correctly remembered that the office contained a desk and a chair. In other regards, however, this office was different from what the participants might have expected. Specifically, participants would expect an academic office to contain shelves filled with books, yet in this particular office no books were in view (see **Figure 8.1**). On this point, the

---

FIGURE 8.1   THE OFFICE USED IN THE BREWER
AND TREYENS STUDY

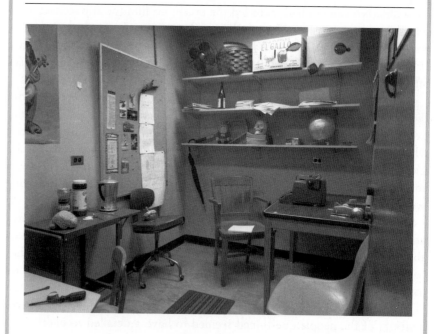

No books were in view in this office, but participants, biased by their expectations of what should be in an academic office, often remembered seeing books.   AFTER BREWER & TREYENS, 1981.

participants' recall was often in line with their expectations and not with reality: Almost one third of them (9 of 30) remembered seeing books in the office, when in fact there were none.

How could this happen? How could so many Dutch participants be wrong in their recall of a significant emotional episode? How could intelligent, alert college students fail to remember what they'd seen in an office just moments earlier?

Memory Errors: A Hypothesis

In Chapters 6 and 7, we emphasized the importance of memory connections, linking each bit of knowledge in your memory to other bits. Sometimes these connections tie together similar episodes, so that a trip to the beach ends up being connected in memory to your recollections of other trips. Sometimes the connections tie an episode to certain ideas—ideas, perhaps, that were part of your *understanding* of the episode, or ideas that were triggered by some element within the episode.

With all of these connections in place, information ends up being stored in memory in a system that looks like a vast spider web, with each bit of information connected by many threads to other bits of information elsewhere in the web. This was the idea that in Chapter 7 we described as a huge *network* of interconnected *nodes*. We need to be clear, though, that within this network there are no boundaries keeping memories of one episode separate from memories of other episodes. The episodes, in other words, aren't stored in separate "files," each distinct from the others. What is it, therefore, that holds together the various elements within each episode? It is simply the density of connections: There are many connections linking the various aspects of your "trip to the beach" to one another; there are fewer connections linking this event to other events.

As we have discussed, these connections play a crucial role in memory retrieval. Imagine, for example, that you're trying to recall the restaurant you ate at during your beach trip. You'll start by activating the nodes in memory that represent some aspect of the trip—perhaps your memory of the rainy weather. Activation will then flow outward from there, through the connections you've established, and this will energize the nodes representing other aspects of the trip. The flow of activation can then continue from there, eventually reaching the nodes you seek. In this way, we've said, the connections serve as *retrieval paths*, guiding your search through memory.

Obviously, then, memory connections are a good thing; without them you might never locate the information you're seeking. However, the connections can also create problems for you. As you add more and more links between the bits of *this* episode and the bits of *that* episode, you're gradually knitting these two episodes together. As a result, you may lose track of the "boundary" between episodes; more precisely, you're likely to lose track of which bits of information were contained within which event. Thus, you become vulnerable to what we might think of as "transplant" errors, in which a bit of information encountered in one context is transplanted into another context.

In the same fashion, as your memory for an episode becomes more and more interwoven with other thoughts you've had about the episode, it becomes difficult to keep track of which elements are linked to the episode because they were, in truth, part of the episode itself, and which are linked merely because they were *associated with* the episode in your thoughts. This, too, can produce transplant errors, in which elements that were part of your thinking get misremembered as if they were actually part of the original experience.

Understanding Both Helps and Hurts Memory

It seems, then, that memory connections both help and hurt recollection. They *help* because the connections, serving as retrieval paths, enable you to locate information in memory. But connections can *hurt* because they sometimes make it difficult to see where the remembered episode stops and other, related knowledge begins. As a result, the connections encourage **intrusion errors**—errors in which other knowledge intrudes into the remembered event.

To see how these points play out, let's look at an early study by Owens, Bower, and Black (1979). In this study, half of the participants read the following passage:

> Nancy arrived at the cocktail party. She looked around the room to see who was there. She went to talk with her professor. She felt she had to talk to him but was a little nervous about just what to say. A group of people started to play charades. Nancy went over and had some refreshments. The hors d'oeuvres were good, but she wasn't interested in talking to the rest of the people at the party. After a while she decided she'd had enough and left the party.

Other participants read the same passage, but with a prologue that set the stage:

> Nancy woke up feeling sick again, and she wondered if she really was pregnant. How would she tell the professor she had been seeing? And the money was another problem.

All participants were then given a recall test in which they were asked to remember the sentences as exactly as they could. **Table 8.1** shows the results; as can be seen, the participants who had read the prologue (the "theme condition") recalled much more of the original story. This is consistent with claims made in Chapter 6: The prologue provided a meaningful context for the remainder of the story, and this helped understanding. Understanding, in turn, promoted recall.

TABLE 8.1 NUMBER OF PROPOSITIONS REMEMBERED BY PARTICIPANTS

STUDIED PROPOSITIONS (THOSE IN STORY)		INFERRED PROPOSITIONS (THOSE NOT IN STORY)	
Theme Condition	Neutral Condition	Theme Condition	Neutral Condition
29.2	20.2	15.2	3.7

In the *theme* condition, a brief prologue set the theme for the passage that was to be remembered.   AFTER OWENS ET AL., 1979.

At the same time, the story's prologue also led participants to include elements in their recall that were not mentioned in the original episode. In fact, participants who had seen the prologue made *four times* as many intrusion errors as did participants who had not seen the prologue. For example, they might recall, "The professor had gotten Nancy pregnant." This is not part of the story but is certainly implied, and so it will probably be part of the participants' understanding of the story. It's then this understanding (including the imported element) that is remembered.

The DRM Procedure

Similar effects, with memory connections *helping* and *hurting* memory, can even be demonstrated with simple word lists, provided that the lists are arranged so that they make appropriate contact with prior knowledge. For example, in many experiments, participants have been presented with lists like this one: "bed, rest, awake, tired, dream, wake, snooze, blanket, doze, slumber, snore, nap, peace, yawn, drowsy." Immediately after hearing this list, participants are asked to recall as many of the words as they can.

As you surely noticed, all of the words in this list are associated with sleep, and the presence of this theme helps memory: The words that are on the list are relatively easy to remember. It turns out, though, that the word "sleep" is not itself included in the list. Nonetheless, research participants spontaneously make the connection between the list words and this associated word, and this connection almost invariably leads to a memory error: When the time comes for recall, participants are extremely likely to recall that they heard "sleep." In fact, they are just as likely to recall "sleep" as they are to recall the actual words on the list (see **Figure 8.2**). When asked how confident they are in their memories, participants are just as confident in their (false) recall of "sleep" as they are in their (correct) memory of genuine list words (Gallo, 2010; for earlier and classic papers in this arena, see Deese, 1957; Roediger & McDermott, 1995, 2000).

This paradigm is referred to as the **DRM procedure**, in honor of the investigators who developed it (Deese, Roediger, and McDermott). The procedure yields a large number of memory errors, even if participants are put on their guard before the procedure begins (i.e., told explicitly about the nature of the lists and the frequency with which these lists produce errors; Gallo,

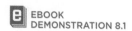
EBOOK
DEMONSTRATION 8.1

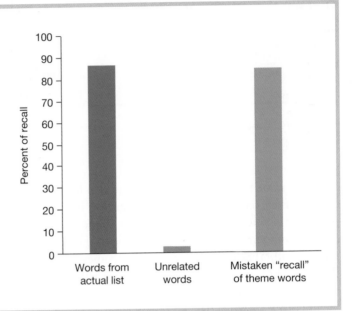

FIGURE 8.2 THE EFFECTS OF THE DRM PARADIGM

Because of the theme uniting the list, participants can remember almost 90% of the words they encountered. However, they're just as likely to "recall" the list's theme word—even though it was not presented.

Roberts, & Seamon, 1997; McDermott & Roediger, 1998). Apparently, the mechanisms leading to these errors are quite automatic and not mechanisms that people can somehow inhibit.

Schematic Knowledge

Imagine that you go to a restaurant with a friend. This setting is familiar for you, and you have some commonsense knowledge about what normally happens here. You'll be seated; someone will bring menus; you'll order, then eat; eventually, you'll pay the check and leave. Knowledge like this is often referred to with the Greek word **schema** (plural: *schemata*). Schemata summarize the broad pattern of what's normal in a situation, and so your kitchen schema tells you that a kitchen is likely to have a stove in it but no piano; your dentist's office schema tells you that there are likely to be magazines in the waiting room, that you'll probably be given a new toothbrush when you leave, and so on.

Schemata help you in many ways. In a restaurant, for example, you're not puzzled by the fact that someone keeps filling your water glass or that someone drops by the table to ask, "How is everything?" Your schema tells you that these are normal occurrences in a restaurant, and you instantly understand how they fit into the broader framework.

Schemata also help when the time comes to *recall* how an event unfolded. This is because there are often gaps in your recollection—either because there were things you didn't notice in the first place, or because you have gradually forgotten some aspects of an experience. (We will say more about forgetting later in the chapter.) In either case, you can rely on your schemata to fill in these gaps. Thus, in thinking back to your dinner at Chez Pierre, you might not remember anything about the menus. Nonetheless, you can be reasonably sure that there were menus and that they were given to you early on and taken away after you placed your order. On this basis, you're likely to include menus within your "recall" of the dinner, even if you have no memory of seeing the menus for this particular meal. In other words, you'll (unwittingly) supplement what you actually remember with a plausible reconstruction based on your schematic knowledge. And in most cases this after-the-fact reconstruction will be correct, since schemata do, after all, describe what happens most of the time.

Evidence for Schematic Knowledge

Clearly, then, schematic knowledge helps you—guiding your understanding and enabling you to reconstruct things you cannot remember. But schematic knowledge can also hurt you, promoting errors in perception and memory. Moreover, the *types* of errors produced by schemata are quite predictable: Bear in mind that schemata summarize the broad pattern of your experience, and so they tell you, in essence, what's typical or ordinary in a given situation. Any reliance on schematic knowledge, therefore, will be shaped by this information about what's "normal." Thus, if there are things you don't notice while viewing a situation or event, your schemata will lead you to fill in these "gaps" with knowledge about what's normally in place in that setting. Likewise, if there are things you can't recall, your schemata will fill in the gaps with knowledge about what's typical in that situation. As a result, a reliance on schemata will inevitably make the world seem more "normal" than it really is and will make the past seem more "regular" than it actually was.

Imagine, for example, that you visit a dentist's office, and this one happens not to have any magazines in the waiting room. It's possible that you won't notice this detail or that you'll forget about it after a while. What will happen, therefore, if you later try to recall this trip to the dentist? Odds are good that you'll rely on your schematic knowledge and "remember" that there were magazines (since, after all, there usually are some scattered around a waiting room). In this way, your recollection will make this dentist's office seem more typical, more ordinary, than it truly was.

This tendency toward "regularizing" the past is easily demonstrated in research. The classic demonstration, however, comes from studies published long ago by British psychologist Frederick Bartlett, the first professor of experimental psychology at the University of Cambridge. Bartlett presented his participants with a story taken from the folklore of Native Americans (the story is shown in **Figure 8.3A**; Bartlett, 1932). When tested later, the participants did reasonably well in recalling the gist of the story, but they made many errors in recalling the particulars (Figure 8.3B shows an example of participants' recall). The pattern of errors, though, was quite systematic: The details omitted tended to be ones that made little sense to Bartlett's British participants. Likewise, aspects of the story that were unfamiliar were changed into aspects that were more familiar; steps of the story that seemed inexplicable were supplemented to make the story seem more logical.

FIGURE 8.3 THE WAR OF THE GHOSTS

One night two young men from Egulac went down to the river to hunt seals, and while they were there it became foggy and calm. Then they heard war cries, and they thought; "Maybe this is a war party." They escaped to the shore and hid behind a log. Now canoes came up, and they heard the noise of paddles and saw one canoe coming up to them. There were five men in the canoe, and they said:

"What do you think? We wish to take you along. We are going up the river to make war on the people."

One of the young men said: "I have no arrows." "Arrows are in the canoe," they said. "I will not go along. I might be killed. My relatives do not know where I have gone. But you," he said, turning to the other, "may go with them."

So one of the young men went, but the other returned home. And the warriors went on up the river to a town on the other side of Kalama. The people came down to the water and they began to fight, and many were killed. But presently the young man heard one of the warriors say: "Quick, let us go home; that Indian has been hit." Now he thought, "Oh, they are ghosts." He did not feel sick, but they said he had been shot.

So the canoes went back to Egulac, and the young man went ashore to his house and made a fire. And he told everybody and said: "Behold I accompanied the ghosts, and we went to fight. Many of our fellows were killed, and many of those who attacked us were killed. They said I was hit, and I did not feel sick."

He told it all, and then he became quiet. When the sun rose, he fell down. Something black came out of his mouth. His face became contorted. The people jumped up and cried. He was dead. (Bartlett, 1932, p. 65)

A

EXAMPLE OF STORY RECALL

Indians were out fishing for seals in the Bay of Manpapan, when along came five other Indians in a war-canoe. They were going fighting. "Come with us," said the five to the two, "and fight." "I cannot come," was the answer of the one, "for I have an old mother at home who is dependent upon me." The other also said he could not come, because he had no arms. "That is no difficulty" the others replied, "for we have plenty in the canoe with us"; so he got into the canoe and went with them. In a fight soon afterwards this Indian received a mortal wound. Finding that his hour was come, he cried out that he was about to die. "Nonsense," said one of the others, "you will not die." But he did.

B

Bartlett presented his British participants with the story, shown in Panel A, drawn from Native American folklore. Later, when the participants tried to remember the story, they did well in recalling the broad gist but tended to alter the story so that it made more sense from their perspective. Specifically, they either left out or distorted elements that did not fit with their schema-based understanding. A typical recall version is shown in Panel B.

Overall, then, the participants' memories seem to have "cleaned up" the story they had read—making it more coherent (from their perspective), more sensible, than it first seemed. This is exactly what we would expect if the memory errors derived from the participants' attempts to understand the story and, with that, their efforts toward fitting the story into a schematic frame. Elements that fit within the frame remained in their memories (or could be reconstructed later). Elements that did not fit dropped out of memory or were changed.

In the same spirit, consider the Brewer and Treyens study we mentioned at the start of this chapter—the study in which participants remembered seeing shelves full of books, even though there were none. This error was produced by schematic knowledge: During the event itself (i.e., while the participants were sitting in the office), schematic knowledge told the participants that academic offices usually contain many books, and this knowledge biased what the participants paid attention to. (If you're already certain that the shelves contain books, why should you spend time looking at the shelves? This would only confirm something you already know—cf. Vo & Henderson, 2009.) Then, when the time came to recall the office, participants used their schema to reconstruct what the office *must have* contained—a desk, a chair, and of course lots of books. In this fashion, the memory for the actual office was eclipsed by generic knowledge about what a "normal" office contains.

Likewise, think back to our other early example—the misremembered plane crash. Here, too, the memory error distorted reality by making the past seem more regular, more typical, than it really was. After all, the Dutch survey respondents probably hear about most major news events via a television broadcast, and these broadcasts typically include vivid video footage. So here, too, the past as remembered seems to have been assimilated into the pattern of the ordinary. The event as it unfolded was unusual, but the event *as remembered* is quite typical of its kind—just as we would expect if understanding and remembering were guided by our knowledge of the way things generally unfold.

The Cost of Memory Errors

There's clearly a "good news, bad news" quality to our discussion so far. On the positive side, we've noted that memory connections serve as retrieval paths, allowing you to locate information in storage. The connections also enrich your understanding, because they highlight how each of your memories is related to other things you know. The links to schematic knowledge also enable you to supplement your (often incomplete) recollection with well-informed (and usually accurate) inference.

On the negative side, though, the same memory connections can undermine memory accuracy. We've now seen that the connections can lead you to remember things as more regular than they were, in some cases adding elements to a memory and in other cases "subtracting" elements, so that (in either case) the memory ends up making more sense (i.e., fitting better with your schemata).

These errors are troubling. As we've discussed in other contexts, you rely on memory in many aspects of life, and it's unsettling that the memories you rely on may be *wrong*—misrepresenting how the past unfolded. To make matters worse, the mistakes seem surprisingly frequent—with two thirds of the participants in one study remembering a nonexistent film, with one third of the participants in another study remembering books that weren't there at all, and so on. Perhaps worst of all, we can easily find circumstances in which these memory errors are deeply consequential. For example, memory errors in eyewitness testimony (e.g., in identifying the wrong person as the culprit or in misreporting how an event unfolded) can potentially send an innocent person to jail and allow a guilty person to go free.

Eyewitness Errors

How often do eyewitnesses make mistakes? A possible answer comes from U.S. court cases in which DNA evidence, not available at the time of the trial, shows that the courts had convicted people who were, in truth, not guilty. There are now over 320 cases of these DNA exonerations—cases in which the courts have acknowledged their tragic error. The exonerees had (on average) spent more than a dozen years in jail for crimes they did not commit; many of them were on death row, awaiting execution.

When closely examined, these cases yield a clear message. Some of these men were convicted because of dishonest informants; some because analyses of forensic evidence had been botched. But by far the most common concern is eyewitness errors. Indeed, according to most analyses, eyewitness errors account for three quarters of these false convictions, more than all other causes combined (e.g., Garrett, 2011; Reisberg, 2014).

Cases like these make it plain that memory errors, including misidentifications, are profoundly important. We're therefore led to ask: Are there ways to avoid these errors? Or, perhaps, are there ways to *detect* the errors, so that we can decide which memories are correct and which are not?

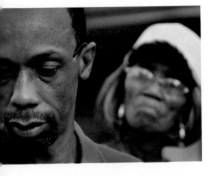

EXONERATION OF THE INNOCENT

Michael Anthony Green spent more than 27 years in prison for a rape he did not commit. He is one of the 300 people who were convicted in U.S. courts but then proven innocent by DNA evidence. Mistaken eyewitness evidence accounts for more of these false convictions than all other causes combined.

Planting False Memories

An enormous number of studies have examined eyewitness memory—the sort of memory that police rely on when investigating crimes. For example, Loftus and Palmer (1974) showed participants a series of pictures depicting an automobile collision. Sometime later, half the participants were asked, "How fast were the cars going when they hit each other?" Others were asked, "How fast were the cars going when they smashed into each other?" The difference between these questions ("hit" vs. "smashed") was slight, but it was enough to bias the participants' estimates of speed. Participants in the first group ("hit") estimated the speed to have been 34 miles per hour; participants in the second group ("smashed") estimated 41 miles per hour—20%

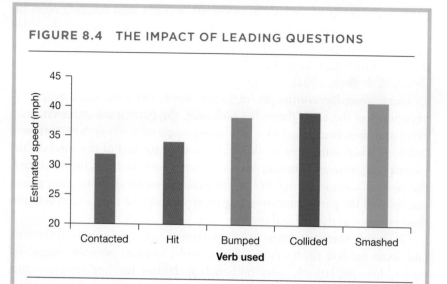

FIGURE 8.4   THE IMPACT OF LEADING QUESTIONS

Witnesses who were asked how fast cars were going when they "hit" each other reported (on average) a speed of 34 miles per hour. Other witnesses, asked how fast the cars were going when they "smashed" into each other, gave estimates 20% higher. When all participants were later asked whether they'd seen broken glass at the scene, participants who'd been asked the "smashed" question were more likely to say yes—even though there was no broken glass.   AFTER LOFTUS & PALMER, 1974.

higher (see **Figure 8.4**). But what is critical comes next: One week later, the participants were asked in a perfectly neutral way whether they had seen any broken glass in the pictures. Participants who had initially been asked the "hit" question tended to remember (correctly) that no glass was visible; participants who had been asked the "smashed" question, though, often made this error. It seems, therefore, that the change of just one word within the initial question can have a significant effect—in this case, more than doubling the likelihood of memory error.

Other studies have varied this procedure. Sometimes participants are asked questions that contain misinformation about an event. For example, they might be asked, "How fast was the car going when it raced by the barn?" when, in truth, no barn was in view. In other studies, participants are exposed to descriptions of the target event allegedly written by "other witnesses." They might be told, for example, "Here's how someone else recalled the crime; does this match what you recall?" Of course, the "other witness" descriptions contained some misinformation, enabling us to ask if participants "pick up" the false leads (e.g., Paterson & Kemp, 2006; also Edelson, Sharon, Dolan, & Dudai, 2011). In still other studies, researchers ask questions that require the participants themselves to *make up* some bit of misinformation. For example, participants could be asked, "In the video, was the man bleeding from his knee or from his elbow after the fall?" Even though it was clear in the video that the man wasn't bleeding at all, participants are forced to choose one of these options (e.g., Chrobak & Zaragoza, 2008; Zaragoza, Payment, Ackil, Drivdahl, & Beck, 2001).

These procedures differ in important ways, but even so, they are all variations on the same theme. In each case, the participant experiences an event and then is exposed to a misleading suggestion about how the event unfolded. Then some time is allowed to pass. At the end of this interval, the participant's memory is tested. And in each of these variations, the outcome is the same: A substantial number of participants—in some studies, more than one third of the participants—end up incorporating the false suggestion into their memory of the original event.

Of course, some attempts at manipulating memory are more successful, and some are less so. It's easier, for example, to plant *plausible* memories rather than implausible ones (although memories for implausible events can also be planted—see Hyman, 2000; Mazzoni, Loftus, & Kirsch, 2001; Pezdek, Blandon-Gitlin, & Gabbay, 2006; Scoboria, Mazzoni, Kirsch, & Jimenez, 2006; Thomas & Loftus, 2002). False memories are also more easily planted if the research participants don't just *hear* about the false event but, instead, are urged to *imagine* how the suggested event unfolded—an effect referred to as "imagination inflation." In one study, for example, participants were given a list of possible childhood events (going to the emergency room late at night; winning a stuffed animal at a carnival game; getting in trouble for calling 911). Participants were asked to "picture each event as clearly and completely" as they could, and this simple exercise was enough to increase participants' confidence that the event had really occurred (Garry, Manning, Loftus, & Serman, 1996; also Mazzoni & Memon, 2003; Sharman & Barnier, 2008; also see Shidlovski, Schul & Mayo, 2014).

Even acknowledging these variations, though, let's emphasize the consistency of these findings. We can use subtle procedures (with slightly leading questions) to plant false information in someone's memory, or we can use a more blatant procedure (demanding that the person make up the bogus facts). We can use printed stories, or movies, or live events as our to-be-remembered materials. In all cases, it is remarkably easy to alter someone's memory, with the result that the past as the person remembers it can differ from the past as it really was. We can alter memories in highly intelligent people and in less intelligent people. We can even alter memories, using these procedures, in the individuals described at this chapter's start who seem otherwise to have "perfect" autobiographical recall (Pathis et al., 2013). Plainly this is a widespread pattern, with numerous implications for how we think about the past and how we think about our *reliance* on our own memories. (For more on research in this domain, see Chan, Thomas, & Bulevich, 2009; Frenda, Nichols, & Loftus, 2011; Laney, 2012; Laney & Loftus, 2010; Seamon, Philbin, & Harrison, 2006.)

Are There Limits on the Misinformation Effect?

The studies just described all fall under the rubric of the **misinformation effect**—a term referring to memory errors that result from some form of post-event misinformation. But what sorts of memory errors can be planted in this way?

We've mentioned studies in which researchers have led participants to remember broken glass when really there was none and to remember a barn when there was no barn in view. Similar procedures have altered how *people* are remembered—so that with just a few "suggestions" from the experimenter, people remember clean-shaven men as bearded, young people as old, and fat people as thin (e.g., Christiaansen, Sweeney, & Ochalek, 1983; Frenda et al., 2011).

It is remarkably easy to produce these errors—with just one word ("hit" vs. "smashed") sometimes being enough to alter an individual's recollection. What happens, though, if we ramp up our efforts to plant false memories? Can we plant larger-scale errors? In one study, college students were told that the investigators were trying to learn how different people remember the same experience. The students were then given a list of events that (they were told) had been reported by their parents; the students were asked to recall these events as well as they could, so that the investigators could compare the students' recall with their parents' (Hyman, Husband, & Billings, 1995).

Some of the events on the list actually had been reported by the participants' parents. Other events were bogus—made up by the experimenters. One of the bogus events was an overnight hospitalization for a high fever; in a different experiment, the bogus event was attending a wedding reception and accidentally spilling a bowlful of punch on the bride's parents.

The college students were easily able to remember the genuine events (i.e., the events actually reported by their parents). In an initial interview, more than 80% of these events were recalled, but none of the students recalled the bogus events. However, repeated attempts at recall changed this pattern: By a third interview, 25% of the participants were able to remember the embarrassment of spilling the punch, and many were able to supply the details of this (entirely fictitious) episode. Other studies have yielded similar results, with participants being led to recall details of particular birthday parties that, in truth, they never had (Hyman et al., 1995) or an incident of being lost in a shopping mall even though this event never took place, or a (fictitious) event in which they were the victim of a vicious animal attack (Loftus, 2003, 2004; also see Chrobak & Zaragoza, 2008; Geraerts et al., 2009; Laney & Loftus, 2010; and many more).

Errors Encouraged through "Evidence"

Other researchers have taken a further step and provided participants with "evidence" in support of the bogus memory. In one procedure, researchers

FIGURE 8.5 THE BALLOON RIDE THAT NEVER WAS

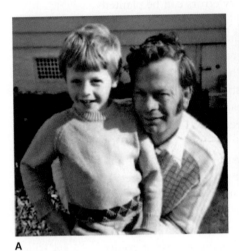
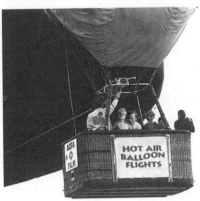

A   B

In this study, participants were shown a faked photo (Panel B) created from a real childhood snapshot (Panel A). With this prompt, many participants were led to a vivid, detailed recollection of the balloon ride—even though it never occurred!

obtained a real childhood snapshot of the participant (see **Figure 8.5A** for an example) and, with a few clicks of a computer mouse, created a fictitious picture like the one shown in Figure 8.5B. With this prompt, many participants were led to a vivid, detailed recollection of the hot-air balloon ride—even though it never occurred (Wade, Garry, Read, & Lindsay, 2002). Another study used an *unaltered* photo, showing the participants' second-grade class (see **Figure 8.6**). This was apparently enough to persuade participants that the experimenters really did have information about the participants' childhood. Thus, when the experimenters "reminded" the participants of an episode of their childhood misbehavior, the participants took this reminder seriously. The result: Almost 80% of the participants were able to "recall" the episode, often in detail, even though it had never happened (Lindsay, Hagen, Read, Wade, & Garry, 2004).

The same sort of result has been documented with children. In one study, children participated in an event with "Mr. Science," a man who showed them a number of fun demonstrations. Afterward, the parents (who were not at the event) were asked to discuss the event with their children—and were, in particular, urged to discuss several elements that (unbeknownst to the parents) actually had never occurred. Later on, the children were interviewed about their visit with Mr. Science, and many of them confidently remembered the (fictitious) elements they had discussed with their

FIGURE 8.6 PHOTOGRAPHS CAN ENCOURAGE MEMORY ERRORS

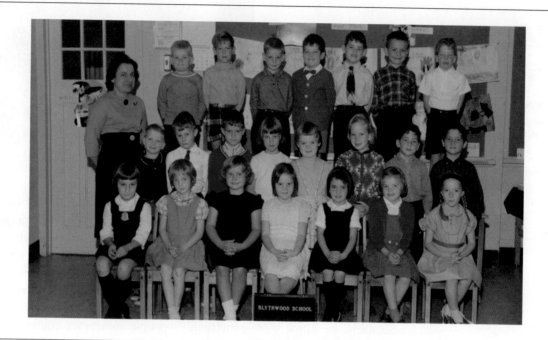

In one study, participants were "reminded" of a (fictitious) stunt they'd pulled while in the second grade. Participants were much more likely to "remember" the stunt (and so more likely to develop a false memory) if the experimenter showed them a copy of their actual second-grade class photo. Apparently, the photo convinced the participants that the experimenter really did know what had happened, and this made the experimenter's (false) suggestion much more persuasive.   LINDSAY ET AL., 2004.

parents—including a time (that never happened) in which Mr. Science put something "yucky" in their mouths or a time in which Mr. Science hurt the child's tummy (by pressing too hard when applying a sticker; Poole & Lindsay, 2001). Such results echo the misinformation results with adults, but they are also important for their own sake because (among other concerns) these results are relevant to children's testimony in the courtroom (Bruck & Ceci, 1999, 2009; Reisberg, 2014).

False Memories Outside the Laboratory

What, then, are the limits of false memory? It seems clear that your memory can sometimes be mistaken on small details (was there broken glass in view?), but memory can also fool you in larger ways: You can remember entire events that never took place. You can remember emotional episodes (like being lost in a shopping mall) that never happened. You can remember your own transgressions (spilling the punch bowl, misbehaving in the second grade), even when they never occurred.

False memories can be quite consequential. In one study, participants were led to believe that as children they had gotten ill after eating egg salad. This "memory" then changed the participants' eating habits—over the next four months, they ended up eating less egg salad. Obviously, false memories can persist and have lasting behavioral effects.   GERAERTS ET AL., 2008.

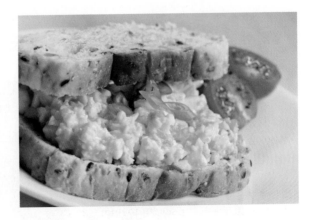

These results fit well with our theorizing and (more specifically) with our claims about how memory errors arise. But these results also have pragmatic implications. As one example, participants changed their eating habits after a researcher persuaded them that as children they had become ill after eating egg salad (Geraerts et al., 2008). Or, as an extremely troubling example, studies of the justice system confirm that children sometimes accuse adults of abuse even when other evidence makes it clear the abuse never happened. Similarly, we know that—remarkably—people sometimes confess to (and apparently "remember") crimes that they did not commit (cf. Kassin et al., 2010; Lassiter & Meissner, 2010; Leo, 2008). It can be no surprise, therefore, that researchers continue to be deeply engaged in exploring how and when these false memories occur.

Avoiding Memory Errors

In light of the discussion so far, it's worth emphasizing that our memories are generally accurate. In other words, we can usually trust our memories because more often than not, our recollection is complete, detailed, long-lasting, and *correct*. The fact remains, however, that errors do occur, and they can be both large and consequential. Is there anything we can do, therefore, to avoid being misled by memory errors? Can we perhaps figure out which memories we can rely on and which ones we can't?

Memory Confidence

People sometimes announce that they're highly confident in their recall ("I distinctly remember her yellow jacket; I'm sure of it"), and sometimes they say the opposite ("Gee, I think she was wearing yellow, but I'm not certain"). And these assessments *matter*, because people put more trust in confident memories than hesitant ones. In a courtroom, for example, juries place much more weight on a witness's evidence if the witness expresses confidence during the testimony; conversely, juries are often skeptical about testimony that is hesitant or hedged (Brigham & Wolfskiel, 1983; Cutler, Penrod, & Dexter, 1990; Loftus, 1979; Wells, Lindsay, & Ferguson, 1979).

This is an issue, however, on which jurors' commonsense view is mistaken, because there's little relationship between how *certain* someone says he is, in recalling the past, and how *accurate* that recollection is likely to be. Any attempt to categorize memories as correct or incorrect, based on someone's confidence, will therefore be riddled with errors. (For some of the evidence, see Busey, Tunnicliff, Loftus, & Loftus, 2000; Roediger & McDermott, 1995; Sporer, Penrod, Read, & Cutler, 1995; Wells & Quinlivan, 2009.)

How can this be? How can we be so poor in evaluating our own memories? One reason is that our confidence in a memory is often influenced by factors that have no impact on memory accuracy. When these factors are present, confidence can shift (sometimes upward, sometimes downward) with no change in the accuracy level, undermining any correspondence between confidence and accuracy.

For example, participants in one study witnessed a (simulated) crime and later were asked if they could identify the culprit from a group of pictures. Some of the participants were then given feedback ("Good, you identified the suspect"); others were not. This feedback could not possibly influence the accuracy of the identification, because the feedback arrived only after the identification had occurred. But the feedback did influence confidence, and witnesses who had received the feedback expressed a much higher level of confidence in their choice than did witnesses who received no feedback (see **Figure 8.7**; Douglas, Neuschatz, Imrich, & Wilkinson, 2009; Semmler & Brewer, 2006; Wells, Olson, & Charman, 2002, 2003; Wright & Skagerberg, 2007; for similar data with *children* as eyewitnesses, see Hafstad, Memon, & Logie, 2004). Thus, with confidence inflated but

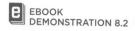
EBOOK
DEMONSTRATION 8.2

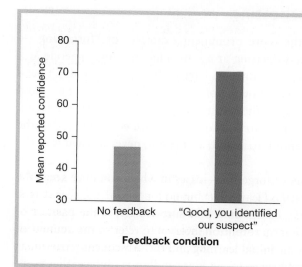

FIGURE 8.7 CONFIDENCE MALLEABILITY

In one study, participants first tried to identify a culprit from a police lineup and then indicated (on a scale of 0 to 100) their level of confidence in their selection. Some participants were given no feedback about their choice; others were given feedback after they'd made their selection but before they indicated their confidence level. This feedback couldn't possibly influence accuracy (because the selection was already done!), but it dramatically increased confidence. AFTER WELLS & BRADFIELD, 1998.

accuracy unchanged, the linkage between confidence and accuracy was diminished. (For other factors contributing to the disconnection between accuracy and confidence, see Heathcote, Freeman, Etherington, Tonkin, & Bora, 2009; Lampinen, Meier, Arnal, & Leding, 2005; Sampaio & Brewer, 2009; Sharman, Manning, & Garry, 2005.)

Researchers continue to seek other ways of distinguishing accurate memories from inaccurate ones. Some studies look at the *emotion* an individual feels when recalling a memory (e.g., McNally et al., 2004). Other investigators have examined the way a memory *feels*, relying on the "remember/know" distinction that we met in Chapter 7 (e.g., Frost, 2000; Holmes, Waters, & Rajaram, 1998; Roediger & McDermott, 1995). Still other studies have looked at *response speed*, on the idea that accurate memories will (on average) be recalled more rapidly than false memories (Dunning & Perretta, 2002; but also Weber, Brewer, Wells, Semmler, & Keast, 2004). Evidence tells us, though, that there is (at best) only a weak linkage between memory accuracy and any of these markers. In the end, therefore, we have no indicators that can reliably guide us in deciding which memories to trust and which ones not to trust. For now, it seems that memory errors, when they occur, are likely to be undetectable.

Forgetting

We've been discussing the errors people sometimes make in recalling the past, but, of course, there's another way your memory can let you down: Sometimes you *forget*. You try to recall what was on the shopping list, or the name of an acquaintance, or what happened last week, and you simply draw a blank. Why does this happen? Are there things you can do to diminish forgetting?

The Causes of Forgetting

Let's start with one of the more prominent examples of "forgetting"—which turns out not to be forgetting at all. Imagine meeting someone at a party, being told his name, and moments later realizing that you don't have a clue what his name is—even though you just heard it. This common (and embarrassing) experience is not the result of ultra-rapid forgetting. Instead, the experience stems from a failure in acquisition. You were exposed to the name but barely paid attention to it and, as a result, never learned it in the first place.

What about "real" cases of forgetting—cases in which you once knew the information (and so plainly *had* learned it) but no longer do? For these cases, one of the best predictors of forgetting (not surprisingly) is the passage of time. Psychologists use the term **retention interval** to refer to the amount of time that elapses between the initial learning and the subsequent retrieval; as this interval grows, you're likely to forget more and more of the earlier event (see **Figure 8.8**).

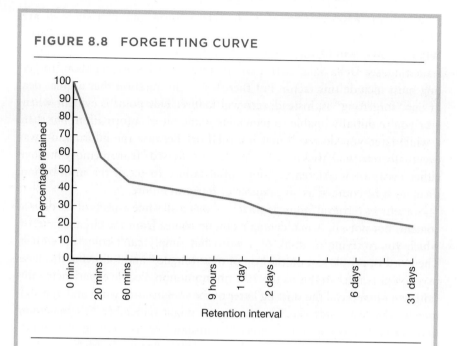

FIGURE 8.8 FORGETTING CURVE

The figure shows retention after various intervals since learning. The data shown here are from classic work by Hermann Ebbinghaus, so the pattern is often referred to as an "Ebbinghaus forgetting curve." The actual speed of forgetting (i.e., how "steep" the "drop-off" is) depends on how well learned the material was at the start. Across most situations, though, the pattern is the same—with the forgetting being rapid at first but then slowing down. Mathematically, this pattern is best described by an equation framed in terms of "exponential decay."

One explanation for this pattern is **decay**. With the passage of time, memories can fade or erode. Perhaps this is because the relevant brain cells die off. Or perhaps the connections among memories need to be constantly refreshed—so that if they're not refreshed, the connections gradually weaken.

A different possibility is that new learning somehow interferes with older learning. This view is referred to as **interference theory**; according to this view, the passage of time is *correlated* with forgetting but does not *cause* forgetting. Instead, the passage of time simply creates the opportunity for new learning, and it is the new learning that disrupts the older memories.

A third hypothesis blames **retrieval failure**. After all, the retrieval of information from memory is far from guaranteed, and we argued in Chapter 7 that retrieval is more likely if your perspective at the time of retrieval matches that in place at the time of learning. If we now assume that your perspective is likely to change as time goes by, we can make a prediction about forgetting: The greater the retention interval, the greater the likelihood that your perspective has changed, and therefore the greater the likelihood of retrieval failure.

EBOOK
DEMONSTRATION 8.3

Which of these hypotheses is correct? It turns out that they all are. Memories do decay with the passage of time (e.g., Altmann & Schunn, 2012; Wixted, 2004; also Hardt, Nader, & Nadel, 2013; for a general overview of forgetting, see Della Sala, 2010), and therefore any theorizing about forgetting must include this factor. But there's also no question that a great deal of our "forgetting" is, instead, retrieval failure. This point is evident whenever you're initially unable to remember some bit of information, but then, a while later, you do recall that information. Because the information was eventually retrieved, we know that it was not "erased" from memory through either decay or interference. Your initial failure to recall the information, then, must be counted as an example of retrieval failure.

Sometimes retrieval failure is *partial*—you recall some aspects of the desired content, but not all. A maddening example comes from the circumstance in which you're trying to think of a word but simply can't come up with it. The word is, people say, on the "tip of their tongue," and following this lead, psychologists refer to this as the **TOT phenomenon**. People experiencing this state can often recall the starting letter of the sought-after word and approximately what it sounds like. Thus, a person might remember "it's something like *Sanskrit*" in trying to remember "scrimshaw" or "something like *secant*" in trying to remember "sextant" (Brown, 1991; Brown & McNeill, 1966; Harley & Brown, 1998; James & Burke, 2000; Schwartz & Metcalfe, 2011).

What about interference? In one early study, Baddeley and Hitch (1977) asked rugby players to recall the names of the other teams they had played against over the course of a season. The key here is that not all players made it to all games (because of illness, injuries, or schedule conflicts), and this allows us to compare players for whom "two games back" means two weeks ago, to players for whom "two games back" means four weeks ago. Thus, we can look at the effects of retention interval (two weeks vs. four) with the number of intervening games held constant. Likewise, we can compare players for whom the game a month ago was "three games back" to players for whom a month ago means "one game back." Now, we have the retention interval held constant, and we can look at the effects of intervening events. In this setting, Baddeley and Hitch reported that the mere passage of time accounts for very little; what really matters is the number of intervening events (see **Figure 8.9**). This is just what we would expect if interference, and not decay, is the major contributor to forgetting.

But *why* does memory interference occur? Why can't the newly acquired information coexist with older memories? The answer has several parts, but a key element is linked to issues we've already discussed: In many cases, newly arriving information gets interwoven with older information, producing a risk of confusion about which bits are old (i.e., the event you're trying to remember) and which are new (i.e., information that you picked up after the event). This confusion is, of course, central for the misinformation effect, described earlier. In addition, in some cases, new information seems literally to replace old information—much as you no longer save the rough draft of one of your papers once the final draft is done. In this situation, the new information isn't woven into the older memory; instead, it erases it.

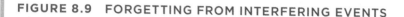

FIGURE 8.9 FORGETTING FROM INTERFERING EVENTS

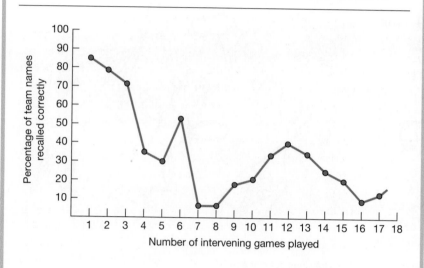

Members of a rugby team were asked to recall the names of teams they had played against. Overall, the broad pattern of the data shows that memory performance was powerfully influenced by the number of games that intervened between the game to be recalled and the attempt to remember. This pattern fits with an interference view of forgetting. AFTER BADDELEY & HITCH, 1977.

Undoing Forgetting

Is there any way to *undo* forgetting and to recover seemingly lost memories? One option, often discussed, is *hypnosis*, with the idea that under hypnosis a person can "return" to an earlier event and remember virtually everything about the event, including aspects the person didn't even notice (much less think about) at the time. Similar claims have been made about certain drugs—sodium amytal, for example—with the idea that these, too, can help people remember things they otherwise never could.

However, as we mentioned in the end-of-chapter essay for Chapter 7, neither of these techniques improves memory. Hypnotized participants often do give detailed reports of the target event, but this isn't because they remember more; instead, they're just willing to *say* more in order to comply with the hypnotist's instructions. As a result, their "memories" are a mix of recollection, guesses, and inferences—and, of course, the hypnotized individual cannot tell which of these are which (Lynn, Neuschatz, Fite, & Rhue, 2001; Mazzoni & Lynn, 2007; Spiegel, 1995). Likewise, the drugs sometimes given to improve memory work largely as sedatives, putting an individual in a less guarded, less cautious state of mind. This state allows people to report more

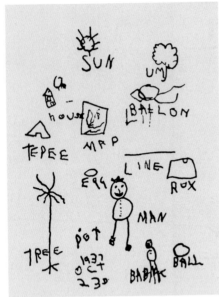

A Drawings done by hypnotized adult told that he was 6 years old

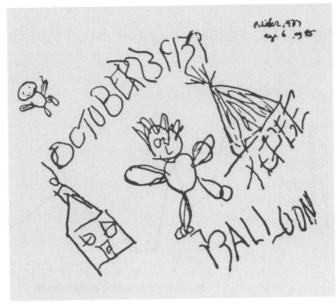

B Drawings done at age 6

HYPNOTIC AGE REGRESSION

In one study, participants were asked to draw a picture while mentally "regressed" to age 6. At first glance, their drawings (see Panel A for an example) looked remarkably childlike. But when compared to the participants' own drawings made at that age (see Panel B for an example), it's clear that the hypnotized adults' drawings were much more sophisticated. They represent an adult's conception of what a childish drawing is, rather than being the real thing.

about the past—not because they remember more, but simply because in this relaxed condition they're willing to say more.

On the positive side, though, there are procedures that do seem to diminish forgetting, including a procedure we mentioned in the end-of-chapter essay for Chapter 7, the "Cognitive Interview." This procedure was designed to help police in their investigations and, more specifically, is aimed at maximizing the quantity and accuracy of information obtained from eyewitnesses to crimes (Fisher & Schreiber, 2007). The cognitive interview builds on the simple fact that retrieval of memories from long-term storage is more likely if a suitable cue is provided. The interview therefore offers a diverse set of retrieval cues on the idea that the more cues provided, the greater the chance of finding a successful one. The cognitive interview is quite successful (both in the laboratory and in real crime investigations), a point that has implications for practical matters as well as for theory. As a pragmatic matter, this procedure genuinely helps law enforcement in the collection of evidence. For theory, the success of this interview technique confirms the notion that forgetting is often due to retrieval failure, and can be undone simply by providing more support for retrieval.

In addition, rather than *undoing* forgetting, perhaps we can *avoid* forgetting: The passage of time has a much smaller impact on memory if you simply "revisit" the memory periodically. Each "visit" seems to refresh the memory, with the result that forgetting is much less likely. Researchers have examined this effect in several contexts, including one that is both theoretically interesting and pragmatically useful: Students often have to take exams, and this forces them to "revisit" the course materials. These revisits, we've just suggested, should slow forgetting, and on this basis, exams can help students hang on to the material they've learned! Several studies have confirmed this optimistic suggestion—that is, have shown that the step of taking a college exam can promote long-term retention (e.g., Carpenter, Pashler, & Cepeda, 2009; Halamish & Bjork, 2011; Karpicke, 2012; Karpicke & Blunt, 2011; McDaniel, Anderson, Derbish, & Morrisette, 2007; Pashler, Rohrer, Cepeda, & Carpenter, 2007; Rowland, 2014).

Memory: An Overall Assessment

Let's pause to recap our main themes. We've now seen that people sometimes recall with confidence events that never took place, and they sometimes forget information they'd hoped to remember. But we've also mentioned the positive side of things: how much people *can* recall, and the key fact that your memory is accurate far more often than not. Most of the time, it seems, you do recall the past as it truly was.

Perhaps most important, we've also suggested that memory's "failings" are simply the price you pay in order to gain crucial advantages. For example, we've argued that memory errors arise because the various episodes in your memory are densely interconnected with one another; it's these interconnections that allow elements to be transplanted from one remembered episode to another. But these connections are there for a purpose: They're the retrieval paths that make memory search possible. Thus, to avoid the errors, you would need to restrict the connections; but if you did that, you would lose the ability to locate your own memories within long-term storage.

The memory connections that lead to error also help you in other important ways. Our environment, after all, is in many ways predictable, and it's enormously useful for you to exploit that predictability. There's little point, for example, in scrutinizing a kitchen to make sure there's a stove in the room, because in the vast majority of cases there is. Why take the time, therefore, to confirm the obvious? Likewise, there's little point in taking special note that, yes, this restaurant does have menus and that, yes, people in the restaurant are eating and not having their cars repaired. These, too, are obvious points, and it would be a waste of effort to give them special notice.

On these grounds, reliance on schematic knowledge is a good thing. Schemata guide your attention to what's informative in a situation, rather than what's self-evident (e.g., Gordon, 2006), and they guide your inferences at the time of recall. If this use of schemata sometimes leads you astray, that is a small price to pay for the gain in efficiency that schemata allow. (For similar points, see Chapter 4.)

In the same fashion, the blurring together of episodes may be a blessing, not a problem. Think, for example, about all the times in your life when you've been with a particular friend. These episodes are related to one another in an obvious way, and so they're likely to become interconnected in your memory. This will cause difficulties if you want to remember which episode is which and whether you had a particular conversation in this episode or in that one. But rather than lamenting this, perhaps we should *celebrate* what's going on here: Because of the "interference," all of the episodes will merge together in your memory, so that what resides in memory is one integrated package, containing in united form all of your knowledge about your friend. Thus, rather than complaining about memory confusion, we should rejoice over the memory *integration* and "cross-referencing."

In these ways, our overall assessment of memory can be rather upbeat. We have, to be sure, discussed a range of memory errors, but the errors are in most cases a side product of mechanisms that otherwise help you—to locate your memories within storage, to be efficient in your contact with the world, and to form general knowledge. Thus, even with the errors, even with forgetting, it seems that human memory functions in a fashion that serves us extraordinarily well. (For more on the benefits produced by memory's apparent limitations, see Howe, 2011; Schacter, Guerin, & St. Jacques, 2011.)

Autobiographical Memory

Most of the evidence in Chapters 6 and 7 was concerned with memory for simple stimuli—word lists, for example, or short sentences. In this chapter, we've considered memories for more complex materials, and this has drawn our attention to the ways in which your knowledge (whether knowledge of a general sort or knowledge about related episodes) can both improve memory and also interfere with it.

In making these points, we've considered memories in which the person was actually involved in the remembered episode, and not just an external witness (e.g., the false memory that you spilled that bowl of punch). We've also looked at studies that involved memories for emotional events (e.g., the plane crash we discussed at the chapter's start) and memory over the very long term (e.g., memories for childhood events "planted" in adult participants).

Do these three factors—involvement in the remembered event, emotion, and long delay—matter in any way, changing how or how well someone remembers? These factors are surely relevant to the sorts of remembering people do outside the laboratory, and indeed, all three are central for **autobiographical memory**. This is the memory that each of us has for the events of our lives, and we've argued (e.g., in Chapters 1 and 7) that this sort of memory plays a central role in shaping how each of us thinks about ourselves and, thus, how we behave. (For more on the importance of autobiographical memory, see Baddeley, Aggleton, & Conway, 2002. For more on the distinction between these types of memory, including *biological* differences between auto-biographical memory and "lab memory," see Cabeza & St. Jacques, 2007; Hodges & Graham, 2001; Kopelman & Kapur, 2001; Tulving, 1993, 2002.)

Let's look, therefore, at how the three factors we've mentioned, each seemingly central for autobiographical memory, influence what we remember.

Memory and the Self

Having some involvement in an event, rather than passively witnessing the event, turns out to have a large effect on memory. In part, this is because information relevant to the self is better remembered than information that's not self-relevant (e.g., Symons & Johnson, 1997; also Westmacott & Moscovitch, 2003). This contrast emerges in many forms, including an advantage in remembering things you have said as opposed to things others have said, better memory for adjectives that apply to you relative to adjectives that do not, better memory for names of places you have visited relative to names of places you've never been, and so on (see **Figure 8.10**).

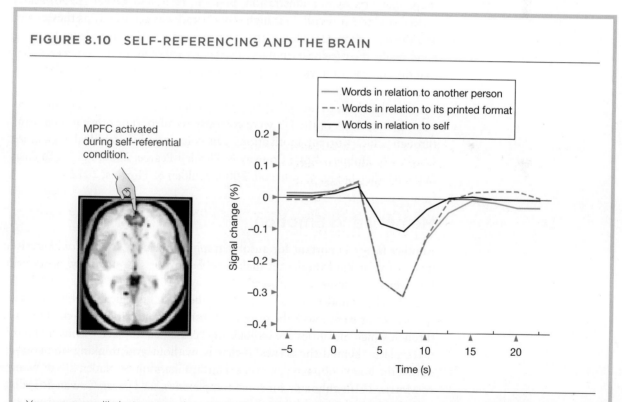

FIGURE 8.10 SELF-REFERENCING AND THE BRAIN

MPFC activated during self-referential condition.

Legend:
— Words in relation to another person
--- Words in relation to its printed format
— Words in relation to self

You are more likely to remember words that refer to *you*, in comparison to words in other categories. Here, participants were asked to judge adjectives in three conditions: answering questions like "Does this word describe the president?" or "Is this word printed in capital letters?" or "Does this word describe you?" Data from fMRI recordings showed a distinctive pattern of processing when the words were "self-referential." This extra processing is part of the reason why self-referential words are better remembered. AFTER KELLEY ET AL., 2002.

But here, too, we can find memory errors, in part because your "memory" for your own life is (just like other memories) a mix of genuine recall and some amount of schema-based reconstruction. Consider the fact that most adults believe they've been reasonably consistent, reasonably stable, over their lifetimes. They believe, in other words, that they've always been pretty much the same as they are now. This notion of consistency is part of their **self-schema**. When the time comes to remember the past, therefore, people will rely to some extent on this belief, and so they will reconstruct their own history in a biased fashion—one that maximizes the (apparent) stability of their lives. As a result, people often misremember their past attitudes and the past status of their romantic relationships, unwittingly distorting their personal history in a fashion that makes the past look more like the present than it really was (Conway & Ross, 1984; Holmberg & Homes, 1994; for related results, see Levine, 1997; Marcus, 1986; McFarland & Buehler, 2012; Ochsner & Schacter, 2000; Ross & Wilson, 2003).

It's also true that most of us would prefer to have a positive view of ourselves, including a positive view of how we've acted in the past. This, too, can shape memory. As one illustration, Bahrick, Hall, and Berger (1996) asked college students to recall their high school grades as accurately as they could, and the data showed a clear pattern of self-service. When students forgot a good grade, their (self-serving) reconstruction led them to the (correct) belief that the grade must have been a good one; consistent with this, 89% of the A's were correctly remembered. But when students forgot a poor grade, reconstruction led them to the (false) belief that the grade must have been okay; as a result, only 29% of the D's were correctly recalled. (For other mechanisms through which current motivations can color autobiographical recall, see Conway & Holmes, 2004; Conway & Pleydell-Pearce, 2000; Forgas & East, 2003; Mather, Shafir, & Johnson, 2000; Molden & Higgins, 2012.)

Memory and Emotion

Another factor important for autobiographical memory is *emotion*, because many of your life experiences make you happy, or sad, or angry, or afraid. How does this influence memory?

In general, emotion helps you to remember. At a biological level, emotional arousal seems to promote the process of memory **consolidation**—the process through which memories are biologically "cemented in place." Consolidation takes place "behind the scenes"—that is, without you thinking about it—during the hours following an event (Hardt, Einarsson & Nader, 2010; Wang & Morris, 2010; although, for some complexities, see Dewar, Cowan & Della Sala, 2010). If the consolidation is interrupted for some reason (e.g., because of fatigue, or injury, or even extreme stress), no memory is established and recall later will be impossible. (That's because there's no information in memory for you to retrieve; you can't read text off a blank page!)

A number of factors can promote consolidation—making it more likely that the memories will be firmly established and, hence, retrievable later.

For example, evidence is increasing that key steps of consolidation take place while you're asleep—and so a good night's rest actually helps you, later on, to remember things you learned while awake the day before (e.g., Tononi & Cirelli, 2013; Zillmer, Spiers, & Culbertson, 2008). For present purposes, though, let's emphasize that emotion also enhances consolidation. Specifically, emotional events trigger a response in the amygdala, and the amygdala in turn increases activity in the hippocampus. The hippocampus is, as we've seen, crucial for getting memories established (see Chapter 7; for reviews of emotion's biological effects on memory, see Buchanan, 2007; Dudai, 2004; Hamann, 2001; Hoschedidt, Dongaonkar, Payne, & Nadel, 2010; Joels, Fernandez, & Roosendaal, 2011; Kensinger, 2007; LaBar, 2007; LaBar & Cabeza, 2006; Öhman, 2002; Phelps, 2004; for a complication, though, see **Figure 8.11**).

FIGURE 8.11 INDIVIDUAL DIFFERENCES IN EPISODIC MEMORY

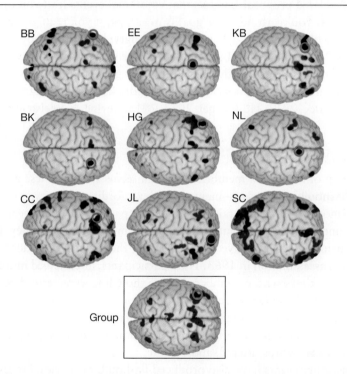

Researchers have made enormous progress in explaining the brain mechanisms that support memory. One complication, though, is that the brain mechanisms may differ from one individual to the next. This figure shows data from nine different people (and then an average of the nine) engaged in a task requiring the retrieval of episodic memories. As you can see, the pattern of brain activation differs somewhat from person to person. AFTER MILLER ET AL., 2002.

Emotion also shapes memory through other mechanisms. An emotional event is likely to be important to you, virtually guaranteeing that you'll pay close attention as the event unfolds, and we've seen (e.g., in Chapter 6) that attention and thoughtful processing help memory. Moreover, you tend to mull over emotional events in the minutes (or hours) following the event, and this is tantamount to memory rehearsal. For all of these reasons, it's not surprising that emotional events are well remembered (Reisberg & Heuer, 2004; Talmi, 2013).

In addition, emotion often changes what you pay attention to within an event, and this will alter the pattern of what is and is not remembered from an emotional episode. In many settings, emotion can lead to a "narrowing" of attention, so that all of your attention will be focused on just a few aspects of the scene (Easterbrook, 1959). This narrowing helps guarantee that these attended aspects will be firmly placed into memory, but it also implies that the rest of the event, excluded from this narrowed focus, won't be remembered later (e.g., Gable & Harmon-Jones, 2008; Reisberg & Heuer, 2004; Steblay, 1992). A related proposal suggests that emotional events lead you to set certain *goals*: If you're afraid, your goal is to escape; if you're angry, your goal is to deal with the person who's made you angry; if you're happy, your goal may be to relax and enjoy! In each case, you're more likely to pay attention to aspects of the scene directly relevant to your goal, and this, too, will color how you remember the emotional event (Fredrickson, 2000; Harmon-Jones, Gable, & Price, 2013; Huntsinger, 2012, 2013; Levine & Edelstein, 2009).

Flashbulb Memories

One group of emotional memories, though, seems special. These are the so-called **flashbulb memories**—memories of extraordinary clarity, typically for highly emotional events, retained despite the passage of many years. When Brown and Kulik (1977) introduced the term "flashbulbs," they pointed to the memories people have of first hearing the news of President John F. Kennedy's assassination in 1963. Their participants, interviewed more than a decade after that event, remembered it "as though it were yesterday," recalling details of where they were at the time, what they were doing, and whom they were with. Many participants were certain they'd never forget that awful day; indeed, they were able to recall the clothing worn by people around them, the exact words uttered, and the like.

Many other events have also produced flashbulb memories. For example, most Americans can clearly recall where they were when they first heard about the attack on the World Trade Center in 2001; many young people vividly remember what they were doing in 2009 when they first heard that Michael Jackson had died; many Italians have clear memories of their country's victory in the 2006 World Cup; and so on (see Pillemer, 1984; Rubin & Kozin, 1984; also see Weaver, 1993; Winograd & Neisser, 1993; for an indication, though, that flashbulb memories may be less likely with emotionally *positive* events, see Kraha, Talarico, & Boals, 2014).

Remarkably, though, these vivid, high-confidence memories can contain substantial errors. Thus, when people say, "I'll never forget that day…" they're sometimes *wrong*. For example, Hirst et al. (2009) interviewed more than 3,000 people soon after the September 11 attack on the World Trade Center, asking them questions designed to probe the usual content of flashbulb memories: How had they first heard about the attack? Who brought them the news? What they were doing at the time? These individuals were then re-interviewed a year later, and more than a third of the participants (37%) provided a substantially different account in this follow-up. Even so, the participants were strongly confident in their recollection (rating their degree of certainty, on a 1-to-5 scale, at an average of 4.41). The picture was the same for participants interviewed three years after the attack—with 43% of these participants offering different accounts from those they had given initially. (For similar data, see Neisser & Harsch, 1992; see also Rubin & Talarico, 2007; Schmidt, 2012; Talarico & Rubin, 2003; Wagenaar & Groeneweg, 1990; **Figure 8.12**.)

Other data, though, tell a different story, suggesting that some flashbulb memories are entirely accurate. Why should this be? Why are some flashbulb events remembered well, while others are not? The answer involves several

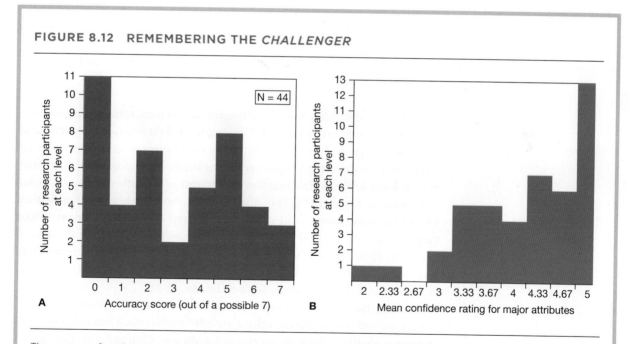

FIGURE 8.12 REMEMBERING THE *CHALLENGER*

Three years after the tragic explosion of the space shuttle *Challenger*, research participants had very poor memories of the event—but high confidence in their (false) recollections. Panel A shows how many of the 44 participants obtained each of the possible accuracy scores (11 participants had a score of 0, four had a score of 1, and so on). Panel B shows a parallel breakdown for confidence ratings (one participant had a confidence level, averaged across questions, of 2.0; two had an average confidence level of 3.0, and so on). While 25% of the participants got a 0 score on the memory test, and half of them got a score of 2 or lower, confidence ratings were generally at the high end of the scale. AFTER NEISSER & HARSCH, 1992.

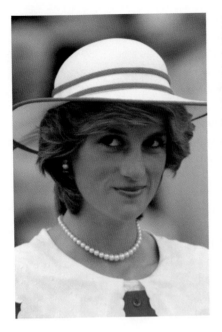
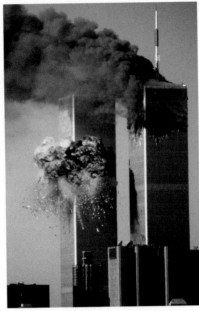
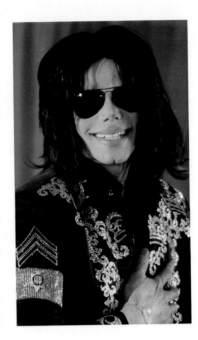

FLASHBULB MEMORIES

People often have especially clear and long-lasting memories for events like their first hearing about Princess Diana's death in 1997, the attack on the World Trade Center in September 2001, or the news of Michael Jackson's death in 2009. These memories—called "flashbulb memories"—are vivid and compelling, but they are not always accurate.

elements, including how, and how often, and with whom, someone discusses the flashbulb event. In many cases, this discussion will serve as memory rehearsal, a process that (as we have discussed) promotes memory accuracy (see Schmidt, 2012). In other cases, this discussion will introduce new information—an inadvertent form of the misinformation effect. And in still other cases, discussion may motivate people to "polish" their reports—so that they are offering their audience a better, more interesting narrative, and eventually this new version may supplant the original memory. (For more on these issues, see Conway et al., 1994; Hirst et al., 2009; Luminet & Curci, 2009; Neisser, Winograd, & Weldon, 1991; Palmer, Schreiber, & Fox, 1991; Tinti, Schmidt, Sotgiu, Testa, & Curci, 2009; Tinti, Schmidt, Testa & Levine, 2014).

Overall, though, let's not lose track of the fact that some flashbulb memories are marvelously accurate; others are filled with error. Therefore, the commonsense idea that these memories are somehow "burned into the brain," and thus always reliable, is surely mistaken. In addition, let's emphasize that from the point of view of the person who has a flashbulb memory, there's no detectable difference between an accurate and an inaccurate one: Either will be recalled with great detail; either will be recalled with enormous confidence. In each case, the memory can be intensely emotional. Apparently, then, memory errors can occur even in the midst of our strongest, most vivid recollection.

Traumatic Memories

Flashbulb memories usually concern events that were strongly emotional. Sadly, though, we can also find cases in which people experience truly *extreme* emotion, and this leads us to ask: How are *traumatic* events remembered? If someone has witnessed wartime atrocities, can we count on the accuracy of their testimony in a war crimes trial? If someone suffers through the horrors of a sexual assault, will the painful memory eventually fade? Or will the memory remain as a horrific remnant of the brutal experience?

Evidence suggests that most traumatic events are well remembered for many years; indeed, victims of atrocities often seem plagued by a cruel enhancement of memory, leaving them with extra-vivid and long-lived recollections of the terrible event (e.g., Alexander et al., 2005; Goodman et al., 2003; Peace & Porter, 2004; Porter & Peace, 2007; Thomsen & Berntsen, 2009). In fact, people who have experienced trauma sometimes complain about having "too much" memory and wish they remembered *less*.

This enhanced memory is best understood in terms of a mechanism we've already mentioned: consolidation. This process is promoted by the conditions that accompany bodily arousal, including the extreme arousal typically present in a traumatic event (Buchanan & Adolphs, 2004; Hamann, 2001). But this does not mean that traumatic events are always well remembered. There are, in fact, cases in which people who have suffered through extreme events have little or no recall of their experience (e.g., Arrigo & Pezdek, 1997). In addition, we can sometimes document substantial errors in someone's recall of a traumatic event (Paz-Alonso & Goodman, 2008).

Why are traumatic events sometimes *not* remembered? In some cases, these events are accompanied by sleep deprivation, head injuries, or substance abuse, each of which can disrupt memory (McNally, 2003). In other cases, the stress associated with the event will disrupt consolidation. As a result, stress can lead to gaps or distortions in the memory and, in truly extreme cases, stress can utterly derail the consolidation process, so that no memory is ever established (Brand & Markowitsch, 2010; Hasselmo, 1999; Joels et al., 2011; McGaugh, 2000; Payne, Nadel, Britton, & Jacobs, 2004).

Repression and "Recovered" Memories

A different mechanism, however, is highly controversial. Some authors have argued that highly painful memories will be *repressed*—pushed out of awareness as a step toward self-protection. Repressed memories, it is claimed, will not be consciously available but will still exist in a person's long-term storage and, in suitable circumstances, may be "recovered"—that is, made conscious once again. (See, for example, Belli, 2012; Freyd, 1996, 1998; Terr, 1991, 1994.)

Most memory researchers, however, are skeptical about the repression idea. As one consideration, painful events—including events that seem likely candidates for repression—are typically well remembered, and this is, of course, not at all what we would expect if repression is in place as a self-protective mechanism. In addition, at least some of the memories reported as "recovered" may, in fact, have been remembered all along, and so they provide no evidence of repression. In these cases, the memories had appeared to be "lost" because the person refused to discuss the memories for many years; the "recovery" of these memories simply reflects the fact that the person is at last willing to discuss them out loud. This sort of "recovery" can be extremely consequential—emotionally and perhaps legally—but it does not tell us anything about how memory works.

Sometimes, though, memories do seem to be genuinely lost for a while and then recovered. But this pattern may not reveal the operation (and, eventually, the "lifting") of repression. Instead, this pattern may simply be the result of retrieval failure. As we've discussed, this mechanism can "hide" memories for long periods of time, only to have the memories reemerge once a suitable retrieval cue is available. Here, too, the recovery is of enormous importance for the person finally remembering the long-lost episodes; but again, this merely confirms the role of an already documented memory mechanism, with no need for theorizing about repression.

In addition, we need to acknowledge the possibility that at least some "recovered memories" may, in fact, be false memories. After all, we know that false memories occur and that they are more likely when one is recovering the distant past than when one is trying to remember recent events. It is also relevant that many recovered memories emerge only with the assistance of a therapist who is genuinely convinced that a client's psychological problems stem from long-forgotten episodes of childhood abuse. Even if therapists scrupulously avoid leading questions, bias might still lead them to shape their clients' memory in other ways—by giving signs of interest or concern if the clients hit on the "right" line of exploration, by spending more time on topics related to the alleged memories, and so forth. In these ways, the climate within a therapeutic session could guide the client toward finding exactly the "memories" the therapist expects to find.

These are, of course, difficult issues, especially when we bear in mind that recovered memories usually involve the recall of horrible experiences. And we also need to be clear that in many cases, these memories do turn out to be accurate—perhaps entirely or in part—and provide evidence for repugnant crimes. But, as in all cases, the veracity of recollection cannot be taken for granted. This caveat is important in evaluating any memory, and it is far more so for anyone wrestling with this sort of traumatic recollection. (For recent discussions of this difficult—and sometimes angrily debated—issue, see, among others, Belli, 2012; Brewin & Andrews, 2014; Dalenberg et al., 2012; Geraerts et al., 2007; Geraerts et al., 2009; Ghetti et al., 2006; Giesbrecht, Lynn, Lilienfeld, & Merckelbach, 2008; Kihlstrom, 2006; Küpper, Benoid, Dalgleish & Anderson, 2014; Patihis, Lilienfeld, Ho, & Loftus, 2014.)

Long, Long-Term Remembering

In the laboratory, a researcher might ask you to recall a word list you read just minutes ago or perhaps a film you saw a week ago. Away from the lab, however, people routinely try to remember events from years—perhaps decades—back. We've mentioned that these longer *retention intervals* are, in general, associated with a greater amount of forgetting. But, impressively, memories from long ago can sometimes turn out to be wonderfully accurate.

We've discussed the fact that flashbulb memories can be long-lasting, but memory across very long intervals can also be observed with mundane materials. For example, Bahrick, Bahrick, and Wittlinger (1975; also Bahrick, 1984; Bahrick & Hall, 1991) tracked down the graduates of a particular high school—people who had graduated in the previous year, and the year before, and the year before that, and ultimately, people who had graduated 50 years earlier. All of these alumni were shown photographs from their own year's high school yearbook. For each photo, they were given a group of names and had to choose the name of the person shown in the picture. The data for this "name matching" task show remarkably little forgetting; performance was approximately 90% correct if tested 3 months after graduation, the same after 7 years, and the same after 14 years. In some versions of the test, performance was still excellent after 34 years (see **Figure 8.13**).

FIGURE 8.13   MEMORY OVER THE VERY LONG TERM

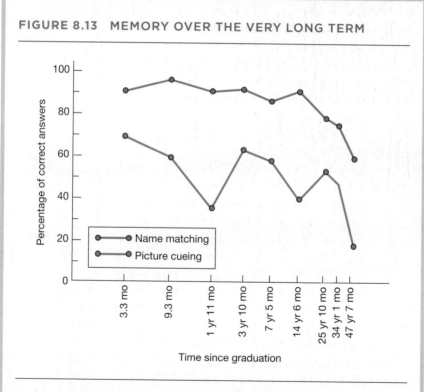

People were tested for how well they remembered names and faces of their high school classmates; memory was remarkably long-lasting. (See the text for a description of the tasks.) The data do show a drop-off after 47 years, but it is unclear whether this reflects an erosion of memory or a more general drop-off in performance caused by the normal process of aging.
AFTER BAHRICK, BAHRICK, & WITTLINGER, 1975.

As a different example, what about the material you're learning right now? Five years from now, will you still remember what you've learned? How about a decade from now? Conway, Cohen, and Stanhope (1991, 1992) explored these questions, testing students' retention of a cognitive psychology course taken years earlier. The results broadly echo the pattern we've already seen: Some forgetting of names and specific concepts was observed during the first 3 years after the course. After the third year, however, performance stabilized, so that students tested after 10 years still remembered a fair amount and, indeed, remembered just as much as students tested after 3 years (see **Figure 8.14**). Memory for more general facts and memory for research methods showed even less forgetting.

In an earlier section, we argued that the retention interval is crucial for memory and that memory gets worse and worse as times goes by. The data now in front of us, though, make it clear that *how much* the interval matters—that is, how *quickly* memories "fade"—may depend on how well

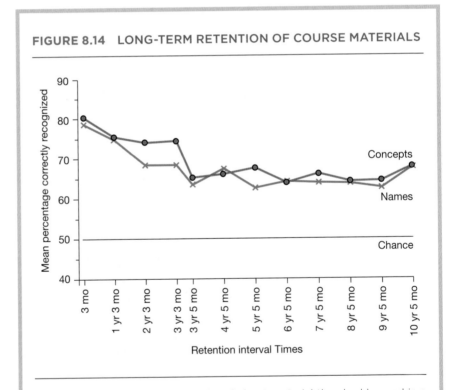

FIGURE 8.14   LONG-TERM RETENTION OF COURSE MATERIALS

Participants in this study were quizzed about material they had learned in a college course taken as recently as 3 months ago or as far back as a decade ago. The data showed some forgetting, but then performance leveled off; memory seemed remarkably stable from three years onward. Note that in a recognition task, memory is probed with "familiar-or-not" questions, so someone with no memory, responding at random, would get 50% right just by chance.   AFTER CONWAY, COHEN, & STANHOPE, 1991.

established the memories were in the first place. Thus, the high school students in the Bahrick et al. study had seen their classmates day after day, for (perhaps) several years. Hence, they knew their classmates' names very, very well—and this is why the passage of time had only a slight impact on their memories for the names. Likewise, students in the Conway et al. study had, apparently, learned their psychology quite well—and so they retained what they'd learned for a very long time. Indeed, we first met this study in Chapter 6, when we mentioned that students' *grades* in the course were good predictors of how much the students would still remember many years after the course was done. Here, too, the better the original learning, the slower the forgetting.

We can maintain our claim, therefore, that the passage of time is the enemy of memory: Longer retention intervals produce lower levels of recall. However, if the material is very well learned at the start, and also if you periodically "revisit" the material, you can dramatically diminish the impact of the passing years.

How General Are the Principles of Memory?

There is certainly more to be said about autobiographical memory. For example, there are clear patterns for how well each of us remembers specific portions of our lives. People tend to remember very little from the early years of childhood (before age 3 or so; e.g., Akers et al., 2014; Bauer, 2007; Hayne, 2004; Howe, Courage, & Rooksby, 2009; Morrison & Conway, 2010). In contrast, people tend to have clear and detailed memories of their late adolescence and early adulthood, a pattern known as the *reminiscence bump* (see **Figure 8.15**; Conway & Haque, 1999; Conway, Wang, Hanyu, & Haque 2005; Dickson, Pillemer, & Bruehl, 2011; Rathbone, Moulin, & Conway, 2008). Thus, for many Americans, the last years of high school and the years they spend in college are likely to be the most memorable period of their lives.

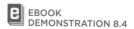

EBOOK
DEMONSTRATION 8.4

But with an eye on the broader themes of this chapter, where does our brief survey of autobiographical memory leave us? In many ways, this form of memory is similar to other sorts of remembering. Autobiographical memories can last for years and years, but so can memories that do not refer directly to your own life. Autobiographical remembering is far more likely if the person occasionally revisits the target memories; these rehearsals dramatically reduce forgetting. But the same is true in nonautobiographical remembering.

Autobiographical memory is also open to error, just as other forms of remembering are. We saw this in cases of flashbulb memories that turn out to be false. We've also seen that misinformation and leading questions can plant false autobiographical memories—about birthday parties that never happened and trips to the hospital that never took place (also see Brown & Marsh, 2008). Misinformation can even reshape memories for traumatic events, just as it can alter memories for trivial episodes in the laboratory (Paz-Alonso & Goodman, 2008).

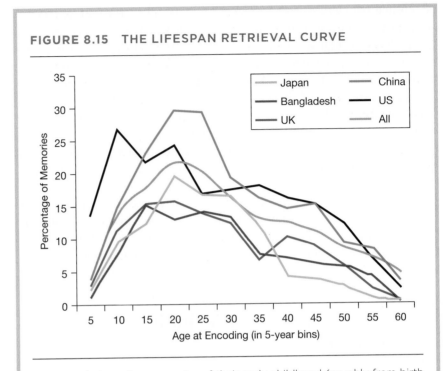

FIGURE 8.15 THE LIFESPAN RETRIEVAL CURVE

Most people have few memories of their early childhood (roughly from birth to age 4 or 5); this pattern is referred to as "childhood amnesia." In contrast, the period from age 10 to 30 is well remembered; a pattern called the "reminiscence bump." The reminiscence bump has been observed in multiple studies and in diverse cultures. In many countries, the data suggest people are more likely to recall events that took place when they were young adults. These events are remembered more often and in more detail (although perhaps less *accurately*) than more recent events.

These facts strengthen a claim that has emerging in our discussion over the last three chapters: Certain principles seem to apply to memory in general, independent of what is being remembered. All memories depend on connections. The connections promote retrieval. The connections also facilitate interference, because they allow one memory to blur into another. The connections can fade with the passage of time, producing memory gaps, and the gaps are likely to be filled via reconstruction based on generic knowledge. All of these things seem to be true whether we're talking about relatively recent memories or memories from long ago, emotional memories or memories of calm events, memories for complex episodes or memories for simple word lists.

But this does not mean that all principles of memory apply to all types of remembering. As we saw in Chapter 7, the rules that govern implicit memory may be different from those that govern explicit memory. And as we've now seen, some of the factors that play a large role in shaping autobiographical remembering (e.g., the role of emotion) may be irrelevant to other sorts of memory.

In the end, therefore, our overall theory of memory is going to need more than one level of description. We will need some principles that apply to only certain types of memory (e.g., principles specifically aimed at emotional remembering). But we'll also need broader principles, reflecting the fact that some themes apply to memory of all sorts (e.g., the importance of memory connections). As we have seen over the last three chapters, these more general principles have moved us forward considerably in our understanding of memory in many different domains and have enabled us to illuminate many aspects of learning, of memory retrieval, and of the sources of memory error.

Remembering for the Long Term

Sometimes you need to recall things after a short delay—a friend tells you her address, and you drive to her house an hour later; or you study for a quiz that you'll take tomorrow morning. Sometimes, however, you want to remember things over a much longer time span—perhaps trying to recall things you learned months or even years ago. This longer-term retention is certainly important, for example, in educational settings. Facts that you learn in high school may be crucial for your professional work later in life. Likewise, facts that you learn in your first year at your university, or in your first year in a job, may be crucial in your third or fourth year. How, therefore, can we help people to remember things for the very long term?

The answer has two parts. First (and not surprisingly), you're more likely to hang on to material that you learned very well in the first place. This chapter mentions one study in which people tried to recall the material they'd learned in a college course a decade earlier. In that study, students' *grades* in the course were good predictors of how much the students would remember many years after the course was done, and so, apparently, the better the original learning, the slower the forgetting.

But long-term retention also depends on another factor that we mentioned in the chapter—whether you occasionally "revisit" the material you learned earlier. In fact, even a brief refresher can help enormously. In one study, students were quizzed on little factoids they had learned at some prior point in their lives (Berger, Hall & Bahrick, 1999). ("Who was the first astronaut to walk on the moon?"; "Who wrote the fable about the fox and the grapes?") In many cases, the students couldn't remember these little facts, so they were given a quick reminder. The correct answer was shown to them for 5 seconds, with the simple instruction that they should look at the answer because they'd need it later on.

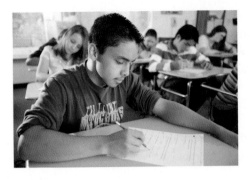

Memory research provides powerful lessons for students hoping
to retain what they are learning in
their courses.

Without this reminder, participants couldn't recall these answers at all. But
nine days after the quick reminder, they were able to remember roughly half
the answers. This isn't perfect performance, but it's surely an enormous return
from a very small investment. And it's likely that a *second* reminder a few days
later, again lasting just 5 seconds, would have lifted their performance still
further and enabled them to recall the items after an even longer delay.

One suggestion, then, is that testing yourself (perhaps with flashcards—with
a cue on one side and an answer on the other) can be quite useful. Flashcards
are often a poor way to *learn* material, because (as we've seen) learning requires
thoughtful and meaningful engagement with the materials you're trying to memorize, and running through a stack of flash cards probably won't promote that
thoughtful engagement. But using flashcards may be an excellent way to review
material that is already learned—and thus a way to avoid forgetting this material.

Other, more substantial, forms of testing can also be valuable. Think about
what happens each time you take a vocabulary quiz in your Spanish class.
A question like "What's the Spanish word for 'bed'?" gives you practice in
retrieving the word, and that practice promotes fluency in retrieval. In addition,
seeing the word (*cama*) can itself refresh the memory, promoting retention.

Consistent with these ideas, several studies have shown that students who
have taken a test will have better retention later on, in comparison to students
who didn't take the initial test (e.g., Carpenter, Pashler, & Cepeda, 2009;
Halamish & Bjork, 2011; Karpicke, 2012; McDermott, Agarwal, D'Antonio,
Roediger, & McDaniel, 2014; and many others). This pattern has been documented with students of various ages (including high school students and
college students) and with different sorts of material.

The implications for students should be clear. It really does pay to go back
periodically and review what you've learned—including material you've learned
earlier this academic year as well as the material you learned in previous years.
The review does not have to be lengthy or intense; in the first study described
here, just a 5-second exposure was enough to decrease forgetting dramatically.

In addition, you shouldn't complain if a teacher insists on frequent quizzes. These quizzes can, of course, be a nuisance, but apparently they serve
two functions: They help you assess your learning, and they can actually help
you to hold on to what you've learned—for days, and probably months, and
perhaps even decades after you've learned it.

chapter summary

- Your memory is usually accurate, but errors do occur and can be quite significant. In general, these errors are produced by the connections that link your memories to one another and link memories for specific episodes to other, more general knowledge. These connections help you because they serve as retrieval paths. But the connections can also "knit" separate memories together, making it difficult to keep track of which elements belong in which memory.

- Some memory errors arise from your understanding of an episode. The understanding promotes memory for the episode's gist but also encourages memory errors. A similar pattern emerges in the DRM procedure, in which a word related to other words on a list is (incorrectly) recalled as being part of the list. Closely related effects arise from schematic knowledge. This knowledge helps you understand an episode, but at the same time a reliance on schematic knowledge can lead you to remember an episode as being more "regular," more "normal," than it actually was.

- Memory errors can also arise through the misinformation effect, in which people are exposed to some (false) suggestion about a previous event. Such suggestions can easily change the details of how an event is remembered and can, in some cases, plant memories for entire episodes that never occurred at all.

- People seem genuinely unable to distinguish their accurate memories from their inaccurate ones. This is because false memories can be recalled with just as much detail, emotion, and confidence as historically accurate memories. Nor can we reliably detect false memories by relying on the contrast between whether people say they "remember" the past or merely "know" what happened in the past. The absence of a connection between memory accuracy and memory confidence contrasts with the commonsense belief that you should rely on someone's degree of certainty in assessing their memory. The problem in this commonsense notion lies in the fact that confidence is influenced by factors (such as feedback) that have no impact on accuracy, and this influence undermines the linkage between accuracy and confidence.

- While memory errors are easily documented, cases of accurate remembering can also be observed, and they are probably more numerous than cases involving memory error. Memory errors are more likely, though, in recalling distant events rather than recent ones. One reason for this is decay of the relevant memories; another reason is retrieval failure. Retrieval failure can be either complete or partial; the tip-of-the-tongue pattern provides a clear example of partial retrieval failure. Perhaps the most important source of forgetting, though, is interference.

- People have sought various means of undoing forgetting, including hypnosis and various drugs. These approaches, however, seem ineffective. Forgetting can be diminished, though, through procedures that provide a rich variety of retrieval cues, and it can be avoided through occasional revisits to the target material.

- Although memory errors are troubling, they may simply be the price you pay in order to obtain other advantages. For example, many errors result from the dense network of connections that link your various memories. These connections sometimes make it difficult to recall which elements occurred in which setting, but the same connections serve as retrieval paths, and without the connections you might have great difficulty in locating your memories in long-term storage. Even forgetting may have a positive side, by virtue of trimming details from memory in a fashion that may foster abstract thinking.

- Autobiographical memory is influenced by the same principles as any other form of memory, but it is also shaped by its own set of factors. For example, episodes connected to the self are, in general, better remembered—a pattern known as the self-reference effect.

- Autobiographical memories are also often emotional, and this has multiple effects on memory. Emotion seems to promote memory consolidation, but it may also produce a pattern of memory narrowing. Some emotional events give rise to very clear, long-lasting memories called "flashbulb memories." Despite their subjective clarity, these memories, like memories of any other sort, can contain errors and in some cases can be entirely inaccurate.

At the extreme of emotion, trauma has mixed effects on memory. Some traumatic events are not remembered, but most traumatic events seem to be remembered for a long time and in great detail.

- Some events can be recalled even after many years have passed. In some cases, this is because the knowledge was learned very well in the first place. In other cases, occasional rehearsals preserve a memory for a very long time.

eBook Demonstrations & Essays

Online Demonstrations:
- Demonstration 8.1: Associations and Memory Error
- Demonstration 8.2: Memory Accuracy and Confidence
- Demonstration 8.3: The Tip-of-the-Tongue Effect
- Demonstration 8.4: Childhood Amnesia

Online Applying Cognitive Psychology Essays:
- Cognitive Psychology and Education: Overconfidence
- Cognitive Psychology and the Law: Jurors' Memory

ZAPS 2.0 Cognition Labs

- Go to http://digital.wwnorton.com/cognition6 for the online labs relevant to this chapter.

part 4

Knowledge

I n Parts 2 and 3, we saw case after case in which your interactions with the world are guided by knowledge. In perceiving, for example, you make inferences guided by knowledge about the world's regular patterns. In attending, you anticipate inputs guided by your knowledge about what's likely to occur. In learning, you connect new information to things you already know. And so on. But what is knowledge? How is knowledge represented in your mind? How do you locate knowledge in memory when you need it?

We've already taken some steps toward answering these questions—by arguing in previous chapters that knowledge is represented in the mind by means of a network of interconnected nodes. In this section, we'll flesh out this proposal in important ways. In Chapter 9, we'll describe the basic building blocks of knowledge—individual concepts—and consider several hypotheses about how concepts are represented in the mind. We'll see that each hypothesis captures a part of the truth, and so we'll be driven toward a several-part theory combining the various views. We'll also see that knowledge about individual concepts depends on linkages to other, related concepts. Thus, you cannot know what a "dog" is without also understanding what an "animal" is, what a "living thing" is, and so on. As a result, connections among ideas will be crucial for us here, just as they were in previous chapters.

Chapters 10 and 11 then focus on two special types of knowledge: knowledge about language and knowledge about visual images. In Chapter 10, we'll see that your knowledge of language is highly creative in the sense that you can produce new words and new sentences that no one has ever used before. But at the same time, the creativity is constrained, so there are some words and sequences of words that are considered unacceptable by virtually any speaker. In order to understand this pattern of "constrained creativity," we'll consider the possibility that language knowledge involves abstract rules that are, in some fashion, known and honored by every user of the language.

In Chapter 11, we'll discuss the fact that mental images seem to involve representations that are distinct from those involved in other forms of knowledge, but we'll also consider some of the ways in which memory for visual appearances is governed by the same principles as other forms of knowledge.

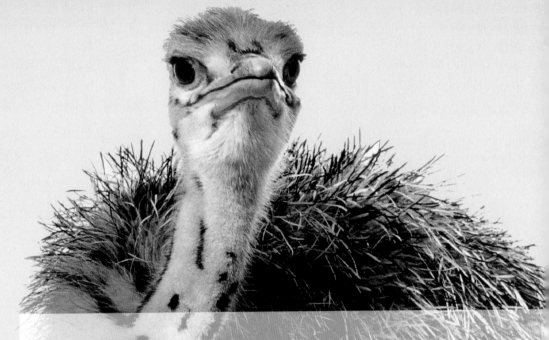
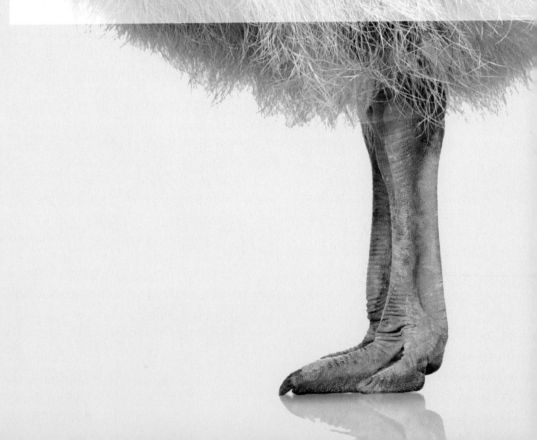

chapter 9

Concepts and Generic Knowledge

what if... In Chapter 8, we mentioned people who have "superior autobiographical recall." It is remarkable how much these individuals can remember—but some people, it turns out, can remember even more. Indeed, one might say that these people have "perfect memories," but this terminology would surely be misleading.

We begin with a work of fiction. In a wonderful short story titled "Funes the Memorious," the Argentine writer Jorge Luis Borges describes a character named Funes who never forgets anything. But rather than being proud of his capacity, Funes is immensely distressed by his own memorial prowess: "My memory, sir, is like a garbage heap." Among other problems, Funes complains that he is incapable of thinking in general terms; he remembers so much about how individuals *differ* that he has a hard time focusing on what these individuals might *have in common*: "Not only was it difficult for him to comprehend that the generic symbol *dog* embraces so many unlike individuals of diverse size and form; it bothered him that the dog at 3:14 (seen from the side) should have the same name as the dog at 3:15 (seen from the front)" (Borges, 1964).

Funes is a fictional character, but consider the actual case of Solomon Shereshevsky (Luria, 1968). Shereshevsky—like Funes—never forgot anything. After hearing a lengthy speech, he could repeat it back word for word. If shown a complex mathematical formula (even one that had no meaning at all for him), he could reproduce it perfectly months later. He effortlessly memorized poems written in languages he did not understand. And let's be clear that Shereshevsky's flawless retention was not the result of some deliberate trick or strategy. Just the opposite: Shereshevsky seemed to have no choice about his level of recall.

Like Funes, Shereshevsky was not well served by his extraordinary memory. He was so alert to the literal form of his experiences that he could not remember the deeper implications of these experiences. Similarly, he had difficulty recognizing faces because he was so alert to the *changes* in a face from one view to the next. And, like Funes, Shereshevsky was often distracted by the detail of his own recollections, and so he found it difficult to think in abstract terms.

Basic concepts—like "chair" and "dog"—are the building blocks of all knowledge. However, attempts at *defining* these concepts usually fail because we easily find exceptions to virtually any definition that might be proposed.

This leads to a suggestion that knowledge of these concepts is cast in terms of *probabilities*, so that a creature that has wings and feathers, and that flies and lays eggs, is *probably* a bird.

Many results are consistent with this probabilistic idea and show that the more a test case resembles the "prototype" for a category, the more likely people are to judge the case as being in that category.

Other results, however, indicate that conceptual knowledge includes other beliefs—beliefs that link a concept to other concepts and also specify why the concept is as it is.

These beliefs may be represented in the mind as propositions encoded in a network structure; alternatively, they may be represented in a distributed form in a connectionist network.

We are driven, therefore, to a multipart theory of concepts. Your conceptual knowledge must include a prototype for each category and also a set of remembered exemplars. But you also seem to have a broad set of beliefs about each concept—beliefs that provide a "theory" for why the concept takes the form it does, and you use this theory in a wide range of judgments about the concept.

Unmistakably, there are settings in which you do want to remember the specific episodes of your life. You want to recall what you saw at the crime scene, holding to the side (as best you can) the information you picked up in your conversation with the police. You hope to remember what you read in your textbook, trying to ignore the (possibly bogus) information you heard from your roommate. Funes and Shereshevsky obviously excel in this type of memory, but their limitations remind us that there are also disadvantages for this type of particularized recall. In many settings, you want to set aside the details of this or that episode and, instead, weave your experiences together so that you can pool information received from various sources. This allows you to create a more complete, more integrated type of knowledge, one that enables you to think (for example) about dogs in general, rather than focusing on *this* view of *that* dog; or one that enables you to remember what your friend's face generally looks like rather than concentrating on what she looked like, say, yesterday at noon. This more general type of knowledge is surely drawn from your day-to-day experience, but it is somehow abstracted away from that experience. What is this more general type of knowledge?

Understanding Concepts

Concepts like "shoe" or "house" or "tree" are so ordinary, so common, that there seems to be nothing special about knowing—and being able to think about—these simple ideas. However, ordinary concepts like these are, in an important way, the building blocks out of which all your knowledge is created, and as we've seen in previous chapters, you depend on your knowledge in many aspects of your day-to-day functioning. Thus, you know what to pay attention to in a restaurant because you understand the basic concept of "restaurant." You're able to understand a simple story about a child checking her piggy bank because you understand the concepts of "money," "shopping," and so on.

The idea, then, is that you need concepts in order to have knowledge, and you need knowledge in order to function. In this way, your understanding of ideas like "shoe" and "house" might seem commonplace, but it is an ingredient without which cognition cannot proceed.

But what exactly does it mean to understand simple concepts like these? How is this knowledge represented in the mind? In this chapter, we'll begin with the obvious hypothesis: that understanding a concept is analogous to knowing a dictionary definition, and so, if someone knows what a "house" is, or a "taxi," he or she can offer something like a definition for these terms—and likewise for all the other concepts in each person's knowledge base. As we will see, though, this hypothesis quickly runs into problems, so we'll need to turn to a richer—and more complicated—proposal.

Definitions: What Is a "Dog"?

You know perfectly well what a dog is. You have some knowledge that represents this concept for you and contains what you know about the dogs. But what is that knowledge?

One possibility is that you know something akin to a dictionary definition. That is, what you know is of this form: "A dog is a creature that (a) is mammalian, (b) has four legs, (c) barks, (d) wags its tail." You could then use this definition in straightforward ways: When asked whether a candidate creature is a dog, you could use the definition as a checklist, scrutinizing the candidate for the various defining features. When told that "a dog is an animal," you would know that you hadn't learned anything new, because this information is already contained, presumably, within the definition. If you were asked what dogs, cats, and horses have in common, you could scan your definition of each one looking for common elements.

This proposal is surely correct in some cases, and so, for example, you certainly know definitions for concepts like "triangle" and "even number." But what about more commonplace concepts? The concern here was brought to light by the 20th-century philosopher Ludwig Wittgenstein, who argued (e.g., Wittgenstein, 1953) that the simple terms we all use every day actually don't have definitions. For example, consider the word "game." You know

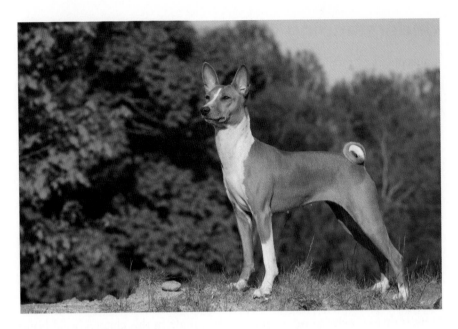

THE HUNT FOR DEFINITIONS

It is remarkably difficult to define even very familiar terms. For example, what is a "dog"? Most people include "has fur" in the definition, but what about the hairless Chihuahua? Many people include "communicates by barking" in the definition, but what about the Basenji (one of which is shown here)—a breed of dog that does not bark?

this word and can use it sensibly, but what is a game? As an approach to this question, we could ask, for example, about the game of hide-and-seek. What makes hide-and-seek a "game"? Hide-and-seek (a) is an activity most often practiced by children, (b) is engaged in for fun, (c) has certain rules, (d) involves several people, (e) is in some ways competitive, and (f) is played during periods of leisure. All these are plausible attributes of games, and so we seem well on our way to defining "game." But are these attributes really part of the *definition* of "game"? What about the Olympic Games? The competitors in these games are not children, and runners in marathon races don't look like they're having a great deal of fun. Likewise, what about card games played by one person? These are played alone, without competition. For that matter, what about the case of professional golfers?

It seems that for each clause of the definition, we can easily find an exception: an activity that we call a game but that doesn't have the relevant characteristic. And the same is true for almost any concept. We might define "shoe" as an item of apparel made out of leather, designed to be worn on the foot. But what about wooden shoes? What about a shoe designed by a master shoemaker, intended only for display and never for use? What about a shoe filled with cement, which therefore cannot be worn? Similarly, we might define "dog" in a way that includes four-leggedness, but what about a dog that has lost a limb in some accident? We might specify "communicates by

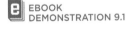

EBOOK
DEMONSTRATION 9.1

barking" as part of the definition of dog, but what about the African Basenji, which has no bark? Examples like these make it clear that even simple terms, terms denoting concepts we use easily and often, resist being defined. In each case, we can come up with what seems to be a plausible definition, but then it's easy to find exceptions to it.

Family Resemblance

Plainly, then, we can't say things like, "A dog is a creature that has fur and four legs and barks." That's because, as we've seen, it's easy to find exceptions to this rule (a hairless Chihuahua? a three-legged dog? the barkless Basenji?). But surely we *can* say, "Dogs *usually* are creatures that have fur, four legs, and bark, and a creature without these features is *unlikely to be* a dog." This probabilistic phrasing preserves what's good about definitions—the fact that they do name sensible, relevant features, shared by most members of the category. But this phrasing also allows a degree of uncertainty, some number of exceptions to the rule.

In a similar spirit, Wittgenstein proposed that members of a category have a **family resemblance** to one another. To understand this term, think about the resemblance pattern in an actual family—your own, perhaps. There are probably no "defining features" for your family—features that every family member has. Nonetheless, there are features that are common in the family, and so, if we consider family members two or even three at a time, we can usually find some shared attributes. Thus, you, your brother, and your mother might all have the family's beautiful red hair and the same wide lips; as a result, you three look alike to some extent. Your sister, however, doesn't have these features. Nonetheless, she's recognizable as a member of the family because (like you and your father) she has the family's typical eye shape and the family's distinctive chin. Thus, there are common features, but the identity of those common features depends on what "subgroup" of the family you're considering—hair color shared for *these* family members; eye shape shared by *those* family members; and so on.

One way to think about this pattern is by imagining the "ideal" for each family—someone who has *all* of the family's features. (In our example, this would be someone who is a wide-lipped redhead with the right eye and chin shapes.) In many families, this person may not exist, and there may be no one who has all of the family's features, so no one who looks like the "perfect Jones" (or the "perfect Martinez" or the "perfect Goldberg"). Nonetheless, each member of the family has at least some features in common with this ideal—and therefore some features in common with other family members. This is why the family members resemble one another, and it's how we manage to recognize these individuals as being within the family.

Wittgenstein proposed that ordinary categories like "dog" or "game" or "furniture" work the same way. There may be no features that are shared by all dogs or all games, but even so, we can identify "characteristic features" for each category—features that many (and perhaps most) category members

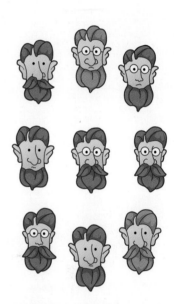

TYPICALITY IN FAMILIES

In the Smith family, many (but not all) of the brothers have dark hair, so dark hair is typical for the family (i.e., is found in *many* family members) but does not define the family (i.e., is not found in *all* family members). Likewise, wearing glasses is typical for the family but not a defining feature; so is having a mustache and a big nose. Many concepts have the same character—with many features shared among the instances of the concept, but no features shared by all of the instances.

have. And the more of these features an object has, the more likely you are to believe it is in the category. Family resemblance is a matter of degree, not all-or-none.

There are several ways we might translate all of these points into a psychological theory, but one influential translation was proposed by psychologist Eleanor Rosch in the mid-1970s (Rosch, 1973, 1978; Rosch & Mervis, 1975; Rosch, Mervis, Gray, Johnson, & Boyes-Braem, 1976). Rosch had focused her undergraduate thesis on Wittgenstein, before launching her formal training as a psychologist; she was, therefore, well positioned to develop Wittgenstein's ideas into a set of scientific hypotheses. Let's look at her model.

Prototypes and Typicality Effects

One way to think about definitions is that they set the "boundaries" for a category. If a test case has certain attributes, then it's "inside" the boundaries. If a test case doesn't have the defining attributes, then it's "outside" the category. **Prototype theory**, in contrast, begins with a different tactic: Perhaps the best way to identify a category is to specify the "center" of the category, rather than the boundaries. Just as we spoke earlier about the "ideal" family member, perhaps the concept of "dog" (for example) is represented in the mind by some depiction of the "ideal" dog, and all judgments about dogs are made with reference to this ideal; likewise for "bird" or "house" or any other concept in your repertoire—in each case, the concept is represented by the appropriate prototype.

In most cases, this "ideal"—the prototype—will be an average of the various category members you've encountered. Thus, the prototype dog will be the average color of the dogs you've seen, the average size of the dogs you've seen, and so forth. (Notice, then, that different people, each with their own experiences, will have slightly different prototypes.) No matter what the specifics of the prototype, though, you'll use this "ideal" as the anchor, the benchmark, for your conceptual knowledge; as a result, whenever you use your conceptual knowledge, your reasoning is done with reference to the prototype.

Prototypes and Graded Membership

To make these ideas concrete, consider a simple task of categorization: deciding whether something is or is not a dog. To make this decision, you compare the creature currently before your eyes with the prototype in your memory. If there's no similarity between them, the creature standing before you is probably not in the category; if there's considerable similarity, you draw the opposite conclusion.

This sounds plausible enough, but note an important implication: Membership in a category depends on resemblance to the prototype, and resemblance is a matter of degree. (After all, some dogs are likely to resemble the prototype rather closely, while others will have less in common with this ideal.) As a result, membership in the category is not a simple "yes or no"

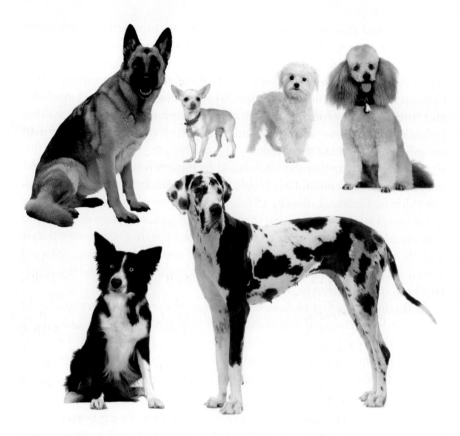

CATEGORIES HAVE PROTOTYPES

As the text describes, people seem to have a prototype in their minds for a category like "dog." For many people, the German shepherd shown here is close to that prototype, and the other dogs depicted are more distant from the prototype.

decision; instead, it's a matter of "more" or "less." In technical terms, we'd say that categories, on this view, have a **graded membership**, such that objects closer to the prototype are "better" members of the category than objects farther from the prototype. Or, to put this concretely, some dogs are "doggier" than others, some books "bookier" than others, and so on for all the other categories you can think of.

Testing the Prototype Notion

In a **sentence verification task**, research participants are presented with a succession of sentences; their job is to indicate (by pressing the appropriate button) whether each sentence is true or false. In this procedure, participants' response is slower for sentences like "A penguin is a bird" than for sentences like "A robin is a bird"; slower for "An Afghan hound is a dog" than for "A German shepherd is a dog" (Smith, Rips, & Shoben, 1974).

Why should this be? According to a prototype perspective, participants choose their response ("true" or "false") by comparing the thing mentioned (e.g., penguin) to their prototype for that category (i.e., their bird prototype). When there is close similarity between the test case and the prototype, participants can make their decisions quickly; judgments about items more distant from the prototype take more time. And given the results, it seems that penguins and Afghans are more distant from their respective prototypes than are robins and German shepherds.

Other results can also be understood in these terms. For example, in a **production task** we simply ask people to name as many birds or dogs as they can (Mervis, Catlin, & Rosch, 1976). According to a prototype view, they will do this task by first locating their bird or dog prototype in memory and then asking themselves what resembles this prototype. In essence, they'll start with the center of the category (the prototype) and work their way outward from there. Thus, birds close to the prototype should be mentioned first; birds farther from the prototype, later on.

By this logic, the first birds to be mentioned in the production task should be the birds that yielded fast response times in the verification task; that's because what matters in both tasks is proximity to the prototype. Likewise, the birds mentioned later in production should have yielded slower response times in verification. This is exactly what happens.

TABLE 9.1 PARTICIPANTS' TYPICALITY RATINGS FOR THE CATEGORY "FRUIT" AND THE CATEGORY "BIRD"

Fruit	Rating	Bird	Rating
Apple	6.25	Robin	6.89
Peach	5.81	Bluebird	6.42
Pear	5.25	Seagull	6.26
Grape	5.13	Swallow	6.16
Strawberry	5.00	Falcon	5.74
Lemon	4.86	Mockingbird	5.47
Blueberry	4.56	Starling	5.16
Watermelon	4.06	Owl	5.00
Raisin	3.75	Vulture	4.84
Fig	3.38	Sandpiper	4.47
Coconut	3.06	Chicken	3.95
Pomegranate	2.50	Flamingo	3.37
Avocado	2.38	Albatross	3.32
Pumpkin	2.31	Penguin	2.63
Olive	2.25	Bat	1.53

Ratings were made on a 7-point scale, with 7 corresponding to the highest typicality. Note also that the least "birdy" of the birds isn't (technically speaking) a bird at all! AFTER MALT & SMITH, 1984.

In fact, this outcome sets the pattern of evidence for prototype theory: Over and over, in category after category, members of a category that are "privileged" on one task (e.g., yield the fastest response times) turn out also to be privileged on other tasks (e.g., are most likely to be mentioned). As a further illustration of this pattern, consider the data from **rating tasks**. In these tasks, participants are given instructions like these (Rosch, 1975; also Malt & Smith, 1984): "We all know that some birds are 'birdier' than others, some dogs are 'doggier' than others, and so on. I'm going to present you with a list of birds or of dogs, and I want you to rate each one on the basis of how 'birdy' or 'doggy' it is."

People are easily able to render these judgments, and quite consistently they rate items as being very "birdy" or "doggy" when these instances are close to the prototype (as determined in the other tasks). They rate items as being less "birdy" or "doggy" when these are farther from the prototype. This finding suggests that once again, people perform the task by comparing the test item to the prototype (see **Table 9.1**).

EBOOK DEMONSTRATION 9.2

Basic-Level Categories

It seems, then, that certain category members are indeed "privileged," just as the prototype theory proposes. It turns out, in addition, that certain *types of category* are also privileged—in their structure and the way they are used. Thus, imagine that we show you a picture like the one in **Figure 9.1** and simply ask, "What is this?" You're likely to say "a chair" and unlikely to offer a more specific response ("upholstered armchair") or a more general one ("an item of furniture"). Likewise, we might ask, "How do people get to work?" In responding, you're unlikely to say, "Some people drive Fords; some drive Toyotas." Instead, your answer is likely to use more general terms, such as "cars," "trains," and "buses."

In keeping with these observations, Rosch and others have argued that there is a "natural" level of categorization, neither too specific nor too general,

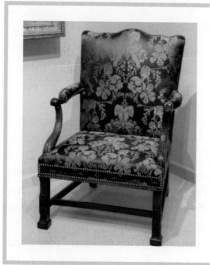

FIGURE 9.1 BASIC VERSUS SUPERORDINATE LABELING

What is this? The odds are good that you would answer by saying "It's a chair," using the basic-level description, rather than the superordinate label ("It's a piece of furniture") or a more specific description ("It's an upholstered armchair"), even though these other descriptions would certainly be correct.

that people tend to use in their conversations and their reasoning. The special status of this **basic-level categorization** can be demonstrated in many ways. Basic-level categories are usually represented in our language via a single word, while more specific categories are identified only via a phrase. Thus, "chair" is a basic-level category, and so is "apple." The more specific (subordinate) categories of "lawn chair" or "kitchen chair" are not basic level; neither is "Granny Smith apple" or "Golden Delicious apple."

We've already suggested that if you're asked to describe an object, you're likely to use the basic-level term. In addition, if asked to explain what members of a category have in common with one another, you have an easy time with basic-level categories ("What do all chairs have in common?") but some difficulty with more encompassing (superordinate) categories ("What does all furniture have in common?"). Moreover, children learning to talk often acquire basic-level terms earlier than either the more specific subcategories or the more general, more encompassing categories. In these (and other) ways, basic-level categories do seem to reflect a natural way to categorize the objects in our world. (For more on basic-level categories, see Corter & Gluck, 1992; Pansky & Koriat, 2004; Rosch et al., 1976; Rogers & Patterson, 2007.)

EBOOK
DEMONSTRATION 9.3

Exemplars

Let's return, though, to our main agenda. As we've seen, a broad spectrum of tasks reflects the "graded membership" of mental categories. In other words, some members of the categories are "better" than others, and the better members are recognized more readily, mentioned more often, judged to be more typical, and so on. (For yet another way you're influenced by typicality, see **Figure 9.2**.) All of this fits well with the notion that conceptual knowledge is represented via a prototype and that we categorize by making comparisons to that prototype. It turns out, though, that prototype theory isn't the only way you can think about these data.

Analogies from Remembered Exemplars

Imagine that we place a wooden object in front of you and ask, "Is this a chair?" According to the prototype view, you'll answer this question by calling up your chair prototype from memory and then comparing the candidate to that prototype. If the resemblance is great, you'll announce, "Yes, this is a chair."

But you might make this decision in a different way. You might notice that the object is very similar to an object in your Uncle Jerry's living room, and you know that Uncle Jerry's object is a chair. (After all, you've seen Uncle Jerry sitting in the thing, reading his newspaper; you've heard Jerry referring to the thing as "my chair," and so on.) These points allow an easy inference: If the new object resembles Jerry's, and if Jerry's object is a chair, then it's a safe bet that the new object is a chair too.

The idea here is that in some cases categorization relies on knowledge about specific category members ("Jerry's chair") rather than the prototype (e.g., the

FIGURE 9.2 TYPICALITY AND ATTRACTIVENESS

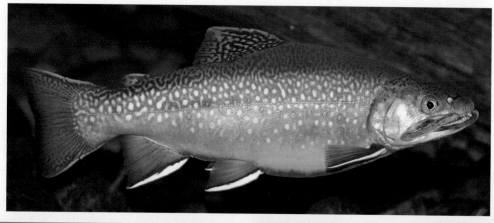

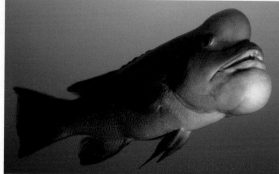
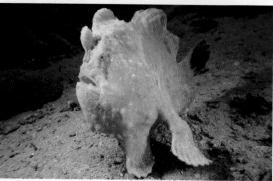

Typicality influences many judgments about category members, including attractiveness. Which of these pictures shows the most attractive-looking fish? Which shows the least attractive-looking? In several studies, participants' ratings of attractiveness have been closely related to (other participants') ratings of typicality—so that people seem to find more-typical category members to be more attractive (e.g., Halberstadt & Rhodes, 2003). Plainly, the influence of typicality is rather broad.

ideal chair). This process is referred to as **exemplar-based reasoning**, with an exemplar being defined as a specific remembered instance—in essence, an example.

The exemplar-based approach is in many ways similar to the prototype view. According to each of these proposals, you categorize objects by comparing them to a mentally represented "standard." The difference between the views lies in what that standard is: For prototype theory, the standard is the prototype—an average representing the entire category; for exemplar theory, the standard is provided by whatever example of the category comes to mind (and, of course, different examples may come to mind on different occasions). In either case, though, the process is then the same. You assess the similarity between a candidate object and the standard. If the resemblance is great, you judge the candidate as being within the relevant category; if the resemblance is minimal, you seek some alternative categorization.

Explaining Typicality Data with an Exemplar Model

Consider a task in which we show people a series of pictures and ask them to decide whether each picture shows a fruit or not. We already know that they'll respond more quickly for typical fruits (apple, orange, banana) than for less typical fruits (kiwi, olive, cranberry), and we've seen how this result is handled by a prototype account. It turns out, however, that an exemplar-based account can also explain this result, so this result favors neither the prototype nor the exemplar theory; instead, it's fully compatible with both.

How would an exemplar-based account handle this result? Let's imagine that you're trying to decide whether a picture shows a fruit or not. To make your decision, you'll try to think of a fruit exemplar (again: a memory for a particular fruit) that resembles the object in the picture. If you find a memory that's a good match to the object, then you know the object in the picture is indeed a fruit. No match? Then it's not a fruit.

How this sequence will play out, however, depends on the picture. If the picture shows, say, an apple, then your memory search will be extremely rapid: Apples are common in your experience (often seen, often mentioned), so

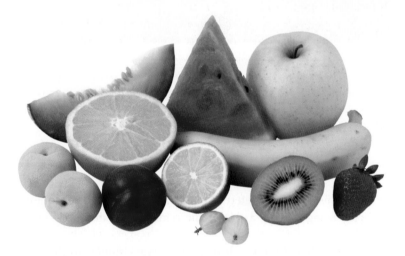

WHICH ARE THE TYPICAL FRUITS?

If asked to name fruits, you're more likely to name typical fruits (apples, oranges) than atypical fruits (figs, starfruit). According to a prototype account, this result occurs because you start your memory search with the prototype and "work outward" from there. According to an exemplar account, the result occurs because you have many memories of apples and oranges, and these are well primed; it's no surprise, therefore, that these are the fruit memories that come easily to mind for you.

you've had many opportunities to establish apple memories. As a result, you'll easily find a memory that matches the picture, so you will swiftly respond that, yes, the picture does show a fruit. But if the picture shows, say, a fig or a star-fruit, then your memory search will be more difficult: You probably don't have many memories that will match these pictures, so your response will be slow.

A similar argument will handle the other tasks showing the graded-membership pattern, and so the results we've reviewed so far favor neither theory over the other. We'll need other evidence, therefore, to decide which theory is correct, but it turns out that this framing of the issue is misleading. The reason, in brief, is that *both* theories are correct.

A Combination of Exemplars and Prototypes

There's reason for you to rely *both* on prototypes *and* on exemplars in your thinking about categories. Prototypes provide an economical representation of what's typical for a category, and there are many circumstances in which this quick summary is quite useful. But exemplars, for their part, provide information that's lost from the prototype—including information about the variability within the category.

Consider the fact that people routinely "tune" their concepts to match the circumstances. Thus, they think about birds differently when thinking about Chinese birds than when thinking about American birds; they think about gifts differently when thinking about gifts for a student rather than gifts for a faculty member (Barsalou, 1988; Barsalou & Sewell, 1985). In fact, people can adjust their categories in fairly precise ways: not just "gift," but "gift for a 4-year-old" or "gift for a 4-year-old who recently broke her wrist" or "gift for a 4-year-old who likes sports but recently broke her wrist."

This pliability in concepts is easy to understand if people are relying on exemplars; after all, different settings, or different perspectives, would trigger different memories and thus bring different exemplars to mind. If people then rely on these exemplars in their reasoning, it makes sense that reasoning will vary as someone moves from one circumstance to the next or when someone shifts perspective.

It's useful, then, that conceptual knowledge includes prototypes *and* exemplars, because each carries its own advantages. And, in fact, the mix of exemplar and prototype knowledge may vary from person to person and from concept to concept. One person, for example, might have extensive knowledge about individual horses, so she has many exemplars in memory; the same person might have only general information (a prototype, perhaps) about snowmobiles. Some other person might show the reverse pattern. And for all people, the pattern of knowledge might depend on the size of the category and on how confusable the category memories are with one another (with exemplars being used when the individuals are more distinct; for further discussion of how the mix of exemplars and prototypes is shaped by various factors, see Brooks, Norman, & Allen, 1991; Homa, Dunbar, & Nohre, 1991; Minda & Smith, 2001; Rips, Smith, & Medin, 2012; Rouder & Ratcliff, 2006; Smith, 2002, 2014; Vanpaemel & Storms, 2008; also see **Figure 9.3**).

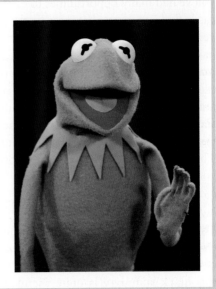

FIGURE 9.3 DISTINCTIONS WITHIN CATEGORIES

The chapter suggests that you have knowledge of both exemplars and prototypes. As a further complication, though, you also have special knowledge about distinctive individuals within a category. Thus, you know that Kermit has many frogly properties (he's green, he eats flies, he hops) but also has unusual properties that make him a rather unusual frog (since, after all, he can talk, he can sing, and he's in love with a pig).

Overall, though, it cannot be surprising that we have the option of *combining* prototype and exemplar models, because, as we've said, the two types of model are similar in crucial ways. In either case, an object before your eyes triggers some information in memory (either a specific instance, according to exemplar theory, or the prototype, according to prototype theory). In either case, you assess the resemblance between this conceptual knowledge, supplied by memory, and the novel object now before you: "Does this object resemble my sister's couch?" If so, the object is a couch. "Does the object resemble my prototype for a soup bowl?" If so, it's probably a soup bowl.

Given these similarities, it seems sensible that we might merge the models, with each of us on any particular occasion relying on whichever sort of information (exemplar or prototype) comes to mind more readily.

The Difficulties with Categorizing via Resemblance

We are moving, it seems, toward a relatively clear-cut set of claims. For most concepts, definitions are not available. For many purposes, though, you don't need a definition and can rely instead on a mix of prototypes and exemplars. In addition, there's no question that **typicality** does play a role in people's thinking, with more-typical category members being "privileged" in many regards. And typicality is exactly what we would expect if category knowledge does, in fact, hinge on prototypes and exemplars.

All of this reasoning seems straightforward enough. However, there are some results that do not fit into this picture, so the time has come to broaden our conception of concepts.

The Differences between Typicality and Categorization

In the view we've been developing, judgments of *typicality* and judgments of *category membership* both derive from the same source: resemblance to an exemplar or to a prototype. If the resemblance is great, then a test case will be judged to be typical and will be judged to be a category member. If the resemblance is small, the test case will be judged atypical and probably not a category member. Thus, typicality and category membership should go hand in hand.

It turns out, though, that typicality and category membership sometimes *don't* go hand in hand. Armstrong, Gleitman, and Gleitman (1983), for example, gave their participants this peculiar instruction: "We all know that some numbers are even-er than others. What I want you to do is to rate each of the numbers on this list for how good an example it is for the category 'even number.'" Participants were then given a list of numbers (4, 16, 32, and so on) and had to rate "how even" each number was. The participants thought this was a strange task but were nonetheless able to render these judgments—and, interestingly, were just as consistent with one another using these stimuli as they were with categories like "dog" or "bird" or "fruit" (see **Table 9.2**).

Of course, participants responded differently (and correctly!) if asked directly which numbers on the list were even and which were odd. Therefore, the participants could judge category membership as easily as they could judge typicality, but, importantly, these judgments were entirely independent of each other: Participants believed that 4 is a more typical even number than 7534, but also knew this has nothing to do with the fact that both are unmistakably in the category *even number*. Clearly, therefore, there's some

TABLE 9.2 PARTICIPANTS' TYPICALITY RATINGS FOR WELL-DEFINED CATEGORIES

EVEN NUMBER		ODD NUMBER	
Stimulus	Typicality Rating	Stimulus	Typicality Rating
4	5.9	3	5.4
8	5.5	7	5.1
10	5.3	23	4.6
18	4.4	57	4.4
34	3.6	501	3.5
106	3.1	447	3.3

Participants rated each item on "how good an example" it was for its category. Ratings were on a scale from 0 to 7, with 7 meaning the item was a "very good example." Participants rated some even numbers as being "better examples" of even numbers than others, although mathematically this is absurd: Either a number is even (divisible by 2 without a remainder) or it is not. The same remarks apply to the category of odd numbers. Either a number is odd or it is not, but even so, participants rated some odd numbers as being "odder" than others. AFTER ARMSTRONG ET AL., 1983.

basis for judging category membership that's separate from the assessment of typicality, and we obviously need some explanation for this point.

One might argue, though, that mathematical concepts like "even number" are somehow special, and so their status doesn't tell us much about other, more "ordinary" concepts. However, this suggestion is quickly rebutted, because many other concepts show a similar distinction between category membership and typicality. Thus, robins strike us as being closer to the typical bird than penguins do; even so, most of us are certain that both robins and penguins are birds. Likewise, Moby Dick was definitely not a typical whale, but he certainly was a whale; Abraham Lincoln was not a typical American, but he was an American. These informal observations, like the even-number result, drive a wedge between typicality and category membership—a wedge that does not fit with our theory so far.

How are category judgments made when they *don't* rely on typicality? As an approach to this question, let's think through an example. Consider a lemon. Paint the lemon with red and white stripes. Is it still a lemon? Most people believe that it is. Now, inject the lemon with sugar water, so it has a sweet taste. Then, run over the lemon with a truck, so that it's flat as a pancake. What have we got at this point? Do we have a striped, artificially sweet, flattened lemon? Or do we have a non-lemon? Most people still accept this poor, abused fruit as a lemon, but consider what this judgment entails. We've taken steps to make

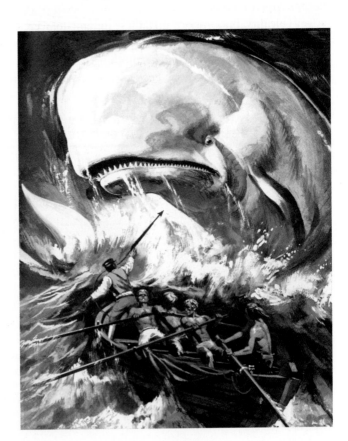

CATEGORIZATION OUTSIDE OF TYPICALITY

Moby Dick is not a typical whale, but he unmistakably is a whale, even so. Clearly, then, typicality can, in some settings, be separated from category membership.

this object more and more distant from the prototype and also very different from any specific lemon you've ever encountered (and thus very different from any remembered exemplars). But this seems not to shake your faith that the object remains a lemon. To be sure, we have a not-easily-recognized lemon, an exceptional lemon, but it's still a lemon. Apparently, something can be a lemon with virtually no resemblance to other lemons.

Related points emerge in research with children. In an early study, preschool children were asked what makes something a "coffeepot," a "raccoon," and so on (Keil, 1986). As a way of probing their beliefs, the children were asked whether it would be possible to turn a toaster into a coffeepot. Children often acknowledged that this would be possible. We would have to widen the holes in the top of the toaster and fix things so that the water wouldn't leak out of the bottom. We'd also need to design a place to put the coffee grounds. But the children saw no obstacles to these manipulations and were quite certain that with these adjustments in place, we would have created a bona fide coffeepot.

Things were different, though, when the children were asked a parallel question—whether one could, with suitable adjustments, turn a skunk into a raccoon. The children understood that we could dye the skunk's fur, teach it to climb trees, and, in general, teach it to behave in a raccoon-like fashion. Even with these provisions, the children steadfastly denied that we would have created a raccoon. A skunk that looks, sounds, and acts just like a raccoon might be a very peculiar skunk, but it would be a skunk nonetheless. (For related data, see Gelman & Wellman, 1991; Keil, Smith, Simons, & Levin, 1998; Walker, 1993. For other evidence suggesting that people reason differently about *naturally occurring items* like raccoons and *manufactured items* like coffeepots, see Caramazza & Shelton, 1998; Estes, 2003; German & Barrett, 2005; Levin, Takarae, Miner, & Keil, 2001; also see "Different Profiles for Different Concepts" section on p. 330.)

What lies behind all of these judgments? If people are asked why the abused lemon still counts as a lemon, they're likely to mention the fact that it grew on a lemon tree, is genetically a lemon, and so on. It's these "deep" features that matter, not the lemon's current properties. And so, too, for raccoons: In the child's view, being a raccoon is not merely a function of having the relevant features; instead, in the eyes of the child, the key to being a raccoon involves (among other things) having a raccoon mommy and a raccoon daddy. Thus, a raccoon, just like a lemon, is defined in ways that refer to deep properties and not to mere appearances.

We need to be clear, however, that these claims about an object's "deep" properties depend, in turn, on a web of other beliefs—beliefs that are, in each case, "tuned" to the category being considered. Continuing the example, you're more likely to think that a creature is a raccoon if you're told that it has raccoons as parents. But this is true only because you have some ideas about how a creature comes to be a raccoon—ideas that are linked to your broader understanding of biological categories and inheritance; it's this understanding that tells you that parentage

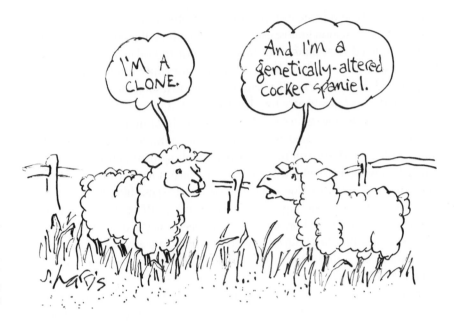

Both of these creatures resemble the prototype for sheep, and both resemble many sheep exemplars you've seen (or perhaps read about). But are they really sheep?

is relevant here. If this isn't clear, consider, as a contrasting case, the steps you'd go through in deciding whether Judy really is a doctor. In this case, you're unlikely to worry about whether Judy has a doctor mommy and a doctor daddy, because your other beliefs tell you, of course, that for this category parentage doesn't matter.

As a different example, think about the category of *counterfeit money*. A counterfeit bill, if skillfully produced, will bear a nearly perfect resemblance to the prototype for legitimate money. Despite this resemblance, you understand that a counterfeit bill is not in the category of legitimate money, so here, too, your categorization doesn't depend on typicality. Instead, your categorization depends on a web of other beliefs, including beliefs about circumstances of printing: A $20 bill is legitimate, you believe, only if it was printed with the approval of, and under the supervision of, the relevant government agencies. And once again, these beliefs arise only because you have a broader understanding of what money is and how government regulations apply to monetary systems. In other words, you consider circumstances of printing only because your understanding tells you that the circumstances are relevant here, and you won't consider circumstances of printing in a wide range of other cases. If asked, for example, whether a copy of the Lord's Prayer is "counterfeit" or not, your beliefs tell you that the Lord's Prayer is the Lord's Prayer no matter where (or by whom) it was printed. Instead, what's crucial for the prayer's "authenticity" is simply whether the words are the correct words.

The Complexity of Similarity

Let's pause to take stock. Judgments about categories are often influenced by typicality, and we'll need to account for this fact in our theorizing.

Sometimes, though, category judgments are independent of typicality: You judge some candidates to be category members even though they bear no resemblance to the prototype (think about Moby Dick or the abused lemon). You judge some candidates not to be in the category even though they do resemble the prototype (think about counterfeit money or the disguised skunk).

We need to ask, therefore, how you think about categories when you're not guided by typicality. The answer, it seems, is that you focus on attributes that you believe are essential for each category. Your judgments about what's essential depend, in turn, on your *beliefs* about that category. Thus, you consider parentage when you're thinking about a category (like skunk or raccoon) for which you believe biological inheritance is important. You consider circumstances of printing when you're concerned with a category (like counterfeit money) that's shaped by your beliefs about economic systems. And so on.

Is it possible, though, that we're pushed into these complexities only because we've been discussing oddball categories such as abused citrus fruits and transformed forest animals? The answer is no, because similar complexities emerge in less exotic cases. The reason is that the prototype and exemplar views both depend, at their base, on judgments of *resemblance*—resemblance to the prototype or to some remembered instance—and resemblance, in turn, is itself a complex notion.

Imagine you're in the grocery store, and you decide to purchase some apples. According to prototype theory, you find these fruits by looking around in the produce section, seeking objects that resemble your apple prototype. But what exactly does this involve? More specifically, how do you assess this resemblance? The obvious suggestion is that objects will resemble each other if they share properties, and the more properties shared, the greater the resemblance. Let's say, then, that the items in the store share with your apple prototype a shape (round), a color (red), and a size (about 4 inches in diameter). That seems like a good basis for deciding the objects are apples, and so you're ready for your purchase.

But, in fact, this notion of "resemblance from shared properties" won't work. To see why, consider plums and lawn mowers; how much do these two things resemble each other? Common sense says they don't resemble each other all that much, but we'll reach the opposite conclusion if we simply count "shared properties" (Murphy & Medin, 1985). After all, both weigh less than a ton, both are found on Earth, both have a detectable odor, both are used by people, both can be dropped, both cost less than a thousand dollars, both are bigger than a grain of sand, both are unlikely birthday presents for your infant daughter, both contain carbon molecules, both cast a shadow on a sunny day. And on and on and on. With a little creativity, you could probably count thousands of properties shared by these two objects—but that doesn't change the basic assessment that there's not a close resemblance here. (For discussion, see Goldstone & Son, 2012; Goodman, 1972; Markman & Gentner, 2001; Medin, Goldstone, & Gentner, 1993.)

The solution to this puzzle is easy: Resemblance *does* depend on shared properties, but—more precisely—resemblance depends on whether the objects share *important, essential* properties. On this basis, you regard plums and lawn mowers as different from each other because the features they share are trivial or inconsequential. But, of course, this demands a question: How do you decide which features to ignore when assessing similarity and which features to consider? How do you decide, in comparing a plum and a lawn mower, which features are relevant and which ones can be set aside?

The answers to these questions bring us back to familiar territory, because your decisions about which features are important depend on your beliefs about the concept in question. Thus, in judging the resemblance between plums and lawn mowers, you were unimpressed that they share the feature "cost less than a thousand dollars." This is because you believe cost is irrelevant for these categories. (Imagine a lawn mower covered with diamonds; it would still be a lawn mower, wouldn't it?) But, of course, guided by other beliefs, you do consider cost for other categories. (Consider a necklace selling for $1; you're unlikely to categorize this necklace as a "luxury item.") Likewise, you don't perceive plums to be similar to lawn mowers even though both weigh less than a ton, because you know this attribute, too, is irrelevant for these categories. But you do consider weight in thinking about other categories. (Does a sumo wrestler resemble a hippopotamus? In this case, you might be swayed by weight.)

Overall, then, the idea here is that prototype use depends on judgments of resemblance, and these judgments depend in turn on your being able to focus on the features that are essential, so that you're not misled by trivial features. This point is in place when we're thinking about oddball judgments (like that mutilated lemon) or ordinary cases (plums, lawn mowers, or apples). And as we've seen, your decisions about which features are essential (cost or weight or whatever) vary from category to category, and they vary, in particular, according to your beliefs about what matters for that category.

BLUE GNU

Imagine that you encounter a creature and wonder what it is. Perhaps you reason, "This creature reminds me of the animal I saw in the zoo yesterday. The sign at the zoo indicated that the animal was a gnu, so this must be one, too. Of course, the gnu in the zoo was a different color and slightly smaller. But I bet that doesn't matter. Despite the new blue hue, this is a gnu, too." In this example, you've decided that color isn't a critical feature, and you categorize despite the contrast on this dimension. But you also know that color does matter for other categories, and so you know that something's off if a jeweler tries to sell you a green ruby or a red emerald. In case after case, therefore, whether in judging resemblance or in deciding on categorization, the features that you consider depend on the specific category.

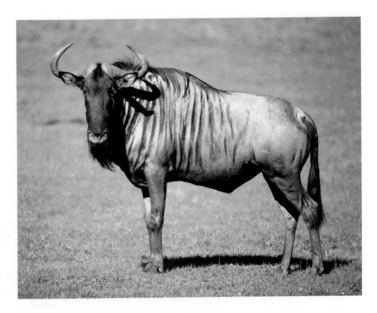

Concepts as Theories

Clearly, then, our theorizing needs to include more than prototypes and exemplars. Several pieces of evidence point this way, including the fact that whenever you *use* a prototype or exemplar, you're relying on a judgment of resemblance, and resemblance, we've now seen, depends on other knowledge—knowledge about which attributes to pay attention to in judging resemblance, and which ones to regard as trivial. But what is this other knowledge?

Explanatory Theories

In many of the cases we've discussed, your understanding of a concept seems to involve a network of interwoven beliefs linking the target concept to other concepts. To understand what counterfeit is, you need to know what money is, and probably what a government is, and what crime is. To understand what a raccoon is, you need to understand what parents are, and with that, you need to know some facts about life cycles, heredity, and the like.

Perhaps, therefore, we need to change our overall approach. We've been trying throughout this chapter to characterize concepts one by one, as though each concept could be characterized independently of other concepts. We talked about the prototype for bird, for example, without any thought about how this prototype is related to the animal prototype or the egg prototype. Maybe, though, we need a more holistic approach, one in which we place more emphasis on the interrelationships among concepts. This would enable us to include in our accounts the wide network of beliefs in which concepts seem to be embedded.

To see how this might play out, let's again consider the concept "raccoon." Your knowledge about this concept probably includes a raccoon prototype and some exemplars, and you rely on these representations in many settings. But your knowledge also includes your belief that raccoons are biological creatures (and therefore the offspring of adult raccoons) and also your belief that raccoons are wild animals (and therefore usually not pets, usually living in the woods). These various beliefs may not be sophisticated, and they may sometimes be inaccurate, but nonetheless they provide you with a broad cause-and-effect understanding of why raccoons are as they are. (Various authors have suggested different proposals for how we should conceptualize this web of beliefs. See, among others, Bang, Medin, & Atran, 2007; Keil, 1989, 2003; Lakoff, 1987; Markman & Gentner, 2001; Murphy, 2003; Rips et al., 2012.)

Guided by these considerations, many authors have suggested that each of us has something that we can think of as a "theory" about raccoons—what they are, how they act, and why they are as they are—and likewise a "theory" about most of the other concepts we hold. The theories are less precise, less elaborate, than a scientist's theory, but they serve the same function: They provide a crucial knowledge base that we rely on in our thinking about an object, event, or category; and they enable us to understand new facts we might encounter about the object or category.

The Function of Explanatory Theories

We've already suggested that your implicit "theories" influence how you *categorize* things—that is, your decisions about whether a test case is or is not in a particular category. This was crucial, for example, in our discussion of the abused lemon, the transformed raccoon, and the counterfeit bill. In each case, you relied on your background knowledge in deciding which features were crucial for the categorization and which one were not; then, with the features "selected" in this fashion, the new case before your eyes could be categorized appropriately.

As a different example, imagine that you see someone at a party jump fully clothed into a pool. Odds are good that you would decide this person belongs in the category "drunk," but why? Jumping into a pool in this way is surely not part of the *definition* of being drunk, and it's also unlikely to be part of the *prototype* (Medin & Ortony, 1989). But each of us has certain beliefs about how drunks behave; we have, in essence, a "theory" of drunkenness. This theory enables us to think through what being drunk will cause someone to do and not to do, and on this basis we would decide that, yes, someone who jumped into the pool fully clothed probably was inebriated.

You also draw on a "theory" when thinking about new possibilities for a category. For example, could an airplane fly if it were made of wood? What if it were ceramic? How about one made of whipped cream? You immediately reject this last option, because you know that a plane's function depends on its aerodynamic properties, and those, in turn, depend on the plane's shape. Whipped cream wouldn't hold its shape, and so it isn't a candidate for airplane construction. This is an easy conclusion to draw—but

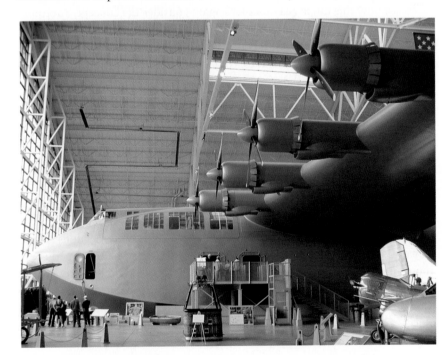

A WOODEN AIRPLANE?

Could an airplane be made of wood? Made from ceramic? Made from whipped cream? You immediately reject the last possibility, because your implicit "theory" about airplanes tells you that planes can fly only because of their wings' shape, and whipped cream wouldn't maintain this shape. Planes can, however, be made of wood—and this one (the famous *Spruce Goose*) was.

only because your concept "airplane" contains some ideas about why airplanes are as they are.

Your "theories" also affect how quickly you learn new concepts. Imagine that you're given a group of objects and must decide whether each belongs in Category A or Category B. Category A, you are told, includes all the objects that are metal, have a regular surface, are of medium size, and are easy to grasp. Category B, in contrast, includes objects that are not made of metal, have irregular surfaces, and are small and hard to grasp. This sorting task would be difficult—unless we give you another piece of information: namely, that Category A includes objects that could serve as substitutes for a hammer. With this clue, you immediately draw on your other knowledge about hammers, including your understanding of what a hammer is and how it's used. This understanding enables you to see why Category A's features aren't an arbitrary hodgepodge; instead, the features form a coherent package. And once you see this point, learning the experimenter's task (distinguishing Category A from Category B) is easy (Medin, 1989; Wattenmaker, Dewey, Murphy, & Medin, 1986; for related findings, see Heit & Bott, 2000; Kaplan & Murphy, 2000; Rehder & Ross, 2001).

Inferences Based on Theories

Here's another way in which theories guide your everyday concept use. If you meet my pet, Boaz, and decide that he's a dog, then you instantly know a great deal about Boaz—the sorts of things he's likely to do (bark, beg for treats, chase cats) and the sorts of things he's unlikely to do (climb trees, play chess, hibernate all winter). Likewise, if you learn some new fact about Boaz, you'll be able to make broad use of that knowledge—applying it to other creatures of his kind. If, for example, you learn that Boaz has sesamoid bones, you'll probably conclude that all dogs have sesamoid bones—and that perhaps other animals do, too.

These examples remind us of one of the reasons that categorization is so important: Categorization enables you to apply your general knowledge (e.g., knowledge about dogs) to new cases you encounter (e.g., Boaz). Conversely, categorization enables you to draw broad conclusions from your experience (so that things you learn about Boaz can be applied to other dogs you meet). All of this is possible, though, only because you realize that Boaz *is a dog*; without this simple realization, you wouldn't be able to use your knowledge in this way. But how exactly does this use-of-knowledge proceed?

Early research indicated that inferences about categories were guided by typicality. In one study, participants who were told a new fact about robins were willing to infer that the new fact would also be true for ducks. If they were told a new fact about ducks, however, they would not extrapolate to robins (Rips, 1975). Apparently, people were willing to make inferences from the typical case to the whole category, but not from an atypical case to the category. (For discussion of *why* people are more willing to draw conclusions from typical cases, see Murphy & Ross, 2005.)

WHY IS CATEGORIZATION SO IMPORTANT?

If you decide that Boaz is a dog, then you instantly know a great deal about him (e.g., that he's likely to bark and chase cats, unlikely to climb trees or play chess). In this way, categorization enables you to apply your general knowledge to new cases. And if you learn something new about Boaz (e.g., that he's at risk for a particular virus), you're likely to assume the same is true for other dogs. Thus, categorization also enables you to draw broad conclusions from specific experiences.

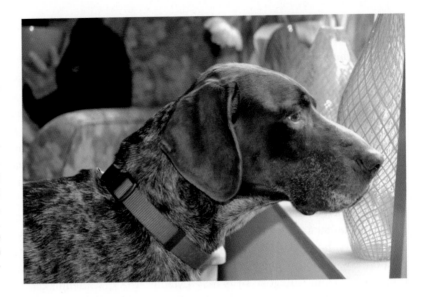

However, your inferences are also guided by your broader set of beliefs, and so, once again, we meet a case of concept use being shaped by the background knowledge that accompanies each concept. For example, if told that gazelle's blood contains a certain enzyme, people are willing to conclude that lion's blood contains the same enzyme. However, if told that lion's blood contains the enzyme, people are less willing to conclude that gazelle's blood does, too. The obvious explanation is that in the first case, people find it easy to imagine the property being transmitted from gazelles to lions via the food chain. Likewise, if told that grass contains a certain chemical, people are willing to believe that cows have the same chemical inside them. This makes perfect sense if people are thinking of the inference in terms of cause and effect, relying on their beliefs about how these concepts are related to each other (Medin, Coley, Storms, & Hayes, 2003; also see Heit, 2000; Heit & Feeney, 2005; Rehder & Hastie, 2004).

Different Profiles for Different Concepts

This proposal about "theories" and background knowledge has another important implication: People may think about different concepts in different ways. For example, most people believe that *natural kinds* (groups of objects that exist naturally in the world, such as bushes or alligators or stones or mountains) are as they are because of forces of nature, which are consistent across the years. As a result, the properties of these objects are relatively stable. There are, in effect, certain properties that a bush must have in order to survive as a bush; certain properties that a stone must have because of its chemical composition. Things are different, though, for *artifacts*, objects made by human beings. If we wished to make a table with 15 legs rather than 4, or one made of gold, we could do this. The design of tables, after all, is up to us; and the same is true for most artifacts.

This leads to the proposal that people will reason differently about natural kinds and artifacts—because they have different beliefs about why categories of either sort are as they are. We have already seen one result consistent with this idea: the finding that children would agree that toasters could be turned into coffeepots but not that skunks could be turned into raccoons. Plainly, the children had different ideas about artifacts (like toasters) than they had about animate objects (like skunks). Other results confirm this pattern: In general, people tend to assume more stability and more homogeneity when reasoning about natural kinds than when reasoning about artifacts (Atran, 1990; Coley, Medin, & Atran, 1997; Rehder & Hastie, 2001).

The diversity of concepts, as well as the role of beliefs, is also evident in another context: Many concepts can be characterized in terms of their features (e.g., the features that most dogs have, or the features that chairs usually have, and so on; after Markman & Rein, 2013). Other concepts, though, involve *goal-derived categories*, like "diet foods" or "exercise equipment" (Barsalou, 1983, 1985). Your understanding of concepts like these surely depends on your understanding of the goal (e.g., "losing weight") and some cause-and-effect beliefs about how a particular food might help you achieve that goal. Similar points apply to *relational categories* ("rivalry," "hunting") and *event categories* ("visits," "dates," "shopping trips"); here, too, you are plainly influenced by a web of beliefs about how various elements (the predator and the prey; the shopper and the store) are related to each other.

The contrasts among different types of concepts can also be detected in neuroscience evidence. For example, fMRI scans tell us that in healthy, intact brains, different sites are activated when people are thinking about living things than when they're thinking about nonliving things (e.g., Chao, Weisberg, & Martin, 2002), and likewise different sites are activated when people are thinking about manufactured objects (like tools) rather than natural objects (like rocks; Gerlach et al., 2002; Kellenbach et al. 2003).

Related evidence comes from cases in which people who have suffered brain damage. In some cases, these people lose the ability to name certain objects or to answer simple questions about these objects ("Does a whale have legs?") and often the problem is specific to certain categories. Thus some patients lose the ability to name living things but not nonliving things; other patients show the reverse pattern (Mahon & Caramazza, 2009; for an alternative conception of these data, though, see Warrington & Shallice, 1984; also Peru & Avesani, 2008; Phillips, Noppeney, Humphreys, & Price, 2002; Rips et al., 2012). Sometimes the symptoms caused by brain damage are even more specific, with some patients losing the ability to answer questions about fruits and vegetables but still being able to answer questions about other objects, living or nonliving (see **Figure 9.4**). These data certainly suggest that separate brain systems are responsible for different types of conceptual knowledge—with the result that damage to a particular brain area disrupts one type of knowledge but not others.

Let's also note that brain scans of healthy, intact brains often reveal activation in *sensory* and *motor* areas when people are thinking about various

FIGURE 9.4 DIFFERENT BRAIN SITES SUPPORT DIFFERENT CATEGORIES

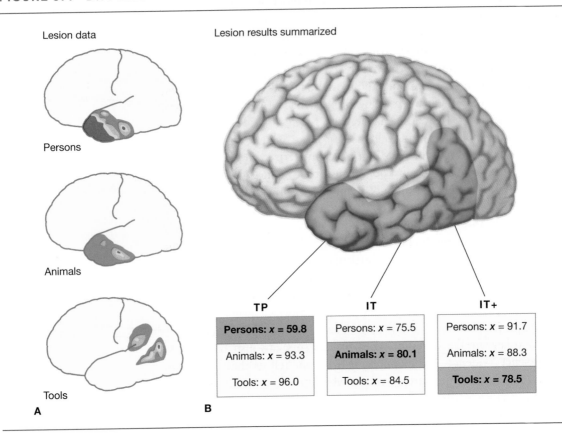

Brain damage often causes **anomia**—an inability to name common objects. But the specific loss depends on where exactly the brain damage has occurred. Panel A summarizes lesion data for patients who had difficulty naming persons (top), animals (middle), or tools (bottom). The colors indicate the percentage of patients with damage at each site: red, most patients; purple, few. Panel B offers a different summary of the data: Patients with damage in the brain's temporal pole (TP, shown in blue) had difficulty naming persons (only 59.8% correct) but were easily able to name animals and tools. Patients with damage in the inferotemporal region (IT, shown in red) had difficulty naming persons and animals but did somewhat better naming tools. Finally, patients with damage in the lateral occipital region (IT+) had difficulty naming tools but did reasonably well naming animals and persons.   AFTER DAMASIO, GRABOWSKI, TRANEL, HICHWA, & DAMASIO, 1996.

concepts (Mahon & Caramazza, 2009; McRae & Jones, 2012). This finding suggests that our seemingly abstract conceptual knowledge is intertwined with knowledge about what particular objects look like (or sound like or feel like) and also with knowledge about how one might interact with the object. (For related data, see Binder & Desai, 2011.) This point fits well with another theme we have been developing—namely, that conceptual knowledge has many elements.

The Knowledge Network

Overall, then, our theorizing is going to need some complexities. We need to distinguish between categories that represent natural kinds and categories of artifacts, and perhaps offer a different account for concepts that are goal-derived or relational. We may need to include, in a category's representation, "sensory knowledge" and "muscular" knowledge. Across all of this diversity, though, one idea emerges again and again: How you think about your concepts, how you use your concepts, and indeed, what your concepts *are*, are all shaped by a broad web of beliefs and background knowledge. But what does this "web of beliefs" involve?

Traveling through the Network to Retrieve Knowledge

In earlier chapters, we explored the notion that information in long-term memory is represented by means of a network, with associative links connecting nodes to each other. Let's now carry this proposal one step further: The associative links don't just tie together the various bits of knowledge; they also help *represent* the knowledge. For example, you know that George Washington was an American president. As a first approximation, this simple idea can be represented as an associative link between a node representing WASHINGTON and a node representing PRESIDENT. In other words, the link itself is a constituent of the knowledge.

If knowledge is stored via the memory network, then, whenever you draw on your knowledge, you're retrieving information from the network, and this retrieval presumably uses the processes we've already described—with activation spreading from one node to the next. This spread of activation is quick, but it does take time, and the further the activation must travel, the more time needed. Therefore, you'll need less time to retrieve knowledge involving closely related ideas, more time to retrieve knowledge about more distant ideas.

Collins and Quillian (1969) tested this prediction many years ago, using the *sentence verification task* described earlier in this chapter. Their participants were shown sentences such as "A robin is a bird" or "Cats have claws" or "Cats have hearts." Mixed together with these obviously true sentences were a variety of false sentences (e.g., "A cat is a bird"). In response to each sentence, participants had to hit a "true" or "false" button as quickly as they could.

Participants presumably perform this task by "traveling" through the network, seeking a connection between nodes. Thus, when the participant finds the connection from, say, the ROBIN node to the BIRD node, this confirms that there is, in fact, an associative path linking these nodes, which tells the participant that the sentence about these two concepts is true. This travel should require little time if the two nodes are directly linked by an association, as ROBIN and BIRD probably are (see **Figure 9.5**). In this case, we'd expect participants to answer "true" rather quickly. The travel will require more time, however, if the two nodes are connected only indirectly (e.g., ROBIN and

FIGURE 9.5   HYPOTHETICAL MEMORY STRUCTURE FOR KNOWLEDGE ABOUT ANIMALS

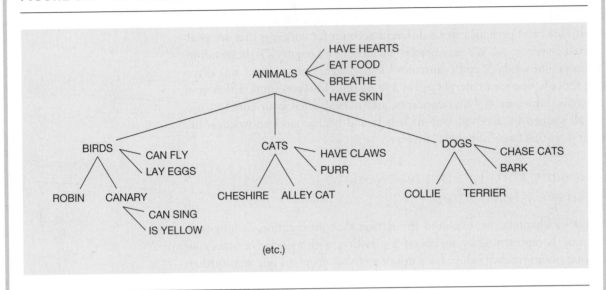

Collins and Quillian proposed that the memory system avoids redundant storage of connections between CATS and HAVE HEARTS, and between DOGS and HAVE HEARTS, and so on for all the other animals. Instead, HAVE HEARTS is stored as a property of all animals. To confirm that cats have hearts, therefore, you must traverse two links: from CATS to ANIMALS, and from ANIMALS to HAVE HEARTS.   AFTER COLLINS & QUILLIAN, 1969.

ANIMAL), and so we'd expect slower responses to sentences that require a "two-step" connection than to sentences that require a single connection.

In addition, Collins and Quillian argued that there is no point in storing in memory the fact that cats have hearts *and* the fact that dogs have hearts *and* the fact that squirrels have hearts. Instead, they proposed, it would be more efficient just to store the fact that these various creatures are animals, and then the separate fact that animals have hearts. Hence, the property "has a heart" would be associated with the ANIMAL node rather than the nodes for each individual animal, and the same is true for all the other properties of animals, as shown in the figure. According to this logic, we should expect relatively slow responses to sentences like "Cats have hearts," since, to choose a response, a participant must locate the linkage from CAT to ANIMAL and then a second linkage from ANIMAL to HEART. We would expect a quicker response to "Cats have claws," because here there would be a direct connection between CAT and the node representing this property: All cats have claws, but other animals do not, and so this information could not be entered at the higher level.

As **Figure 9.6** shows, these predictions are borne out. Responses to sentences like "A canary is a canary" take approximately 1 second (1,000 ms). This is presumably the time it takes just to read the sentence and to move your finger on the response button. Sentences like "A canary can sing" require an additional

FIGURE 9.6 TIME NEEDED TO CONFIRM VARIOUS
SEMANTIC FACTS

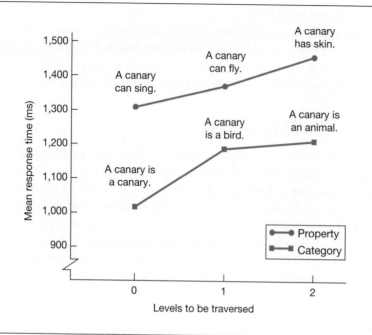

In a sentence verification task, participants' responses were fastest when the test required them to traverse zero links in memory ("A canary is a canary"), slower when the necessary ideas were separated by one link, and slower still if the ideas were separated by two links. Responses were also slower if participants had to take the additional step of traversing the link from a category label ("bird") to the node representing a property of the category ("can fly").   AFTER COLLINS & QUILLIAN, 1969.

step of traversing one link in memory and yield slower responses. Sentences like "A canary can fly" require the traversing of two links, from CANARY to BIRDS and then from BIRDS to CAN FLY, so they are correspondingly slower.

More recent data, however, add some complications. For example, we saw earlier in the chapter that verifications are faster if a sentence involves creatures close to the prototype—and so responses are faster to, say, "A canary is a bird" than to "An ostrich is a bird." This difference isn't reflected in Figure 9.6, nor is it explained by the layout in Figure 9.5. Clearly, then, the Collins and Quillian view is incomplete.

In addition, the principle of "nonredundancy" proposed by Collins and Quillian doesn't always hold. For example, the property of "having feathers" should, on their view, be associated with the BIRDS node rather than (redundantly) with the ROBIN node, the PIGEON node, and so forth. This fits with the fact that responses are relatively slow to sentences like "Sparrows have feathers." However, it turns out that participants respond rather quickly to a sentence like "Peacocks have feathers." This is because in observing peacocks, you often think about their prominent tail feathers (Conrad, 1972). Thus, even though it is informationally redundant, a strong association between PEACOCK and FEATHERS is likely to be established.

Even with these complications, the fact remains that we can often predict the speed of knowledge access by counting the number of nodes participants must traverse in answering a question. This observation powerfully confirms the claim that associative links play a pivotal role in knowledge representation.

Propositional Networks

To represent the full fabric of your knowledge, however, we'll need more than simple associations. After all, we need somehow to represent the contrast between "Sam has a dog" and "Sam is a dog." If all we had is an association between SAM and DOG, we wouldn't be able to tell these two ideas apart. Early theorizing sought to deal with this problem by introducing different types of associative links, with some representing equivalence (or partial equivalence) relations and others representing possessive relations. These links were termed *isa* links, as in "Sam *isa* dog," and *hasa* links, as in "A bird *hasa* head" or "Sam *hasa* dog" (Norman, Rumelhart, & Group, 1975).

Later theorists, however, have sought ways in which networks can represent more complex ideas. One proposal was developed by John Anderson (1976, 1980, 1993; Anderson & Bower, 1973), and at the center of this conception is the idea of **propositions**, defined in this setting as the smallest units of knowledge that can be either true or false. For example, "Children love candy" is a proposition, but "Children" is not; "Susan likes blue cars" is a proposition, but "blue cars" is not. Propositions are easily represented as sentences, but this is merely a convenience. Propositions can also be represented in various nonlinguistic forms, including a structure of nodes and linkages, and that is exactly what Anderson's model does.

Figure 9.7 provides an example. Here, the ellipses identify the propositions themselves (thus, each ellipse identifies a new proposition). Associations connect an ellipse to the ideas that are the proposition's constituents. The associations are labeled, but only in general terms—terms that specify the constituent's role within that proposition. This enables us to distinguish, say, the proposition "Dogs chase cats" (shown in the figure) from the proposition "Cats chase dogs" (not shown). (For more on how this network can store information, see **Figure 9.8**.)

Anderson's model shares many claims with the network theorizing we discussed in earlier chapters: Nodes are connected by associative links. Some of these links are stronger than others. The strength of a link depends on how frequently and recently it has been used. Once a node is activated, the process of spreading activation causes nearby nodes to become activated as well. The model is distinctive, however, in its attempt to represent knowledge in terms of propositions, and the promise of this approach has attracted the support of many researchers.

FIGURE 9.7 NETWORK REPRESENTATIONS OF SOME OF YOUR KNOWLEDGE ABOUT DOGS

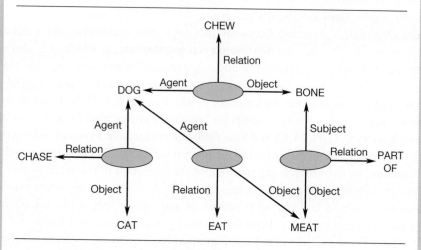

Your understanding of dogs—what dogs are, what they are likely to do—is represented by an interconnected network of propositions, with each proposition being indicated by an ellipse. Labels on the arrows indicate each node's role within the proposition. AFTER ANDERSON, 1980.

FIGURE 9.8 REPRESENTING EPISODES WITHIN A PROPOSITIONAL NETWORK

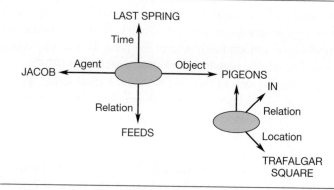

In order to represent episodes, the propositional network includes time and location nodes. This fragment of a network represents two propositions: the proposition that Jacob fed pigeons last spring, and the proposition that the pigeons are in Trafalgar Square. Note that no time node is associated with the proposition about pigeons being in Trafalgar Square. Therefore, what is represented is that the feeding of the pigeons took place last spring but that the pigeons are always in the square.

Distributed Processing

In a model like Anderson's, individual ideas are represented with **local representations**: Each node represents one idea, so that when that node is activated, you're thinking about that idea, and when you're thinking about that idea, that node is activated. **Connectionist networks**, in contrast, take a different approach. They rely on **distributed representations**, in which each idea is represented, not by a certain set of nodes, but instead by means of a specific pattern of activation across the network. To take a simple case, the concept "birthday" might be represented by a pattern in which nodes B, F, H, N, P, and R are firing, whereas the concept "computer" might be represented by a pattern in which nodes C, G, H, M, O, and S are firing. Note that node H is part of both of these patterns and probably part of the pattern for many other concepts as well. Therefore, we can't attach any meaning or interpretation to this node by itself; we can only learn what is being represented by looking at many other nodes simultaneously to find out what pattern of activation exists across the entire network. (For more on local and distributed representations, see Chapter 4.)

This reliance on distributed representation has important consequences for how a connectionist network functions. Imagine being asked what sort of computer you use. For you to respond, the idea "computer" needs to trigger the idea "MacBook" (or "Toshiba" or whatever it is you have). In a distributed network, this means that the many nodes representing "computer" have to manage collectively to activate the many nodes representing "MacBook." To continue our simple illustration, node C has to trigger node L at the same time that node G triggers node A, and so on, leading ultimately to the activation of the L-A-F-J-T-R combination that, let's say, represents "MacBook." In short, a network using distributed representations must use processes that are similarly distributed, so that one widespread activation pattern can have broad enough effects to evoke a different (but equally widespread) pattern. In addition, the steps bringing this about must all occur simultaneously—in parallel—with each other, so that one entire representation can smoothly trigger the next. This is why connectionist models are said to involve **parallel distributed processing (PDP)**.

Many argue that models of this sort make biological sense. We know that the brain relies on parallel processing, with ongoing activity in many regions simultaneously. We also know that the brain uses a "divide and conquer" strategy, with complex tasks being broken down into small components, and with separate brain areas working on each component. In addition, PDP models are remarkably powerful: According to many researchers, computers relying on this sort of processing have learned the rules of English grammar, have learned how to read, and have even learned how to play strategic games like backgammon (e.g., MacDonald, 1995; Marcus, 2001; Rogers & McClelland, 2014). Related, PDP models have an excellent capacity for detecting *patterns* in the input they receive, despite a range of variations in how the pattern is implemented. Thus, the models can recognize a variety of different sentences as all having the same structure, and a variety of game positions as all inviting the same next move. As a result, these models are impressively able to generalize what they have "learned" to new, never-seen-before variations on the pattern.

Learning as the Setting of Connection Weights

How do PDP models manage to detect patterns? How do these models "learn"? Recall that in any associative network, knowledge is represented by the associations themselves. To return to an earlier example, the knowledge that "George Washington was president" is represented via a link between the nodes representing WASHINGTON and those representing PRESIDENT. When we first introduced this example, we phrased it in terms of local representations, with individual nodes having specific referents. The idea, however, is the same in a distributed system. What it means to know this fact about Washington is to have a pattern of connections among the many nodes that together represent "Washington" and the many nodes that together represent "president." Once these connections are in place, activation of either of these patterns will lead to the activation of the other.

Notice, then, that knowledge refers to a *potential* rather than to a *state*. If you know that Washington was a president, then the connections are in place so that if the "Washington" pattern of activations occurs, this will lead to the "president" pattern of activations. And, of course, this state of readiness will remain even if you happen not to be thinking about Washington right now. In this way, "knowing" something, in network terms, corresponds to how the activation will flow *if* there is activation on the scene. This is different from "thinking about" something, which corresponds to which nodes are active at a particular moment, with no comment about where that activation will spread next.

In this view, "learning" must involve some sort of adjustments of the connections among nodes, so that after learning, activation will flow in a fashion that can represent the newly gained knowledge. Technically, we would say that learning involves the adjustment of **connection weights**—the strength of the individual connections among nodes. Moreover, in this type of modeling, learning requires the adjustment of *many* connection weights: We need to adjust the connections, for example, so that the thousands of nodes representing "Washington" manage, together, to activate the thousands of nodes representing "president." Thus, learning, just like everything else in the connectionist scheme, is a distributed process involving thousands of changes across the network.

Concepts: Putting the Pieces Together

We have now covered a lot of ground—discussing both individual concepts and also how these concepts might be woven together, via the network, to form larger patterns of knowledge. We've also talked a bit about how the network itself might be set up—with knowledge perhaps being represented by propositions, or perhaps via a connectionist network. But in the end, where does all of this leave us?

You might think that there's nothing glorious or complicated about knowing what a dog is, or a lemon, or a fish. Your use of these concepts is effortless and ubiquitous, and so is your use of thousands of other concepts. No one over the age of 4 takes special pride in knowing what an odd number is, nor do people find it challenging to make the elementary sorts of judgments we've considered throughout this chapter.

As we've seen, though, human conceptual knowledge is impressively complex. At the very least, this knowledge contains several parts. People probably have a prototype for most of their concepts, as well as a set of remembered exemplars, and use them for a range of fast and easy judgments about the relevant category. People also seem to have a set of beliefs about each concept they hold, and (among other points) these beliefs reflect the person's understanding of cause-and-effect relationships in the world—and so why it is that drunks act as they do, or how it could be that enzymes found in gazelles might be transmitted to lions. These beliefs, in turn, are woven into the broader network that manages to store all the information in your memory, and that network influences how you categorize items and also how you reason about the objects in your world.

Apparently, then, even our simplest concepts require a multifaceted representation in our minds, and at least part of this representation (the "theory") seems reasonably sophisticated. It is all this richness, presumably, that makes human conceptual knowledge extremely powerful and flexible—and so easy to use in a remarkable range of circumstances.

COGNITIVE PSYCHOLOGY AND THE LAW

Defining Legal Concepts

In many court cases, the judge's or jury's task lies in categorizing someone's actions. A jury might need to decide, for example, whether a defendant's actions fall into the category of "sexual harassment." (If the defendant was offensive in some way, but his actions don't fit into the category of "harassment," then he isn't guilty of harassment.) Or, as a different example, a jury might be certain that the defendant caused someone's death, but they still need to decide whether the crime should be categorized as "first-degree murder" or "second-degree," a categorization with large implications for the likely punishment.

To help with this categorization, laws define each crime in precise terms, so that there is a careful definition of "robbery," a clear definition of "trespassing" or "first-degree murder," and so on. Even with these definitions, though, the courts regularly encounter ambiguous cases, raising questions about whether the person's actions satisfy the definition of the crime the person is charged with. At the least, this reminds us how difficult it is to find satisfactory, broadly useful definitions for concepts, a point that was important throughout Chapter 9. But, in addition, we need to ask: How do the courts proceed when they encounter one of these ambiguous cases?

We've seen that people have prototypes in mind for their various concepts, and so, in day to day life, they often assess a new case by asking how closely it resembles that prototype. It turns out that, in the courts, jurors do the same in making legal judgments, and so they're more likely to convict someone if the trial facts fit with their prototype for the crime—if the facts fit the jurors' notion of, say, a "typical bank robbery" or a "typical hit-and-run violation." Put differently, a "typical" crime with weak evidence is more likely to lead to a conviction than an unusual crime with similarly weak evidence. Of course, this is legally nonsensical: Jury decisions should depend on the quantity and quality of the evidence, and on the legal definition of the crime. The jurors' ideas about what's typical for that crime should play no role at all—especially when we acknowledge that these ideas are shaped more by TV crime shows than by actual crime statistics. Nonetheless, the prototypes do influence the jury, and so legal judgments (like concept use in general) are plainly shaped by typicality.

In addition, we've seen that concept users often seem to have a "theory" in mind about why a concept is as it is, and they use the theory in reasoning about the concept. The chapter used the example of someone jumping into a pool fully clothed. You're likely to categorize this person as a "drunk," not because the person fits your definition for being drunk or even fits your prototype, but because you have a set of beliefs about how drunks are likely to act. Based on those beliefs (i.e., based on your "theory"), you decide that drunkenness is the most plausible explanation for the behavior you just observed, and you categorize accordingly.

Similar categorization strategies are evident in the courtroom. For example, consider the crime of stalking. This crime is difficult to define in a crisp way; in fact, it is defined in different ways in different states. Often, though, the definition includes the notion that the stalker intended to force some sort of relationship with the victim—perhaps a relationship involving intimacy or a relationship in which the victim feels fear. It's often the case, however, that there's no direct evidence of this intention, so the jury needs to infer the intention from the defendant's behaviors, or from the context.

In making these inferences, juries rely on their "theory" of stalking—their beliefs about how and why one individual might stalk another. This helps us understand why juries are more likely to convict someone of stalking if (for example) the defendant was a former intimate of the person being "stalked." Apparently, jurors are guided by their ideas about how former (but now rejected) lovers behave—even if these ideas have nothing to do with the legal definition of stalking.

How should we think about these points? On one side, we want jurors to be guided by the law, and not by their (perhaps idiosyncratic, perhaps uninformed) intuitions about the crime at issue in a trial. On the other side, the U.S. criminal justice system relies on the good sense and good judgment of juries—so plainly we want jurors to use their judgment. How best to balance these points isn't clear, but the tension between these points is perhaps inevitable, given what we know about human concepts and human categorization.

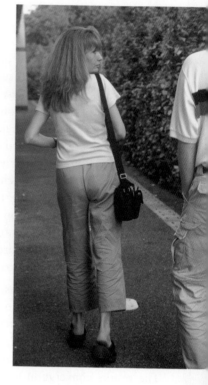

STALKING

The crime of stalking is difficult to define, and in court cases involving stalking, juries are often influenced by their commonsense beliefs about what stalking "typically" involves.

chapter summary

● People cannot provide definitions for most of the concepts they use; this suggests that knowing a concept and being able to use it competently do not require knowing a definition. However, when trying to define a term, people mention properties that are indeed closely associated with the concept. One proposal, therefore, is that your knowledge specifies what is typical for each concept, rather than naming properties that are truly definitive for the concept. Concepts based on typicality will have a family resemblance structure, with different category members sharing features but with no features being shared by the entire group.

● Concepts may be represented in the mind via prototypes, with each prototype representing what is most typical for that category. This implies that categories will have graded membership, and many research results are consistent with this prediction. The results converge in identifying some category members as "better" members of the category. This is reflected in sentence verification tasks, production tasks, explicit judgments of typicality, and so on.

● In addition, basic-level categories seem to be the categories we learn earliest and use most often. Basic-level categories (like "chair") are more homogeneous than their superordinate categories ("furniture") and much broader than their subordinate categories ("armchair"), and they are also usually represented by a single word.

● Typicality results can also be explained with a model that relies on specific category exemplars, and with category judgments made by the drawing of analogies to these remembered exemplars. The exemplar model can explain your ability to view categories from a new perspective. Even so, prototypes provide an efficient summary of what is typical for the category. Perhaps it is not surprising, therefore, that your conceptual knowledge includes exemplars and prototypes.

● Sometimes categorization does not depend at all on whether the test case resembles a prototype or a category exemplar. This is evident with some abstract categories ("even number") and some weird cases (a mutilated lemon), but it is also evident with more mundane categories ("raccoon"). In these examples, categorization seems to depend on knowledge about a category's essential properties.

● Knowledge about essential properties is not just a supplement to categorization via resemblance. Instead, knowledge about essential properties may be a *prerequisite* for judgments of resemblance. With this knowledge, you are able to assess resemblance with regard to just those properties that truly matter for the category and not be misled by irrelevant or accidental properties.

● The properties that are essential for a category vary from one category to the next. The identification of these properties seems to depend on beliefs held about the category, including causal beliefs that specify why the category features are as they are. These beliefs are implicit theories, and they describe the category not in isolation but in relation to various other concepts.

● Researchers have proposed that knowledge is stored within the same memory network that we have discussed in earlier chapters. Searching through this network seems to resemble travel in the sense that greater travel distances (more connections to be traversed) require more time.

● Early proposals tried to represent knowledge with a small number of types of associative links, including *isa* and *hasa* links. However, to store all of knowledge, the network may need more than simple associations. One proposal is that the network stores propositions, with different nodes each playing the appropriate role within the proposition.

● A different proposal is that knowledge is contained in memory via distributed representations. These representations require distributed processes, including the processes that adjust connection weights to allow the creation of new knowledge.

ⓔ eBook Demonstrations & Essays

Online Demonstrations:
- Demonstration 9.1: The Search for Definitions
- Demonstration 9.2: Assessing Typicality
- Demonstration 9.3: Basic-Level Categories

Online Applying Cognitive Psychology Essays:
- Cognitive Psychology and Education: Learning New Concepts

ZAPS 2.0 Cognition Labs

- Go to **http://digital.wwnorton.com/cognition6** for the online labs relevant to this chapter.

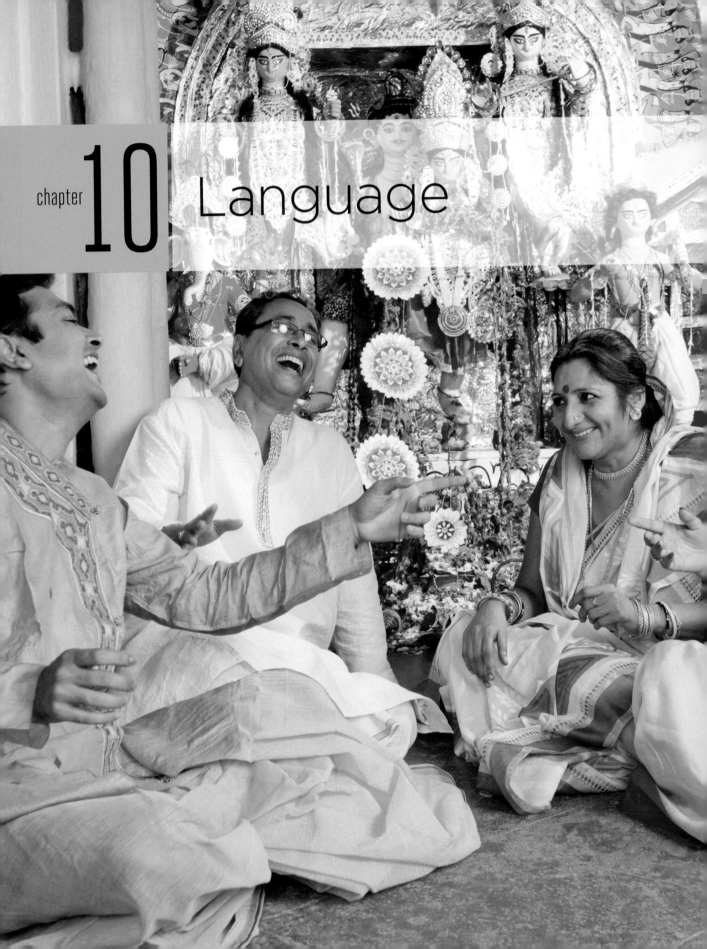

chapter 10

Language

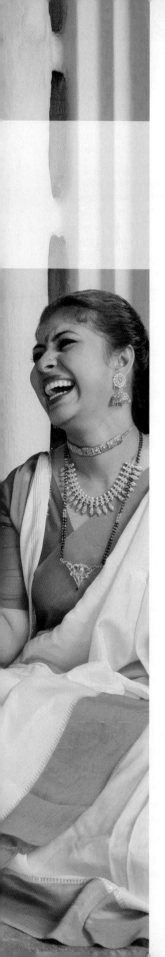

what if...

On January 8, 2011, Congresswoman Gabby Giffords was meeting with citizens outside a Safeway grocery store near Tucson, Arizona. A man ran up to the crowd and began shooting. Six people were killed; Giffords was among the others who were wounded. A bullet had passed through her head, traveling the length of her brain's left side and causing extensive damage.

As a result of her brain injury, Giffords has suffered from many profound difficulties, including a massive disruption of her language capacity, and her case has brought enormous public attention to the disorder termed "aphasia"—a loss of the ability to produce and understand ordinary language. In the years since the shooting, Giffords has shown a wonderful degree of recovery—but she will never recover fully. Just five months after the injury, an aide announced that her ability to *comprehend* language had returned to a level that was "close to normal, if not normal." Her progress has been slower for language *production*. Consider an interview she gave in early 2014. Giffords had, on the third anniversary of her shooting, decided to celebrate life by skydiving. In a TV interview, she described the experience: "Oh, wonderful sky. Gorgeous mountain. Blue skies. I like a lot. A lot of fun. Peaceful, so peaceful."

Giffords's recovery is remarkable but—sadly—not typical. The outcome for patients with aphasia is highly variable, and many patients recover far less of their language ability than Giffords has. Her case is typical, though, in other ways: Different brain areas control the comprehension and the production of speech, so it is common for one of these capacities to be spared while the other is damaged, and the prospects for recovery are generally better for language comprehension than for production. And like Giffords, many patients with aphasia retain the ability to *sing* even if they have lost the ability to *speak*, a clear indication that these seemingly similar activities are controlled by different processes.

Giffords also shares with other aphasic patients the horrific frustration of aphasia. Aphasia is, after all, a disorder of *language*, not a disorder of *thought*. Thus, patients with aphasia can think normally but (with great difficulty, and often only later) complain that they are "trapped" in their own heads, unable to express what they are thinking. They are

• Language can be understood as having a hierarchical structure—with units at each level being assembled to form the larger units at the next level.

• At each level in the hierarchy, we can endlessly combine and recombine units, but the combinations seem to be governed by rules of various sorts. The rules provide the explanation of why some combinations of elements are rare and others seem prohibited outright. Within the boundaries created by these rules, though, language is *generative*, so any user of the language can create new forms (new sound combinations, new words, new phrases).

• A different set of principles describes how, moment by moment, people interpret the sentences they hear or read; in this process, people are guided by many factors, including syntax, semantics, and contextual information.

• In interpreting sentences, people seem to use a "compile as you go" strategy, trying to figure out the role of each word the moment it arrives. This approach is efficient but can lead to error.

• Our extraordinary skill in using language is made possible in part by the fact that large portions of the brain are specialized for language use, making it clear that we are, in a literal sense, a "linguistic species."

• Finally, language surely influences our thoughts, but in an indirect fashion: Language is one of many ways to draw our attention to this or that aspect of the environment. This shapes our experience, which in turn shapes our cognition.

sometimes forced to grunt and point in hopes of conveying their meaning; in other cases, their speech is so slurred that others cannot understand them, so they are caught in a situation of trying again and again to express themselves—but often without success.

To understand this deep frustration, bear in mind that we use language (whether it's the spoken language most of us use or the sign language of the deaf) to convey our ideas to one another, and our wishes and our needs. Without language, cooperative endeavors would be a thousand times more difficult—if possible at all. Without language, the acquisition of knowledge would be enormously impaired. Plainly, then, language capacity is crucial for us all, and in this chapter we'll consider the nature of this extraordinary and uniquely human skill.

The Organization of Language

Language use involves a special type of translation. I might, for example, want to tell you about a happy event in my life, and so I need to translate my ideas about the event into sounds that I can utter. You, in turn, detect those sounds and need to convert them into some sort of comprehension. How does this translation—from ideas to sounds, and then back to ideas—take place?

The answer lies in the fact that language relies on well-defined patterns— patterns in how individual words are used, patterns in how words are put together into phrases. I follow those patterns when I express my ideas, and the same patterns guide you when you're figuring out what I just said. In essence, then, we're both using the same "codebook," with the result that (most of the time) you can understand my messages, and I yours.

But where does this "codebook" come from? And what's in the codebook? More concretely, what are the patterns of English (or whatever language you speak) that—apparently—we all know and use? As a first step toward tackling these issues, let's note that language has a structure, as depicted in **Figure 10.1**. At the highest level of the structure (not shown in the figure) are the ideas intended by the speaker, or the ideas that the listener derives from the input. These ideas are typically expressed in **sentences**— coherent sequences of words that express the intended meaning of a speaker. Sentences, in turn, are composed of phrases, which are in turn composed of words. Words are composed of **morphemes**, the smallest language units that carry meaning. Some morphemes, like "umpire" or "talk," are units that can stand alone, and they typically refer to particular objects, ideas, or actions. Other morphemes get "bound" onto these "free" morphemes and add information crucial for interpretation. Examples of bound morphemes in Figure 10.1 are the past-tense morpheme "ed" and the plural morpheme "s." Then, finally, in spoken language, morphemes are conveyed by sounds called **phonemes**, defined as the smallest unit of sound that can serve to distinguish words in language.

FIGURE 10.1 THE HIERARCHY OF LINGUISTIC UNITS

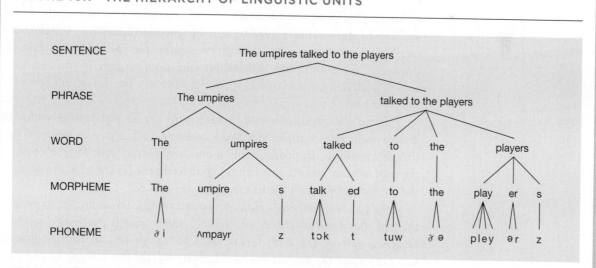

It is useful to think of language as having a hierarchical structure. At the top of the hierarchy, there are sentences. These are composed of phrases, which are themselves composed of words. The words are composed of morphemes, and when the morphemes are pronounced, the units of sound are called "phonemes." In describing phonemes, the symbols correspond to the actual sounds produced, independent of how these sounds are expressed in ordinary writing.

Language is also organized in another way: Within each of these levels, people can combine and recombine the units to produce novel utterances—assembling phonemes into brand-new morphemes or assembling words into brand-new phrases. Crucially, though, not all combinations are possible—so that a new breakfast cereal (for example) might be called "Klof" but would probably seem strange to English speakers if it were called "Ngof." Likewise, someone might utter the novel sentence "I admired the lurking octopi" but almost certainly would not say, "Octupi admired the I lurking." What lies behind these points? Why are some sequences acceptable—even if strange—while others seem awkward or even unacceptable?

Phonology

Let's use the hierarchy in Figure 10.1 as a way to organize our examination of language. We'll start at the bottom of the hierarchy—with the sounds of speech.

The Production of Speech

In ordinary breathing, air flows quietly out of the lungs and up through the nose and mouth (see **Figure 10.2**). Noise is produced, however, if this airflow is interrupted or altered, and this capability enables humans to produce a wide range of different sounds.

For example, within the larynx there are two flaps of muscular tissue called the "vocal folds." (These structures are also called the "vocal cords," although they're not cords at all.) The vocal folds can be rapidly opened and closed, producing a buzzing sort of vibration known as **voicing**. You can feel this vibration by putting your palm on your throat while you produce a [z] sound. You will feel no vibration, though, if you hiss like a snake, producing a sustained [s] sound. (Try it!) The [z] sound is voiced; the [s] is not.

You can also produce sound by narrowing the air passageway within the mouth itself. For example, hiss like a snake again and pay attention to your tongue's position. To produce this sound, you placed your tongue's tip near the roof of your mouth, just behind your teeth; the [s] sound is the sound of the air rushing through the narrow gap you created.

If the gap is elsewhere, a different sound results. For example, to produce the [sh] sound (as in "shoot" or "shine"), the tongue is positioned so that it creates a narrow gap a bit further back in the mouth; air rushing through this gap causes the desired sound. Alternatively, the narrow gap can be more toward the front. Pronounce an [f] sound; in this case, the sound is produced by air rushing between your bottom lip and your top teeth.

These various aspects of speech production provide a basis for categorizing speech sounds. We can distinguish sounds, first, according to how the airflow is restricted; this is referred to as **manner of production**. Thus, air is allowed to move through the nose for some speech sounds but not others. Similarly, for some speech sounds, the flow of air is fully stopped for a moment (e.g., [p], [b], and [t]). For other sounds, the air passage is restricted, but air continues to flow (e.g., [f], [z], and [r]).

Second, we can distinguish between sounds that are voiced—produced with the vocal folds vibrating—and those that are not. The sounds of [v], [z], and [n] (to name a few) are voiced; [f], [s], [t], and [k] are unvoiced. (You can confirm this by running the hand-on-throat test while producing each of these sounds.) Finally, sounds can be categorized according to where the airflow is restricted; this is referred to as **place of articulation**. Thus, you close your lips to produce "bilabial" sounds like [p] and [b]; you place your top teeth close to your bottom lip to produce "labiodental" sounds like [f]

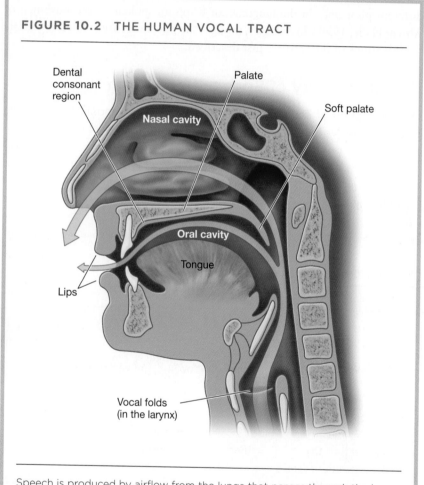

FIGURE 10.2   THE HUMAN VOCAL TRACT

Dental
consonant
region

Palate

Soft palate

Nasal cavity

Oral cavity

Tongue

Lips

Vocal folds
(in the larynx)

Speech is produced by airflow from the lungs that passes through the larynx and from there through the oral and nasal cavities. Different vowels are created by movements of the lips and tongue that change the size and shape of the vocal cavity. Consonants are produced by movements that temporarily obstruct the airflow through the vocal tract.

and [v]; and you place your tongue just behind your upper teeth to produce "alveolar" sounds like [t] and [d].

This categorization scheme enables us to describe any speech sound in terms of a few simple features. For example, what are the features of a [p] sound? First, we specify the manner of production: This sound is produced with air moving through the mouth (not the nose) and with a full interruption to the flow of air. Second, voicing: The [p] sound happens to be unvoiced. Third, place of articulation: The [p] sound is bilabial. These features are all we need to identify the [p], and if any of these features changes, so does the sound's identity.

In English, these features of sound production are combined and recombined to produce 40 or so different phonemes. Other languages use as few as a dozen phonemes; still others, many more. (For example, there are 141 different phonemes in the language of Khoisan, spoken by the Bushmen of Africa; Halle, 1990.) In all cases, though, the phonemes are created by simple combinations of the features just described.

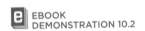

EBOOK
DEMONSTRATION 10.1

The Complexity of Speech Perception

Our description of speech sounds invites a simple proposal about speech *perception*. We've just said that each speech sound can be defined in terms of a small number of features. Perhaps, then, all a perceiver needs to do is detect these features, and with this done, the speech sounds are identified.

EBOOK
DEMONSTRATION 10.2

It turns out, though, that speech perception is more complicated than this. Consider **Figure 10.3**, which shows the moment-by-moment sound amplitudes

FIGURE 10.3 THE ACTUAL PATTERN OF SPEECH

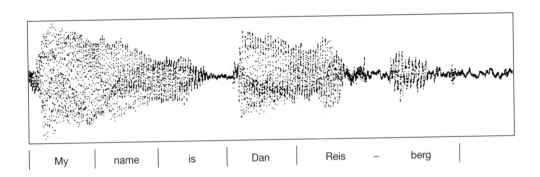

| My | name | is | Dan | Reis | – | berg | |

Shown here are the moment-by-moment sound amplitudes produced by the author uttering a greeting. Notice that there is no gap between the sounds carrying the word "my" and the sounds carrying "name." Nor is there a gap between the sounds carrying "name" and the sounds carrying "is." Therefore, the listener needs to figure out where one sound stops and the next begins, a process known as "segmentation."

produced by a speaker uttering a brief greeting. It's these amplitudes, in the form of air-pressure changes, that reach the ear, and so, in an important sense, the figure shows the pattern of input with which "real" speech perception begins.

Notice that within this stream of speech there are no markers to indicate where one phoneme ends and the next begins. Likewise, there are, for the most part, no gaps to indicate the boundaries between successive syllables or successive words. Therefore, as a first step prior to phoneme identification, you need to "slice" this stream into the appropriate segments—a step known as **speech segmentation.**

For many people, this pattern comes as a surprise. Most of us are convinced that there are pauses between words in the speech that we hear, and it's these pauses, we assume, that mark the word boundaries. This perception, however, turns out to be an illusion, and we are "hearing" pauses that, in truth, aren't there. This is evident when we "hear" the pauses in the "wrong places" and thus segment the speech stream in a way the speaker didn't intend (see **Figure 10.4**). The illusion is also revealed when we physically measure the speech stream (as we did in order to create Figure 10.3) or when we listen to speech we can't understand—for example, speech in a foreign language.

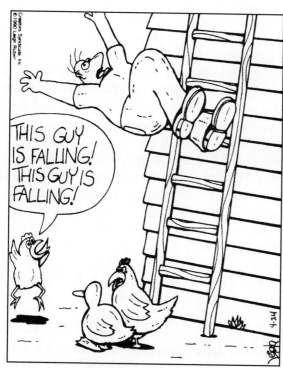

"Boy, he must think we're pretty stupid to fall for that again."

FIGURE 10.4 AMBIGUITY IN SEGMENTATION

Virtually every child has heard the story of Chicken Little. No one believed this poor chicken when he announced, "The sky is falling." It turns out, though, that the acoustic signal—the actual sounds produced—would have been the same if Chicken Little had said, "This guy is falling." The difference between these utterances ("The sky..." vs. "This guy...") is not in the input. Instead, the difference lies in how the listener segments the sounds.

In the latter circumstance, we lack the skill needed to segment the stream, so we are unable to "supply" the word boundaries. As a consequence, we hear what is really there: a continuous, uninterrupted flow of sound. That is why speech in a foreign language often sounds so fast.

Speech perception is further complicated by a phenomenon known as **coarticulation** (Liberman, 1970; also Daniloff & Hammarberg, 1973). This term refers to the fact that in producing speech, you don't utter one phoneme at a time. Instead, the phonemes "overlap," and so, while you're producing the [s] sound in "soup" (for example), your mouth is getting ready to say the vowel. While uttering the vowel, you're already starting to move your tongue, lips, and teeth into position for producing the [p].

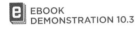
EBOOK
DEMONSTRATION 10.3

This overlap helps to make speech production faster and considerably more fluent. But the overlap also has consequences for the sounds produced, so that the [s] you produce while getting ready for one upcoming vowel is actually different from the [s] you produce while getting ready for a different vowel. As a result, we can't point to a specific acoustical pattern and say, "This is the pattern of an [s] sound." Instead, the acoustical pattern is different in different contexts. Speech perception therefore has to "read past" these context differences in order to identify the phonemes produced.

Aids to Speech Perception

The need for segmentation in a continuous speech stream, the variations caused by coarticulation, the variations from speaker to speaker—all make speech perception rather complex. Nonetheless, you manage to perceive speech accurately and easily. How do you do it?

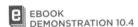
EBOOK
DEMONSTRATION 10.4

Part of the answer lies in the fact that the speech you encounter, day by day, is surprisingly limited in its range. Each of us knows tens of thousands of words, but most of these words are rarely used. In fact, it has been estimated that the 50 most commonly used words in English make up more than half of the words you actually hear (Miller, 1951).

In addition, the perception of speech shares a crucial attribute with all other types of perception: You don't rely only on the stimuli you receive; instead, you *supplement* this input with other knowledge, guided by the context in which a word appears. This is evident, for example, in the **phonemic restoration effect**. To demonstrate this effect, researchers start by recording a bit of speech, and then they modify what they've recorded. For example, they might remove the [s] sound in the middle of "legislatures" and replace the [s] with a brief burst of noise. This now-degraded stimulus can then be presented to participants, embedded in a sentence such as

The state governors met with their respective legi*latures.

When asked about this stimulus, participants insist that they heard the *complete* word, "legislatures," accompanied by a burst of noise. Apparently, they use the context to figure out what the word must have been, and so, in essence, they supply the missing sound on their own (Repp, 1992; Samuel, 1987, 1991).

How much does the context in which we hear a word help us? Pollack and Pickett (1964) recorded a number of naturally occurring conversations. From these recordings, they spliced out individual words and presented them in isolation to their research participants. With no context to guide them, participants were able to identify only half of the words. If restored to their original context, though, the same stimuli were easy to identify. Apparently, the benefits of context are considerable.

Categorical Perception

Speech perception also benefits from a pattern called **categorical perception.** This term refers to the fact that people are much better at hearing the differences *between* categories of sounds than they are at hearing the variations *within* a category of sounds. Said differently, you're very sensitive to the differences between, say, a [g] sound and a [k], or the differences between a [d] and a [t]. But you're surprisingly insensitive to differences within each of these categories, so you have a hard time distinguishing, say, one [p] sound from another, somewhat different [p] sound. And, of course, this pattern is precisely what you want, because it enables you to hear the differences that matter without hearing (and being distracted by) inconsequential variations within the category.

Demonstrations of categorical perception generally rely on a series of stimuli, created by computer. The first stimulus in the series might, for example, be a [ba] sound. Another stimulus might be a [ba] that has been distorted a tiny bit, to make it a little bit closer to a [pa] sound. A third stimulus might be a [ba] that has been distorted a bit more, so that it's a notch closer to a [pa], and so on. In this fashion we create a series of stimuli, each slightly different from the one before, ranging from a clear [ba] sound at one extreme, through a series of "compromise" sounds, until we reach at the other extreme a clear [pa] sound.

How do people perceive these various sounds? **Figure 10.5A** shows the pattern we might expect. After all, our stimuli are gradually shading from a clear [ba] to a clear [pa]. Therefore, as we move through the series, we might expect people to be less and less likely to identify each stimulus as a [ba], and correspondingly more and more likely to identify each as a [pa]. In the terms we used in Chapter 9, this would be a "graded-membership" pattern: Test cases close to the [ba] prototype should be reliably identified as [ba]; as we move away from this prototype, cases should be harder and harder to categorize.

However, the actual data, shown in Figure 10.5B, don't fit with this prediction. Even though the stimuli are gradually changing from one extreme to another, participants "hear" an abrupt shift, so that roughly half the stimuli are reliably categorized as [ba] and half are reliably categorized as [pa]. Moreover, participants seem indifferent to the differences *within* each category. Across the first dozen stimuli, the syllables are becoming less and less [ba]-like, but this is not reflected in how the listeners identify the sounds. Likewise, across the last dozen stimuli, the syllables are becoming more and

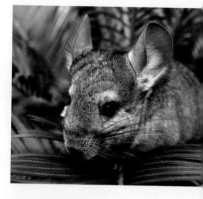

CATEGORICAL
PERCEPTION IN
OTHER SPECIES

The pattern of categorical perception is not limited to language—or to humans. A similar pattern, for example, with much greater sensitivity to between-category differences than to within-category variations has been documented in the hearing of the chinchilla.

FIGURE 10.5 CATEGORICAL PERCEPTION

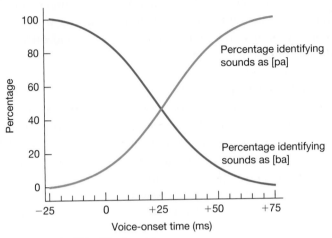

Percentage identifying sounds as [pa]

Percentage identifying sounds as [ba]

A Hypothetical identification data

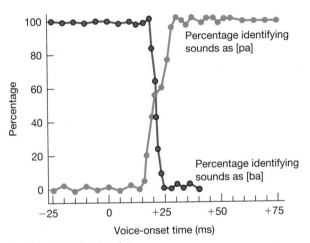

Percentage identifying sounds as [pa]

Percentage identifying sounds as [ba]

B Actual identification data

With computer speech, we can produce a variety of compromises between a [pa] and a [ba] sound, differing only in when the voicing begins (i.e., the **voice-onset time**, or **VOT**). Panel A shows a plausible prediction about how these sounds will be perceived: As the sound becomes less and less like an ordinary [ba], people should be less and less likely to perceive it as a [ba]. Panel B, however, shows the actual data: Research participants seem indifferent to small variations in the [ba] sound, and they categorize a sound with a 10 ms or 15 ms VOT in exactly the same way that they categorize a sound with a 0 VOT. The categorizations also show an abrupt categorical boundary between [pa] and [ba], although there is no corresponding abrupt change in the stimuli themselves. AFTER LISKER & ABRAMSON, 1970.

more [pa]-like, but again, this trend has little effect. What listeners seem to hear is either a [pa] or a [ba], with no gradations inside of either category (Liberman, Harris, Hoffman, & Griffith, 1957; for reviews, see Handel, 1989; Yeni-Komshian, 1993).

It seems, then, that your perceptual apparatus is "tuned" to provide you just the information you need. After all, you want to know whether someone advised you to "take a path" or "take a bath." You certainly care whether a friend said, "You're the best" or "You're the pest." Plainly, the difference between [b] and [p] matters to you, and this difference is clearly marked in your perception. In contrast, you usually don't care how exactly the speaker pronounced "path" or "best"—that's not information that matters for getting the meaning of these utterances. And here too, your perception serves you well by largely ignoring these "subphonemic" variations. (For more on the broad issue of speech perception, see Mattys, 2012.)

Combining Phonemes

English relies on just a few dozen phonemes, but these sounds can be combined and recombined to produce thousands of different morphemes, which can themselves be combined to create word after word after word. It turns out, though, that there are rules governing these combinations, and users of the language reliably respect these rules. Thus, in English, certain sounds (such as the final sound in "going" or "flying") can occur at the end of a word but not at the beginning. Other combinations seem prohibited outright. For example, the sequence "tlof" seems anomalous to English speakers; indeed, no words in English contain the "tl" combination within a single syllable. (The combination can, however, occur at the boundary between syllables—as in "motley" or "sweetly.") These limits, however, are simply facts about English; they are not at all a limit on what human ears can hear or human tongues can produce, and other languages routinely use combinations that for English speakers seem unspeakable.

There are also rules governing the adjustments that occur when certain phonemes are uttered one after another. For example, consider the "s" ending that marks the English plural—as in "books," "cats," and "tapes." In these cases, the plural is pronounced as an [s]. In other contexts, though, the plural ending is pronounced differently. Say these words out loud: "bags," "duds," "pills." If you listen carefully, you will realize that these words actually end with a [z] sound, not an [s] sound.

English speakers all seem to know the rule that governs this distinction. (The rule hinges on whether the base noun ends with a voiced or an unvoiced sound; Chomsky & Halle, 1968; Halle, 1990.) Moreover, they obey this rule even with novel, made-up cases. For example, I have one wug, and now I acquire another. Now, I have two . . . what? Without hesitation, people pronounce "wugs" using the [z] ending—in accord with the standard pattern. Indeed, even young children pronounce "wugs" with a [z], and so, it seems, they too have internalized—and obey—the relevant principles (Berko, 1958).

Morphemes and Words

A typical college graduate in the United States knows between 75,000 and 100,000 different words (e.g., Oldfield, 1963; Zechmeister, Chronis, Cull, D'Anna, & Healy, 1995). For each word, the speaker knows the word's *sound* (the sequence of phonemes that make up the word) and its *orthography* (the sequence of letters that spell the word). The speaker also knows how to use the word within various phrases, governed by the rules of syntax (see **Figure 10.6**). Finally—and obviously—the speaker knows the meaning of a word; he must have a *semantic representation* for the word to go with the *phonological representation*.

Building New Words

Estimates of someone's vocabulary size, however, need to be interpreted with caution, because the size of an individual's vocabulary is actually quite fluid. One reason is that new words are created all the time. For example, the world of computers has demanded many new terms—with the result that someone who wants to know something will often *google* it; many of us get information from *blogs*; and most of us are no longer fooled by the *phishing* we sometimes find in our *email*. The terms *software* and *hardware* have been around for a while, but *spyware* and *malware* are relatively new.

Moreover, let's be clear that these new words don't arrive in the language as isolated entries, because language users immediately know how to create variations on each by adding the appropriate morphemes. Imagine, for example, that you have just heard the word "hack" for the first time. You know instantly that someone who does this activity is a

---

FIGURE 10.6   KNOWING A WORD

(1)	She can place the books on the table.
(2)	* She can place on the table.
(3)	* She can sleep the books on the table
(4)	She can sleep on the table.

Part of what it means to "know a word" is knowing how to use a word. For example, a word like "place" demands an object—so that Sentence 1 (with an object) sounds fine, but Sentence 2 is anomalous. Other words have other demands. "Sleep," for example, does not take an object—so Sentence 3 is anomalous, but Sentence 4 is fine.

"hacker" and that the activity itself is "hacking," and you understand someone who says, "I've been hacked." In these ways, the added morphemes enable you to use these words in new ways—and in some cases to create entirely new words.

Once again, therefore, let's highlight the **generativity** of language—that is, the capacity to create an endless series of new combinations, all built from the same set of fundamental units. Thus, someone who "knows English" (or, for that matter, someone who knows *any* language) has not just memorized the vocabulary of the language and some set of phrases. Instead, someone who "knows English" knows how to create new forms within the language: He knows how to combine morphemes to create new words, knows how to "adjust" phonemes when they're put together into novel combinations, and so on. This knowledge isn't conscious—and so most English speakers could not (for example) articulate the principles governing the sequence of morphemes within a word, or why they pronounce "wugs" with a [z] sound rather than an [s]. Nonetheless, speakers honor these principles with remarkable consistency in their day-by-day use of the language and in their day-to-day *creation* of novel words.

EBOOK DEMONSTRATION 10.5

Syntax

The incredible potential for producing new forms is even more salient when we consider the upper levels in the language hierarchy—the levels of *phrases* and *sentences*. After all, you can combine production features to create a few dozen phonemes, and you can combine these to produce thousands of morphemes and words. But think about what you can do with those words: If you have 40,000 words in your vocabulary, or 60,000, or 80,000, how many sentences can you build from those words?

Sentences range in length from the very brief ("Go!" or "I do") to the absurdly long. Most sentences, though, contain 20 words or fewer. With this length limit, it has been estimated that there are 100,000,000,000,000,000,000 possible sentences in English (Pinker, 1994). For comparison, if you could read off sentences at the insane rate of 1,000 per second, you'd still need over 30,000 *centuries* to read through this list!

Once again, though, there are limits on which combinations (i.e., which sequences of words) are acceptable and which ones are not. Thus, in English you could say, "The boy hit the ball" but not "The boy hit ball the." Likewise, you could say, "The moose squashed the car" but not "The moose squashed the" or just "Squashed the car." Virtually any speaker of the language would agree that these sequences have something wrong in them, suggesting that speakers somehow respect the rules of **syntax**—rules governing the sequence of words in a phrase or sentence.

One might think that the rules of syntax depend on *meaning*, so that meaningful sequences are accepted as "sentences" while meaning*less* sequences are rejected as nonsentences. This suggestion, though, is plainly wrong. As one

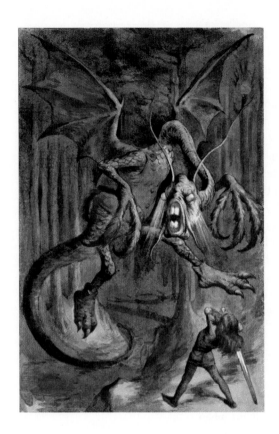

In the poem "Jabberwocky," Lewis Carroll relies on proper syntax and appropriate use of morphemes to create gibberish that is wonderfully English-like. "He left it dead, and with its head / He went galumphing back."

concern, many nonsentences do seem meaningful ("Me Tarzan"). In addition, consider these two sentences:

'Twas brillig, and the slithy toves did gyre and gimble in the wabe.

Colorless green ideas sleep furiously.

(The first of these is from Lewis Carroll's famous poem "Jabberwocky"; the second was penned by the important linguist Noam Chomsky.) These sentences are, of course, without meaning: Colorless things aren't green; ideas don't sleep; toves aren't slithy. Nonetheless, speakers of English, after a moment's reflection, regard these sequences as grammatically acceptable in a way that "Furiously sleep ideas green colorless" is not. It seems, therefore, that we need principles of syntax that are separate from considerations of semantics or sensibility.

Phrase Structure

What are the principles of syntax? Part of the answer involves **phrase structure rules.** These are stipulations that list the elements that must appear in a phrase and (for some languages) specify the sequence of those elements. The rules also determine the overall organization of the sentence—how the various elements are linked to one another.

FIGURE 10.7 A PHRASE STRUCTURE TREE

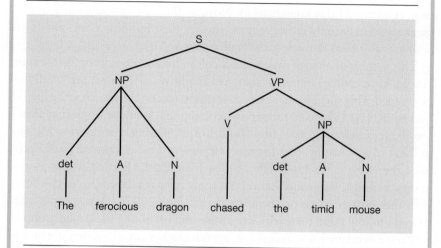

The diagram shows that the overall sentence itself (S) consists of a **noun phrase (NP)** plus a **verb phrase (VP)**. The noun phrase is composed of a determiner (det) followed by an adjective (A) and a noun (N). The verb phrase is composed of a verb (V) followed by a noun phrase (NP).

One way to depict these rules is with a **tree structure** like the one shown in **Figure 10.7**. You can read the structure from top to bottom, and as you move from one level to the next, you can see that each element has been "expanded" in a fashion that's strictly governed by the phrase structure rules.

Prescriptive Rules, Descriptive Rules

We need to be clear, though, about what sorts of rules we're discussing here. Let's begin with the fact that most of us were taught, at some stage of our education, how to talk and write "properly." We were taught never to say "ain't." Many of us were scolded for writing in the passive voice or starting a sentence with "And." Injunctions like these are the result of **prescriptive rules**—rules describing how language is "supposed to be." Language that doesn't follow these rules, it's claimed, is "improper" or maybe just "wrong."

We should be skeptical, however, about these prescriptive rules. After all, languages change with the passage of time, and what's "proper" in one period is often different from what seems right at other times. A generation back, for example, many people insisted it was wrong to end a sentence with a preposition; modern speakers think this prohibition is silly. Likewise, consider the split infinitive. Prominent writers of the 18th and 19th centuries (e.g., Ben Franklin, William Wordsworth, Henry James) commonly split their infinitives; grammarians of the early 20th century, in contrast, energetically condemned this construction. Now, in the 21st century, most English speakers seem entirely indifferent to whether their infinitives are split or not (and may not even know what a "split infinitive" *is*).

This pattern of change makes it difficult to justify prescriptive rules. Many people, for example, still insist that split infinitives are "improper" and must be avoided. This suggestion, however, seems to rest on the idea that the English spoken in, say, 1926 was proper and correct, and that the English spoken a few decades before or after this "Golden Age" is somehow inferior. It's hard to think of any justification for this assessment. The selection of prescriptive rules, therefore, may simply reflect the preferences of a particular group—and in most settings, the group that defines these rules will of course be the group with the most prestige or social cachet (Labov, 2007). Thus, people often strive to follow these rules with the simple aim of joining these elite groups.

Phrase structure rules, in contrast, are not at all prescriptive; they are instead **descriptive rules**—that is, rules characterizing the language as it is ordinarily used by fluent speakers and listeners. There are, after all, strong regularities in the way English is used, and the rules we are discussing here describe these patterns. No value judgment is offered (nor should one be) about whether these patterns constitute "proper" or "good" English. These patterns simply describe how English is structured—or perhaps we should say, *what English is*.

The Function of Phrase Structure

The idea here is not that people are consciously aware of their language's phrase structure rules. But it does seem that in some fashion we have all internalized these rules; this is evident in the fact that many aspects of language use are reliably in line with the rules.

For example, people have clear intuitions about how the words in a sentence should be grouped. As an illustration, consider the simple sentence "The boy loves his dog." The sentence seems to break naturally into two parts: The first two words, "the boy," identify what the sentence is about; the remaining three words ("loves his dog") then supply some information about the boy. These latter words, in turn, also break easily into two parts: the verb, "loves," and then two more words ("his dog") identifying what is loved. These groups are precisely what we would expect based on the phrase structure rules. The first grouping ("The boy" and "loves his dog") respects the boundary between the sentence's noun phrase (NP) and its verb phrase (VP). The next group ("loves" and "his dog") respects the main components of the VP.

Perhaps more important, phrase structure rules help us *understand* the sentences we hear or read, because syntax in general specifies the relationships among the words in each sentence. For example, the NP + VP sequence typically divides a sentence into the "doer" (the NP) and some information about that doer (the VP). Likewise, the V + NP sequence usually indicates the action described by

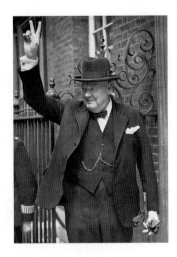

THE (SOMETIMES) PECULIAR NATURE OF PRESCRIPTIVE RULES

According to an often-repeated story, an editor had rearranged one of Winston Churchill's sentences to bring it into alignment with "proper" English. Specifically, the editor rewrote the sentence to avoid ending it in a preposition. In response, the prime minister, proud of his style, scribbled this note: "This is the sort of English up with which I will not put." (Often repeated or not, though, we note that there's some debate about the historical roots of this story!)

FIGURE 10.8 PHRASE STRUCTURE ORGANIZATION AIDS THE READER

Panel A shows a sentence written so that the breaks between lines correspond to breaks between phrases; this makes reading easier because the sentence has, in effect, been visually "pre-organized." In Panel B, the sentence has been rewritten so that the visual breaks don't correspond to the boundaries between phrases. Reading is now slower and more difficult.

the sentence and then the recipient of that action. In this way, the phrase structure of a sentence provides an initial "road map" that is useful in understanding the sentence. Thus (to take a simple case), it's syntax that tells us who's doing what when we hear "The boy chased the girl." Without syntax (if, for example, our sentences were merely lists of words, such as "boy, girl, chased"), we'd have no way to know who was the chaser and who was chased. (Also see **Figure 10.8**.)

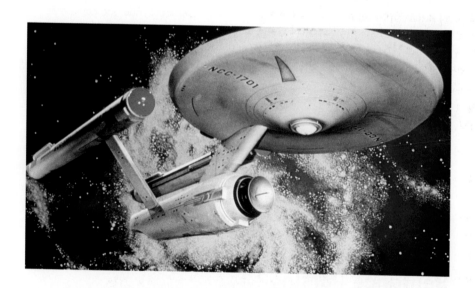

THE (OBSOLETE?) PROHIBITION ON SPLIT INFINITIVES

"To boldly go where no man has gone before." A split infinitive is a construction in which some word (usually an adverb) comes between the "to" and the base form of the verb. For many years, grammatical authorities were horrified by the opening sequence of the *Star Trek* TV series, in which "boldly" split the infinitive "to go."

FIGURE 10.9 PHRASE STRUCTURE AMBIGUITY

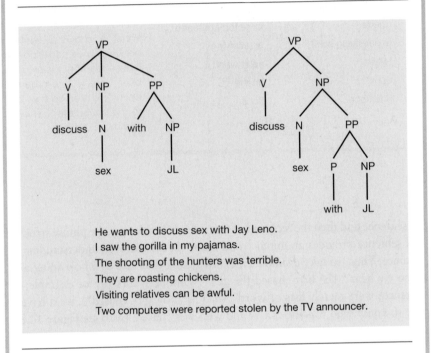

He wants to discuss sex with Jay Leno.
I saw the gorilla in my pajamas.
The shooting of the hunters was terrible.
They are roasting chickens.
Visiting relatives can be awful.
Two computers were reported stolen by the TV announcer.

Often, the words of a sentence are compatible with more than one phrase structure; in such cases, the sentence will be ambiguous. Thus, you can understand the first sentence here either as describing a *discussion with Leno* or as describing *sex with Leno*; both analyses of the verb phrase are shown. Can you find both interpretations for the remaining sentences?

EBOOK
DEMONSTRATION 10.6

Confirmation for the role of phrase structure comes from cases in which two different phrase structures can lead to the same sequence of words; if you encounter one of these sequences, you may not know which phrase structure was intended. How will this affect you? If, as we've suggested, phrase structures guide interpretation, then with multiple phrase structures available, there should be more than one way to interpret the sentence. This turns out to be correct—often, with comical consequences (see **Figure 10.9**).

Sentence Parsing

A sentence's phrase structure, we've said, conveys crucial information about who did what to whom, and so, once you know the phrase structure, you're well on your way to understanding the sentence. But how do you figure out the phrase structure in the first place? This would be an easy question if sentences were uniform in their structure: "The boy hit the ball. The girl drove

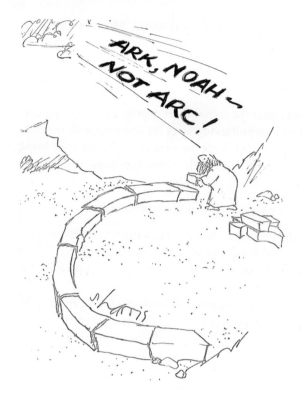

the car. The elephant trampled the geraniums." But, of course, sentences are more variable than this, a fact that makes the identification of a sentence's phrase structure appreciably more difficult.

How, therefore, do you **parse** a sentence—that is, figure out each word's syntactic role? One possibility is that you wait until the sentence's end and only then go to work on figuring out the structure. With this strategy, your comprehension might be slowed a little (because of the wait for the sentence's end), but you'd avoid errors, because your interpretation could be guided by full information about the sentence's content.

It turns out, though, that people don't use this wait-for-all-the-information strategy. Instead, they seek to parse sentences as they hear them, trying to figure out the role of each word the moment it arrives (e.g., Marcus, 2001; Savova, Roy, Schmidt, & Tenenbaum, 2007; Tanenhaus & Trueswell, 2006). This approach is efficient (since there's no waiting) but, as we'll see, can lead to errors.

Garden Paths

Even simple sentences can be ambiguous if you're open-minded (or perverse) enough:

Mary had a little lamb. (But I was quite hungry, so I had the lamb and also a bowl of soup.)

Time flies like an arrow. (But fruit flies, in contrast, like a banana.)

Temporary ambiguity is also common inside a sentence. More precisely, the early part of a sentence is often open to multiple interpretations, but then the later part of the sentence clears things up. For instance, consider this example:

The old man the ships.

In this sentence, most people read the initial three words as a noun phrase: "the old man." However, this interpretation leaves the sentence with no verb, so a different interpretation is needed, with the subject of the sentence being "the old" and with "man" being the verb. (Who mans the ships? It is the old, not the young. The old man the ships.) Likewise:

The secretary applauded for his efforts was soon promoted.

Here, one tends to read "applauded" as the sentence's main verb, but it isn't. Instead, this sentence is just a shorthand way of answering the question, "Which secretary was soon promoted?" (Answer: "The one who was applauded for his efforts.")

These examples are referred to as **garden-path sentences**: You are initially led to one interpretation (you are, as they say, "led down the garden path"), but this interpretation then turns out to be wrong. Hence, you need to reject your first construal and seek an alternative. Here are two more examples:

Fat people eat accumulates.

Because he ran the second mile went quickly.

Garden-path sentences highlight the risk attached to the strategy of interpreting a sentence as it arrives: The information you need in order to understand these sentences arrives only late in the sequence, and so, to avoid an interpretive dead end, you'd be well advised to remain neutral about the sentence's meaning until you've gathered enough information. That way, you'd know that "the old man" couldn't be the sentence's subject, that "applauded" couldn't be the sentence's main verb, and so on. But this is not what you do. Instead, you commit yourself fairly early to one interpretation and then try to "fit" subsequent words, as they arrive, into that interpretation. This strategy is often effective, but it does lead to the "double-take" reaction when late-arriving information forces you to abandon your initial interpretive efforts (Grodner & Gibson, 2005).

Syntax as a Guide to Parsing

What is it that leads you down the garden path? More specifically, why do you initially choose one interpretation of a sentence, one parsing, rather than another? Many cues are relevant, because many types of information influence parsing (see **Figure 10.10**). For one, people usually seek the simplest phrase structure that will accommodate the words heard so far. This strategy is fine if the sentence structure is indeed simple; the strategy produces problems, though, with more complex sentences. To see how this plays out, consider the earlier sentence, "The secretary applauded for his efforts was soon promoted." As you read "The secretary applauded," you had the

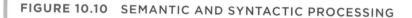

FIGURE 10.10   SEMANTIC AND SYNTACTIC PROCESSING

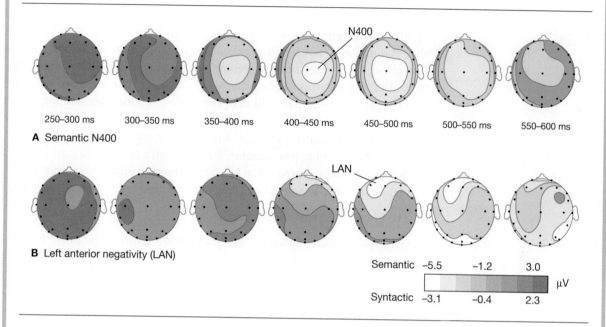

A Semantic N400

250–300 ms   300–350 ms   350–400 ms   400–450 ms   450–500 ms   500–550 ms   550–600 ms

N400

B Left anterior negativity (LAN)

LAN

| Semantic | −5.5 | −1.2 | 3.0 | μV |
| Syntactic | −3.1 | −0.4 | 2.3 | |

Many types of information influence parsing. The figures here show patterns of electrical activity on the scalp (with different voltages represented by different colors). If the person hears a sentence that violates *semantic* expectations (e.g., a sentence like, "He drinks his coffee with cream and dog"), this triggers a brain wave termed the N400 (so-called because the wave involves a negative voltage roughly 400 ms after the trigger ("dog") is encountered. If the person hears a sentence that violates *syntactic* expectations, though, (e.g., a sentence like, "He prefers to solve problems herself"), a different brain wave is observed—the so-called left anterior negativity (LAN).

option of interpreting this as a noun phrase plus the beginning of a separate clause modifying "secretary." This is, of course, the correct construal and is demanded by the way the sentence ends. However, you ignored this possibility, at least initially, and went instead with a simpler interpretation—of a noun phrase plus verb, with no idea of a separate embedded clause.

People also tend to assume that they'll be hearing (or reading) *active-voice* sentences rather than *passive-voice* sentences, so they generally interpret a sentence's initial noun phrase as the "doer" of the action and not the recipient. As it happens, most of the sentences you encounter are active, not passive, so this assumption is usually correct (Svartik, 1966). However, this assumption can slow you down when you do encounter a passive sentence (Hornby, 1974; Slobin, 1966). And, of course, this assumption added to your difficulties with the "secretary" sentence: The embedded clause in this sentence is in the passive voice (the secretary was applauded by someone else); your tendency to assume active voice, therefore, works against the correct interpretation of this sentence.

Not surprisingly, parsing is also influenced by the function words that appear in a sentence and by the various morphemes that signal syntactic role (Bever, 1970). Thus, for example, people easily grasp the structure of "He gliply rivitched the flidget." That's because the "-ly" morpheme indicates that "glip" is an adverb; the "-ed" identifies "rivitch" as a verb; and "the" signals that "flidget" is a noun—all excellent cues to the sentence structure. This factor, too, is relevant to the "secretary" sentence, which included none of the helpful function words. Notice that we didn't say, "The secretary who was applauded . . ."; if we had said that, the chance of misunderstanding would have been much reduced.

With all these factors stacked against you, it's no wonder you were (temporarily) confused about "the secretary." Indeed, with all these factors in place, garden-path sentences can sometimes be enormously difficult to comprehend. For example, spend a moment puzzling over this (fully grammatical) sequence:

The horse raced past the barn fell.

(If you get stuck with this sentence, try adding the word "that" after "horse.")

Background Knowledge as a Guide to Parsing

Parsing is also guided by background knowledge, and in general, people try to parse sentences in a way that makes sense to them. Thus, for example, readers are unlikely to misread the headline *Drunk Gets Six Months in Violin Case* (Gibson, 2006; Pinker, 1994; Sedivy, Tanenhaus, Chambers, & Carlson, 1999). And this point, too, matters for the "secretary" sentence: Your background knowledge tells you that women secretaries are more common than men, and this likely added to your confusion in figuring out who was applauding and who was applauded.

How can we document these knowledge effects? Several studies have tracked how people move their eyes while reading, and these movements can tell us when the reading is going smoothly and when the reader is confused. Let's say, for example, that we ask someone to read a garden-path sentence. The moment the person realizes he has misinterpreted the words so far, he'll backtrack and reread the sentence's start. With appropriate instruments, we can easily detect these backwards eye movements (MacDonald, Pearlmutter, & Seidenberg, 1994; Trueswell, Tanenhaus, & Garnsey, 1994).

Using this technique, investigators have examined the effects of *plausibility* on readers' interpretations of the words they're seeing. For example, participants might be shown a sentence beginning "The detectives examined . . . "; upon seeing this, the participants sensibly assume that "examined" is the sentence's main verb and are therefore puzzled when the sentence continues "by the reporter . . ." (see **Figure 10.11**). We detect this puzzlement in their eye movements: They pause and look back at "examined," realizing that their initial interpretation was wrong. Then, after this recalculation, they press onward.

Things go differently, though, if the sentence begins "The evidence examined . . . " Here, readers can draw on the fact that "evidence" can't

FIGURE 10.11 INTERPRETING COMPLEX SENTENCES

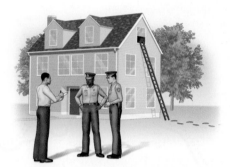

A The detectives examined by the reporter revealed the truth about the robbery.

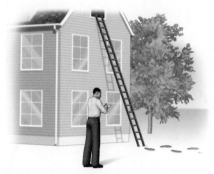

B The evidence examined by the reporter revealed the truth about the robbery.

Readers are momentarily confused when they reach the "by the reporter" phrase in Sentence A. That is because they initially interpreted "examined" as the sentence's main verb. Readers aren't confused by Sentence B, though, because their background knowledge told them that "examined" couldn't be the main verb (because evidence is not capable of examining anything). Notice, though, that readers *won't* be confused if the sentences are presented as they are here—with a picture. In that case, the "extralinguistic context" guides interpretation, and helps readers avoid the garden path.

examine anything, so "examined" can't be the sentence's main verb. Hence, they're quite unsurprised when the sentence continues "by the reporter . . . " Their understanding of the world had already told them that the first three words were the start of a passive sentence, not an active one. (Also see **Figure 10.12.**)

The Extralinguistic Context

We've now mentioned several strategies that you use in parsing the sentences you encounter. The role of these strategies is obvious when the strategies mislead you, as they do with garden-path sentences, but that doesn't change the fact that these strategies are used for *all* sentences and, in truth, usually lead to the correct parsing.

It turns out, though, that our catalogue of strategies isn't done, because you also make use of another factor: the *context* in which you encounter sentences, including the conversational context. Thus, the garden-path problem is much less likely to occur in the following setting:

Jack: Which horse fell?

Kate: The horse raced past the barn fell.

FIGURE 10.12   N400 BRAIN WAVE

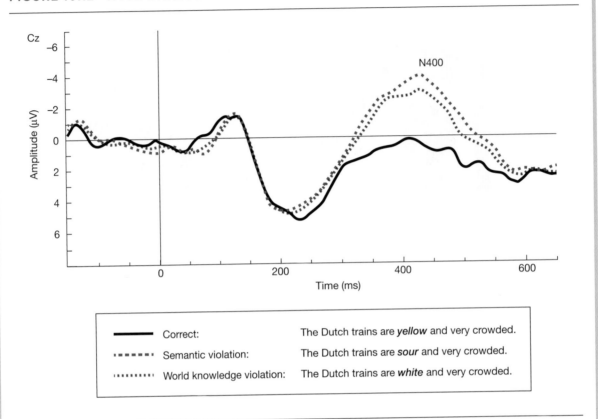

In parsing a sentence, you rely on many cues—including your (nonlinguistic) knowledge about the world. This point is evident in a study of electrical activity in the brain while people were hearing different types of sentences. Some of the sentences were sensible and true ("The Dutch trains are yellow and very crowded"). Other sentences contained a semantic anomaly ("The Dutch trains are sour and very crowded") and this peculiarity produced the N400 brain wave. The key, though, is that a virtually identical N400 was produced in a third condition in which sentences were perfectly sensible but false: "The Dutch trains are white and very crowded." (The falsity was immediately obvious to the Dutch participants in this study.) Apparently, world knowledge (including knowledge about train color) is a part of sentence processing from a very early stage.

FIG. 1 FROM HAGOORT ET AL., "INTEGRATION OF WORD MEANING AND WORLD KNOWLEDGE IN LANGUAGE COMPREHENSION," *SCIENCE* 304 (APRIL 2004): 438–441. © 2004 AAAS. REPRINTED WITH PERMISSION FROM AAAS.

Just as important is the **extralinguistic context**—the physical and social setting in which you encounter sentences. To see how this factor matters, consider the following sentence:

Put the apple on the towel into the box.

At its start, this sentence seems to be an instruction to put an apple onto a towel; this interpretation must be abandoned, though, when the words "into the box" arrive. Now, you realize that the box is the apple's destination; "on

FIGURE 10.13 THE EXTRALINGUISTIC CONTEXT

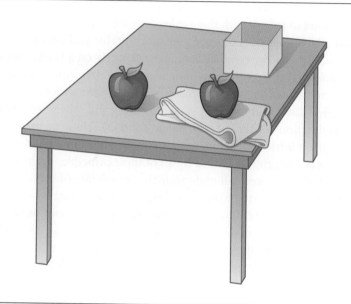

"Put the apple on the towel into the box." Without the setting shown here, this sentence causes momentary confusion: The listener will initially think she is supposed to put the apple onto the towel and is then confused by the sentence's last three words. If the sentence is presented together with this picture, however, there's no confusion. Now, the listener immediately sees the potential for confusion (which apple is being discussed?), counts on the speaker to provide clarification for this point, and immediately understands "on the towel" as specification, not a destination.

the towel" is simply a specification of which apple is to be moved. (Which apple should be put into the box? The one that is on the towel.) In short, this is another garden-path sentence—initially inviting one analysis but eventually demanding another.

This confusion is avoided, however, if the sentence is uttered in the appropriate setting. Imagine that two apples are in view, as shown in **Figure 10.13**. In this context, a listener hearing the sentence's start ("Put the apple . . .") would immediately see the possibility for confusion (which apple is being referred to?) and so would expect the speaker to specify which one is to be moved. When the phrase "on the towel" is uttered, the listener immediately understands it (correctly) as the needed specification. Hence, there is no confusion and no garden path (Eberhard, Spivey-Knowlton, Sedivy, & Tanenhaus, 1995; Tanenhaus & Spivey-Knowlton, 1996).

The Use of Language: What Is Left Unsaid

What does it mean to "know a language"—to "know English," for example? As we've discussed, each language user seems somehow to know (and obey) a rich set of rules—with these rules determining which sound combinations and which sequences of words seem acceptable and which ones do not. In addition, we've now seen that language users rely on a further set of principles whenever they perceive and understand linguistic inputs. Some of these principles are rooted in syntax; others depend on semantics (e.g., knowing that detectives can "examine" but evidence can't); still others seem pragmatic (e.g., considerations of the extralinguistic context). These factors then seem to interact in an intricate fashion, so that your understanding of the sentences you hear (or see in print) is guided by all of these principles at the same time.

These points, however, still *understate* the complexity of language use and, with that, the complexity of the knowledge someone must have in order to "know a language." For illustration, note that we have said nothing about another source of information that is useful in parsing: the rise and fall of speech intonation and the pattern of pauses. These rhythm and pitch cues, together called **prosody**, play an important role in speech perception. Prosody can reveal the mood of a speaker; it can also direct the listener's attention by, in effect, specifying the focus or theme of a sentence (Jackendoff, 1972). Prosody can also render unambiguous a sentence that would otherwise be entirely confusing (Beach, 1991). (Thus, garden-path sentences and ambiguous sentences are much more effective in print, where prosody provides no information.)

Likewise, we have not even touched on several other puzzles: How is language produced? How does one turn ideas, intentions, and queries into actual sentences? How does one turn the sentences into sequences of sounds? These are important issues, but we have held them to the side here.

Finally, what happens after one has parsed and understood an individual sentence? How is the sentence integrated with earlier sentences or subsequent sentences? Here, too, more theory is needed to explain the inferences you routinely make in ordinary conversation. If you are asked, for example, "Do you know the time?" you understand this as a request that you report the time—despite the fact that the question, understood literally, is a yes/no question about the extent of your temporal knowledge. In the same vein, consider this bit of conversation (Pinker, 1994):

> Woman: I'm leaving you.
>
> Man: Who is he?

We easily provide the soap-opera script that lies behind this exchange, but we do so by drawing on a rich fabric of additional knowledge, including knowledge of **pragmatics** (i.e., of how language is ordinarily used), and, in this case, also knowledge about the vicissitudes of romance. (For discussion, see Ervin-Tripp, 1993; Graesser, Millis, & Zwaan, 1997; Hilton, 1995; Kumon-Nakamura, Glucksberg, & Brown, 1995; Noveck & Reboul, 2008; Noveck & Sperber, 2005.)

These other topics—prosody, production, and pragmatics—are central concerns within the study of language, but for the sake of brevity we have not tackled them here. Even so, we mention these themes to emphasize a key message of this chapter: Each of us uses language all the time—to learn, to gossip, to instruct, to persuade, to warn, to express affection. We use this tool as easily as we breathe; we spend more effort in choosing our clothes in the morning than we do in choosing the words we will utter. But these observations must not hide the facts that language is a remarkably complicated tool and that we are all exquisitely skilled in its use.

The Biological Roots of Language

How is all of this possible? How is it that ordinary human beings—indeed, ordinary two-and-a-half-year-olds—manage the extraordinary task of mastering and fluently using language? According to many authors, the answer lies in the fact that humans are equipped with sophisticated neural machinery specialized for learning, and then using, language. Let's take a quick look at this machinery.

Aphasias

As we saw early in the chapter, damage to specific parts of the brain can cause a disruption of language known as **aphasia**. Damage to the left frontal lobe of the brain, especially a region known as **Broca's area** (see **Figure 10.14**), usually produces a pattern of symptoms known as **nonfluent aphasia**. People with this disorder have adequate verbal comprehension but are unable to produce language. In extreme cases, a patient with this disorder is unable to utter or write any words at all. In less severe cases, only a part of the patient's vocabulary is lost, but the patient's speech becomes labored and fragmented, and articulating each word requires special effort. The resulting speech can sound something like "Here . . . head . . . operation . . . here . . . speech . . . none . . . talking . . . what . . . illness" (Luria, 1966, p. 406).

Different symptoms are associated with damage to a brain site known as **Wernicke's area** (again see Figure 10.14) and usually involve a pattern known as **fluent aphasia**. In these cases, patients seem able to talk freely but they actually say very little. One patient, for example, uttered, "I was over the other one, and then after they had been in the department, I was in this one" (Geschwind, 1970, p. 904). Or another patient: "Oh, I'm taking the word the wrong way to say, all of the barbers here whenever they stop you it's going around and around, if you know what I mean, that is tying and tying for repucer, repuceration, well, we were trying the best that we could while another time it was with the beds over there the same thing" (Gardner, 1974, p. 68)

This distinction between fluent and nonfluent aphasia, however, captures the data only in the broadest sense. One reason lies in the fact that—as we've seen—language use involves the coordination of many different steps, many

FIGURE 10.14 BRAIN AREAS CRUCIAL FOR THE PERCEPTION AND PRODUCTION OF LANGUAGE

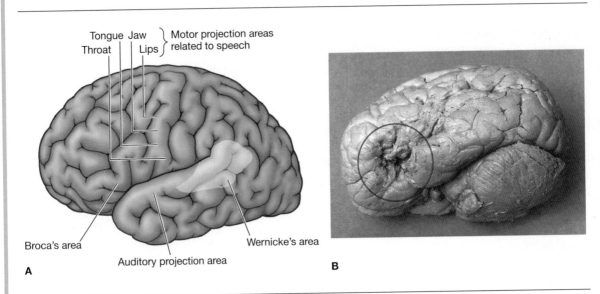

Panel A shows some of the many brain regions that are crucial in supporting the comprehension and production of language. For most individuals, most of these regions are in the left cerebral hemisphere (as shown here). Broca's area is heavily involved in language production; Wernicke's area plays a crucial role in language comprehension. Panel B shows an actual photograph of Broca's patient "Tan." Because of his brain damage, this patient was no longer able to say anything other than the syllable "Tan"—and hence the nickname often used for him. This pattern (along with observations gained through Tan's autopsy) led Broca to propose that a specific brain region is crucial for speech.

different processes. These include processes needed to "look up" word meanings in your "mental dictionary," processes needed to figure out the structural relationships within a sentence, processes needed to integrate information about a sentence's structure with the meanings of the words within the sentence, and so on. Each of these processes relies on its own set of brain pathways, so damage to those pathways disrupts the process. As a result, the language loss observed in aphasia can sometimes be quite specific, with impairment just to one particular processing step (Cabeza & Nyberg, 2000; Demonet, Wise, & Frackowiak, 1993; Martin, 2003). Related, various brain sites other than Broca's area and Wernicke's area play a role in language processing, and it will likely be some years before researchers have catalogued the full set of brain areas crucial for language (e.g., Dronkers, Wilkins, Van Valin, Redefern, & Jaeger, 2004; Poeppel & Hickok, 2004).

Even with these complexities, the point here is that humans have a considerable amount of neural tissue that is specialized for language. Damage to this tissue can disrupt language understanding, language production, or both. And in all cases, the data make it clear that our skill in using language rests in part on the fact that we have a lot of neural apparatus devoted to precisely this task.

The Biology of Language Learning

The biological roots of language also show up in another way—in the way that language is learned. This learning occurs remarkably rapidly: By the age of 3 or 4, almost every child is able to converse at a reasonable level. Moreover, this learning can proceed in an astonishingly wide range of environments. Children who talk a lot with adults learn language, and so do children who talk very little with adults. Indeed, children learn language even if their communication with adults is strictly limited. Evidence on this last point comes from children who are born deaf and with no opportunity to learn sign language. (In some cases, this is because their caretakers don't know how to sign; in other cases, it's because their caretakers choose not to teach signing.) Even in these extreme cases, language emerges: Children in this situation *invent* their own gestural language (usually called "home sign") and teach the language to the people in their surroundings. Remarkably, the language they invent shows many of the formal structures routinely seen in the world's existing languages (Feldman, Goldin-Meadow, & Gleitman, 1978; Goldin-Meadow, 2003; Senghas, Román, & Mavillapalli, 2006).

How should we think about this? According to many psychologists, the answer lies in highly sophisticated learning capacities that all humans share, capacities that have specifically evolved for language learning. Support for this claim comes from many sources, including observations of **specific language impairment (SLI)**. Children with this disorder have normal intelligence and no problems with the muscle movements needed to produce language. Nonetheless, they are slow to learn language and, throughout their lives, have difficulty in understanding and producing many sentences. They are also impaired on tasks designed to test their linguistic knowledge. They have difficulty, for example, completing passages like this one: "I like to blife. Today I blife. Tomorrow I will blife. Yesterday I did the same thing. Yesterday I _____." Most 4-year-olds know that the answer is "Yesterday I blifed." But adults with SLI cannot do this task—apparently having failed to learn the simple rule of language involved in forming the past tense of regular verbs (Bishop & Norbury, 2008; Lai, Fisher, Hurst, Vargha-Khadem, & Monaco, 2001; van der Lely, 2005; van der Lely & Pinker, 2014).

Claims about SLI remain controversial, but many authors point to this disorder as evidence for brain mechanisms that are somehow specialized for language learning. Disruption to these mechanisms throws language off track but, remarkably, seems to leave other aspects of the brain's functioning undisturbed.

The Processes of Language Learning

Even with these biological contributions, there's no question that learning does play a crucial role in the acquisition of language. After all, children who grow up in Paris learn to speak French; children who grow up in Beijing learn to speak Chinese. In this rather obvious way, language learning depends on the child's picking up information from her environment.

But what learning mechanisms are involved here? Part of the answer rests on the fact that children are exquisitely sensitive to patterns and regularities in what they hear, as though each child were an astute statistician, keeping track of the frequency-of-occurrence of this form or that. In one study, 8-month-old infants heard a 2-minute tape recording that sounded something like "bidakupadotigolabubidaku." These syllables were spoken in a monotonous tone, with no difference in stress from one syllable to the next and no pauses in between any of the syllables. But there was a pattern. The experimenters had decided in advance to designate the sequence "bidaku" as a word. Therefore, they arranged the sequences so that if the infant heard "bida," then "ku" was sure to follow. For other syllables, there was no such pattern. For instance, "daku" (the end of the nonsense word "bidaku") would sometimes be followed by "go," sometimes by "pa," and so on. The babies reliably detected these patterns, a point that was evident in a subsequent test: In the test, babies showed no evidence of surprise if they heard the string "bidakubidakubidaku." From the babies' point of view, these were simply repetitions of a word they already knew. However, the babies did show surprise if they were presented with the string "dakupadakupadakupa." This was not a "word" they had heard before, although of course they had heard each of its syllables many times. Thus, the babies had learned the vocabulary of this made-up language. They had detected the statistical pattern of which syllables followed which, despite their rather brief, entirely passive exposure to these sounds and despite the absence of any supporting cues such as pauses or shifts in intonation (Aslin, Saffran, & Newport, 1998; Marcus, Vijayan, Rao, & Vishton, 1999; Saffran, 2003; Xu & Garcia, 2008).

In addition, it's important that children don't just detect (and echo) patterns in the speech they hear. Children also seem to derive broad principles from what they hear. Consider, for example, how English-speaking children learn to form the past tense. Initially, they proceed in a word-by-word fashion, so they memorize that the past tense of "play" is "played," the past tense of "climb" is "climbed," and so on. By age 3 or so, however, children seem to realize that they don't have to memorize each word's past tense as a separate vocabulary item. Instead, they realize they can produce the past tense by manipulating morphemes—that is, by adding the "-ed" ending onto a word. Once children make this discovery, they're able to apply this principle to many new verbs, including verbs they've never encountered before.

However, children over-rely on this pattern, and their speech at this age contains **overregularization errors:** They say things like "Yesterday we goed" or "Yesterday I runned." The same thing happens with other morphemes, so that children of this age also overgeneralize their use of the plural ending—they say things like "I have two foots" or "I lost three tooths" (Marcus et al., 1992). They also generalize on contractions; having heard "she isn't" and "you aren't," they say things like "I amn't."

It seems, then, that children (even young infants) are keenly sensitive to patterns in the language that they are learning, and they are able to figure out the (sometimes rather abstract) principles that govern these patterns. In addition, language learning relies on a theme that has been in view throughout this chapter: Language has many elements (syntax, semantics, phonology, prosody, etc.), and these elements interact in ordinary language use (thus, you rely on a sentence's syntactic form to figure out its meaning; you rely on semantic cues in deciphering the syntax). In the same fashion, language learning also relies on all these elements in an interacting fashion. Thus, children rely on prosody (again: the rise and fall of pitch, the pattern of timing) as clues to syntax, and adults speaking to children helpfully exaggerate these prosodic signals, easing the children's interpretive burden. Children also rely on their vocabulary, listening for words they already know as clues helping them to process more complex strings. Likewise, children rely on their knowledge of semantic relationships as a basis for figuring out syntax—a process known as **semantic bootstrapping** (Pinker, 1987). In this way, the very complexity of language is both a burden for the child (because there's so much to learn in "learning a language") and an aid (because the child can use each of the elements as sources of information in trying to figure out the other elements).

Animal Language

We've suggested that humans are biologically prepared for language learning, and this claim has many implications. Among other points, can we locate the genes that underlie this preparation? Many researchers claim that we can, and they point to a gene dubbed "FOXP2" as crucial; people who have a mutated form of this gene are markedly impaired in their language learning (e.g., Vargha-Khadem, Gadian, Copp, & Mishkin, 2005).

As a related point, if language learning is somehow tied to human genetics, then we might expect *not* to find language capacity in other species—no matter how the other species is trained or encouraged to use language. Of course, other species do have sophisticated communication systems—including the songs and clicks of dolphins and whales, the dances of honeybees, and the various forms of alarm calls used by monkeys. These naturally occurring systems, however, are extremely limited—with small vocabularies and little (or perhaps nothing) that corresponds to the rules of syntax that are plainly evident in human language. These systems will certainly not support the sort of *generativity* that is a prominent feature of human language—and so these other species don't have anything approaching our capacity to produce an unending variety of new sentences or our ability to understand an unending variety of new ideas.

Perhaps, though, these naturally occurring systems understate what animals can do. Perhaps animals can do more if only we help them a bit. To explore this issue, researchers have tried to train animals to use more sophisticated forms of communication. Some of the projects have tried to train dolphins to communicate with humans; one project involved an African grey parrot; other projects have focused on primates—asking what a chimpanzee,

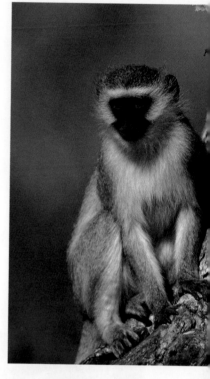

COMMUNICATION AMONG VERVET MONKEYS

Animals of many species communicate with each other. For example, Vervet monkeys give alarm calls when they spot a nearby predator. But they have distinct alarm calls for different types of predator—and so their call is different when they see a leopard than it is when they see an eagle or a python. The fact remains, though, that no naturally occurring animal communication system comes close to human language in richness or complexity.

gorilla, or bonobo might be capable of. The results from these studies are impressive, but it is notable that the greatest success involves animals that are quite similar to humans genetically (e.g., Savage-Rumbaugh & Lewin, 1994; Savage-Rumbaugh & Fields, 2000). For example, Kanzi, a male bonobo, seems to understand icons on a keyboard as *symbols* that refer to other ideas, and he also has some mastery of syntax—so he responds differently and (usually) appropriately, using stuffed animals, to the instructions "Make the doggie bite the snake" or "Make the snake bite the doggie."

Kanzi's abilities, though, after an enormous amount of careful training, are way below those of the average 3- or 4-year-old human who has received no explicit language training. (For example, as impressive as Kanzi is, he has not mastered the distinction between present, past, and future tense, although every human child effortlessly learns this basic aspect of language.) Thus, it seems that other species (especially those closely related to us) can learn the rudiments of language, but nothing in their performance undercuts the amazing differences between human language capacity and that in other organisms.

"Wolf Children"

Before moving on, we should address one last point—one that concerns the *limits* on our "biological preparation" for language. To put the matter simply, our human biology gives us a fabulous start on language learning, but to turn this "start" into "language capacity," we also need a communicative partner.

In 1920, villagers in India discovered a wolf mother in her den together with four cubs. Two were baby wolves, but the other two were human

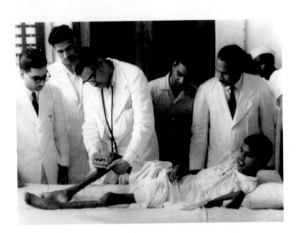 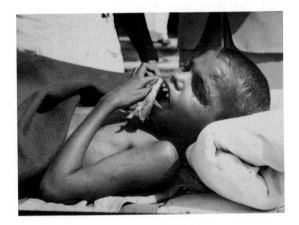

A MODERN WILD BOY

Ramu, a young boy discovered in India in 1976, appears to have been raised by wolves. He was deformed, apparently from lying in cramped positions, as in a den. He could not walk, and he drank by lapping with his tongue. His favorite food was raw meat, which he seemed to be able to smell at a distance. After he was found, he lived at the home for destitute children run by Mother Teresa in Lucknow, Uttar Pradesh. He learned to bathe and dress himself but never learned to speak. He continued to prefer raw meat and would often sneak out to prey upon fowl in the neighbor's chicken coop. Ramu died at the age of about 10 in February 1985.

children, subsequently named Kamala and Amala. No one knows how they got there or why the wolf adopted them. Roger Brown (1958) tells us what these children were like:

> Kamala was about eight years old and Amala was only one and one-half. They were thoroughly wolfish in appearance and behavior: Hard callus had developed on their knees and palms from going on all fours. Their teeth were sharp edged. They moved their nostrils sniffing food. Eating and drinking were accomplished by lowering their mouths to the plate. They ate raw meat. . . . At night they prowled and sometimes howled. They shunned other children but followed the dog and cat. They slept rolled up together on the floor. . . . Amala died within a year but Kamala lived to be eighteen. . . . In time, Kamala learned to walk erect, to wear clothing, and even to speak a few words. (p. 100)

The outcome was similar for the 30 or so other wild children for whom researchers have evidence. When found, they were all shockingly animal-like. None could be rehabilitated to use language normally, although some (like Kamala) did learn to speak a few words.

Of course, the data from these wild children are difficult to interpret, in part because we do not know why the children were abandoned in the first place. (Is it possible, for example, that these children were abandoned because their human parents detected some sign of mental retardation or some other birth defect? If so, these children likely were impaired in their functioning from the start.) Nonetheless, the consistency of these findings underscores an important point: Language learning may depend on both a human genome and a human environment.

Language and Thought

Virtually every human knows and uses a language. Indeed, to find people who cannot use language, we need to focus on truly extreme circumstances—individuals who have suffered serious brain damage, or (as we just discussed) people who have grown up completely isolated from other humans. In addition, we've also seen that no other species has a language comparable to ours in complexity or communicative power. In a real sense, then, knowing a language is a key part of being human—a nearly universal achievement in our species, yet unknown in its full form in any other species.

But it's also important that people speak *different* languages—some of us speak English, others German, and still others Abkhaz or Choctaw or Kanuri or Quanzhou. How do these differences matter? Is it possible that people who speak different languages end up somehow different in their thought processes?

Linguistic Relativity

Anthropologist Benjamin Whorf was a strong proponent of the view that the language you speak forces you into certain modes of thought—a claim

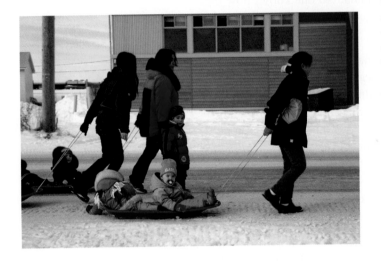

MYTHS ABOUT LANGUAGE AND THOUGHT

Many people believe that the native peoples of the far north (including the Inuit) have an enormous number of terms for the various forms of snow and are correspondingly skilled in discriminating types of snow. It turns out, though, that the initial claim (the number of terms for snow) is wrong; the Inuit have roughly the same number of snow terms as do people living further south. In addition, if the Inuit people are more skilled in discriminating snow types, is this because of the language that they speak? Or is it because their day-to-day lives demand that they stay alert to the differences among snow types?   AFTER ROBERSON, DAVIES, & DAVIDOFF, 2000.

usually known as **linguistic relativity** (Whorf, 1956). Thus, he claimed, people who speak a different language from the one you do inevitably *think* differently than you do. How can we test this claim?

One line of work has examined how people perceive colors, building on the fact that some languages have many terms for colors (red, orange, mauve, puce, salmon, fawn, ocher, etc.) and others have few (see **Figure 10.15**). Do these differences among languages affect perception? Recent findings suggest, in fact, that people who speak languages with a richer color vocabulary may perceive colors differently—making finer and more sharply defined distinctions (Özgen, 2004; Roberson, Davies, & Davidoff, 2000).

Other studies have focused on other ways in which languages differ. Some languages, for example, emphasize absolute directions (terms defined independently of which way the speaker happens to be facing at the moment). Other languages emphasize relative directions (these *do* depend on which way the speaker is facing). Research suggests that these language differences can lead to corresponding differences in how people remember—and perhaps how they perceive—position (Majid, Bowerman, Kita, Haun, & Levinson, 2004; Pederson et al., 1998).

Languages also differ in how they describe events. In English, we tend to use active-voice sentences that name the agent of the action, even if the action was accidental ("Sam made a mistake"). It sounds awkward or evasive to describe these events in other terms ("Mistakes were made"). In other languages, including Japanese or Spanish, it's common *not* to mention the agent for an accidental event, and this in turn can shape memory: After viewing videos of accidental events, Japanese and Spanish speakers are less likely than English speakers to remember the person who triggered the accident (Boroditsky, 2011).

How should we think about all of these results? One possibility—in line with Whorf's original hypothesis—is that language has a direct impact on cognition, so that the categories recognized by your language become the

FIGURE 10.15   COLORS IN DIFFERENT LANGUAGES

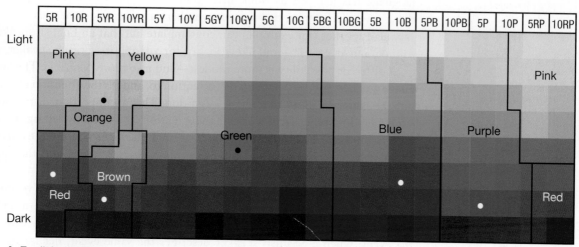

A English naming

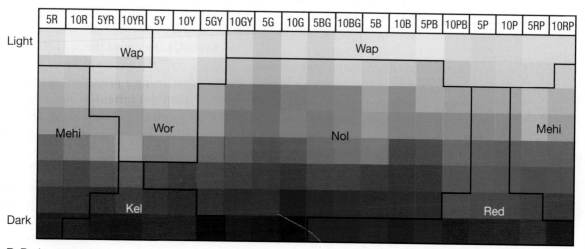

B Berinmo naming

The Berinmo people, living in Papua New Guinea, have only five words for describing colors, and so, for example, they use a single word ("nol") to describe colors that English speakers call "green" and colors we call "blue." (The letters and numbers in these panels refer to a system often used for classifying colors.) These differences, from one language to the next, have an impact on how people perceive and remember colors. This effect is best understood, however, in terms of attention: Language can draw our attention to some aspect of the world and in this way can shape our experience and, thus, our cognition.   AFTER ROBERSON, DAVIES, & DAVIDOFF, 2000.

categories used in your thought. In this view, language has a unique effect on cognition (because no other factor can shape cognition in this way). And because language's influence is unique, it is also irreversible: Once your language has led you to think in certain ways, you will forever think in those ways. Thus, from this perspective, there are literally some ideas that a Japanese speaker (for example) can contemplate but that an English speaker cannot, and vice versa—and likewise, say, for a Hopi or a French speaker.

A different possibility is more modest—and also more plausible: The language you hear guides what you pay attention to, and it's the attention effects, not the language itself, that shape cognition. This an important distinction simply because other factors also shape attention, and in many settings these factors will erase any impact that language might have. As a result, the effects of language on cognition are important but not irreversible, and they are certainly not as fundamental as Whorf proposed.

To see how these points play out, let's look at a concrete case. We've mentioned that when English speakers describe an event, our language usually demands that we name (and thus pay attention to) the actor who caused the event; when a Spanish speaker describes the same event, her language doesn't have this requirement, and so doesn't force her to think about the actor. In this fashion, the structure of each language influences what you'll pay attention to, and the data tell us that this difference in focus can have consequences for thinking and for memory.

But, of course, we could, if we wished, simply give the Spanish speaker an instruction: "Pay attention to the actor." Or we could make sure that the actor is wearing a brightly colored coat, using a perceptual cue to guide attention. These simple steps can (and often do) offset the bias created by language. For this reason, an effect of language on cognition is often not observed and is surely not a permanent effect, forever defining (and perhaps limiting) how someone thinks.

The logic is similar for the effect of language on color perception. If you're a speaker of Berinmo (a language spoken in New Guinea), your language makes no distinction between "green" and "blue," so your language never leads you to think about these as separate categories. If you're an English speaker, your language does make this distinction, and this can draw your attention to what all green objects have in common and what all blue objects have in common. If your attention is drawn to this point again and again, you'll gain familiarity with the distinction and eventually become better at making the distinction. Once more, therefore, language does matter—but it matters because of language's impact on attention.

Again, let's be clear on the argument here: If language directly and uniquely shapes thought, then the effects of language on cognition will be systematic and permanent. But the alternative is that it's your *experience* that shapes thought, and your experience depends on what you pay attention to, and (finally) language is just one of the factors guiding what you pay attention to. On this basis, the effects of language will be detectable but inconsistent and certainly not permanent. This latter view fits better with the evidence (e.g., Boroditsky, 2001; but then Chen, 2007, or January & Kako, 2007). Indeed, even within a single experiment, it's possible to undo the effects of language by using some other means to redirect the participants' attention. Thus, for example, English speakers and speakers of Mandarin Chinese seem initially to think about spatial relations differently—because their languages bias them toward different interpretive habits. But the difference between English and Chinese speakers can be eradicated by a brief conversation, leading them to consider other ways one might think about space (Li & Gleitman, 2002; also Li, Abarbanell, Gleitman, & Papafragou, 2011).

A half-century ago, Whorf argued for a strong claim—that the specific language you speak plays a unique role in shaping your thought and has a lifelong impact in determining what you can or cannot think, what ideas you can or cannot entertain. There is an element of truth here, because language can shape cognition. But language's impact is neither profound nor permanent, and there is no reason to accept Whorf's ambitious proposal. (For more on these issues, see Gleitman & Papafragou, 2012; Hanako & Smith, 2005; Hermer-Vazquez, Spelke, & Katsnelson, 1999; Kay & Regier, 2007; Özgen & Davies, 2002; Papafragou, Li, Choi, & Han, 2007; Stapel & Semin, 2007.)

Bilingualism

There's one more—and intriguing—way that language is said to influence cognition. It comes from cases in which someone knows more than one language.

Children who are raised in bilingual homes generally learn both languages as quickly and as well as monolingual children learn their single language (Kovelman, Shalinksy, Berens, & Petitto, 2008). Bilingual children do tend to have smaller vocabularies, compared to monolingual children, but this contrast is evident only at an early age, and bilingual children soon catch up on this dimension (Bialystok, Craik, Green, & Gollan, 2009).

These findings surprise many people, on the expectation that bilingual children would become confused—blurring together their languages and getting mixed up about which words and which rules belong in each language. But, remarkably, this confusion seems not to occur. In fact, children who are raised bilingually seem to develop skills that specifically help them avoid this sort of confusion—so that they develop a skill of (say) turning off their French-based habits in *this* setting so that they can speak uncompromised English, and then turning off their English-based habits in *that* setting so that they can speak fluent French. This skill obviously supports their language learning, but it may also help them in other settings (Bialystok et al., 2009; Calvo & Bialystok, 2013; Engel de Abreu, Cruz-Santos, Tourinho, Martion, & Bialystok, 2012; Hernández, Costa, & Humphreys, 2012; Hilchey & Klein, 2011; Kroll, Bobb, & Hoshino, 2014; Pelham & Abrams, 2014; Zelazo, 2006). In Chapter 5 we introduced the idea of executive control, and the suggestion here is that being raised bilingually may encourage *better* executive control. As a result, bilinguals may be better at avoiding distraction, switching between competing tasks, or holding information in mind while working on some other task.

There has, however, been some debate about these findings, and not all experiments find a bilingual advantage in executive control (e.g., Costa, Hernández, Costa-Faidella, & Sebastián-Galés, 2009; de Bruin, Treccani, & Della Salla, 2015). There is some suggestion that this advantage only emerges with certain tasks or in certain age groups (perhaps: children, but not adults). There is also some indication that other forms of training can also improve executive control—and so bilingualism may be just one way to achieve this goal. Obviously, further research is needed in this domain, especially since the (alleged and often-observed) benefits of bilingualism have important implications—for public policy, for education, and for parenting. These implications become all the more intriguing when we bear in mind that roughly a fifth of the population in the United States speaks a language at home that is different from the English they use in other settings; the proportion is even higher in some states, including California, Texas, New Mexico, and Nevada (Shin & Kominski, 2010). These points to the side, though, research on bilingualism provides one more (and perhaps a surprising) arena in which scholars continue to explore the ways in which language use may shape cognition.

COGNITIVE PSYCHOLOGY AND THE LAW

Remembering Conversation

Many legal cases hinge on a witness reporting details of how a conversation unfolded. Did the shooter say, "Die, fool," just before pulling the trigger? If so, this provides evidence that the murder was (at least briefly) premeditated. Did Fred tell Jim about the new product when they were together at the business meeting? If so, this might indicate that Jim is guilty of insider trading.

How accurate is memory for conversation? The answer grows out of two themes. First, in most conversations, people have no reason to care about the exact sequence of words or how exactly the ideas are expressed. Instead, what people usually care about and pay attention to is the "propositional content" of the conversation—the underlying gist.

If people are focused on the gist and remember what they have paid attention to, then we should expect them to remember the gist and not the wording. Put differently, we should expect from the outset that people will have difficulty recalling how utterances were phrased or how exactly a conversation unfolded.

Second, in most conversations, a lot of information goes unsaid, but the conversational participants effortlessly make inferences to fill in the bits not overtly expressed. This filling-in is made possible by the fact that participants in a conversation draw on their "common ground"—that is, beliefs shared by the individuals taking part in that conversation. When there is no common ground, the risk of misunderstanding is increased.

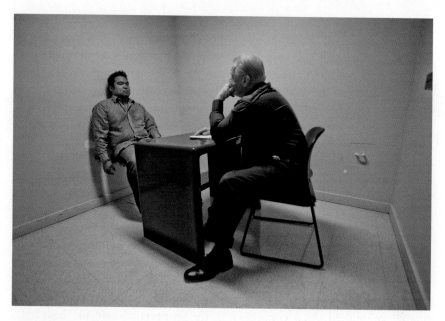

INTERROGATION

Police interrogations are often conducted in a bare, windowless room; the suspect sits in an uncomfortable (unpadded, armless) chair. Crucially, though, the police and the suspect often bring different assumptions to the interrogation. The police are alert to the exact words spoken (and so they are careful not to offer promises, although they may *imply* promises). The suspect, however, may not be alert to the exact words, and so may understand merely implied promises as actual promises.

Again, note the implication. We've just said that the gist of a conversation depends on inferences and assumptions. We've also said that people tend to remember the gist of a conversation, not the actual words spoken. Putting these pieces together, we're led to the expectation that people will often blur together in their recall the propositions that were actually expressed and those that were merely implied. Said differently, people will often recall fragments of conversation that were not spoken at all.

A range of evidence supports these claims. In one study, mothers had a conversation with their 4-year-old daughters and then, three days later, were asked to recall exactly how the conversation had unfolded. The mothers' memories for the exact words spoken were quite poor, and they had difficulty recalling (among other points) whether their child's statements were spontaneous or prompted by specific questions; they even had difficulty recalling which utterances were spoken by them and which ones by the children.

This study (and others making the same point) is worrisome for law enforcement. In evaluating a child's report, we want to know if the report was spontaneous or prompted; we want to know if the details in the report came from the child or were suggested by an adult. Unfortunately, evidence suggests that memory for these crucial points is quite poor.

Here's a different line of evidence, with its own implications for the justice system. Memory for conversations, we've said, usually includes many points that were actually absent from the conversation but were instead supplied by the conversational participants, based on the "common ground" these individuals brought to the conversation. But what happens if there is no common ground—if the individuals bring different assumptions to the conversation?

Think about the "conversation" that takes place between a police detective and a suspect in an interrogation room. The suspect's statement will be inadmissible at trial if the detectives make any promises or threats during the interrogation, but detectives can (and often do) imply promises or threats. The result is a situation in which the investigator and the suspect are "playing by different rules." The investigator's perspective emphasizes the specific words spoken (words that do not contain an overt promise or threat). The suspect, in contrast, will likely adopt a perspective that's sensible in most settings—one that (as we've said) focuses on the gist of the exchange, with minimal attention to how that gist is expressed. The suspect, in other words, has no reason to focus on whether a promise was expressed or merely implied. As a consequence, the suspect is likely to "hear" the (implied) promise or threat, even though the investigator uttered neither.

All of these results are, from a research perspective, virtually inevitable, given what we know about how conversations proceed and how memory functions. Once we acknowledge these points, though, the obvious conclusion must be that electronic recording is essential whenever we draw evidence from (or about) a conversation. In the absence of that recording, we need to be careful (and perhaps skeptical) in drawing evidence from remembered conversations.

chapter summary

• All speech is built up from a few dozen phonemes, although the selection of phonemes varies from language to language. Phonemes in turn are built up from a small number of production features, including voicing, place of articulation, and manner of production. Phonemes can be combined to form more complex sounds, but combinations are constrained by a number of rules.

• Speech perception is more than a matter of detecting the relevant features in the input sound stream. The perceiver needs to deal with speaker-to-speaker variation in how sounds are produced; she also needs to segment the stream of speech and cope with coarticulation. The process of speech perception is helped enormously by context, but we also have the impressive skill of categorical perception, which makes us keenly sensitive to differences between categories of speech sounds but insensitive to distinctions within each category.

• People know many thousands of words, and for each one they know the sound of the word, its syntactic role, and its semantic representation. Our understanding of words is also generative, enabling us to create limitless numbers of new words. Some new words are wholly made up (e.g., "geek"), but many new words are created by combining familiar morphemes.

• The rules of syntax govern whether a sequence of words is grammatical. One set of rules governs phrase structure, and the word groups identified by these rules do correspond to natural groupings of words. Phrase structure rules also guide interpretation. Like all the rules discussed in this chapter, though, phrase structure rules are descriptive, not prescriptive.

● To understand a sentence, a listener or reader needs to parse the sentence, determining each word's syntactic role. Evidence suggests that people parse a sentence as they see or hear each word, and this approach sometimes leads them into parsing errors that must be repaired later; this outcome is revealed by garden-path sentences. Parsing is guided by syntax, semantics, and the extralinguistic context.

● The biological roots of language are revealed in many ways. The study of aphasia makes it clear that some areas of the brain are specialized for learning and using language. The rapid learning of language also speaks to the biological basis for language.

● Processes of imitation and direct instruction play relatively small parts in language learning. This is evident in the fact that children produce many forms (often, overregularization errors) that no adult produces; these forms are obviously not the result of imitation. Language learning is, however, strongly influenced by children's remarkable sensitivity to patterns in the language they hear. Children can also use their understanding of one aspect of language (e.g., phonology or vocabulary) to help learn about other aspects (e.g., syntax).

● There has been considerable discussion about the ways in which thought might be shaped by the language one speaks. Language certainly guides and influences your thoughts, and the way a thought is formulated into words can have an effect on how you think about the thought's content. In addition, language can call your attention to a category or to a distinction, which makes it likely that you will have experience in thinking about the category or distinction. This experience, in turn, can promote fluency in these thoughts. However, these effects are not unique to language (because other factors can also draw your attention to the category), nor are they irreversible. Hence, there is no evidence that language can shape what you *can* think.

● Research shows that children raised in bilingual homes learn both languages as quickly and as well as monolingual children learning their single language. In fact, bilingual children seem to develop an impressive ability to switch between languages, and this ability may also help them in other settings that demand executive control of mental processes.

⒠ eBook Demonstrations & Essays

Online Demonstrations:
● Demonstration 10.1: Phonemes and Subphonemes
● Demonstration 10.2: The Speed of Speech
● Demonstration 10.3: Coarticulation
● Demonstration 10.4: The Most Common Words
● Demonstration 10.5: Patterns in Language
● Demonstration 10.6: Ambiguity

Online Applying Cognitive Psychology Essays:
● Cognitive Psychology and Education: Writing
● Cognitive Psychology and the Law: Jury Instructions

ZAPS 2.0 Cognition Labs

● Go to **http://digital.wwnorton.com/cognition6** for the online labs relevant to this chapter.

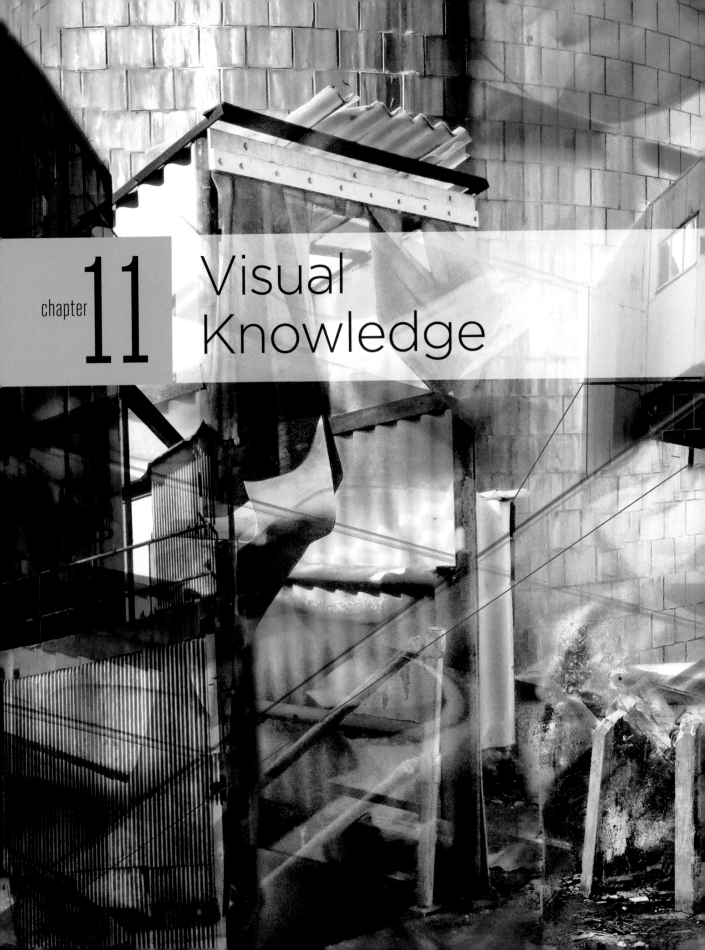

11

Visual
Knowledge

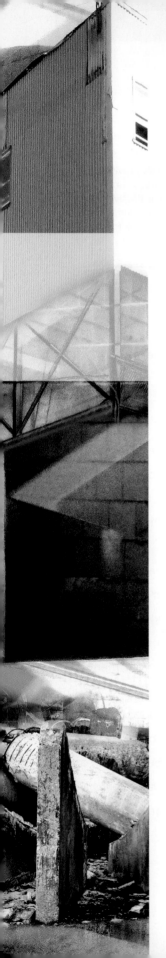

what if... Researchers use many means to study *dreams*. The most obvious path, though, is simply to ask people about the content of their dreams. For example, consider this exchange. E is the experimenter; S is the person reporting the dream, which was about a cancer clinic (Kerr, 1983, p. 276).

S: I was in a room that looked similar to my instant banker at work, but it was a big machine with lots of buttons, like a car machine.

E: Like an instant banker machine?

S: Right, at [name of bank]. And I don't know why I was there, but I guess there was a screen and there were other buttons you could push, you could look in and see how different cancer patients are doing.

E: Was this visual, could you see anything?

S: I couldn't, but I stood by the screen and I knew that *others* could see what was going on through all the little panels.

. . .

S: I guess I imagined the board with the buttons. Maybe because I imagined them in my mind, it was not that I could really see them with my eyes, but I know what that board looks like, and the only reason I know what it looks like is by touch, and I could remember where the buttons were without touching them on the boards.

. . .

E: Okay. Where did the events in this experience seem to be taking place? What were the settings?

S: It seemed to be a large room that was oblong in shape, and there seemed to be an X-ray machine's work. I felt like it was in an office building where I worked.

E: And you mentioned something before about the bank?

S: Uh huh, it looked like the bank where I do my instant banking (E: Okay.), except it was larger and more oblong.

E: And is that more like where you worked?

S: No, where I do work, the room is smaller, just large enough for that little instant banker machine.

. . . .

- In important ways, mental images are picturelike, representing in a direct fashion the spatial layout of the represented scene. It's not surprising, therefore, that there is considerable overlap between imagery and perception—in how each functions and also in their neural bases.

- People can also use spatial imagery, which is not visual and may instead be represented in the mind in terms of movements or perhaps in some more abstract format.

- Although they are picturelike, images (visual or spatial) are plainly not pictures; instead, images seem to be organized and already interpreted in a fashion that pictures are not.

- Even though images in working memory provide a distinctive form of representation, information about appearances in long-term memory may not be distinctive. In fact, long-term memory for sensory information seems to obey all the principles we described, in earlier chapters, for verbal or symbolic memories.

This dream report seems in most ways unremarkable—other people, describing their own dreams, offer reports that are similar. What is remarkable, though, is that this report was offered by someone who had been blind since birth.

The dreamer's blindness helps us understand some aspects of this report (e.g., she says that she only knew what the board looked like *by touch*). But how should we think about other aspects of the report: How could she know "what that board *looks like*"? What was it, in the dream, that told her the room was large and oblong?

Of course, close reading of her dream reveals the absence of truly "visual" properties: There are no mentions of colors or visible textures on surfaces. This pattern—an absence of visual descriptions—is typical for individuals who were blinded before the age of 5 or so (e.g., Kerr & Domhoff, 2004). You might wonder, therefore, what your mental life would be like—in your dreams and while you're awake—if you had lost the sense of sight at an early age. But, in addition, we need to confront several questions: What does it mean for something to be "truly visual"? How should we think about reports from the blind about their dreams? What is the nature of their experience? To work our way toward these issues, let's start with a much more familiar case—the sort of visual imagery that most sighted people have all the time.

Visual Imagery

We all have knowledge of many different types. For example, you know what a fish is, but you also know what fish smells like when it's cooking and what a fish looks like. You know what a guitar is, but you also know what one sounds like. Likewise, people describe their *thoughts* in a variety of ways: Sometimes, they claim, their thoughts seem to be formulated in words. Sometimes their thoughts seem more abstract—a sequence of ideas that lacks any concrete form. But sometimes, people claim, their thoughts involve a sequence of *pictures* or *sounds* or other sensory impressions.

What can we say about this variety? How are specific sights or sounds or smells represented in the mind? How should we think about the proposal that people sometimes "think in pictures"? In this chapter, we'll focus largely on *visual* knowledge and *visual* thoughts (and so, for now, our focus will be on sighted individuals, not the blind). It's clear, though, that other forms of knowledge do exist—for example, many of us have vivid imagery for sounds (e.g., Pfordresher & Halpern, 2013) and for tastes and smells (e.g., Carrasco & Ridout, 1997; Drummond, 1995; Lyman & McDaniel, 1986). These other forms of knowledge are part of both our waking thoughts and our dreams (e.g., Antonio, Neilsen & Donderi, 1998). As we proceed, therefore, you should keep an eye on how the questions we're asking might be applied to other forms of nonverbal knowledge.

The Mind's Eye

How many windows are there in your house or your apartment? Who has bushier eyebrows—Justin Bieber or Simon Cowell? For most people, questions like these seem to elicit "mental pictures." You know what Bieber and Cowell look like, and you call a "picture" of each before your "mind's eye" in order to make the comparison. Likewise, you call to mind a "map" of your apartment and count the windows by inspecting this map. Many people even trace the map in the air when they're counting the windows, moving their finger around to follow the imagined map's contours.

Various practical problems also seem to evoke images. There you are in a store, trying on a new sweater. Will the sweater look good with your blue pants? To decide, you'll probably try to visualize the blue of the pants, using your "mind's eye" to ask how they'll look with the sweater. Similarly, if a friend asks you, "Was David in class yesterday?" you might try to recall by visualizing what the room looked like during the class; is David "visible" in your image?

These examples illustrate the common, everyday use of visual images—as a basis for making decisions, as an aid to remembering. But surely there is no tiny eye somewhere deep in your brain; thus, the phrase "mind's eye" cannot be taken literally. Likewise, mental "pictures" cannot be actual pictures; with no eye deep inside the brain, who or what would inspect such pictures? In light of these puzzles, what *are* images?

Introspections about Images

People have written about imagery (and the "mind's eye") for hundreds of years, but the first systematic research in this domain was conducted in the late 1800s by Francis Galton. He was an important figure and made contributions as an inventor, explorer, statistician, and meteorologist. (He also happened to be Charles Darwin's cousin.) But, as part of his work in psychology, he explored the nature of visual imagery. His method was simple: He asked various people simply to describe their images and rate them for vividness (Galton, 1883). In other words, he asked his research participants to *introspect*, or "look within" (a method that we first met in Chapter 1), and to report on their own mental contents. The **self-report data** he obtained fit well with common sense: The participants reported that they could "inspect" their images much as they would inspect a picture. Their descriptions also made it clear that they were "viewing" their images from a certain position and a certain distance—just as they'd look at an actual scene from a specific viewing perspective. They also reported that they could "read off" from the image details of color and texture. All of this implies a mode of representation that is, in many ways, picturelike—and that is, of course, consistent with our informal manner of describing mental images as "pictures in the head," to be inspected with the "mind's eye."

There was also another side of these early data: Galton's participants differed widely from one another in their self-reports. Many described images of photographic clarity, rich in detail, almost as if they were actually *seeing* the imaged scene rather than visualizing it. Other participants, in contrast, reported very sketchy images or no images at all. They were able to think about the scenes or objects Galton named for them, but they insisted that in no sense were they "seeing" these scenes. Their reports rarely included mention of color or size or viewing perspective; indeed, their reports were devoid of *any* visual qualities.

These observations suggest that people differ enormously in the nature of their imagery—so that some people are "visualizers" and others are not. Indeed, these observations invite the notion that some people may be *incapable* of forming visual images; but if so, what consequences does this notion have? Are there tasks that the visualizers can do that the "nonvisualizers" cannot (or vice versa)?

Before we can answer these questions, we need to address a methodological concern raised by Galton's data, and it's a concern that probably occurred to you right at the start of this chapter. (We also met this issue in Chapter 1.) When someone who is blind says that a room in her dream "looked similar" to her instant banker machine, how should we think about this report? It seems plausible that this person would mean something different by the phrase "looked similar" than a sighted person might mean. Indeed, blind people routinely talk about "watching TV" or "taking a look at something," and they know that a star "appears" as a small spot in the night sky (Kerr & Domhoff, 2004). These phrases are surely metaphorical when used by the blind, and obviously the subjective experience of someone blind "watching TV" is different from the experience of someone with full vision.

Points like these remind us that there is, in essence, a "translation step" involved whenever people translate their subjective inner experience into a verbal report, and there's no guarantee that everyone translates in the same way. Returning to Galton's study, it's therefore possible that all of his participants had the *same* imagery skill but varied in how they described their experience (i.e., in how they translated the experience into words). Perhaps some were cautious and therefore kept their descriptions brief and undetailed, while others were more extravagant and took pleasure in providing elaborate and flowery reports. In this way, Galton's data might reveal differences in how people *talk about* their imagery, not differences in imagery per se.

To address this concern, what we need is a more objective means of assessing imagery—one that does not rely on the subjectivity inherent in self-reports. With this more objective approach, we could assess the differences, from one individual to the next, suggested by Galton's data. Indeed, with this more objective approach we could hope to find out exactly what images *are*. Let's look at the data, and then, from that base, we'll return to the intriguing differences in imagery experience from one person to the next; this framework will also help us to return to the puzzle we met at the chapter's start: the imagery experience of the blind.

Chronometric Studies of Imagery

Imagery researchers are keenly sensitive to the concerns we've just described regarding self-report, and this is why imagery experiments usually don't have participants *describe* their images. Instead, to gain more objective data, experiments have people *do something* with their images—usually, make a judgment based on the image. We can then examine how fast people are in making these judgments, and with appropriate comparisons we can use these measurements as a basis for testing hypotheses about imagery. In other words, the data are generally chronometric ("time measuring") and give us a much more accurate portrait of imagery than could ever be obtained with self-report.

Mental Images as "Picturelike"

For example, **chronometric studies** allow us to ask what sorts of information are prominent in a mental image and what sorts are not; we can then use these evaluations as a basis for asking how "picturelike" mental images really are. To see the logic, think about how actual, out-in-the-world pictures are different from verbal descriptions. Concretely, consider what would happen if you were asked to *write a paragraph* describing a cat. It seems likely that you'd mention the distinctive features of cats—their whiskers, their claws, and so on. Your paragraph probably wouldn't include the fact that cats have heads, since this is too obvious to be worth mentioning. But now consider, in contrast, what would happen if we asked you to *draw a picture* of a cat. In this format, the cat's head would be prominent, for the simple reason that the head is relatively large and up front. The claws and whiskers might be less salient, because these features are small and so would not take up much space in your drawing.

The point here is that the pattern of *what information is included*, as well as what information is prominent, depends on the mode of presentation. For a description, features that are prominent will be those that are distinctive and strongly associated with the object being described. For a *depiction*, in contrast, size and position will determine what's prominent and what's not.

Against this backdrop, let's now ask what information is available in a visual image. Is it the pictorially prominent features, which would imply a depictive mode of representation, or is it the verbally prominent ones, implying a descriptive mode? Self-reports about imagery surely indicate a picture-like representation; is this confirmed by the data?

In an early study by Kosslyn (1976), research participants were asked to form a series of mental images and to answer yes/no questions about each. For example, they were asked to form a mental image of a cat and then were asked: "Does the cat have a head? Does the cat have claws?" Participants responded to these questions quickly, but—crucially—responses to the head question were quicker than those to the claws question. This difference suggests that information quickly available in the image follows the rules for pictures, not paragraphs. For comparison, though, a different group of participants was asked merely to think about cats (with no mention of imagery). These participants, when asked the same questions, gave quicker responses about claws than about head—the reverse pattern of the first group. Thus, it seems that people have the option of thinking about cats via imagery

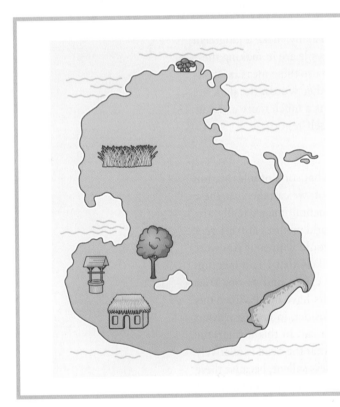

FIGURE 11.1 FICTIONAL ISLAND USED IN IMAGE-SCANNING EXPERIMENTS

Participants in the study first memorized this map, including the various landmarks (the hut, the well, the patch of grass, and so on). They then formed a mental image of this map for the scanning procedure. AFTER KOSSLYN, 1983.

and also the option of thinking about cats without imagery; as the mode of representation changes, so does the pattern of information availability.

In a different experiment, participants were asked to memorize the fictional map shown in **Figure 11.1** and, in particular, to memorize the locations of the various landmarks: the well, the straw hut, and so on (Kosslyn, Ball, & Reiser, 1978). The experimenters made sure participants had the map memorized by asking them to draw a replica of it from memory; once they could do this, the main experiment began. Participants were asked to form an image of the island and to point their "mind's eye" at a specific landmark—let's say, the well. Another landmark was then mentioned, perhaps the straw hut, and participants were asked to imagine a black speck moving in a straight line from the first landmark to the second. When the speck "reached" the target, participants pressed a button, stopping a clock. This action provided a measure of how long the participants needed to "scan" from the well to the hut. The same was done for the well and the tree, and the hut and the patch of grass, so that the researchers ended up with scanning times for each of the various pairs of landmarks.

Figure 11.2 shows the results. The data from this **image-scanning procedure** clearly suggest that participants scan across their images at a constant rate, so that doubling the scanning "distance" doubles the time required for the scan, and tripling the distance triples the time required.

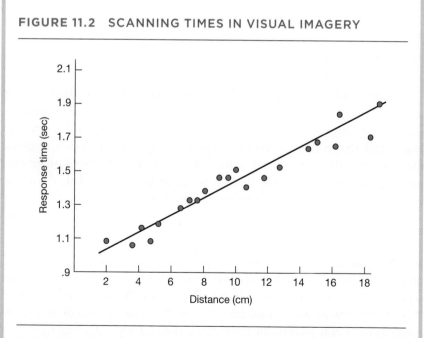

FIGURE 11.2   SCANNING TIMES IN VISUAL IMAGERY

Participants had to "scan" from one point on their mental image to another point; they pressed a button to indicate when their "mind's eye" had arrived at its destination. Response times were closely related to the "distance" participants had to scan across on the image.   AFTER KOSSLYN, 1983.

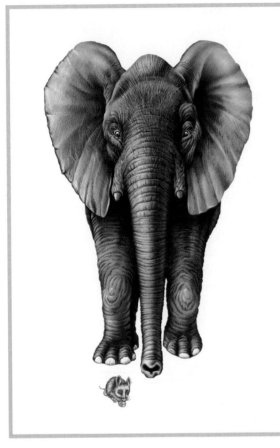

FIGURE 11.3 ZOOMING IN ON MENTAL PICTURES

Just as it takes time to "scan across" a mental image, it also takes time to "zoom in" on one. Thus, participants respond slowly if they are instructed to imagine a mouse standing with an elephant, and then are asked: Does the mouse have whiskers? To answer this question, participants need a bit of time (which we can measure) to zoom in on the mouse, in order to bring the whiskers "into view." Responses were faster if participants were initially asked to imagine the mouse standing next to a paper clip. For this image, participants started with a "close-up" view, so no zooming was needed to "see" the whiskers.

Similar results emerge if participants are given a task that requires them to "zoom in" on their images (e.g., a task that requires them to inspect the image for some small detail) or a task that requires them to "zoom out" (e.g., a task that requires a more global judgment). In these studies, response times are directly proportional to the amount of zoom required, suggesting once again that travel in the imaged world resembles travel in the actual world, at least with regard to timing (**Figure 11.3**).

Depictions versus Descriptions

Whether you're scanning across a mental image, therefore, or zooming in on one, "traveling" a greater "distance" requires more time. This is the same relationship we would observe if we asked research participants to move their eyes across an actual map (rather than an image of one) or literally to zoom in on a real picture. In these cases, too, traveling a greater distance would require more time. All of this points toward the similarity between mental images and actual out-in-the-world pictures.

More precisely, though, the data are telling us a great deal about the nature of mental images. According to these results, images represent a scene in a fashion that preserves all of the distance relationships within that scene: Points close to one another in the scene are somehow "close" to one another in the image; points that are farther apart in the scene are somehow "farther apart" in the image. Thus, in a very real sense, the image preserves the spatial layout of the represented scene and, therefore, rather directly represents the *geometry* of the scene. It's in this way that images *depict* the scene rather than describing it; thus, they are much more similar to pictures or maps than they are to descriptions.

Mental Rotation

In a series of experiments by Shepard, Cooper, and Metzler, participants were asked to decide whether displays like the one in **Figure 11.4A** showed two different shapes or just one shape viewed from two different perspectives (Cooper & Shepard, 1973; Shepard & Metzler, 1971; Shepard & Cooper, 1982). In other words, is it possible to "rotate" the form shown on the left in Figure 11.4A so that it will end up looking just like the form on the right? What about the two shapes shown in Figure 11.4B or the two in 11.4C?

To perform this **mental rotation** task, participants seem first to imagine one of the forms rotating into alignment with the other. Then, once the forms are oriented in the same way, participants can make their judgment. This step of imagined rotation takes some time; in fact, the amount of time depends on how much rotation is needed. **Figure 11.5** shows the data pattern, with response times clearly being influenced by how far apart the two forms were in their initial orientations. Thus, once again, imagined "movement" resembles actual movement: The farther you have to imagine a form rotating, the longer the evaluation takes. (Also see **Figure 11.6**.)

FIGURE 11.4 STIMULI FOR A MENTAL ROTATION EXPERIMENT

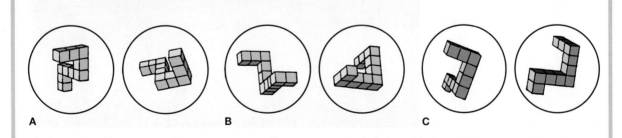

A   B   C

Participants had to judge whether the two stimuli shown in Panel A are the same as each other but viewed from different perspectives, and likewise for the pairs shown in Panels B and C. Participants seem to make these judgments by imagining one of the forms rotating until its position matches that of the other form.   FIG. 1 FROM SHEPARD & METZLER, "MENTAL ROTATION OF THREE-DIMENSIONAL OBJECTS," *SCIENCE* 171 (FEBRUARY 1971): 701-703. © 1971 AAAS. REPRINTED WITH PERMISSION FROM AAAS.

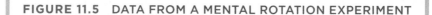

FIGURE 11.5 DATA FROM A MENTAL ROTATION EXPERIMENT

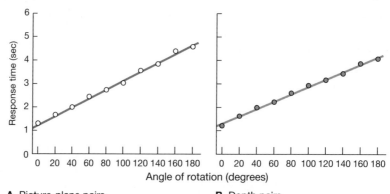

A Picture-plane pairs   **B** Depth pairs

Panel A shows data from stimulus pairs requiring mental rotation in two dimensions, so that the imaged forms stay within the imagined picture plane. Panel B shows data from pairs requiring an imagined rotation in depth. The data are similar, indicating that participants can imagine three-dimensional rotations as easily as they can imagine two-dimensional rotations. AFTER SHEPARD & METZLER, 1971.

FIGURE 11.6 BRAIN ACTIVITY IN MENTAL ROTATION

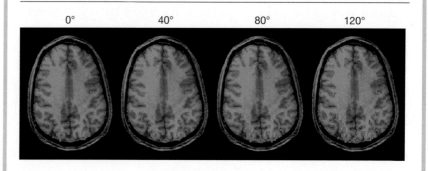

As the text describes, it takes more time to imagine something rotating, say, 80 degrees, than it does to imagine it moving 40 degrees. Related data comes from brain scans—with more brain activity needed for a 40-degree rotation than for no rotation at all, and even more activity needed for an 80-degree or 120-degree rotation. AFTER CARPENTER ET AL., 1999.

This task can also be used to answer some further questions about imagery. For example, notice that if you were to cut out the left-hand drawing in Figure 11.4A and spin it around while leaving it flat on the table, you could align it with the drawing on the right. The relevant rotation, therefore, is one that leaves the pictures within the two-dimensional plane in which they are drawn. In contrast, the two forms shown in Figure 11.4B are identical except for a rotation in depth. No matter how you spin the *picture* on the left, it will not line up with the picture on the right. You can align these forms, but to do so you need to spin them around a vertical axis, in essence lifting them off the page.

People have no trouble with mental rotation in depth. Their accuracy level in these judgments is around 95%, and the data resemble those obtained with picture-plane rotation (compare Figures 11.5A and 11.5B). Apparently, participants can represent three-dimensional forms in their images, and they can imagine these forms moving in depth. In some circumstances, therefore, visual images are not mental pictures; they are more like mental sculptures.

The Concern about Demand Character

In both mental rotation and mental scanning, the farther the imagined "travel," the longer it takes. We've interpreted these results as revealing the way in which images represent spatial layout—with points that are more distant in the represented scene being somehow farther apart in the image. But there's another way one might try to interpret the data. Participants in these studies obviously know that movement through the world takes time and that moving a longer distance takes more time. Perhaps, therefore, the participants simply control the timing of their responses in order to re-create this "normal" pattern.

This proposal can be fleshed out in a variety of ways; but to phrase things strongly, perhaps participants in these studies are not imagining rotations or scanning across an image at all. Instead, they might be thinking, "The experimenter just asked me to scan a long way, and I'd like to make it look like I'm obeying. I know that a long scan takes a long time, so let me wait a moment before hitting the response button."

Why should participants act in this way? One reason is that research participants usually want to be helpful, and they do all they can to give the experimenter "good" data. As a result, they are very sensitive to the **demand character** of the experiment—that is, cues that might signal how they are "supposed to" behave in that situation (Intons-Peterson, 1983, 1999; Intons-Peterson & White, 1981).

A different possibility is that this sort of "simulation" is, in fact, what imagery is really all about. Perhaps whenever someone tries to "imagine" something, he draws on his knowledge about how an event in the world would actually unfold, and then he does his best to simulate this event. In this case, a longer scan or a greater rotation requires more time, not because there really is some "travel" involved but because people know that these manipulations should take more time and do their best to simulate the process (Pylyshyn, 1981).

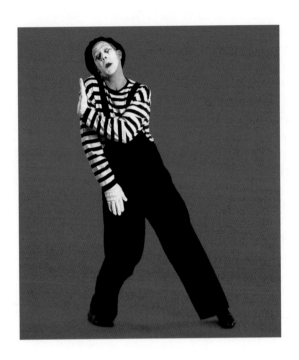

IMAGERY AS "SIMULATION"

There is, of course, no "box" trapping this mime. Instead, the mime is simulating what would happen if he were trapped in a box. In the same fashion, researchers have asked whether study participants, guided by an experiment's demand character, are simply simulating (re-creating?) how they'd act if they were looking at a picture.

As it turns out, though, we can set aside these concerns, allowing us to maintain the claims we've already sketched—namely, that the scanning and rotation data are as they are, not through simulation but, indeed, *because of how images represent spatial layout*. Several lines of evidence support this claim, including (crucially) data we will turn to, later in the chapter, examining the neural bases for imagery. But we can also tackle concerns about demand character directly. In several studies, the experimenters have asked participants to make judgments about spatial layout but have taken care never to mention that imagery might be relevant to the task (e.g., Finke & Pinker, 1982). This procedure avoids any suggestion to participants that they should simulate some sort of "mental travel." Even so, participants in these procedures spontaneously form images and scan across them, and their responses show the standard pattern: longer response times observed with longer scans. Apparently, this result emerges whenever participants are using visual imagery—whether the result is encouraged by the experimenters' instructions or not.

Interactions between Imagery and Perception

It seems that there really are parallels between visual images and actual visual stimuli, and this leads to a question: If images are so much like pictures, then are the mental processes used to inspect images similar to those used to inspect stimuli? To put it more broadly, what is the relation between imaging and perceiving?

In a study by Segal and Fusella (1970, 1971), participants were asked to detect very faint signals—either dim visual stimuli or soft tones. On each trial, the task was merely to indicate whether a signal had been presented

FIGURE 11.7 CAN YOU VISUALIZE AND SEE AT THE SAME TIME?

Percentage of Detections

	Visual signal	Auditory signal
While visualizing	61%	67%
While maintaining an auditory image	63%	61%

Percentage of False Alarms

	Visual signal	Auditory signal
While visualizing	7.8%	3.7%
While maintaining an auditory image	3.6%	6.7%

Participants were less successful in detecting a weak visual signal if they were simultaneously maintaining a visual image than if they were maintaining an auditory image. (The effect is small but highly reliable.) The reverse is true with weak auditory signals: Participants were less successful in this detection if maintaining an auditory image than if visualizing. In addition, visual images often led to "false alarms" for participants trying to detect visual signals; auditory images led to false alarms for auditory signals. AFTER SEGAL & FUSELLA, 1970.

or not. Participants did this in one of two conditions: either while forming a visual image before their "mind's eye" or while forming an auditory image before their "mind's ear." Thus, we have a 2 × 2 design: two types of signals to be detected, and two types of imagery.

Let's hypothesize that there's some overlap between imaging and perceiving—that is, there are mental processes that are involved in both activities. On this basis, we should expect interference if participants try to do both of these activities at once, on the idea that if these processes are occupied with imaging, they're not available for perceiving, and vice versa. That interference is exactly what Segal and Fusella observed. They found that forming a visual image interferes with seeing and that forming an auditory image interferes with hearing (see **Figure 11.7**; also see Farah & Smith, 1983).

You'll notice in the figure that the effect here was relatively small and that error rates were relatively low. (The false alarm rates indicate that participants were rarely fooled into thinking their image was an actual out-in-the-world stimulus.) These points remind us that images are not hallucinations—largely because people are alert to the fact that they have *control* over their images. (For more on hallucinations, see, for example, Billock & Tsou, 2012.) Nonetheless, the pattern in these data is statistically reliable—confirming that there is interference, in line with the claims we are exploring.

The Segal and Fusella participants were trying to visualize one thing while perceiving something altogether different. What happens if participants are contemplating a mental image *related to* the stimulus they're trying to perceive? Can visualizing a possible input "pave the way" for perception? Farah (1985) had participants visualize a form (either an *H* or a *T*). A moment later, either an *H* or a *T* was actually presented—but at a very low contrast, making the letter difficult to perceive. With this setup, perception was facilitated if participants had just been visualizing the target form, and the effect was quite specific: Visualizing an *H* made it easier to perceive an *H*; visualizing a *T* made it easier to perceive a *T*. This result provides further confirmation of the claim that visualizing and perceiving draw on similar mechanisms, so that one of these activities can serve to prime the other. (Also see Heil, Rösler, & Hennighausen, 1993; McDermott & Roediger, 1994.)

More recent studies have explored another way in which imagery can prime perception. **Binocular rivalry** occurs when two different visual stimuli are presented, one stimulus to each eye. (Thus, for example, green vertical stripes might be presented to your left eye and red horizontal stripes to your right eye.) With this setup, your visual system is unable to combine the inputs, and instead you end up being aware of just one of the stimuli for a few moments, then aware of the other for a bit of time, then the first again. How this sequence plays out, though, can be shaped by visualization—and so (for example) if you visualize a specific pattern, the pattern is likely to dominate (to be perceived earlier and for more time) in a subsequent binocular-rivalry presentation (Pearson, 2014; Pearson, Clifford, & Tong, 2008). Moreover, this effect is particularly robust for specific trials in which the research participants described the image as clear and strong, suggesting that the mechanism is indeed mediated by the conscious image itself (Pearson, Rademaker, & Tong, 2011).

Visual Imagery and the Brain

The overlap between imaging and perceiving is also clear in biological evidence. As we discussed in Chapter 3, we know a great deal about the specific brain structures required for vision, and it turns out that many of the same structures are crucial for imagery. This can be documented in several ways, including procedures that rely on neuroimaging techniques (like PET or fMRI) that map the moment-by-moment activity in the brain (see Figure 2.9 in Chapter 2). These techniques confirm that vision relies heavily on tissue located in the occipital cortex (and so these brain areas are highly activated whenever you are examining a visual stimulus). It turns out that activity levels are also high in these areas when participants are visualizing a stimulus before their "mind's eye" (Behrmann, 2000; Isha & Sagi, 1995; Kosslyn, 1994; Miyashita, 1995; Thompson & Kosslyn, 2000).

The biological parallels between imagery and perception can be documented even at a fine grain. Specifically, we know that different areas of the occipital cortex are involved in different aspects of visual perception—and so, for example, Areas V1 and V2 in the cortex are involved in the earliest stages of visual perception, responding to the specific low-level features of the input. It's striking, therefore, that these same brain areas are particularly active whenever participants are maintaining highly detailed images, and that the amount

FIGURE 11.8   IMAGERY FOR FACES AND PLACES IN THE BRAIN

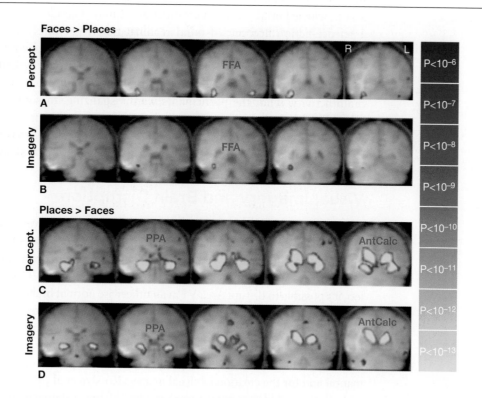

The successive brain pictures in each row show different "slices" through the brain, moving from the front of the brain to the back. To analyze the data, the researchers initially compared brain activity in two conditions: when participants were viewing *faces* and when they were viewing *places* (scenes). Next, the researchers compared brain activity in two more conditions: when the participants were *visualizing* faces or places. The row marked "a" shows brain sites more activated when participants were viewing *faces* than *places*; not surprisingly, activity levels are high in the so-called fusiform face area (FFA). The row marked "b" shows brain sites more activated when participants were *visualizing faces* than when they were visualizing places. The key here is that rows "a" and "b" look rather similar: the pattern of brain activation is roughly the same in the perception and imagery conditions. The bottom two rows show the brain sites that were more activated when participants were viewing (row "c") or visualizing (row "d") *places*, with considerable activity in the so-called parahippocampal place area (PPA). Again, the activity pattern is quite similar for the perception and imagery conditions.

of brain tissue showing activation increases as participants imagine larger and larger objects (Behrmann, 2000; Kosslyn & Thompson, 2003). In a similar fashion, certain areas in the brain are highly sensitive to motion in ordinary visual perception, and it turns out that the same brain areas are particularly activated when participants are asked to *imagine* movement patterns (Goebel, Khorram-Sefat, Muckli, Hacker, & Singer, 1998). Likewise, brain areas that are especially active during the perception of faces are also highly activated when people are imagining faces (O'Craven & Kanwisher, 2000; also see **Figure 11.8**).

In fact, these various parallels have led researchers to develop techniques for "decoding" patterns of brain activation in people who are holding visual images (e.g., Albers, Kok, Toni, Dijkerman, & de Lange, 2013; Pearson, 2014; Schlegel et al., 2013; Thirion et al., 2006). The idea here sounds like a science-fiction account of mind reading, but it is entirely real. Research participants are asked to create and maintain a visual image while investigators record brain activity. The activity (an fMRI pattern) is then subjected to mathematical analysis, allowing computers to figure out, based on the brain activity, what the participants were visualizing. In some studies, this "decoding" is based on a comparison between participants' brain activity while *visualizing* and their activity while *seeing*, confirming that the activity patterns for images are indeed similar to those evoked by actual visual inputs.

Visual Imagery and Brain Disruption

Further evidence comes from *transcranial magnetic stimulation* (TMS), a technique that we first described in Chapter 2. TMS creates a series of strong magnetic pulses at a specific location on the scalp; this causes a (temporary!) disruption in the brain region directly underneath this scalp area (Helmuth, 2001). In this fashion, it's possible to disrupt Area V1 in an otherwise normal brain. Area V1, recall, is the brain area where axons from the visual system first reach the occipital cortex (see Chapter 2). Not surprisingly, using TMS in this way causes problems in vision, but it also causes parallel problems in visual imagery, providing a powerful argument that Area V1 is important both for the processing of visual information and for the creation of visual images (Kosslyn et al., 1999).

Still more evidence comes from studies of brain damage, and here, too, we find parallels between visual perception and visual imagery. For example, in some patients brain damage has disrupted the ability to perceive color; in most cases these patients also lose the ability to imagine scenes in color. Likewise, patients who, because of brain damage, have lost the ability to perceive fine detail seem also to lose the ability to visualize fine detail; and so on (Farah, Soso, & Dasheiff, 1992; Kosslyn, 1994; let's note, though, that we'll add some complications to this point later in the chapter).

Brain damage also causes parallels in how people *pay attention* to visual inputs and to visual images. In one case, a patient had suffered a stroke and, as a result, had developed the "neglect syndrome" we described in Chapter 5. If this patient was shown a picture, he seemed to see only the right side of it; if asked to read a word, he read only the right half. The same pattern was evident in the patient's imagery. In one test, he was urged to visualize a familiar plaza in his city and to list the buildings "in view" in the image. If the patient imagined himself standing at the northern edge of the plaza, he listed all the buildings on the plaza's western side (i.e., on his right), but none on the eastern. If the patient imagined himself standing on the southern edge of the plaza, he listed all the sights on the plaza's eastern side, but none on the western. In both cases, he neglected half of the imaged scene, just as he did with perceived scenes (Bisiach & Luzzatti, 1978; Bisiach, Luzzatti, & Perani, 1979).

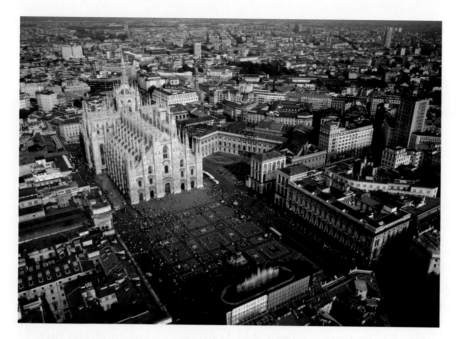

NEGLECT SYNDROME IN VISUAL IMAGERY

Because of brain damage, a patient had developed the pattern (first discussed in Chapter 2) of unilateral neglect—and so he paid attention only to the right half of the visual world. He showed the same pattern in his visual images: When asked to imagine himself standing at the southern edge of the Piazza del Duomo and to describe all he could "see" in his image, he only listed buildings on the piazza's eastern side. When he imagined himself standing at the northern edge of the piazza, he only listed buildings on the western side. In both cases, he neglected the left half of the (visualized) piazza.

Spatial Images and Visual Images

We are building an impressive case for a close relationship between imagery and perception. Indeed, the evidence so far implies that we can truly speak of imagery as being *visual* imagery, drawing on the same mechanisms and having many of the same traits as actual vision. Other results, however, add some complications.

Early in the chapter, we discussed dreams in people who have been blind since birth, and more broadly, many studies have examined imagery in the blind. Obviously, these procedures need to be adapted in important ways—so that (for example) the stimuli to be imaged are initially presented as sculptures to be explored with the hands, rather than as pictures to be examined visually. Once this is done, however, experiments parallel to those we have described can be carried out with the blind—procedures examining how the blind scan across an image, for example, or how they imagine a form in rotation. What are the results? In tests involving mental scanning, blind individuals produce response times proportional to the "distance" traveled in the image—exactly the result we've already seen with sighted people. In tests requiring mental rotation, response times with blind research participants are proportional to the amount of "rotation" needed, just as with participants who have normal vision. Indeed, in procedure after procedure, people blind since birth produce results just like those from people who can see. The blind, in other words, seem to have normal imagery. (For a sampling of the data, see Carpenter & Eisenberg, 1978; Giudice, Betty, & Loomis, 2011; Kerr, 1983; Marmor & Zabeck, 1976; also see Jonides, Kahn, & Rozin, 1975; Paivio & Okovita, 1971; Zimler & Keenan, 1983. For a broad overview of imagery in the blind—including discussion of the important ways in which visually impaired individuals differ from one another—see Heller & Gentaz, 2014.)

What's going on here? It seems unlikely that people blind since birth are using a sense of what things "look like" to perform these tasks. Presumably, therefore, they have some other means of thinking about spatial layout and spatial relations. This "spatial imagery" might be represented in the mind in terms of a series of imagined movements, so that it is body imagery or motion imagery rather than visual imagery. Alternatively, perhaps spatial imagery is not tied to any sensory modality but is instead part of our broader cognition about spatial arrangements and layout.

One way or another, though, it looks like we need to distinguish between *visual* and *spatial* imagery. Blind individuals presumably use spatial imagery to carry out the tasks we have been discussing in this chapter; it seems plausible that sighted people can use either visual or spatial imagery to carry out these tasks. (For a related distinction among several types of imagery, see Kosslyn & Thompson, 1999, 2003; for other data emphasizing the importance of the visual/spatial distinction, see Hegarty, 2004; Hegarty & Stull, 2012; Klauer & Zhao, 2004. For data suggesting that mental rotation in *sighted* participants may involve spatial imagery, not visual, see Liesefeld & Zimmer, 2013.)

This distinction between visual and spatial imagery is confirmed by neuroscience evidence. For example, fMRI data tell us that the brain areas activated for visual tasks are different from those activated by spatial tasks (Thompson, Slotnick, Burrage, & Kosslyn, 2009). Likewise, we've already noted the cases in which brain damage seems to produce similar patterns of disruption in seeing and imaging. Thus, patients who (because of brain damage) have lost their color vision also seem to lose the ability to imagine scenes in color; patients who have lost their ability to perceive motion also lose the ability to imagine movement. However, there are exceptions to this pattern—that is, cases in which brain damage causes problems in imagery but not in perception, or vice versa. (See, for example, Bartolomeo et al., 1998; Behrmann, 2000; Goldenberg, Müllbacher, & Nowak, 1995; Logie & Della Salla, 2005; Servos & Goodale, 1995.) What should we make of this uneven pattern—with brain damage sometimes causing similar problems in imagery and in perception, and sometimes not? The answer lies in the fact that *visual* imagery relies on brain areas also needed for vision, and so damage to these areas disrupts both imagery and vision. *Spatial* imagery, in contrast, relies on different brain areas, and so damage to visual areas won't interfere with this form of imagery, and damage to brain sites needed for this imagery won't interfere with vision (see **Figure 11.9**).

FIGURE 11.9   BRAIN AREAS CRUCIAL FOR VISUAL AND SPATIAL TASKS

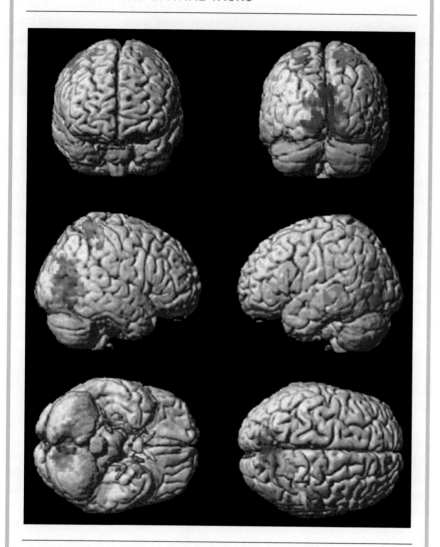

In one condition of this study, participants had to visualize a particular target in a particular location. In the other condition, participants had to imagine a rotation of a target. The authors refer to these conditions as "spatial location" and "spatial transformation," but the distinction at issue obviously parallels the distinction made here between visual and spatial tasks. The two types of tasks clearly relied on distinct brain regions, providing further evidence that we must distinguish between visual and spatial imagery. The blue area in the figure indicates brain regions associated with the spatial location (visual) task; the yellow area indicates brain regions associated with the spatial transformation (spatial) task.

Likewise, consider patient L.H. He suffered brain damage in an automobile accident and, afterward, had enormous difficulty in tasks requiring judgments about visual appearance—for example, judgments about *color* (Farah, Hammond, Levine, & Calvanio, 1988). In contrast, L.H. performed well on tasks like image scanning or mental rotation. More generally, he showed little disruption on tasks requiring spatial manipulations or memory for spatial positions. To make sense of L.H.'s profile, therefore, it seems once again crucial to distinguish between visual tasks (for which he's impaired) and spatial ones (for which he's not) and, correspondingly, between visual imagery and spatial imagery.

Individual Differences

Various lines of evidence, therefore, suggest there are at least two types of imagery—one visual and one spatial—and, presumably, most people have the capacity for both types: They can "visualize" and they can "spatialize." But this invites a new question: When do people use one type of imagery, and when do they use the other?

To some extent, the answer depends on the task. For example, to think about *colors*, you need to imagine exactly what something *looks like*; it won't be enough just to think about shapes or spatial positions. In this case, therefore, you'll need visual imagery, not spatial. Or, as a reverse case, think about tasks that require complex navigation—perhaps navigation through a building or across an entire city. For tasks like these, visualizing the relevant layout may be difficult and would include a lot of detail irrelevant to the navigation. In this setting, spatial imagery, not visual, may be a better option (cf. Hegarty & Stull, 2012).

In many other cases, though, either form of imagery will get the job done. For an image-scanning task, for example, you can think about what a speck would *look like* as it zoomed across an imagined scene, or you can think about what it would *feel like* to move your finger across the scene. In these cases, the choice between visual and spatial imagery will depend on other factors, including your preferences and perhaps the exact instructions you receive.

The choice between these forms of imagery will also be influenced by each individual's ability levels. Some people may be poor visualizers but good "spatializers," and they would surely rely on spatial imagery, not visual, in most tasks. And, of course, for other people, this pattern would be reversed.

With this context, think back to Galton's data, mentioned early on in this chapter. If we take those data at face value, they imply that people differ markedly in their conscious experience of imaging. People with vivid imagery report that their images are truly picturelike—in color, quite detailed, and with all of the depicted objects viewed from a particular distance and a particular viewing angle. People without vivid imagery, in contrast, will say none of these things. Their images, they report, are not at all picturelike, and it's meaningless to ask them whether an image is in color or in black and white; their image simply isn't the sort of thing that could be in color or in black and white. Likewise, it's meaningless to ask whether their image is viewed from a particular perspective; their image is abstract in a way that makes this question inapplicable. In no sense, then, do these "non-imagers" feel like they're "seeing" with the "mind's eye." From their perspective, these figures of speech are (at best) loosely metaphorical. This stands in clear contrast to the reports offered by vivid imagers; for them, mental seeing really does seem like actual seeing.

Roughly 10% of the population will, in this fashion, "declare themselves entirely deficient in the power of seeing mental pictures" (Galton, 1883, p. 110). As William James (1890) put it, they "have no visual images at all worthy of the name" (p. 57). But what should we make of this? Is it truly the case that members of our species differ in whether or not they're capable of experiencing visual images?

To explore this issue, a number of studies have compared "vivid imagers" and "non-imagers" on tasks that depend on mental imagery, with the obvious prediction that people with vivid imagery will do better in these tasks and those with sparse imagery will do worse. The results, however, have often been otherwise, with many studies finding no difference between vivid imagers and sparse imagers in how they do mental rotation, how quickly or accurately they scan across their images, and so on (e.g., Ernest, 1977; Katz, 1983; Marks, 1983; Richardson, 1980).

Notice, though, that when people describe their images as "vivid," they are specifically reporting how much their image experience is *like seeing*, and so the self-report, it seems, provides an assessment of *visual* imagery. In contrast, tasks like mental rotation or scanning can be performed with either spatial imagery or visual imagery. Perhaps it's unsurprising, therefore, that there's no relationship between this self-report and the performance of these tasks: The self-report is reflecting a capacity (visual imagery) that isn't at all necessary for the tasks.

On this basis, there should be a relationship between image vividness and how well people perform on tasks that really do require visual imagery. This prediction turns out to be correct. We can design tasks that require people to make an exact judgment about what an imagined object would look like— for example, what its color would look like or whether a small gap in the object would be "visible" in the image. People who (claim they) have vivid imagery do perform better on these visual tasks—presumably, because their vivid images enable them to "see" exactly what the imagined objects look like (e.g., Cui, Jeter, Yang, Montague, & Eagleman, 2006; Finke & Kosslyn, 1980; Keogh & Pearson, 2011; Kozhevnikov, Kosslyn, & Shephard, 2005; McKelvie, 1995; Pearson, Rademaker & Tong, 2011).

Apparently, then, people really do differ in the quality of—and perhaps the *nature* of—their imagery experience. In some ways, this is a remarkable finding; indeed, people with vivid imagery often have a difficult time conceiving what it would be like to have no visual images, or for that matter, what dreams "feel like" for someone, blind since birth, who has no experience at all with seeing. But these points also invite many questions: How do these differences in experience influence people outside the laboratory, away from experimenters' tasks? What can people "with imagery" do that people "without imagery" cannot? As an illustration for how these issues might unfold, one study indicates a link between imagery prowess and career choice, with visual imagers being more likely to succeed in the arts, while people with spatial imagery are better suited to careers in science or engineering (Kozhevnikov et al., 2005). Another study suggests a strong link between visual imagery and autobiographical memory (with "non-imagers" being much less likely to feel as if they can "relive" their memories; Greenberg & Knowlton, 2014). These are tantalizing suggestions and obviously a target for further research.

Eidetic Imagery

As we just noted, people with vivid imagery are often surprised to hear that other individuals (including the author of this book!) lack this capacity. But the differences among people are just as striking if we consider variation in the other direction: people who have "super-skills" in imagery.

There is a lot of folklore associated with the idea of "photographic memory," but this term needs to be defined carefully. Some people have fabulously detailed, wonderfully long-lasting memories, but without any "photographic" quality in their memory. These people often use careful rehearsal, or complex, well-practiced mnemonics, to remember the value of pi to a hundred decimal places, or the names of a hundred people they've just met—but these memories are not in any way "visual," and imagery is not necessary for these memorization strategies.

Other people, in contrast, do seem to have exquisitely detailed imagery that can indeed be described as "photographic," and researchers refer to this type of imagery as **eidetic imagery**. People with this skill are called "eidetikers." This form of imagery is sometimes found in people who have been diagnosed as autistic: These individuals can briefly glance at a complex scene and then draw incredibly detailed reproductions of the scene, as though they really had taken a "photograph" of the scene when first viewing it. But similar capacities can be documented with no link to autism. For example, Stromeyer (1982) described a woman who could recall poetry written in a language she did not understand, even years after she'd seen the poem; she was also able to recall complicated random dot patterns after viewing them only briefly. Similarly, Haber (1969; also Haber & Haber, 1988) showed a picture like **Figure 11.10** to a 10-year-old eidetiker for just 30 seconds. After the picture was taken away, the boy was unexpectedly asked detail questions: How many stripes were there on the cat's back? How many leaves on the front flower? The child was able to give completely accurate answers, as though his memory had perfectly preserved the picture's content.

However, we know relatively little about this form of imagery. We do know that this capacity is rare. We know that some people who claim to have this capacity do not: They often *do* have fabulous memories, but they rely on mnemonics, not on some special form of imagery. But beyond these obvious points, this remains a truly intriguing phenomenon in need of further research.

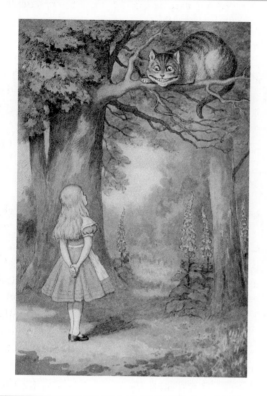

FIGURE 11.10 EIDETIC IMAGERY

Eidetic imagery is vastly more detailed than ordinary imagery. In one study (Haber, 1969), a 10-year-old was shown a picture like this one for 30 seconds. After the picture was taken away, the boy was unexpectedly asked detail questions: How many stripes were there on the cat's back? How many leaves on the front flower? The child was able to give completely accurate answers, as though his memory had perfectly preserved the picture's content.

Images Are Not Pictures

Let's return, though, to more "normal" (at least, more ordinary) forms of imagery. At many points in this chapter, we've referred to mental images (especially *visual* images) as "mental pictures." That comparison is hardly new; the phrase "the mind's eye" was popularized by Shakespeare five centuries ago and is embedded in the way most of us talk about our imagery. And as we've seen, the comparison is in several ways appropriate. Visual images do depict a scene in a fashion that seems quite pictorial. In other ways, though, this comparison may be misleading.

We've already seen that mental images can represent three-dimensional figures, and so they may be more like mental sculptures than mental pictures. We've also distinguished visual images and spatial images, and so *some* images are like pictures to be explored with the mind's eye, and other images are not. But on top of these points, there is a further complication. To introduce this issue, let's review some points we first raised in Chapter 3 and with that, an example we first met in that chapter. **Figure 11.11A** shows the figure known as the Necker cube (see also Figure 3.11). The drawing of this cube—the stimulus itself—is ambiguous: It can be understood as a depiction of a cube viewed from above or as a depiction of a cube viewed from below. The picture itself, in other words, doesn't specify in any way which of these two cubes it shows, and so, in this sense, the picture is neutral with regard to interpretation—and fully compatible with either interpretation.

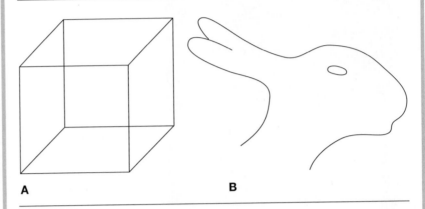

FIGURE 11.11   THE NECKER CUBE AND THE DUCK/RABBIT

A   B

(Panel A) The cube can be perceived as if viewed from above or below. (Panel B) This figure can be perceived as a duck facing left or a rabbit facing right. If people are visualizing this ambiguous figure, they have great difficulty reinterpreting it. Of course, once they know that both interpretations are possible, they can hop from one to the other. What seems enormously difficult, though, is discovering the alternative interpretation of the imaged figure in the first place.

Unlike the picture, though, your *perception* of the cube is not neutral, is not indeterminate with regard to depth. Instead, at any moment in time you perceive the cube as having one arrangement in depth or another. Your perception, in other words, "goes beyond the information given" by specifying a configuration in depth, a specification that in this case supplements an ambiguous drawing in order to create an unambiguous perception.

As we discussed in Chapter 3, the configuration in depth is just one of the ways that perception goes beyond the information given in a stimulus. Your perception of a stimulus also specifies a figure/ground organization, the form's orientation (e.g., identifying the form's "top"), and so on. These specifications serve to organize the form and have a powerful impact on the subjective appearance of the form—and with that, what the form is seen to resemble and what the form will evoke in memory.

Let's be clear, then, that our **percepts** (i.e., our mental representations of the stimuli we're perceiving) are in some ways similar to pictures, but in other ways different. Like pictures, percepts are *depictions*, representing key aspects of the three-dimensional layout of the world. Percepts, in other words, are not descriptions of a stimulus; instead, percepts, just like pictures, show directly what a stimulus looks like. At the same time, percepts are in some ways different from pictures: They are organized and unambiguous in a fashion that pictures are not.

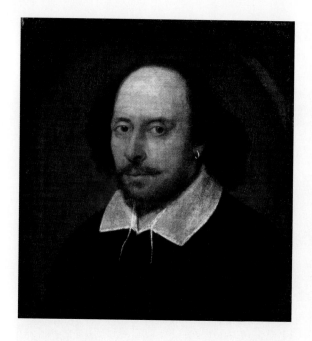

Hamlet: My father—methinks I see my father—
Horatio: Where, my lord?
Hamlet: In my mind's eye, Horatio.
(*Hamlet,* act 1, scene 2)

William Shakespeare is credited with popularizing the phrase "the mind's eye."

What about visual images? Are they just like pictures—neutral with regard to organization, and thus open to different interpretations? Or are they organized in the way percepts seem to be, and so, in a sense, already interpreted? One line of evidence comes from studies of ambiguous figures. In one experiment, participants were first shown a series of practice stimuli to make sure that they understood what it meant to reinterpret an ambiguous figure (Chambers & Reisberg, 1985). They were then shown a drawing of one more ambiguous figure (such as the Necker cube or the duck/rabbit in Figure 11.11); then, after this figure had been removed from view, they were asked to form a mental image of it. Once the image was formed, they were asked if they could reinterpret this image, just as they had reinterpreted the practice figures.

Across several experiments, not one of the participants succeeded in reinterpreting his or her images: They reliably failed to find the duck in a "rabbit image" or the rabbit in a "duck image." Is it possible that they didn't understand their task or perhaps didn't remember the figure? To rule out these possibilities, participants were given a blank piece of paper immediately after their failure at reinterpreting their images and were asked to draw the figure based on their image. Now, looking at their own drawings, all of the participants were able to reinterpret the configuration in the appropriate way. Thus, we have 100% failure in reinterpreting these forms with images and 100% success a moment later with drawings.

Apparently, therefore, what participants "see" in their image (even if it's a *visual* image, not a spatial one) is not a "picture"—neutral with regard to interpretation, and thus open to new interpretations. Instead, images are inherently organized, just as percepts are. As such, images are entirely unambiguous and strongly resistant to reinterpretation. (For more on these issues, see Peterson, Kihlstrom, Rose, & Glisky, 1992; Thompson, Kosslyn,

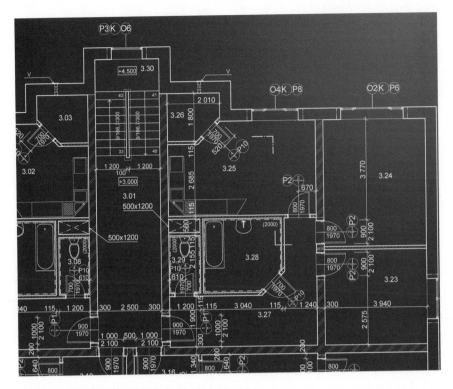

CHANGING A FRAME OF REFERENCE

In many professions—architecture, for example—designers visualize the early stages of their ideas without needing to sketch the designs on paper. Research suggests, though, that there may be limits on this image-based process and that some discoveries are much more likely if the designers put their ideas down on paper and then inspect the drawings. This is because the drawing, on its own, has no interpretive "reference frame," making it much easier for the designer to impose a new reference frame.

Hoffman, & Kooij, 2008; for a discussion on how image-based discovery is used in a real-world setting, see Verstijnen, Hennessey, van Leeuwen, Hamel, & Goldschmidt, 1998; Verstijnen, van Leeuwen, Goldschmidt, Hamel, & Hennessey, 1998).

Images and Pictures: An Interim Summary

Images, both visual and spatial, provide a distinctive means of representing the world, and so *visualizing* a robot (for example) is quite different from thinking about the word "robot" or merely contemplating the idea "robot." As one key difference, images are, without question, like pictures in the fact that images show exactly what a form looks like. Visualizing a robot, therefore, will highlight the robot's appearance in your thoughts and make it much more likely that you'll be reminded of other forms having a similar appearance. Thinking about the robot without an image might not highlight appearance and so will probably call different ideas to mind.

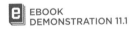

EBOOK
DEMONSTRATION 11.1

Creating an image will also make some attributes of a form more prominent and others less so (the cat's head, for example, rather than its whiskers). This, too, can influence what further ideas the image calls to mind, and so, again, putting your thoughts into imagery can literally shape the flow and sequence of your ideas.

At the same time, we've highlighted ways in which images are *not* picturelike. Images, it seems, are inherently organized in a fashion that pictures are not, and this organization can itself influence the sequence of your thoughts—with your understanding of the image (your understanding of where its "top" and "front" are, your understanding of its figure/ground organization, etc.) guiding which discoveries will, and which will not, easily flow from an image.

Where does all this leave us? Images have a great deal in common with pictures, but they are also different from pictures. Thus, the common phrase "mental pictures" is misleading, and it would be more accurate to say that mental images are picturelike. In addition, we need to keep track of the contrast between visual images and spatial images. As we have seen, this contrast shows up in many aspects of the data, and it must be part of our theorizing if we are going to explain what imagery is, how it is supported by the brain, and how it functions in shaping our thoughts.

Long-Term Visual Memory

So far, our discussion has focused on "active" images—images that you're currently contemplating, images presumably held in working memory. What about visual information in long-term memory? For example, if you wish to form an image of an elephant, you need to draw on your knowledge of what an elephant looks like. What is this knowledge, and how is it represented in long-term storage? Likewise, if you recognize a picture as familiar, this is probably because you've detected a "match" between it and some memory of an earlier-viewed picture. What is the nature of this memory?

Image Information in Long-Term Memory

In earlier chapters, we suggested that your concept of "birthday" (for example) is represented by some number of nodes in long-term memory. Perhaps we can adapt this proposal to account for long-term storage of visual information (and likewise information for the other sensory modalities).

One possibility is that nodes in long-term memory represent entire, relatively complete pictures. Thus, to form a mental image of an elephant, you would activate the ELEPHANT PICTURE nodes; to scrutinize an image of your father's face, you would activate the FATHER'S FACE nodes; and so on.

However, evidence speaks against this idea (e.g., Kosslyn, 1980, 1983). Instead, images seem to be stored in memory in a piecemeal fashion. To form an image, therefore, you first have to activate the nodes specifying the "image frame," which depicts the form's global shape. Then, elaborations can be added to this frame, if you wish, to create a full and detailed image.

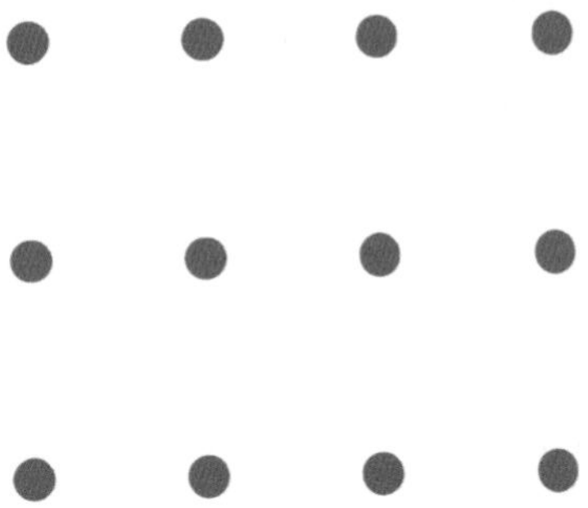

FIGURE 11.12   COLUMNS OR ROWS?

This picture shows "three rows of dots." The same picture also shows "four columns of dots." There is, in short, no difference between a picture of rows and a picture of columns. There is a difference, however, between a mental image of "three rows of dots" and a mental image of "four columns of dots." The latter image, for example, takes longer to generate and is more difficult to maintain, presumably because it contains a larger number of units—four columns, rather than three rows.

In support of this claim, images containing *more parts* take longer to create, just as we would expect if images are formed on a piece-by-piece basis (see **Figure 11.12**). In addition, images containing *more detail* also take longer to create, in accord with this hypothesis. Third, we know that imagers have some degree of control over how complete and detailed their images will be, so that (depending on the task, the imagers' preferences, etc.) images can be quite sketchy or quite elaborate (Reisberg, 1996). This variation is easily explained if imagers first create an image frame and only then add as much detail as they want.

But how does the imager know *how to* construct the image—what its form should be and what it should include? The relevant information is drawn from **image files** in long-term memory. Each file contains the information needed in order to create a mental image—information about how to create the image frame, and then information about how to elaborate the frame in this way or that, if desired. How is this information represented within the image file? One proposal is that the image files contain something like a set of instructions, or even a "recipe," for creating an image. By analogy, someone could instruct you in how to create a picture by uttering the appropriate sentences: "In the top left, place a circle. Underneath it, draw a line, angling down. . . ." Such instructions would enable you to create a picture, but notice that there is nothing pictorial about the instructions themselves; they are sentences, not pictures. In the same way, the instructions within an image file allow you to create a representation that, as we have repeatedly seen, is picturelike in important ways. In long-term memory, however, this information may not be at all picturelike.

Verbal Coding of Visual Materials

The proposal before us, therefore, is that visual information is represented in long-term memory in a fashion that isn't itself "visual." Instead, visual information may be represented in long-term memory via propositions that provide a "recipe" to be used, when needed, for creating an image.

In some cases, though, visual information is represented in long-term storage in an even simpler format: a verbal label. This point is relevant to issues we met in Chapter 10, concerning the interplay between language and thought. Specifically, evidence tells us that individuals with large color vocabularies have better color memories, probably because they're remembering the verbal label for the color rather than the color itself, and it's *easier* to remember a word than it is to recall a tint.

A related point was made in a classic study by Carmichael, Hogan, and Walters (1932). Their research participants were shown pictures like those in the center column of **Figure 11.13**. Half of the participants were shown the top form and told, "This is a picture of eyeglasses." The other half were told, "This is a picture of a barbell." Later, the participants were asked to reproduce these pictures as carefully as they could, and those who had understood the picture as eyeglasses produced drawings that resembled eyeglasses; those who understood the picture as weights distorted their drawings appropriately. This is again what one would expect if the participants had memorized the description rather than the picture itself and were re-creating the picture on the basis of this description.

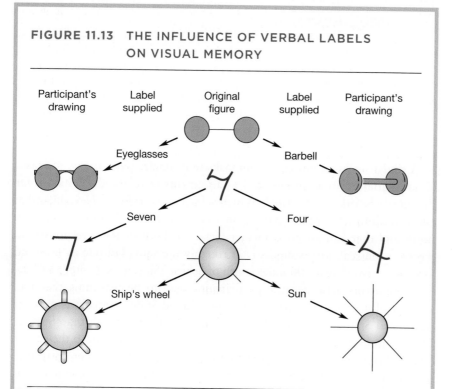

FIGURE 11.13   THE INFLUENCE OF VERBAL LABELS
ON VISUAL MEMORY

Participants were shown the figures in the middle column. If the top figure was presented with the label "eyeglasses," participants were later likely to reproduce the figure as shown on the left. If the figure was presented with the label "barbell," they were likely to reproduce it as shown on the right. (And so on for the other figures.) One interpretation of these data is that participants were remembering the verbal label and not the drawing itself.   AFTER CARMICHAEL, HOGAN, & WALTERS, 1932.

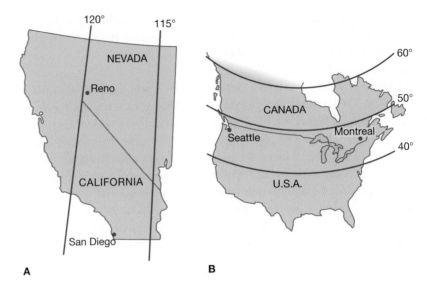

CONCEPTUAL MENTAL MAPS

Research participants tend to judge San Diego to be west of Reno and Montreal to be north of Seattle. But these judgments are in error. (Panel A) A map of California and Nevada with lines of longitude, which show that in fact San Diego is east of Reno. (Panel B) A map of the United States and southern Canada with lines of latitude, which show that Seattle is slightly north of Montreal.

A similar message emerges from tasks that require participants to reason about spatial position. In one study, participants were asked, "Which is farther north: Seattle or Montreal? Which is farther west: Reno, Nevada; or San Diego, California?" Many participants responded that Montreal is farther north and that San Diego is farther west, but both of these responses are wrong. Montreal, for example, is at roughly the same latitude as Portland, Oregon, a city almost 200 miles south of Seattle (Stevens & Coupe, 1978).

These errors arise because participants seem to be reasoning this way: "Montreal is in Canada; Seattle is in the United States. Canada is north of the United States. Therefore, Montreal must be farther north than Seattle." This kind of reasoning is sensible, since it will often bring you to the correct answer. (That's because most parts of Canada are, in fact, farther north than most parts of the United States.) Even so, this reasoning will sometimes lead to error, and it does so in this case. (The logic is the same for the Reno/San Diego question.)

Of course, what is of interest here is not the participants' knowledge about the longitude and latitude of these particular cities. What is important is that the sort of reasoning revealed in these studies hinges on propositional knowledge, not on any sort of mental images or maps. Apparently, at least some of our spatial knowledge relies on a symbolic/propositional code. (For more on reasoning about geography, see Friedman & Brown, 2000a, 2000b.)

Imagery Helps Memory

No matter how images are stored in long-term memory, however, it's clear that images influence memory in important ways and, in general, imagery improves memory. For example, materials that evoke imagery are considerably easier to remember than materials that do not evoke imagery. This can be demonstrated in many ways, including the following two-step procedure. First, participants are presented with a list of nouns and asked to rate each noun, on a scale from 1 to 7, for how readily it evokes an image (Paivio, 1969; Paivio, Yuille, & Madigan, 1968). Examples of words receiving high ratings are "church," with an average rating of 6.63, and "elephant," rated at 6.83. Words receiving lower ratings include "context" (2.13) and "virtue" (3.33).

As a second step, we ask whether these imagery ratings, generated by one group of participants, can be used to predict memory performance with a new group of participants. The new participants are asked to memorize lists of words, and the data reliably indicate that participants learn high-imagery words more readily than low-imagery words (Paivio, 1969; Paivio, Smythe, & Yuille, 1968).

EBOOK DEMONSTRATION 11.2

In the same fashion, memory can be enormously aided by the use of imagery mnemonics. In one study, some participants were asked to learn pairs of words by rehearsing each pair silently. Other participants were instructed to make up a sentence for each pair of words, linking the words in some sensible way. Finally, other participants were told to form a mental image for each pair of words, with the image combining the words in some interaction. The results showed poorest recall performance by the rehearsal group and intermediate performance by the group that generated the sentences. Both of these groups, though, did appreciably worse than the imagery group (Bower & Winzenz, 1970; for discussion of other mnemonic techniques, see Chapter 6).

In order to be helpful, though, imagery mnemonics need to do more than depict the objects side by side. These mnemonics are helpful only if they show the objects to be remembered *interacting* in some way (Wollen, Weber, & Lowry, 1972). This is not surprising: As we saw in Chapter 6, memory is improved in general if you can find ways to organize the material; interacting images provide one means of achieving this organization.

There are, in fact, many ways in which imagery can help you organize the materials you're learning; one of those ways is concerned with issues of *timing* and *sequence*. Let's say, for example, that you want to learn several facts about Marta, with some of the facts being concerned with Marta's past and some with her future. Perhaps you want to remember that a week ago Marta was in a great mood, that two months ago she bought a new car, and that next month she'll be going to Atlanta. To learn these various facts, you might imagine them arranged in a line—with past events off to the left and future events, in proper sequence, arrayed to the right.

Do people use this strategy? One study examined patients with neglect syndrome. As we mentioned in Chapter 5, these patients attend only to the right side of space and consistently overlook stimuli on their left. We then saw in this chapter (p. 402) that these patients show a corresponding pattern in their *imagery*, consistently overlooking objects that might be depicted on the left in an image. How will this matter if these patients are using the mnemonic strategy just described? If they are imagining events on a line, they'll likely overlook events on the left—that is, past events. And, in fact, that is the pattern of the results: Patients with left spatial neglect have a harder time remembering *past* facts about Marta (in the example we sketched) and an easier time remembering future facts. As the study's authors put it, these patients seem to neglect the "left side" of time—just what we would expect if they're using the strategy we've outlined (Saj, Fuhrman, Vuilleumier, & Boroditsky, 2014).

Dual Coding

There's no question, then, that imagery improves memory. But why is this? What memory aid does imagery provide? The answer has at least two parts. First, we've just suggested that imagery provides a means of organizing materials, and of course organization helps memory. But, second, another mechanism also contributes. Imageable materials, such as high-imagery words, will likely be doubly represented in memory: The word itself will be remembered, and so will the corresponding picture. This pattern is referred to as **dual coding**, and its advantage should be obvious: When the time comes to retrieve these memories, either record—the verbal or the image—will provide the information you seek. This gives you a double chance of locating the information you need, thereby easing the process of memory search.

Of course, framing things in this way builds on the idea that you have (at least) two types of information in long-term storage: memories that represent the content of symbolic (and perhaps verbal) materials, and memories that represent imagery-based materials. Paivio (1971), the source of the dual-coding proposal, argues that these two types of memory differ from each other in important ways—including the information that they contain and the ways they are accessed. Access to symbolic memories, he suggests, is easiest if the cue provided is a word, as in, "Do you know the word 'squirrel'?" Access to an image-based memory, in contrast, is easiest if one begins with a picture: "Do you recognize this pictured creature?"

Memory for Pictures

Paivio (1971) also proposed that there are two separate memory systems: one containing the symbolic memories, the other containing images. However, many psychologists are skeptical about this claim, arguing instead that there's just one long-term memory, holding both of these types of information (and perhaps other types as well). Within this single memory, each type of content does have its own traits, its own pattern of functioning. But even with these differences, the two types of information are contained in a unified memory—much as a single library building, with one indexing system and one set of rules, can hold both books and photographs, sound recordings as well as videos. (For discussion of this point, see Heil, Rösler, & Hennighausen, 1994.)

On this basis, we would expect the two types of memory to have many traits in common, thanks to the fact that both reside within a single memory system. This expectation turns out to be correct, and so many of the claims we made in Chapters 6, 7, and 8 apply with equal force to visual memories and verbal memories. Recall of both memory types, for example, is dependent on memory connections; priming effects can be observed with both types of memory; encoding specificity is observed in both domains; and so on.

Likewise, visual memory (like memory in general) is heavily influenced by schema-based, generic knowledge—knowledge about how events unfold in general. Chapter 8 described how these knowledge effects influence memory for sentences and stories, but similar effects can easily be demonstrated with pictures. In an early study, Friedman (1979) showed participants pictures of scenes such as a typical kitchen or a typical barnyard. In addition, the pictures also contained some unexpected objects. The kitchen picture, for example, included some items rarely found in a kitchen, such as a fireplace. Participants were later given a recognition test in which they had to discriminate between pictures they'd actually seen and altered versions of these pictures in which something had been changed.

Participants' memories were plainly influenced by their broader knowledge of what "should be" included in a kitchen picture. Thus, in some of the test pictures, one of the ordinary, expected objects in the scene had been changed—for example, participants might be shown a test picture in which a different kind of stove appeared in place of the original stove, or one in which a radio replaced the toaster on the counter. Participants rarely noticed these changes and thus tended (incorrectly) to respond that this new picture was in fact "old"—that is, had been seen before. This is sensible on schema grounds: Both the original and altered pictures were fully consistent with the kitchen schema, so both would be compatible with a schema-based memory.

However, participants almost always noticed changes to the unexpected objects in the scene. If the originally viewed kitchen had a fireplace and the test picture did not, participants consistently detected this alteration. Again, this is predictable on schema grounds: The fireplace did not fit with the kitchen schema and so was likely to be specifically noted in memory. In fact, Friedman recorded participants' eye movements during the original presentations of the pictures. Her data showed that participants tended to look twice as long at the unexpected objects as they did at the expected ones; clearly, these objects did catch the participants' attention. (For more on schema guidance of eye movements, see Henderson & Hollingworth, 2003; Vo & Henderson, 2009.)

A different line of evidence also shows schema effects in picture memory. Recall our claim that in understanding a story people place the story within a schematic frame. As we saw in Chapter 8, this can often lead to intrusion errors, as people import their own expectations and understanding into the story and thus end up remembering the story as including more than it actually did.

A similar pattern can be demonstrated with picture memory, in a phenomenon known as **boundary extension** (Intraub & Bodamer, 1993; Intraub & Dickinson, 2008; Intraub, Gottesman, & Bills, 1998; Intraub, Hoffman, Wetherhold, & Stoehs, 2006; McDunn, Siddiqui, & Brown, 2014). That is, people remember a picture as including more than it actually did, in effect

FIGURE 11.14 BOUNDARY EXTENSION IN PICTURE MEMORY

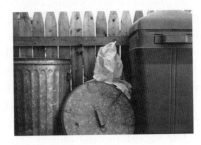

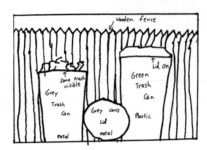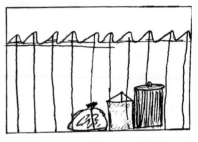

Participants were initially shown the photograph on the top of this picture. The two panels below show the scene as drawn from memory by two different participants. The participants clearly recalled the scene as a wide-angle shot, revealing more of the background than it actually did. AFTER INTRAUB & RICHARDSON, 1989.

extending the boundaries of the remembered depiction. For example, participants who were shown the top panel in **Figure 11.14** were later asked to sketch what they had seen. Two of the participants' drawings are shown at the bottom of Figure 11.14, and the boundary extension is clear: Participants remember the scene as less of a close-up view than it actually was, and correspondingly they remember the scene as containing more of the backdrop than it did. This effect is observed whether participants initially see a few pictures or many, whether they are tested immediately or after a delay, and even when they are explicitly warned about boundary extension and urged to avoid this effect.

Intraub has argued that this boundary extension arises from the way in which people perceive these pictures in the first place. People understand a picture, she claims, by means of a perceptual schema. This schema places the picture in a larger context, informing the perceiver about the real-world scene only partially revealed by the picture. Intraub suggests that this leads people to a series of expectations about what they might see if they could somehow look beyond the picture's edges, and these expectations become part of the experience of viewing the picture. It's then the *experience* that is remembered—and so your memory includes both the picture itself and also your understanding of what you'd see if you explored further, leading to the boundary extension that reliably emerges in the data.

Overall, then, it looks like picture memory follows the same rules, and is influenced by the same factors, as memory for verbal materials. Schema effects, we've just seen, can be found in both domains. Similarly, participants show primacy and recency effects when they learn a series of pictures (Tabachnick & Brotsky, 1976), just as they do when they learn a series of words (Chapter 6). Spread of activation can be demonstrated with nonverbal materials (Kroll & Potter, 1984), just as it can be with verbal materials (Chapter 9). In short, there's considerable commonality between picture memory and memory of other sorts, confirming our suggestion of a single memory system—a system that holds diverse contents but with a uniform set of operating principles.

The Diversity of Knowledge

Notice, then, where the data are leading us. When you're thinking about an image—and thus holding the image in working memory—there's no question that you're considering a distinctive form of mental representation. Images in working memory contain different information than other representations do; they make different information prominent; they require a set of operations (like scanning, or rotation, or zooming) that are irrelevant to other sorts of memory contents. Hence, our theorizing about active images has to be different from our theorizing about other forms of representation.

The situation changes, however, when we turn to long-term memory and consider your long-term retention for what a circus clown looks like or your recollection of what an earlier-viewed picture contained. The *content* of these memories is different from, say, your memory for stories. But even so, the image-based memories seem to be stored in the same memory system as every other memory—and so they are influenced by exactly the same principles. In support of this claim, we can find many commonalities in the ways people remember diverse types of knowledge. We've mentioned some of these commonalities already, but in addition let's add that memory for faces benefits from rehearsal (Sporer, 1988), just as memory for stories does. Similarly, a separation between *familiarity* and *source memory* (see Chapter 7) can be demonstrated for remembered music or remembered faces (Brigham & Cairns, 1988; Brown, Deffenbacher, & Sturgill, 1977), just as it can be for remembered words. And so on.

It would appear, therefore, that there really is just one long-term memory, with a set of rules consistently applicable to all its diverse contents. However, we should attach one caution to this claim. In this chapter, we've focused on visual memories, and one might well ask whether similar conclusions would emerge with other categories of knowledge. For example, do memories for tastes or smells benefit from rehearsal, show schema effects, and the like? Do memories for emotions or for pain benefit from deep processing? Do they show the effects we called (in Chapter 7) "implicit memory" effects? Relatively little research speaks to these issues.

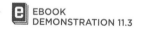 EBOOK DEMONSTRATION 11.3

It's on this basis, then, that the claims about the singularity of long-term memory should remain tentative, and that is one of the reasons that throughout this chapter our agenda has been both substantive and methodological. We've obviously surveyed what is known about visual imagery and visual memory, but at the same time we've tried to illustrate the questions that you might ask and the methods that you might use in exploring other types of knowledge—asking whether the content is distinctive in working memory and what evidence we'd need in order to propose a separate system within long-term memory. We've seen how things stand on these issues with regard to visual materials. However, the field awaits additional data before these issues can be resolved for other modalities.

COGNITIVE PSYCHOLOGY AND EDUCATION

Using Imagery

Visual imagery can serve as a powerful aid to memory, and so visualization is often helpful when you're trying to learn new materials. It's often useful, in other words, to form "mental pictures" of the materials you're studying.

You should, however, be careful about how and when you rely on visualization. Mental images do an excellent job of representing what something looks like, so imagery mnemonics can help you a lot if you want to remember appearances—how a visualized scene looked and what it included. But at the same time, appearances can mislead you. Let's say that you hope to remember the term "Korsakoff syndrome" (a form of amnesia discussed in Chapter 7). You therefore form a mental picture of someone standing on a race course and coughing. Later, when you're trying to recall the term, you call this mental picture to mind, and after examining the picture (with your "mind's eye"), you confidently announce, "I remember—the term is Race-cough syndrome" (or "Track-sick syndrome" or some such). These responses are, of course, consistent with the picture, a point that reminds us that pictures (mental or otherwise) are often not specific enough to provide the information you need.

Likewise, in forming a mnemonic picture you're likely to think about what the to-be-remembered items look like, and this may distract you from thinking about what these items mean. Imagine, for example, that you want to remember that a hypothesis was offered by the important psychologist Henry Roediger. To remember this name, you might playfully convert it to "rod-digger" and form a mental picture of someone digging in the earth with a fishing rod. This will help you remember the name, but it will promote no insights into what Roediger's hypothesis was, or how it relates to other aspects of his theorizing, or to other things you know. Images, in other words, are excellent for remembering some things, but often what you need (or want) to remember goes beyond this.

These points are not meant to warn you against using image-based mnemonics. In fact, let's again emphasize how effective these mnemonics are.

However, it's important to understand why these mnemonics work as they do, because with that knowledge you can avoid using the mnemonics in circumstances in which they might not serve you well.

In the same fashion, imagery can be a powerful aid to problem solving and can sometimes be more helpful than an actual out-in-the-world drawing. Images can, for example, represent movement and 3-D in ways that a drawing cannot. Mental images can also be more easily adjusted than a drawing (if, for example, you want to alter the size or position of one of the image's elements).

Sometimes, though, images are less helpful than a drawing. If the scene you're contemplating is complex, it may be difficult to maintain all of the scene's elements in a mental image, so in this case a drawing would be better. In addition, the chapter argues that mental images are understood within a certain framework—one that indicates the imager's understanding of the image's figure/ground organization and its orientation in space. This framework helps the imager interpret the depicted form but can also limit what the imager will discover from a given mental picture. (This is, for example, why imagers routinely fail to find a "duck" in a "rabbit image" and vice versa, as described in the chapter.)

People can, however, often escape these limits by drawing a picture, based on their own mental image. The picture depicts the same form as the image; but because the picture is not linked to a particular reference frame, it will often support new discoveries that the original image would not. We can demonstrate this in the laboratory (e.g., in people discovering the duck in their own drawing of the duck/rabbit form, even though they couldn't make this discovery from their image). We can also demonstrate this point in real-world settings (e.g., in architects who cannot reconceptualize a building plan by scrutinizing their mental image of the plan, but who then make striking new discoveries once they draw out the plan on paper).

Overall, then, we can again see the benefits of understanding the limits of your own strategies. Once you understand those limits, you can find ways to make full use of these strategies to improve your problem-solving skills, your memory, and your comprehension of new materials—but without falling into traps created by the strategies' limits.

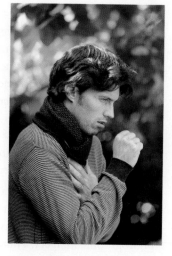

THE HAZARDS OF IMAGERY MNEMONICS?

To remember the name *Korsakoff*, you might visualize someone near a race *course* who is *coughing*. This mnemonic may be effective . . . but may mislead you. Later, when you recall the image, you might decide the name was "Coursick" or "Racecold."

chapter summary

● People differ enormously in how they describe their imagery experience, particularly the vividness of that experience. However, concerns about how we should interpret these self-reports have led investigators to seek more objective means of studying mental imagery.

● Chronometric studies indicate that the pattern of what information is more available and what is less available in an image closely matches the pattern of what is available in an actual picture. Likewise, the times needed to scan across an image, to zoom in on an image to examine detail, or to imagine the form rotating, all correspond closely to the times needed for these operations with actual pictures. These results emerge even when the experimenter makes no mention of imagery, ruling out an account of these data in terms of the demand character of the experiments.

● In many settings, visual imagery seems to involve mechanisms that overlap with those used for visual perception. This is reflected in the fact that imaging one thing can make it difficult to perceive something else, or that imaging the appropriate target can prime a subsequent perception. Further evidence comes from neuroimaging and studies of brain damage; this evidence confirms the considerable overlap between the biological basis for imagery and that for perception.

- Not all imagery, however, is visual, so that we need to distinguish between *visual* and *spatial* imagery. This proposal is confirmed by studies of individuals with brain damage, some of whom seem to lose the capacity for visual imagery but retain their capacity for spatial imagery. This proposal may also help us understand the pattern of individual differences in imagery ability, with some individuals being particularly skilled in visual imagery and some in spatial.

- Just as some individuals seem to have little or no visual imagery, other individuals—called "eidetikers"—seem to have fabulously detailed, photographic imagery. There is no question that this astonishingly vivid imagery exists in some people, but the mechanisms behind it remain unknown.

- Even when imagery is visual, mental images are picturelike—they are not actually pictures. Unlike pictures, mental images seem to be accompanied by a perceptual reference frame that guides the interpretation of the image and also influences what can be discovered about the image.

- To create a mental image, you draw on information stored in an image file in long-term memory.

These image files can be thought of as "recipes" for the construction of a mental image, usually by first constructing a frame and then by elaborating the frame as needed. In addition, at least some information about visual appearance or spatial arrangement is stored in long-term memory in terms of verbal labels or conceptual frameworks. For example, information about the locations of cities may be stored in terms of propositions ("Montreal is in Canada; Canada is north of the United States") rather than being stored in some sort of mental map.

- Imagery helps people to remember, so word lists are more readily recalled if the words are easily imaged; similarly, instructions to form images help people to memorize. These benefits may be the result of dual coding: storing information in both a verbal format and a format that encodes appearances; this approach doubles the chances of recalling the material later on.

- When you're trying to remember combinations of ideas, it is best to imagine the objects to be remembered interacting in some way.

- Memory for pictures can be accurate, but it follows most of the same rules as any other form of memory; for example, it is influenced by schematic knowledge.

- It is unclear what other categories of memory there might be. In each case, other kinds of memory are likely to have some properties that are distinctive and also many properties that are shared with memories of other sorts.

eBook Demonstrations & Essays

Online Demonstrations:
- Demonstration 11.1: Imaged Synthesis
- Demonstration 11.2: Mnemonic Strategies
- Demonstration 11.3: Auditory Imagery

Online Applying Cognitive Psychology Essays:
- Cognitive Psychology and the Law: Lineups

ZAPS 2.0 Cognition Labs

- Go to **http://digital.wwnorton.com/cognition6** for the online labs relevant to this chapter.

Thinking

Many people believe that the capacity for complex *thought* is what makes us human. And there's no question that we rely on this capacity all the time. We draw conclusions; we make choices; we solve problems. But how do we achieve these things? How do we think? And how *well* do we think?

In this section, we'll see that human thinking is often flawed, and we'll encounter examples of bad judgment, improper reasoning, and highly inefficient problem solving. As we'll see, though, this poor performance is usually not the product of laziness or stupidity. The explanation lies instead in a theme that has already arisen in our discussion: In a wide range of settings, humans rely on mental shortcuts—strategies that are efficient but that risk error. These shortcuts played an important part in Chapter 4, when we discussed object recognition, and in Chapter 8, when we discussed memory errors. Similar shortcuts will emerge in this section, and as we'll see, they play a central role in guiding human thought.

However, it's clear that in many circumstances people rise above these shortcuts and think carefully and well. This will, at the least, drive us toward a multilayered conception of thinking, because we'll need to describe both the shortcuts that people use and also the more careful strategies that people often turn to. In addition, we'll need to tackle the obvious questions of *why* and *when* people rely on one sort of thinking or the other. What are the circumstances, or the reasons, that lead to efficient-but-risky thinking, and what are the triggers for slower-but-better thinking?

It's also important that people seem to differ in their thinking. Some people are wonderfully logical; others seem capricious. Some people are creative problem solvers; others are stymied by even simple problems. Some people seem fabulously intelligent; others seem less so. In this section, we'll examine these differences as well.

Finally, one other set of issues will arise in this section: How much of thought is conscious? Are there benefits associated with conscious thought, as opposed to unconscious thought? We will tackle these questions in the book's final chapter, but we'll do this largely by pulling together points we've made in earlier chapters. In this way, the final chapter will provide something of a review for the text at the same time that it explores a series of enormously important theoretical questions.

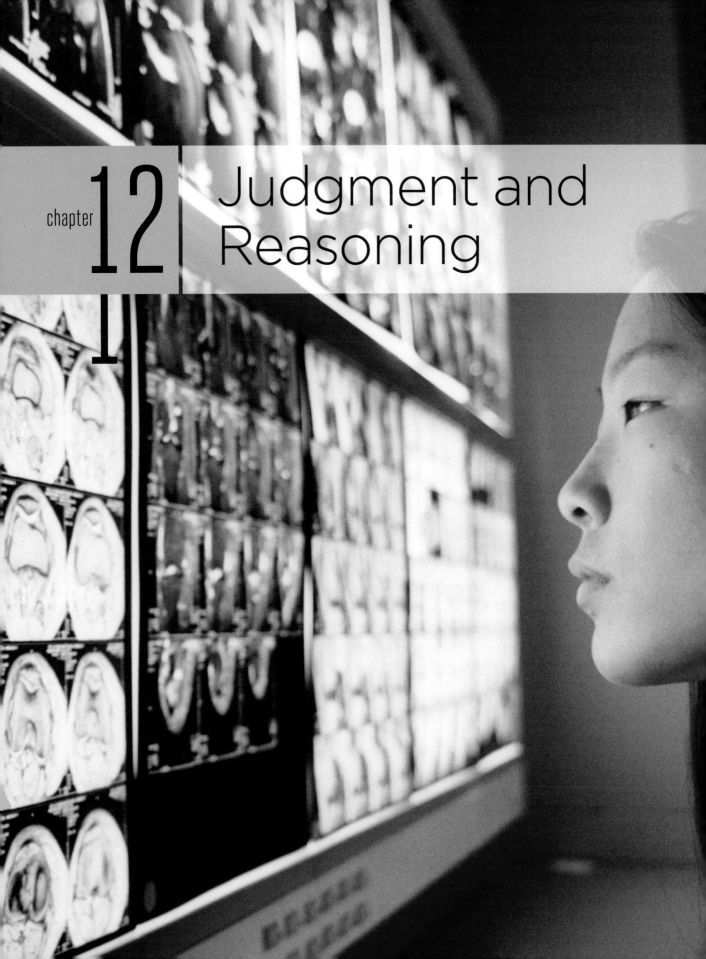

12

Judgment and Reasoning

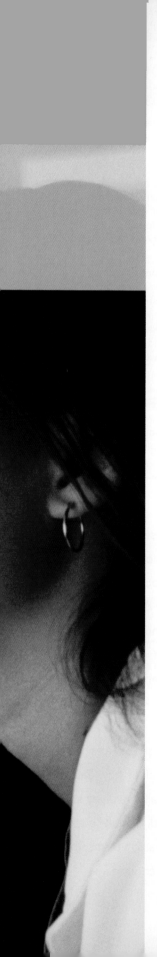

what if... The activity we call "thinking" involves many processes, and this simple point blocks us from asking in a general way, "What would happen if you lost the ability to think?" We can, however, ask what would happen if you lost *this* aspect of thinking or *that* aspect—and the answers are often intriguing.

Many of us regard *emotion* as a force that disrupts thinking. We say things like "I was so angry I couldn't think straight" or "I knew I'd regret the choice, but at that moment I was listening more to my heart than to my head." These sentiments capture important truths, but they surely overstate the separation between "heart" and "head," because emotion turns out to play a huge role in our ordinary thinking. We see this if we ask: "What if someone loses *the capacity for ordinary emotion*?" Consider Elliot, a patient whose case is discussed in detail by Antonio Damasio (1994). Elliot had undergone surgery to remove a small brain tumor, and the surgery seemed to have little impact on his intellect; his IQ score was just as high after the operation as it was before. But after the operation, Elliot became hopelessly indecisive. In scheduling an appointment, for example, he needed 30 minutes, staring at his calendar, to decide which of two days would be better for him. He'd spend an entire afternoon deciding whether to classify a set of records by "place" or by "date." He needed so much time to choose where he'd eat lunch that he was likely to miss lunchtime. In choosing a restaurant, he'd scrutinize each place's menu, its lighting, and its seating patterns; he'd drive to each restaurant to see how busy it was—but he still couldn't decide where to eat. Even the simplest of decisions—whether to use a blue or black pen for office paperwork—was paralyzing for him.

Because of damage to a part of the brain called the "orbitofrontal cortex" (see **Figure 12.1**), Elliot seemed to have lost emotions; Damasio reports that he "never saw a tinge of emotion" in his hours of conversation with Elliot. When tested in the laboratory, Elliot showed no bodily response at all if shown pictures depicting tragedy or aggression; he did not react to sexual images, or gruesome pictures of wounds, or any other image that for other people cause a powerful emotional response.

preview of chapter themes

- In a wide range of circumstances, people use cognitive shortcuts, or "heuristics," to make judgments. These heuristics tend to be relatively efficient and often lead to sensible conclusions. However, heuristic use sometimes can lead to error.

- People use heuristics even when they're trying to be careful in their judgment and even when they're highly motivated to be accurate. The heuristics are used both by experts and by ordinary people, and so expert judgments, too, are vulnerable to error.

- However, heuristic use is far from inevitable, and in some circumstances people rely on more sophisticated forms of reasoning—with the result that they judge covariation accurately, are sensitive to base rates, are alert to the problems of drawing a conclusion from a small sample of evidence, and so on.

- We will consider when people use their more sophisticated ("Type 2") reasoning and when they rely on heuristics ("Type 1"). Evidence suggests that Type 2 is likely to come into play only if the circumstances are right and only if the case being judged contains the appropriate triggers for this form of reasoning.

- The quality of people's thinking is also uneven when we turn to the broad domain of deduction. For example, people often show a pattern of "confirmation bias" and so are more sensitive to, and more accepting of, evidence that supports their beliefs than they are of evidence that challenges their beliefs.

- Errors in logical reasoning are easy to document, and these errors follow patterns suggesting that people are guided by principles other than those of logic. In fact, in a fashion distinct from the pattern set by formal logic, people's reasoning is heavily influenced by the *content* of what they're reasoning about.

- People seem not to base their decisions on utility calculations; this is evident in the fact that many factors (including the decision's frame) have a strong impact on decisions even though these factors do not change utilities in any way. Instead, people seem to make decisions that they feel they can explain and justify, and so they are influenced by factors that make one choice or another seem more compelling.

- Another factor influencing decision making is emotion. Here, the complication is that people are often inept in predicting their future emotions and so work hard to avoid regret that they wouldn't have felt anyhow, and spend money for things that provide only short-term pleasure.

But why did Elliot's lack of emotion lead to paralysis in his decision making? Part of the answer lies in the fact that decisions often involve some element of risk ("Will this dinner taste as good as the menu description implies?"). To evaluate these (and other) risks, people rely heavily on emotion—and so, if thinking about the dinner fills you with joyful anticipation, you'll judge the risk to be low (cf. Slovic & Peters, 2010). Or, as a contrasting case, if thinking about a terrorist attack fills you with dread, you'll likely judge the risk of an attack to be high. It's processes like these that were unavailable for Elliot.

Emotion also plays a role in *evaluating our options*. In choosing whether to eat at this restaurant or that one, we often ask ourselves how each of the options makes us feel, and often this activity literally involves some monitoring of our own bodies: Do I feel a little excited, or a little tense, when I think about another lunch at Carl's Café? In Damasio's terms, these *somatic markers* play an important role in guiding our choices.

FIGURE 12.1 ORBITOFRONTAL CORTEX

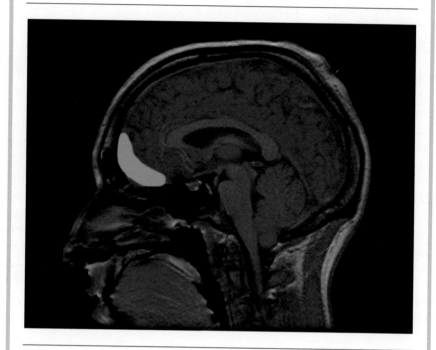

The area highlighted in green is the orbitofrontal cortex—the portion of the brain just behind your eyeballs. Many researchers argue that this brain region plays a crucial role in the processes through which we detect and interpret our own emotions.

There are surely occasions in which emotions disrupt your thinking. But, apparently, there are many occasions in which emotions *contribute* in important ways to your thinking. We'll need to address this contribution before we're through.

Diverse Forms of Thinking

The activity of "thinking" takes many forms. We *draw conclusions* from the evidence we encounter (often, evidence provided by life experiences). We *consider the implications* of our various beliefs. We *make decisions*—some trivial (soup or salad? Coke or Pepsi?) and some consequential ("Should I quit my job and go to school?"; "Should I get married to my partner?").

In this chapter, we'll ask how these various processes unfold, and we'll also ask how *well* people think—that is, how well people do in drawing conclusions or reasoning things through. This evaluation will lead us to consider what steps we can take to make people better, more critical, more astute thinkers.

Judgment

Experience is an extraordinary teacher, and so you're likely to believe the sports coach who, after many seasons, tells you which game strategies work and which ones don't. Likewise, you trust the police detective who asserts that over the years he's learned how to tell whether a suspect is lying. You welcome the advice of the hair stylist who says, "I can tell you from the hair I cut every day; this shampoo repairs split ends."

But we can also find cases in which people *don't* learn from experience: "He's getting married *again*? Why does he think this one will last longer than the last four?"; "I can't believe you bought another European car; didn't you learn from the last one?"; "He's so biased! It doesn't matter how many polite New Yorkers he meets; he's *still* convinced that everyone in New York is rude."

What's going on here? More broadly, since experience seems not to be an infallible teacher, can we really trust the conclusions that people draw from experience?

Attribute Substitution

Let's start with the *information* you use when drawing a conclusion from experience. Imagine that you're shopping for a car and trying to decide if European cars are reliable or not. Surely, you'd want to know how often these cars break down and need repair. Or, as a different example, imagine that you want to take Professor Jones's course next year, but you've heard that grades in his class tend to be very low, and you want to find out if that's true. Again, the information you want concerns frequencies: How many students in the class get B's? How many get C's? How many get lower grades?

Examples like these remind us that judgments often begin with a **frequency estimate**—an assessment of how often various events have occurred in the past. For many of the judgments you make in day-to-day life, though, you don't have direct access to frequency information. Imagine, for example, that you're trying to choose an efficient route for your morning drive to work. Here you might ask, "When I've gone down 4th Avenue, how often was I late? How often was I late when I stayed on Front Street instead?" If you had a detailed list of your various commute times, you'd soon have the answers you seek. Chances are, though, that you don't have this list, so what can you do instead? You're likely to do a quick scan through memory, looking for relevant cases. If you can immediately think of three occasions in which you got caught in a traffic snarl on 4th Avenue and can't think of any similar occasions on Front Street, you'll probably decide that Front Street is the better bet. In contrast, if you can recall two horrible traffic jams on Front Street but only one on 4th Avenue, you'll draw the opposite conclusion.

The strategy you're using here is known as **attribute substitution**—a strategy in which you rely on easily assessed information as a proxy for the information you really need. In this judgment about traffic, you're relying on a specific form of attribute substitution known as the **availability heuristic** (Tversky & Kahneman, 1973). The information you need is *frequency* (how often you're late when you've taken one route or the other), but you don't have access to this information. As a substitute, you base your judgment on *availability*—how easily and how quickly you can come up with relevant examples. The logic, in essence, is this: "Examples leap to mind? Must be a common, often-experienced event. A struggle to come up with examples? Must be a rare event."

Here's a different type of attribute substitution: Imagine that you're applying for a job. You hope that the employer will examine your credentials carefully and make a thoughtful judgment about whether you'd be a good hire. It's likely, though, that the employer will rely on a faster, easier strategy. Specifically, he may barely glance at your résumé and instead ask himself how much you resemble other people he's hired who have worked out well. Do you have the same mannerisms, the same look as Joan, say, an employee that he's very happy with? If so, you're likely to get the job. In this case, the employer wants to judge a *probability* (namely, the probability that you'd work out well if hired) and instead relies on *resemblance*. This particular substitution is referred to as the **representativeness heuristic**. Let's look at these two heuristics—availability and representativeness—in more detail. (See **Table 12.1** for a summary comparison of these two heuristics; for a broad discussion of heuristics, see Griffin, Gonzalez, Koehler, & Gilovich, 2012.)

TABLE 12.1   DIFFERENT TYPES OF ATTRIBUTE SUBSTITUTION

You want to judge . . .	Instead you rely on . . .	This usually works because . . .	But this strategy can lead to error because . . .
Frequency of occurrence in the world	Availability in memory: How easily can you think of cases?	Events that are frequent in the world are likely to be more available in memory.	Many factors *other than* frequency in the world can influence availability from memory!
Probability of an event being in a category or having certain properties	Resemblance between that event and other events that are in the category	Many categories are homogeneous enough so that the category members do resemble one another.	Many categories are not homogeneous!

The Availability Heuristic

Heuristics are efficient strategies that usually lead to the right answer. The key word, however, is "usually," because heuristics allow errors. That's the price you pay in order to gain the efficiency.

The availability and representativeness heuristics both fit this profile. In each case, you're relying on an attribute (availability or resemblance) that's easy to assess, and that's the source of the efficiency. And in each case, the attribute is in fact correlated with the target dimension, so that it can serve as a reasonable proxy for the target: Events or objects that are frequent in the world are, in most cases, likely to be easily available in memory, and so generally you'll be fine if you rely on availability as an index for frequency. And many categories are homogeneous enough so that members of the category do resemble one another; that's why you can often rely on resemblance as a way of judging probability of category membership.

Nonetheless, these strategies can lead to error. To take a simple case, ask yourself, "Are there more words in the dictionary beginning with the letter *R* ('rose,' 'rock,' 'rabbit') or more words with an *R* in the third position ('tarp,' 'bare,' 'throw')?" Most people assert that there are more words beginning with *R* (Tversky & Kahneman, 1973, 1974), but the reverse is true—by a margin of at least two to one.

Why do people get this wrong? The answer lies in availability. If you search your memory for words starting with *R*, many will come to mind. (Try it: How many *R*-words can you name in 10 seconds?) But if you search your memory for words with an *R* in the third position, fewer will emerge. (Again, try this for 10 seconds.) This difference, favoring the words beginning with *R*, arises because your memory is organized roughly like a dictionary, with words that share a starting sound all grouped together. As a consequence, it's easy to search memory using "starting letter" as your cue; a search based on "*R* in third position" is more difficult. Thus, the organization of memory creates a bias in what's easily available, and this bias in availability leads to an error in frequency judgment.

The Wide Range of Availability Effects

The *R*-word example is not very interesting on its own—how often do you need to make judgments about spelling patterns? But the example is, as they say, the tip of a large iceberg, because people rely on availability in a wide range of other cases, including cases in which they're making judgments of some importance.

For example, people regularly overestimate the frequency of events that are, in actuality, quite rare (Attneave, 1953; Lichtenstein, Slovic, Fischhoff, Layman, & Combs, 1978). This probably plays a part in people's willingness to buy lottery tickets; they overestimate the likelihood of winning. Likewise, physicians often overestimate the likelihood of a rare disease and, in the process, fail to pursue other, more appropriate, diagnoses (e.g., Elstein et al., 1986; Obrecht, Chapman, & Gelman, 2009).

What causes this pattern? There's little reason to spend time thinking about familiar events ("Oh, look—that airplane has wings!"), but you're likely to notice and think about rare events, especially rare *emotional* events ("Oh, God—that airplane crashed!"). As a result, rare events are likely to be well recorded in memory, and this will, in turn, make these events easily available to you. As a consequence, if you rely on the availability heuristic, you'll overestimate the frequency of these distinctive events and, correspondingly, overestimate the likelihood of similar events happening in the future.

Here's a different example. Participants in one study were asked to think about episodes in their lives in which they'd acted in an assertive fashion (Schwarz et al., 1991; also see Raghubir & Menon, 2005). Half of the participants were asked to recall 6 of these episodes; half were asked to recall 12 episodes. Then, all the participants were asked some general questions, including how assertive overall they thought they were.

Participants in this study had an easy time coming up with 6 episodes, and so, using the availability heuristic, they concluded, "Those cases came quickly to mind; therefore, there must be a large number of these episodes; therefore, I must be an assertive person." In contrast, participants who were asked for 12 episodes had some difficulty generating the longer list, and so they concluded, "If these cases are so difficult to recall, I guess the episodes can't be typical for how I act."

Consistent with these suggestions, participants who were asked to recall fewer episodes judged themselves to be more assertive. Notice, ironically, that the participants who tried to recall more episodes actually ended up with more evidence in view for their own assertiveness. But it's not the quantity of evidence that matters. Instead, what matters is the ease of coming up with the episodes. Participants who were asked for a dozen episodes had a hard time with the task *because they'd been asked to do something difficult*—namely, to come up with a lot of cases. But the participants seemed not to realize this. They reacted only to the fact that the examples were difficult to generate, and using the availability heuristic, they concluded that being assertive was relatively infrequent in their past.

The Representativeness Heuristic

Similar points can be made about the representativeness heuristic. Just like availability, this strategy is efficient and often leads to the correct conclusion. But here, too, the strategy can lead you astray.

How does the representativeness heuristic work? Let's start with the fact that many of the categories you encounter are relatively homogeneous. The category "birds," for example, is reasonably uniform with regard to the traits of *having wings, having feathers,* and so on. Virtually every member of the category has these traits, and so, in these regards, each member of the category resembles all the others. Likewise, the category "motels" is homogeneous with regard to traits like *has beds in each room, has a Bible in each*

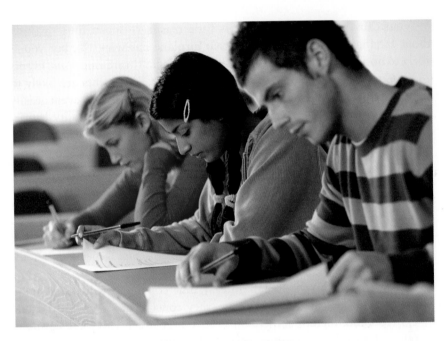

ABUSE OF THE AVAILABILITY HEURISTIC?

Imagine a diabolical college professor who wants to improve student evaluations of his teaching. A possible strategy is suggested by a study in which students were asked to list ways a particular course could be improved (Fox, 2006). Students were then asked for an overall rating of how good the course was. Students in one group were asked to list just two potential improvements to the course. These students had an easy time generating this short list, and guided by the availability heuristic, they seemed to reason this way: "It surely was easy to come up with possible improvements for the course. I guess, therefore, that the course must have many flaws and so isn't very good." As a result, they gave the course lower ratings than students who were asked to do a more difficult task—to come up with ten potential improvements for the course. Students in the latter group ended up with much more evidence in their view for the course's problems, but that's not what mattered. Instead, these students seemed to be thinking: "It was hard to produce this list. I guess, therefore, the course doesn't have many flaws; if it did, I'd have had an easier time thinking of improvements. So, I'll give the course a high rating." Of course, no professor would ever think about exploiting this pattern to manipulate student evaluations. . .

room, and *has an office*, and so, again, in these regards each member of the category (each motel) resembles all the others.

The representativeness heuristic capitalizes on this homogeneity. We expect each individual to resemble the other individuals in the category (i.e., we expect each individual to be *representative* of the category overall). As a result, we can use resemblance as a basis for judging the likelihood of category membership. Thus, if a creature resembles other birds you've seen, you conclude that the creature probably is a bird. We first met this approach in Chapter 9, when we were discussing simple categories like "dog" and "fruit." But the same approach can be used more broadly—and this is the heart of the representativeness strategy. Thus, if a job candidate resembles successful hires you've made, you conclude that the person will probably be a successful hire; if someone you meet at a party resembles engineers you've known, you assume that the person is likely to be an engineer.

Of course, since many categories *are* homogeneous, reasoning in this fashion will often lead you to sensible judgments. Even so, the use of this heuristic can lead to error. Imagine, for example, tossing a coin over and over; let's say that the coin has landed heads up six times in a row. Many people believe that on the next toss the coin is more likely to come up tails. But this conclusion, called the "gambler's fallacy," is wrong. The "logic" leading to this fallacy seems to be that if the coin is fair, then a series of tosses should contain equal numbers of heads and tails. If no tails have appeared for a while, then some are "overdue" to bring about this balance.

But of course a coin has no "memory," so it has no way of knowing (or being influenced by) how long it has been since the last tails. Therefore, the likelihood of a tail occurring on any particular toss must be independent of what has happened on previous tosses; there's no way that the previous tosses could influence the next one. Hence, the probability of a tail on toss number 7 is .50, just as it was on the first toss—and on every toss.

What produces the gambler's fallacy? The explanation lies in the assumption of category homogeneity. We all know that in the long run, a fair coin will produce equal numbers of heads and tails. Thus, the category of "all tosses" has this property. Our assumption of homogeneity, though, leads us to expect that any "representative" of the category will also have this property—that is, any sequence of tosses will also show the 50-50 split. But this isn't true: Some sequences of tosses are 75% heads; some are 5% heads. It is only when we combine these sequences that the 50-50 split emerges.

EBOOK DEMONSTRATIONS 12.1 AND 12.2

Reasoning from a Single Case to the Entire Population

The assumption of homogeneity can also lead to a different error—an expectation that the entire category will have the same properties as the individual category members. Hamill, Wilson, and Nisbett (1980) showed their participants a videotaped interview in which a prison guard discussed his job. In one condition, the guard was compassionate and kind; in another condition, the guard expressed contempt for the prison inmates and scoffed at the idea of rehabilitation. Before seeing either video, though, some participants were told that this guard was *typical* of those at the prison; other participants were told that he was quite *atypical*, chosen for the interview precisely because of his extreme views.

Participants were later questioned about their own views of the criminal justice system, and they were plainly influenced by the interview they'd just seen. Those who had seen the compassionate guard indicated that they believed prison guards in general were decent people; those

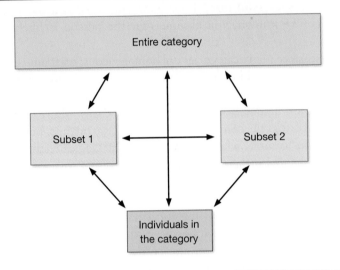

FIGURE 12.2 IMPLICATIONS OF ASSUMING CATEGORY HOMOGENEITY

If a category is truly homogeneous, then we know what the category's subsets will be like, based on information about the overall category, and we know what the category will be like, based on the subsets. Likewise, if the category is truly homogeneous, then we know what the individual category members will be like, based on information about the category, and vice versa. Unfortunately, though, people are far too quick to assume that categories are homogeneous, and so they make all these inferences even when they shouldn't!

who had seen the contemptuous guard reported more negative views of guards. What's remarkable, though, is that participants seemed to ignore the information about whether the interviewed guard was typical or not. Those who were explicitly told that the guard was atypical were influenced by the interview just as much as those who were told that the guard was typical.

In this study, participants drew a conclusion about an entire category ("prison guards") based on a single case—and they did so even when explicitly warned *against* this extrapolation. Similarly, imagine that you're shopping for a new cell phone. You've read various consumer magazines and decided, based on their test data, that you'll buy a Smacko brand phone. You report this to a friend, who is aghast. "Smacko? You must be crazy. Why, I know a man who bought a Smacko, and the case fell apart two weeks after he got it. Then, the wire for the headphones went. Then, the charger failed. How could you possibly buy a Smacko?"

In this instance, your friend is offering a "man who" argument (a term proposed by Nisbett & Ross, 1980). What should you make of this argument? The consumer magazines tested many phones and reported that, say, 2% of all Smackos have repair problems. In your friend's "data," 100% of the Smackos (one out of one) broke. Should this "sample of one" outweigh the much larger sample tested by the magazine? Your friend presumably believes he's offering a persuasive argument; but if so, your friend must be assuming that the category will resemble the instance. Only in that case would reasoning from a single instance be appropriate (see **Figure 12.2**).

If you listen to conversations around you, you'll regularly hear "man who" (or "woman who") arguments. "What do you mean, cigarette smoking causes cancer?! I have an aunt who smoked for 50 years, and she runs in marathons!" Often, these arguments seem persuasive. But they have force only by virtue of the representativeness heuristic—and thus your willingness to extrapolate from a tiny sample.

Detecting Covariation

It cannot be surprising that people often rely on mental shortcuts. After all, you don't have unlimited time, and many of the judgments you make are far from life-changing. It's unsettling, though, that people use the same shortcuts when making deeply consequential judgments. And to make things worse, the errors caused by the heuristics can trigger other sorts of errors, including errors in judgments about **covariation**. This term has a technical meaning, but for our purposes we can define it this way: X and Y "covary" if X tends to be on the scene whenever Y is, and if X tends to be absent whenever Y is absent. For example, exercise and stamina covary: People who do the first tend to have a lot of the second. Owning audio CDs and going to concerts also covary, although less strongly than exercise and stamina. (Some people own many CDs but rarely go to concerts.) Thus, covariation can be strong or weak, and it can also be negative or positive. Exercise and stamina, for example, covary positively (as exercise increases, so does stamina). Exercise and risk of heart attacks covary negatively (because exercise strengthens the heart muscle, decreasing the risk).

Covariation is important for many reasons—including the fact that it's what you need to consider when checking on a belief about cause and effect. Does education lead to a higher-paying job? If so, then degree of education and salary should covary. Likewise, do you feel better on days when you eat a good breakfast? If so, then the presence or absence of a good breakfast in the morning should covary with how you feel as the day wears on. Similarly: Are you more likely to fall in love with someone tall? Does your car start more easily if you pump the gas pedal? These, too, are questions that hinge on covariation, leading us to ask: How accurately do people judge covariation?

Illusions of Covariation

People routinely "detect" covariation even where there is none. For example, many people are convinced there's a relationship between a person's astrological sign (e.g., whether the person is a Libra or a Virgo) and their personality, yet no serious study has documented this covariation. Likewise, many people believe they can predict the weather by paying attention to their arthritis pain ("My knee always acts up when a storm is coming"). This belief, too, turns out to be groundless. Other examples concern social stereotypes (e.g., the idea that being "moody" covaries with gender), superstitions (e.g., the idea that Friday the 13th brings bad luck), and more. (For some of the evidence, see Arkes & Harkness, 1983; Chapman & Chapman, 1971; King & Koehler, 2000; Redelmeier & Tversky, 1996; Schustack & Sternberg, 1981; Shaklee & Mims, 1982; Smedslund, 1963.)

Further examples include some commonsense beliefs about psychology that, when examined, turn out to be mistaken. In Chapter 8, for example, we noted that people believe that *confidence that a memory is correct* covaries with the likelihood that the memory is, in fact, correct. However, this belief is to a large extent groundless. People also believe that certain cues covary with lying ("I could tell he was lying by the way he was jiggling his foot"), although the evidence is otherwise (DePaulo, Lindsay, Malone, Muhlenbruck, Charlton & Cooper, 2003; Reisberg, 2014). And on and on.

What causes illusions like these? One proposal focuses on the evidence that people consider in judging covariation, because in making these judgments people seem to consider only a *subset* of the evidence, and it's a subset that's skewed by their prior expectations (Baron, 1988; Evans, 1989; Gilovich, 1991; Jennings, Amabile, & Ross, 1982). This virtually guarantees mistaken judgments, since even if the judgment process were 100% fair, a biased input would lead to a biased output.

Specifically, when judging covariation, your selection of evidence is likely to be guided by **confirmation bias**—a tendency to be more responsive to evidence that *confirms* your beliefs rather than to evidence that might *challenge* your beliefs (Nisbett & Ross, 1980; Tweney, Doherty, & Mynatt, 1981). We'll have more to say about confirmation bias later; for now, note how confirmation bias could distort the assessment of covariation. Let's say, for example, that you have the belief that big dogs tend to be vicious. With this belief, you're more likely to notice big dogs that are, in fact, vicious and little dogs that are friendly. As a result, a biased sample of dogs is available to you, in the dogs you perceive and the dogs you remember. Therefore, if you're asked to estimate covariation between dog size and temperament, you'll probably overestimate the covariation. This isn't because you're ignoring the facts, nor is it because you're incompetent in thinking about covariation. The problem instead lies in your "data"; if the data are biased, so will be your judgment.

Base Rates

Assessment of covariation can also be pulled off track by another problem: neglect of **base-rate information**—information about how frequently something occurs in general. To make this point concrete, imagine that we're testing a new drug in hopes that it will cure the common cold. Here, we're trying to find out if taking the drug covaries with a better medical outcome, and let's say that our study tells us that 70% of the patients taking the drug do recover from their illness within 48 hours. This result is uninterpretable on its own, because we need the base rate: We need to know how often *in general* people recover from their colds in the same time span. If it turns out (for example) that the overall recovery rate within 48 hours is 70%, then our new drug is having no effect whatsoever.

Similarly, do good-luck charms help? Let's say that you wear your lucky socks whenever your favorite team plays, and the team has won 85% of its games. Here, too, we need to ask about base rates: How many games has your team won over the last few years? Perhaps the team has won 90% overall. In that case, your socks are actually a jinx (also see **Table 12.2**).

Despite the importance of base rates, people often ignore them. In a classic study, Kahneman and Tversky (1973) asked participants this question: If someone is chosen at random from a group of 70 lawyers and 30 engineers, what is his profession likely to be? Participants understood perfectly well that in this setting the probability of the person being a lawyer is .70. Hence, people can use base-rate information sensibly.

TABLE 12.2 THE IMPORTANCE OF BASE RATES: AN EXAMPLE

DO LEECHES CURE FEVER?

	Fever cured	Fever not cured
Patients treated with leeches	195	105
Patients not treated with leeches	130	70

Years ago, physicians believed that attaching leeches to the body would cure fever. Here, we've provided some *fictitious data* to illustrate why many people believed this claim—and also why the claim is *false*. Notice that in these data, 195 people treated with leeches were cured. If we focus on just these cases, we might decide that leeches are effective ("I know a man who . . ."). In addition, among people treated this way, two thirds (roughly 200 out of 300) were cured. If we focused on this fact, we might again be impressed with leeches' efficacy. We draw the opposite (and correct) conclusion, though, when we consider the base rate: The overall cure rate in these data is also two thirds, so your chances of cure are the same with leeches or without. Can you think of modern examples of bogus cures that show the same data pattern?

Other participants were given a similar task, but they were given the same base rates *and also* brief descriptions of certain individuals. Based on this information, they were asked whether each individual was more likely to be a lawyer or an engineer. Some of the descriptions had been crafted (based on common stereotypes) to suggest that the person was a lawyer; some suggested engineer; some were relatively neutral.

Participants understand the value of these descriptions and—as we've just seen—also seem to understand the value of base rates: They're responsive to base-rate information if this is the only information they have. When given both types of information, therefore, we should expect that the participants will combine these inputs as well as they can. If both the base rate and the diagnostic information favor the lawyer response, participants should offer this response with confidence. If the base rate indicates one response and the diagnostic information the other response, participants should temper their estimates accordingly.

However, this is not what participants did. When provided with both types of information, participants relied only on the descriptive information about the individual. Indeed, they responded the same way if the base rates were as already described (70 lawyers, 30 engineers) or if the base rates were reversed (30 lawyers, 70 engineers). This reversal had no impact on participants' judgments, confirming that they were indeed ignoring the base rates.

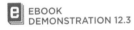
EBOOK
DEMONSTRATION 12.3

What produces this neglect of base rates? The answer, in part, is attribute substitution. When asked whether a particular person—Tom, let's say—is a lawyer or an engineer, people seem to turn this question about category membership into a question about resemblance. (In other words, they rely on the representativeness heuristic.) Thus, to ask whether Tom *is* a lawyer, they ask themselves how much Tom *resembles* (their idea of) a lawyer. This substitution is (as we've discussed) often helpful, but the strategy provides no role for base rates—and this guarantees that people will routinely ignore base rates. Consistent with this claim, base-rate neglect is indeed widespread and can be observed both in laboratory tasks and in many real-world judgments (Dawes, 1988; Griffin et al., 2012; Klayman & Brown, 1993; Pennycook, Trippas, Handley, & Thompson, 2014).

Dual-Process Models

We seem to be painting a grim portrait of human judgment. There are several sources of error, and even experts make the errors—for example, skilled financial managers making claims about investments (e.g., Hilton, 2003; Kahneman, 2011) and physicians diagnosing cancer (but ignoring base rates; Eddy, 1982; also see Koehler, Brenner, & Griffin, 2002). These errors occur even when people are doing their best to be careful. Indeed, in some studies participants have been offered substantial cash bonuses if they perform accurately. Even with these bonuses, errors are frequent (Arkes, 1991; Gilovich, 1991; Hertwig & Ortmann, 2003).

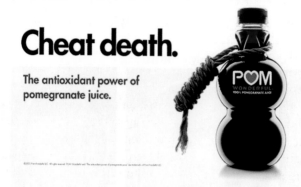

Cheat death.

The antioxidant power of pomegranate juice.

POM
WONDERFUL
100% POMEGRANATE JUICE

FTC Complaint Charges Deceptive Advertising by POM Wonderful

Agency Proceedings Will Determine Whether Health Claims for Products Pomegranate Are False and Not Supported by Scientific Evidence

As part of its ongoing efforts to uncover over-hyped health claims in food advertising, the Federal Trade Commission has issued an administrative complaint charging the makers of POM Wonderful 100% Pomegranate Juice and POMx supplements with making false and unsubstantiated claims that their products will prevent or treat heart disease, prostate cancer, and erectile dysfunction.

MIRACLE CURES?

People are remarkably ready to believe in a variety of "miracle cures," and advertisers are certainly ready to take advantage of these beliefs. One seller of pomegranate juice, for example, made extraordinary claims about the health benefit of its product . . . until the Federal Trade Commission stepped in. Because of the FTC ruling, POM is no longer allowed to make these (unsubstantiated) claims about its product's benefits.

Could it be, then, that human judgment is fundamentally flawed? If so, this might explain why people are so ready to believe in telepathy, astrology, and a variety of bogus cures (Gilovich, 1991; King & Koehler, 2000). Indeed, perhaps these points help us understand why warfare, racism, neglect of poverty, and environmental destruction are so widespread; perhaps these ills are the inevitable outcome of people's inability to understand facts and to draw decent conclusions.

Before we make these claims, however, let's acknowledge—and celebrate—another side to our story: Sometimes human judgment rises above the heuristics we've described so far. Thus, people often rely on availability in judging frequency, but sometimes they seek other (more accurate) bases for making their judgments (Oppenheimer, 2004; Schwarz, 1998; Winkielman & Schwarz, 2001). Likewise, people often rely on the representativeness heuristic, and so (among other concerns) they draw conclusions from "man who" stories. But in other settings people are keenly sensitive to sample size, and they draw no conclusions if their sample is small or possibly biased (e.g., Nisbett, Krantz, Jepson, & Kunda, 1983). How can we make sense of this mixed pattern?

Ways of Thinking: Type 1, Type 2

A number of authors have proposed that people have two distinct ways of thinking. One type of thinking is fast and easy; the heuristics we've described fall into this category. The other type is slower and more effortful, but also

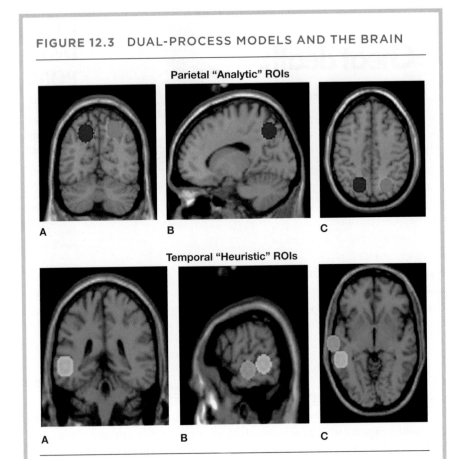

FIGURE 12.3 DUAL-PROCESS MODELS AND THE BRAIN

Parietal "Analytic" ROIs

A   B   C

Temporal "Heuristic" ROIs

A   B   C

Most dual-process models focus on the functioning of the two modes of thinking—How accurate are they? How fast? How much effort do they take? But we can also ask about the neural basis for these two modes of thinking. Here, the colored patches highlight "regions of interest" (ROIs) when participants were relying on Type 2 ("Analytic") thinking and when they were relying on Type 1 ("Heuristic") thinking.

more accurate, and when people rely on this type of thinking they're unlikely to make heuristic-based errors.

Researchers have offered various versions of this **dual-process** proposal (Evans, 2003, 2006, 2012a; Ferreira, Garcia-Marques, Sherman, & Sherman, 2006; Kahneman, 2011; Pretz, 2008; Shafir & LeBoeuf, 2002; for some concerns, though, about dual-process models, see De Neys, Vartanian, & Goel, 2008; Evans, 2008; Evans & Stanovich, 2013; Griffin et al., 2012; Keysers et al., 2008; Kruglanski & Orehek, 2007; Osman, 2004). The various models differ in their specifics and use different terminology. We'll rely, though, on rather neutral terms (initially proposed by Stanovich and West, 2000; Stanovich, 2012), so we'll use **Type 1** as the label for the fast, easy sort of thinking and **Type 2** as the label for the slower, more effortful thinking. (Also see **Figure 12.3**.)

When do people use Type 1, and when do they use Type 2? One hypothesis is that people *choose* when to rely on each system; presumably, they shift to the less efficient, more accurate Type 2 when making a judgment that really matters. As we've seen, however, people rely on Type 1's heuristics even when incentives are offered for accuracy, even when making important professional judgments, even when making medical diagnoses that may, in some cases, literally be matters of life and death. Surely people would choose to use Type 2 in these cases if they could, yet they still rely on Type 1 and fall into error. On these grounds, it's difficult to argue that using Type 2 is a matter of deliberate choice.

Instead, evidence suggests that Type 2 is likely to come into play only if triggered by certain cues and only if the circumstances are right. We've already suggested, for example, that Type 2 judgments are slower than Type 1, and on this basis it's not surprising that heuristic-based judgments (and, thus, heuristic-based *errors*) are more likely when judgments are made under time pressure (Finucane, Alhakami, Slovic, & Johnson, 2000). We've also said that Type 2 judgments require *effort*, so this form of thinking is more likely if the person can focus attention on the judgment being made (De Neys, 2006; Ferreira et al., 2006; Gilbert, 1989; for some complexity, though, see Chun & Kruglanski, 2006).

Sophisticated Type 1 Thinking

Factors like time pressure and focus, however, cannot be the whole story, because sometimes our fast "intuitive" judgments are quite accurate. Plainly, then, we cannot equate "Type 1 thinking" with "bad" or "sloppy thinking." (For an *endorsement* of Type 1 thinking and a celebration of "the power of thinking without thinking," see Gladwell, 2007. But for a reminder that Type 1 thinking often leads to error, see, among others, Ferreira et al., 2006.)

In fact, intuitive judgments can sometimes be quite sophisticated (e.g., Kahneman & Klein, 2009). For example, studies of skilled firefighters, anticipating how flames will spread through a building or judging the risk of the building collapsing, have shown that these professionals make judgments that are fast, apparently effortless, and quite accurate. The firefighters themselves often don't know how they've made their judgment—they say they looked at the fire and "just knew." Similar observations come from studies of nurses who are often able to look at a patient and detect life-threatening infections almost immediately (and well before blood tests were concluded).

What enables firefighters or nurses to make these swift, effortless judgments? Three factors seem to be crucial. First, these professionals are working in environments that contain informative cues that can in fact guide their judgments. Second, these professionals have had plenty of opportunity to observe these cues; third, they also get feedback when their initial assessment is mistaken. Over time, then, they learn to detect the relevant cues, so that they can recognize specific types of situation and react accordingly.

Triggers for Skilled Intuition

But it's not just skilled professionals who are capable of high-quality Type 1 thinking. This type of thinking is, in general, responsive to cues and triggers in the immediate environment, so Type 1 thinking can be quite sophisticated if the environment contains the "right sort" of triggers. Consider base-rate neglect. We have already said that people often ignore base rates—and, as a result, often misinterpret the evidence they encounter. But *sensitivity* to base rates can also be demonstrated, even in cases involving Type 1 thinking (cf. Pennycook et al., 2014). This mixed pattern is attributable, in part, to how the base rates are presented. Base-rate neglect is more likely if the relevant information is cast in terms of probabilities or proportions: "There is a .01 chance that people like Mary will have this disease"; "Only 5% of the people in this group are lawyers." But base-rate information can also be conveyed in terms of *frequencies*, and it turns out that people often use the base rates if they're conveyed in this way. Thus, people are more alert to a base rate phrased as "12 out of every 1,000 cases" than they are to the same information cast as a percentage (1.2%) or a probability (.012) (Gigerenzer & Hoffrage, 1995; also Brase, 2008; Cosmides & Tooby, 1996).

EBOOK
DEMONSTRATION 12.4

There is debate about why this "frequency format" is advantageous (Evans, Handley, Perham, Over, & Thompson, 2000; Fiedler, Brinkmann, Betsch, & Wild, 2000; Girotto & Gonzalez, 2001; Lewis & Keren, 1999; Mellers, Hertwig, & Kahneman, 2001), but there's no question that participants' performance in dealing with judgment problems is improved if the data are cast in this way. Much depends, therefore, on how the problem is presented, with some presentations being more "user friendly" than others.

Codable Data

Better-quality judgments (both more sophisticated Type 1 judgments and also the use of Type 2) are more likely if the role of *random chance* is conspicuous in a problem. If this role is salient, people are more likely to realize that the "evidence" they're considering may just be a fluke or an accident, not an indication of a reliable pattern. With this, people are more likely to pay attention to the *quantity* of evidence, on the (sensible) idea that a larger set of observations is less vulnerable to chance fluctuations. In one study, for example, participants were asked about someone who assessed a restaurant based on just one meal (Nisbett, Krantz, Jepson, & Kunda, 1983). The participants were more alert to considerations of sample size if the diner had chosen his entrée by blindly dropping a pencil onto the menu (presumably, because participants realized that a different sample, and perhaps different views of the restaurant, might have emerged if the pencil had fallen on a different selection). (Also see Baratgin & Noveck, 2000; Gigerenzer, 1991; Gigerenzer, Hell, & Blank, 1988; Tversky & Kahneman, 1982.)

Likewise, people are more accurate in their judgments, and less prone to heuristic use, when confronting evidence that is easily understood in statistical terms (Holland, Holyoak, Nisbett, & Thagard, 1986; Kunda & Nisbett, 1986). The suggestion here is that people do have some understanding of basic statistical concepts (e.g., the importance of sample size) but often don't realize these concepts are applicable to a judgment they're trying to make.

Thus, they might not realize that the evidence they're contemplating can be understood as a *sample of data* drawn from a larger set of potential observations. If they do have this insight, however, their judgment is improved.

For example, it's clear that an athlete's performance in a game's first quarter is just a sample of evidence and may or may not reflect his performance in other samples (other quarters or other games). It's also clear how to measure performance (via points or other sports statistics). For these reasons, the evidence is already "packaged" in a way that leads people to think in statistically sophisticated terms, and this explains why people are better at judging covariation—and more likely to be sensitive to the size of the sample of evidence—when thinking about sports (Jepson, Krantz, & Nisbett, 1983) than when thinking about many other domains.

Education

The quality of our thinking therefore depends on many factors—including the pattern of our experiences (think about those firefighters)—and also on how a problem is presented (probabilities vs. frequencies). Our thinking is also shaped by the background knowledge that we bring to a judgment (**Figure 12.4**; Nisbett et al., 1983).

In addition—and optimistically—the quality of thinking is influenced by *education*. For example, Fong, Krantz & Nisbett (1986) conducted a telephone survey of "opinions about sports," calling students who were taking an undergraduate course in statistics. Half of the students were contacted during the first week of the semester; half were contacted during the last week. There was no indication to the students that the telephone interview was connected to their course; as far as they knew, they had been selected entirely at random.

In their course, these students had learned about the importance of sample size. They'd been reminded that accidents do happen, but that accidents don't keep happening over and over. Therefore, a small sample of data might be the result of some accident, but a large sample probably isn't. Consequently, large samples are more reliable, more trustworthy, than small samples.

This classroom training had a broad impact. In the phone interview (which, again, was—as far as the students knew—unconnected to their course), one of the questions involved a comparison between how well a baseball player did in his first year and how well he did in the remainder of his career. This is, in effect, a question about sample size (with the first year being just a sample of the player's overall performance). Did the students realize that sample size was relevant here? For those contacted early in the term, only 16% gave answers that showed any consideration of sample size. For those contacted later, the number of answers influenced by sample size more than doubled (to 37%). The quality of the answers also increased, with students being more likely to articulate the relevant principles correctly at the end of the semester than at the beginning.

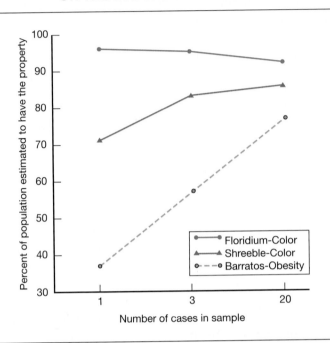

FIGURE 12.4 THE IMPACT OF SAMPLE SIZE DEPENDS ON THE JUDGMENT DOMAN

Participants were told that they were visitors to an island and that they had viewed one native (from the Barratos tribe) and had observed that he was obese. They were then asked how likely they thought it was that all Barratos were obese. Other participants were asked whether they would draw a conclusion after seeing *three* Barratos, or *twenty*. Participants were also asked whether they would draw conclusions after observing one Shreeble (a type of bird on the island) or three, or twenty. Participants were likewise asked whether they would draw conclusions after observing samples of a new mineral, Floridium. The data show that participants' willingness to draw conclusions depended heavily on the category—presumably, because participants were guided by background knowledge that samples of minerals tend to resemble one another; individual birds, however, can differ from one another; and certainly, tribal members can differ from one another. Hence, with the more diverse groups, participants insisted on gaining more evidence before drawing any conclusions.   AFTER NISBETT, KRANTZ, JEPSON, & KUNDA, 1983.

It seems, then, that how well people think about evidence can be improved, and that the improvement applies to problems in new domains and in new contexts. (Also see **Figure 12.5;** Fong & Nisbett, 1991.) Training in statistics, it appears, can have widespread benefits. (For more on education effects, see Ferreira et al., 2006; Gigerenzer, Gaissmaier, Kurz-Milcke, Schwartz, & Woloshin, 2008; Lehman & Nisbett, 1990; Schunn & Anderson, 1999.)

FIGURE 12.5   THE IMPACT OF STATISTICAL TRAINING

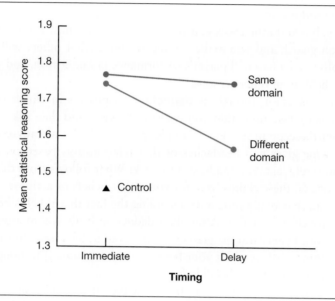

Participants were given brief training in statistics and then were tested later to see if they could apply this new training to new problems. The benefit of training was greater if the new problems came from the same domain as the original problems (thus, students trained with sports problems did better if later tested with sports problems). The benefit was also greater if participants were tested immediately, rather than at a delay. What is most important, though—and quite encouraging—is that the benefit of training (relative to a control condition, which involved no training) emerged even with a delay and a shift in domain. Participants were plainly able to use (and generalize from) what they had learned!   AFTER FONG & NISBETT, 1991.

We close this section, then, on an optimistic note, because we've now considered multiple factors that can improve the quality of someone's thinking. We can change features of the environment (e.g., recasting numbers as frequencies rather than proportions), so that we design what one paper calls "environments that make us smart" (Todd & Gigerenzer, 2007). And, it seems, *training* can improve judgment and so, for example, education helps you to see that an athlete's rookie year, or a brief interview, should be thought of as a small sample of data and perhaps trusted less than other sources of information based on a larger sample of evidence.

Of course, no one has uncovered a means of eliminating judgment errors, nor is there a way to guarantee the triumph of Type 2 thinking. But we do know how to decrease the danger of someone making the errors we've catalogued so far.

Confirmation and Disconfirmation

So far in this chapter, we've been looking at judgments that fall within the domain of **induction**—the process through which you make forecasts about new cases, based on the cases you've observed so far. Thus, you've observed one prison guard, and you make a forecast about what others will be like. You've observed a baseball player's performance in one season, and you predict how he'll do in other seasons.

Just as important, though, is **deduction**—a process in which you start with claims or assertions that you count as "given" and then ask what follows from these premises. For example, perhaps you're already convinced that red wine gives you headaches or that relationships based on physical attraction rarely last. You might want to ask: What follows from this? What implications do these claims have for your other beliefs or actions?

Deduction has many functions, including the fact that it helps keep your beliefs in touch with reality. After all, if deduction leads you to a prediction based on your beliefs and the prediction turns out to be *wrong*, this indicates that something is off track in your beliefs—so that claims you thought were solidly established aren't so solid after all.

Does human reasoning respect this principle? If you encounter evidence confirming your beliefs, does this strengthen your convictions? If evidence challenging your beliefs should come your way, do you adjust?

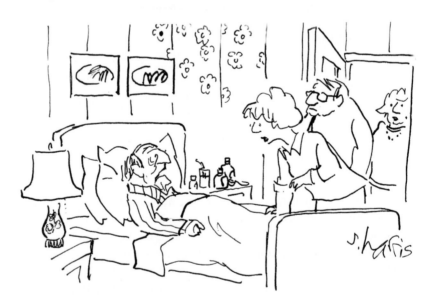

"MY PARENTS DIED. THEIR PARENTS DIED. THEIR PARENTS DIED... IT RUNS IN THE FAMILY."

DRAWING CONCLUSIONS FROM EVIDENCE

We rely on induction in many settings. Sometimes we misread the pattern. Sometimes we detect the pattern but draw the wrong conclusions.

Confirmation Bias

It seems sensible that in evaluating any belief, you'd want to take a balanced approach—considering evidence that supports your belief, and weighing that information against other evidence that might challenge the belief. And, in fact, the latter type of evidence (evidence that challenges you) is especially valuable; many authors argue that this type evidence is more informative than evidence that seems to support you. (For the classic statement of this position, see Popper, 1934.)

There's a substantial gap, however, between these suggestions about what people *should* do in evaluating their beliefs and what they actually do. Specifically, people routinely display a pattern we've already mentioned, *confirmation bias*: a greater sensitivity to confirming evidence and a tendency to neglect disconfirming evidence. Let's be clear, however, that this is an "umbrella" term, because confirmation bias can take many different forms (see **Figure 12.6**). What all the forms have in common, though, is the capacity to protect your beliefs from challenge (see, among others, Bilalic´, McLeod, & Gobet, 2010; Evans, 1982; Gilovich, 1991; Kassin, Bogart, & Kerner, 2012; Schulz-Hardt, Frey, Lüthgens, & Moscovici, 2000; Stangor & McMillan, 1992).

FIGURE 12.6   CONFIRMATION BIAS

Confirmation bias takes many forms:

- First, when people are assessing a belief or a hypothesis, they're more likely to seek evidence that might confirm the belief than evidence that might disconfirm it.

- Second, when disconfirming evidence is made available to them, people often fail to use it in adjusting their beliefs.

- Third, when people encounter confirming evidence, they take it at face value; when they encounter disconfirming evidence, they reinterpret the evidence to diminish its impact.

- Fourth, people often show better memory for confirming evidence than for disconfirming evidence, and, if they do recall the latter, they remember it in a distorted form that robs the evidence of its force.

- Finally, people often fail to consider alternative hypotheses that might explain the available data just as well as their current hypothesis does.

"Confirmation bias" is a blanket term that refers to many specific effects: We've listed some of these effects here. Confirmation bias is often a *good thing*; it helps you to maintain stability in your understanding of the world, and it often leads you to overrule evidence that should, in fact, be overruled. (For example, if someone told you she saw a unicorn yesterday, would you believe her?) But confirmation bias can also create many problems.

In an early demonstration of confirmation bias, Wason (1966, 1968) presented research participants with a series of numbers, such as "2, 4, 6." The participants were told that this trio of numbers conformed to a specific rule, and their task was to figure out what the rule was. Participants were allowed to propose their own trios of numbers ("Does '8, 10, 12' follow the rule?"), and in each case the experimenter responded appropriately ("Yes, it does follow the rule" or "No, it doesn't"). Then, once participants were satisfied that they had discovered the rule, they announced their "discovery."

The rule was, in fact, quite simple: The three numbers had to be in ascending order. Thus, "1, 3, 5" follows the rule, but "6, 4, 2" does not, and neither does "10, 10, 10." Despite this simplicity, participants had difficulty discovering the rule, often requiring many minutes. This was largely due to the type of information they requested as they sought to evaluate their hypotheses: To an overwhelming extent, they sought to *confirm* the rules they had proposed; requests for disconfirmation were relatively rare. And, we should note, those few participants who did seek out disconfirmation for their hypotheses were more likely to discover the rule. It seems, then, that confirmation bias was strongly present in this experiment, and it interfered with performance. (For related data, see Mahoney & DeMonbreun, 1978; Mitroff, 1981; Mynatt, Doherty, & Tweney, 1977, 1978.)

Reinterpreting Disconfirming Evidence

It's also the case that when people encounter confirmation for their beliefs, they're likely to take it at face value. When they encounter disconfirming evidence, they're often skeptical about it and scrutinize this new evidence, seeking flaws or ambiguities.

As an illustration, one study examined gamblers who bet on professional football games (Gilovich, 1983; also Gilovich & Douglas, 1986). These people all believed they had good strategies for picking winning teams, and their faith in these strategies was undiminished by a series of losses. Why is this? It's because the gamblers didn't remember their losses as "losses." Instead, they remembered them as flukes or oddball coincidences: "I was right. New York was going to win if it hadn't been for that crazy injury to their running back"; "I was correct in picking St. Louis. They would have won except for that goofy bounce the ball took after the kickoff." In this way, winning bets were remembered as wins, but losing bets were remembered as "near wins" (Gilovich, 1991). No wonder, then, that the gamblers maintained their views despite the (seemingly) contrary evidence provided by their own empty wallets.

Belief Perseverance

Even when disconfirming evidence is undeniable, people sometimes don't use it, leading to a phenomenon called **belief perseverance**. Participants in one study were asked to read a series of suicide notes; their task was to figure out which notes were authentic, collected by the police, and which were fake, written by other students as an exercise. As participants offered their judgments, they received feedback about how well they were doing—that is, how accurate they were in detecting the authentic notes. The trick, though, was that the feedback was predetermined and had nothing to do with the participants' actual judgments. By prearrangement, some participants were told that they were performing at a level well above average in this task; other participants were told the opposite—that they were performing far below average (Ross, Lepper, & Hubbard, 1975; also Ross & Anderson, 1982).

Later on, participants were debriefed. They were told that the feedback they had received was bogus and had nothing to do with their performance. Indeed, they were shown the experimenter's instruction sheet, which had assigned them in advance to the *success* or *failure* group. They were then asked a variety of additional questions, including some for which they had to assess their own "social sensitivity." Specifically, they were asked to rate their actual ability, as they perceived it, in tasks like the suicide-note task.

Let's emphasize that participants were making these judgments about themselves after they'd been told explicitly that the feedback they'd received was randomly determined and had no credibility whatsoever. Nonetheless, participants were influenced by the feedback: Those who had received the "above average" feedback continued to think of their social sensitivity as being above average, and likewise their ability to judge suicide notes. Those who had received the "below average" feedback showed the opposite pattern. All participants, in other words, persevered in their beliefs even when the basis for the belief had been completely discredited.

What was going on here? Imagine yourself as one of the participants, and let's say that we've told you that you're performing rather poorly at the suicide-note task. As you digest this new "information" about yourself, you'll probably wonder, "Could this be true? Am I less sensitive than I think I am?" To check on this possibility, you might search through your memory, looking for evidence that will help you evaluate this suggestion.

What sort of evidence will you seek? This is where confirmation bias comes into play. Because of this bias, chances are good that you'll check on the researcher's information by seeking other facts or other episodes in your memory that might confirm your lack of social perception. As a result, you'll soon have two sources of evidence for your social insensitivity: the (bogus) feedback provided by the researcher, and the supporting information you came up with yourself, thanks to your (selective) memory search. Thus, even if the researcher discredits the information he provided, you still have the information you provided, and on this basis you might maintain your belief. (For discussion, see Nisbett & Ross, 1980; also Johnson & Seifert, 1994.)

Of course, in this experiment, participants could be led either to an enhanced estimate of their own social sensitivity or to a diminished estimate, depending on which false information they were given in the first place.

Presumably, this is because the range of episodes in participants' memories is rather wide: In some previous episodes they've been sensitive, and in some they haven't been. Therefore, if they search through their memories seeking to confirm the hypothesis that they've been sensitive in the past, they will find confirming evidence. If they search through memory seeking to confirm the opposite hypothesis, this too will be possible. In short, they can confirm either hypothesis via a suitably selective memory search. This outcome highlights the dangers built into a selective search of the evidence and, more broadly, the danger associated with confirmation bias.

Logic

In displaying confirmation bias, people sometimes seem to defy logic. "If my gambling strategy is good, then I'll win my next bet. But I lose the bet. Therefore, my strategy is good." How widespread a pattern is this? In general, do people understand—and, better, *follow*—the rules of *logic*?

Reasoning about Syllogisms

A number of theorists have proposed that human thought is governed by the rules of logic, and so, if people make reasoning errors, the problem must lie elsewhere: carelessness, perhaps, or a misinterpretation of the problem (Boole, 1854; Henle, 1962, 1978; Mill, 1874; Piaget, 1952). It turns out, however, that errors in logical reasoning are ubiquitous. If people are careless or misread problems, they do so with great frequency. This is evident, for example, in studies using **categorical syllogisms**—a type of logical argument that begins with two assertions (the problem's **premises**), each containing a statement about a category, as shown in **Figure 12.7**. The syllogism can then be completed with a conclusion that may or may not follow from these premises. The cases shown in the figure are all **valid syllogisms**—that is,

FIGURE 12.7 EXAMPLES OF CATEGORICAL SYLLOGISMS

All of the syllogisms shown here are valid; that is, if the two premises are true, then the conclusion must be true.

All M are B.
All D are M.
    Therefore, all D are B.

All X are Y.
Some A are X.
    Therefore, some A are Y.

Some A are not B.
All A are G.
    Therefore, some G are not B.

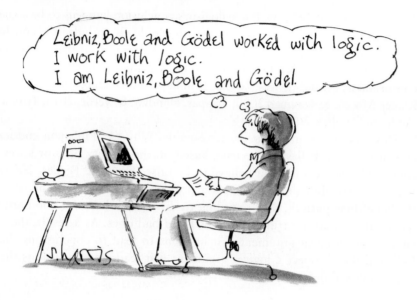

HOW LOGICAL ARE WE?

Errors in logic are extraordinarily common—in adults and in children, and even when we are contemplating very simple logical arguments.

the conclusion *does* follow from the premises stated. In contrast, here is an example of an **invalid syllogism**:

All P are M.

All S are M.

Therefore, all S are P.

To see that this is invalid, try translating it into concrete terms, such as "All plumbers are mortal" and "All sadists are mortal." Both of these are surely true, but it doesn't follow from this that "All sadists are plumbers."

Research participants who are asked to reason about syllogisms do remarkably poorly—a fact that has been clear in the research for many years. Chapman and Chapman (1959), for example, gave their participants a number of syllogisms, including the one just discussed, with premises of "All P are M," and "All S are M." The vast majority of participants, 81%, endorsed the invalid conclusion "All S are P." Another 10% endorsed other invalid conclusions; only 9% got this problem right. Other studies, with other problems, yield similar data—with error rates regularly as high as 70% to 90%. (Khlemani & Johnson-Laird, 2012, provide a review.)

Belief Bias

Errors in logical reasoning are also quite *systematic* and so don't look at all like the product of mere carelessness. For example, people often show a pattern dubbed **belief bias:** If a syllogism's conclusion happens to be something people believe to be true anyhow, they're likely to judge the conclusion as following logically from the premises. Conversely, if the conclusion happens to be something they believe to be false, they're likely to reject the conclusion as invalid (Evans, 2012b; Handley, Newstead, & Trippas, 2011; Klauer, Musch, & Naumer, 2000; Trippas, Handley, & Verde, 2013; Trippas, Verde, & Handley, 2014).

This strategy at first appears reasonable. Why wouldn't you endorse conclusions you believe to be true, based on the totality of your knowledge, and reject claims you believe to be false (Evans & Feeney, 2004)? Let's be clear, though, that there's a problem here: When people show the belief-bias pattern, they're failing to distinguish between good arguments (those that are truly persuasive) and bad ones. As a result, they'll endorse an illogical argument if it happens to lead to conclusions they like, and they'll reject a logical argument if it leads to conclusions they have doubts about.

FIGURE 12.8   ERRORS IN LOGIC

Affirming the consequent
(1)   If A is true, then B is true.
        B is true.
        Therefore, A is true.

Denying the antecedent
(2)   If A is true, then B is true.
        A is not true.
        Therefore, B is not true.

Many people accept these arguments as valid, but they are not. To see this, consider some concrete cases:

(3)   If the object in my hand is a frog, then the object is green.
        The object in my hand is green.
        Therefore, it is a frog.
(4)   If the object in my hand is a frog, then the object is green.
        The object in my hand is not a frog.
        Therefore, it is not green.

People commonly make the errors called "affirming the consequent" and "denying the antecedent." However, a moment's reflection, guided by a concrete case, makes it clear that reasoning in these patterns is, in fact, incorrect.

The Four-Card Task

Similar conclusions derive from research on a different aspect of logic: reasoning about **conditional statements**. These are statements of the familiar "If X, then Y" format, with the first statement providing a *condition* under which the second statement is guaranteed to be true.

Overall, reasoning about conditionals is quite poor, with error rates again as high as 80% or 90% (Evans, 1982; Evans, Newstead, & Byrne, 1993; Rips, 1990; Wason & Johnson-Laird, 1972; see **Figure 12.8**). And here, too, belief bias plays a role: People will endorse a conclusion if they happen to believe it to be true, even if the conclusion doesn't follow from the stated premises. Conversely, people will reject a conclusion if they happen to believe it to be false, even if the premises logically lead to the conclusion.

Often, psychologists study conditional reasoning directly: "If Q is true, then R is true. R is not true. What follows from this?" More commonly, though, researchers have turned to the **selection task** (sometimes called the **four-card task**). In this task, participants are shown four playing cards, as in **Figure 12.9**

FIGURE 12.9   THE FOUR-CARD TASK

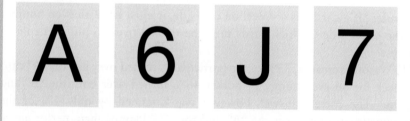

Which cards would you turn over to test this rule: "If a card has a vowel on one side, it must have an even number on the other side"? If we turn over the "A" card and find an even number, that's consistent with the rule. But if we turn it over and find an odd number, that's inconsistent. Therefore, by turning over the "A," we'll discover if this card is consistent with the rule or not. In other words, there's something to be learned by turning over this card. What about the "J"? The rule makes no claims about what is on the flip side of a consonant card, so no matter what we find on the other side, it will not challenge the rule. Therefore, there's nothing to be learned by turning over this card; we already know (without flipping the card over) that it's consistent with the rule. By similar reasoning, we'll learn nothing by turning over the "6"; no matter what we find, it satisfies the rule. Finally, if we turn over the "7" and a consonant is on the other side, this fits with the rule. If there's a vowel on the other side, this doesn't fit. Therefore, we do want to turn over this card, because there is a chance that we might find something informative.

FIGURE 12.10 AN EASIER VERSION OF THE FOUR-CARD TASK

DRINKING A BEER	22 YEARS OF AGE	DRINKING A COKE	16 YEARS OF AGE

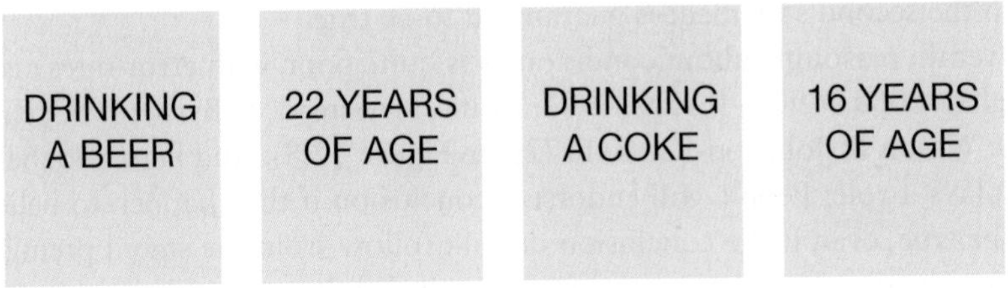

Participants do reasonably well with this version of the four-card task. Here, each card has a person's age on one side and what the person is drinking on the other side. The participants' task is to select the cards that one would have to turn over in order to test the following rule: "If a person is drinking beer, then the person must be over 21 years of age."

(after Wason, 1966, 1968). The participants are told that each card has a number on one side and a letter on the other. Their task is to evaluate this rule: "If a card has a vowel on one side, it must have an even number on the other side." Which cards must be turned over to put this rule to the test?

In Wason's research, 33% of the participants turned over just the "A" card to check for an even number. Another 46% turned over both the "A" and the "6." The correct answer, however, was obtained by only 4% of the participants—turning over the "A" and the "7." Plainly, then, performance is atrocious in this problem, with 96% of the participants giving wrong answers. (See the caption for Figure 12.9 for an explanation of why turning over the "A" and the "7" is the right answer.)

Performance is much better, though, with some variations of the four-card task. For example, Griggs and Cox (1982) asked their participants to test rules like this one: "If a person is drinking beer, then the person must be at least 21 years old." As in the other studies, participants were shown four cards and asked which cards they would need to turn over to test the rule (see **Figure 12.10**). In this version, participants did quite well: 73% (correctly) selected the card labeled "Drinking a beer" and also the card labeled "16 years of age." They did not select "Drinking a Coke" or "22 years of age."

It seems, then, that how *well* you think depends on what you're thinking about. The problems posed in Figures 12.9 and 12.10 have the same logical structure, but they yield very different performances. Researchers have offered a variety of explanations for this pattern, but so far the data don't allow us to choose which account is preferable. (For a hypothesis cast in terms of evolution, see Cosmides, 1989; Cummins, 2004; Cummins & Allen, 1998; Gigerenzer & Hug, 1992. For a hypothesis cast in terms of day-to-day learning, see Cheng & Holyoak, 1985; Cheng, Holyoak, Nisbett, & Oliver, 1986; Nisbett, 1993, also see **Figure 12.11**. For other options, see Almor & Sloman, 2000; Girotto, 2004; Oaksford & Chater, 1995; Polk & Newell, 1995; Sperber, Cara, & Girotto, 1995.)

Even with this unsettled issue, it's important to note the parallels between these points and our earlier discussion of how people make judgments about the evidence they encounter. In both domains (inductive judgments and deductive reasoning), it's easy to document errors in people's thinking. But in both domains we can also document higher-quality, more-sophisticated thinking. This more-sophisticated thinking seems to play a role, however, only in the "right" circumstances. When we were discussing judgment, we listed several factors that can trigger better thinking. In our discussion of logic, we've now seen that a problem's *content* can sometimes trigger more accurate reasoning. Thus, the quality of thinking is certainly uneven—but with the right triggers (and, it turns out, proper education), it can be improved.

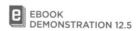

EBOOK
DEMONSTRATION 12.5

Decision Making

We turn now to a different type of thinking: the thinking that underlies *choices*. Choices, big and small, fill your life, whether you're choosing what courses to take next semester, which candidate to support in an election, or whether to stay with your current partner. How do you make any of these decisions?

Costs and Benefits

Each of us has our own values—things we like, things we prize, or conversely, things we hope to avoid. Likewise, each of us has a series of goals—things we hope to accomplish or things we hope to see. The obvious suggestion, then, is that we use these values and goals in making decisions. In choosing courses for next semester, for example, you'll choose classes that are interesting (something you value) and also those that help fill the requirements for your major (one of your goals). In choosing a medical treatment, you hope to avoid pain and you also hope to retain your physical capacities as long as possible.

To put this a bit more formally, each decision will have certain costs attached to it (consequences that will carry you farther from your goals) as well as benefits (consequences moving you toward your goals and providing you with things you value). In deciding, you weigh the costs against the benefits and seek a path that will minimize the former and maximize the latter. When you have several options, you choose the one that provides the best balance of benefits and costs.

Economists cast these ideas in terms of **utility maximization**. The word "utility" simply refers to the value that you place on a particular outcome—some people gain utility from eating in fancy restaurants; others gain utility from watching their savings accumulate in a bank account; other people gain utility from giving away their money to charity. No matter how you gain utility, though, the proposal is that you try to make decisions that will bring you as much utility as possible. (For discussion, see von Neumann & Morgenstern, 1947; also see Baron, 1988; Speekenbrink & Shanks, 2012.)

Framing of Outcomes

It's remarkably easy, however, to find cases in which decision making is not guided by the principle of utility maximization. Part of the reason is that we're all powerfully influenced by factors having nothing to do with utilities.

Consider the problem posed in **Figure 12.12**. In this choice, a huge majority of people—72%—choose Program A, selecting the sure bet rather than the gamble (Tversky & Kahneman, 1987; also Willemsen, Böckenholt, & Johnson, 2011). But now consider the problem in **Figure 12.13**. Here, an

FIGURE 12.12 THE ASIAN DISEASE PROBLEM: POSITIVE FRAME

Imagine that the United States is preparing for the outbreak of an unusual Asian disease, which is expected to kill 600 people. Two alternative programs to combat the disease have been proposed. Assume that the exact scientific estimates of the consequences of the programs are as follows:

If Program A is adopted, 200 people will be saved.

If Program B is adopted, there is a one-third probability that 600 people will be saved, and a two-thirds probability that no people will be saved.

Which program would you prefer? There is clearly no right answer to this question; one could defend selecting the "risky" choice (Program B) or the less-rewarding but less-risky choice (Program A). The clear majority of respondents, however, lean toward Program A, with 72% choosing it over Program B. Note that this problem is "positively" framed in terms of lives "saved."

FIGURE 12.13 THE ASIAN DISEASE PROBLEM: NEGATIVE FRAME

Imagine that the United States is preparing for the outbreak of an unusual Asian disease, which is expected to kill 600 people. Two alternative programs to combat the disease have been proposed. Assume that the exact scientific estimates of the consequences of the programs are as follows:

If Program A is adopted, 400 people will die.

If Program B is adopted, there is a one-third probability that nobody will die, and a two-thirds probability that 600 people will die.

Which program would you prefer? This problem is identical in content to the one shown in Figure 12.12: 400 dead out of 600 people is the same as 200 saved out of 600. Nonetheless, respondents react to the problem shown here rather differently than they do to the one in Figure 12.12. In the "lives saved" version, 72% choose Program A. In the "will die" version, 78% choose Program B. Thus, by changing the phrasing we reverse the pattern of respondents' preferences.

enormous majority—78%—choose Program B, this time preferring the gamble rather than the sure bet. The puzzle lies in the fact that the two problems are objectively identical: 200 people saved out of 600 is the same as 400 dead out of 600. Nonetheless, this change in how the problem is phrased—that is, the **frame** of the decision—has an enormous impact, turning a 3-to-1 preference (72% to 28%) in one direction into a 4-to-1 preference (78% to 22%) in the opposite direction.

Let's emphasize that there's nothing wrong with participants' individual choices. In either Figure 12.12 or Figure 12.13, there's no "right answer," and you can persuasively defend either the decision to avoid risk (by selecting Program A) or the decision to gamble (by choosing Program B). The problem lies in the contradiction created by choosing Program A in one context and Program B in the other context. Indeed, if a single participant is given both frames on slightly different occasions, the participant is quite likely to contradict himself. For that matter, if you wanted to manipulate someone's evaluation of these programs (e.g., if you wanted to manipulate voters or shoppers), then framing effects provide an effective way to do this.

Related effects are easy to demonstrate. Consider the two problems shown in **Figure 12.14.** When participants are given the first problem, almost three quarters of them (72%) choose Option A—the sure gain of $100. Participants contemplating the second problem generally choose Option B, with 64% going for this choice (Tversky & Kahneman, 1987). Note, though,

---

FIGURE 12.14   FRAMING EFFECTS IN MONETARY CHOICES

Problem 1

Assume yourself richer by $300 than you are today. You have to choose between:

A. a sure gain of $100

B. 50% chance to gain $200 and 50% chance to gain nothing

Problem 2

Assume yourself richer by $500 than you are today. You have to choose between:

A. a sure loss of $100

B. 50% chance to lose nothing and 50% chance to lose $200

These two problems are identical. In both cases, the first option leaves you with $400, while the second option leaves you with an even chance between $300 and $500. Despite this identity, respondents prefer the first option in Problem 1 (72% select this option) and the second option in Problem 2 (64% select this option). Once again, by changing the frames we reverse the pattern of preferences.

that the problems are once again identical. Both pose the question of whether you'd rather end up with a certain $400 or with an even chance of ending up with either $300 or $500. Despite this equivalence, participants treat these problems very differently, preferring the sure thing in one case and the gamble in the other.

In fact, there's a reliable pattern in these data. If the frame casts a choice in terms of *losses*, decision makers tend to be **risk seeking**—that is, they prefer to gamble, presumably because they hope to avoid or reduce the loss. (This pattern is especially strong when people contemplate *large* losses— see Harinck, Van Dijk, Van Beest, & Mersmann, 2007; also see LeBoeuf & Shafir, 2012; for an alternative view of framing, however, see Mandel, 2014.) Thus, when the Asian disease problem (for example) is cast in terms of lives lost, people choose Program B, apparently attracted by the (slim) possibility that with this program they may avoid the loss. Likewise, Problem 2 in Figure 12.14 casts the options in terms of financial losses, and this, too, triggers risk seeking: Here, people reliably choose the 50-50 gamble over the sure loss.

In contrast, if the frame casts the choice in terms of gains, decision makers tend to demonstrate **risk aversion**: They refuse to gamble, choosing instead to hold tight to what they already have. Thus, Figure 12.12 casts the Asian disease problem in terms of gains (the number of people saved), and this leads people to prefer the risk-free choice (Program A) over the gamble offered by Program B. (And likewise for Problem 1 in Figure 12.14.)

Again, let's emphasize that there's nothing wrong with either of these strategies by itself: If someone prefers to be risk seeking, this is fine; if someone prefers to be risk averse, this is okay too. The problem arises, though, when people flip-flop between these strategies, depending on how the problem is framed. The flip-flopping, in brief, leaves people wide open to manipulation, inconsistency, and self-contradiction.

Framing of Questions and Evidence

So far, we've considered changes in the way your *options* are framed. Related effects emerge with changes in how a *question* is framed. For example, imagine that you're on a jury in a messy divorce case; the parents are battling over who will get custody of their only child. The two parents have the attributes listed in **Figure 12.15**. To which parent will you award sole custody of the child?

Research participants who are asked this question tend to favor Parent B by a 64% to 36% margin. After all, this parent does have a close relationship with the child and has a good income. Note, though, that we asked to which parent you would *award* custody. Results are different if we ask participants to which parent they would *deny* custody. In this case, 55% of the participants choose to deny custody to Parent B (and so, by default, end up awarding custody to Parent A). Thus, the decision is simply reversed: With the "award" question, the majority of participants award custody to Parent B. With the

EBOOK DEMONSTRATION 12.6

FIGURE 12.15 THE INFLUENCE OF HOW A QUESTION IS FORMED

Imagine that you serve on the jury of an only-child sole-custody case following a relatively messy divorce. The facts of the case are complicated by ambiguous economic, social, and emotional considerations, and you decide to base your decision entirely on the following few observations. To which parent would you award sole custody of the child?

Parent A   average income
average health
average working hours
reasonable rapport with the child
relatively stable social life

Parent B   above-average income
very close relationship with the child
extremely active social life
lots of work-related travel
minor health problems

When asked the question shown here, 64% of the research participants decided to award sole custody to Parent B. Other participants, however, were asked a different question: "To which parent would you deny sole custody?" Asked this question, 55% of the participants chose to deny sole custody to Parent B (and so, by default, to award custody to Parent A). Thus, with the "award" question, a majority votes for granting custody to Parent B; with the "deny" question, a majority votes for granting custody to Parent A.

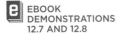

EBOOK DEMONSTRATIONS 12.7 AND 12.8

"deny" question, the majority deny custody to Parent B—and so give custody to Parent A. (Also see Downs & Shafir, 1999; Shafir, 1993.)

People are also influenced by how *evidence* is framed. Thus, they rate a basketball player more highly if the player has made 75% of his free throws, compared to their ratings of a player who has missed 25% of his free throws. They're more likely to endorse a medical treatment with a "50% success rate" than they are to endorse one with a "50% failure rate." And so on (Levin & Gaeth, 1988; Levin, Schnittjer, & Thee, 1988; also Dunning & Parpal, 1989).

None of this makes sense from the perspective of utility maximization, since these differences in framing should, on most accounts, have no impact on the expected utilities of the options. Yet these differences in framing can dramatically change people's choices. (For further, related evidence, see Lichtenstein & Slovic, 2006; Mellers, Chang, Birnbaum, & Ordóñez, 1992; Schneider, 1992; Schwarz, 1999.)

Maximizing Utility versus Seeing Reasons

In explaining these data, one possibility is that people are trying to use (something like) utility calculations when making decisions, but they aren't very good at it. As a result, they're pulled off track by various distractions, including how the decision is framed.

A different possibility, though, is more radical. Perhaps we're not guided by utilities at all. Instead, suppose our goal is simply to make decisions that we feel good about, decisions that we think are reasonable and justified. This view of decision making is called **reason-based choice**. To see how the account plays out, let's go back to the divorce/custody case just described. Half of the participants in this study were asked to which parent they would *award* custody. These participants therefore asked themselves: "What would justify giving custody to one parent or another?" and this drew their attention to each parent's positive traits. As a result, they were swayed by Parent B's above-average income and close relationship with the child. The other participants were asked to which parent they would *deny* custody, and this led them to ask: "What would justify this denial?" This approach drew attention to the parents' negative attributes—thus, Parent B's heavy travel schedule and health problems.

In both cases, then, the participants relied on *justification* in making their decision. As it turns out, though, the shift in framing caused a change in the factors relevant to that justification, and this is why the shift in framing reversed the pattern of decisions.

For a different example, consider a study in which medical doctors were asked how they would treat a particular patient. Half of the doctors were given a choice between surgery and one option for medication, and roughly half of them recommended surgery. Other doctors, though, were given the same two options plus one more choice—their options were surgery, the same medication as before, and a different option for medication. Now, with two choices for nonsurgical treatment (including the choice that many doctors preferred in the first scenario), most doctors chose neither. Specifically, the proportion of doctors opting for surgery jumped from 53% (in the first condition, with one nonsurgery choice) to roughly 75% in the condition with two nonsurgery choices (see **Figure 12.16**).

This outcome makes little sense from a utility perspective. The result is easy to understand, though, if we assume that the doctors are looking for reasons for their decisions. When only one medication is available, there may be persuasive arguments for using it. But when two medications are available, it's harder to find persuasive arguments for preferring one rather than the other—each drug has its advantages and disadvantages. And with no good reasons for choosing either one, the physicians choose neither—and send the patient off to the operating room. (For related data, see Hadar & Sood, 2014; Iyengar & Lepper, 2000; Schwartz, Chapman, & Brewer, 2004.)

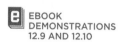

EBOOK
DEMONSTRATIONS
12.9 AND 12.10

Emotion

There's still another factor that needs to be included in our theorizing. For many people, the idea of *utility maximization* makes it sound like

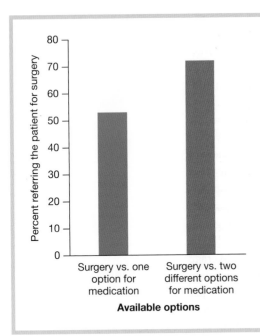

FIGURE 12.16   THE COST OF TOO MANY OPTIONS

Practicing physicians were given a description of a patient and were asked to choose a treatment. For one group of physicians, the choices offered were surgery and a specific medication. For a second group, the choices included surgery, the same medication, and a different medication. When doctors were choosing between one drug and surgery, many thought the drug was worth a try, and only 53% referred the patient for surgery. When the doctors had three choices, though, they found it difficult to justify choosing either drug over the other, and so most— 72%—opted for surgery instead. When the doctors couldn't justify one drug option over the other, they chose neither. AFTER REDELMEIER & SHAFIR, 1995.

their decisions are governed by calm and dispassionate calculations. To be sure, the assessment of utilities is a subjective matter, but once the utilities are "measured," the rest of the decision depends largely on arithmetic. Likewise, an emphasis on *reasons* seems to suggest that decision making is a cold, intellectual exercise. But despite these implications, it's clear that people's decisions are powerfully influenced by *emotion*. (See, among others, Kahneman, 2003; Loewenstein, Weber, Hsee, & Welch, 2001; Medin, Schwartz, Blok, & Birnbaum, 1999; Slovic, Finucane, Peters, & MacGregor, 2002; Weber & Johnson, 2009.)

The importance of emotion was in our view early in the chapter, when we saw that Elliot, unable to feel emotion, seems unable to make decisions. But what exactly is the linkage between emotion and decision making? At the chapter's start, we pointed out that many decisions involve an element of risk. (Should you try out a new, experimental drug? Should we rely more on nuclear power? Should you sign up for the new professor's course, even though you don't know much about her?) In cases like these, we suggested, people seem to assess the risk in emotional terms. Specifically, they ask themselves (for example) how much dread they experience when thinking about a nuclear accident, and they use that dread as an indicator of risk (Fischhoff, Slovic, & Lichtenstein, 1978; Slovic et al., 2002; also Pachur, Hertwig, & Steinmann, 2012).

At the chapter's start, we also mentioned another way in which emotion influences decisions. We know that *memories* can cause a strong bodily reaction. In remembering a scary movie, for example, you once again become tense and your palms might begin to sweat. In remembering a romantic encounter, you once again become aroused. In the same fashion, *anticipated events* can also produce bodily arousal, and Damasio (1994) suggests that you use these sensations—**somatic markers**, as he calls them—as a guide to decision making. In making a choice, he argues, you literally rely on your "gut feelings" to assess your various options, and this approach pulls you toward options associated with positive feelings and away from ones that trigger negative feelings.

Damasio argues, in addition, that a particular region of the brain—the orbitofrontal cortex (at the base of the frontal lobe, just behind your eyeballs)—is crucial in your use of these somatic markers, because it is this brain region that enables you to interpret your emotions. Evidence comes from patients who (like Elliot, whom we met earlier) have suffered damage to the orbitofrontal cortex. In one study, participants were required to choose cards from one stack or another; each card, when turned over, showed the amount of money the participant had won or lost on that trial. The cards in one stack often showed large payoffs, but sometimes they showed huge penalties; thus, overall, it was better to choose cards from the other stack (which had smaller payoffs but much smaller penalties).

Participants *without* orbitofrontal damage figured out this pattern as they worked their way through the task, so they ended up making most of their choices from the less risky stack (and thus earned more overall; see **Figure 12.17**). Participants *with* orbitofrontal damage, in contrast, continued (unwisely) to favor the risky deck. Because of their brain damage, they were unable to use the somatic markers normally associated with risk—so they failed to heed the "gut feeling" that could have warned them against a dangerous choice (Damasio, 1994; Naqvi, Shiv, & Bechara, 2006; also see Bechara, Damasio, Tranel, & Damasio, 2005; Coricelli, Dolan, & Sirigu, 2007; Dunn et al., 2010; Jones et al., 2012; Maia & McClelland, 2005).

Predicting Emotions

Emotion also plays another role in decision making, because many decisions depend on a *forecast* of future emotions. Thus, when people assess the risk associated with nuclear power, they seem to be asking themselves how they would react if, someday, there were a nuclear accident. Or, as a different example, imagine that you're choosing between two apartments that you might rent for next year. One is cheaper and larger but faces a noisy street. Will you just grow used to the noise, so that it ceases to bother you? If so, then you should take the apartment. Or will the noise grow more and more obnoxious to you as the weeks pass? If so, you should pay the extra money for the other apartment. Here, too, your decision depends on a prediction about the future—in this case, a prediction about how your likes and dislikes will change as time goes by.

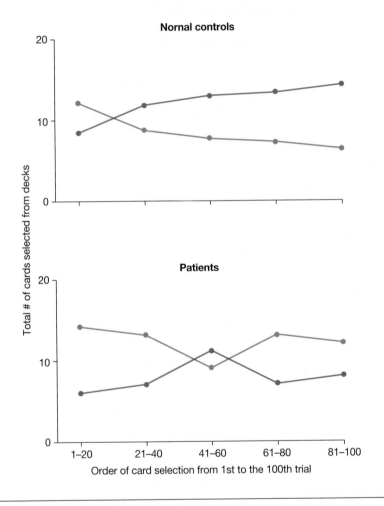

FIGURE 12.17 EMOTION AND DECISION MAKING

In this study, participants had to choose cards from one of two decks. One deck (the "disadvantageous" one) offered large payoffs but also large penalties; so, in the long run, it was better to choose from the other ("advantageous" deck), which provided smaller payoffs but also smaller penalties. "Normal control" participants—people with no brain damage—quickly learned about the decks, and were soon making most of their choices from the advantageous deck. Participants with brain damage, in contrast, continued making choices from the disadvantageous deck.

How accurate are people in making these predictions about their own feelings? Research suggests that this **affective forecasting**—the ability to predict one's own emotions—is in fact often inaccurate. For example, people tend to overestimate how much they'll regret their errors later (Gilbert, Morewedge, Risen, & Wilson, 2004), so they give more weight to "regret avoidance" than they should, since they're working to avoid something that, in the end, really won't be that bad.

People are also quite poor in predicting how they'll react to various life events. In various studies, people have been asked how they will feel after a significant event; the events at issue include "breaking up with a romantic partner, losing an election, receiving a gift, learning they have a serious illness, failure to secure a promotion, scoring well on an exam," and so on (Gilbert & Ebert, 2002, p. 503; Kermer, Driver-Linn, Wilson, & Gilbert, 2006; see also **Figure 12.18**). People can usually predict the "valence" of their reaction—that is, whether the reaction will be positive or negative—and so they realize that scoring well on an exam will make them feel good and that a romantic breakup will make them feel bad. But people consistently overestimate how long these feelings will last—apparently underestimating their ability to adjust to changes in fortune, and also underestimating how easily they'll find excuses and rationalizations for their own mistakes.

As a related matter, people generally believe that their *current* feelings will last longer than they actually will—so they seem to be convinced that things that bother them now will continue to bother them in the future, and that things that please them now will continue to bring pleasure in the future. In both directions, people underestimate their own ability to adapt; as a result, they work to avoid things that they'd soon get used to anyhow and spend money for things that provide only short-term pleasure.

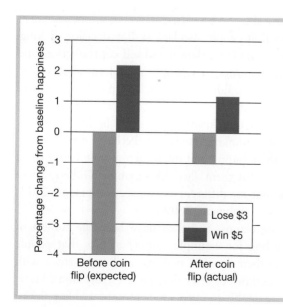

FIGURE 12.18 OVERPREDICTING EMOTIONS

People are often inaccurate in predicting their own emotions. Here, people sensibly predicted that they'd be unhappy if a gamble caused a $3 loss, but the sadness they actually experienced after the coin flip (right side) was much less than the sadness they'd predicted before the coin flip (left side). Likewise, people knew they'd be happy if they won $5, but the happiness they experienced was less than the happiness they'd predicted. AFTER KERMER ET AL., 2006, IN E. BRUCE GOLDSTEIN, 2011.

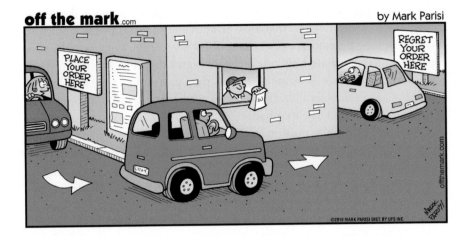

off the mark.com — by Mark Parisi

PLACE YOUR ORDER HERE

REGRET YOUR ORDER HERE

©2010 MARK PARISI DIST. BY UFS INC.

THE ROLE OF REGRET

In making decisions, people are powerfully motivated to avoid decisions they might regret later. It turns out, though, that when decisions work out badly, people generally experience far less regret over their choice than they'd anticipated.

(For glimpses of the data, see Hsee & Hastie, 2005; Kahneman & Snell, 1992; Loewenstein & Schkade, 1999; Sevdalis & Harvey, 2007; Wilson, Wheatley, Meyers, Gilbert, & Axsom, 2000. For some further complications regarding how people *remember* emotional experiences, see Chajut, Caspi, Chen, Hod & Ariely, 2014.)

Research on Happiness

Earlier in this chapter, we saw that people often make errors in judgment and reasoning. It now appears that people also lack skill in decision making. Framing effects leave them open to manipulation and self-contradiction, and errors in affective forecasting guarantee that people will often take steps to avoid regrets that in reality they wouldn't have felt, and pay for expensive toys that they'll soon lose interest in.

Some investigators draw strong conclusions from these findings. Perhaps people really are incompetent in making decisions. Perhaps people really don't know what will make them happy and might actually be better off if someone else made their choices for them. (See, for example, Gilbert, 2006; Hsee, Hastie, & Chen, 2008; but for different views, see Kahneman, 2011; Keys & Schwartz, 2007; Weber & Johnson, 2009.)

These are, of course, strong claims, and they have been the subject of considerable debate. One author, for example, simply asserts that people are "predictably irrational" in their decision making, and we're stuck with that (Ariely, 2009). Another author suggests that people truly don't know what's best for them, so they're unable to move efficiently toward happiness;

the best they can do is "stumble on happiness" (Gilbert, 2006). Yet another author notes that we all like to have choices but argues that having too many choices actually makes us less happy—a pattern he calls the "paradox of choice" (Schwartz, 2003).

Plainly, these are issues that demand scrutiny, with implications for how each of us lives and also, perhaps, implications that might guide government policies or business practices, helping people to become happy (Layrd, 2010; Thaler & Sunstein, 2009). Indeed, the broad study of "subjective well-being"—what it is, what promotes it—has become an active and exciting area of research. In this way, the study of *how* people make decisions has led to important questions—and, perhaps, some helpful answers—regarding how they *should* make decisions. In the meantime, the research certainly highlights some traps to avoid and suggests that each of us should be a bit more careful in making the choices that shape our lives.

COGNITIVE PSYCHOLOGY AND THE LAW

Confirmation Bias in Police Investigation

Overall, the police do a fine job in an extremely difficult task—apprehending criminals and keeping us all safe. But sometimes police investigations go off track, and we need to ask why this happens, with the obvious goal of helping the police do an even better job.

Police officers are human, and they work under considerable pressure with heavy caseloads and limited resources. Under these circumstances, it's inevitable that police will be vulnerable to the cognitive errors and illusions described in this chapter—and will, for example, be vulnerable to the pattern of confirmation bias. To see how this bias emerges, let's focus on confession evidence.

We're well served when people who are guilty of crimes confess what they have done. Their confessions ensure an efficient prosecution, helping us to achieve justice and promote public safety. But there's another side to this story, because sometimes it's innocent people who confess, and the power of confession evidence makes it likely that the innocent party will end up in jail and will simultaneously allow the actual perpetrator to escape punishment.

How often do false confessions occur? No one really knows, but one insight comes from the cases (mentioned in Chapter 8) of people who have been convicted in U.S. courts but then exonerated, years later, when DNA evidence finally showed that they were not guilty at all. Scrutiny of these cases indicates that roughly 25% of the exonerees had offered confessions—and since the DNA evidence tells us they were not guilty, we know these confessions were false.

Police understand these issues and certainly don't assume that every confession is truthful. Instead, they seek further evidence to corroborate (or, in some cases, undermine) a confession. The problem, though, is that this collection of further evidence can be biased by the confession itself. In other words, the confession can lead the police officer to believe a suspect is guilty and, at that point, confirmation bias enters the scene and can shape the subsequent investigation.

In one study, Kassin et al. (2012) examined all of the DNA exoneration cases that included a confession (again, the DNA evidence makes it clear that these confessions are false) and found that these cases tended to contain other errors as well. Specifically, these confession cases tended also to include invalid forensic evidence, mistaken eyewitness identifications, and false testimony from snitches or informants. Each of these types of errors was more common in the false-confession cases than in cases without confessions. And in a troubling discovery, the police records from these cases indicate that the confessions were obtained early in the investigation, before the other errors occurred. The suggestion, then, is that the false confessions may have encouraged these other errors.

Other studies show directly that hearing about a confession can influence the judgment of experienced fingerprint experts. Dror and Charlton (2006) presented six experts with pairs of fingerprints (one print from a

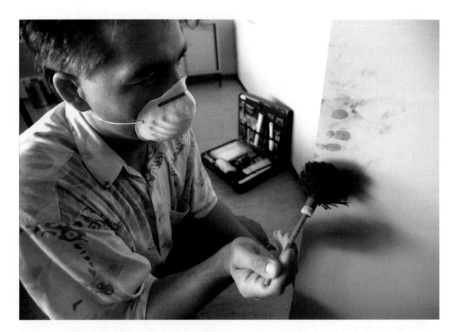

THE POWER OF CONFIRMATION BIAS

Fingerprint evidence is often persuasive to juries. The *interpretation* of this evidence, however, is tricky. Often, fingerprints at a crime scene are partial, or smudged, requiring a fingerprint expert to use some judgment in deciding whether the print "matches" the suspect's or not. Recent studies suggest, however, that these judgments can be swayed by various forms of bias, including confirmation bias.

crime scene, one from the suspect) and asked the experts whether the fingerprints in each pair were a "match." In some cases, the fingerprint examiners were told that the suspect had already confessed. This contextual information shouldn't have influenced the examiners' judgment (which should have depended only on the fingerprints themselves). Nonetheless, the examiners—carefully trained, experienced professionals—were more likely to "perceive" a match after they'd learned about the confession. In fact, they were likely to "perceive" a match even though they'd earlier seen the same fingerprints and decided the prints weren't a match.

Similar patterns have been observed with other forms of evidence. In a study by Hasel and Kassin (2009), witnesses were asked to identify a thief in a lineup. Once the witnesses had made their selection, they were sent home. Two days later, the witnesses were told that someone else in the lineup (not the person the witness had selected) had actually confessed. With this new information, almost two thirds of the witnesses abandoned their first selection and chose the confessor. ("Now that I think about it, I'm sure it was number 4, and not the person I chose two days ago.")

What should we do with these results? At the least, it seems important to get these findings into the view of the police, in the hope that they can somehow guard against this type of bias. It's also important to get these findings into a jury's view, with the goal of helping the jury interpret confession evidence. More broadly, these results provide a compelling indication of the power of confirmation bias—a form of bias that can even influence trained professionals and can certainly influence people making highly consequential judgments.

chapter summary

- Induction often relies on attribute substitution, so that (for example) people estimate frequency by relying on availability. Thus, they judge an observation to be frequent if they can easily think of many examples of that observation. The more available an observation is, the greater the frequency is judged to be.

- Judgments based on the availability heuristic are often accurate, but they do risk error. The risk derives from the fact that many factors influence availability, including the pattern of what is easily retrievable from memory, bias in what you notice in your experiences, and bias in what the media report.

- People also use the representativeness heuristic, relying on the assumption that categories are relatively homogeneous, so that any case drawn from the category will be representative of the entire group. Because of this assumption, people expect a relatively small sample of evidence to have all the properties that are associated with the entire category; one example of this is the gambler's fallacy. Similarly, people seem insensitive to the importance of sample size, so they believe that a small sample of observations is just as informative as a large sample. In the extreme, people are willing to draw conclusions from just a single observation, as in "man who" arguments.

- People are likely to make errors in judging covariation. In particular, their beliefs and expectations sometimes lead them to perceive illusory covariations. These errors have been demonstrated not just in novices working with unfamiliar materials but also in experts dealing with the sorts of highly familiar materials they encounter in their professional work. The errors are probably attributable to the fact that confirmation bias causes people to notice and remember a biased sample of the evidence, which leads to inaccurate covariation judgments.

● People often seem insensitive to base rates. Again, this can be demonstrated both in novices evaluating unfamiliar materials and in experts making judgments in their professional domains.

● Use of heuristics is widespread, and so are the corresponding errors. However, we can also find cases in which people rely on more-sophisticated judgment strategies, and thus are alert to sample size and sample bias, and do consider base rates. This has led many theorists to propose dual-process models of thinking. One process (Type 1) relies on fast, effortless shortcuts; another process (Type 2) is slower and more effortful but is less likely to lead to error.

● Type 1 thinking is more likely when people are pressed for time or distracted. However, Type 1 thinking can be observed even in the absence of time pressure or distraction, and even when the matter being judged is both familiar and highly consequential.

● Better quality thinking seems more likely when the data are described in terms of frequencies rather than probabilities and also when the data are easily coded in statistical terms (as a *sample* of data, with *chance* playing a role in shaping the sample). Type 2 thinking is also more likely if people bring to a situation background knowledge that helps them to code the data and to understand the cause-and-effect role of sample bias or base rates. Training in statistics also makes Type 2 thinking more likely, leading us to the optimistic view that judging is a *skill* that can be improved through suitable education.

● Reasoning often shows a pattern of confirmation bias. People tend to seek evidence that might confirm their beliefs rather than evidence that might challenge their beliefs. When evidence challenging a belief is in view, it tends to be underused or reinterpreted. One manifestation of confirmation bias is belief perseverance, a pattern in which people continue to believe a claim even after the basis for the claim has been thoroughly discredited. This probably occurs because people engage in a biased memory search, seeking to confirm the claim. The evidence provided by this search then remains even when the original basis for the claim is removed.

● People's performance with logic problems such as categorical syllogisms or problems involving conditional statements is often quite poor. The errors are not the product of carelessness but often derive from belief bias or a primitive matching strategy.

● How well people reason depends on what they are reasoning about. This is evident in the four-card task, in which some versions of the task yield reasonably good performance, even though other versions yield enormous numbers of errors.

● According to many economists, people make decisions by calculating the expected utility of each of their options. Evidence suggests, however, that decisions are often influenced by factors that have nothing to do with utilities—for example, how the question is framed or how the possible outcomes are described. If the outcomes are described as potential gains, decision makers tend to be risk averse; if outcomes are described as potential losses, decision makers tend to be risk seeking.

● Some investigators have proposed that people's goal in making decisions is not to maximize utility but, instead, to make decisions that they think are reasonable or justified. When people cannot justify a decision, they sometimes decide *not* to decide.

● Decisions are also clearly influenced by emotion. This influence is evident in decision makers' efforts toward avoiding regret; it is also evident in decision makers' reliance on their own bodily sensations as a cue for evaluating various options. Decision makers are surprisingly inept, however, at predicting their own future reactions. This is true both for predictions of regret and for predictions of future enjoyment or future annoyance.

ⓔ eBook Demonstrations & Essays

Online Demonstrations:
- Demonstration 12.1: Sample Size
- Demonstration 12.2: Relying on the Representativeness Heuristic
- Demonstration 12.3: Applying Base Rates
- Demonstration 12.4: Frequencies versus Percentages
- Demonstration 12.5: The Effect of Content on Reasoning
- Demonstration 12.6: Wealth versus Changes in Wealth
- Demonstration 12.7: Probabilities versus Decision Weights
- Demonstration 12.8: Framing Questions
- Demonstration 12.9: Mental Accounting
- Demonstration 12.10: Seeking Reasons

Online Applying Cognitive Psychology Essays:
- Cognitive Psychology and Education: Making People Smarter
- Cognitive Psychology and Education: The Doctrine of Formal Disciplines
- Cognitive Psychology and the Law: Pretrial Publicity

ＺＡＰＳ 2.0 Cognition Labs

- Go to **http://digital.wwnorton.com/cognition6** for the online labs relevant to this chapter.

13

Problem Solving and Intelligence

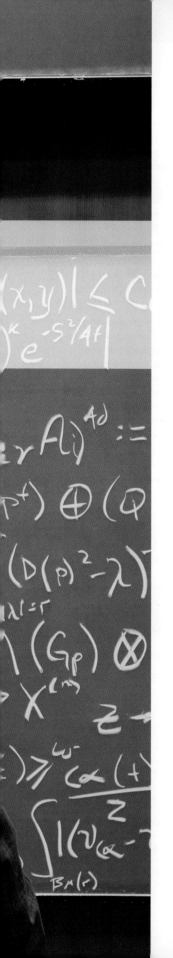

what if...

Which of your acquaintances do you consider really smart? Which of them do you think of as being relatively slow? Most people can easily answer these questions—and so apparently they have intuitions about who's more intelligent and who's less so. But how should we think about this? What does it mean to be "intelligent"?

Researchers have developed various tests for measuring intelligence, and as we will see, there are powerful reasons to take these tests seriously—they do measure something important. But people with very *low* scores often have amazing abilities, and a consideration of these individuals can provide insights into what intelligence is and when intelligence is needed.

Alonzo Clemons suffered a traumatic brain injury when he was a child, and test scores indicate that he has an IQ score of 40—way below the score of 70 often used as an indication of disability. But Clemons is considered by some people to be a "genius" as a sculptor. He swiftly produces incredibly accurate clay sculptures of animals—usually, animals he has seen only in books. With remarkable skill, he effortlessly transforms these two-dimensional depictions into perfect three-dimensional forms. (For more on cases like Clemons's, see Treffert, 2014.)

Stephen Wiltshire's IQ score has been measured at 52, but he also is a gifted artist and has a near-perfect visual memory. Stephen has been called the "Living Camera," and it's easy to see why: After a 30-minute helicopter ride over London, he was able to draw (entirely from memory) an exquisitely detailed aerial view of the city. He's done the same for Rome, New York City, and Tokyo. The resulting drawings (more than 15 feet across) take him days to complete, and, when carefully checked, the drawings turn out to be remarkably accurate, with a precise correspondence between his artwork and the actual view. Stephen creates an error-free reproduction of building positions and sizes, and even the correct number of windows shown in each building, the correct number of columns on each building's façade, and more.

preview of chapter themes

- Often, people solve problems by using general heuristics that help them narrow their search for the problem's solution. In other cases, people solve problems by drawing analogies based on problems they've solved in the past. As helpful as they are, however, analogies are often underused.

- Training can improve a person's skill in problem solving. The training can draw someone's attention to a problem's deep structure, which promotes analogy use. Training can also help someone see how a problem can be divided into subproblems. Experts consistently attend to a problem's deep structure and are quite sensitive to a problem's parts. Experts also benefit from their highly cross-referenced knowledge in their domain of expertise.

- Problem solving is often stymied by how people approach the problem in the first place, and that leads to a question of how people find new and creative approaches to problems.

- When closely examined, creative approaches seem to be the result of the same processes that are evident in "ordinary" problem solving—processes hinging on analogies, heuristics, and the like. Hence, the creative *product* is often extraordinary, but the creative *process* may not be.

- Measures of intelligence turn out to be both reliable and valid, and so, if we know someone's score on an intelligence test, we can predict that person's performance in a wide range of settings (both academic and otherwise). Thus, intelligence tests seem to be measuring a capacity that is associated with many important life outcomes.

- The data also suggest that we can truly speak of "intelligence-in-general"—intelligence that applies to a wide range of tasks. This general intelligence may be a result of mental speed and may be a result of better executive control, with some people being better able than others to control their own thoughts.

- We can easily demonstrate that genetic and environmental factors both matter for intelligence, but, crucially, these factors interact in producing a person's level of intelligence.

- There has been much discussion (and much debate) about how *groups* differ in their average level of performance. For example, American Whites and American Blacks differ in the average scores for each group, and at least part of the explanation lies in the inferior nutrition, inferior health care, and inferior education available to many American Blacks. In addition, social stereotypes play a large role in how individuals are trained and encouraged, as well as in the expectations individuals hold for their own performance.

People like Alonzo and Stephen are termed "autistic savants." This label refers to a condition in which someone with a mental disability nonetheless shows some remarkable talent. Perhaps the most famous autistic savant was Kim Peek (the inspiration for the Hollywood movie *Rain Man*). Kim had an extraordinary memory and could apparently read both pages of an open book at once and retain virtually all of what he had read. He could also do calendar calculations (What day of the week was December 19, 1401?), and he remembered a vast range of political and historical facts (including old baseball scores).

Scholars estimate that worldwide there are fewer than 100 autistic savants at this level of talent, and the achievements of these individuals remain deeply puzzling to science. We certainly do not know why one autistic savant becomes a sculptor, another becomes a calendar calculator, and other shows musical talent. Even with these mysteries in view, though, these cases are a powerful reminder that there can sometimes be a huge separation between being intelligent and having a specialized talent. In addition, let's emphasize that the talents shown by these savants are indeed specialized and so their disability becomes evident the moment we step away from their extraordinary gift. This point raises the possibility that one important benefit of intelligence may be the flexibility to perform a wide range of mental tasks and not to be limited to one talent (no matter how amazing that talent is). These are intriguing suggestions that we'll explore in this chapter.

Of Course, People Differ

In many ways, humans are remarkably alike. We all have two arms, one nose. We all have roughly the same biochemistry, and to a large extent we all have roughly the same brains, with the structures inside your skull being virtually identical to the ones inside mine. Perhaps it's no surprise, then, that throughout this book we've been able to discuss truths that apply to all of us—the ways in which we all pay attention, the ways in which we all learn and remember.

But people also differ—in their personalities, their values, and their cognition. We've occasionally mentioned these differences, but the time has come to focus on these differences more directly. In this chapter, we'll start with a skill that we all rely on every day: our ability to solve problems, large and small. We'll ask why some people are especially good problem solvers, and we'll look at some of the factors that can make someone an *expert* problem solver and also a *creative* problem solver. Then, we'll turn to the topic of intelligence. We all know people who seem amazingly smart and people we regard as slow. But what do these differences amount to? What is "intelligence"? Can it be measured? Can it be improved? We'll address all these questions before we're done.

General Problem-Solving Methods

People solve problems all the time. Some problems are pragmatic ("I want to go to the store, but Tom borrowed my car. How can I get there?"). Others are social ("I really want Amy to notice me; how should I arrange it?"). Others are academic ("I'm trying to prove this theorem. How can I do it, starting from these axioms?"). What all these situations share, though, is that in each case the person has a goal and is trying to figure out how to reach that goal—a configuration that defines what we call **problem solving**. How do people solve problems?

Problem Solving as Search

Researchers often compare problem solving to a process of *search*, as though you were navigating through a maze, seeking a path toward your goal (cf. Newell & Simon, 1972; also Bassok & Novick, 2012; Mayer, 2012). To make this point concrete, consider the Hobbits and Orcs problem in **Figure 13.1**. For this problem, you have choices for the various moves you can make (transporting creatures back and forth), but you also have two limits: the size of the boat and the requirement that Hobbits can never be outnumbered (lest they be eaten). This setup leaves you with a set of options shown graphically in **Figure 13.2**. More precisely, the figure shows the moves available early in the solution and depicts the options as a tree, with each step leading to more branches. All the branches together form the **problem space**—that is, the set of all states that can be reached in solving the problem.

To solve this problem, one strategy would be to trace through the entire problem space, exploring each branch in turn. This would be akin to exploring every possible corridor in a maze, an approach that would guarantee that you'd eventually find the solution. For most problems, however, this "brute force" approach would be hopeless. Consider, for example, the game of chess: In chess, which move is best at any point in the game depends in part on what your opponent will be able to do in response to your move, and then what you'll do next. To make sure you're choosing the best move, therefore, you need to think through a few cycles of play, so that you can select as your current move the one that leads to the best sequence.

Let's imagine, therefore, that you decide to look ahead just three cycles of play—three of your moves and three of your opponent's. Some quick

---

FIGURE 13.1 THE HOBBITS AND ORCS PROBLEM

Five Orcs and five Hobbits are on the east bank of the Muddy River. They need to cross to the west bank and have located a boat. In each crossing, at least one creature must be in the boat, but no more than three creatures will fit in the boat.

And, of course, if the Orcs ever outnumber the Hobbits in any location, they will eat the Hobbits! Therefore, in designing the crossing we must make certain that the Hobbits are never outnumbered, either on the east bank of the river or on the west.

How can the creatures get across without any Hobbits being eaten?

This problem has been used in many studies of problem-solving strategies. Can you solve it?

calculation, however, tells us that for three cycles of chess play there are roughly 700 million possibilities for how the game could go; this number immediately rules out the option of considering every possibility. If you could evaluate 10 sequences per second, you'd still need more than 2 years, on a 24/7 schedule, to evaluate the full set of options each time you wanted to select a move.

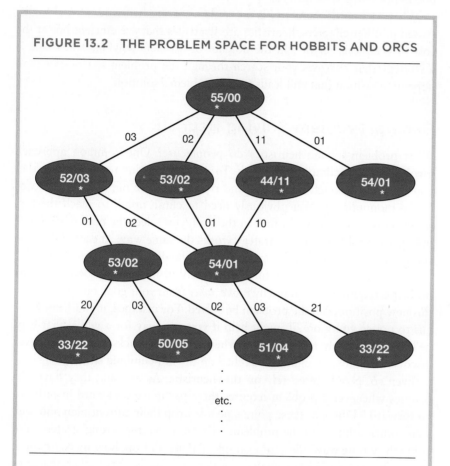

FIGURE 13.2 THE PROBLEM SPACE FOR HOBBITS AND ORCS

Each circle shows a possible problem state. The state 54/01, for example, indicates that five Hobbits and four Orcs are on the east bank; there are no Hobbits, but one Orc, on the west bank. The star shows the position of the boat. The numbers alongside each line indicate the number of creatures in the boat during each river crossing. The move 02, for example, transports no Hobbits, but two Orcs. The problem states shown here are all the legal states. (Other states and other moves would result in some of the Hobbits being eaten.) Thus, there are four "legal" moves one can make, starting from the initial state. From these, there are four possible moves one can make, but these lead to just two problem states (53/02 and 54/01). From these two states, there are four new states that can be reached, and so on. We have here illustrated the first three moves that can be made in solving this problem; the shortest path to the problem's solution involves 11 moves.

And, of course, there's nothing special here about chess, because most real-life problems offer so many options that you couldn't possibly explore every one.

Plainly, then, you somehow need to narrow your search through a problem space, but this involves an element of risk: If you don't consider every option, there's a chance you'll miss the *best* option. However, you have no choice about this, since the alternative—the strategy of considering each possibility—would be absurd.

What you need, therefore, is a problem-solving heuristic. As we've discussed in other chapters, heuristics are strategies that are efficient but at the cost of occasional errors. In the domain of problem solving, a heuristic is a strategy that narrows your search through the problem space—but (you hope) in a fashion that still leads to the problem's solution.

General Problem-Solving Heuristics

What problem-solving heuristics do people use? One common approach involves the **hill-climbing strategy**. To understand this term, imagine that you're hiking through the woods and trying to figure out which trail leads to the mountaintop. You obviously need to climb uphill to reach the top, so whenever you come to a fork in the trail, you select the path that's going uphill. The problem-solving strategy works the same way: At each point, you simply choose the option that moves you in the direction of your goal.

This strategy is often helpful but is surely of limited use, because many problems require that you briefly move *away* from your goal; only then, from this new position, can the problem be solved. For instance, if you want Mingus to notice you more, it might help if you go away for a while; that way, he'll be more likely to notice you when you come back. You would never discover this ploy, though, if you relied on the hill-climbing strategy.

Even so, people often rely on this heuristic. As a result, they have difficulties whenever a problem requires them to "move backward in order to go forward." Often, at these points, people drop their current plan and seek some other solution to the problem: "This must be the wrong strategy; I'm going the wrong way." (See, for example, Jeffries, Polson, Razran, & Atwood, 1977; Thomas, 1974.) Fortunately, though, people also have other heuristics available to them. For example, people often rely on **means-end analysis**. To use this strategy, you compare your current state to the goal state, and then you ask, "What means do I have to make these more alike?" **Figure 13.3** offers a commonsense example of how this strategy plays out.

Pictures and Diagrams

People also have other options in their mental toolkit. For example, it's often helpful to translate a problem into concrete terms, relying on a mental image or a picture. Indeed, the histories of science, art, and engineering are filled with instances in which great discoveries emerged in this way (Hegarty & Stull, 2012; Miller, 1986; Reed, 1993; Shepard, 1988).

FIGURE 13.3   EXAMPLE OF MEANS-END ANALYSIS

I want to take my son to nursery school. What's the difference between what I have and what I want? One of distance. What changes distance? My automobile. My automobile won't work. What is needed to make it work? A new battery. What has new batteries? An auto repair shop.

I want the repair shop to put in a new battery; but the shop doesn't know I need one. What is the difficulty? One of communication. What allows communication? A telephone . . .

People use a variety of heuristics to solve problems, but one common strategy is means-end analysis. To use this strategy, you compare your current status to your desired status and ask: "What means do I have to make these more alike?" Among its other benefits, this strategy helps you to break a problem into small subproblems.   NEWELL & SIMON, 1972, P. 416.

As a simple illustration, consider the problem described in **Figure 13.4**. Most people try an algebraic solution to this problem (width of each volume, multiplied by the number of volumes, divided by the worm's eating rate) and end up with the wrong answer. People generally get this problem right, though, if they start by visualizing the arrangement. Now, they can discern the actual positions of the worm's starting point and end point, and this

FIGURE 13.4   THE BOOKWORM PROBLEM

Solomon is proud of his 26-volume encyclopedia, placed neatly, with the volumes in alphabetical order, on his bookshelf. Solomon doesn't realize, though, that there's a bookworm sitting on the front cover of the *A* volume. The bookworm begins chewing his way through the pages on the shortest possible path toward the back cover of the *Z* volume.

Each volume is 3 inches thick (including pages and covers), so that the entire set of volumes requires 78 inches of bookshelf. The bookworm chews through the pages and covers at a steady rate of ¾ of an inch per month. How long will it take before the bookworm reaches the back cover of the *Z* volume?

People who try an algebraic solution to this problem often end up with the wrong answer.

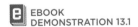

FIGURE 13.5 DIAGRAM FOR THE BOOKWORM PROBLEM

When the bookworm problem is illustrated, as shown here, people solve it more easily. Notice that a worm starting on the front cover of the *A* volume would not have to chew through volume *A*'s pages in moving toward the *Z* volume. Likewise, at the end of the worm's travel, he would reach the back cover of the *Z* volume before penetrating the *Z* volume!

usually takes them to the correct answer (see **Figure 13.5**; also see Anderson, 1993; Anderson & Helstrup, 1993; Reed, 1993; Reisberg, 2000; Verstijnen, Hennessey, van Leeuwen, Hamel, & Goldschmidt, 1998).

Drawing on Experience

Where do these points leave us with regard to the questions with which we began—and, in particular, the ways in which people differ from one another in their mental abilities? There's actually little difference from one person to the next in the use of strategies like hill climbing or means-end analysis—most people can and do use these strategies. People do differ, of course, in their drawing ability and in their imagery prowess (see Chapter 11), but these points are relevant only for some problems. Where, then, do the broader differences in problem-solving skill arise?

Problem Solving via Analogy

Often, a problem reminds you of other problems you've solved in the past, and so you can rely on your past experience in tackling the current challenge. In other words, you solve the current problem by means of an analogy with other, already solved, problems.

Analogies have certainly been helpful in the history of science—with scientists furthering their understanding of the heart by comparing it to a

EBOOK
DEMONSTRATION 13.1

pump, and extending their knowledge of gases by comparing molecules to billiard balls. Analogies are also useful in the classroom—with the atom being described to students as (roughly) resembling the solar system, or with memory being compared to a library (Donnelly & McDaniel, 1993; for more on the powerful effects of analogy use, see Chan, Paletz, & Schunn, 2012; Gentner & Smith, 2012; Holyoak, 2012).

What about ordinary problem solving? The tumor problem (see **Figure 13.6A**) is difficult, but people generally solve it if they're able to use an analogy. Gick and Holyoak (1980) first had their participants read about

FIGURE 13.6 THE TUMOR PROBLEM

Suppose you are a doctor faced with a patient who has a malignant tumor in his stomach. To operate on the patient is impossible, but unless the tumor is destroyed the patient will die. A kind of ray, at a sufficiently high intensity, can destroy the tumor. Unfortunately, at this intensity the healthy tissue that the rays pass through on the way to the tumor will also be destroyed. At lower intensities the rays are harmless to healthy tissue but will not affect the tumor. How can the rays be used to destroy the tumor without injuring the healthy tissue?

A

A dictator ruled a country from a strong fortress, and a rebel general, hoping to liberate the country, vowed to capture the fortress. The general knew that an attack by his entire army would capture the fortress, but he also knew that the dictator had planted mines on each of the many roads leading to the fortress. The mines were set so that small groups of soldiers could pass over them safely, since the dictator needed to move his own troops to and from the fortress. However, any large force would detonate the mines, blowing them up and also destroying the neighboring villages.

The general knew, therefore, that he couldn't just march his army up one of the roads to the fortress. Instead, he devised a simple plan. He divided his army into small groups and dispatched each group to the head of a different road. When all were ready, he gave the signal and each group marched up a different road to the fortress, with all the groups arriving at the fortress at the same time. In this way, the general captured the fortress and overthrew the dictator.

B

The tumor problem, designed by Duncker (1945) and presented in Panel A, has been studied extensively. Can you solve it? One solution is to aim multiple low-intensity rays at the tumor, each from a different angle. The rays will meet at the site of the tumor and so, at just that location, will sum to full strength. People are much more likely to solve this problem if encouraged to use the hint provided by the problem shown in Panel B.

a related situation (see Figure 13.6B) and then presented them with the tumor problem. When participants were encouraged to use this hint, 75% were able to solve the tumor problem. Without the hint, only 10% solved the problem.

However, despite the clear benefit of using analogies, people routinely fail to use them. Gick and Holyoak had another group of participants read the "general and fortress" story, but no further hints were given. In particular, these participants were not told that this story was relevant to the tumor problem. Only 30% of this group solved the tumor problem (see **Figure 13.7**). (Also see Hayes & Simon, 1977; Ross, 1984, 1987, 1989; Weisberg, DiCamillo, & Phillips, 1978.)

Apparently, then, people benefit from analogies if suitably instructed, but spontaneous, uninstructed use of analogies is surprisingly rare. One reason lies in how people search through memory when seeking an analogy. In solving a problem about tumors, people seem to ask themselves, "What else do I know

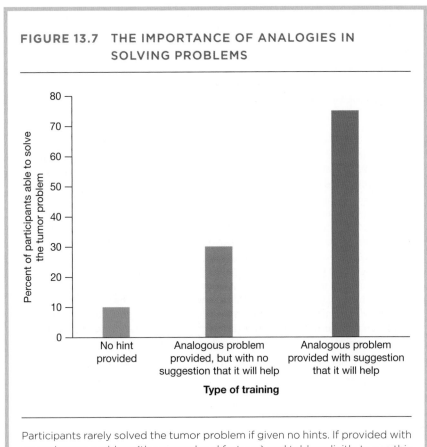

FIGURE 13.7   THE IMPORTANCE OF ANALOGIES IN SOLVING PROBLEMS

Participants rarely solved the tumor problem if given no hints. If provided with an analogous problem (the general and fortress) and told explicitly to use this problem as a guide, most solved the tumor problem. Surprisingly, though, participants often failed to make use of the analogy unless they were specifically encouraged to do so.   AFTER GICK & HOLYOAK, 1980.

about tumors?" This search will help them remember other situations in which they thought about tumors, but of course it won't lead them to the "general and fortress" problem (e.g., Bassok, 1996; Cummins, 1992; Hahn, Prat-Sala, Pothos, & Brumby, 2010; Wharton, Holyoak, Downing, & Lange, 1994). This (potential) analogue will therefore lie dormant in memory and provide no help.

Thus, to locate helpful analogies in memory, people often need to get beyond the superficial features of the problem and think instead about the principles governing the problem—focusing on what's sometimes called the problem's "deep structure" rather than its "surface structure." As a related point, people can use analogies only if they figure out how to map the prior case onto the problem now being solved—only if they realize, for example, that converging groups of soldiers correspond to converging rays and that a fortress-to-be-captured corresponds to a tumor-to-be-destroyed. This **mapping** process can be difficult (Holyoak, 2012), and failures to figure out the mapping are another reason that people regularly fail to find and use analogies.

Strategies to Make Analogy Use More Likely

Perhaps, then, we have our first suggestion about why people differ in their problem-solving ability. Perhaps the people who are better problem solvers are those who make better use of analogies—plausibly, because they pay attention to a problem's dynamic rather than its superficial traits, and this helps them both to find analogies and to master the mapping.

Consistent with these claims, it turns out that we can *improve* problem solving by encouraging people to pay attention to the problems' underlying dynamic. For example, Cummins (1992) instructed participants in one group to analyze a series of algebra problems one by one. Participants in a second group were asked to *compare* the problems to one another, describing what the problems had in common. The latter instruction forced participants to think about the problems' underlying structure; guided by this perspective, the participants were more likely, later on, to use the training problems as a basis for forming and using analogies.

Likewise, Needham and Begg (1991) presented participants with a series of training problems. Some participants were told that they'd need to recall the problems later and were encouraged to work at memorizing them. Other participants were encouraged to work at *understanding* each solution, so that they'd be able to explain it later to another person. When the time came for the test problems, participants in the second group were more likely to transfer what they'd learned earlier. As a result, those who had taken the "understand" approach were able to solve 90% of the test problems; participants who had taken the "memorize" approach solved only 69%. (For related data, see Catrambone, Craig, & Nersessian, 2006; Chen & Daehler, 2000; Kurtz & Loewenstein, 2007; Lane & Schooler, 2004; Pedrone, Hummel, & Holyoak, 2001.)

Expert Problem Solvers

How far can we go with these points? Can we use these simple ideas to explain the difference between ordinary problem solvers and genuine experts? To some extent, we can.

We've claimed, for example, that it's helpful to think about problems in terms of their deep structure, and this is, it seems, the way experts think about problems. In one study, participants were asked to categorize simple physics problems (Chi, Feltovich, & Glaser, 1981). Novices tended to place together all the problems involving river currents, all the problems involving springs, and so on, in each case focusing on the surface form of the problem, independent of what physical principles were needed to solve the problem. In contrast, experts (Ph.D. students in physics) ignored these details of the problems and, instead, sorted according to the physical principles relevant to the problems' solution. (For more on expertise, see Ericsson & Towne, 2012.)

We've also claimed that attention to a problem's structure promotes analogy use, so if experts are more attentive to this structure, they should be more likely to use analogies—and they are (e.g., Bassok & Novick, 2012). Experts' reliance on analogies is evident both in the laboratory (e.g., Novick and Holyoak, 1991) and in real-world settings. Christensen and Schunn (2007) recorded work meetings of a group of expert engineers who were trying to create new products for use in the medical world. As the engineers discussed their options, analogy use was frequent—with an analogy being offered in the discussion every 5 minutes!

Setting Subgoals

Experts have another advantage: For many problems, it's helpful to break a problem into subproblems, so that the problem can be solved part by part rather than all at once. This, too, is a technique that experts often use.

What is a "subproblem"? The answer depends on what the overall problem is, and it takes knowledge to recognize how a problem can be broken into meaningful parts. Classic evidence on this point comes from studies of chess experts (de Groot, 1965, 1966; also see Chase & Simon, 1973). The data show that these experts are particularly skilled in organizing a chess game—in seeing the structure of the game, understanding its parts, and perceiving how the parts are related to one another. This skill is revealed in how chess masters remember board positions. In one procedure, chess masters were able to remember the positions of 20 pieces after viewing the board for just 5 seconds; novices remembered many fewer (see **Figure 13.8**). In addition, there was a strong pattern to the experts' recollection: In recalling the layout of the board, the experts would place four or five pieces in their proper positions, then pause, then recall another group, then pause, and so on. In each case, the group of pieces was one that made "tactical sense"—for example, the pieces involved in a "forked" attack, a chain of mutually defending pieces, and the like.

FIGURE 13.8 EXPERTS REMEMBERING PATTERNS

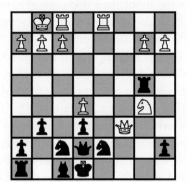

A Actual position

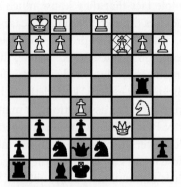

B Typical master player's performance

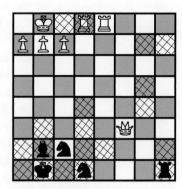

C Typical average player's performance

Experienced chess players who viewed the pattern in Panel A for 5 seconds were easily able to memorize it; average players could not, and performance from outright novices was even worse. This is because the experts were able to organize the pattern into meaningful chunks, thereby lightening their memory load. Cross-hatched squares indicate memory errors.　FIG. 8.15 FROM R. BOOTZIN, *PSYCHOLOGY TODAY: AN INTRODUCTION*, 4TH ED. © 1979 MCGRAW-HILL EDUCATION. REPRINTED WITH PERMISSION.

It seems, then, that the masters had memorized the board in terms of higher-order units, defined by their strategic function within the game. Consistent with this suggestion, the masters showed no memory advantage if they were asked to memorize random configurations of chess pieces. Here, there were no sensible groupings, and so the masters were unable to organize (and thus memorize) the board. (For similar data with other forms of expertise, see Egan & Schwartz, 1979; Tuffiash, Roring, & Ericsson, 2007.)

This perception of higher-order units helps to organize an expert's thinking. By focusing on the units and how they're related to one another, the expert keeps track of broad strategies without getting bogged down in the details. Likewise, these units set subgoals for the expert. Having perceived a group of pieces as a coordinated attack, the expert sets the subgoal of preparing for the attack. Having perceived another group of pieces as the early development of a pin, a situation in which a player cannot move without exposing a more valuable piece to an attack, the expert creates the subgoal of avoiding the pin.

Can nonexperts be trained to use subgoals in this way? Participants in one study were shown a new mathematical procedure. For some participants, key steps of the procedure were labeled in a fashion that highlighted the function of those steps; for other participants, no labels were provided (Catrambone, 1998). The idea here is that the labels can help participants to divide the procedure into meaningful parts; and, it turns out, participants who were given the labels were better able to use this new procedure in solving novel problems.

Let's be clear, though, that experts also have other advantages, including the simple fact that they know much more about their domains of expertise than novices do. Experts in many cases have also received feedback or explicit instruction, thereby improving their performance (Campitelli & Gobet, 2011; Ericsson, 2005, Ericsson & Towne, 2012; Ericsson & Ward, 2007). Experts also organize their knowledge more effectively than novices. In particular, studies indicate that experts' knowledge is heavily cross-referenced, so that each bit of information has associations to many other bits (e.g., Bédard & Chi, 1992; Heller & Reif, 1984). As a result, experts have better access to what they know.

Thus, overall there are multiple factors separating novices from experts, but these factors all hinge on the processes we've already discussed—with an emphasis on analogies, subproblems, and memory search. Apparently, then, we can use our theorizing so far to describe how people (in particular, novices and experts) differ from one another.

Defining the Problem

Experts, we've said, define problems in their area of expertise in terms of the problems' underlying dynamic. As a result, the experts are more likely to break a problem into meaningful parts, more likely to realize what other problems are analogous to the current problem, and so more likely to benefit from analogies.

Apparently, then, there are better and worse ways to define a problem— ways that will lead to a solution and ways that will obstruct it. But what does it mean to "define" a problem? And what determines how people define the problems they encounter?

Ill-Defined and Well-Defined Problems

For many problems, the goal and the options for solving the problem are clearly stated at the start: Get all the Hobbits to the other side of the river, using the boat. Solve the math problem, using the axioms stated. Many of the problems you encounter, though, are rather different. For example, we all hope for peace in the world, but what exactly will this goal involve? There will be no fighting, of course, but what other traits will the goal have? Will the nations currently on the map still be in place? How will disputes be settled? It's also unclear what steps should be tried in an effort toward reaching this goal. Would diplomatic negotiations work? Or would economic measures be more effective?

Problems like this one are said to be **ill-defined**, with no clear statement at the outset of how the goal should be characterized or what operations might be used to reach that goal. Other examples of ill-defined problems include "having a good time while on vacation" and "saving money for college" (Halpern, 1984; Kahney, 1986; Schraw, Dunkle, & Bendixen, 1995; Simon, 1973). When confronting ill-defined problems, your best bet is often to create subgoals, because many ill-defined problems have reasonably well-defined parts, and by solving each of these you can move toward solving the overall problem. A different strategy is to add some structure to the problem by including extra constraints or extra assumptions. In this way, you gradually render the problem well defined instead of ill defined—perhaps with a narrower set of options in how you might approach the problem, but with a clearly specified goal state and, eventually, with a manageable set of operations to try.

Functional Fixedness

Even for well-defined problems, however, there's often more than one way to understand the problem. We've already considered the contrast between superficial and deeper-level descriptions of a problem, but other examples are easy to find.

Consider the problem in **Figure 13.9**. To solve it, you need to cease thinking of the box as a container and instead think of it as a potential platform. Thus, your chances of solving the problem depend on how you represent the

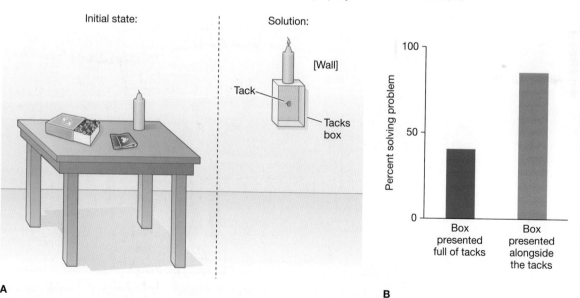

FIGURE 13.9   THE CANDLE PROBLEM

You are given the objects shown: a candle, a book of matches, and a box of tacks. Your task is to find a way to attach the candle to the wall of the room, at eye level, so that it will burn properly and illuminate the room.

Initial state:

Solution:

[Wall]

Tack

Tacks box

Percent solving problem

Box presented full of tacks

Box presented alongside the tacks

A

B

What makes this problem so difficult is the tendency to think of the box of tacks as a box—that is, as a container. The problem is readily solved, though, once you think of the box as a potential platform. However, this approach is less likely if the box is presented initially *full of tacks*. Such presentation emphasizes the usual function of the box (as a container for tacks), making it less likely that participants will think of an alternative function.

box in your thoughts, and we can show this by *encouraging* one representation or another. In one study, participants were given the equipment shown in Figure 13.9A: some matches, a box of tacks, and a candle. This configuration (implicitly) underscored the box's conventional function. As a result, the configuration increased **functional fixedness**—the tendency to be rigid in how one thinks about an object's function. With fixedness in place, the problem was rarely solved (Duncker, 1945; Fleck & Weisberg, 2004).

Other participants were given the same tools, but configured differently. They were given some matches, a pile of tacks, the box (now empty), and a candle. In this setting, the participants were less likely to think of the box as a container for the tacks, so they were less likely to think of the box *as a container*. As a result, they were more likely to solve the problem (Duncker, 1945). (For a similar problem, see **Figure 13.10**; for more on escaping the limits imposed by fixedness, see McCaffrey, 2012.)

FIGURE 13.10   THE TWO-STRING PROBLEM

You enter a room in which two strings are hanging from the ceiling and a pair of pliers is lying on a table. Your task is to tie the two strings together. Unfortunately, though, the strings are positioned far enough apart so that you can't grab one string and hold on to it while reaching for the other. How can you tie them together?

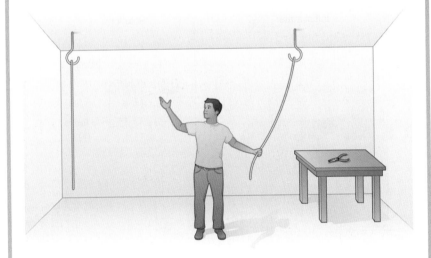

The two-string problem is difficult—because of functional fixedness. The trick here is not to think of the pliers in terms of their usual function—squeezing or pulling. Instead, the trick is simply to think of the pliers as a weight. The solution to the puzzle is to tie the pliers to one string and push the pliers away from the other string. While this pendulum is in motion, go and grab the second string, and then, when the pendulum swings back toward you, grab it and you're all set.

Einstellung

A related obstacle to problem solving arises when people start work on a problem and, because of their early steps, get locked in to a particular line of thinking. In this case, too, people can end up being the victims of their own assumptions, rigidly following a path that no longer serves them well.

Some investigators describe this rigidity as a **problem-solving set**—the collection of beliefs and assumptions a person makes about a problem. Other investigators use the term **Einstellung**, the German word for "attitude," to describe the problem solvers' perspective (their beliefs, habits, preferred strategies, etc.).

A classic demonstration of Einstellung involves the water jar problem, illustrated in **Figure 13.11**. Most participants find the solution, and once they do so, we give them some new problems. Crucially, though, all of the problems in this series can be solved in the same way, using the "formula" shown in the figure.

After solving several problems with this design, participants are given one more problem: Jar A holds 18 ounces; Jar B holds 48 ounces; Jar C holds 4 ounces. The goal is 22 ounces. Participants generally solve this problem in the same way they've solved the previous problems, failing to see that a more direct route to the goal is possible—by filling A, filling C, and combining them (18 + 4). Their prior success in using the same procedure over and over renders them blind to the more efficient alternative (Luchins, 1942; Luchins & Luchins, 1950, 1959).

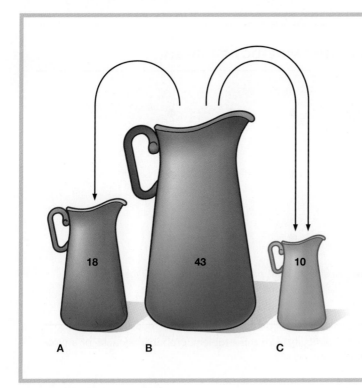

FIGURE 13.11 THE WATER JAR PROBLEM

You're given these three jars, an unlimited supply of water, and an uncalibrated bucket. You want to pour exactly 5 ounces of water into the bucket; how can you do it? The solution is shown here, and can be summarized by formula B-A-2C. Once participants have solved a couple of problems, though, each of which can be solved in the same way, they seem to grow blind to other solution paths.

Let's be clear that in a way, participants are doing something sensible here: Once they've discover a strategy that "gets the job done," they might as well use that strategy and they have no reason to hunt for an alternative plan. It's unsettling, though, that this mechanization of problem solving can interfere with subsequent performance.

"Thinking Outside the Box"

Another often-discussed example of a problem-solving set involves the nine-dot problem (see **Figure 13.12**). People routinely fail to solve this problem, because—according to some interpretations—they (mistakenly) assume that the lines they draw need to stay inside the "square" defined by the dots. In fact, this problem is probably the source of the cliché "You need to think outside the box."

Ironically, though, this cliché may be misleading. In one study, participants were told explicitly that in order to solve the problem their lines would need to go outside the square. The hint provided little benefit, and most participants still failed to find the solution (Weisberg & Alba, 1981). Apparently, beliefs about "the box" are not the obstacle here; even when we eliminate these beliefs, performance remains poor.

Nonetheless, the expression "think outside the box" does get the broad idea right, because to solve this problem people do need to jettison their initial approach. Specifically, most people assume that the lines they draw

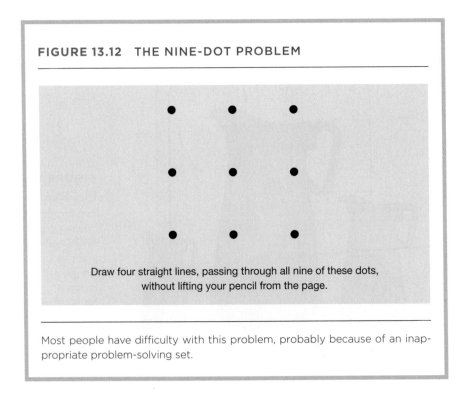

FIGURE 13.12   THE NINE-DOT PROBLEM

Draw four straight lines, passing through all nine of these dots, without lifting your pencil from the page.

Most people have difficulty with this problem, probably because of an inappropriate problem-solving set.

must begin and end on dots. People also have the idea that they'll need to maximize the number of dots "canceled" with each move; as a result, they seek solutions in which each line cancels a full row or column of dots. It turns out, though, that these assumptions are wrong; and so, guided by these mistaken beliefs, people find this problem quite hard to solve (Kershaw & Ohlsson, 2004; MacGregor, Ormerod, & Chronicle, 2001; also Öllinger, Jones, Faber, & Knoblich, 2013).

Once again, therefore, people seem to be victims of their own problem-solving set; to find the problem's solution, they need to change that set. This phrasing, however, makes it sound like a set is a bad thing, blocking the discovery of a solution, so it's important once more to remind ourselves that sets also provide a benefit. This is because (as we mentioned early on) most problems offer a huge number of options as you seek the solution—an enormous number of moves you might try or approaches you might consider. A problem-solving set helps you, therefore, by narrowing your options, which in turn eases the search for a solution. Thus, in solving the nine-dot problem, you didn't waste any time wondering whether you should try drawing the lines while holding the pencil between your toes or whether the problem

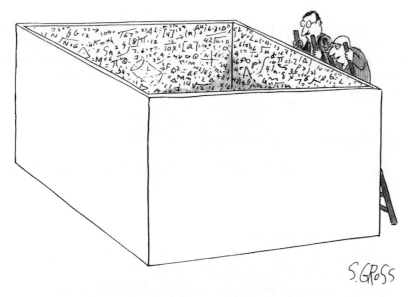

"Actually, I got some pretty good ideas when I was in the box."

THINKING OUTSIDE THE BOX

The expression "thinking outside the box" captures an important truth: Often, our problem solving is limited by unnecessary or misleading assumptions, and it's helpful to break free of those assumptions. However, the likely source of this expression (the nine-dot problem; see Figure 13.12) involves far more than just thinking outside the box (i.e., the square formed by the dots).

was hard because you were sitting down while you worked on it instead of standing up. These are foolish ideas, so you brushed past them. But what identifies them as foolish? It is your problem-solving set, which tells you, among other things, which options are plausible, which ones are physically possible, and the like.

In short, there are costs and benefits to a problem-solving set. A set can blind you to important options, and in this way it can be an obstacle. But a set can also blind you to a wide range of futile strategies, and this is a good thing: It enables you to focus, much more productively, on options that are likely to work out. Indeed, without a set, you might be so distracted by silly notions that even the simplest problem would become insoluble.

Creativity

Problem-solving sets are helpful, we've just argued, but there's no question that your efforts toward a problem solution are often *hindered* by your set, and this observation points us toward another important way in which people differ. Some people are remarkably flexible in their approaches to life's problems; they seem easily able to "think outside the box." Other people, in contrast, seem far too ready to rely on routine, so they're more vulnerable to the obstacles we've just described.

How should we think about these differences? Why do some people reliably produce novel and unexpected solutions, while other people offer only mundane and familiar solutions? This is, in effect, a question of why some people are *creative* and others are not—a question that forces us to ask: What is creativity?

Case Studies of Creativity

One way to approach this issue is by examining individuals who've been enormously creative—artists like Pablo Picasso and Johann Sebastian Bach, or scientists like Charles Darwin and Marie Curie. By studying these giants, perhaps we can draw hints about the nature of creativity when it arises, on a much smaller scale, in day-to-day life—when, for example, you find a creative way to begin a conversation or to repair a damaged friendship. As some researchers put it, we may be able to learn about "little-c creativity" (the everyday sort) by studying "Big-C Creativity" (the sort shown by people we count as scientific or artistic geniuses—cf. Simonton & Damian, 2012).

Research suggests, in fact, that highly creative people like Bach and Curie tend to have certain things in common, and perhaps we can think of these shared elements as "prerequisites" for creativity (e.g., Hennessey & Amabile, 2010). These individuals, first of all, generally have great knowledge and skills in their domain. (This point can't be surprising: If you don't know a lot of chemistry, you can't be a creative chemist. If you're not a skilled storyteller, you can't be a great novelist.) Second, to be creative, it seems that you need certain personality traits: a willingness to take risks, a willingness to ignore criticism, an ability to tolerate ambiguous findings or situations, and an inclination not to "follow the crowd." Third, highly creative people tend to be motivated by the pleasure of their work rather than by the promise of external rewards. With this, highly creative people tend to work extremely hard on their endeavors and to produce a lot of their product, whether these products are poems, paintings, or scientific papers. Fourth, these highly creative people have generally been "in the right place at the right time"—that is, in environments that allowed them freedom, provided them with the appropriate supports, and offered them problems "ripe" for solution with the resources available.

Of course, we need to be cautious in drawing conclusions about "little-c creativity" based on these observations of "Big-C Creativity." As one concern, we just suggested that external rewards play little role in encouraging "Big-C Creativity," but the evidence is mixed on whether rewards can encourage smaller-scale creativity (e.g., Byron & Khazanchi, 2012). Even so, it's important to emphasize that these observations highlight the contribution of factors outside the person, as well as the person's own capacities and skills. The external environment, for example, is the source of crucial knowledge and resources, and it often defines the problem itself; this is why many authors have suggested that we need a systematic "sociocultural approach" to creativity—one that considers the social and historical context, as well as the processes unfolding inside the creative individual's mind (e.g., Sawyer, 2006).

We still need to ask, however: What does go on in a creative mind? If a person has all the prerequisites just listed, what happens next to produce the creative step forward? In truth, there is wide disagreement on these points. One review, for example, celebrates a diversity of approaches to creativity but describes the theoretical options as "plentiful but murky" (Hennessey & Amabile, 2010, p. 576; also Mumford & Antes, 2007). It will be instructive, though, to examine a proposal offered years ago by Wallas (1926). As we'll see, Wallas's notion fits well with some commonsense ideas about creativity, and this is one of the reasons his framework continues to guide modern research. Nonetheless, we'll soon see that the evidence forces us to question several of Wallas's claims.

The Moment of Illumination

According to Wallas, creative thought proceeds through four stages. In the first stage, **preparation**, the problem solver gathers information about the problem. This stage is characterized by periods of effortful, often frustrating work on the problem, but with little progress. In the second stage, **incubation**, the problem solver sets the problem aside and seems not to be working on it. Wallas argued, though, that the problem solver continues to work on the problem during this stage, albeit unconsciously. Thus, the problem's solution is continuing to develop, unseen, just as a baby bird develops, unseen, inside the egg. This period of incubation leads to the third stage, **illumination**, in which some key insight or new idea emerges, paving the way for the fourth stage, **verification**, in which the person confirms that the new idea really does lead to a problem solution and works out the details.

Was Wallas right? Historical evidence suggests that many creative discoveries don't include the steps he described or, if they do, include these steps in a complex, back-and-forth sequence (Weisberg, 1986). Likewise, the moment of great illumination celebrated in Wallas's proposal may be more myth than reality: When we examine creative discoveries (Watson and Crick's discovery of the double helix, Calder's invention of the mobile as a form of sculpture, etc.), we find that these ideas developed through a succession of "mini-insights," each moving the process forward in some way rather than springing forth, full-blown, from some remarkable "Aha!" moment (Klein, 2013; Sawyer, 2006).

For that matter, what exactly does the "Aha!" experience—the moment in which people feel they've made a great leap forward—involve? To explore this issue, Metcalfe (1986; Metcalfe & Weibe, 1987) gave her participants a series of "insight problems" like those shown in **Figure 13.13A**. As participants worked on each problem, they rated their progress by using a judgment of "warmth" ("I'm getting warmer . . . , I'm getting warmer . . ."), and these ratings did capture the "moment of insight": Initially, the participants didn't have a clue how to proceed and gave warmth ratings of 1 or 2; then, rather abruptly, they saw a way forward, and at that instant their warmth ratings shot up to the top of the scale.

To understand this pattern, though, we need to look separately at those participants who subsequently announced the correct solution to the problem and those who announced an *incorrect* solution. Remarkably, the pattern is the same for the two groups (see Figure 13.13B). Thus, some participants abruptly announced that they were getting "hot" and, moments later, solved the problem. Other participants made the same announcement and, moments later, slammed into a dead end.

Apparently, then, when you say "Aha!" it means only that you've discovered a new approach, one that you've not yet considered. This is by itself important, because often a new approach is just what you need. But there's nothing magical about the "moment of illumination." This moment doesn't signal the fact that you have at last discovered a path leading to the solution. Instead, it means only that you've discovered something new to try, with no guarantee that this "something new" will be helpful. (For more on these issues, see Bassok & Novick, 2012; Chronicle, MacGregor, & Ormerod, 2004; Fleck, Beeman, & Kounios, 2012; Jones, 2003; Knoblich, Ohlsson, & Raney, 2001; Smith & Ward, 2012; Topolinski & Reber, 2010; van Steenburgh, Fleck, Beeman, & Kounios, 2012; for a discussion of neural mechanisms underlying insight, see Kounios & Beeman, 2014, and also **Figure 13.14**.)

FIGURE 13.13 INSIGHT PROBLEMS

Problem 1
A stranger approached a museum curator and offered him an ancient bronze coin. The coin had an authentic appearance and was marked with the date 544 B.C. The curator had happily made acquisitions from suspicious sources before, but this time he promptly called the police and had the stranger arrested. Why?

Problem 2
A landscape gardener is given instructions to plant four special trees so that each one is exactly the same distance from each of the others. How should the trees be arranged?

A

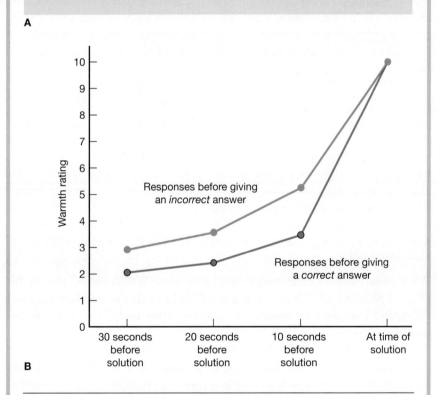

B

As participants worked on these problems, they were asked to judge their progress by using an assessment of "warmth" ("I'm getting warmer . . . , I'm getting warmer . . . , I'm getting hot!"). For Problem 1, you must realize that no one in the year 544 B.C. knew that it was 544 B.C.; that is, no one could have known that Christ would be born exactly 544 years later. For Problem 2, the gardener needs to plant one of the trees at the top of a tall mound and then plant the other trees around the base of the mound, with the three together forming an equilateral triangle and with the four forming a triangle-based pyramid (i.e., a tetrahedron).   AFTER METCALFE, 1986.

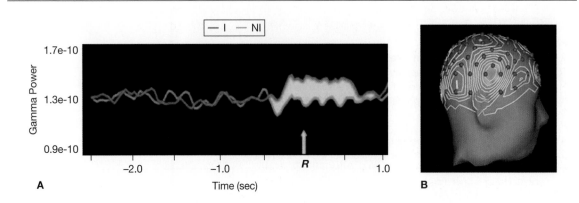

FIGURE 13.14 NEURAL CORRELATES OF INSIGHT

There is no question that problems requiring some insight involve a distinctive set of brain processes. In Panel A, the yellow *R* indicates the moment at which the research participant announced that he or she had figured out the problem solution, either for a problem requiring some insight (red line, keyed "I") or for a problem not requiring a special insight (blue line, keyed "NI"). To make the difference between these lines easily visible, the difference is shaded in yellow. The time axis shows the time relative to the participants' announcement that an insight had emerged. The measure of "gamma power" is derived from EEG procedures, and it represents the square of the voltage measured in brain waves. Panel B shows the spatial focus of this distinctive brain process—called "gamma-band activity." The red dots in Panel B show where the EEG electrodes were placed.

Incubation

What about Wallas's claims regarding incubation? Wallas argued that in this stage of problem solving the person seems to have set the problem aside but (allegedly) continues to work on it unconsciously and, as a result, makes considerable progress.

Many people find this to be an appealing idea, since most of us have had an experience along these lines: You're working on a problem but getting nowhere. After a while, you give up and turn your thoughts to other matters. Sometime later, though, you're thinking about something altogether different when the solution suddenly pops into your thoughts.

Many examples of this pattern have been recorded, and a number of authors point out that great scientific discoveries seem often to have been made in this manner (e.g., Kohler, 1969). However, more-systematic data tell us that the incubation effect is (at best) unreliable: Some studies do show that time away from a problem helps in finding the problem's solution, but many studies find no effect (see Baird et al., 2012; Dodds, Ward, & Smith, 2007, 2012; Gilhooly, Georgiou, Garrison, Reston, & Sirota, 2012; Hélie & Sun, 2010; Segal, 2004; Sio & Ormerod, 2009).

How should we think about this mixed pattern? Some researchers argue that timing is the key, on the idea that incubation effects will be stronger if the incubation happens right after you've set the problem aside (e.g., Gilhooly et al., 2012). Other studies focus on how you spend your time during the incubation period, with a suggestion that problem solving will be promoted only if the circumstances allow your thoughts to "wander" during this period (Baird et al., 2012).

Why should "mind wandering" be relevant here? As one option, recall that in Chapter 9 we described the process of *spreading activation* through which one memory can activate related memories. It seems likely that when you're carefully working on a problem, you try to direct this flow of activation—and perhaps end up directing it in unproductive ways. When you simply allow your thoughts to wander, though, the activation can flow wherever the memory connections take it, and this may lead to new ideas being activated (cf. Ash & Wiley, 2006; Bowden, Jung-Beeman, Fleck, & Kounios, 2005; Radel, Davaranche, Fournier, & Dietrick, 2015; Smith & Ward, 2012). This process provides no guarantee that *helpful* or *productive* ideas will come to mind, only that *more* (and perhaps unanticipated) ideas will be activated. In this way, incubation is like illumination—a source of new possibilities that may or may not pay off.

Other authors, though, offer a more mundane explanation of "incubation" effects. They note that your early efforts with a problem may have been tiring or frustrating, and if so, the interruption simply provides an opportunity for the frustration or fatigue to dissipate. Likewise, your early efforts with a problem may have been dominated by a particular approach, a particular set. If you put the problem aside for a while, it's possible you'll forget about these earlier tactics, freeing you to explore other, more productive avenues (Smith & Blankenship, 1989, 1991; Storm, Angello, & Bjork, 2011; Storm & Patel, 2014; Vul & Pashler, 2007).

For the moment, there is no consensus in the field about which of these proposals is best, and it seems plausible that each captures part of the truth. Likewise, it remains unclear why time away from a problem sometimes helps and sometimes doesn't. To put the matter bluntly, sometimes when you're stymied by a problem, it does help to walk away from it for a while. But sometimes your best bet is just to keep plugging away, doggedly trying to move forward. For now, research provides less guidance than we'd like in choosing which of these is the better plan.

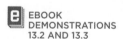

EBOOK
DEMONSTRATIONS
13.2 AND 13.3

The Nature of Creativity

Where does all of this discussion leave us with regard to our overarching question—the question of how people differ in their cognitive abilities? In discussing *expertise*, we saw that experts in a domain have a stack of advantages: a tendency to think about problems in terms of their structure rather than their surface form, a broad knowledge base deriving from their experience in a field, heavily cross-referenced memories, and so on. Now, in

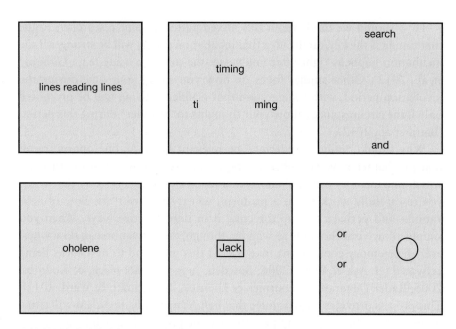

AN INCUBATION BENEFIT FROM SIMPLE FORGETTING

Shown here are the problems used in a study of incubation. Each panel refers to a familiar word or phrase, and participants had to figure out what the word or phrase was. Clues were given for each problem, but for many of the problems the clues were designed to be misleading. Control participants had a minute to work on each puzzle; other participants worked on each puzzle for 30 seconds, then were interrupted, and later returned to the puzzle for an additional 30 seconds. This interruption did improve performance, so that problem solution was more likely for the "incubation" group. Crucially, though, the researchers tested participants' memory for the misleading clues, and they found that the incubation participants were less likely to remember the clues. The researchers argued that this forgetting is what created the "incubation" advantage: After the interruption, participants were no longer misled by the bad clues, and their performance improved accordingly. (The solutions to these puzzles are given at the end of the chapter.)   SMITH & BLANKENSHIP, 1991.

discussing *creativity*, we've seen a similar pattern: Highly creative people tend to have certain personality traits (e.g., a willingness to take risks), a lot of knowledge, intense motivation, and some amount of luck. But what mental processes do they rely on? When we examine Darwin's notebooks or Picasso's early sketches, we discover that these creative giants relied on analogies, hints, heuristics, and a lot of hard work, just as the rest of us do (Gruber, 1981; Sawyer, 2006; Weisberg, 1986). In some cases, creativity may even depend on blind trial and error (e.g., Klein, 2013; Simonton, 2011); with this sort of process, the great artist or great inventor is simply someone who's highly discriminating—and thus able to discern which of the randomly produced products actually have value.

Some research suggests in addition that highly creative people may be especially skillful in how they search through their memories. For example, some authors emphasize the skill of "divergent thinking"—the ability to spot novel connections among ideas, connections that others had missed (Guilford, 1967, 1979; also see Beaty, Silvia, Nusbaum, Jauk, & Benedek, 2014; Carson, Peterson, & Higgins, 2005; Vartanian, Martindale, & Matthews, 2009; see **Figure 13.15**). Other authors showcase the ability to hunt through memory for ideas that will satisfy multiple requirements—an ability sometimes measured through the Remote Associates Test (Mednick, 1962; Mednick & Mednick, 1967; also Smith, Huber, & Vul, 2013; **Figure 13.16**). In all cases, though, the mechanism of memory search is the same one we have met in other contexts—spreading activation flowing through the memory network (for more on the link between creativity and memory search, see Smith & Ward, 2012).

Notice, then, that there's no evidence that Darwin or Picasso, Rachel Carson or Georgia O'Keeffe possessed some special "creativity mechanism." Instead, they seem to have been relying on the same processes, the same strategies, as ordinary problem solvers (cf. DeHaan, 2011; Goldenberg, Mazursky, & Solomon, 1999; Klahr & Simon, 2001; Simonton, 2003, 2009; Simonton & Damian, 2012; Weisberg, 2006). There may be one regard, though, in which these extraordinary individuals were distinctive: Many of us are smart or particularly skillful in memory search; many of us are

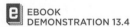
EBOOK
DEMONSTRATION 13.4

FIGURE 13.15   CREATIVITY AS DIVERGENT THINKING

Tests of divergent thinking require you to think of new uses for simple objects or new ways to think about familiar ideas. How many different uses can you think of for a brick?

As a paperweight.
As the shadow-caster in a sundial (if positioned appropriately).
As a means of writing messages on a sidewalk.
As a stepladder (if you want to grab something just slightly out of reach).
As a nutcracker.
As a pendulum useful for solving the two-string problem.

Choose five names, at random, from the telephone directory. In how many different ways could these names be classified?

According to the number of syllables.
According to whether there is an even or odd number of vowels.
According to whether their third letter is in the last third of the alphabet.
According to whether they rhyme with things that are edible.

Guilford (1967, 1979) argued that creativity lies in the ability to take an idea in a new, unprecedented direction. Among its other items, his test of creativity asks people to think of new uses for a familiar object. Some possible responses are listed here.

willing to take risks and to ignore criticism; many of us live in a cultural setting that might support a new discovery. What may distinguish creative geniuses, though, is that they are the special few people who have *all* of these ingredients—the right intellectual tools, the right personality characteristics, living in the right context, and so on. It's a rare individual who has all of these elements, and it is the convergence of these elements that seems to be the recipe for monumental creativity.

Intelligence

We turn now to another—and equally important—way in which people differ: in their *intelligence*. Common sense tells us that differences in intelligence exist, and we all celebrate those people whom we count as wonderfully smart, and express concerns about (and try to help) those whom we consider intellectually dull. But what exactly is "intelligence"? Is there a proper way to measure it? And, crucially, should we be focused on *intelligence* (singular) or *intelligences* (plural)? In other words, is there such a thing as "intelligence-in-general," so that someone who has this intelligence will be better off in all mental endeavors? Or should we instead talk about different types of intelligence, so that someone might be "smart" in some domains but less so in others? We'll tackle all of these questions in this section.

Defining and Measuring Intelligence

More than a dozen years ago, a group of 52 experts offered their consensus definition of intelligence: "the ability to reason, plan, solve problems, think abstractly, comprehend complex ideas, learn quickly and learn from experience," an ability that must be distinguished from "book learning . . . or test-taking smarts." The experts also noted that this is an ability crucial for "'catching on,' 'making sense' of things, or 'figuring out' what to do" (Gottfredson, 1997a, p. 13).

This many-part definition, however, played no role in the early efforts toward measuring intelligence. Instead, Alfred Binet (1857–1911) and his colleagues began with the simple idea that intelligence is a capacity that matters for many aspects of cognitive functioning. They therefore created a test that included a range of tasks: copying a drawing, repeating a string of digits, understanding a story, doing arithmetic, and so on. Performance was then assessed with a composite score, summing across these various tasks.

In its original form, the test score was computed as a ratio between a child's "mental age" (the level of development reflected in the test performance) and his or her chronological age. (The ratio was then multiplied by 100 to get the final score.) This ratio—or *quotient*—was the source of the test's name: The test evaluated the child's "intelligence quotient," or IQ.

Modern forms of the test no longer calculate this ratio, but they're still called IQ tests. One commonly used test is the Wechsler Intelligence Scale for Children (WISC; Wechsler, 2003); adult intelligence is often evaluated with the Wechsler Adult Intelligence Scale (WAIS). Like Binet's original test, these modern tests rely on numerous subtests. In the WAIS, for example, there are tests to assess general knowledge, vocabulary, and comprehension (see **Figure 13.17A**); a perceptual-reasoning scale includes visual puzzles like the one shown in Figure 13.17B. Separate subtests assess working memory and speed of intellectual processing. (Other commonly used tests include the fifth edition of the Stanford Binet test [Roid, 2003] and the Kaufman Assessment Battery for Children, or KABC [Kaufman & Kaufman, 2004].)

Other intelligence tests have different formats. For example, the Raven's Progressive Matrices Test (Figure 13.17C; Raven & Raven, 2008) hinges entirely on a person's ability to analyze figures and detect patterns. This test presents the test taker with a series of grids (these are the "matrices"), and he or she must select an option that sensibly completes the pattern in each grid. This test is designed to minimize any influence from verbal skills or background knowledge.

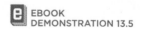

EBOOK
DEMONSTRATION 13.5

Reliability and Validity

Whenever we design a test—to assess intelligence, personality, mental health, or anything else—we need to determine whether the test is *reliable* and *valid*. **Reliability** refers to how consistent a measure is, and one aspect of reliability is *consistency from one occasion to another*. In other words, if we give you a test, wait a while, and then give it again, do we get essentially the same outcome? The issue here is called **test-retest reliability**.

FIGURE 13.17 INTELLIGENCE TEST ITEMS

- Vocabulary
  Presents a series of words of increasing difficulty; asks for a definition of each word: "What is a lute?" or "What does solitude mean?"
- Comprehension
  Asks the test-taker to explain why certain social practices are followed or the meaning of common proverbs: "What does it mean to say, 'Don't judge a book by its cover'?"
- Similarities
  Presents pairs of objects and asks how the items in each pair are alike: "In what ways are an airplane and a car alike?"
- Information
  Asks whether the test-taker knows various bits of information, with each bit being something that is widely known in our culture: "Who is the president of Russia?"

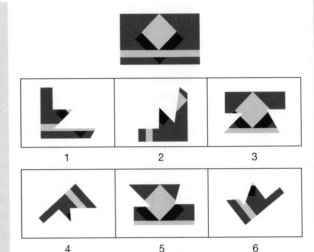

A Sample questions from verbal scale of the WAIS

B WAIS visual puzzle

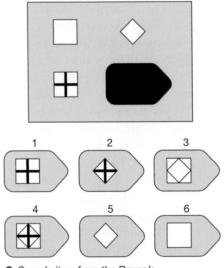

C Sample item from the Raven's Progressive Matrices

Panel A shows questions used in some of the subtests of the Wechsler Adult Intelligence Scale (WAIS). Panel B shows a sample item used in the perceptual-reasoning portion of the WAIS; the task is to assemble some of the parts to form the pattern shown. Panel C shows an easy item from the Raven's Progressive Matrices; the task is to identify the figure that completes the pattern. The test items get harder and harder as the test progresses.

Research indicates that intelligence tests have strong test-retest reliability. There is, for example, a high correlation between measurements of someone's IQ at, say, age 6 and measurements of IQ when she's 18. For that matter, if we know someone's IQ at age 11, we can predict with reasonable accuracy what his IQ will be at age 80 or 90 (e.g., Deary, 2014; Deary, Pattie, & Starr, 2013; Plomin & Spinath, 2004).

We should mention that someone's IQ score can change—especially if there's a substantial change in the person's environment. (We'll return to this point later in the chapter; also see Ramsden et al., 2011.) Nonetheless, the data show remarkable stability in IQ scores, even over spans as long as 70 or 80 years.

What about the validity of the IQ test? In general, the term "validity" refers to whether a test actually measures what it is intended to measure, and one way to approach this issue is via an assessment of **predictive validity**. Thus, if intelligence tests truly measure what they're supposed to, then someone's score on the test should enable us to predict how well that person will do in settings that require intelligence. And here, too, the results are impressive. For example, there's at least a .50 correlation between a person's IQ and measures of academic performance (e.g., grade-point average; Arneson, Sackett, & Beatty, 2011; Deary, 2012; Kuncel, Hezlett, & Ones, 2004; Strenze, 2007).

Let's pause to emphasize that this is far from a perfect correlation, but that cannot be a surprise, because of course other factors beyond intelligence matter for performance. For example, how well you'll do in school also depends—rather obviously—on your motivation, whether you get adequate amounts of sleep, whether your friends encourage you to study or instead go to a party, and dozens of other factors. These points make it inevitable that intelligence levels won't be a perfect predictor of your academic achievements. Or, to put this more bluntly, these points make it inevitable that some high-IQ people will perform poorly in school, while some low-IQ people will excel. (Clearly, therefore, an IQ score does not define your destiny.) Even so, there's no question that the correlation between IQ and school performance is strong—in fact, it is stronger than the correlation for any other predictor. It seems plain, then, that the capacities measured by the IQ test play a powerful role in shaping your performance—just as we would expect if the test scores are a valid measure of intelligence.

IQ scores are also correlated with performance outside of the academic world. For example, an IQ score is a strong predictor of how someone will perform on the job, although—sensibly—the data indicate that IQ matters more for some jobs than for others (Sackett et al., 2008; Schmidt & Hunter, 1998, 2004). Jobs of low complexity require relatively little intelligence, so, not surprisingly, the correlation between IQ and job performance is small (although still positive) for such jobs—for example, a correlation of .20 between IQ and performance on an assembly line. As jobs become more complex, intelligence matters more, so the correlation between IQ and performance gets stronger (Gottfredson, 1997b). For example, we find

TABLE 13.1   THE RELATION BETWEEN IQ
AND HIGHWAY DEATHS

IQ	Death Rate per 100,000 Drivers
>115	51.3
100–115	51.5
85–99	92.2
80–84	146.7

Holden, C. (2003). The practical benefits of general intelligence. Science, 299, 192–193.

correlations between .50 and .60 when we look at IQ scores and people's success as accountants or shop managers.

IQ scores are also correlated with other life outcomes. For example, people with higher IQ tend, overall, to earn more money during their lifetime, end up with higher-prestige careers, and are less likely to suffer various life problems (and so are less likely to end up in jail, less likely to become pregnant as teens, and more). Higher-IQ people even live longer—with various mechanisms contributing to this longevity. Among other considerations, higher-IQ individuals are less likely to die in automobile accidents (see **Table 13.1**) and less likely to have difficulty following a doctor's instructions (see, among others, Deary, Weiss, & Batty, 2010; Gottfredson, 2004; Kuncel et al., 2004; Lubinski, 2004; Murray, Pattie, Starr, & Deary, 2012.)

Let's note once again, though, that all of these correlations are appreciably less than +1.00, a consequence of the fact that many other factors also matter for job performance, longevity, and so on. Even so, the data are clear that IQ tests do have impressive predictive validity—with the clear implication that these tests are measuring something interesting, important, and consequential.

General versus Specialized Intelligence

If—as it seems—IQ tests are measuring something important, what is this "something"? This question is often framed in terms of two broad options. One proposal is that the tests measure a singular ability that can apply to any content. The idea, in other words, is that someone's score on an IQ test reveals the person's *general* intelligence, a capacity that provides an advantage on virtually any mental task. (This notion was proposed early on by the English psychologist Charles Spearman, 1904, 1927; for a more recent treatment, see Kaufman, Kaufman, & Plucker, 2012.)

In contrast, many authors argue that there's no such thing as being intelligent in a general way. Instead, they claim, each person has a collection of more specific talents—and so you might be "math smart" but not strong with language, or "highly verbal" but not strong with tasks requiring visualization. From this perspective, if we represent your capacities with a single number—an IQ score—this is only a crude summary of what you can do, because it averages together the things you're good at and the things you're not.

Which proposal is correct? One way to find out relies on the fact that, as we've said, many intelligence tests include numerous subtests. It's therefore instructive to compare a person's score on each subtest with his or her scores on other subtests. In this way, we can ask: If someone does well on one portion of the test, is she likely to do well across the board? If someone does poorly on one subtest, will he do poorly on other subtests as well? If we observe these patterns, this would indicate that there is such a thing as intelligence-in-general, a cognitive capacity that shapes how well someone does no matter what the specific task might be.

More than a century ago, Spearman developed a statistical procedure that enables us to pursue this issue in a precise, quantitative manner. The procedure is called **factor analysis**; as the name implies, this procedure looks for common factors—elements that contribute to multiple subtests and which therefore link those subtests. And, in fact, factor analysis confirms that there is a common element shared by all the components of the IQ test; indeed, this common element seems to account for roughly half of the overall data pattern (Arnau & Thompson, 2000; Carroll, 1993; Deary, 2012; Johnson, Carothers, & Deary, 2008; Watkins, Wilson, Kotz, Carbone, & Babula, 2006). Some of the subtests (e.g., someone's comprehension of a simple story) depend heavily on this general factor; others (e.g., someone's ability to recall a string of digits) depend less on the factor. Nonetheless, this general factor matters across the board, and that's why all the subtests end up being correlated with one another.

Spearman named this common element **general intelligence**, usually abbreviated with the letter *g*. Spearman (1927) proposed that *g* is called on for virtually any intellectual task—and so an individual with a high level of *g* will have an advantage in every intellectual endeavor; if *g* is in short supply, the individual will do poorly on a wide range of tasks.

A Hierarchical Model of Intelligence

Spearman's data, however, made it clear that *g* is not the whole story, because people also have more specialized skills. One of these skills, for example, involves aptitude for verbal and linguistic tasks, so performance on (say) a reading comprehension test depends on how much *g* a person has *and also* on the strength of these verbal skills. A second specialized ability involves quantitative or numerical aptitude, so performance on an arithmetic test depends on how much *g* a person has and also the strength of these skills.

Putting these pieces together, we can think of intellectual performance as having a hierarchical structure as shown in **Figure 13.18**. Researchers disagree about the details of this hierarchy; but by most accounts, *g* is at the top of the hierarchy and contributes to virtually all tasks. At the next level down are the abilities we just described—linguistic and numerical—and several more,

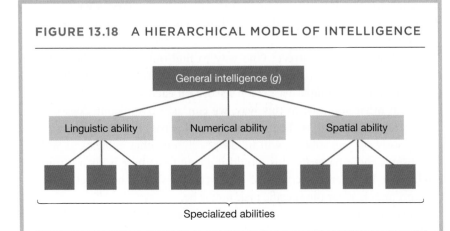

FIGURE 13.18   A HIERARCHICAL MODEL OF INTELLIGENCE

Most modern researchers regard intelligence as having a hierarchical structure. General intelligence (*g*) is an ability called on to some extent by virtually all mental tasks. At the next level, broad linguistic, numerical, and spatial ability are each called on by a wide range of tasks of a certain type; other abilities at this level include an ability to handle fast-paced tasks and also to memorize new material. At the next level down, more than 80 specialized abilities have been identified, each applicable to a certain type of task.

including spatial skill, an ability to handle fast-paced mental tasks, and an ability to learn new and unfamiliar materials. Then, at the next level are even more specific capacities—at least 80 have been identified—each useful for a narrow and specialized set of tasks (Carroll, 1993; Flanagan, McGrew, & Ortiz, 2000; Johnson, Nijenhuis, & Bouchard, 2007; McGrew, 2009; Snow, 1994, 1996).

This hierarchical conception leads to a prediction that if we choose tasks from two different categories—say, a verbal task and one requiring arithmetic—we should find a correlation in performance. This is because no matter how different these tasks seem, they do have something in common: They both draw on *g*. If we choose tasks from the *same* category, though—say, two verbal tasks or two quantitative tasks—we should find a *higher* correlation because these tasks have two things in common: They both draw on *g*, and they both draw on the more specialized capacity needed for just that category. The data confirm both of these predictions—moderately strong correlations among all of the IQ test's subtests, and even stronger correlations among subtests in the same category.

It seems, then, that both of the broad hypotheses we introduced earlier are correct: There is some sort of general capacity that is useful for all mental endeavors, but there are also various forms of more-specialized intelligence. Each person has some amount of the general capacity and draws on it in all tasks; this is why there's an overall consistency in each person's performance. At the same time, the consistency isn't perfect, because each task also requires more specialized abilities. Each of us has our own profile of strengths and weaknesses for these skills, and thus there are things we do relatively well and things we do less well.

Fluid and Crystallized Intelligence

We need one more complication in our theorizing, though, because it's also important to distinguish *fluid intelligence* and *crystallized intelligence* (Carroll, 2005; Horn, 1985; Horn & Blankson, 2005). **Fluid intelligence** refers to the ability to deal with novel problems. It's the form of intelligence you need when you have no well-practiced routines you can bring to bear on a problem. **Crystallized intelligence**, in contrast, refers to your acquired knowledge, including your verbal knowledge and your broad repertoire of skills—skills useful for dealing with problems similar to those already encountered.

Fluid and crystallized intelligence are highly correlated (e.g., if you have a lot of one, you're likely to have a lot of the other). Nonetheless, these two aspects of intelligence differ in important ways. Crystallized intelligence usually increases with age, but fluid intelligence reaches its peak in early adulthood and then, for most of us, declines steadily across the lifespan (see **Figure 13.19**; Horn, 1985; Horn & Noll, 1994; Salthouse, 2004, 2012). Similarly, many factors—including alcohol consumption, fatigue, and depression—cause more impairment in tasks requiring fluid intelligence

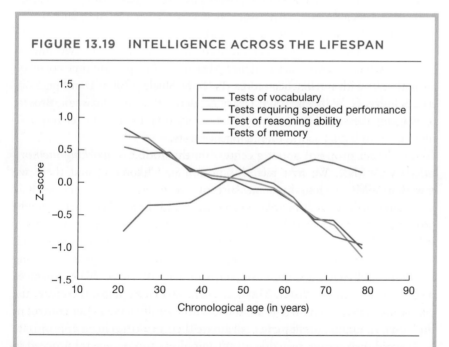

FIGURE 13.19   INTELLIGENCE ACROSS THE LIFESPAN

Tests that involve crystallized intelligence (like tests of vocabulary) often show a genuine improvement in test scores across the lifespan, declining only when—at age 70 or so—the person's overall condition starts to deteriorate. In contrast, tests that involve fluid intelligence (like tests requiring speeded performance) peak at age 20 or so and decline thereafter. The "Z-scores" used here are a common statistical measure used for comparing tests with disparate scoring schemes.

than in those dependent on crystallized intelligence (Duncan, 1994; Hunt, 1995). Thus, someone who is tired will probably perform adequately on tests involving familiar routines and familiar facts. The same individual, however, may be markedly impaired if the test requires quick thinking or a novel approach—earmarks of fluid intelligence.

The Building Blocks of Intelligence

It's clear, then, that intelligence has many components. However, one component—*g*—is crucial, for the simple reason that this aspect of intelligence is relevant to virtually all mental activities. But what exactly is *g*? What gives a person more *g* or less?

One proposal is simple: Mental processes are quick but do take some time, and perhaps the people we consider intelligent are those who are especially fast in these processes. This speed would enable them to perform intellectual tasks more quickly; it also would give them time for more steps in comparison with those of us who aren't so quick (Coyle, Pillow, Snyder, & Kochunov, 2011; Deary, 2012; Eysenck, 1986; Nettelbeck, 2003; Sheppard, 2008; Vernon, 1987). (For discussions of the possible biological basis for this speed, see Miller, 1994; Penke et al., 2012; Rae, Digney, McEwan, & Bates, 2003.)

Many studies support this idea, including those that involve measures of **inspection time**—the time a person needs to decide which of two lines is longer or which of two tones is higher. Measures of inspection time correlate around −.30 with intelligence scores (Bates & Shieles, 2003; Danthiir, Roberts, Schulze, & Wilhelm, 2005; Deary & Derr, 2005; Ravenzwaaij, Brown, & Wagenmakers, 2011); the correlation is negative because lower response times go with higher scores on intelligence tests.

A different proposal about *g* centers on the notion of *working-memory capacity* (WMC). We first met this notion in Chapter 6, and there we saw that WMC is actually a measure of *executive control*—and so it is a measure of how well people can monitor and direct their own thought processes. We mentioned in the earlier chapter that people with a larger WMC do better on many intellectual tasks, including, we can now add, tests specifically designed to measure *g*; this linkage is especially strong for *fluid* intelligence (Burgess, Braver, Conway, & Gray, 2011; Engel & Kane, 2004; Fukuda, Vogel, Mayr, & Awh, 2011). Perhaps, therefore, the people we consider intelligent are those who literally have better control of their own thoughts, so they can coordinate their priorities in an appropriate way, avoid distraction, override errant impulses, and in general proceed in a deliberate manner when making judgments or solving problems. (For a complication, though, see Redick et al., 2013. For more on executive control, see Chuderiski & Necka, 2012; Diamond, 2013; Kane & McVay, 2012. For a different view of how working memory might shape intelligence, see Duncan et al., 2008; Duncan, Schramm, Thompson, & Dumontheil, 2012; for a different conception of the mechanisms crucial for intelligence, see **Figures 13.20** and **13.21**.)

FIGURE 13.20   THE P-FIT MODEL

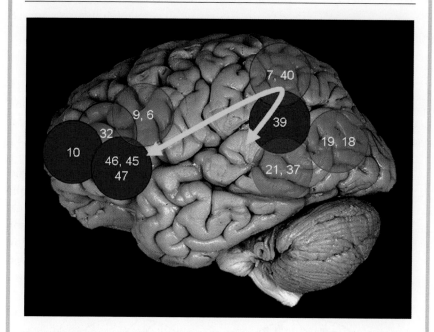

What is it in the brain that makes intelligence possible? One view is the parieto-frontal integration theory (P-FIT), suggested by Jung & Haier, 2007. Their theory identifies a network of brain sites that seem crucial for intellectual performance. Some of the sites are in the parietal lobe and are heavily involved in the control of attention. Other sites are in the frontal lobe and are essential for working memory. Still other important sites are crucial for language processing. (The dark circles in the figure indicate brain areas that are especially relevant in the left hemisphere; the light circles indicate brain areas that are relevant in both hemispheres. The numbers refer to a scheme—so-called Brodmann areas—commonly used for labeling brain regions.) The P-FIT conception emphasizes, though, that what really matters for intelligence is the integration of information from all of these sites—and thus the coordinated functioning of many cognitive components.

Intelligence Beyond the IQ Test

In the previous section, we asked what it is that gives someone more *g* or less. But we can also ask what forms of intelligence there might be *in addition to g*—aspects of intelligence separate from the capacities measured with conventional intelligence tests.

Practical Intelligence

Psychologist Robert Sternberg has emphasized the importance of **practical intelligence**, the kind of intelligence needed for skilled reasoning in

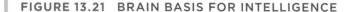

FIGURE 13.21 BRAIN BASIS FOR INTELLIGENCE

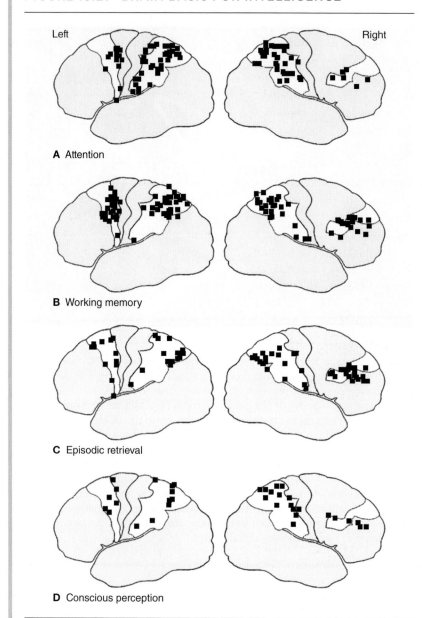

Researchers disagree with some of the specific claims in the P-FIT theory (described in Figure 13.20), but there is no disagreement about the fact that many brain sites in the frontal and parietal areas are involved in the mental processes needed for intelligence. The data shown here are derived from fMRI and PET studies; they show some of the sites associated with four different mental achievements. AFTER NAGHAVI & NYBERG, 2005.

day-to-day settings. The idea here is that someone might be "street-smart" or "savvy" even if she or he lacks the sort of analytical skill needed in a classroom. Sternberg and his associates have explored this issue extensively, including research on whether *teaching* is more effective when instruction is matched to students' abilities (with different forms of instruction for students high in practical ability, students high in analytical ability, and students high in creative ability). Evidence suggests that "tuning" the curriculum in this fashion can be helpful (Grigorenko, Jarvin, & Sternberg, 2002; Sternberg & Grigorenko, 2004; also see Sternberg, 1985; also see Henry, Sternberg, & Grigorenko, 2005; Sternberg, Kaufman, & Grigorenko, 2008; Wagner, 2000).

It is unclear, however, whether practical intelligence is truly distinct from intelligence as measured in traditional intelligence tests. As one concern, Gottfredson (2003) reminds us that traditional IQ scores are good predictors of many real-world outcomes. (We noted earlier, for example, that IQ scores are predictive of job performance, occupational prestige, and even the ability to stay out of jail or to stay alive.) On this basis, she argues, IQ tests do measure the ability to handle practical matters—so there may be no need for a separate category of "practical intelligence."

Measures of Rationality?

A different sort of complexity has been highlighted by Keith Stanovich, who argues that there are aspects of cognition untapped by the standard intelligence tests. As part of his evidence, Stanovich reminds us that we all know people who are very smart according to their test scores but who nonetheless ignore facts, are overconfident in their judgment, are insensitive to inconsistencies in their views, and more. As a result, they are especially prone to the reasoning errors we described in the last chapter—including belief perseverance and confirmation bias. (It's for people like these that you find yourself asking, "How could someone that smart be so stupid?") In light of such cases (and a great deal of other evidence), Stanovich (2009) argues that we need separate measures of *intelligence* and *rationality*, with the latter term being defined (in Stanovich's view) roughly as the capacity for critically assessing information as it is gathered in the natural environment. (Also see DeNeys & Bonnefon, 2013; Stanovich, West, & Toplak, 2013.)

Other Types of Intelligence

Still other authors highlight a capacity they call **emotional intelligence**—the ability to understand one's own emotions and others', and also the ability to control one's emotions when appropriate (Mayer, Roberts, & Barsade, 2008; Salovey & Mayer, 1990; also Brackett et al., 2006). Tests have been constructed to measure this capacity, and people who score well on these tests are judged to create a more positive atmosphere in the workplace and to have more leadership potential (Grewal & Salovey, 2005; Lopes, Salovey, Côté, & Beers, 2005). Likewise, college students who score well on these tests are rated by their friends as being more caring and more supportive; they're also less likely to experience conflict with peers (Brackett & Mayer, 2003; Mayer, et al., 2008).

Perhaps the best-known challenge to IQ testing, however, comes from Howard Gardner's theory of **multiple intelligences.** Gardner (1983, 2006) argues for *eight* types of intelligence: Three of these are assessed in standard IQ tests: linguistic intelligence, logical-mathematical intelligence, and spatial intelligence. But Gardner also argues that we should acknowledge musical intelligence, bodily-kinesthetic intelligence (the ability to learn and create complex patterns of movement), interpersonal intelligence (the ability to understand other people), intrapersonal intelligence (the ability to understand ourselves), and naturalistic intelligence (the ability to understand patterns in nature).

Some of Gardner's evidence comes from the study of people with so-called **savant syndrome,** including the individuals we mentioned at the very start of this chapter. These individuals have a single extraordinary talent even though they're otherwise disabled to a profound degree. Some display unusual artistic talent (see **Figure 13.22**). Others are "calendar calculators," able to answer immediately when asked questions like "What day of the week was March 19 in the year 1642?" Still others have remarkable musical skills and can effortlessly memorize lengthy and complex musical works (Hill, 1978; Miller, 1999).

Apparently, it's possible to have extreme talent that is separate from intelligence as it's measured on IQ tests. But beyond this intriguing point, how should we think about Gardner's claims? First, there is no question that Gardner (as well as the researchers working on "emotional intelligence") reminds us that a broad range of human achievements are of great value, and surely we should celebrate the skill displayed by an artist at her canvas, a skilled dancer in the ballet, or an empathetic clergyman in a hospital room. These are certainly talents to be acknowledged and, as much as possible, nurtured and developed.

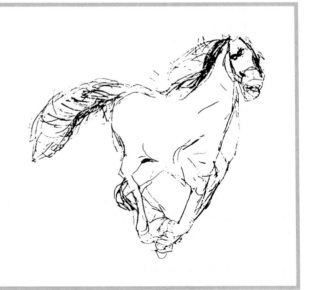

FIGURE 13.22 AN "AUTISTIC SAVANT"

Nadia is an often-mentioned example of a child who, on the one hand, appears to be severely retarded but, on the other hand, has remarkable drawing skill. This horse was drawn when Nadia was 4 years old. She preferred to draw in fine-point pen and showed little interest in the use of color. The pattern of her artistic production was also unusual: Rather than beginning with an outline, Nadia would begin with details (such as a hoof or the horse's mane) and only later connect these features.

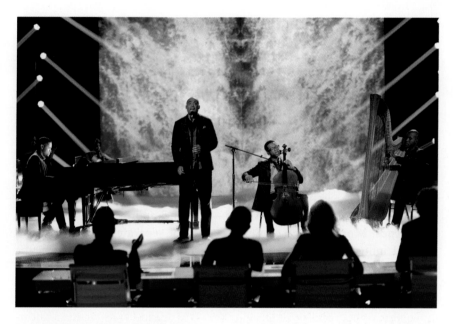

"AMERICA'S GOT TALENT"

Many types of performance can reveal "talent," and so are eligible for the TV show America's Got Talent. Even so, most people make a distinction between "talent" and "intelligence," and Gardner's proposal for "multiple intelligences" deliberately blurs this distinction.

But let's also be clear that Gardner's conception shouldn't be understood as a challenge to conventional intelligence testing. Some of the capacities he highlights are measured by standard tests. More broadly, IQ tests were never designed to measure all human talents—and so it is no surprise that, say, these tests tell us little about musical intelligence or bodily-kinesthetic intelligence. These other talents are themselves important, but that takes nothing away from the importance of the capacities measured by IQ tests—capacities that (as we've seen) are needed for many aspects of life.

Finally, there's room for debate about whether the capacities showcased by Gardner (or, for that matter, the capacity labeled "emotional intelligence") should be thought of as forms of "intelligence." In ordinary conversation, we mean something different if we talk about an "intelligent" athlete in contrast to a "talented" athlete; likewise, various television shows seek performers with *talent* rather than performers with *intelligence*. Should we step away from this commonsense usage of these terms and follow Gardner's lead? His use of the term "intelligence" does encourage us to give these other pursuits the esteem they surely deserve. At the same time, his terminology may lead us to ignore distinctions we might otherwise need. (For more on Gardner's claims, see Cowan & Carney, 2006; Deary, 2012; Thioux, Stark, Klaiman, & Shultz, 2006; Visser, Ashton, & Vernon, 2006; White 2008.)

The Roots of Intelligence

Differences in intelligence, we've suggested, may be the result of variations in mental speed or in the functioning of working memory. But what causes those differences? Why does one person end up with a high level of intelligence, while other people end up with a lower level?

Discussions of these questions often frame the issue as if it were a choice between two alternatives—"nature versus nurture." In other words, should our explanation emphasize genetics and heredity, or should we focus on learning and the environment? Let's be clear from the start, though, that this framing of the issue is misleading: Both types of influence—one rooted in genetics, one rooted in experience—play an important role in shaping intelligence. Moreover, these influences are not separate; instead, the two types of influence actually *depend* on each other. As we'll see, then, the "competition" that's implied by the "nature versus nurture" phrase really makes no sense.

Genetic Influences on IQ

A traditional method for assessing genetic influences begins by asking whether people who resemble each other genetically also resemble each other in terms of the target trait. Often, the evidence on this point comes from a comparison between the two types of twins. **Identical**, or **monozygotic (MZ), twins** originate from a single fertilized egg. Early in development, that egg splits into two exact replicas, which develop into two genetically identical individuals. In contrast, **fraternal**, or **dizygotic (DZ), twins** arise from two different eggs, each fertilized by a different sperm cell. As a result, fraternal twins share only half of their genetic material, just as ordinary (non-twin) siblings do (see **Figure 13.23**).

Identical twins, therefore, resemble each other genetically more than fraternal twins do. It turns out that identical twins also resemble each other in their IQs more than fraternal twins do—just as we'd expect if genetic factors play a role in shaping IQ. In one early data set, for example, the correlation for identical twins was .86; the correlation for fraternal twins was notably lower, around .60 (Bouchard & McGue, 1981). More recent data confirm this pattern (see **Figure 13.24**), strongly suggesting a genetic component in the determination of IQ, with greater genetic similarity (in identical twins) leading to greater IQ similarity.

Further evidence comes from identical twins who were separated soon after birth, adopted by different families, and reared in different households. The data show a correlation for these twins of about .75 (Bouchard, Lykken, McGue, Segal, & Tellegen, 1990; McGue, Bouchard, Iacono, & Lykken, 1993; Plomin & Spinath, 2004). It seems, then, that identical genetic profiles lead to highly similar IQs even when the individuals grow up in different environments. (For other data confirming the influence of genetic factors, see Plomin, Fulker, Corley, & DeFries, 1997; Plomin & Spinath, 2004; for some

FIGURE 13.23 MONOZYGOTIC AND DIZYGOTIC TWINS

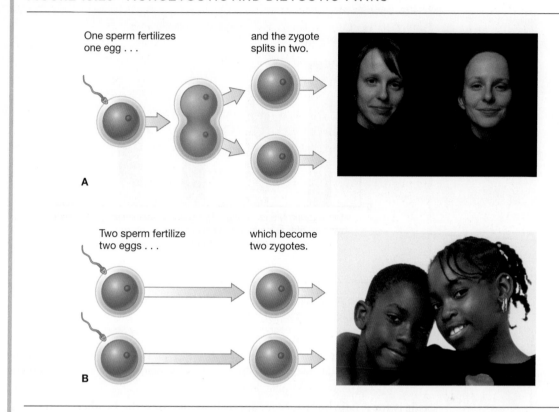

One sperm fertilizes one egg . . .

and the zygote splits in two.

A

Two sperm fertilize two eggs . . .

which become two zygotes.

B

(Panel A) Sometimes a woman releases a single egg that is fertilized and then splits into two. This sequence results in monozygotic (identical) twins with 100% overlap in their genetic pattern. (Panel B) Sometimes a woman releases two eggs in the same month, and both are fertilized. The result is dizygotic twins—conceived at the same time and born on the same day, but with only 50% overlap in their genetic pattern (the same overlap as ordinary siblings).

possible limits on these data, though, see Nisbett, 2009. Researchers have also been making impressive progress in exploring DNA patterns associated with intelligence differences; see, for example, Benyamin et al., 2013; Payton, 2009; Plomin et al., 2013; Rizzi & Posthuma, 2012.)

Environmental Influences on IQ

There's no question, though, that environmental factors also matter for intelligence. For example, one study examined the intelligence scores for pairs of brothers and found that the correlation between the brothers' scores was *smaller* for brothers who were widely separated in age (Sundet, Eriksen, & Tambs, 2008). This result is difficult to explain genetically, because the genetic resemblance is the same for a pair of brothers born, say, 1 year apart

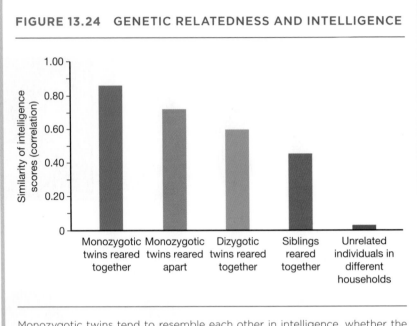

FIGURE 13.24   GENETIC RELATEDNESS AND INTELLIGENCE

Monozygotic twins tend to resemble each other in intelligence, whether the twins are raised together or not; dizygotic twins show less resemblance, although they resemble each other more than randomly selected (unrelated) individuals do.

as it is for a pair born 5 years apart. In both cases, the brothers share 50% of their genetic material. However, this result makes sense on environmental grounds. The greater the age difference between the brothers, the more likely it is that the family circumstances changed between the years of one brother's childhood and the years of the other's. Thus, a greater age difference would increase the probability that the brothers grew up in different environments, and to the degree that these environments shape intelligence, we would expect the more widely spaced brothers to resemble each other less than the closely spaced siblings do—just as the data show.

We've also known for years that impoverished environments impede intellectual development, and these effects are cumulative: The longer the child remains in such an environment, the greater the harm. This point emerges in the data as a negative correlation between IQ and age. That is, the older the child (the longer she had been in the impoverished environment), the lower her IQ (Asher, 1935; Gordon, 1923; also see Heckman, 2006). Related results come from communities where schools have closed and educational services have been unavailable. These circumstances typically lead to a decline in intelligence test scores—with a drop of roughly 6 points for every year of school missed (Green, Hoffman, Morse, Hayes, & Morgan, 1964; see also Ceci & Williams, 1997; Neisser et al., 1996).

Let's also emphasize, however, the optimistic finding that *improving* the environment can *increase* IQ. In one study, researchers focused on cases in

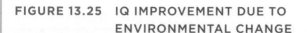

FIGURE 13.25   IQ IMPROVEMENT DUE TO ENVIRONMENTAL CHANGE

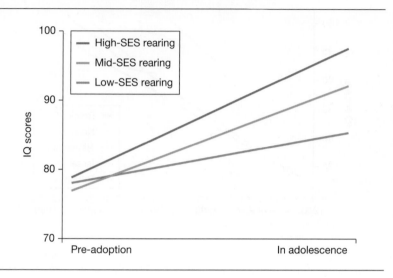

Researchers examined the IQ scores of children who were adopted out of horrible environments in which they had been abused or neglected. After the adoption (when the children were in better environments), the children's IQ scores were markedly higher—and all the more so if the children were adopted into a family with higher socioeconomic status (SES). AFTER DUYME, DUMARET, & TOMKIEWICZ, 1999.

which the government had removed children from their biological parents because of abuse or neglect (Duyme, Dumaret, & Tomkiewicz, 1999). The researchers compared the children's "pre-adoption IQ" (when the children were living in a high-risk environment) with their IQ in adolescence—after years of living with adoptive families. The data showed substantial improvements in the children's scores, thanks to this environmental change (see **Figure 13.25**). (Also see Diamond & Lee, 2011; Grotzer & Perkins, 2000; Martinez, 2000; Nisbett, Aronson, Blair, Dickens, Flynn, Halpern & Turkheimer, 2012; Protzko, Aronson, & Blair, 2012.)

The impact of environmental factors is also undeniable in another fact. Around the globe, scores on intelligence tests have been increasing over the last few decades, at a rate of approximately 3 points per decade. This pattern is known as the **Flynn effect**, after James Flynn (1984, 1987, 1999, 2009), one of the first researchers to note this effect. (See also Daley, Whaley, Sigman, Espinosa, & Neumann, 2003; Kanaya, Scullin, & Ceci, 2003; Trahan, Stuebing, Fletcher, & Hiscock, 2014; Waj, Putallaz, & Makel, 2012.) This improvement has been documented in relatively affluent nations (see **Figure 13.26**) and also in impoverished third-world nations. Moreover, the effect is stronger in measures of fluid intelligence—such as the Raven's Matrices—so it seems to reflect

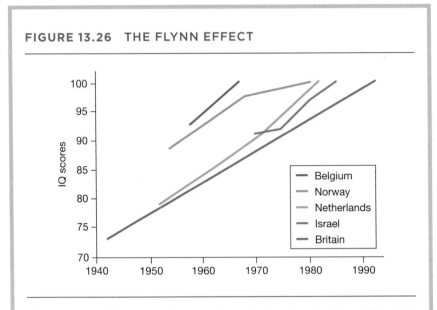

FIGURE 13.26   THE FLYNN EFFECT

IQ scores have been improving worldwide, in developed nations (like those shown here) and also in third-world nations. There's debate over the cause of this improvement, but there's no question that the improvement must be explained largely in environmental (not genetic) terms.

a genuine change in how quickly and flexibly people can think, and not just a worldwide increase in how much information people have.

There's disagreement about the causes of the Flynn effect (Daley et al., 2003; Dickens & Flynn, 2001; Flynn, 2009; Fox & Mitchum, 2013; Greenfield, 2009; Nisbett et al., 2012), and it's likely that several factors contribute. In third-world nations, improvements in nutrition and health care are surely relevant. In affluent nations, some scholars propose, intelligence is promoted by the "information complexity" of our world: Whether we're browsing the Internet or reading the back of a cereal box, we often encounter complicated displays containing many bits of information, and it's plausible that our experience with this complexity is what's helping us all to grow smarter. Whatever the explanation, though, the Flynn effect cannot be explained genetically. While the human genome does change, it doesn't change at a pace commensurate with this effect. Therefore, this worldwide improvement becomes part of the package of evidence documenting that intelligence can indeed be improved by suitable environmental conditions.

The Interaction among Genetic Factors, Environment, and IQ

We've now established two simple points: Genetic factors matter for IQ, and so do environmental factors. But how do we put these pieces together? The key here is that genetic and environmental effects don't just "add"

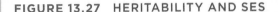

FIGURE 13.27   HERITABILITY AND SES

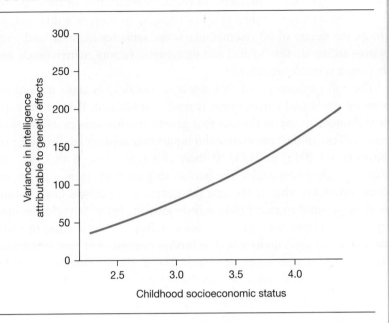

People vary in their IQ scores, and researchers have found ways to measure how much of this variance can be understood in genetic terms. The data plot here is a summary of the Bates et al. (2013) results—with variation in the genes having a much greater impact at higher levels of socioeconomic status (SES). SES was measured here in terms of parental income and occupational status.

together. Instead, these influences interact in crucial ways. This point is especially clear when we consider the impact of *poverty*.

There's no question that poverty interferes with intellectual development (Hackman & Farah, 2009; Lubinski, 2004; Raizada & Kishiyama, 2010), and children who live in poverty during their preschool years are more at risk than children who live in poverty in middle or late childhood (Duncan, Yeung, Brooks-Gunn, & Smith, 1998; Farah et al., 2006). Apparently, then, the harmful effects of poverty aren't due only to inferior education. Instead, the effects derive from many factors, including exposure to toxins found in lower-quality housing, lack of stimulation, poor nutrition, and inferior health care. All of these factors interfere with the normal development of the brain, with tragic consequences for intellectual functioning.

If you live in poverty, that's a fact about your environment. But this environmental influence interacts with genetic influences (Turkheimer, Haley, Waldron, D'Onofrio, & Gottesman, 2003; also Bates, Lewis, & Weiss, 2013; Tucker-Drob, Rhemtulla, Harden, Turkheimer, & Fask, 2011; also see **Figure 13.27**). Specifically, we've already discussed the fact that identical twins tend to resemble each other in their IQ scores more than fraternal twins do. This observation, we've said, provides powerful evidence that genetic factors play an important role here, so that people who resemble each other genetically are likely to resemble each other in their test scores. If we focus on impoverished families, though, the pattern is different. In this group, the degree of IQ resemblance is the *same* for identical and fraternal twins—telling us that in this setting, genetic factors matter much less for shaping a person's intelligence.

The full explanation of this result is complex, because the interaction between genes and environment is itself complicated. Part of the explanation, though, hinges on the fact that genetic mechanisms enable someone to make full use of the "environmental inputs that support intellectual growth" (Bates et al., 2013, p. 2111). If there is a rich fabric of these inputs, the genetic mechanisms enable the person to gain from them and flourish. If these inputs are absent, though, the genetic mechanisms have nothing to work with—and so they produce little growth. Put differently, the machinery that could promote growth is present, but with little input to work on, the machinery can't do its job. (For further discussion of how environmental factors interact with genes, see Davis, Hayworth, & Plomin, 2009; Taylor, Roehrig, Hensler, Connor, & Schatschneider, 2010; also Vinkhuyzen, van der Sluis, & Posthuma, 2011.)

Comparisons between Groups

Most research on intelligence has focused on the differences from one person to the next. There has also been discussion, though, about the differences between *groups*, with much of the debate centered on a comparison between American Whites and American Blacks. (We'll hold to the side a parallel debate about comparisons between *men* and *women*, although we do note that there's no reliable difference between the average male IQ score and the average female IQ score—e.g., Blinkhorn, 2005; Deary, 2012; Johnson, Segal, & Bouchard, 2008; Miller & Halpern, 2013.)

Studies indicate that the average intelligence score of American (and European) Whites is higher than the average score of African Americans (Dickens & Flynn, 2006; Jencks & Phillips, 1998; Jensen, 1985; Loehlin, Lindzey, & Spuhler, 1975; Reynolds, Chastain, Kaufman, & McLean, 1987; Rushton & Jensen, 2005). Let's emphasize that this is a point about averages, and there is, in fact, a huge amount of overlap between the full set of scores for American Whites and American Blacks. Nonetheless, there is a detectable difference between the averages, leading us to ask what's going on here. A large part of the answer is surely economic, because Blacks and Whites in the United States do not have the same opportunities or access to the same resources. On average, African Americans have lower incomes than Whites and live in less affluent neighborhoods. A higher proportion of Blacks than Whites are exposed to poor nutrition, low-quality educational resources, and poor health care, and as we've already mentioned, these environmental

ⓔ eBook Demonstrations & Essays

Online Demonstrations:
- Demonstration 13.1: Analogies
- Demonstration 13.2: Incubation
- Demonstration 13.3: Verbalization and Problem Solving
- Demonstration 13.4: Remote Associates
- Demonstration 13.5: IQ Testing

Online Applying Cognitive Psychology Essays:
- Cognitive Psychology and the Law: Problem Solving in the Courts
- Cognitive Psychology and the Law: Intelligence and the Legal System

ZAPS 2.0 Cognition Labs

- Go to **http://digital.wwnorton.com/cognition6** for the online labs relevant to this chapter.

The solutions to the puzzles on **p. 500** are: reading between the lines, split-second timing, search high and low, hole in one, Jack in the Box, and double or nothing.

The solutions to the puzzles on **p. 502** are: spin (spinoff, topspin, tailspin), heart (heartache, sweetheart, heartburn), glasses (dark glasses, shot glasses, sunglasses), pit (armpit, coil pit, peach pit), boat (tugboat, gravy boat, showboat).

chapter 14

Conscious Thought, Unconscious Thought

what if... This is a chapter about *consciousness*—what it is and what it's for. We can learn a great deal about this topic, though, by considering the opposite: the processes in your mind that you're not conscious of, and the mental steps you can accomplish without conscious supervision or control. For example, consider the achievement of *seeing* something, out in plain view in front of your eyes.

Imagine that your friend René puts a red rose on the table in front of you and asks, "What color is this?" You'd likely be puzzled by this question, but you could still answer, "It's red, obviously." Now, imagine that René asks, "How do you know?" Again, this seems an odd question, but with a bit of impatience in your voice you'd probably say, "Because I can see it." René, however, is still not satisfied and asks, "But how do you know you can see it?" This question is even odder. After all, how could you *not* know what you're seeing?

This (fictitious) exercise reminds us of the commonsense point that "seeing" involves some sort of "visual awareness." Indeed, think about the sentence "Linda was looking right at the moose, but somehow she didn't see it." This sentence seems to indicate that Linda wasn't aware of the moose's presence, and that's why the sentence offers a contrast between "looking" and "seeing."

But what if these commonsense claims are mistaken? Consider patient D.B., who developed a tumor in his occipital cortex and underwent surgery to remove the tumor and, with it, a significant amount of brain tissue. As a result, D.B. became partially blind and was unable to see anything in the left half of the world in front of him. Careful testing, though, revealed a surprising pattern. In one study, D.B. sat in front of a computer screen while a target on the screen's left side moved in some trials and was still in others. D.B. insisted he could not see the target at all, but when forced to guess, he generally guessed correctly whether the target was moving. Likewise, if asked to reach toward an object off to his left, he insisted he couldn't—but when forced to reach, he generally moved his hand toward the proper location. Later, when researchers showed the results of these studies to D.B., he was bewildered by his own performance and had no idea how his guessing could have been so accurate.

preview of chapter themes

- Throughout this text, we have discussed processes that provide an unnoticed support structure for cognition. We begin, therefore, by reviewing themes from earlier chapters, in order to ask what sorts of things are accomplished within the "cognitive unconscious."

- Overall, it appears that you can perform a task unconsciously if you arrive at the task with a routine that can be guided by strong habits or powerful cues within the situation. With this constraint, unconscious processes can be remarkably sophisticated.

- Unconscious operations are fast and efficient, but they are also inflexible and difficult to control. They free you to pay attention to higher-order aspects of a task but leave you ignorant about the sources of your ideas, beliefs, and memories.

- From a biological perspective, we know that most operations of the brain are made possible by highly specialized modules. These modules can be interrelated by means of workspace neurons, literally connecting one area of the brain to another and allowing the integration of different processing streams.

- The workspace neurons create a "global workspace," and this is what makes consciousness possible; the operations of this workspace fit well with many things we know to be true about consciousness.

- However, profound questions remain about how (or whether) the global workspace makes possible the subjective experience that for many theorists is the defining element of consciousness.

Patient G.Y. showed a similar pattern. G.Y. was involved in a traffic accident when he was 8 years old and (like D.B.) suffered damage to the occipital cortex. As a result, G.Y. was blind—he insisted he couldn't see, and he failed to react to visual inputs. Yet, in one study G.Y. was asked to move his arm in a fashion that matched the motion of a moving target (a point of light). G.Y.'s performance was quite accurate even though he said he couldn't see the target at all. He said that he only had an "impression" of motion and that he was "aware there was an object moving." But it's hard to interpret these remarks, because G.Y. insisted he had no idea what the moving object looked like.

To describe patients like these, Weiskrantz and Warrington coined the term "blind sight" (see, for example, Weiskrantz, 1986, 1997). Blindsight patients are, by any conventional definition, truly blind, but even so they are generally able to "guess" the color of targets that (they insist) they cannot see; they can "guess" the shape of a form (*X* or *O*, square or circle); they can also "guess" the orientation of lines. Some of these patients can even "guess" the emotional expression of faces that (apparently) they cannot see at all.

Patients with blind sight force us to distinguish between "seeing" and "having visual awareness"—because they apparently can do one but not the other. This separation in turn demands new questions about what "seeing" is and why (at least) some aspects of seeing can go forward without consciousness. In addition, what might these observations tell us about consciousness itself? If consciousness isn't needed for visual perception, then when is it needed?

The Study of Consciousness

The field of psychology emerged as a separate discipline, distinct from philosophy and biology, in the late 1800s, and in those early years of our field, the topic of consciousness was a central concern. In Wilhelm Wundt's laboratory in Germany, researchers sought to understand the "elements" of consciousness; William James, in America, sought to understand the "stream" of consciousness.

The young field of psychology, however, soon rejected this focus on consciousness, arguing that this research was subjective and unscientific. By the early 20th century, therefore, the topic of consciousness was largely gone from mainstream psychological research (although theorizing about consciousness, without much experimentation, continued, particularly among clinical psychologists). Over the last few decades, however, researchers have made enormous advances in their understanding of what consciousness is, how it functions, and how the brain makes consciousness possible. Indeed, these advances have been woven into the material we've already covered, and so this chapter can do two things at once: describe what's known about consciousness, but also review where we've been for the last thirteen chapters.

Of course, questions about consciousness are extraordinarily difficult, because we are asking about a phenomenon that is subjective and invisible to anyone other than the experiencer. Indeed, in Chapter 1 we discussed concerns about *introspection* as a research tool, and consciousness researchers take those concerns seriously. Nonetheless, we now know a lot about consciousness—and so we have made considerable progress in exploring one of the mind's greatest mysteries.

Even so, let's acknowledge at the start that there's still much about consciousness that we don't understand; indeed, there's still disagreement about how consciousness should be defined. We'll return to this conceptual issue later in the chapter. For now, we'll proceed with this rough definition: Consciousness is a state of awareness of sensations or ideas, such that you can reflect on those sensations and ideas, know what it "feels like" to experience these sensations and ideas, and can, in many cases, report to others that you are aware of the sensations and ideas. As we'll see later, this broad definition has certain problems, but it will serve us well enough as an initial guide for our discussion.

The Cognitive Unconscious

Activities like thinking, remembering, and categorizing all feel quick and effortless. You instantly recognize the words on this page; you easily remember where you were this morning; you have no trouble deciding to have Cheddar on your sandwich, not Swiss. As we've seen throughout this book, however, these (and other) intellectual activities are possible only because of an elaborate "support structure"—processes and mechanisms working "behind the scenes." Indeed, describing this behind-the-scenes action has been one of the main concerns of this text.

Psychologists refer to this behind-the-scenes activity as the **cognitive unconscious**—mental activity that you're not aware of but that makes possible your ordinary interactions with the world. The processes that unfold in the cognitive unconscious are sophisticated and powerful, and as we'll see, it's actually quite helpful that a lot of mental work can take place without conscious supervision. At the same time, we also need to discuss the ways in which the absence of supervision can, in some cases, be a problem for you.

Unconscious Processes, Conscious Products

For many purposes, it is useful to distinguish the *products* created within your mind (beliefs you have formed, conclusions you have reached) from the *processes* that led to these products. This distinction isn't always clearcut, and so, in some cases, we can quibble about whether a particular mental step counts as "product" or "process" (see, for early discussion, Miller, 1962; Neisser, 1967; Nisbett & Wilson, 1977; Smith & Miller, 1978; White, 1988). Even so, this distinction allows an important rule of thumb—namely, that you're generally aware of your mental products but unaware of your mental processes.

For example, we saw in Chapter 8 that your memories of the past seamlessly combine genuine recall with some amount of after-the-fact reconstruction. Thus, when you "remember" your restaurant dinner last month, you're probably weaving together elements that were actually recorded into memory at the time of the dinner, along with other elements that are just inferences or assumptions. In that earlier chapter, we argued that this weaving together is a good thing, because (among its other benefits) it enables you to fill in bits that you've forgotten or bits that you didn't notice in the first place. But this weaving together also creates a risk of error: If, for example, the dinner you're trying to recall was somehow unusual, then assumptions based on the more typical pattern may be misleading.

Let's be clear, though, about what's conscious here and what's not. Your recollection of the dinner is a mental *product* and is surely something you're aware of. Thus, you can reflect on the dinner if you wish and can describe it if someone asks you. You're unaware, though, of the *process* that brought you this knowledge, so you have no way of telling which bits are supplied by memory retrieval and which bits rest on inference or assumption. And, of course, if you can't determine which bits are which, there's no way for you to reject the inferences or to avoid the (entirely unnoticed) assumptions. That's why memory errors, when they occur, are undetectable: Since the process that brings you a "memory" is unconscious, you can't distinguish genuine recall from (potentially misguided) assumption.

Here's a different example. In Chapter 4, we considered a case in which people were briefly shown the stimulus "CORN"; we also considered a case in which people were shown "CQRN." Despite the different stimuli, both groups of people perceived the input to be "CORN"—a correct perception for the first group, but an error for the second.

For reasons we described in that earlier chapter, though, people won't be able to tell whether they're in the first group or the second, so they won't be able to tell whether they're perceiving correctly or *mis*-perceiving. Both groups are aware of the product created by their minds, so both groups have the conscious experience of "seeing" the word "CORN." But they're unaware of the processes and, specifically, are clueless about whether the stimulus was actually perceived or merely inferred. These processes unfold in (what we're now calling) the cognitive unconscious and, as such, are entirely hidden from view.

Unconscious Reasoning

The role of the cognitive unconscious is also evident in other settings, and here we meet another layer of complexity—because in many cases participants seem to be engaging in a process of unconscious *reasoning*.

In Chapter 7, for example, we discussed a study in which participants convinced themselves that several utterly fictitious names were actually the names of famous people. In this procedure, participants were apparently aware of the fact that some of the names they were reading were distinctive; their conscious experience told them that these names somehow "stood out" from other names on the list. But to make sense of the data from this study, we need to take a further step and argue that thoughts roughly like these were going through the participants' minds: "That name rings a bell, and I'm not sure why. But the experimenter is asking me about famous names, and there are other famous names on this list in front of me. I guess, therefore, that this one must also be the name of some famous person." This surely sounds like something that we want to count as "thinking," but it's thinking, the evidence suggests, of which the participants were entirely unaware—thinking that took place in their cognitive unconscious.

Similarly, imagine that someone is an eyewitness to a crime. The police might show this person a lineup, and let's say that the witness chooses Number Two as the robber. In Chapter 8, we explored what happens if the witness now gets *feedback* about this identification—if, for example, the police say something like, "Good; the person you've chosen is our suspect." In one study, witnesses who received no feedback said that their confidence in their lineup selection was (on average) 47%; witnesses who got the feedback, though, expressed much greater confidence: 71%. Of course, this leap in confidence makes no sense, because there's no way for the feedback to have "strengthened" the witnesses' memory or to have influenced their selection. (Bear in mind that the feedback arrived only after the witnesses had made the selection.) So why did the feedback elevate confidence? It seems that the witnesses must have been thinking something like, "The police say I got the right answer, so I guess I can set aside my doubts." Of course, witnesses aren't aware of making this adjustment—and so the thought process here is again unconscious.

But the effects of feedback don't stop there. Witnesses who receive this sort of feedback also end up "remembering" that they got a closer, longer, clearer view of the perpetrator, that the lighting was good, and so on (see **Figure 14.1**). Here, the witnesses seem to be thinking something like, "I chose the right person, so I guess I must have gotten a good view after all." Once more, however, these aren't conscious thoughts, and in this case the witnesses are being misled by some after-the-fact reconstruction.

Interpretation and Inference

These examples make it plain that unconscious processes can sometimes involve *interpretation* and *inference*. And in some settings this unconscious thinking can be rather sophisticated. In an early experiment by Nisbett and Schachter (1966), participants were asked to endure a series of electric shocks, with each shock being slightly more severe than the one before. The question of interest was how far into the series the participants would go. What was the maximum shock they would voluntarily accept?

Before beginning the series of shocks, some of the participants were given a pill that, they were told, would diminish the pain but would also have several side effects: It would cause trembling in the hands, butterflies in the stomach, irregular breathing, and the like. Of course, none of this was true. The pill was a placebo and had no analgesic properties, nor did it produce any of these side effects. Even so, taking this inert pill was remarkably effective: Participants who took the pill were willing to accept four times as much amperage as control participants.

Why was the placebo so effective? Nisbett and Schachter proposed that their control participants noticed that their hands were shaking, that their stomachs were upset, and so on. (These are, of course, common manifestations of fear—including the fearful anticipation of electric shock.) The participants then used these self-observations as evidence in judging their own states, drawing on what (in Chapter 12) we called "somatic markers." It is as if participants said to themselves, "Oh, look, I'm trembling! I guess I must be scared. Therefore, these shocks must really be bothering me." This led them to terminate the shock series relatively early. Placebo participants, in contrast, attributed the same physical symptoms to the pill. "Oh, look, I'm trembling! That's just what the experimenter said the pill would do. I guess I can stop worrying, therefore, about the trembling. Let me look for some other indication of whether the shock is bothering me." As a consequence, these participants were less influenced by their own physical symptoms. They detected these symptoms but discounted them, attributing them to the pill and not to the shock. In essence, they overruled the evidence of their own anxiety and so misread their own internal state. (For related studies, see Nisbett & Wilson, 1977; Wilson, 2002; Wilson & Dunn, 2004.)

FIGURE 14.1 THE (MANY) EFFECTS OF FEEDBACK

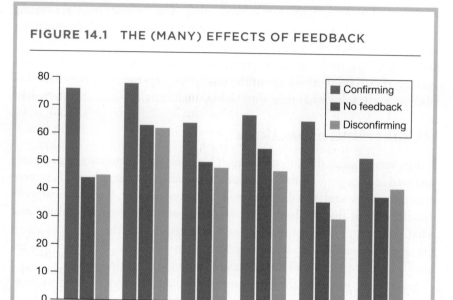

Participants in this study viewed a (videotaped) crime and then attempted to pick the perpetrator's picture out of a lineup. Later, participants were either given confirming feedback for their choice ("Good, you identified the actual suspect"), disconfirming feedback ("Actually, the suspect was . . ."), or no feedback. Then, participants were asked further questions about the video. (Confidence was assessed on a 0 to 100 scale, and so the numbers shown on the y-axis correspond to the actual responses from the research participants. The other questions were answered with a 0 to 10 scale.) Crucially, the feedback arrived well after participants had viewed the crime and after they'd made their ID selection. Therefore, the feedback couldn't possibly have changed the original event ("how good a view did you get?" or "how well did you see his face?"), nor could it have changed the experience of making the identification ("how easy was it for you to choose?"). Nonetheless, the feedback altered participants' memory for these earlier events: Those who had received confirming feedback now recalled that they'd gotten a better view of the crime, including a better view of the face, even though all participants got the same view! They also recalled that their ID had been fast and easy, even though in truth their IDs had been no easier, or faster, than anyone else's. AFTER WELLS, OLSON, & CHARMAN, 2003.

Let's emphasize, though, that this reasoning about the pill was entirely unconscious for the participants. In fact, the participants in this study were specifically asked why they had accepted so much shock, and in responding they never mentioned the pill. When asked directly, "While you were taking the shock, did you think about the pill at all?" participants consistently said things like, "No, I was too worried about the shock to think of anything else."

Apparently, then, participants were observing "symptoms," generating hypotheses about those symptoms, drawing conclusions, and then making decisions based on these conclusions; they were, however, aware of none of these steps. As it turns out, these participants reached erroneous conclusions, because they'd been misled about the pill by the experimenter. But that takes nothing away from what they were doing intellectually—and unconsciously.

Mistaken Introspections

It does seem useful, then, to distinguish between the (unconscious) processes involved in thought and the (conscious) products that result from these processes. As we've said, this distinction isn't always clearcut, but it does support a useful rule of thumb about what you're aware of in your mental life and what you're not. Thus, you arrive at a conclusion, but the steps leading to the conclusion are hidden from view. You reach a decision, but again, you are unable to introspect about the processes leading to that decision.

Sometimes, however, the processes of thought do seem to be conscious, and you feel like you can voice the reasons for your decision or the basis for your conclusion, if anyone asks. This surely sounds like a situation in which your thoughts *are* conscious. Remarkably, though, this sense of knowing your own thoughts may, in many cases, be an illusion.

We've just discussed one example of this pattern: In the Nisbett and Schachter (1966) study, participants steadfastly denied that their willingness to accept shock was influenced by the pill they'd taken. Instead, they offered other explanations—explanations that had nothing to do with the pill. Apparently, then, the participants had some beliefs about why they had acted as they did, but their beliefs were *wrong*—systematically ruling out a factor (the supposed effect of the pill) that, in truth, was having an enormous impact.

Related examples are easy to find. Participants in one study read a brief excerpt from a novel, and then they were asked to describe what emotional impact the excerpt had on them and also *why* the excerpt had the impact it did: Which sentences or which images, within the excerpt, led to the emotional "kick"? The participants were impressively consistent in their judgments, with 86% pointing to a particular passage (describing the messiness of a baby's crib) as playing an important role in creating the emotional tone of the passage. However, it appears that the participants' judgments were simply wrong. Another group of participants read the same excerpt, but without the bit about the crib. These participants reacted to the overall excerpt in exactly the same way as the earlier group did. Apparently, the bit about the crib wasn't crucial at all (Nisbett & Wilson, 1977; for other, more recent data, see Bargh, 2005; Custers & Aarts, 2010).

In studies like these, participants think they know why they acted as they did, but they're mistaken. Their self-reports are offered with full confidence, and in many cases the participants tell us that they carefully and deliberately thought about their actions, so that the various causes and influences were, it seems, out in plain view. Nonetheless, from our perspective as researchers,

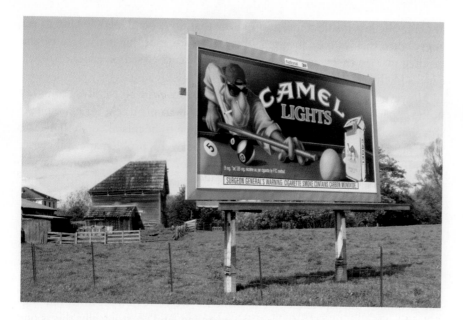

DO WE KNOW WHY WE DO WHAT WE DO?

For years, there has been debate over whether the government should regulate (and limit) cigarette advertising, based on the idea that we don't want to lure people into this unhealthy habit. In response, the tobacco industry has sometimes offered survey data, asking people: "Why did you start smoking?" The industry notes that in some of these surveys the respondents do not attribute their start to the ads; therefore, the ads do no harm; therefore, the ads should not be regulated. Let's be clear, though, that this argument assumes that people know why they do what they do, and this assumption is often mistaken.

we can see that these introspective reports are wrong—ignoring factors we know to be crucial, highlighting factors we know to be irrelevant.

After-the-Fact Reconstructions

How could these introspections get so far off track? The answer starts with a fact that we've already showcased—namely, that the processes of thought are often unconscious. People seeking to introspect, therefore, have no way to inspect these processes, and so, if they're going to explain their own behavior, they need some other source of information, and in most cases that other source is likely to be an *after-the-fact reconstruction*. Roughly put, people reason in this fashion: "Why did I act that way? I have no direct information, but perhaps I can draw on my broad knowledge about why, in general, people might act in certain ways in this situation. From that base, I can make some plausible inferences about why I acted as I did." Thus, for example: "I know that, in general, passages about babies or passages about squalor can be emotionally moving; I bet that's what moved me in reading this passage."

These after-the-fact reconstructions will often be correct, because people's beliefs about why they act as they do are generally sensible: "Why am I angry at Gail? She just insulted me, and I know that, in general, people tend to get angry when they've been insulted. I bet, therefore, that I'm angry because she insulted me." In cases such as this one, an inference based on generic knowledge is likely to be accurate.

However, in other cases these reconstructions will be totally wrong (as in the experiments we've mentioned). They will go off track, for example, if someone's beliefs about a specific setting happen to be mistaken; in that case, inferences based on those beliefs will obviously be problematic. Likewise, the reconstructions will go off track if the person didn't notice some relevant factor in the setting; here, too, inferences not taking that factor into account will likely yield mistaken interpretations.

But let's also be clear that these after-the-fact reconstructions don't "feel like" inferences. When research participants (or people in general) explain their own behaviors, they're usually convinced that they're simply *remembering* their own mental processes based on some sort of direct inspection of what went on in their own minds. These reconstructions, in other words, feel like genuine "introspections." The evidence we've reviewed, however, suggests that these subjective feelings are mistaken, and so, ironically, this is one more case in which people are conscious of the product and not the process. They are aware of the conclusion ("I acted as I did because . . .") but not aware of the process that led them to the conclusion. Hence, they continue to believe (falsely) that the conclusion rests on an introspection, when, in truth, it rests on an after-the-fact reconstruction. Hand in hand with this, they continue to believe confidently that they know themselves, even though, in reality, their self-perception is (in these cases at least) focusing on the wrong factors. (For more on this process of "self-interpretation," see Cooney & Gazzaniga, 2003.)

Unconscious Guides to Conscious Thinking

Many people find these claims to be troubling. Each of us likes to believe that we know ourselves reasonably well. Each of us likes to believe that we typically know why we've acted as we have or why we believe what we do. The research we're considering, though, challenges these ideas. Often, we don't know where our beliefs, emotions, or actions came from. We don't know which of our "memories" are based on actual recall and which ones are inferences. We don't know which of our "perceptions" are mistaken. And even when we insist that we do know why we acted in a certain way and are sure we remember the reasoning that led to our actions, we can be wrong.

Sometimes, though, you surely are aware of your own thoughts. Sometimes you make decisions based on a clear, well-articulated "inner dialogue" with yourself. Sometimes you make discoveries based on a visual image that you carefully (and consciously) scrutinized. Even here, though, there's a role for the cognitive unconscious, because even here a support structure is needed—one that exists at (what philosophers have called) the "fringe" or the "horizon" of your conscious thoughts (Husserl, 1931; James, 1890).

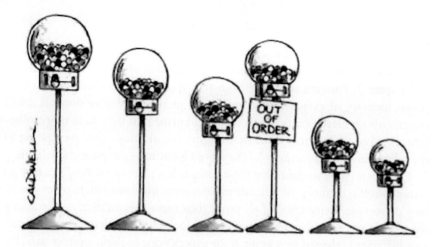

CONSCIOUSNESS IS GUIDED BY UNCONSCIOUS FRAMEWORKS

Language understanding provides another example in which your conscious experience is guided by unconscious processes. It's striking, for example, that you often fail to detect the ambiguity you encounter—such as the two ways to interpret "Out of Order." You choose one interpretation ("needs repair") so rapidly that you are generally unaware that another interpretation ("in the wrong position in the series") is even possible.

Evidence for this unnoticed fringe comes from a wide variety of cases in which your thoughts are influenced by an "unseen hand." For example, in our description of problem solving (Chapter 13), we emphasized the role of a problem-solving *set*—unnoticed assumptions and definitions that guide your search for the problem's solution. Even when the problem solving is conscious and deliberate, even when you "think out loud" about the steps of the problem solution, you are guided by a set. For the most part this is a good thing, because (as we argued in the earlier chapter) the set keeps you focused, protecting you from distracting and unproductive lines of thought. But the set can sometimes be an obstacle to problem solving, and the fact that the set is unconscious makes it all the more difficult to overcome the obstacle: A problem solver cannot easily pause and reflect on the set, so she cannot alter the problematic beliefs or abandon the misleading assumptions.

Similarly, in our discussion of decision making (Chapter 12), we emphasized the importance of a decision's *frame*. You might be completely focused on the decision and fully aware of your options. Nonetheless, you'll be influenced by the (unnoticed) framing of the decision—the way the options are described and the way the question itself is posed. You don't think about the framing itself, but the framing unmistakably colors your thoughts about the decision and plays a large role in determining which option you'll choose.

In these ways, then, an unnoticed framework guides your deliberate, conscious thinking—about problems, decisions, and more. In each case, this framework protects you from uncertainty and ambiguity, but it also governs the content and the sequence of your thoughts.

Amnesia and Blind Sight

Another line of evidence for unconscious processes comes from patients who have suffered brain damage. Consider the discussion of Korsakoff's syndrome in Chapter 7. Patients suffering from this syndrome seem to have no conscious memory of events they've witnessed or things they've done. If asked directly about these events, the patients will insist that they have no recollection. If asked to perform tasks that require recollection—like navigating to the store, based on a memory of the store's location—the patients will fail.

Even so, it's false to claim that these patients have "no memories," because on tests of *implicit* memory the amnesic patients seem quite normal. In other words, they do seem to "remember" if we probe their memories indirectly—not asking them explicitly what they recall, but instead looking for evidence that their current behavior is shaped by specific prior experiences. In these indirect tests, the patients are plainly influenced by memories they don't know they have, and so, apparently, some aspects of remembering—and some influences of experience—can go smoothly forward even in the absence of a conscious memory. (For similar data from people with intact, healthy brains, see Chapter 7. There, we saw that people can show the effects of implicit memory even when they have no conscious recollection of the event that gave rise to the memory, a pattern that Jacoby & Witherspoon [1982] refer to as "memory without awareness.")

Parallel claims can be made for *perception*. As we said at the chapter's start, the phenomenon of **blind sight** is sometimes observed in patients who have suffered damage to the visual cortex. For all practical purposes, these patients are blind: If asked what they see, they insist they see nothing. They do not react to flashes of bright light. They hesitate to walk down a corridor, convinced they will collide with whatever obstacles lie in their path. Tests reveal, however, that these patients can respond with reasonable accuracy to questions about their visual environment (de Gelder, 2010; Rees, Kreiman, & Koch, 2002; Weiskrantz, 1986, 1997). Thus, they can answer questions about the shape and movement of visual targets, the orientation of lines, and even the emotional expression (sad vs. happy vs. afraid) on faces. If an experimenter requires them to reach toward an object, the patients tend to reach in the right direction and with a hand position (e.g., fingers pinched together or wide open) that's appropriate for the shape and size of the target. In all cases, though, the patients insist they can't see the targets, and they can offer no explanation for why their "guesses" are consistently accurate. Apparently, therefore, these patients are not aware of seeing but, even so, can in some ways "see."

How is this possible? Part of the answer lies in the fact that there may be "islands" of intact tissue within the brain area that's been damaged in these patients (Fendrich, Wessinger, & Gazzaniga, 1992; Gazzaniga, Fendrich, & Wessinger, 1994; Radoeva, Prasad, Brainard, & Aguirre, 2008.) In other patients, the explanation rests on the fact that there are several neural pathways carrying information from the eyeball to the brain. Damage to one of these pathways is the reason that these patients seem (on many measures) to be blind. However, information flow is still possible along some of the other pathways (including a pathway through a brain area called the "superior colliculus" in the midbrain; Leh, Johansen-Berg, & Ptito, 2006; Tamietto et al., 2010), and this is what enables these patients to use visual information that they cannot (consciously) see. One way or the other, though, it's clear that we need to distinguish between "perception" and "conscious perception," because unmistakably it is possible to perceive in the absence of consciousness. (For more data, also showing a sharp distinction between a patient's conscious perception of the world and her ability to gather and use visual information, see Goodale & Milner, 2004; Logie & Della Salla, 2005; and also **Figure 14.2**.)

FIGURE 14.2 CONSCIOUS SEEING, UNCONSCIOUS SEEING

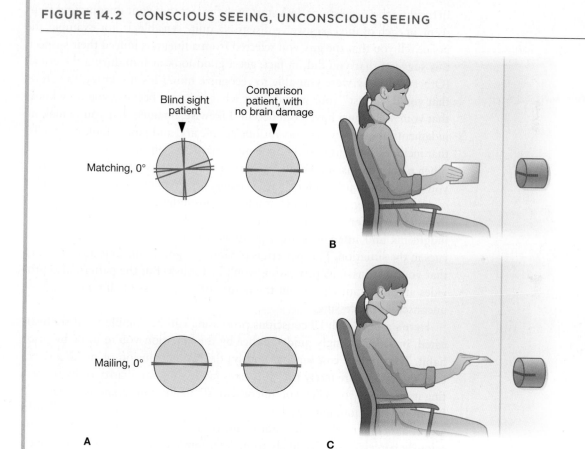

In one condition (Panel B), a blind-sight patient was instructed to hold a piece of cardboard so that its orientation "matched" the orientation of the slot. As Panel A shows, she had considerable difficulty in this task and often held the card at an angle far from the correct angle. This performance confirms the blind-sight diagnosis. In another condition, though, the patient was asked to imagine that she was "mailing" the card, placing it into a "mailslot" (Panel C). In this condition, her performance was perfect, and she consistently matched the card's orientation to the orientation of the slot. It would seem, then, that the patient is (consciously) blind but is able to see and to use the information that she sees in guiding her own actions.   AFTER GOODALE, MILNER, JACOBSON, & CAREY, 1991.

Consciousness and Executive Control

Where, then, does all of this discussion leave us? Clearly, a huge range of activities, including complex activities, can be accomplished unconsciously. You can see, you can remember, you can interpret, you can infer—all without any awareness of these activities (and for still another example, see Mudrik, Faivre & Koch, 2014). So why do you need consciousness at all? What function does it serve? And related to this, what things *can't* you do unconsciously?

The Limits of Unconscious Performance

In tackling these questions, let's start with the fact that your unconscious steps seem, in each of the cases we've discussed, quite sensible. If, for example, the police tell you that the guy you selected from a lineup is indeed their suspect, this suggests that you did, in fact, get a good look at him during the crime. (Otherwise, how were you able to recognize him?) It's not crazy, therefore, that you'd "adjust" your memory for what you saw, because you now know that your view must have been decent. Likewise, imagine that you're making judgments about how famous various people are, and you're looking at a list that includes some unmistakably famous names. If, in this setting, one of the other names seems somehow familiar, it again seems entirely sensible that you'd (unconsciously) infer that this name, too, belongs to someone famous.

Over and over, therefore, your unconscious judgments and inferences tend to be fast, efficient, and also *reasonable*. In other words, your unconscious judgments and inferences are well tuned to, and appropriately guided by, cues in the situation. This pattern is obviously a good thing, because it means that your unconscious processing won't be foolish. But the pattern also provides an important clue about the nature of—and possible limitations on—unconscious processing.

Here's a proposal: Unconscious processing can be complex and sophisticated, but it is strongly guided either by the situation you're in or by prior habit. Thus, when you (unconsciously) draw a conclusion or make a selection, these steps are likely to be the ones favored by familiarity or by the setting itself. Similarly, when you unconsciously make some response—whether it's an overt action, like reaching for an object that you cannot consciously see, or a mental response, like noting the meaning of a word you did not consciously perceive—you're likely to make a familiar response, one that's well practiced in that situation.

If this proposal is right, then unconscious processing will usually be uncontrollable—governed by habit or by the setting, not by your current plans or desires. And, in fact, this is correct. For example, think about the inferences that you rely on to fill in the gaps in what you remember. These inferences, we've said, are often helpful, but we've discussed how they can lead to errors—and, in some cases, to large and consequential errors. Knowing these facts about memory, however, is no protection at all. Just as you cannot choose to avoid a perceptual illusion, you also cannot choose to avoid

FIGURE 14.3 OUT OF CONTROL

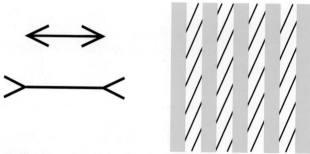
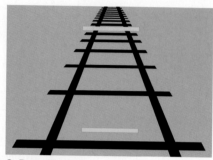

A Müller–Lyer illusion   **B** Poggendorff illusion   **C** Ponzo illusion

The inferences you make in perception and memory are automatic and unconscious—and so they are not something you can "turn off" when you want to. Hence, any errors produced by these inferences are akin to perceptual illusions—shaping your reality whether you like it or not. In Panel A, the two horizontals are the same length. In Panel B, the black segments are perfectly aligned, and so if you could remove the yellow bars, you'd see perfectly straight black lines. In Panel C, the two yellow horizontals are the same length. Knowing these facts, however, does not in any way protect you from the illusions. (These illusions are named, by the way, in honor of the people who created them.)

memory error, and (more specifically) you cannot "turn off" your inferences even when you want to. The process of making inferences is automatic and effortless, and it's also irresistible (see **Figure 14.3**).

In the same way, the inferences and assumptions that are built into object recognition (Chapter 4) are usually helpful, enabling you to identify objects even if your view is brief and incomplete. Sometimes, though, you want to shut off these inferences, but you can't. If, for example, you're proofreading something you've written, you want to be alert to what's actually on the page and not be fooled by your ideas about what *should* be there. Plainly, though, proofreading is very hard—and you (unconsciously) "correct" what's on the page whether you want to or not, and so you often fail to see the misspelling or the missing letter. (Also see **Figure 14.4**.)

Similarly, the inflexibility in routine makes it all too easy for you to become a victim of habit, relying on customary thought patterns even when you hope to avoid them. This is evident, for example, in **action slips**—cases in which you do something different from what you intend. In most cases, these slips involve your doing what's *normal* in a situation, rather than what you want to do on that occasion. For example, you're in the car, driving to the store. You intend to turn left at the corner, but, distracted for a moment, you turn right, taking the route that you usually take on your way to school (Norman, 1981; Reason, 1990; also see Langer, 1989). This observation is just as we'd expect if routine is forceful, automatic, and uncontrolled.

FIGURE 14.4   COUNT THE F'S

FINISHED FILES ARE THE RESULT
OF YEARS OF SCIENTIFIC STUDY
COMBINED WITH THE EXPERIENCE
OF YEARS.

In ordinary reading, you skip over many of the letters on the page, and rely on inferences to "fill in" what you've skipped. This process is automatic and essentially uncontrollable—and so it's hard to avoid the skipping even when you want to. Count the appearances here of the letter F. For this task, you want to read in a letter-by-letter fashion, but this turns out to be difficult. How many F's are there? Did you find all six?

The Role for Control

The idea, then, is that unconscious processes—in perception, memory, and reasoning—serve as a sophisticated and highly useful set of "mental reflexes." These "reflexes" are guided by the circumstances and are therefore generally appropriate for the circumstances. But at the same time, the "reflexes," because they are guided by the circumstances, are inflexible. (For a related view, see Kahneman, 2011; Stanovich, 2009, 2012; for an alternative view, though, see Hassin, 2013.)

In many regards, though, it's *helpful* not to have control. Since unconscious processes can operate without "supervision," you can run many of these processes at the same time—thereby increasing the speed and efficiency of your mental life. In addition, since you're not supervising these unconscious processes, you're free to devote your attention to other, more pressing matters.

But how could it be that these often-complex processes can run without supervision? Part of the answer is straightforwardly biological, and the sequence of events for some unconscious processing (e.g., the steps needed for perception) is likely built into the essential structure of the nervous system. Hence, no supervision, no attention, was ever required for these steps. For other sorts of unconscious processing, the answer is different, and it's an answer we first met in Chapter 5. There, we argued that when learning a new task you need to monitor each step so that you'll know when it's time to start the next step. Then, you need to *choose* what the next step will be and get it started. This combination of monitoring, choosing, and launching does give you close control over how things proceed, but it can also make the performance quite demanding.

After some practice, however, things are different. The steps needed for the task are still there, but you don't think about them one by one. That's because you have stored in memory a complete routine that specifies what all the

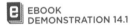
EBOOK
DEMONSTRATION 14.1

steps should be and when each step should be initiated. All you need to do, therefore, is launch the overall routine, and from that point forward you let the familiar sequence unfold. Thus, with no need for monitoring or decisions, you can do the task without paying close attention to it.

The Prerequisites for Control

In Chapter 5, we described these changes, made possible by practice, in terms of *executive control*, and that notion is still important here. Unconscious actions (whether rooted in biology or created through practice) go forward without executive control. When you need to direct your own mental processes—to rise above habit or to avoid responding to salient cues in your surrounding—you need executive control. (For related claims, see Lapate, Rokers, Li, & Davidson, 2014. For some complications, though, see Cohen, Cavanagh, Chun, & Nakayama, 2012; Feldman Barrett, Tugade, & Engle, 2004.) But what does executive control involve?

In order to perform its function, executive control needs, first of all, a means of launching desired actions and overriding unwanted actions. In other words, the executive needs an "output" side—things it can do, actions it can initiate. Second, the executive needs some means of representing its goals and subgoals so that they can serve as guides to action; as a related point, the executive needs some means of representing its plan or "agenda" (Duncan et al., 2008; Duncan, Schramm, Thompson, & Dumonthell, 2012). Then, third, on the "input" side, the executive needs to know what's going on in the mind: What bits of information are coming in? How can these bits of information be integrated with one another? Is there any conflict among the various elements of the arriving information, or conflict between the information and the current goals? Fourth, it also seems plausible that the executive needs to know how easily and how smoothly current processes are unfolding. If the processes are proceeding without difficulties, there's no need to make adjustments; but if the processes are somehow stymied, the executive would probably seek an alternative path toward the goal.

As it turns out, these claims about the prerequisites for control fit well with the traits of conscious experience and also with current claims about the biological basis for consciousness. Before we turn to those claims, though, let's consider a slightly different perspective on issues of mental control.

Metacognition

Some years back, developmental psychologist John Flavell noted that as children grow up they need to develop (what Flavell called) **metacognitive skills**—skills in *monitoring* and *controlling* their own mental processes (e.g., Flavell, 1979). Metacognition matters for many domains but is especially important for memory, and so researchers often focus on **metamemory**—people's knowledge about, awareness of, and control over their own memory.

Metacognition (and metamemory in particular) is crucial for adults as well. Imagine that you're studying for an exam. As you look over your notes, you might decide that some facts will be easy to remember, and so you'll devote little study time to them. Other facts, though, will be more challenging, and so you'll give them a lot of time. Then, while you're studying, you'll need to make further decisions: "Okay, I've got this bit under control; I can look at something else now" versus "I'm still struggling with this; I guess I should give it more time." In all of these ways, you're making metamemory judgments—forecasts for your own learning and assessments of your learning so far. Metamemory also includes your *beliefs* about memory—for example, your belief that mnemonics can be helpful or your belief that "deep processing" is an effective way to memorize (see Chapter 6). Another aspect of metamemory is your ability to *control* your own studying—so that you use your beliefs to guide your own behavior (Nelson & Narens, 1990; also Dunlosky & Bjork, 2008).

There's an obvious link between these claims about metacognition and our broader claims about executive control. In both cases, there's a need for self-monitoring; in both cases, there's a need for self-control and self-direction. In both cases, you're guided by a sense of goals—whether those goals are generated on the spot or derived from your long-standing beliefs about how your own memory functions.

Our emphasis here, however, will be on executive control, largely because it's the more inclusive process—concerned with all sorts of self-monitoring and self-control, not just the monitoring and control of, say, your own memory. Nonetheless, the notion of metacognition (and metamemory in particular) provides further illustration of the ways in which executive control matters for you and how important it is. But how are these points related to consciousness? Let's start with the relevant biology.

The Cognitive Neuroscience of Consciousness

In the last decade or so, there has been an avalanche of intriguing research on the relationship between consciousness and brain function. Some of this research has focused on cases of brain damage, including the cases of amnesia or blind sight mentioned earlier in this chapter. Other research has scrutinized people with normal brains and has asked, roughly, what changes we can observe in the brain when someone becomes conscious of a stimulus. In other words, what are the **neural correlates** of consciousness (Atkinson, Thomas, & Cleeremans, 2000; Baars & Franklin, 2003; Bogen, 1995; Chalmers, 1998; Crick & Koch, 1995; Dehaene & Naccache, 2001; Kim & Blake, 2005; Rees et al., 2002)? As we'll see, consideration of these neural correlates will lead us directly back to the questions we've just been pondering.

The Many Brain Areas Needed for Consciousness

To explore the neural correlates of consciousness, researchers rely on the recording techniques we described in Chapter 2. Thus, some studies use neuroimaging (PET or fMRI) to assess activity at specific brain locations. Other studies use EEG to track the brain's electrical activity. With all of these methods, researchers can ask how the pattern of brain activity changes when someone shifts attention from one idea to another. Researchers can also track the changes that occur in brain activity when someone first becomes aware of a stimulus that's been in front of her eyes all along.

Research in this arena makes it clear that many different brain areas are crucial for consciousness. In other words, there is no group of neurons or some place in the brain that's the "consciousness center." There is no brain site that functions as if it's a light bulb that "turns on" when you're conscious and then changes its brightness when your mental state changes.

It's helpful, though, to distinguish two broad categories of brain sites, corresponding to two aspects of consciousness (see **Figure 14.5**). First, some brain sites are crucial for your level of alertness or sensitivity, independent of what you're currently sensitive *to*. The difference here is (roughly) the difference that ranges from being sleepy and dimly aware of a stimulus (or an idea or a memory), at one extreme, and being fully awake, highly alert, and totally focused on a stimulus, at the other extreme. This aspect of consciousness is compromised when someone suffers damage to certain sites in either the thalamus or the *reticular activating system* in the brain stem—a system that controls the overall arousal level of the forebrain and that also helps control the cycling between sleep and wakefulness (e.g., Koch, 2008).

Second, a different (and broader) set of brain sites matter for the *content* of consciousness. This content can, of course, vary widely. Sometimes you're thinking about your immediate environment; sometimes you're thinking about past events. Sometimes you're focused on a current task, and sometimes you're dreaming about the future. These various contents for consciousness rely on different brain areas—and so cortical structures in the visual system are especially active when you're consciously aware of sights in front of your

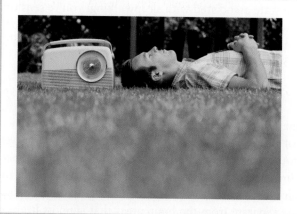

FIGURE 14.5 TWO SEPARATE ASPECTS OF CONSCIOUSNESS

At any given moment, a radio might be receiving a particular station either dimly or with a clear signal. Likewise, at any given moment the radio might be receiving a rock station, a jazz station, or the news. These two dimensions—the clarity of the signal and the station choice—correspond roughly to the two aspects of consciousness described in the text.

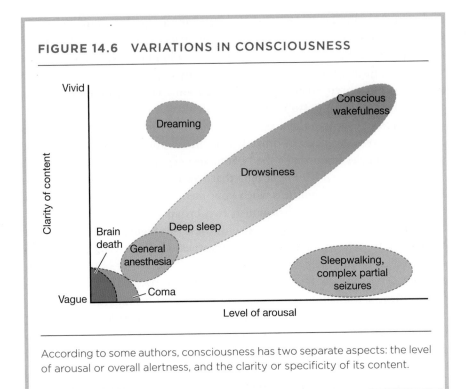

FIGURE 14.6 VARIATIONS IN CONSCIOUSNESS

According to some authors, consciousness has two separate aspects: the level of arousal or overall alertness, and the clarity or specificity of its content.

eyes (or aware of a visual image that you have created); cortical structures in the forebrain are essential when you're thinking about a stimulus that is no longer present in your environment; and so on.

The broad distinction between the *degree of awareness* and the *content of consciousness* is helpful, therefore, when we consider the diversity of brain areas involved in consciousness. This distinction is also useful in thinking about *variations* in consciousness, as suggested by **Figure 14.6** (after Laureys, 2005; also Koch, 2008). In dreaming, for example, you are conscious of a richly detailed scene, with its various sights and sounds and events, and so there is a well-defined content, but your sensitivity to the environment is low. In contrast, in the mental state associated with sleepwalking, you're sensitive to certain aspects of the world so that you can, for example, navigate through the environment, but you seem to have no particular thoughts in mind, and so the content of your consciousness is not well defined.

The Neuronal Workspace

But what is it in the brain that makes consciousness possible at all? Researchers have offered a variety of proposals, but many investigators endorse one version or another of the **neuronal workspace hypothesis.** In broad outline, here is the proposal. As we first discussed in Chapter 2, different areas within the brain seem highly specialized in their function. The brain areas that make vision possible, for example, are separate from the brain areas that support hearing.

Even within vision, the various aspects of perception each depend on their own brain sites, with one area being specialized for the perception of color, another for the perception of movement, another for the perception of faces, and so on.

We have already said, though, that these various brain sites need somehow to communicate with one another, so that the elements processed by different sites can be assembled into an integrated package. After all, you don't perceive *round + red + moving*; you instead perceive *falling apple*. You don't perceive *rectangular + white + still*; you instead perceive *book page*. In earlier chapters, we referred to this as the *binding problem*—the task of linking together the different aspects of experience in order to create a coherent whole.

We also said early on that attention plays a key role in this integration—that is, in solving the binding problem. Thus, a moving stimulus in front of your eyes will trigger a response in one brain area; a red stimulus will trigger a response in another area. In the *absence* of attention, these two neural responses will be independent of each other. However, if you're paying attention to a single stimulus that is red and moving, the neurons in these two systems fire in synchrony (see Chapter 3; also Kolb & Whishaw, 2008; Salazar, Dotson, Bressler, & Gray, 2012; Thompson & Varela, 2001). When neurons fire in this coordinated fashion, the brain seems to register this activity as a linkage among the different processing areas. As a result, these attributes are bound together, so that you end up correctly perceiving the stimulus as a unified whole.

This synchronization requires communication, so that neurons in one brain area can influence (and be influenced by) neurons in other, perhaps distant, brain areas. This communication is made possible by "workspace neurons," neurons that literally connect one area of the brain to another. Let's emphasize, though, that the process of carrying information back and forth via the workspace neurons is selective, so it's certainly not the case that every bit of neural activity gets linked to every other bit. Instead, various mechanisms create a *competition* among different brain processes, and the "winner" in this competition (typically, the most active process) is communicated to other brain areas, while other information is not.

Which elements will "win" in this competition? Again, attention is crucial: When you pay attention to a stimulus, this involves (among other neural steps) activity in the prefrontal cortex that can *sustain* and *amplify* the activity in other neural systems (Maia & Cleeremans, 2005). This will obviously shape how the competition plays out. By increasing activity in one area or another, attention ensures that this area wins the competition—and thus ensures that information from this area is broadcast to other brain sites.

Notice, then, that the information flow from each brain area to all the others is *limited*; this point is guaranteed by the competition. At the same time, the information flow is also *controllable*, by virtue of what you choose to pay attention to.

With this backdrop, we're ready for our hypothesis: The integrated activity, made possible by the workspace neurons, provides the biological basis for consciousness. The workspace neurons themselves don't carry the *content* of

FIGURE 14.7 THE CENTERPIECE OF THE WORKSPACE?

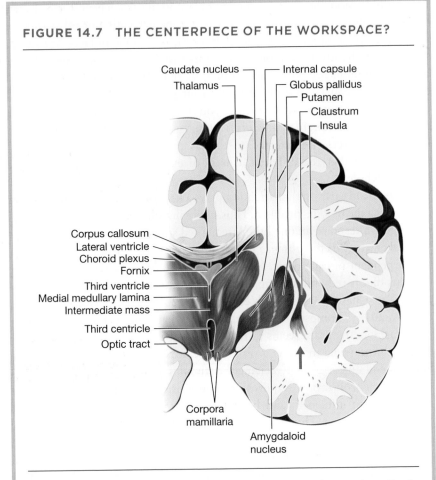

Researchers have offered several versions of the workspace hypothesis. According to one version, a brain structure called the *claustrum* (shown in blue) is crucial for the workspace. The claustrum is a structure that receives input from, and sends signals back to, virtually all regions of the cortex. This structure is therefore a plausible candidate for a structure that serves to integrate information from many different sites in the brain.

consciousness; the content—the sense of seeing something red, the sense of seeing something moving—is represented in the same neurons, the same processing modules, that analyzed the perceptual information in the first place. But what the workspace neurons do is glue these bits together, creating a unified experience and promoting the exchange of information from one module to the next. (For some of the specific versions of this hypothesis, see Baars, 2005; Baars & Franklin, 2003; Cooney & Gazzaniga, 2003; Crick & Koch, 2003; Dehaene & Changeux, 2011; Dehaene & Naccache, 2001; Engel & Singer, 2001; Maia & Cleeremans, 2005; Roser & Gazzaniga, 2004; also see **Figure 14.7**. We should mention, though, that some researchers have offered alternatives to the workspace conception, although most of these alternatives also emphasize mechanisms that can coordinate and integrate distinct processing modules; see, for example, Morsella & Bargh, 2011; Morsella, Krieger, & Bargh, 2010.)

The Function of the Neuronal Workspace

Again, let's pause to outline the proposal that's before us. Any idea—whether it's an idea about a stimulus in front of your eyes or an idea drawn from memory—is represented in the brain by means of a widespread pattern of activity, with different parts of the brain each representing just one of the idea's elements. You become *aware of* that idea, though, when these various elements are linked to one another in a single overarching representation made possible by the workspace.

What does this linkage do for you? What does it make possible? And how is all of this related to our earlier comments about executive control or metacognition? Let's start with some basic facts about conscious experience. It's important, first, that your experience feels unitary and coherent: As we've noted in other contexts, you're not aware of orange and also aware of movement, and of roundness, and of closeness. Instead, you are aware of a single experience in which the basketball is flying toward you. This integrated coherence, of course, is just what the workspace allows: one representation, constructed from the coordinated activity of many processing components (Roser & Gazzaniga, 2004).

Likewise, we emphasized in Chapter 5 that conscious experience is *selective*. In other words, you're conscious of only a narrow slice of the objects and events in your world, so that you might focus on the rose's color but fail to notice its thorns, or a driver might be so absorbed in a phone call that he misses his exit. Moreover, you can typically *choose* what you're going to focus on (so that you might, when picking up the rose, decide to pay attention to those thorns). These observations, too, are easily accommodated by the workspace model: The information carried by the workspace neurons is, we've said, governed by a competition (and so is limited) and also shaped by how you focus attention. In this way, the properties of the workspace readily map onto the properties of your experience.

Let's also note that attention both amplifies *and sustains* neural activity. As a result, the workspace, supported by attention, enables you to maintain mental representations in an active state for an extended period of time. Thus, the workspace makes it possible for you to continue thinking about a stimulus or an idea even after the specific trigger for that idea has been removed. This point enables us to link the workspace proposal to claims about working memory (Chapter 6) and to the brain areas associated with working memory's function—specifically, the prefrontal cortex (or PFC; Goldman-Rakic, 1987). (For other evidence linking activation in the PFC to conscious awareness, see McIntosh, Rajah, & Lobaugh, 1999; Miller & Cohen, 2001.) This connection seems appropriate, since working memory is, of course, the memory that holds materials you're currently *working on*, and this presumably means materials currently within your conscious awareness. (For some possible complications, though, in the linkage between consciousness and working memory, see Soto & Silvanto, 2014.)

The Neuronal Workspace and Executive Control

What is the connection between the neuronal workspace and executive control? Bear in mind that the workspace enables you to integrate what's going on in one neural system with what's going on in others. This integration allows you to reflect on relationships among various inputs or ideas; it also allow you to produce new combinations of ideas and new combinations of operations. Thus, the neural mechanisms underlying consciousness are just the right sort to help you to produce novel thoughts, thoughts in which you can rise above habit or routine. In this way, the workspace provides a plausible neural basis for executive functioning and, with this, enables you to escape the *limits* (discussed earlier) that seem to characterize unconscious processing.

The workspace also provides another crucial function. As we've noted, unconscious processes are generally inflexible, and so (for example) if there's a conflict between habit and current goals, this has little influence on the process. In contrast, conscious thought *is* guided by a sense of your goals, and it can launch exactly the behavior that will lead to those goals.

How does the workspace support this sensitivity to current goals? By linking the various processing modules, the workspace makes it possible to compare what's going on in one module with what's going on elsewhere in the brain, and this activity allows you to detect conflict—if, for example, two simultaneous stimuli are triggering incompatible responses, or if a stimulus is triggering a response incompatible with your goals. This detection, in turn, enables you to shift processing in one system (again, by adjusting how you pay attention) in light of what is going on in other systems.

In fact, this capacity to detect conflict may itself be supported by brain mechanisms specialized for just this function. One area that is crucial for this conflict detection is the **anterior cingulate cortex (ACC)**, a structure linked to (and slightly behind) the frontal cortex and also connected to structures (including the amygdala, nucleus accumbens, and hypothalamus) that play pivotal roles in emotion, motivation, and feelings of reward (Botvinick, Cohen, & Carter, 2004; van Veen & Carter, 2006). (For more on the link between the ACC and conscious awareness, see Dehaene et al., 2003; but for some complications, see Mayr, 2004.)

The neuronal workspace idea also helps us with another puzzle—a shift in consciousness that every one of us experiences virtually every day: specifically, the difference between being *awake* and being *asleep*. When you're asleep (and not dreaming), you're not conscious of the passing of time, not conscious of any ongoing stream of thought, and not conscious of many events taking place in your vicinity. This is not, however, because the brain is inactive during sleep; activity in the sleeping brain is, in fact, quite intense. What, then, is the difference between the sleeping brain and the "awake brain"? Evidence suggests that when you're asleep (and not dreaming), communication breaks down among different parts of the cortex, so that the brain's various activities are not coordinated with one another. The obvious suggestion, then, is that this communication (mediated by the neuronal

FIGURE 14.8   VARIOUS "NON-CONSCIOUS" STATES

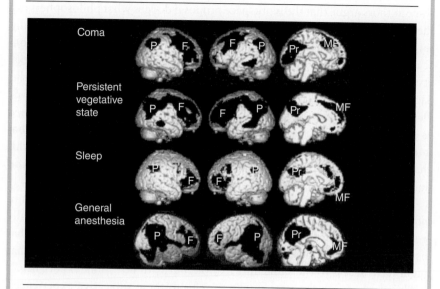

Coma

Persistent vegetative state

Sleep

General anesthesia

There are many states in which a person suffers an interruption of consciousness. Researchers have therefore asked: What brain sites are compromised in these various states? As can be seen, wide tracts of the brain are involved, including prefrontal tissue (F), parietal tissue (P), and other regions as well.

workspace) is crucial for consciousness, so it makes sense that sleeping people, having temporarily lost this communication, are not conscious of their state or their circumstances (Massimini et al., 2005). (For a similar account of the loss of consciousness during surgical anesthesia, see Alkire, Hudetz, & Tononi, 2008; for more on other "states" of consciousness, see Gleitman, Gross, & Reisberg, 2011; also see **Figure 14.8**.)

The Role of Phenomenal Experience

In several ways, therefore, we can draw parallels between the functioning of the neuronal workspace and the traits and capacities of consciousness. We can also link our claims about the workspace to the needs of executive control. The workspace, for example, supports the comparisons among processing streams that enable the executive to monitor mental processes; the workspace also supports the sustained neural activity that makes it possible for the executive to keep its goals and plans in view. The mechanisms involved in the workspace can also amplify certain types of activity, and this allows the executive to take control of mental events—ramping up desired activities and allowing distractions to languish.

Qualia

All of these suggestions, though, leave a substantial puzzle untouched; in fact, some authors argue that the workspace proposal dodges what philosophers call the "hard problem" of consciousness (e.g., Chalmers, 1996, 1998). Specifically, several authors have claimed that we need to distinguish between "access consciousness" and "phenomenal consciousness" (e.g., Block, 1997, 2005; Block et al., 2014; Bronfman, Brezis, Jacobson, & Usher, 2014; Koulder, de Gardelle, Sackur & Dupoux, 2010; Paller & Suzuki, 2014; but also see Cohen & Dennett, 2011; Lau & Rosenthal, 2011). Access consciousness can be defined as one's sensitivity to certain types of information (and thus one's *access* to that information). Discussions of consciousness (like our discussion so far in this chapter) generally emphasize the function of this access—that is, what you can do if you have this access, and what you can't do *without* this access.

Phenomenal consciousness, in contrast, isn't about the use or function of information. Instead, this sort of consciousness centers on what it actually *feels like* to have certain experiences—that is, the subjective experience that distinguishes a conscious being from a "zombie" (or robot or computer) that might have access to the same information, but with no "inner experience."

Philosophers use the term **qualia** to refer to these subjective experiences. ("Qualia" is the plural form of the word; the singular is "quale," pronounced KWAH-lee.) As an example, imagine meeting some unfortunate soul who has never tasted chocolate. You could offer this person a detailed and vivid description of what chocolate tastes like. You could compare chocolate's flavor to various other flavors. You might even provide this person with a full account of chocolate's impact on the nervous system (which receptors on the tongue are activated, and so on). What you could not do, however, is convey the subjective first-person experience of just what chocolate tastes like. In other words, you could provide this person with lots of information, but not the *quale* of chocolate taste.

There are many questions to ask about qualia. For example, philosophers have wondered whether any one of us can ever understand the qualia experienced by other people—a question, in essence, about whether you experience the world in the same way I do (see **Figure 14.9**). Neuroscientists might ask how the nervous system produces qualia—how does biological tissue give rise to subjective states? But a cognitive psychologist might ask: How do qualia matter in shaping mental processes?

Processing Fluency

In truth, we know relatively little about how people are influenced by the subjective experience of consciousness. We've argued in this chapter that the *information content* of consciousness is crucial, but does it matter how this content "feels" from a first-person perspective?

Research provides some intriguing hints about these issues—but let's be clear that these are *hints*, and claims here must be somewhat speculative.

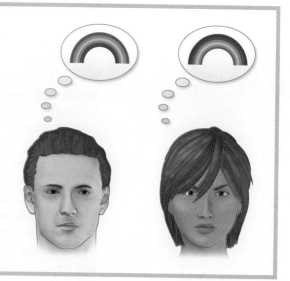

FIGURE 14.9   THE INVERTED SPECTRUM

Does each of us experience the world in the same way? Philosophers sometimes cast this question in terms of the "inverted spectrum" problem. Imagine that your nervous system is somehow "wired differently" than mine. When you perceive red, the color you're experiencing is the color I call "violet." When you perceive blue, the color you're experiencing is the color I call "yellow." Of course, you and I have both learned to call the color of stoplights "red," even though we have very different experiences when looking at a stoplight. We've both learned that mixing yellow and red paints creates orange, even though we have different experiences of this "orange." How, then, would we ever find out if your color experience differs from mine?

Surely, though, this is no surprise: Qualia are, by their nature, undetectable by anyone other than the person who experiences them, so they are obviously difficult to study. It is also possible that some qualia matter deeply in shaping a person's thoughts and actions, while others do not; as a result, research in this arena has to pursue leads wherever we can find them.

Consider, as an illustration, the experience of *processing fluency*. In Chapter 7, we discussed the fact that the steps of perception sometimes proceed swiftly and with little effort but at other times proceed more slowly and only with a lot of effort. The same is true for the steps of remembering, or deciding, or any other mental process. Thus, overall, mental processing is sometimes more fluent and sometimes less so, and people seem sensitive to this degree of fluency: They know when their steps have gone easily, and when not.

We've discussed the fact, though, that people don't detect the fluency *as* fluency. They do not have the experience of "Boy, that object sure was easy to perceive." Instead, people simply have a broad sense that their processing was, on this occasion, somehow special—and then they try to figure out *why* the processing was special. Hence, they might decide that the input is one they've met recently (and so the fluency leads to a subjective sense of *familiarity*). Or they might conclude that the name they're considering belongs to someone famous. And so on.

Fluency effects can be demonstrated in many arenas. For example, the confidence expressed in a particular memory is influenced by the fluency of retrieval, apparently based on reasoning along the lines of "That memory came to mind easily; I guess it must be a strong memory and therefore an *accurate* memory, so I can be confident that the memory is right." This reasoning is often sensible—but it can be misleading. For example, if you retrieve a memory over and over, the retrieval becomes more fluent because of this "practice," quite independent of how firmly established the memory was at the start. As a result, repeated retrieval increases memory confidence—whether the memory is accurate or not.

Likewise, in Chapter 12, we discussed the *availability heuristic*—the strategy of judging how frequent something is in the world by relying on how easily you can think of relevant examples. For example, are you in general an assertive person? People seem to answer this question by trying to think of events in the past in which they've been assertive, and if the examples come easily to mind, they decide that, yes, they are frequently assertive (Schwarz et al., 1991). So here, too, fluency of retrieval guides your thoughts. (For more on fluency, including the diversity of fluency effects, see Alter & Oppenheimer, 2006; Besken & Mulligan, 2014; Griffin, Gonzalez, Koehler, & Gilovich, 2012; Kahneman, 2011; Lanska, Old, & Westerman, 2013; Oppenheimer, 2005, 2008; Oppenheimer & Alter, 2014; Oppenheimer & Frank, 2007.)

Fluency is certainly different from the more commonly discussed examples of qualia: the raw experience of tasting chocolate, or the experience of itch, or red. Even so, you do notice and react to your own fluency—and so this does seem to be an element of your mental life that you're conscious of. And just as with other qualia, you can experience your own fluency but no one else can, and you can't experience anyone else's fluency. It's also important that we can describe the subjective experience of fluency only in rough terms—talking about someone "resonating" to an input or suggesting that a visual stimulus somehow "rings a bell." To go beyond these descriptions, we need to rely on the fact that each of us knows what fluency feels like, because we've all experienced fluent processing and we've all experienced processing that's not fluent. Each of these points is a trait of qualia, so research on fluency may provide important insights about how and when people are influenced by this entirely personal, entirely subjective, aspect of conscious experience.

Consciousness as Justification for Action

Other evidence hints at a different role for the actual experience of consciousness—a role in promoting, and perhaps allowing, *spontaneous* and *intentional* behavior (Dehaene & Naccache, 2001). To understand this point, consider the blind-sight patients. We've emphasized the fact that these patients are sensitive to visual information, and this tells us something important: Apparently, some aspects of vision can go forward with no conscious awareness and with no conscious supervision. But it's also striking that these patients insist that they are blind, and their behaviors are consistent with this self-assessment: They are fearful of walking across a room (lest they bump into something), they fail to react to many stimuli, and so on.

Note the puzzle here. If, as it seems, these patients can see (at least to some extent), why don't they *use* the information that they gain by vision—for example, to guide their reaching or to navigate across the room? The evidence suggests that these patients see enough so that they reach correctly when they do reach. Why, then, don't they reach out on their own? Why do they reach (in the right direction, with the right hand shape) only when the experimenter insists that they try? Is it possible that perceptual information has to be *conscious* before a person puts that information to use? (For further discussion of this puzzle, see Dennett, 1992; Goodale & Milner, 2004; Weiskrantz, 1997.)

Roughly the same questions can be asked about people who suffer from amnesia. We've emphasized how much amnesic patients do remember, when properly tested (i.e., with tests of implicit memory). But it's also important that people with amnesia do not use this (implicitly) remembered information. Thus, for example, amnesic patients will insist that they don't know the route to the hospital cafeteria, so they won't go to the cafeteria on their own. However, if we demand that they *guess* which way to turn to get to the cafeteria, they typically guess correctly. Once again, therefore, we might ask: Why don't the amnesic patients spontaneously use their (implicit) memories? Why do they reveal their knowledge only when we insist that they guess? Is it possible that remembered information has to be conscious before it is put to use?

Similar questions arise when we consider data from people with no brain damage—such as ordinary college students. Participants in one study were shown a list of words and then, later, were tested in either of two ways (Graf, Mandler, & Haden, 1982). Some were explicitly asked to recall the earlier list and were given word stems as cues: "What word on the prior list began 'CLE'?" Other participants were tested indirectly: "Tell me the first word that comes to mind beginning 'CLE.'"

The results show rather poor memory in the explicit test but much better performance in the implicit test. This observation echoes many findings we have reviewed. You often have implicit memories for episodes you have explicitly forgotten. But note that there's something peculiar in this result. In the explicit test, participants could, in principle, have proceeded this way: "I don't recall any words from the list beginning with 'CLE.' Perhaps I'll just guess. Let's see: What words come to mind that begin with 'CLE'?" In this way, participants could use their implicit memory to supplement what they remember explicitly. If they did this, the performance difference between the two conditions would be erased; performance on the explicit test would be just as good as performance on the implicit test. Given the results, however, participants are obviously not using this strategy. For some reason, participants in this situation seem unable or unwilling to use their implicit memories to guide explicit responding.

What is going on in all of these cases? Here is one plausible answer. In many situations, you need to take action based on remembered or perceived information. In some settings, the action is overt (walking across the room or making a verbal response); at other times, the action is mental (reaching a decision or drawing a conclusion). In all cases, though, it seems not enough merely to have access to the relevant information. In addition, you also seem to need some justification, some reason, to take the information seriously.

To make this point concrete, imagine that you're trying to remember some prior event, and some misty thoughts about that event come to mind. You vaguely recall that friends were present on the target occasion; you have a dim idea that food was served. You might hesitate to voice these thoughts, though, because you're not convinced that these thoughts are *memories*. (Perhaps they're chance associations or dreams you once had.) Thus, you will report your memory only if you're satisfied that you are, in fact, remembering. In other words, in order to report on your recollection, you need more than the remembered information. You also need some reason to believe that the remembered information is credible.

How do you decide whether to trust your recollection or not? The answer, perhaps, is conscious experience. In other words, perhaps you'll take action based on some information only if the information "feels right"—that is, only if it has the right qualia. If the experience has these qualities, this convinces you that the presented information is more than a passing fantasy, more than a chance association, and so you take the information seriously. However, if the conscious presentation is impoverished (as it seems to be in blind sight or in amnesia), you may not trust the information provided by your own eyes or your own memory, so you're paralyzed into inactivity. (For related discussion, see Johnson, 1988; Johnson, Hashtroudi, & Lindsay, 1993.)

In fact, these points can be linked to our earlier claims about the neuronal workspace. Bear in mind that the workspace allows an integration from multiple brain areas, and it's plausible that this integration is essential when you're trying to decide whether to take a memory (or a perception) seriously. The integration enables you to see, among other points, that the information provided by vision is confirmed by touch, that the information gained from your senses is consistent with your other beliefs, and so on. This convergence of cues may play a key role in persuading you that the perception or memory is real, not just a passing thought.

In one of Shakespeare's plays, Macbeth asks himself whether the dagger he sees is real or a hallucination—"a dagger of the mind, a false creation proceeding from a heat-oppressed brain" (act 2, scene 1). He tries to decide by checking the visual information against other cues, asking whether the dagger is "sensible to feeling as to sight." The idea we're discussing here is similar: The confluence of inputs provided by the neuronal workspace helps provide the richness—and, plausibly, the conscious experience itself—that you use in deciding whether your ideas and perceptions and memories are "false creations" or true to reality. And it's only after you decide that they're real that you use them as a basis for action.

Consciousness: What Is Left Unsaid

The cognitive unconscious is remarkably sophisticated—able to recognize objects in the world, to reason, to draw conclusions, to retrieve information from memory. As a result, you often have no direct information about why you decided what you did or acted as you did. We've seen throughout this book, however, that careful research can reveal these processes, leaving us with an understanding of these processes that is both theoretically rich and pragmatically useful.

The fact remains, though, that you *are* aware of some things in your mind, and as we've now seen, researchers have also made progress in describing the function of this awareness and also its biological underpinnings. There is, however, still a lot that we don't know about consciousness. Our remarks about qualia have been speculative, and debate continues about the completeness (or accuracy) of theorizing about the neuronal workspace. In this chapter, we've also held other issues to the side: Can we specify what it is that changes in conscious experience during meditation or when someone is taking drugs? And how should we think about an issue of consciousness that emerged in Chapter 11 in our discussion of visual imagery? There, we saw that individuals may *differ* in their conscious experience, with some people apparently enjoying rich, detailed visual images (so that their conscious experience often includes "mental pictures") but with other people insisting they have no mental imagery at all. This is plainly a point in need of investigation—investigation that might illuminate the functional consequences of these differences and also their biological roots.

A different—and immensely difficult—puzzle centers on how the 3 pounds of the human brain make consciousness possible. The brain, after all, is a physical object with a certain mass, a certain temperature (a degree or two warmer than the rest of the body), and a certain volume (a bit less than a half gallon). It occupies a specific position in space. Our conscious thoughts and experiences, in contrast, aren't physical objects and have none of these properties. An idea, for example, doesn't have mass or a specific temperature; a feeling of sadness or fear has neither volume nor a location in space.

EBOOK
DEMONSTRATION 14.2

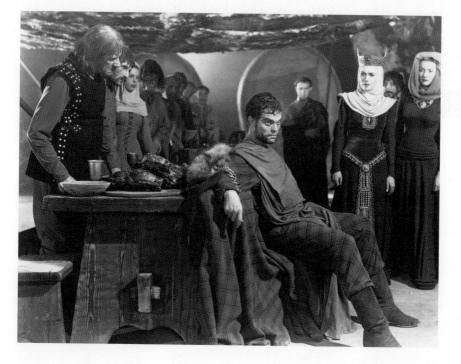

A DAGGER OF THE MIND?

In act 2, scene 1, Macbeth asks himself whether he sees a real dagger or "a dagger of the mind, a false creation . . . [of] a heat-oppressed brain." He tries to decide by checking the visual information against other cues. The proposal we're considering is that this is a common pattern—in which you check the credibility of your own thoughts by considering the qualia associated with those thoughts.

How, therefore, is it possible for a physical entity like the brain to give rise to nonphysical thoughts and feelings? Conversely, how can your thoughts and feelings *influence* your brain or your body? Imagine that you want to wave to a friend, and so you do. Your arm, of course, is a physical object with an identifiable mass. To move your arm, therefore, you need some physical force. But your initial idea ("I want to wave to Dan") is not a physical thing with a mass or a position in space. How, then, could this (nonphysical) idea produce a (physical) force to move your arm?

The puzzles in play here stem from a quandary that philosophers refer to as the **mind-body problem**. The term refers to the fact that the mind (and the ideas, thoughts, and feelings it contains) is an entirely different sort of entity from the physical body, and yet the two, somehow, can influence each other. How can this be? The mind-body problem remains a mystery. In this chapter, we've discussed the *correlation* between brain states and conscious states, but we've left untouched the much harder question of how either of these states *causes* changes in the other.

Thus, we leave this chapter acknowledging that our discussion has only tackled *part of* the problem of consciousness and has left other parts untouched. Indeed, it's possible that only some aspects of consciousness can be studied by means of scientific research, while other aspects require other forms of inquiry (e.g., philosophical analysis—see, for example, Dehaene & Changeux, 2004). Nonetheless, the data we have reviewed in this chapter, as well as the conclusions that flow from these data, do provide powerful insights into the nature of consciousness, and these data will certainly inform future discussions of this profound and complex issue. This by itself—the mere fact that research can address these extraordinarily difficult issues—has to be a source of enormous satisfaction for investigators working on these intriguing problems.

COGNITIVE PSYCHOLOGY AND EDUCATION

Mindfulness

As we have discussed in this chapter, you're able to accomplish a great deal through unconscious processing, and in many ways this is a good thing. With no attention paid to the low-level details of a task, and with no thought given to the exact processes needed for the task, you're able to focus attention instead on other priorities—on your broader goals or on the products (the ideas, memories, and beliefs) resulting from these unconscious, unnoticed processes.

The chapter makes it clear, though, that there's a cost associated with these benefits, because this state of affairs leaves you less able to control some of your own mental processes. The role of unconscious processes also guarantees that you end up being less well informed and less insightful about why you believe what you believe, perceive what you perceive, feel what you feel. As a result, with less control and less information about your own mental life, you end up more likely to rely on habit or routine, and more vulnerable to the pressures or cues built into the situations you encounter. You're also more likely to be influenced by chance associations and by the relatively primitive thought processes that in Chapter 12 we referred to as Type 1 thinking.

It's not surprising, therefore, that some people urge us all to be more mindful of our actions and, in general, to seek a state of mindfulness. Sports coaches, piano teachers, writing instructors, and many others urge us to "pay attention" to what we're doing—on the sports field, at the piano, at the word processor—with the clear notion that by paying attention we'll be able to rise above old habits and adjust (and improve) our performance. In the same spirit, instructors sometimes complain about their students performing a task in a "mechanical" fashion or "on autopilot," with the broad suggestion that a thoughtful, more mindful performance would be better—more alert to the circumstances, better tuned to the situation. Likewise, commonsense wisdom urges us to "Look before you leap" or sometimes just to "Think!"—apparently based on the idea that some forethought or some thought during an action might help us to be more aware of, and therefore wiser about, what we are doing.

These various suggestions—all celebrating the advantages of mindfulness—fit well with the argument that unconscious processes tend to be inflexible and rigidly controlled by situational cues or prior patterns. But how should you use this information? How should you try to be more mindful? You might start by asking yourself: "What is my usual practice in taking notes in class? What is my usual strategy when the time comes to prepare for an exam? What does the rhythm of my typical day look like?" In each case, you might pause to ask whether these practices and strategies developed for good reasons or simply arose out of habit. In each case, you might ask yourself whether, on reflection, you might want to modify your practices to take advantage of suggestions you've read about in these chapters or found in other sources.

It's also worth mentioning that an emphasis on mindfulness is prominent in some forms of psychotherapy. In some types of therapy, people are encouraged to pause and pay attention to—and perhaps savor—their current state, with a nonjudgmental focus on their thoughts and feelings at just that moment. This notion of mindfulness is related to (and probably derived from) meditation practices in some forms of Buddhism, and the emphasis on mindfulness seems to have various benefits—helping people to reduce stress, to deal with some forms of mental illness, and more broadly to improve the quality of their lives.

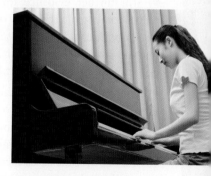

"PAY ATTENTION!"

Piano teachers, sports coaches, and many other instructors often urge their students to "pay attention." The idea here is that we often need to "rise above" our habits to improve performance.

In all of these ways, therefore, we can celebrate how much is accomplished through unconscious thought, but we should also acknowledge the potential benefits of sometimes shifting to conscious thought. Apparently, there are circumstances in which thoughtful, mindful reflection on your thoughts and behaviors may lead you to some improvements in how you think, what you think, and how you feel and how you act.

chapter summary

• An enormous amount of cognitive processing happens "behind the scenes," in the cognitive unconscious. In many cases, you are conscious only of the products that result from your mental processes; the processes themselves are unconscious. This is reflected in the fact that you are not conscious of searching through memory; you are aware only of the results produced by that search. Similarly, you cannot tell when you have truly perceived a word and when you have merely inferred the word's presence.

• Unconscious processing can be rather sophisticated. For example, implicit memory influences you without your being aware that you are remembering at all, and this influence is typically mediated by a complex process through which you attribute a feeling of fluency to a particular cause. Unconscious attributions can also shape how you interpret and react to your own bodily states.

• Even when your thinking is conscious, you are still influenced by unconscious guides that shape and direct your thought. This is evident in the effects of framing in decision making and in the effects of sets in guiding your problem-solving efforts.

• Still further evidence for unconscious achievements comes from the study of blind sight and amnesia; in both cases, patients seem to have knowledge (gained from perception or from memory) but no conscious awareness of that knowledge.

• The cognitive unconscious allows enormous efficiency, but at the cost of flexibility or control. Likewise, the cognitive unconscious keeps you from being distracted by the details of your mental processes, but in some cases there is a cost to your ignorance about how your mental processes unfolded and how you arrived at a particular memory or a particular perception. These trade-offs point the way toward the function of consciousness: Conscious thinking is less efficient but more controllable, and it is also better informed by information about process.

• The neuronal workspace hypothesis begins with the fact that most of the processing in the brain is carried out by separate, specialized modules. When you pay attention to a stimulus, however, the neurons in the various modules are linked by means of workspace neurons. This linkage amplifies and sustains the processing within individual modules, and it allows integration and comparison of the various modules. The integration, it is proposed, is what makes consciousness possible. The integration provides the basis for the unity in your experience; it also enables flexibility and the detection of conflict.

• Consciousness may give you a sense that you have adequate justification for taking an action. This may be why amnesic patients seem unable to take action based on what they (unconsciously) recall and why blind-sight patients seem unable to respond to what they (unconsciously) see.

• Several theorists have argued that we must distinguish types of conscious experience. The considerations in this chapter bear more directly on "access consciousness," which is a matter of how information is accessed and used within the mind. The chapter has had less to say about "phenomenal consciousness," which is concerned with the subjective experience of being conscious. Even so, research on mental *fluency* provides an intriguing hint both of how you are guided by qualia and how we can do research on the effects of qualia.

e eBook Demonstrations & Essays

Online Demonstrations:
- Demonstration 14.1: Practice and the Cognitive Unconscious
- Demonstration 14.2: The Quality of Consciousness

Online Applying Cognitive Psychology Essays:
- Cognitive Psychology and the Law: Unconscious Thinking

ZAPS 2.0 Cognition Labs

- Go to **http://digital.wwnorton.com/cognition6** for the online labs relevant to this chapter.

Appendix
Research Methods

Research in cognitive psychology yields results that are intriguing and useful. These results have value, however, only if they're based on sound methods and good science. If not, we may be offering practical suggestions that do more harm than good, and making theoretical claims that lead us away from the truth, not toward it.

It's therefore important to understand the methods that make our science possible. This understanding will enable you to see why our results are compelling and why we can, with confidence, draw the conclusions that we do. For this reason, this appendix contains a series of Research Methods "modules," each one highlighting a methodological issue or focusing on a research example.

Let's make a few quick points, though, about this presentation. First, these modules are no substitute for a full research methods course, a course of considerable value on its own. Even so, the methodological concepts covered here are crucial—not just for students who want to become scientists, but for anyone hoping to understand evidence (whether it's the evidence presented in this text, or the evidence you read about in the newspaper, or the evidence you hear in a conversation).

Second, each of the modules in this appendix is linked to a specific chapter. This linkage will allow you to read the modules (usually, one per chapter) in parallel with your reading of the text. I hope this configuration will help you see how these methodological points apply to concrete examples, which will, in turn, help you see why these points are so important. But, third, I don't want to distract those readers who want to focus exclusively on our field's content—and that's why these modules are in an appendix: easily available for readers who want them, but not a distraction for those who don't.

Chapter 1:   Testable Hypotheses
Chapter 2:   Control Groups
Chapter 3:   The Proper N

Chapter 1: The Science of the Mind

Testable Hypotheses

What is "science," and what is it about cognitive psychology that makes it count as a science? The key lies in the idea that science cannot be based just on someone's opinions about the world or on someone's (perhaps biased) interpretation of the facts. Instead, science needs to be based on the facts themselves, and that means the scientific community needs to check every one of its claims against the facts, to find out with certainty whether each claim is correct. If we learn that the evidence for a claim is weak or ambiguous, then we need to seek more evidence in order to achieve certainty. And, of course, if we learn that a claim does not fit with the facts, then we're obligated to set the claim aside, to make sure we only offer claims that we know are in line with reality.

Clearly, then, the notion of *testing* our claims, to make sure they match the facts, is essential for science, and this has a powerful implication for how we formulate our claims in the first place. Specifically, we need to make sure that all of our claims are formulated in a way that will allow the testing that is central to the scientific enterprise.

A scientist therefore begins by offering a *hypothesis*—a supposition about the facts that may or may not turn out to be true. Crucially, though, the hypothesis must be stated in a fashion that makes it **testable**. But how do we ensure testability? How do we ensure that it will be possible to confront our claims with the facts? Among other considerations, we need to make certain our claims never rely on ambiguous terms or vague phrasing; we also need to avoid escape clauses like "Maybe this will happen" or "Sometimes we'll observe X and sometimes we won't."

To see how this plays out, consider the claim "No matter what day of the year you pick, a famous psychologist was born on that day." To test this claim, you might hop onto the Internet and, with a bit of searching, assemble a long list of who was born on which day. Then let's imagine that as you look over this list, you realize that Daniel Reisberg is the most prominent psychologist born on December 19. Does this observation support the initial claim, because Reisberg is famous? (After all, thousands of students have read his books.) Or does it contradict the claim, because Reisberg isn't famous? (After all, most people have never heard of him.) Both of these positions seem plausible, and so your "test" of this claim about birthdays turns out to depend on opinion, not fact: If you hold the opinion that Reisberg is famous, then the evidence about the December 19 birthday confirms the claim; if you hold the opposite opinion, the same evidence doesn't confirm the claim. As a result, this claim is not testable—there's no way to say with certainty whether it fits with the facts or not.

Of course, we could make this claim testable if we could find a suitable definition of "famous." In that case, we could, with some certainty, decide whether Reisberg is famous or not, and then we could use this point to test our claim about birthdays. But until that is done, there is no way to test this claim in the fashion, not dependent on opinion, that science requires.

This example illustrates why a scientific hypothesis must be framed precisely—so that we can check the facts and then say with certainty whether the hypothesis is correct. But how do we check the facts? We'll explore this question in upcoming sections of this appendix.

Chapter 2: The Neural Basis for Cognition

Control Groups

In several passages in Chapter 2, we talk about this or that brain area as being activated during a particular activity—so that certain areas in the occipital lobe (for example) are especially active when someone is examining a visual stimulus, certain areas of the frontal lobe are especially active when someone is listening to a verbal input, and so on. We need to be clear, though, about what these claims really mean.

All cells in the brain are active all the time. When they receive some input, however, or when they are involved in a particular process, the brain cells *change* their activation level. Therefore, when we talk about, say, the occipital lobe's response to a visual input, we do not mean that the cells are active when an input arrives and dormant the rest of the time. Instead, we're saying that when a visual input arrives, the activity in the occipital lobe increases from its prior **baseline level**.

To measure these increases, we need a basis for comparison, and in fact this is a feature of virtually all scientific investigation: Usually, we can interpret a measurement or an observation only with reference to some appropriate baseline. This is true outside of science as well. Imagine that a TV ad boasts that 90% of the people who use Yippee toothpaste have no cavities when they see their dentists. Does this mean the toothpaste is effective? We'd need to ask how often people who use *other* toothpastes have cavity-free checkups. If that number is also 90%, then Yippee brings no benefits. If the number is 95%, then Yippee might actually be bad for your teeth.

In scientific research, our basis for comparison in evaluating data is typically provided by a **control condition**—a condition that enables us to see how things unfold in the absence of the experimental manipulation. If, therefore, we want to understand how the brain responds to visual inputs, we need to compare a condition with a visual input (the **experimental condition**) with a control condition lacking this input. The difference between the conditions is the **independent variable**—the factor that's varying and that differentiates the two conditions.

In our toothpaste example, the independent variable was the presence or absence of Yippee toothpaste. Let's be clear that there's just one thing that's varying in this comparison—whether Yippee is in use or not—and so there is just one independent variable. However, there are two options for this variable (with Yippee vs. without), so the one independent variable creates two conditions. (Technically, we'd say that this is one variable with two "levels.")

Likewise, if we are asking how visual stimulation changes brain activity, there is again just one factor that's varying: whether the stimulus is present or absent. But here, too, there are two options for this variable, so the single independent variable leaves us with two conditions. (In other, more complicated experiments, there might be three or more options for a variable—perhaps no visual input vs. dim input vs. bright input. Likewise, there might be more than one independent variable. We'll hold these complications to the side for now.)

The independent variable is sometimes called the "predictor variable," because our comparison is asking, in effect, whether we can use this variable to predict the experiment's outcome. (Does the use of Yippee toothpaste predict a greater chance of a good checkup? Is the presence of a visual input associated with greater brain activity, so that when the input is on the scene we can predict that the activity will increase?)

The variable we measure in our data collection is called the **dependent variable**, so that our study is asking, in essence, whether this variable depends on the predictor variable. In many cases, the dependent variable is straightforward (How many cavities did you have? What is the level of brain activity?), but sometimes it is not. We will return to this topic in a Research Methods module for Chapter 13.

We still need to ask, however, exactly how we should set up our study of brain activity, and how in particular we should set up the control condition. Imagine, as one possibility, that participants in our experimental condition are staring attentively at a computer screen, eagerly awaiting (and eventually seeing) a visual stimulus, while participants in our control condition are told merely to hang out, so that we can observe the functioning of their brains. If we found differences between these two conditions, we could draw no conclusions. That's because any differences we observe might be due to the presence of the visual stimulus in one condition and not the other, or they might be due to the fact that participants in one condition are attentive while those in the other condition are relaxed. With no way to choose between these options, we'd have no way to interpret the data.

Clearly, then, our control condition must be carefully designed so that it differs from the experimental condition in just one way (in our example, in the presence or absence of the visual stimulus). We want to make sure that the two conditions are essentially identical in all other regards. As part of this concern, we want to make sure that participants in the two conditions get similar instructions and have similar expectations for the experiment. Only then, with the independent variable being "isolated" in this fashion, will the contrast between the conditions be meaningful, enabling us to interpret the data and thus to properly test our hypothesis.

Chapter 3: Visual Perception

The Proper *N*

A researcher wonders: Who's better at crossword puzzles, men or women? To find out, the researcher recruits two friends, Jeff and Jane, and gives them each a puzzle to work on. Jane finishes 3 minutes sooner than Jeff, so the researcher concludes: Women are better.

It should be obvious, though, that this conclusion is silly. Among other problems, we've only considered two people, and perhaps Jane just happens to be extraordinarily skilled in puzzles (and not representative of women in general), or perhaps Jeff happens to be particularly inept. At the very least, we'd want more data before we draw any conclusions. In other words, we'd need an adequate number of research participants, and this number is usually referred to with the single (and capitalized) letter N.

But what is the proper N for a study? How many observations do we need? The answer varies. It depends (among other considerations) on how consistent the data are or, conversely, how *variable* the data are—that is, how much difference there is from one observation to the next. In the study of perception, for example, researchers often rely on a small N, and the reason is straightforward: Your eyes have two types of photoreceptors (rods and cones), just like everyone else's eyes. Your cones are concentrated in your eyeballs' foveas, just like everyone else's cones are. We could, therefore, just study your eyeballs and draw broad conclusions from our data.

In other cases, though, we do need more data. For example, some people wear eyeglasses (or contact lenses); others do not. Therefore, if we were studying, say, how well people can recognize a face at certain distances, we'd need to study an adequate number of cases in order to accommodate this variation.

The decision about a proper N is therefore made on a case-by-case basis. It's common, though, for studies of visual perception to rely on just a half dozen research participants, while a study of memory accuracy might rely on 40 or 50, and a study of intelligence might rely on 100 participants or more.

But how exactly do we choose an N? Sometimes we have detailed information in advance about how variable the data will be, and we can use that information to choose our N. Specifically, statisticians recommend that we perform what's called a "power calculation," which will tell us what N we'd need in order to have a specified probability of detecting an effect of a specified size. Often, though, researchers take a different path: They go ahead and gather the data, then measure (with some straightforward arithmetic) how variable the observations are, and use this as a basis for deciding, with the data now in hand, whether the N was adequate. More precisely, researchers evaluate the variability relative to other factors, including the size of the effect they're trying to evaluate. The idea here is that we can tolerate greater variability if we're trying to detect a large difference. (Fleas vary in their weight, and so do elephants. But this variability won't be a problem if we're trying to document that elephants weigh more than fleas, so our comparison will be fine with a small N—maybe just one flea and one elephant. The same level of variability might be a problem, though, if we were asking whether fleas were heavier than mosquitoes.) We also need more observations if our measurements are imprecise or relatively insensitive (and so, for example, we'll need a larger N if we're relying on a "yes or no" measure, rather than a measure that can pick up gradations that are more finely grained).

Of course, we don't just want an adequately sized N. We also need to ensure that we've included the right observations in our data set. Specifically, we usually want a **representative sample**, but on this point, too, our methods must be chosen on a case-by-case basis. If we are studying some issue for which there is little variability, then it matters less who's in our **sample**. For example, the visual system of an American college student works the same way as it does in any other human, so a sample of college students *is* representative. In contrast, a sample of students might be inappropriate if we wanted to study how people in general make decisions or solve problems.

Researchers use several techniques to create a representative sample, but a crucial tool is the use of **random sampling**—a procedure in which every member of the **population** being studied has an equal chance of being picked for inclusion in the study. With random sampling (especially if the sample is large), the investigators hope to ensure that the diversity in the population is mirrored within their sample, so that the sample really can inform them about the properties of the overall population.

Chapter 4: Recognizing Objects

Dealing with Confounds

Imagine an experiment in which research participants are asked to recognize letter strings briefly presented on a computer screen—let's say for 30 milliseconds—followed by a mask. In the first 50 trials, the letter strings are random sequences (like "OKBO" or "PMLA"). In the next 50 trials, the letter strings are all common words ("BOOK," "LAMP," "TREE"). Let's say that the participants are able, on average, to identify 30% of the random sequences and 65% of the words. This is a large difference; what should we conclude from it?

In fact, we can conclude nothing from this (fictitious) experiment, because the procedure just described is flawed. The data tell us that participants did much better with the words, but why did this happen? One possibility is that words are, in fact, easier to recognize than nonwords. A different possibility, however, is that we are instead seeing an effect of *practice*: Maybe the participants did better with the word trials not because words are special, but simply because the words came later in the experiment, after the participants had gained some experience with the procedure. Conversely, perhaps the participants did worse with the nonwords not because they were hard to recognize, but because they were presented before any practice or warm-up.

To put this in technical terms, the experiment just described is **invalid**—that is, it does not measure what it is intended to measure (the difference between words and nonwords). The experiment is invalid because a **confound** is present—an extra variable that could have caused the observed data pattern. The confound in this particular case is the *sequence*, and the confound makes the data ambiguous: Maybe the words were better recognized because they're words, *or* maybe the words were better recognized simply because they came second. With no way in the data to choose between these interpretations, we cannot say which is the correct interpretation; hence, we can draw no conclusions from the experiment.

How should this experiment have been designed? One possibility is to **counterbalance** the sequence of trials: For half of the participants, we would show the words first, then the random letters; for the other half of the participants, we would use the reverse order—random letters, then words. This setup doesn't eliminate the effect of practice, but it ensures that practice has the same impact on both conditions. Specifically, with this setup, practice would favor one condition half the time and the other condition half the time. Thus, the contribution of practice would be the same for both conditions, so it could not be the cause of a *difference* between the conditions.

If this point isn't perfectly clear, consider an analogy. Imagine a championship football game between the Rockets and the Bulldogs. As it turns out, there's a strong wind blowing across the field, and the wind is coming from *behind* the Rockets. The wind helps the Rockets throw and kick the ball farther, giving them an unfair advantage. The referees have no way to eliminate the wind. What they can do, though, is have the teams take turns in which direction they're moving. For one quarter of the game, the Rockets have their backs to the wind; then, in the next quarter, the direction of play is reversed, so it's the Bulldogs who have their backs to the wind; and so on. (This is, of course, how football games operate.) That way, the wind doesn't favor one team over the other, and so, when the Rockets win, we can't say it was because of the wind; in other words, the wind could not have caused the difference between the teams' performance.

Returning to our word/nonword experiment, we know how it would turn out when properly designed: Words are, in fact, easier to recognize than random strings of letters. Our point here, though, lies in what it takes for the experiment to be "properly designed." In this and in all experiments, we need to remove confounds so that we can be sure what lies beneath the data pattern. Several techniques are available for dealing with confounds; we've mentioned just one of them (counterbalancing) here. The key, however, is to remove the confounds; only then can we legitimately draw conclusions from the experiment.

Chapter 5: Paying Attention

The Power of Random Assignment

Is it hazardous to talk on a cell phone while driving? Many people believe it is, and they point to evidence showing that people who use a cell phone while driving are more likely to be involved in accidents than people who do not use a cell phone while driving. This association—between increased accident risk and cell-phone use—stays in place even if we focus only on "hands-free" phones. The problem, it seems, is not that you take one hand off the steering wheel to hold the phone. Instead, the problem seems to be the phone conversation itself. But we need to ask: Is this evidence persuasive?

Actually, the accident statistics are ambiguous—open to more than one interpretation. Being alert to this sort of ambiguity is crucial for science, because if results can be interpreted in more than one way, then we can draw no conclusions from them. What is the ambiguity in this case? Perhaps talking on a cell phone while driving is, in fact, distracting and increases the likelihood of an accident. But, as an alternative, perhaps drivers who use cell phones while on the road are people who, from the start, are less cautious or more prone to take risks. This lack of caution is why these people talk on the phone while driving, and it's also the reason why they're more often involved in accidents. Thus, cell-phone use and accidents go together, but not because either one causes the other. Instead, both of these observations (cell-phone use and having accidents) are the by-products of a third factor: being a risk taker in the first place.

In technical terms, the concern here is called the **third-variable problem**—the possibility that two observations are correlated, not because either one is causing the other but because both are the result of some other (third) factor. The third-variable problem is one of the reasons why a *correlation* (e.g., the finding that cell-phone use and accidents are correlated) cannot, on its own, show *causation* (e.g., the idea that cell-phone use causes accidents).

How can we move forward in understanding the possible dangers involved in cell-phone use? The problem here comes from the fact that the people who drive while on the phone are a **self-selected group**. In other words, they decided for themselves whether they'd be in our "experimental group" (the cell-phone users) or our "control group" (people who don't use phones while they drive). Presumably, people make this choice for some reason—they have some tendency or attributes at the start that lead them to the behavior of using the phone while driving. And the problem, of course, is that it might be these initial attributes, not the cell-phone use itself, that caused the observed outcome—the increased accident rate.

If we really want to examine the effects of cell-phone use on driving, we need to make sure that our "phone group" and our "no-phone group" are equivalent to begin with, before cell phones enter the scene. If we then discover that cell-phone use is associated with more accidents, we'd know that the cell phones are indeed at fault, and not some preexisting difference between the groups.

Psychologists usually achieve this matching of groups by means of **random assignment**. In our example, rather than allowing research participants to sort themselves into a group of phone users and a group of nonusers, the experimenters would assign them to one group or the other on some random basis (perhaps a coin toss). This strategy wouldn't change the fact that some drivers are careful and others are not, or that some are more attentive than others. But our coin toss would ensure that careless drivers have an equal chance of ending up in the phone or no-phone group, and likewise for careful drivers or risky ones. As a result, our two groups would end up being matched to each other, not because all of our participants were alike but instead because each group would contain the same mix of different driver types.

Random assignment is one of the most important tools in a psychologist's research kit, ensuring that groups are matched before an experiment begins. That way, if the groups differ at the *end* of the experiment, we can be sure it's because of our experimental manipulation, and not because of some preexisting difference.

With all of this said, what about cell-phone use? The evidence suggests that talking on a cell phone while driving *is* dangerous, because of the distraction. The evidence comes from laboratory studies, because it would be unethical to require people to use phones while actually driving; this would put them in danger, so it is unacceptable as a research procedure. However, the studies use high-tech, realistic driving simulators, and the data are clear: Having phone conversations while driving increase the risk of accidents. Hence, there is an important message in these data—but it's not a message we can draw from the evidence mentioned at the start of this module (the greater accident frequency among cell-phone users). The properly designed studies, though, using random assignment, make it clear that the bumper stickers have it right when they advise us to "Hang up and drive."

Chapter 6: The Acquisition of Memories and the Working-Memory System

Replication

So far in this appendix, we've talked about some of the steps needed to make sure the results of an experiment are unambiguous. We've talked, for example, about the need for a precise hypothesis, so that there's no question about whether the results fit with the hypothesis. We've talked about the advantages of random assignment, to make certain that the results couldn't be the product of preexisting differences in our comparison groups. We've discussed the need to remove confounds, so that within the experiment there is no ambiguity about what caused the differences we observe.

Notice, though, that all of these points concern the interpretation of individual experiments. However, researchers rarely draw conclusions from individual experiments, no matter how well designed the experiment is. One reason is statistical: A successful **replication**—a reproduction of the result in a new experiment—provides assurance that the original result wasn't just a fluke or a weird accident. Another reason is methodological: If we can replicate a result with a new experimenter, new participants, and new stimuli, this tells us there was nothing peculiar about these factors in the first experiment. This is our guarantee that the result was produced by the factors that we deliberately varied in the experiment and was *not* the chance by-product of some unnoticed factor in the procedure or the context.

In addition, researchers generally don't repeat experiments exactly as they were run the first time. Instead, replications usually introduce new factors into the design, to ask how (or whether) the new factors alter the results. (In fact, many scientific journals are hesitant to publish straight replications, largely because space is limited in the journals; however, they routinely publish studies that include a replication as part of a larger design that also introduces some new variation in the procedure.)

This broad pattern of "replication + variation" enables researchers to refine their hypotheses and to test new hypotheses about a result. We gave one example of this approach in the text chapter: Specifically, if people are asked to recall as many words as they can from a list they just heard, the results show a characteristic U-shaped serial-position curve. This result is easily replicated, so we know it doesn't depend on the specific words that are used in the procedure, or the particular group of participants we recruit, or the time of day in which we run the experiment. This knowledge allows us to move forward, asking the next question: What produces this reliable pattern? One proposal, of course, is provided by the *modal model*, a theoretical account of memory's basic architecture. But is this model correct?

To address this question, researchers have varied a number of factors in the basic list-learning experiment—factors that should, if the hypothesis is correct, alter the results. One factor is speed of list presentation: According to our hypothesis, if we slow down the presentation, this should increase recall for all but the last few words on the list. A different factor is distraction right after the list's end: Our hypothesis predicts that this will decrease the *recency effect* but will have no other effects. These predictions both turn out to be right.

Notice, then, that our claims about the modal model rest on many results, not just on one. This is the typical pattern in any science. Single results are often open to more than one interpretation. Broad *patterns* of results, in contrast, usually allow just one interpretation—and that is what we want. Within the broad data pattern, some of the results show the replicability of the basic findings (e.g., the U-shaped data pattern). Other results provide tests of specific predictions derived from our model. In the end, though, it's the full fabric of results that tells us our explanation is correct, and it's this full fabric that tells us the explanation is powerful—able to explain a wide range of experimental data.

Chapter 7: Interconnections between Acquisition and Retrieval

Chronometric Studies

Our mental processes are usually quite fast, but even so, they do take a measurable amount of time, and by scrutinizing these times we can learn a great deal about the mind. This is why **chronometric studies** (or time-measuring studies) play a key role in cognitive psychology. In these studies, participants are asked a specific question in each trial, and we measure how long they need to respond; hence, our data take the form of **response times (RTs)**. However, we need to be clear about what response-time data really tell us.

Let's take as an example a lexical-decision task. In each trial of this task, a sequence of letters is presented, and the participants must decide whether the sequence forms a word or not. If it does, the participants press one button; if not, then a different button. In this situation, the trials we're interested in are the ones in which the sequence does form a word; those trials tell us how rapidly the participants can "look up" the word in their "mental dictionary." Trials in which the letter sequences *aren't* words are not helpful for this question. Nonetheless, we need to include these nonword trials as **catch trials**. If we don't include them, then the correct answer would be "Yes, this sequence is a word" on every trial. Participants would quickly figure this out and would shift to a strategy of hitting the "yes" button every time without even looking at the stimulus. To avoid this problem, we include nonwords as catch trials to make sure that participants take the task seriously.

But let's focus on the trials that do involve words; those are the trials that provide our data. For these trials, we can, if we wish, think about the task as including several steps: On each trial, the participants first have to perceive the letters on the screen; then, they have to look up this letter sequence in memory. Then, when they locate the relevant information in storage, they must draw the conclusion that, yes, the sequence does form a word. Finally, they must make the physical movement of pressing the appropriate button to indicate their decision.

As it turns out, we're only interested in a part of this sequence—namely, the time needed to locate the word in memory. In other words, the *total* response time isn't useful for us, because it includes many elements that we really don't care about. How, then, can we isolate just that bit of the process that is of interest? The key, quite simply, is *subtraction*. Specifically, let's imagine a comparison between trials in which the target word has been primed and trials in which there has been no priming. Both types of trials include letter reading; both include a decision that, yes, the stimulus is a word; both include the physical movement of a button press. Therefore, if we find *differences* between these two types of trials, the differences cannot be the result of these elements, because these elements are the same in both types. Any differences, then, must be the result of the one stage that *is* different between the two types of trials—a memory look-up in the presence of priming, as opposed to a memory look-up without priming. By examining that difference, we can ask what the effect of priming is—and that, in general, is the key to chronometric studies. We are usually interested in the differences in response times between conditions, not the absolute times themselves; these differences enable us to isolate (and thus to measure) the processes we want to study.

Clearly, then, some craft is involved in the design of chronometric experiments. We must arrange for the proper comparisons so that we can isolate just the processes that we're interested in. But with the appropriate steps taken, chronometric studies can provide enormously useful information about memory, perception, imagery, and many other mental processes.

Double Dissociations

Chapter 7 describes a number of results indicating that implicit memories are different from explicit ones. For example, certain forms of brain damage affect explicit memory but leave implicit memory intact. Likewise, explicit memory is strongly influenced by level of processing during encoding, whereas implicit memory may not be. And so on.

It turns out, though, that these various results are ambiguous, and as we've seen, ambiguity is a problem for science: If a result can be explained in more than one way, then we don't know which explanation is the right one and can draw no conclusions. Hence, many steps within science are aimed precisely at the *removal* of ambiguity.

What's the ambiguity with regard to implicit and explicit memory? On the one side, we can read the results as suggesting that implicit memory is fundamentally different from explicit memory—governed by its own principles and served by separate portions of the brain. But on the other side, perhaps implicit and explicit memory are not different types at all. Perhaps they are fundamentally the same, obeying the same rules and principles. In that case, the memories we call "explicit" might simply be a more fragile version of this single type of memory, and hence they're more easily influenced by external factors such as brain damage or level of processing.

The issue at stake here is whether the difference between the memory types is qualitative or quantitative, and it's important to get this straight. Claiming a *qualitative* difference is making a claim that the two are different "species" of memory. In that case, we will need different theories for implicit and explicit memory, and we'll confuse ourselves by classing the two types of memory together, seeking principles that apply to both. In contrast, claiming a *quantitative* difference is equivalent to saying that the two are fundamentally similar, differing only in some "adjustment" or "parameter." In this case, we'd be wasting our time if we search for separate governing principles, because the same principles apply to both.

How can we resolve this ambiguity? The key lies in realizing that the facts we've mentioned so far (the effects of brain damage or of level of processing) are all concerned with ways we can influence explicit memory with no effect on implicit. It's this "one-sidedness" that allows the possibility that the two forms of memory are basically the same, but with (what we're calling) explicit memory perhaps just a weaker, more fragile, variant of this memory. To demonstrate a qualitative difference, therefore, we also need the reverse result—cases in which we can influence implicit memory but not explicit. The moment we find such a result, we know that explicit memory is not just more easily influenced, more easily disrupted, than implicit memory—because sometimes, with some manipulations, it's implicit memory that's more easily influenced.

This overall pattern of evidence—with some factors influencing one sort of memory but not the other, and some factors doing the reverse—provides what is called a **double dissociation**. A double dissociation enables us to rule out the idea that one type of memory is just a weaker version of the other (because which is "weaker" and which is "stronger" flip-flops as we move from experiment to experiment). Instead, a double dissociation forces us to conclude that the two types are simply different from each other, each open to its own set of influences—and thus *qualitatively* different.

As it turns out, we do have a double dissociation for implicit and explicit memory. Certain factors (including forms of brain damage) influence explicit memory but not implicit. (Those factors provide a *dissociation*.) Other factors (and other forms of brain damage) influence implicit memory but not explicit (so that now we have a dissociation in the opposite direction, and hence a *double* dissociation).

With all these data in view, it's clear that neither type of memory is, in general, easier to influence than the other. Instead, the evidence tells us that each type of memory is indeed affected by its own set of factors. That tells us a lot about these forms of memory, but it also illustrates the power of a double dissociation.

Chapter 8: Remembering Complex Events

External Validity

How accurately do eyewitnesses to crimes remember what they have seen? To find out, many researchers have run "crime-simulation studies" in which they show their participants brief videos depicting a crime and then test the participants' memories for the video. But can we trust this research?

In these studies, we can set things up in just the way we like. We can design the video so that it allows the comparisons crucial for our hypotheses. We can take steps to remove confounds from the procedure and use random assignment to make sure our groups are matched at the experiment's start. Steps like these guarantee that our results will be unambiguous and informative.

But one thing about these studies is worrisome: The laboratory is in many ways an artificial setting, and it's possible that people behave differently in the lab than they do in other environments. In that case, the crime-simulation studies may lack **external validity**—that is, they may not reflect the real-world phenomena that ultimately we wish to understand. As a consequence, we cannot **generalize** the lab results to situations outside of the lab.

How do we decide whether a laboratory result is generalizable or not? This is an issue to be settled by research, not by argument. As one option, we can draw on the "replication + variation" strategy we discussed in the

Research Methods module for Chapter 6. Specifically, we can see whether we get the same result with different participant groups, different stimuli, different instructions, and so on. If the result keeps emerging despite these changes in procedural detail, we can conclude that the result does not depend on these details in any way. This conclusion, in turn, would strengthen the claim that we can extrapolate from the results to new settings and new groups of people, including settings outside of the carefully designed research environment.

Another important strategy involves the effort toward making our controlled studies as realistic as possible—for example, using "live" (staged) crimes rather than videos depicting crimes, or conducting our studies in natural settings rather than in university laboratories. These steps, on their own, diminish the concern about external validity. In addition, these steps enable us to make some crucial comparisons: Does the effect we're interested in grow weaker and weaker as our studies become more and more realistic? If so, this is an argument *against* extrapolating the result to real-world settings. Or does the effect we're interested in hold steady, or perhaps even grow stronger, as our studies become more and more realistic? This pattern, when we observe it, is an argument *supporting* the extrapolation from our current data.

Yet another option is quite powerful but not always available. Sometimes we can collect data from field studies—for example, studies of actual witnesses to actual crimes—and then compare these new data to our controlled experiments. The field studies by themselves are often difficult to interpret. (We obviously can't arrange a crime to remove confounds from our comparisons, nor can we randomly assign witnesses to one condition or another. This means that the field studies by themselves often suffer from the ambiguities described in earlier modules in this appendix.) Nonetheless, we can ask whether the field data are as we would expect, based on the laboratory findings. If so, this increases our confidence that the lab findings must be taken seriously.

How do all of these efforts work out? Are our data, in the end, externally valid? There's no single answer here, because the pattern of the evidence varies, case by case. Some of our claims, based on lab findings, *can* be generalized to real-world settings—and so we can move forward with these claims. (We can, for example, offer these claims to the justice system, to help police and the courts evaluate eyewitness evidence—or, better, to help them collect more reliable evidence.) For other claims, the external validity is less clear; in these cases, we sometimes need to change our research procedures (so that they will be valid), and we often need to figure out which circumstances outside of the lab *will* show the patterns we've seen in our research. Above all, though, let's emphasize that the broad issue here—and the question about external validity—needs to be taken seriously and has to be addressed through research. Only then do we know whether each of our claims, initially rooted in controlled studies, can be applied to the real-world phenomena we eventually want to explain.

Chapter 9: Concepts and Generic Knowledge

Converging Operations

How should we study conceptual knowledge? How can we find out what your concept of "dog" includes, or your concept of "ideal presidential candidate," or your concept of "worst date ever"? As you can see in Chapter 9, our research often begins with a simple task: We can show you various pictures and ask whether each is a dog or not. We can describe various dates and ask which comes closest to your worst-case scenario.

The problem, though, is that results from this task are ambiguous. It's possible that your judgments in this task reflect the pattern of your broad underlying knowledge, but it's also possible that your judgments merely reflect your approach *to this specific task*—a task in which we're explicitly asking you to use your concept to categorize new, unfamiliar cases. Perhaps, therefore, we'd get a different pattern if we give you some other task—for example, one that had you thinking about familiar cases, rather than cases we've made up. If so, then our first data set is providing only a partial portrait of your conceptual knowledge and might not tell us much about how you use this knowledge in other settings.

The issue here is once again ambiguity and the idea (which we've now met many times) that we can draw no conclusions if our results are ambiguous. To address this particular form of ambiguity, though, the path forward should be obvious: We can ask what happens if we give you a new concept task, perhaps one that involves familiar cases or one that doesn't explicitly require categorization. If the data pattern changes, we know that the first data set was shaped by the task itself. If the data pattern holds steady, we draw the opposite conclusion—namely, that we have succeeded in revealing the general character of your conceptual knowledge, a profile that would show up no matter how, on a particular occasion, you were using that knowledge.

This sort of issue arises throughout cognitive psychology. Of course, in some cases we do want to know how people perform a specific task—how they solve a particular type of problem or retrieve a certain type of information from memory. In many other cases, though, we're interested in people's underlying knowledge pattern, independent of how they've accessed the knowledge in a specific setting. Likewise, we're often interested in strategies that (we believe) are used in a wide variety of tasks, not just for the task we've set for our participants in a particular experiment.

These questions are especially prominent in the study of concepts. Here, we're trying to develop theories about conceptual knowledge itself, rather than theories about how this knowledge happens to be used on some special occasion or in some specialized context. It's crucial, therefore, that we test our claims with a diverse set of paradigms and a diverse set of stimuli. What we're hoping for, of course, is that we'll get similar patterns despite this variation in procedures. Technically speaking, we're hoping for **converging operations**—a variety of studies that all point toward (and so "converge on") the same theoretical claims.

Let's put all of this in concrete terms. We know that people rely on typicality when deciding whether newly encountered objects are in a specified category or not—whether a particular animal is a "dog" or a particular utensil is a "spoon." Is this simply the way people approach *this task*? If so, we might see a smaller role (or no role at all) for typicality in other tasks. Or is the typicality result a reflection of the basic nature of people's category knowledge? If so, we would expect a converging pattern of data—with evidence for typicality coming from a wide range of tasks.

As the chapter makes clear, the actual data lie somewhere between these two poles. People do rely on typicality in a range of tasks, and so the data from many tasks do converge on the idea that prototypes are a crucial part of conceptual knowledge. However, people do not rely on typicality in all tasks. And when they *do* rely on typicality, they need to supplement this knowledge with other knowledge. (We made this point in the chapter by arguing that judgments about typicality have to rely on an assessment of *resemblance*—usually, the resemblance between a candidate object and the category prototype. Resemblance, in turn, depends on other knowledge—knowledge about which features matter for judging resemblance and which features can be ignored.)

It seems, therefore, that we do find convergence from a variety of tasks: a data pattern, across different procedures, consistently pointing toward a single conclusion (namely, the centrality of typicality). This is of enormous importance for us, but just as informative is the *limit* on the convergence. This limit tells us that typicality is important—but is not the whole story.

Putting these points into a larger context, the central message here is the importance of multiple experiments, and also *diverse* experiments, in testing our various claims. Indeed, we've mentioned in other modules that it's extremely rare in science that a claim rests on a single study, no matter how compelling that study is. Instead, science relies on a fabric of interwoven studies—drawing insights from the agreements and convergence across studies, but also (as in this case) drawing insights from the disagreements.

Chapter 10: Language

The Broad Variety of Data Types

In most psychological research, we don't ask our research participants to reflect on, and tell us about, their mental processes. The reason (as we discussed in Chapter 1) is that introspection is an unreliable research tool, making investigators wary of the **self-report data** we gain from introspection. However, sometimes we do care how people feel about, and talk about, the workings of their own minds. This was, for example, an issue for us in Chapter 8, where we discussed the assessments each of us makes about the status of our own memories when we decide how certain we are about this or that bit of recall. Self-assessment was also relevant for Chapter 7, where we discussed the ways people notice, and respond to, the *fluency* of their own mental processes.

Self-assessments also play an important role in language research—with participants often being asked to make **metalinguistic judgments**. In these cases, we are not asking people to *use* language as they ordinarily would, but instead we are asking them to *reflect on* and comment on language. Why are these judgments important? Let's start with the fact that for many purposes researchers do want to know what is said and not said in ordinary language use. However, data of this sort are limited in various ways, and so (for example) it's not clear what we should conclude if a word or phrase is *absent* from ordinary usage. If Henry never uses the word "boustrephedon," is it because he doesn't know the word or because he simply has no interest in talking about boustrephedon? If Lila never uses the word "unmicrowavable," is it because she regards the word as illegitimate or merely because she's in the habit of using some other term to convey this idea?

In addition, spontaneous speech is filled with performance errors. Sometimes you start a sentence with one idea in mind, but then you change your idea as you're speaking, perhaps realizing your words need clarification or even realizing you want to say something altogether different. Thus, you might end up saying, "He went my father went yesterday," even though you realize, as you are uttering these words, that this word sequence contains a grammatical error. On other occasions, you slip in your production and end up saying something different from what you had intended. You might say, "They were I mean weren't fine," even though you notice (and regret) the slip the moment you produce it.

These speech errors are of considerable importance if we are studying the ways in which speech is actually produced. However, these slips are a nuisance if we are trying to study the content of your linguistic knowledge. The reason is that in most cases you would agree that you had, in these utterances, made an error. In many cases, you know how to repair the error in order to produce a "correct" sentence. Clearly, therefore, your original performance, with its errors, doesn't reflect the full extent of your knowledge about how English sentences are constructed.

Because of considerations like these, we sometimes need to examine language *competence* rather than language *performance*, with "competence" being defined as the pattern of skills and knowledge that might be revealed under optimal circumstances. One way to reveal this competence is via metalinguistic judgments: People are asked to reflect on one structure or another (a particular word, phrase, or sentence) and to tell us whether they find the structure acceptable or not. Note that we are not asking people whether they find the structure to be clumsy, or pleasing to the ear, or useful. Instead, we are asking them whether the structure is something that one could say, if one wished. Thus, "There's the big blue house" seems fine, but "There's house blue big the" does not. Or, to return to an earlier example, you might slip and say, "He went my father went yesterday," but you certainly know there is something wrong with this sequence. It's often these "acceptability judgments" that reveal linguistic competence.

Let's emphasize that these judgments about language are not our only research tool. Indeed, Chapter 10 covers evidence drawn from a rich set of other measures and other procedures, and in some ways that's our point here: The study of language (like most areas) relies on a wide variety of data types. Within this pattern, though, metalinguistic judgments are an important source of evidence—and they are, in particular, of enormous value when we are trying to understand what's involved in language competence.

Chapter 11: Visual Knowledge

Expectations and Demand

In most research, we're trying to study how people behave under natural circumstances—how they behave when they're just being themselves. As a result, it is crucial that we take steps to minimize the **demand character** of the study.

As Chapter 11 describes, demand character refers to any cues in a procedure (including an experiment, a survey, or an interview) that might signal to participants how they "ought to" behave. In some cases, these cues can indicate to participants what results the researcher hopes for (i.e., results that would confirm the researcher's hypothesis), and this may encourage participants to make the hoped-for response, even if they were, on their own, inclined toward some other option. In other cases, a participant might choose to be defiant or rebellious, so that cues about the researcher's hypothesis might lead the participant to do the opposite of what the researcher wants. In still other cases, a procedure's demand character can somehow suggest that certain responses are more desirable than others—so that, for example, participants perceive some responses as indicating greater intelligence or greater sensitivity. It's then plausible that participants will choose these responses to avoid appearing stupid or insensitive.

What can we do to avoid all of these effects, so that we don't guide participants toward some particular response and, instead, observe them as they normally are? Researchers use several strategies. First, we do all we can to make sure that demand character never arises in the first place. Thus, we make sure that the procedure contains no signals about what the hypothesis is. Likewise, we do what we can to phrase our questions and cast the response options so that no response seems preferable to any others.

Second, it's often a good idea to direct participants' attention *away from* the study's main comparisons or, if the study is an experiment, away from the procedure's key manipulation. That way, the participants won't spend their efforts thinking about the crucial comparison, and this makes it more likely that they'll respond naturally and spontaneously to the variables we hope to understand. Likewise, by diverting attention away from the manipulation, we make it less likely that participants will try to guard against (or somehow tune) their response to the manipulation.

How do we divert the participants' attention in order to achieve these goals? Many procedures contain some sort of "cover story" about what the study is addressing. The cover story is designed, of course, to draw the participants' thinking away from the key aspects of the procedure. But, in addition, a good cover story encourages participants to take the study seriously and also makes it less likely that they'll spend their minutes, during the study, speculating about the procedure's true purpose.

Notice, by the way, that the cover story involves some amount of deception—and this raises an ethical issue: Is it okay to deceive participants? Researchers generally take the position that mild deception is acceptable, provided that there is good scientific reason for the deception and—crucially—that participants be fully "debriefed" at the end of the procedure. In the **debriefing**, the participants are told about the deception and why they were deceived. Participants are also told about the overall aims of the research—and so, in the end, get to learn something about research and research methods.

Finally, it's crucial that we make sure that participants in all conditions receive exactly the same treatment—so that they all have the same expectations about the study and the same motivations. For this purpose, many studies rely on a **double-blind procedure**, in which neither the participant nor the person administering the procedure knows what the study is about or whether a particular trial (or a particular test session) is in the experimental condition or the control condition. All of these steps ensure that the administrator won't be more encouraging or more forceful with one group in comparison with the other or in one condition rather than another. The steps also guarantee that all participants will have the same understanding and beliefs about the study.

With these various safeguards in place, can we be sure that participants' expectations, goals, and hypotheses play no role in shaping our data? Probably not, and this is one more reason why replications (with other participants and other procedures) are so important. Even so, we do what we can to minimize the contribution of these factors, making it far more likely that our results can be understood in the terms we intend.

Chapter 12: Judgment and Reasoning

Systematic Data Collection

As we saw in the chapter, in daily life you frequently rely on judgment *heuristics*—shortcuts that usually lead to the correct conclusion but that sometimes produce error. As a result, you sometimes draw inappropriate conclusions, but these errors are simply the price you pay for the heuristics' efficiency. To avoid the errors, you'd need to use reasoning strategies that would require much more time and effort than the heuristics do.

For scientists, though, efficiency is less of a priority; it's okay if we need months or even years to test a hypothesis. And, of course, accuracy is crucial for scientists: We want to make certain our claims are correct and our conclusions fully warranted. For these reasons, scientists need to step away from the reasoning strategies we all use in our daily lives and to rely instead on more laborious, but more accurate, forms of reasoning.

How exactly does scientific reasoning differ from ordinary day-to-day reasoning? The answer has many parts, but one part is directly relevant to points prominent in Chapter 12. In ordinary reasoning, people are heavily influenced by whatever data are easily available to them—the observations that they can think of first when they consider an issue, or the experiences that happen to be prominent in their memory when they try to think of cases pertinent to some question. This is an easy way to proceed, but it's risky, because the evidence that's easily available to someone may not be representative of the broader patterns in the world. Sometimes evidence is easily available simply because it's more memorable than other (perhaps more common) observations. Sometimes evidence is more available because the media have showcased it.

Yet another problem is that sometimes certain bits of evidence are more available because of the pattern known as **confirmation bias**. This term refers to the fact that when people search for evidence they often look only for evidence that might *support* their views; they do little to collect evidence that might challenge those views. This can lead to a lopsided collection of facts—and an inaccurate judgment.

Scientists avoid these problems by insisting on **systematic data collection**—either recording *all* the evidence or at least collecting evidence in a fashion carefully designed to be independent of the hypothesis being considered (hence, neither biased toward the hypothesis nor against it). Systematic data collection surely rules out consideration of **anecdotal evidence**—evidence that has been informally collected and reported—because an anecdote may represent a highly atypical case or may provide only one person's description of the data, with no way for us to know if the description is accurate or not. Anecdotal evidence is also easily swayed by confirmation bias: The anecdote describes just one observation, raising questions about how the observation was selected. The obvious concern is that the anecdotal case was noticed, remembered, and then reported merely because it fits well with prejudices the reporter had at the outset!

These points seem straightforward, but they have many implications, including implications for how we choose our participants (we can't just gather data from people likely to support our views) and for how we design our procedures. The requirement of systematic data collection also shapes how the data will be recorded. For example, we cannot rely on our memory for the data, because it's possible that we might remember just those cases that fit with our interpretation. Likewise, we cannot treat the facts we like differently from the facts we don't like, so that, perhaps, we're more alert to flaws in the observations that conflict with our hypotheses or less likely to report these observations to others.

Clearly, then, many elements are involved in systematic data collection. But all of these elements are crucial if we are to make certain that our hypotheses have been fully and fairly tested. In this regard, scientific conclusions are on a firmer footing than the judgments we offer as part of our daily experience.

The Community of Scientists

Our Research Methods modules have described many of the steps scientists take to ensure that their data are persuasive and their claims are correct. We need to add to our discussion, though, another important factor that keeps scientific claims on track—the fact that scientists don't work in isolation from one another. To see how this matters, consider the phenomenon of *confirmation bias*. This broad term refers to a number of different effects, all of which have the result of protecting our beliefs from serious challenge. Thus, for example, when we're evaluating beliefs, we tend to seek out information that might confirm the belief rather than information that might undermine it. Likewise, if we encounter information that is at all ambiguous, we are likely to interpret the information in a fashion that brings it into line with our beliefs. And so on.

Individual scientists do what they can to avoid this bias, but even so, scientists are, in the end, human and hence vulnerable to the same problems as everyone else—so it's no surprise that confirmation bias can be detected in scientific reasoning. Thus, when scientists encounter facts that fit with their preferred hypothesis, they tend to accept those facts as they are; when they encounter facts that don't fit, they scrutinize the facts with special care, seeking problems or flaws.

Some scholars, however, have argued that confirmation bias can be a *good thing* for scientists. After all, it takes effort to develop, test, and defend a scientific theory and, eventually, to persuade others to take that theory seriously. All of this effort requires motivation and commitment from the theory's advocates, and confirmation bias may help them to maintain this commitment: Thanks to this bias, the advocates remain certain that they're correct, and this certainty sustains their efforts in developing and promoting the theory. Perhaps it makes sense, therefore, that according to some studies the scientists who are most guilty of confirmation bias are often those who are considered by their peers to be most important and influential.

These points, however, do not diminish the serious problems that confirmation bias can create. How, therefore, do scientists manage to gain the advantages (in motivation) that confirmation bias creates, without suffering the negative consequences of this bias? Part of the answer lies in the fact that science depends on a *community* of scientists, and within this community there is almost always a diversity of views. As a result, the confirmation bias of one researcher can be counteracted by the corresponding bias of other researchers. To put it bluntly, I'll be gentle with the data favoring my view but harsh in scrutinizing the data favoring your claims. You'll be gentle with your data but harsh in scrutinizing mine. In the end, therefore, both your data and mine will receive careful examination—and that's precisely what we want.

To promote this scrutiny, scientists rely on a **peer-review process**. Before a new finding is taken seriously, it must be published in a scientific journal. And before any article can be published, it must be evaluated by the journal's editor (usually, a scientist with impressive credentials) and three or four experts in the field. (These are the "peers" who "review" the paper—hence, the term "peer review.") The reviewers are chosen by the editor to represent a variety of perspectives—including, if possible, a perspective likely to be critical of the paper's claims. If these reviewers find problems in the method or the interpretation of results, the article will not be published by the journal. Thus, any article can appear in print only if it has survived this evaluation—an essential form of quality control.

Then, once the paper is published, the finding is accessible to the broader scientific community and therefore open to scrutiny, criticism, and—if appropriate—attack. In addition, once the details of a study are available in print, other scientists can try to replicate the experiment to make sure that the result is reliable. These are significant long-term benefits from publication.

In short, we take a hypothesis seriously only after it has received the scrutiny of many scientists—both during the (pre-publication) formal process of peer review and in the months after the paper is published. These steps ensure that the hypothesis undergoes examination both by scientists who are inclined to protect the hypothesis and by others who are inclined to reject it. In this way, we can be certain that the hypothesis has been fully and persuasively tested, and thus the scientific community can gain from the commitment and motivation that are the good sides of confirmation bias, without suffering the problems associated with this bias.

Chapter 13: Problem Solving and Intelligence

Defining the Dependent Variable

In the Research Methods module for Chapter 1, we discussed the importance of testable hypotheses—that is, hypotheses framed in a way that makes it clear what evidence will confirm them and what evidence will not. Sometimes, though, it's not obvious how to phrase a hypothesis in testable terms. For example, in Chapter 13 we discuss research on creativity, and in this domain investigators often present hypotheses about the factors that might foster creativity or might undermine it. Thus, one hypothesis might be: "When working on a problem, an interruption (to allow incubation) promotes creativity." To test this hypothesis, we would have to specify what counts as an interruption (5 minutes of working on something else? An hour?). But then, we'd also need some way to measure creativity; otherwise, we couldn't tell if the interruption was beneficial or not.

For this hypothesis, creativity is the dependent variable—that is, the measurement that, according to our hypothesis, might "depend on" the factor being manipulated. The presence or absence of an interruption would be the independent variable—the factor that, according to our hypothesis, influences the dependent variable.

In many studies, it's easy to assess the dependent variable. For example, consider this hypothesis: "Context reinstatement improves memory accuracy." Here, the dependent variable is accuracy, and this is simple to check—for example, by counting up the number of correct answers on a memory test. In this way, we would easily know whether a result confirmed the hypothesis or not. Likewise, consider this hypothesis: "Implicit memories can speed up performance on a lexical-decision task." Here, the dependent variable is response time; again, it is simple to measure, allowing a straightforward test of the hypothesis.

The situation is different, though, for our hypothesis about interruptions and creativity. In this case, people might disagree about whether a particular problem solution (or poem, or painting, or argument) is creative. This will make it difficult to test our hypothesis.

Psychologists generally solve this problem by recruiting a panel of judges to assess the dependent variable. In our example, the judges would review each participant's response and evaluate how creative it was, perhaps on a scale from 1 to 5. By using a panel of judges rather than just one, we can check directly on whether different judges have different ideas about what creativity is. More specifically, we can calculate the **inter-rater reliability** among the judges—the degree to which they agree with one another in their assessments. If they disagree with one another, it would appear that the assessment of creativity really is a subjective matter and cannot be a basis for testing hypotheses. In that case, scientific research on this issue may not be possible. But if the judges do agree to a reasonable extent—if the inter-rater reliability is high—then we can be confident that their assessments are neither arbitrary nor idiosyncratic.

Let's be clear, though, that this is a measure of **reliability**—that is, a measure of how consistent our measurements are. As the text describes, reliability is separate from **validity**—that is, whether we've succeeded in measuring what we intended to measure. It's possible, for example, that all of our judges are reacting to, say, whether they find the responses humorous or not. If the judges all have similar senses of humor, they might agree with one another in this assessment (and so would have a high level of inter-rater reliability), but even so, they would be judging humor, not creativity (and so would not offer *valid* assessments). On this basis, measures of inter-rater reliability are an important step toward establishing our measure—but we still need other steps (perhaps what the chapter calls a **predictive validation**) before we're done.

Notice, in addition, that this way of proceeding doesn't require us to start out with a precise definition of creativity. Of course, a definition would be very useful because (among other benefits) it would enable us to give the judges on our panel relatively specific instructions. Even without a definition, though, we can just ask the judges to rely on their own sense of what's creative. This isn't ideal; we'd prefer to get beyond this intuitive notion. But having a systematic, non-idiosyncratic consensus measurement at least allows our research to get off the ground.

In the same way, consider this hypothesis: "College education improves the clarity of someone's writing." This hypothesis—and many others as well—again involves a complex dependent variable, and it might also require a panel of judges to obtain measurements we can take seriously. But by using these panels, we can measure things that seem at the outset to be unmeasurable, and in that way we appreciably broaden the range of hypotheses we can test.

Correlations

Often in psychology, data are analyzed in terms of **correlations**, and this is certainly true in the study of intelligence. We say that intelligence tests are reliable, for example, because measures of intelligence taken, say, when people are 6 years old are correlated with measures taken from the same people a dozen years later. (This is called **test-retest reliability**.) Likewise, we say that intelligence tests have validity because measures of intelligence are correlated with other performance measures (grades in school or some assessment of performance in the workplace; this is a predictive validation). Or, as one more example, we conclude that g (i.e., *general intelligence*) exists because we can observe correlations among the various parts of the IQ test—so that someone's score on a verbal test is correlated with her score on a spatial test. (This is—roughly—what a *factor analysis* evaluates.)

But what does any of this mean? What is a correlation? The calculation of a correlation begins with a list of *pairs*: someone's IQ score at, say, age 6 and then the same person's score at age 18; the *next person's* scores at age 6 and age 18; the same for the next person and the next after that. A correlation examines these pairs and asks, roughly, how well we can predict the second value within each pair once we know the first value. If we know your IQ score at age 6, how confident can we be in our prediction of your score a dozen years later?

Correlation values—usually abbreviated with the letter r—can fall between +1.0 (a so-called perfect correlation) and –1.0 (a perfect *inverse* correlation). Thus, the strongest possible correlation is *either* +1.0 *or* –1.0. The weakest possible correlation is zero—indicating no relationship. As some concrete examples, the correlation between your height, measured in inches, and your height, measured in centimeters, is +1.0 (because these two measurements are assessing the exact same thing). The correlation between your current distance from the North Pole and your current distance from the South Pole is –1.0 (because each mile you move closer to one pole necessarily takes you one mile away from the other pole). The correlation between your height and your IQ, in contrast, is zero: There's no indication that taller people differ in their intelligence from shorter people.

Most of the r values you'll encounter in psychology, though, are more moderate. For example, the chapter mentions a correlation of roughly $r = +.50$ between someone's IQ and his GPA in college; the correlation between someone's IQ score and the score of her (non-twin) brother or sister is about $r = +.60$. What do these values mean? The full answer is complicated, but here's an approximation.

Researchers routinely report r values, but the really useful statistic is r^2 that is, $r \times r$. Bear in mind here that (as we've said) correlations are based on *pairs* of observations, and the r^2 value literally tells you how much of the overall variation in one measure within the pair can be predicted, based on the other measure in the pair. Thus, let's look at the correlation between IQ and school performance (measured in grade point average). The correlation is +.50, so r^2 is +.25. This means that 25% of the variation in GPA is predictable, if you know students' IQ scores. The remaining 75% of the variation, it seems, has to be explained in other terms.

One way of thinking about these points hinges on the "reduction of uncertainty." To understand this point, imagine that all we know about Kim is that she's a student at your school. If we had to guess Kim's GPA, our best option is just to guess the average for your school—since we have no basis for thinking Kim's above the average or below it. But, of course, we'd have no reason to be confident in this estimate, so we'd probably want to hedge our bets, saying something like "her GPA is likely to be 3.1, plus-or-minus 1."

Now, let's imagine that we receive a new piece of information about Kim—that her IQ score is 118, well above the national average. In this setting, we'd probably estimate that her GPA will be above average as well (and so we'd predict a value greater than 3.1). Crucially, though, we'd also now be a bit more certain in our forecast, because we have more information to go on. Therefore, we might offer a more precise forecast—that is, with a smaller "plus-or-minus" bit. We might say, "her GPA is likely to be 3.5, plus-or-minus .4." We've therefore offered a new forecast *and* decreased our uncertainty (from +/– 1.0 to +/– 0.4). That's exactly what correlations allow us to do—first, to refine our predictions, and second, to decrease uncertainty; and the stronger the correlation, the more it reduces uncertainty. (By the way, if you have a math background, the notion here is that with stronger correlations the individual observations are more tightly clustered around the regression line. But more broadly, what's crucial here is the idea that correlations allow predictions and that stronger correlations allow more precise predictions.)

Let's once again note, though, that we usually find only modest correlations in psychology research. We've said, for example, that the correlation between IQ scores and academic performance is roughly +.50; using the r^2 value, this means that only 25% of the variation from student to student is predictable based on IQ, and the remaining 75% of the variation needs to be explained in other terms. Thus, knowing someone's IQ does decrease our uncertainty in forecasting what that person's academic performance will be—but the IQ score still leaves three quarters of the uncertainty in place. Or, put differently, the data are telling us that IQ is a major contributor to performance, but even so, a large amount of the observed variation—the differences between an A student and a B student, and so on—is influenced by *other* variables, separate from IQ. Some of these other variables, on their own, matter a lot (e.g., the amount of studying, or choice of strategy in studying, or, for that matter, whether the person has stayed healthy throughout the academic year, is getting enough sleep, and so on). Other variables contribute only a little to the overall pattern, but there are many of these variables, and so, in combination they add to the 75% of the variation *not* accounted for by the IQ score. All of this is, again, a way of saying that IQ is a major factor in determining life outcomes, but a long list of other factors also play a role. As we noted in the chapter, IQ does measure something important, but your IQ score does not define your destiny.

Chapter 14: Conscious Thought, Unconscious Thought

Introspection

In Chapter 1, we discussed some of the limits on **introspection** as a research tool, and, in fact, our discussion throughout this book has rarely relied on introspective evidence. This is because, as one concern, introspection relies on what people *remember* about their own mental processes, and we cannot count on these memories being accurate. In addition, introspections are usually reported verbally: The person uses words to describe what happened in his or her own mind. But as we discussed in Chapter 11, some thoughts are nonverbal in content and may not be captured adequately by a verbal description.

As a further problem, your introspections, by definition, involve an "inspection" of your mental life, so this method necessarily rests on the assumption that your mental state is "visible" to you. (You can't inspect something that's invisible.) As Chapter 14 describes, however, a great deal of mental activity goes on outside of awareness and is, in fact, "invisible" to introspection. This provides yet another limit on introspection as a source of scientific evidence—because introspective data will necessarily be incomplete in what they tell us about mental processes.

Let's be careful, though, not to overstate these claims, because unmistakably, introspective reports sometimes do have value. For example, in the study of problem solving, researchers sometimes ask people simply to "think out loud" as a means of discovering what strategies people use as they work on the problem. Likewise, in Chapter 11 we acknowledged the complexities attached to someone's introspective reports about the vividness of his or her own mental images, but we also argued that these vividness reports can be an important source of data about images. And in Chapter 7 we explored the nature of implicit memories; an important source of data there was people's introspective reports about whether a stimulus "felt familiar" or not.

How can we reconcile these uses of introspective data with the concerns we've raised about introspection? How can we argue that introspective data are of questionable value but then turn around and use introspective data? The answer lies in the simple fact that *some* thoughts *are* conscious, memorable, and easily verbalized; for thoughts like these, introspection can provide valuable data. The obvious challenge, therefore, lies in determining which thoughts are in this category—and so available for introspectively based self-report—and which thoughts are not.

How does this determination proceed? Let's say that "think out loud" data indicate that participants are relying on a certain strategy in solving problems. We then need to find *other* evidence that might confirm (or disconfirm) this introspection. We can ask, for example, whether people make the sorts of errors that we'd expect if they are, in fact, using the strategy suggested by the self-report. We can also ask whether people have trouble with problems that can't easily be solved via the strategy suggested by the self-report. In these ways, we can *check on* the introspections and thus find out if the self-reports provide useful evidence.

Likewise, in Chapter 11 we discussed some of the evidence indicating that self-reports of image vividness do have value. Specifically, we described evidence that reveals a relationship between these reports, on the one hand, and how well people do in certain imagery tasks, on the other hand. Other evidence indicates a link between these imagery self-reports and activation levels in the visual cortex. So here, too, we can document the value of the introspective evidence by checking the introspections against other types of data, including behavioral data and data from neuroscience.

The point, then, is that introspection is neither wholly worthless nor wonderfully reliable. Instead, introspection can provide fabulous clues about what's going on in someone's mind—but we then need to find other means of checking on those clues to determine whether they are misleading. But let's note that introspection is not unique in this regard. Any research tool must prove its worth—by means of data that in one fashion or another validate the results obtained with that tool. (Consider our discussion in Chapter 13 of the steps needed to assess the validity of intelligence tests.) In this way, we use our research methods to build our science, but we also use our science to check on and, where possible, refine our research methods.

Key Research Methods Concepts

In this appendix, we have covered many crucial concepts; you should by now be familiar with all of these:

anecdotal evidence

baseline level

catch trials

chronometric studies

confirmation bias

confound

control condition

converging operations

correlations

counterbalancing

debriefing

demand character

dependent variable

double dissociation

double-blind procedure

experimental condition

external validity

generalizability

independent variable

inter-rater reliability

introspection

invalid experiment

metalinguistic judgments

N

peer-review process

population

predictive validation

r (and, related, r^2)

random assignment

random sampling

reliability

replication

representative sample

response times (RTs)

sample (vs. population)

self-report data

self-selected group

systematic data collection

test-retest reliability

testable hypothesis

third-variable problem

validity

Glossary

ACC See *anterior cingulate cortex*.

acquisition The process of placing new information into *long-term memory*.

action potential A brief change in the electrical potential of an *axon*. The action potential is the physical basis of the signal sent from one end of a *neuron* to the other; it usually triggers a further (chemical) signal to other neurons.

action slip An error in which someone performs some behavior or makes some response that is different from the behavior or response intended.

activation level A measure of the current status for a *node* or *detector*. Activation level is increased if the node or detector receives the appropriate input from its associated nodes or detectors; activation level will be high if input has been received frequently or recently.

acuity The ability to discern fine detail.

ad hoc category A mental category made up on the spot in response to a specific question.

affective forecasting The process in which a person predicts how he or she will feel at some future point about an object or state of affairs. It turns out that people are surprisingly inaccurate in these predictions and (for

example) understate their own capacity to adapt to changes.

affirming the consequent An error often made in logical reasoning. The error begins with these two premises: (a) "If A then B," and (b) "B is true." The error consists of drawing the false conclusion that (c) "A must therefore be true." Compare with *denying the antecedent*.

agnosia A disturbance in a person's ability to identify familiar objects.

all-or-none law The principle stating that a *neuron* or *detector* either *fires* completely or does not fire at all; no intermediate responses are possible. (Graded responses are possible, however, by virtue of the fact that a neuron or detector can fire more or less frequently, and for a longer or shorter time.)

ambiguous figure A drawing that can be readily perceived in more than one way. Classic examples include the duck/rabbit and the Necker cube.

amnesia A disruption of memory, often due to brain damage.

amygdala (pl. amygdalae) An almond-shaped structure in the *limbic system* that plays a central role in emotion and in the evaluation of stimuli.

anarthria A disorder characterized by an inability to control the

muscles needed for ordinary speech. Anarthric individuals cannot speak, although other aspects of their language functioning are unimpaired.

anchoring A tendency to use the first available estimate for some fact as a reference point for that fact, and then perhaps to make some (small) adjustment from that reference point in determining your final estimate. As a result of anchoring, the first-available estimate often has a powerful influence on you, even if that estimate comes from a source that gives it little credibility.

anecdotal evidence Data or results collected casually, without documentation, and without any steps that might help you determine if the report is accurate or representative of a broader pattern. This evidence is often presented as an informal report or narrative (i.e., an anecdote) relayed in conversation.

anomia A disruption of language abilities, usually resulting from specific brain damage, in which the individual loses the ability to name objects, including highly familiar objects.

antecedent The formal name for the "if . . ." clause in an "if . . . then . . ." statement. See also *consequent*.

anterior cingulate cortex (ACC)
A brain structure known to play a crucial role in detecting and resolving conflicts among different brain systems.

anterograde amnesia An inability to remember experiences that occurred *after* the event that triggered the memory disruption. Often contrasted with *retrograde amnesia*.

aphasia A disruption to language capacities, often caused by brain damage.

apperceptive agnosia A disorder involving a failure in object recognition apparently caused by difficulties in assembling the parts of an image into an understandable whole.

apraxia A disturbance in the capacity to initiate or organize voluntary action, often caused by brain damage.

Area V1 The site on the *occipital lobe* where axons from the *lateral geniculate nucleus* first reach the cerebral *cortex*. This site is (for one neural pathway) the location at which information about the visual world first reaches the brain.

articulatory rehearsal loop One of the low-level assistants hypothesized as being part of the *working-memory system*. This loop draws on *subvocalized* (covert) speech, which serves to create a record in the *phonological buffer*. Materials in this buffer then fade, but they can be refreshed by another cycle of covert speech.

association cortex The traditional name for the portion of the human *cortex* outside the *motor* and *sensory projection areas*.

associations Functional connections that are hypothesized to link *nodes* within a mental network or *detectors* within a detector network; these associations are often hypothesized as the "carriers" of activation from one node or detector to the next.

associative agnosia A disorder involving a failure in *object recognition* in which perception seems normal but the person is unable to link his or her perception to basic visual knowledge.

associative links See *associations*.

attended channel In *selective attention* experiments, research participants are exposed to simultaneous inputs and are instructed to ignore all of these except one. The attended channel is the input to which participants are instructed to pay attention. Often contrasted with *unattended channel*.

attribute substitution A commonly used strategy in which a person needs one type of information but relies instead on a more accessible form of information. This strategy works well if the more accessible form of information is, in fact, well correlated with the desired information. An example is the case in which someone needs information about how frequent an event is in the world and relies instead on how easily he or she can think of examples of the event.

attribution The step of explaining a feeling or event, usually by identifying the factors (or an earlier event) that are the cause of the current feeling or event. Hence, this term is often elaborated with the more specific term: *causal attribution*.

autobiographical memory The aspect of memory that records the episodes and events in a person's life.

automatic tasks Tasks that are well practiced and that do not require flexibility; these tasks usually require little or no attention, and they can be carried out if the person is also busy with some other task. Usually contrasted with *controlled tasks*.

automaticity A state achieved by some tasks and some forms of processing, in which the task can be performed with little or no attention. Automatized actions can, in many cases, be combined with other activities without interference. Automatized actions are also often difficult to control, leading many psychologists to refer to them as "mental reflexes."

availability heuristic A particular form of *attribute substitution* in which the person needs to judge the frequency of a certain type of object or the likelihood of a certain type of event. For this purpose, the person is likely to assess the ease with which examples of the object or event come to mind; this "availability" of examples is then used as an index of frequency or likelihood.

axon The part of a *neuron* that typically transmits a signal away from the neuron's cell body and carries the signal to another location.

back propagation A learning procedure, common in *connectionist networks*, in which an *error signal* is used to adjust the inputs to a *node* within the network (so that the node will be less responsive in the future to the inputs that led it to the inappropriate response). The error signal is then transmitted to those same inputs, so that they can make their own similar adjustments. In this way, the error signal is transmitted backward through the network, starting with the nodes that immediately triggered the incorrect response, but with each node then passing the error signal back to the nodes that caused it to *fire*.

base-rate information Information about the broad likelihood of a particular type of event (also referred to as "prior probability"). Often contrasted with *diagnostic information*.

baseline level A standard or basis for comparison, often assessed by some measurement before a manipulation takes place, or with a group that never receives the experimental manipulation.

basic-level categorization A level of categorization hypothesized as the "natural" and most informative level, neither too specific nor too general. People tend to use basic-level terms (such as "chair," rather than the more general "furniture" or the more specific "armchair") in their ordinary conversation and in their reasoning.

behaviorist theory Broad principles concerned with how behavior changes in response to different configurations of stimuli (including stimuli that are often called "rewards" and "punishments"). In its early days, behaviorist theory sought to avoid mentalistic terms (terms that referred to representations or processes inside the mind).

belief bias A tendency, within logical reasoning, to endorse a conclusion if the conclusion happens to be something one believes is true anyhow. In displaying this tendency, people seem to ignore both the premises of the logical argument and logic itself, and they rely instead on their broader pattern of beliefs about what is true and what is not.

belief perseverance A tendency to continue endorsing some assertion or claim, even when the clearly available evidence completely undermines that claim.

bigram A pair of letters. For example, the word "FLAT" contains the bigrams *FL*, *LA*, and *AT*.

bigram detectors Hypothetical units in a recognition system that respond, or *fire*, whenever a specific letter pair is in view.

binding problem The problem of reuniting the various elements of a scene, given the fact that these elements are initially dealt with by different systems in the brain.

binocular disparity A distance cue based on the differences between the two eyes' views of the world. This difference becomes less pronounced the farther an object is from the observer.

binocular rivalry A pattern that arises when the input to one eye cannot be integrated with the input to the other eye. In this circumstance, the person tends to be aware of only one eye's input at a time.

bipolar cell A type of *neuron* in the eye. Bipolar cells receive their input from the *photoreceptors* and transmit their output to the retinal *ganglion cells*.

blind sight A pattern resulting from brain damage, in which the person seems unable to see in part of his or her field of vision but can often correctly respond to visual inputs when required to do so by an experimenter.

Boaz The author's exceedingly crazy German short-haired pointer, and arguably the prototype for the category "dog."

BOLD (blood oxygenation level dependent) signal A measure of how much oxygen the brain's hemoglobin is carrying in specific parts of the brain; this measurement provides a quantitative basis for comparing activity levels in different brain areas.

bottom-up influences The term given to effects that are governed by the stimulus input itself and that shape the processing of that input. Often contrasted with *top-down influences*.

bottom-up processing See *data-driven processing* and *bottom-up influences*.

boundary extension A tendency for people to remember pictures as being less "zoomed in" (and thus having wider boundaries) than they actually were.

brightness constancy The achievement of perceiving the constant brightness of objects in the world despite changes in the light reaching the eye that result from variations in illumination.

Broca's area An area in the left *frontal lobe* of the brain; damage here typically causes *nonfluent aphasia*.

Capgras syndrome (proun. CAP-grah) A relatively rare disorder, resulting from specific forms of brain damage, in which the afflicted person recognizes the people in his or her world but denies that they are who they appear to be. Instead, the person insists, these familiar individuals are well-disguised impostors.

catch trials Presentations within a research procedure in which the target stimulus is absent or in which a stimulus requires a "no" response. Catch trials are included within a study to guarantee that the participants are taking the task seriously, not just responding in the same fashion on every trial.

categorical perception The tendency to hear speech sounds "merely" as members of a category—the category of [z] sounds, the category of [p] sounds, and so on. As a consequence, one tends to hear sounds *within* the category as being rather similar to one another; sounds from different categories, however, are perceived as being quite different.

categorical syllogism A logical argument containing two *premises* and a conclusion, and concerned with the properties of, and relations between, categories. An example is "All trees are plants. All plants require nourishment. Therefore, all trees require nourishment." This is a valid syllogism, since the truth of the premises guarantees the truth of the conclusion.

causal attribution An interpretation of a thought or behavior in which one decides what caused the behavior.

ceiling level A level of performance in a task that is near the maximum level possible. (In many tasks, this is performance near 100%.)

cell body The area of a biological cell containing the nucleus and the metabolic machinery that sustains the cell.

center-surround cell A *neuron* in the visual system that has a "donut-shaped" *receptive field*. Stimulation in the center of the receptive field has one effect on the cell; stimulation in the surrounding ring has the opposite effect.

central executive The hypothesized director of the *working-memory system*. This is the component of the system that is needed for any interpretation or analysis; in contrast, mere storage of materials can be provided by *working memory*'s assistants, which work under the control of the central executive. Also see *executive control*.

central fissure The separation dividing the *frontal lobes* on each side of the brain from the *parietal lobes*.

cerebellum The largest area of the *hindbrain*, crucial for the coordination of bodily movements and balance.

cerebral hemisphere One of the two hemispherical brain structures— one on the left side, one on the right—that constitute the major part of the *forebrain* in mammals.

change blindness A pattern in which perceivers either do not see or take a long time to see large-scale changes in a visual stimulus. This pattern reveals how little people perceive, even from stimuli in plain view, if they are not specifically attending to the target information.

childhood amnesia The pattern of not remembering the first 3 or 4 years of life. This pattern is very common; a century ago, it was explained in terms of repression of anxious events in those years; more recent accounts focus on the psychological and biological immaturity of 3- and 4-year-olds, which makes them less able to form new episodic memories.

chronometric study Literally, a "time-measuring" study; generally, a study that measures the amount of time a task takes. Often used as a means of examining the task's components or as a means of

examining which brain events are simultaneous with specific mental events.

chunk The hypothetical storage unit in *working memory*; it is estimated that working memory can hold *7 plus-or-minus 2* chunks. However, an unspecified quantity of information can be contained within each *chunk*, because the content of each chunk depends on how the memorizer has organized the materials to be remembered.

coarticulation A trait of speech production in which the way a sound is produced is altered slightly by the immediately preceding and immediately following sounds. Because of this "overlap" in speech production, the acoustic properties of each speech sound vary according to the context in which that sound occurs.

cocktail party effect A term often used to describe a pattern in which a person seems to "tune out" all conversations reaching his or her ears *except for* the conversation he or she wishes to pay attention to; however, if some salient stimulus (such as the person's name) appears in one of the other conversations, the person is reasonably likely to detect this stimulus.

cognitive neuroscience The study of the biological basis for cognitive functioning.

cognitive unconscious The broad set of mental activities of which people are completely unaware but that make possible ordinary thinking, remembering, reasoning, and so on.

commissure One of the thick bundles of fibers via which information is sent back and forth between the two *cerebral hemispheres*.

competence The pattern of skills and knowledge that might be revealed under optimal circumstances. Often contrasted with *performance*.

computerized axial tomography (CT scan) A *neuroimaging technique* that uses X-rays to construct a precise three-dimensional image of the brain's anatomy.

concept-driven processing A type of processing in which the sequence of mental events is influenced by a broad pattern of knowledge and expectations (sometimes referred to as *top-down processing*). Often contrasted with *data-driven processing*.

concurrent articulation task A requirement that a research participant speak or mime speech while doing some other task. In many cases, the person is required to say "Tah-Tah-Tah" over and over, or "one, two, three, one, two, three." These procedures occupy the muscles and control mechanisms needed for speech, so they prevent the person from using these resources for *subvocalization*.

conditional statement A statement of the format "If X then Y," with the first part (the "if" clause, or *antecedent*) providing a condition under which the second part (the "then" clause, or *consequent*) is guaranteed to be true.

cone A *photoreceptor* that is able to discriminate hues and that has high *acuity*. Cones are concentrated in the *retina*'s *fovea* and become less frequent in the visual periphery. Often contrasted with *rod*.

confirmation bias A family of effects in which people seem more sensitive to evidence that confirms their beliefs than they are to evidence that challenges their beliefs. Thus, if people are given a choice about what sort of information they would like in order to evaluate their beliefs, they request information that is likely to confirm their beliefs. Likewise, if they are presented with both confirming and disconfirming evidence, they are more likely to pay attention to, be influenced by, and remember the confirming evidence, rather than the disconfirming.

confound A variable other than the independent variable that could potentially explain the pattern of observed results. For example, if participants always serve in the *control condition* first and the *experimental condition* second, then any differences between these conditions might be due either to the *independent variable* or to an effect of practice (favoring the experimental condition, which came second). In this case, practice would be a confound.

conjunction error An error in perception in which a person correctly perceives what features are present but misperceives how the features are joined, so that (for example) a red circle and a green square might be misperceived as a red square and a green circle.

connection weight The strength of a connection between two *nodes* in a network. The greater the connection weight, the more efficiently activation will flow from one node to the other.

connectionism An approach to theorizing about the mind that relies on *parallel distributed processing* among elements that provide a *distributed representation* of the information being considered.

connectionist networks See *connectionism*.

consequent The "then . . . " clause in an "If . . . then . . . " statement. Also see *antecedent* and *conditional statement*.

consequentiality The perceived importance of an event, or the perception of how widespread and long-lasting the event's effects will be.

consolidation The biological process through which new memories are "cemented in place," acquiring some degree of permanence through the creation of new (or altered) neural connections.

content morpheme A *morpheme* that carries meaning. Often

contrasted with *function morpheme*.

context reinstatement A procedure in which a person is led to the same mental and emotional state he or she was in during a previous event; context reinstatement can often promote accurate recollection of that event.

context-dependent learning A pattern of data in which materials learned in one setting are well remembered when the person returns to that setting, but are less well remembered in other settings.

contralateral control A pattern in which the left half of the brain controls the right half of the body, and the right half of the brain controls the left half of the body.

control condition A condition in which research participants are not exposed to the experimental manipulation, thereby serving as a basis for comparison with participants in the *experimental condition* (who are exposed to the experimental manipulation).

controlled tasks Tasks that are novel or that require flexibility in one's approach; these tasks usually require attention, so they cannot be carried out if the person is also busy with some other task. Usually contrasted with *automatic tasks*.

convergent data A variety of studies that all point toward (and so "converge on") the same theoretical claims.

convolutions The wrinkles visible in the cerebral *cortex* that allow the enormous surface area of the human brain to be stuffed into the relatively small volume of the skull.

cornea The transparent tissue at the front of each eye that plays an important role in focusing the incoming light.

corpus callosum The largest of the *commissures* linking the left and right *cerebral hemispheres*.

correlations The tendency for two variables to change together. If

one goes up as the other goes up, the correlation is positive; if one goes up as the other goes down, the correlation is negative. A value of +1.00 indicates a perfect positive correlation; a value of −1.00 indicates a perfect negative (or inverse) correlation; a value of 0 indicates that there is no relationship at all between the variables.

cortex The outermost surface of an organ in the body; psychologists are most commonly interested in the brain's cortex and, specifically, the cerebral cortex.

counterbalancing A procedure used to ensure that any potential *confound* will have an equal effect on all the experimental conditions, with the goal of ensuring that any difference between the conditions could not possibly be due to the confound. Thus, an experimenter might expose half of the participants to the *control condition* first and half to the *experimental condition* first. In this case, practice favors the experimental condition for half of the participants and favors the control condition for the other half. Therefore, practice should have an equal impact on the two conditions and so cannot be a source of difference between them, because the experimenter has counterbalanced the effect of practice.

covariation A relationship between two variables such that the presence (or magnitude) of one variable can be predicted from the presence (or magnitude) of the other. Covariation can be positive or negative. If it is positive, then increases in one variable occur when increases in the other occur. If it is negative, then decreases in one variable occur when increases in the other occur.

crystallized intelligence A person's acquired knowledge, including his or her repertoire of verbal knowledge and cognitive skills. See also *fluid intelligence*.

CT scans See *computerized axial tomography*.

data-driven processing A type of processing in which the sequence of mental events is determined largely by the pattern of incoming information (sometimes referred to as *bottom-up processing*). Often contrasted with *concept-driven processing*.

debriefing A step at the end of a study in which the researcher explains the study's purpose and design to each participant, and undoes any manipulations to participants' beliefs or state.

decay theory of forgetting The hypothesis that with the passage of time, memories may fade or erode.

deception In research methods, any procedural step designed to hide the actual purpose of the study, or the exact variables under scrutiny, from the participants; deception is one of the strategies used to diminish a study's *demand character*.

deduction A process through which a person starts with claims, or general assertions, and asks what further claims necessarily follow from these *premises*. Often contrasted with *induction*.

deep processing A mode of thinking in which a person pays attention to the meaning and implications of the material; deep processing typically leads to excellent memory retention. Often contrasted with *shallow processing*.

Deese–Roediger–McDermott procedure See *DRM procedure*.

demand character Cues within an experiment that signal to the participant how he or she is "supposed to" respond.

dendrite The part of a *neuron* that usually detects the incoming signal.

denying the antecedent An error that is often made in logical reasoning. The error begins with these two *premises*: (a) "If A then B," and (b) "A is false." The

error consists of drawing the false conclusion that (c) "B must therefore also be false." Often contrasted with *affirming the consequent*.

dependent variable The variable that the researcher observes or measures to determine if the *independent variable* has an effect or influence. The dependent variable can take many forms (e.g., speed of responding, number of errors, type of errors, a biological measure such as brain activation at a certain site).

descriptive account An account that tells us how things are, as opposed to how they should be. Often contrasted with *normative account*.

descriptive rules Rules that simply describe the regularities in a pattern of observations, with no commentary on whether the pattern is "proper," "correct," or "desirable."

destructive updating The hypothesized mechanism through which new learning or new information on a topic replaces old knowledge or information in memory, so that the old information is erased or destroyed by the new input.

detector A *node* within a processing network that *fires* primarily in response to a specific target contained within the incoming perceptual information.

diagnostic information Information about an individual case indicating whether the case belongs in one category or another. Often contrasted with *base-rate information*.

dichotic listening A task in which research participants hear two simultaneous verbal messages— one presented via headphones to the left ear and a second one presented to the right ear. In typical experiments, participants are asked to pay attention to one of these inputs (the *attended channel*) and are urged to ignore the other.

digit-span task A task often used for measuring *working memory*'s storage capacity. Research participants are read a series of digits (e.g., "8 3 4") and must immediately repeat them back. If they do this successfully, they are given a slightly longer list (e.g., "9 2 4 0"), and so forth. The length of the longest list a person can remember in this fashion is that person's digit span. Also see *operation span*.

direct memory testing A form of memory testing in which people are asked explicitly to remember some previous event. *Recall* and standard *recognition* testing are both forms of direct memory testing. Often contrasted with *indirect memory testing*.

distance cues Sources of information that signal the distance from the observer to some target object.

distributed knowledge Information stored via a *distributed representation*.

distributed representation A mode of representing ideas or contents in which there is no one *node* (or specific group of nodes) representing the content and no one place where the content is stored. Instead, the content is represented via a pattern of simultaneous activity across many nodes. The same nodes will also participate in other patterns, so those nodes will also be part of other distributed representations. Often contrasted with *local representation*.

divided attention The skill of performing multiple tasks simultaneously.

dizygotic twins See *fraternal twins*.

doctrine of formal disciplines In educational philosophy, the notion that the best way to train the mind is to provide education in disciplines such as logic, math, and linguistics (i.e., disciplines that hinge on formal structures).

double dissociation A research strategy used to show that two processes or two structures are truly distinct. To make this argument, one must show that each of the processes or structures can be disrupted without in any way interfering with the other.

double-blind procedure A procedure in which neither the research participant nor the person administering the study knows which condition of the study the participant is in (e.g., receiving medication or a placebo; being in the experimental group or in the control group). In this case, there is no risk that the person administering the study can convey to the participant how the participant is "supposed to" behave in the study.

DRM procedure A commonly used experimental procedure, named after its originators (Deese, Roediger, & McDermott), for eliciting and studying memory errors. In this procedure, a person sees or hears a list of words that are all related to a single theme; however, the word that names the theme is not itself included. Nonetheless, people are very likely to remember later that the theme word was presented.

dual-coding theory A theory that imaginable materials, such as high-imagery words, will be doubly represented in memory: The word itself will be remembered, and so will the corresponding mental image.

dual-process model Any model of thinking that claims people have two distinct means of making judgments—one of which is fast, efficient, but prone to error, and one that is slower, more effortful, but also more accurate.

early selection A proposal that *selective attention* operates at an early stage of processing, so that the unattended inputs receive little analysis.

edge enhancement A process created by *lateral inhibition* in which the *neurons* in the visual system give exaggerated responses to edges of surfaces.

eidetic imagery A relatively rare capacity in which the person can retain long-lasting and detailed visual images of scenes that can be scrutinized as if they were still physically present.

Einstellung The phenomenon in *problem solving* in which people develop a certain attitude or perspective on a problem and then approach all subsequent problems with the same rigid attitude.

elaborative rehearsal A way of engaging materials to be remembered such that one pays attention to what the materials mean and how they are related to one another to other things in the surroundings, or to other things one already knows. Often contrasted with *maintenance rehearsal*.

electroencephalography A recording of voltage changes occurring at the scalp that reflect activity in the brain underneath.

emotional intelligence The ability to understand one's own and others' emotions and to control one's emotions appropriately.

encoding specificity The tendency, when memorizing, to place in memory both the materials to be learned and also some amount of the context of those materials. As a result, these materials will be recognized as familiar, later on, only if the materials appear again in a similar context.

error signal Feedback given to a network to indicate that the network's response was not the desired one. Often, the magnitude of the error signal is proportional to the difference between the response produced and the response that should have been produced. The signal can then be used to adjust the network or system (often, via *back propagation*) so that the error will be smaller in the future.

event-related potential Changes in an *electroencephalogram (EEG)* in the brief period just before, during, and after an explicitly defined event, usually measured by averaging together many trials in which this event has occurred.

excitatory connection A link from one *node*, or one *detector*, to another, such that activation of one node activates the other. Often contrasted with *inhibitory connection*.

executive control The mental resources and processes that are used to set goals, choose task priorities, and avoid conflict among competing habits or responses.

exemplar-based reasoning Reasoning that draws on knowledge about specific category members, rather than drawing on more-general information about the overall category.

expected value An estimate of the subjective gain that will result from choosing a particular option. Expected value is calculated as the likely value of the consequences of that option, if these are obtained, multiplied by the probability of gaining those consequences. (Also referred to as "expected utility.")

experimental condition A condition in which research participants are exposed to an experimental manipulation, thereby serving as a basis for comparison with participants in the *control condition* so that the researcher can learn whether the experimental manipulation changes the participants' thoughts, feelings, or behavior.

explicit memory A memory revealed by *direct memory testing* and typically accompanied by the conviction that one is, in fact, remembering—that is, drawing on some sort of knowledge (perhaps knowledge about a specific prior episode, or perhaps more general knowledge). Often contrasted with *implicit memory*.

external validity The quality of a research design that ensures that the data accurately reflect the circumstances outside of the study that the researcher hopes to understand. External validity requires that the research participants, the research task, and the research stimuli are all appropriately representative of the people, tasks, and stimuli to which the researcher wants to *generalize* the results.

extralinguistic context The social and physical setting in which an utterance is encountered; usually, cues within this setting guide the interpretation of the utterance.

factor analysis A statistical method for studying the interrelations among various tests. The goal is to discover the extent to which the tests are influenced by the same factors.

false alarm A response in which a research participant indicates that he or she has detected a target even though the specified target is actually absent.

false memory A memory, sincerely reported, that misrepresents how an event actually unfolded. In some cases, a false memory can be wholly false and can report an event that never happened at all.

familiarity In some circumstances, the subjective feeling that one has encountered a stimulus before; in other circumstances, the objective fact that one has indeed encountered a stimulus before and is now in some way influenced by that encounter, whether or not one recalls that encounter or feels that the stimulus is familiar.

family resemblance The notion that members of a category (e.g., all dogs, all games) resemble one another. In general, family resemblance relies on some number of *features* being shared by any group of category members, even though these features may not be shared by all members of the category. Therefore, the basis for family resemblance may shift from one subset of the category to another.

feature One of the small set of elements out of which more-

complicated patterns are composed.

feature net A system for recognizing patterns that involves a network of *detectors*, with detectors for features as the initial layer in the system.

figure/ground organization The processing step in which the perceiver determines which aspects of the stimulus belong to the central object (or "figure") and which aspects belong to the background (or "ground").

file-drawer problem The concern that *null findings* or disappointing findings are not published and are, so to speak, placed in a file drawer and forgotten. This problem can create a situation in which the published research is not representative of the full pattern of evidence.

filter A hypothetical mechanism that would block potential distractors from further processing.

fire To respond in a discrete and specific way—as when a *neuron*, after receiving a strong enough stimulus, sends a signal down its *axon*, which in turn causes a release of *neurotransmitter* from the membrane at the end of the axon.

fixation target A visual mark (such as a dot or a plus sign) at which one points one's eyes (or "fixates"). Fixation targets are used to help research participants control their eye position.

flashbulb memory A memory of extraordinary clarity, typically for some highly emotional event, that is retained despite the passage of many years. Despite their remarkable vividness, flashbulb memories sometimes turn out to be inaccurate.

fluent aphasia A disruption of language, caused by brain damage, in which afflicted individuals are able to produce speech but the speech is not meaningful, and the individuals are not able to understand what is said to them. Often contrasted with *nonfluent aphasia*.

fluid intelligence The ability to deal with new and unusual problems. See also *crystallized intelligence*.

Flynn effect A worldwide increase in IQ scores over the last several decades, occurring in both third-world and developed nations, and proceeding at a rate of roughly 3 points per decade.

fMRI scans See *functional magnetic resonance imaging*.

forebrain One of the three main structures (along with the *hindbrain* and the *midbrain*) of the brain; the forebrain plays a crucial role in supporting intellectual functioning.

form perception The process through which people see the basic shape, size, and position of an object.

four-card task See *selection task*.

fovea The center of the *retina* and the region on the eye in which *acuity* is best; when a person looks at an object, he or she is lining up that object with the fovea.

frame In decision making, the aspects of how a decision is phrased that are, in fact, irrelevant to the decision but that influence people's choices nonetheless.

fraternal (dizygotic, DZ) twins Twins that develop from two different eggs that are simultaneously fertilized by two sperm. Like ordinary siblings, they share 50% of their genes. See also *identical twins*.

free recall A method of assessing memory. The person being tested is asked to come up with as many items as possible from a particular source (such as "the list you heard earlier" or "things you saw yesterday"), in any sequence.

frequency estimate People's assessment of how often an event has occurred in the past, or how common an object is in the world.

frontal lobe The lobe of the brain in each *cerebral hemisphere* that includes the prefrontal area and the *primary motor projection area*.

function morpheme A *morpheme* that signals a relation between words within a sentence, such as the morpheme "s" indicating a plural in English, or the morpheme "ed" indicating past tense. Often contrasted with *content morpheme*.

functional equivalence A series of close parallels in how two systems work—how they respond to inputs, what errors they make, and so on. An example is the functional equivalence between vision and visual imagery.

functional fixedness A tendency to be rigid in how one thinks about an object's function. This generally involves a strong tendency to think of an object only in terms of its *typical* function.

functional magnetic resonance imaging (fMRI) A *neuroimaging technique* that uses magnetic fields to construct a detailed three-dimensional representation of the activity levels in different areas of the brain at a particular moment in time.

fusiform face area (FFA) A brain area apparently specialized for the perception of faces.

fuzzy boundary A distinction between categories that identifies each instance only as "more or less likely" to be in a category, rather than specifying whether each instance is or is not included in the category.

gamma-band oscillation A particular rhythm of *firing* hypothesized as the signal within the nervous system that indicates when different parts of the visual system are all responding to the same stimulus.

ganglion cell A type of *neuron* in the eye. The ganglion cells receive their input from the *bipolar cells*, and then the *axons* of the ganglion cells gather together to form the *optic nerve*, carrying information back to the *lateral geniculate nucleus*.

garden-path sentence A sentence that initially leads the reader to one understanding of how the sentence's words are related but then requires a change in this understanding to comprehend the sentence. Examples are "The old man ships" and "The horse raced past the barn fell."

general intelligence (*g*) A mental capacity that is hypothesized as contributing to the performance of virtually any intellectual task. The existence of *g* is documented by the statistical overlap among diverse forms of mental testing.

generalization The step of making claims about people, tasks, and stimuli other than those scrutinized within a research study. This step is legitimate only if the study has *external validity*.

generativity The trait of a system that allows someone to combine and recombine basic units to create (or "generate") new and more-complex entities. Linguistic rules, for example, are generative, because they allow someone to combine and recombine a limited set of words to produce a vast number of sentences.

generic knowledge Knowledge of a general sort, as opposed to knowledge about specific episodes.

geon One of the basic shapes proposed as the building blocks of all complex three-dimensional forms. Geons take the form of cylinders, cones, blocks, and the like, and they are combined to form "geon assemblies." These are then combined to produce entire objects.

glia A type of cell found (along with *neurons*) in the central nervous system. Glial cells have many functions, including the support of neurons, the repair of neural connections in case of damage, and a key role in guiding the initial development of neural connections. A specialized type of glia also provide electrical insulation for some neurons, allowing much faster transmission of neuronal signals.

goal neglect A pattern of behavior in which a person fails to keep his or her goal in mind, so that, for example, the person relies on habitual responses even if those responses will not move him or her toward the goal.

goal state The state a person is working toward in trying to solve a problem. Often contrasted with *initial state*.

graded membership The idea that some members of a category are "better" members and therefore are more firmly in the category than other members.

grammatical Conforming to the rules that govern the sequence of words acceptable within the language. Note that a grammatical sentence can be false or even nonsensical, but nonetheless is well-formed according to the rules of syntax.

heuristic A strategy that is reasonably efficient and works most of the time. In using a heuristic, one is in effect choosing to accept some risk of error in order to gain efficiency.

hill-climbing strategy A commonly used strategy in *problem solving*. If people use this strategy, then whenever their efforts toward solving a problem give them a choice, they will choose the option that carries them closer to the goal.

hindbrain One of the three main structures (along with the *forebrain* and the *midbrain*) of the brain; the hindbrain sits atop the spinal cord and includes several structures crucial for controlling key life functions.

hippocampus (pl. hippocampi) A structure in the *temporal lobe* that is involved in the creation of *long-term memories* and spatial memory.

hypothalamus A small structure at the base of the *forebrain* that plays a vital role in the control of motivated behaviors such as eating, drinking, and sexual activity.

identical (monozygotic, MZ) twins Twins that develop from a single fertilized egg that then splits in half. These twins are genetically identical. See also *fraternal twins*.

ill-defined problem A problem for which the goal state is specified only in general terms and the operators available for reaching the goal state are not obvious at the start. Often contrasted with *well-defined problem*.

illumination The third in a series of stages often hypothesized as crucial for creativity. The first stage is *preparation*; the second, *incubation*. Illumination is the stage in which some new key insight or new idea suddenly comes to mind and is then (on this hypothesis) followed by *verification*.

illusion of truth An effect of *implicit memory* in which claims that are familiar end up seeming more plausible.

illusory covariation A pattern that people "perceive" in data, leading them to believe that the presence of one factor allows them to predict the presence of another factor. However, this perception occurs even in the absence of any genuine relationship between the two factors. As an example, people perceive that a child's willingness to cheat in an academic setting is an indicator that the child will also be willing to cheat in athletic contests. However, this perception is incorrect, and so the *covariation* that people perceive is "illusory."

image file Visual information stored in *long-term memory*, specifying what a particular object or shape looks like. Information within the image file can then be used as a "recipe" or set of instructions for how to construct an active image of this object or shape.

image-scanning procedure An experimental procedure in which participants are asked to form a specific mental image and then are asked to scan, with their "mind's eye," from one point in the image to another. By timing these scans, the experimenter can determine how long "travel" takes across a mental image.

implicit memory A memory revealed by *indirect memory testing* and usually manifested as a *priming* effect in which current performance is guided or facilitated by previous experiences. Implicit memories are often accompanied by no conscious realization that one is, in fact, being influenced by specific past experiences. Often contrasted with *explicit memory*.

inattentional blindness A pattern in which perceivers seem literally not to see stimuli right in front of their eyes; this pattern is caused by the participants' attending to some other stimulus and not expecting the target to appear.

incidental learning Learning that takes place in the absence of any intention to learn and, correspondingly, in the absence of any expectation of a subsequent memory test. Often contrasted with *intentional learning*.

incubation The second in a series of stages that are often hypothesized as crucial for creativity. The first stage is *preparation*; the third, *illumination*; the fourth, *verification*. Incubation is hypothesized to involve events that occur when a person puts a problem out of his or her conscious thoughts but continues nonetheless to work on the problem unconsciously. Many current psychologists are skeptical about this process, and they propose alternative accounts for data that ostensibly document incubation.

independent variable In an experimental study, the variable that the researcher deliberately manipulates to ask whether it has an impact on the target (*dependent*) variable. Outside of experimental studies, the independent variable can involve some preexisting difference (e.g., the participants' age or sex), allowing the researcher to ask if this preexisting difference influences the target variable. Sometimes called the "predictor variable."

indirect memory testing A form of memory testing in which research participants are not told that their memories are being tested. Instead, they are tested in a fashion in which previous experiences can influence current behavior. Examples of indirect tests include *word-stem completion*, the *lexical-decision task*, and *tachistoscopic* recognition. Often contrasted with *direct memory testing*.

induction A pattern of reasoning in which a person seeks to draw general claims from specific bits of evidence. Often contrasted with *deduction*.

information processing A particular approach to theorizing in which complex mental events, such as learning, remembering, and deciding, are understood as being built up out of a large number of discrete steps. These steps occur one by one, with each providing as its "output" the input to the next step in the sequence.

inhibitory connection A link from one *node*, or one *detector*, to another, such that activation of one node decreases the *activation level* of the other. Often contrasted with *excitatory connection*.

initial state The state a person is in at the start of his or her efforts toward solving a problem. *Problem solving* can be understood as the attempt to move, with various operations, from the initial state to the *goal state*.

input node A *node*, within a network, that receives at least part of its activation from *detectors* that are sensitive to events in the external world.

insensitivity A property of an experiment that makes the experiment unable to detect differences. An experiment can be insensitive, for example, if the procedure is too easy, so that performance is at *ceiling levels*.

inspection time The time a person needs to make a simple discrimination between two stimuli; used in some settings as a measure of mental speed, and then used as a way to test the claim that intelligent people literally have faster processing in their brains.

integrative agnosia A disorder caused by a specific form of damage to the *parietal lobe*; people with this disorder appear relatively normal in tasks requiring them to detect whether specific features are present in a display, but they are impaired in tasks that require them to judge how the features are bound together to form complex objects.

intentional learning The acquisition of memories in a setting in which people know that their memory for the information will be tested later. Often contrasted with *incidental learning*.

interactive model A model of cognitive processing that relies on an ongoing interplay between *data-driven* and *concept-driven processing*.

interference theory of forgetting The hypothesis that materials are lost from memory because of interference from other materials that are also in memory. Interference that is caused by materials learned prior to the learning episode is called "proactive interference"; interference that is caused by materials learned after the learning episode is called "retroactive interference."

internal validity A trait of a research study that reflects the study's ability to measure what it intends to measure. A study is internally valid if the *dependent variables* measure what they are intended to measure, and if the pattern of results in the dependent variables can be attributed to the

independent variables (and not to some *confound*).

interposition A monocular cue to distance that relies on the fact that objects farther away are blocked from view by closer objects that happen to be in the viewer's line of sight.

inter-rater reliability The degree of agreement between two or more individuals who have each independently assessed some target quality. Thus, two individuals might judge how beautiful various faces are, and then the degree of agreement between the two raters can be calculated.

introspection The process through which one "looks within," to observe and record the contents of one's own mental life.

intrusion error A memory error in which one recalls elements that were not part of the original episode.

invalid syllogism A syllogism (such as a *categorical syllogism*, or a syllogism built on a *conditional statement*) in which the conclusion is not logically demanded by the premises.

Korsakoff's syndrome A clinical syndrome characterized primarily by dense *anterograde amnesia*. Korsakoff's syndrome is caused by damage to specific brain regions, and it is often precipitated by a form of malnutrition common among long-term alcoholics.

late selection A proposal that *selective attention* operates at a late stage of processing, so that the unattended inputs receive considerable analysis.

lateral fissure The separation dividing the *frontal lobes* on each side of the brain from the *temporal lobes*.

lateral geniculate nucleus (LGN) An important way station in the *thalamus* that is the first destination for visual information sent from the eyeball to the brain.

lateral inhibition A pattern in which cells, when stimulated, inhibit

the activity of neighboring cells. In the visual system, lateral inhibition in the *optic nerve* creates *edge enhancement*.

lens The transparent tissue located near the front of each eye that (together with the *cornea*) plays an important role in focusing the incoming light. Muscles control the degree of curvature of the lens, allowing the eye to form a sharp image on the *retina*.

lesion A specific area of tissue damage.

level of processing An assessment of how "deeply" newly learned materials are engaged; *shallow processing* involves thinking only about the material's superficial traits; *deep processing* involves thinking about what the material means. Deep processing is typically associated with a greater probability of remembering the now-processed information.

lexical-decision task A test in which participants are shown strings of letters and must indicate, as quickly as possible, whether or not each string of letters is a word in English. It is supposed that people perform this task by "looking up" these strings in their "mental dictionary."

LGN See *lateral geniculate nucleus*.

limbic system A set of brain structures including the *amygdala, hippocampus*, and parts of the *thalamus*. The limbic system is believed to be involved in the control of emotional behavior and motivation, and it also plays a key role in learning and memory.

limited-capacity system A group of processes in which resources are limited so that extra resources supplied to one process must be balanced by a withdrawal of resources somewhere else, with the result that the total resources expended do not exceed some limit.

linear perspective A cue for distance based on the fact that parallel lines seem to converge as they get farther away from the viewer.

linguistic relativity The proposal that the language that we speak shapes our thought, because the structure and vocabulary of our language create certain ways of thinking about the world.

linguistic universal A rule that appears to apply to every human language.

local representation A representation in which information is encoded in some small number of identifiable *nodes*. Local representations are sometimes spoken of as "one idea per node" or "one content per location." Often contrasted with *distributed representation*.

localization of function The research endeavor of determining what specific job is performed by a particular region of the brain.

long-term memory (LTM) The storage system in which we hold all of our knowledge and all of our memories. Long-term memory contains memories that are not currently activated; those that are activated are represented in *working memory*.

longitudinal fissure The separation dividing the brain's left *cerebral hemisphere* from the right.

M cells Specialized cells within the *optic nerve* that provide the input for the *magnocellular cells* in the *lateral geniculate nucleus*. Often contrasted with *P cells*.

magnetic resonance imaging (MRI) A *neuroimaging technique* that uses magnetic fields (created by radio waves) to construct a detailed three-dimensional representation of brain tissue. Like *CT scans*, MRI scans reveal the brain's anatomy, but they are much more precise than CT scans.

magnocellular cells Cells in the *lateral geniculate nucleus* specialized for the perception of motion and depth. Often contrasted with *parvocellular cells*.

maintenance rehearsal A rote, mechanical process in which items are continually cycled through *working memory*, merely by being repeated over and over. Also called "item-specific rehearsal," and often contrasted with *elaborative rehearsal*.

manner of production The way in which a speaker momentarily obstructs the flow of air out of the lungs to produce a speech sound. For example, the airflow can be fully stopped for a moment, as it is in the [t] or [b] sound; or the air can continue to flow, as it does in the pronunciation of [f] or [v].

mapping The process of figuring out how aspects of one situation or argument correspond to aspects of some other situation or argument; this process is crucial for a problem solver's ability to find and use analogies.

mask A visual presentation used to interrupt the processing of another visual stimulus.

massed learning A memorization strategy in which a person works on memorizing for a solid block of time. Often contrasted with *spaced learning*; akin to "cramming."

matching strategy A shortcut apparently used in reasoning tasks; to use this strategy, the person selects a conclusion that contains the same words (e.g., "not," "some," "all") as the *premises*.

means-end analysis A strategy used in *problem solving* in which the person is guided, step-by-step, by a comparison of the difference, at that moment, between the current state and the *goal state*, and by a consideration of the *operators* available for reducing that difference.

memory rehearsal Any mental activity that has the effect of maintaining information in *working memory*. Two types of rehearsal are often distinguished: *maintenance rehearsal* and *elaborative rehearsal*.

mental accounting A process that seems to guide decision making, in which different choices and different resources are kept separate, so that gains in one "account" (for example) do not influence choices about a different account.

mental model An internal representation in which an abstract description is translated into a relatively concrete representation, with that representation serving to illustrate how that abstract state of affairs might be realized.

mental rotation A process that participants seem to use in comparing one imagined form to another. To make the comparison, participants seem to imagine one form rotating into alignment with the other, so that the forms can be compared.

metacognitive judgment A judgment in which one stands back from a particular mental activity and comments on the activity, rather than using it or participating in it.

metacognitive skills Skills that allow people to monitor and control their own mental processes.

metalinguistic judgments Judgments in which people reflect and comment on language, rather than simply using language as they ordinarily would. Judgments about whether a sequence of words is grammatical, or whether two sentences mean the same thing, are examples of metalinguistic judgments.

metamemory People's knowledge about, awareness of, and control over their own memory.

midbrain One of the three main structures (along with the *forebrain* and the *hindbrain*) of the brain; the midbrain plays an important role in coordinating movements, and it contains structures that serve as "relay" stations for information arriving from the sensory organs.

mind-body problem The difficulty in understanding how the mind (a nonphysical entity) and the body (a physical entity) can influence each other, so that physical events can cause mental events, and mental events can cause physical ones.

minimal attachment A *heuristic* used in *sentence parsing*. The listener or reader proceeds through the sentence seeking the simplest possible *phrase structure* that will accommodate the words heard so far.

misinformation effect An effect in which reports about an earlier event are influenced by misinformation that the person received after experiencing the event. In the extreme, misinformation can be used to create *false memories* concerning an entire event that, in truth, never occurred.

mnemonic strategy A technique designed to improve memory accuracy and to make learning easier; in general, mnemonic strategies seek in one fashion or another to help memory by imposing an organization on the materials to be learned.

modal model A nickname for a specific conception of the "architecture" of memory. In this model, *working memory* serves both as the storage site for material now being contemplated and as the "loading platform" for *long-term memory*. Information can reach working memory through the processes of perception, or it can be drawn from long-term memory. Once in working memory, material can be further processed or can simply be recycled for subsequent use. This model prompted a large quantity of valuable research, but it has now largely been set aside, with modern theorizing offering a very different conception of working memory.

modus ponens A logical rule stipulating that from the two premises "If P then Q" and "P is true," one can draw the conclusion "Therefore, Q is true." Often contrasted with *modus tollens*.

modus tollens A logical rule stipulating that from the two premises "If P then Q" and "Q is false," one can draw the conclusion "Therefore, P is false." Often contrasted with *modus ponens*.

monocular distance cues Features of the visual stimulus that indicate distance even if the stimulus is viewed with only one eye.

monozygotic twins See *identical twins*.

morpheme The smallest language unit that carries meaning. Psycholinguists distinguish *content morphemes* (the primary carriers of meaning) from *function morphemes* (which specify the relations among words).

motion parallax A depth cue based on the fact that as an observer moves, the retinal images of nearby objects move more rapidly than do the retinal images of objects farther away.

MRI See *magnetic resonance imaging*.

multiple intelligences A proposal put forward by Howard Gardner that there are many forms of intelligence, including linguistic, spatial, musical, bodily-kinesthetic, and personal.

N The conventional abbreviation for the total number of participants in a study or, in some circumstances, the total number of participants in a particular condition.

necessary condition A condition that must be fulfilled in order for a certain consequence to occur. However, necessary conditions may not guarantee that the consequence will occur, since other conditions may also be necessary. Often contrasted with *sufficient condition*.

Necker cube One of the classic *ambiguous figures*; the figure is a two-dimensional drawing that can be perceived as a cube viewed from above or as a cube viewed from below.

neglect syndrome See *unilateral neglect syndrome*.

neural correlate An event in the nervous system that occurs at the same time as, and may be the biological basis of, a specific mental event or state.

neural net model An alternative term for a *connectionist network*. This term is used to emphasize the hypothesized parallels between this sort of computer model and the functioning of the nervous system.

neural synchrony A pattern of *firing* by *neurons* in which neurons in one brain area fire at the same time as neurons in another area; the brain seems to use this pattern as an indication that the neurons in different areas are firing in response to the same stimulus.

neuroimaging technique A method for examining either the structure or the activation pattern within a living brain.

neuron An individual cell within the nervous system.

neuronal workspace hypothesis A specific claim about how the brain makes conscious experience possible; the proposal is that "workspace neurons" link together the activity of various specialized brain areas, and this linkage makes possible integration and comparison of different types of information.

neuropsychology The branch of psychology concerned with the relation between various forms of brain dysfunction and various aspects of mental functioning. Neuropsychologists study, for example, *amnesia*, *agnosia*, and *aphasia*.

neurotransmitter One of the chemicals released by *neurons* to stimulate adjacent neurons. See also *synapse*.

neutral depiction A representation that directly reflects the layout and appearance of an object or scene (and so is, on this basis, a "depiction"), but without adding any specifications about how that depiction is to be understood (and so is, on this basis, "neutral"). Often contrasted with *organized depiction*.

node An individual unit within an associative network. In a scheme using *local representations*, nodes represent single ideas or concepts. In a scheme using *distributed representations*, ideas or concepts are represented by a pattern of activation across a wide number of nodes; the same nodes may also participate in other patterns and therefore in other representations.

nonfluent aphasia A disruption of language, caused by brain damage, in which a person loses the ability to speak or write with any fluency. Often contrasted with *fluent aphasia*.

normative account An account that tells how things ought to be, as opposed to how they are. Also referred to as "prescriptive account"; often contrasted with *descriptive account*.

noun phrase (NP) One of the constituents of a *phrase structure* that defines a *sentence*.

null finding A result showing no difference between groups or between conditions. A null finding is generally ambiguous, because it may indicate either that there is no difference or that the study was simply not sensitive enough to detect a difference.

object recognition The steps or processes through which people identify the objects they encounter in the world around them.

occipital lobe The rearmost lobe in each *cerebral hemisphere*, and the one that includes the primary visual projection area.

operation span A measure of *working memory*'s capacity. This measure turns out to be predictive of performance in many other tasks, presumably because these tasks all rely on working memory. This measure is also the modern replacement for the (less useful) measure obtained from the *digit-span task*.

optic flow The pattern of change in the retinal image in which the image grows larger as the viewer approaches an object and shrinks as the viewer retreats from it.

optic nerve The bundle of nerve fibers, formed from the *retina*'s *ganglion cells*, that carries information from the eyeball to the brain.

organized depiction A representation that directly reflects the layout and appearance of an object or scene (and so is, on this basis, a "depiction") but that also adds some specifications about how the depiction is to be understood (e.g., where the form's top is, what the form's *figure/ground organization* is). Often contrasted with a *neutral depiction*.

overregularization error An error in which a person perceives or remembers a word or event as being closer to the "norm" than it really is. For example, misspelled words are read as though they were spelled correctly; atypical events are misremembered in a fashion that brings them closer to more-typical events; words with an irregular past tense (such as "ran") are replaced with a regular past tense ("runned").

P cells Specialized cells within the *optic nerve* that provide the input for the *parvocellular cells* in the *lateral geniculate nucleus*. Often contrasted with *M cells*.

parahippocampal place area (PPA) A brain area apparently specialized for the perception of places.

parallel distributed processing (PDP) A system of handling information in which many steps happen at once (i.e., in parallel) and in which various aspects of the problem or task are represented only in a distributed fashion.

parallel processing A system in which many steps are going on at the same time. Usually contrasted with *serial processing*.

parietal lobe The lobe in each *cerebral hemisphere* that lies between the *occipital* and *frontal lobes* and that includes some of the *primary sensory projection areas*, as well as circuits that are crucial for the control of attention.

parieto-frontal integration theory (P-FIT) A proposal that emphasizes the close coordination among several brain areas (including areas in the *parietal lobe* and areas in the *frontal lobe*) in making intelligence possible.

parsing The process through which an input is divided into its appropriate elements—for example, dividing the stream of incoming speech into its constituent words—or in which a sequence of words is divided into its constituent phrases.

parvocellular cells Cells in the *lateral geniculate nucleus* that are specialized for the perception of patterns. Often contrasted with *magnocellular cells*.

path constraint A limit that rules out some operation in *problem solving*. Path constraints might take the form of resource limitations (limited time to spend on the problem, or limited money) or limits of other sorts (perhaps ethical limits on what one can do).

peer-review process The process through which scientific papers are evaluated before they are judged to be of high enough quality to be published in the field's scholarly journals. The papers are reviewed by individuals who are experts on the topic—in essence, peers of the authors of the papers being reviewed.

peg-word systems A type of *mnemonic strategy* using words or locations as "pegs" on which to "hang" the materials to be remembered.

percept An internal representation of the world that results from perceiving; percepts are *organized depictions*.

perceptual constancy The achievement of perceiving the

constant properties of objects in the world (their sizes, shapes, etc.) despite changes in the sensory information we receive—changes caused by variations in our viewing circumstances.

perceptual reference frame The set of specifications about how a form is to be understood and that provides the organization in an *organized depiction*.

performance The actual behavior a person produces (including the errors he or she makes) under ordinary circumstances. Often contrasted with *competence*.

permastore A hypothesized state in which individual memories seem to be held in storage forever (hence, the state can be considered "permanent storage").

perseveration error A pattern of responding in which a person produces the same response over and over, even though the person knows that the task requires a change in response. This pattern is often observed in patients with brain damage in the *frontal lobe*.

PET scans See *positron emission tomography*.

P-FIT See *parieto-frontal integration theory*.

phonemes The basic categories of sound that are used to convey language. For example, the words "peg" and "beg" differ in their initial phoneme—[p] in one case, [b] in the other.

phonemic restoration effect A pattern in which people "hear" *phonemes* that actually are not presented but that are highly likely in that context. Thus, if one is presented with the word "legislature" but with the [s] sound replaced by a cough, one is likely to hear the [s] sound anyhow.

phonological buffer A passive storage device that serves as part of the *articulatory rehearsal loop*. The phonological buffer is one of the mechanisms that are ordinarily needed for hearing. In memory rehearsal, however, the buffer is loaded by means of

subvocalization. Materials within the buffer then fade, but they can be refreshed by new covert speech under the control of the *central executive*.

phonology The study of the sounds that are used to convey language.

photoreceptor A cell on the *retina* that responds directly to the incoming light; photoreceptors are of two kinds: *rods* and *cones*.

phrase structure The pattern of requirements and relationships, governed by *phrase structure rules*, that defines the structure of a *sentence* (e.g., dividing the sentence into a *noun phrase* and a *verb phrase*, and then specifying the required contents of each phrase).

phrase structure ambiguity Ambiguity in how a *sentence* should be interpreted, resulting from the fact that more than one phrase structure is compatible with the sentence. An example of such ambiguity is "I saw the bird with my binoculars."

phrase structure rule A constraint that governs the pattern of branching in a phrase structure. Likewise, phrase structure rules govern what the constituents must be for any syntactic element of a *sentence*.

pictorial cues Patterns that can be represented on a flat surface to create the sense of a three-dimensional object or scene.

place of articulation The position at which a speaker momentarily obstructs the flow of air out of the lungs to produce a speech sound. For example, the place of articulation for the [b] sound is the lips; the place of articulation for the [d] sound is where the tongue briefly touches the roof of the mouth.

population The entire group about which an investigator wants to draw conclusions.

positron emission tomography (PET scans) A *neuroimaging technique* that determines how much glucose (the brain's fuel)

is being used by specific areas of the brain at a particular moment in time.

postsynaptic membrane The cell membrane of the *neuron* "receiving" information across the *synapse*. Often contrasted with *presynaptic membrane*.

practical intelligence The ability to solve everyday problems through skilled reasoning that relies on tacit knowledge acquired through experience.

pragmatic reasoning schema A collection of rules, derived from ordinary practical experience, that defines what inferences are appropriate in a specific situation. These reasoning *schemata* are usually defined in terms of a goal or theme, so one schema defines the rules appropriate for reasoning about situations involving "permission," and a different schema defines the rules appropriate for thinking about situations involving cause-and-effect relations.

pragmatics A term referring to knowledge of how language is ordinarily used, knowledge (for example) that tells most English speakers that "Can you pass me the salt?" is actually a request for the salt, not an inquiry about someone's arm strength.

predictive validity As assessment of whether a test measures what it is intended to measure, based on whether the test scores *correlate* with (i.e., can predict) some other relevant criterion.

prefrontal cortex The outer surface (*cortex*) of the frontmost part of the brain (i.e., the frontmost part of the *frontal lobe*). The prefrontal coretx has many functions but is crucial for the planning of complex or novel behaviors, so this brain area is often mentioned as one of the main sites underlying the brain's executive functions.

premise A *proposition* that is assumed to be true in a logic problem; the problem asks what conclusion follows from its premises.

preparation In problem solving, the first in a series of stages often hypothesized as crucial for creativity. The second stage is *incubation*; the third, *illumination*; the fourth, *verification*. Preparation is the stage in which one commences effortful work on the problem, often with little progress.

prescriptive rules Rules describing how things are supposed to be instead of how they are. Often called *normative rules* and contrasted with *descriptive rules*.

presynaptic membrane The cell membrane of the *neuron* "sending" information across the *synapse*. Often contrasted with *postsynaptic membrane*.

primacy effect An often-observed advantage in remembering the early-presented materials within a sequence of materials. This advantage is generally attributed to the fact that a person can focus attention on these items, simply because, at the beginning of a sequence, the person is obviously not trying to divide attention between these items and other items in the series. Often contrasted with *recency effect*.

primary motor projection areas The strip of tissue, located at the rear of the *frontal lobe*, that is the departure point for nerve cells that send their signals to lower portions of the brain and spinal cord, and that ultimately result in muscle movement.

primary projection areas Regions of the *cortex* that serve as the brain's receiving station for sensory information (sensory projection areas) or as a dispatching station for motor commands (motor projection areas).

primary sensory projection areas The main points of arrival in the *cortex* for information arriving from the eyes, ears, and other sense organs.

priming A process through which one input or cue prepares a person for an upcoming input or cue.

problem solving A process in which a person begins with a goal and seeks some steps that will lead toward that goal.

problem-solving protocol A record of how one seeks to solve a problem; the record is created by simply asking the person to think aloud while working on the problem. The written record of this thinking-aloud is the protocol.

problem-solving set The starting assumptions that a person uses when trying to solve a new problem. These assumptions are often helpful, because they guide the person away from pointless strategies. But these assumptions can sometimes steer the person away from worthwhile strategies, so they can be an obstacle to problem solving.

problem space The set of all states that can be reached in solving a problem, as the problem solver moves, by means of the problem's *operators*, from the problem's *initial state* toward its *goal state*.

process-pure task A task that relies on only a single mental process. If tasks are "process-pure," then we can interpret the properties of task performance as revealing the properties of the underlying process. If tasks are not process-pure, however, we cannot interpret performance as revealing the properties of a specific process.

processing fluency An improvement in the speed or ease of processing that results from prior practice in using the same processing steps.

processing pathway The sequence of *detectors* and *nodes*, and the connections among these various units, that activation flows through in dealing with (i.e., recognizing or thinking about) a specific stimulus.

production task An experimental procedure used in studying concepts, in which the person is asked to name as many examples (e.g., as many fruits) as possible.

proposition The smallest unit of knowledge that can be either true or false. Propositions are often expressed via simple *sentences*, but this is merely a convenience; other modes of representation are available.

prosody The pattern of pauses and pitch changes that characterize speech production. Prosody can be used (among other functions) to emphasize elements of a spoken *sentence*, to highlight the sentence's intended structure, or to signal the difference between a question and an assertion.

prosopagnosia A syndrome in which individuals lose their ability to recognize faces and to make other fine-grained discriminations within a highly familiar category, even though their other visual abilities seem relatively intact.

prototype theory The claim that mental categories are represented by means of a single "best example," or prototype, identifying the "center" of the category. In this view, decisions about category membership, and inferences about the category, are made with reference to this best example, which is often an average of the examples of that category that the person has actually encountered.

pseudoword A letter string designed to resemble an actual word, even though it is not. Examples include "BLAR," "PLOME," and "TUKE."

qualia (sing. quale; proun. KWAH-lee) The subjective conscious experiences or "raw feels" of awareness. Examples include the pain of a headache and the exact flavor of chocolate.

r The numerical value used in assessing a correlation, varying from −1.00 (a perfect inverse correlation) to +1.00 (a perfect correlation).

random assignment A procedure in which research participants are assigned on a random basis to one *experimental condition* or another. This ensures that there will be no systematic differences, at the start of the experiment, between the participants in the various conditions. If differences are then observed at the end of the experiment, the researcher knows that the differences were caused by something inside the experiment itself. Random assignment is required because participants inevitably differ from one another in various ways; random assignment ensures, however, that these differences are equally represented in all conditions (i.e., that all conditions have a mix of early-arrived and late-arrived participants, a mix of motivated and less motivated participants, etc.).

random sampling A procedure in which every member of the *population* being studied has an equal chance of being picked for inclusion in the data collection.

rating task A task in which research participants must evaluate some item or category with reference to some dimension, usually expressing their response in terms of some number. For example, participants might be asked to evaluate birds for how *typical* they are within the category "birds," using a "1" response to indicate "very typical" and a "7" response to indicate "very atypical."

reason-based choice A proposal for how people make decisions. The central idea is that people make a choice when—and only when—they detect what they believe to be a persuasive reason for making that choice.

recall The task of memory *retrieval* in which the remember must come up with the desired materials, sometimes in response to a cue that names the context in which these materials were earlier encountered (e.g., "Name the pictures you saw earlier"), and sometimes in response to a

cue that broadly identifies the sought-after information (e.g., "Name a fruit" or "What is the capital of California?"). Often contrasted with *recognition*.

recency effect The tendency to remember materials that occur late in a series. If the series was just presented, the recency effect can be attributed to the fact that the late-arriving items are still in *working memory* (simply because nothing else has arrived after these items to bump them out of working memory).

receptive field The portion of the visual field to which a cell within the visual system responds. If the appropriately shaped stimulus appears in the appropriate position, the cell's *firing* rate will change. The firing rate will not change if the stimulus is of the wrong form or is in the wrong position.

recognition The task of memory *retrieval* in which the items to be remembered are presented and the person must decide whether or not the item was encountered in some earlier circumstance. Thus, for example, one might be asked, "Have you ever seen this person before?" or "Is this the poster you saw in the office yesterday?" Often contrasted with *recall*.

recognition by components model A model (often referred to by its initials, RBC) of *object recognition*. In this model, a crucial role is played by *geons*, the (hypothesized) basic building blocks out of which all the objects we recognize are constructed.

recognition threshold The briefest exposure to a stimulus that still allows accurate recognition of that stimulus. For words, the recognition threshold typically lies between 10 and 40 ms. Words shown for longer durations are usually easily perceived; words shown for briefer durations are typically difficult to perceive.

reconstruction A process in which one draws on broad patterns of knowledge to figure out how a prior event actually unfolded. In some circumstances, people rely on reconstruction to fill gaps in what they recall; in other circumstances, people rely on reconstruction because it requires less effort than actual *recall*.

recursion A property of rule systems that allows a symbol to appear both on the left side of a definition (the part being defined) and on the right side (the part providing the definition). Recursive rules within *syntax*, for example, allow a *sentence* to include another sentence as one of its constituents, as in the following example: "Solomon says that Jacob is a great singer."

referent The actual object, action, or event that a word or phrase refers to.

rehearsal loop See *articulatory rehearsal loop*.

relational rehearsal A form of mental processing in which one thinks about the relations, or connections, among ideas. The connections created (or strengthened) in this way will later guide memory search.

reliability The degree of consistency with which a test measures a trait or attribute. See also *test-retest reliability*.

"remember/know" distinction A distinction between two experiences a person can have in recalling a past event. If you "remember" having encountered a stimulus before, then you usually can offer information about that encounter, including when, where, and how it occurred. If you merely "know" that you encountered a stimulus before, then you are likely to have a sense of familiarity with the stimulus but may have no idea when or where the stimulus was last encountered.

repetition priming A pattern of *priming* that occurs simply because a stimulus is presented a second time; processing is more efficient on the second presentation.

replication A reproduction of a result in a new experiment (often with small variations) to ensure that the result is reliable.

representative sample A sample drawn from a *population* in such a way that the properties of the sample are likely to reflect the properties of the population at large.

representativeness heuristic A strategy that is often used in making judgments about categories. This strategy is broadly equivalent to making the assumption that, in general, the instances of a category will resemble the *prototype* for that category and, likewise, that the prototype resembles each instance.

research literature The term scientists use to describe the papers published on a particular topic in *peer-reviewed* technical journals. These papers are usually referred to via citations of a particular format, such as "Monk, 2012," referring perhaps to a paper published in a technical journal by Peter Monk.

response selector A (hypothesized) mental resource needed for the selection and initiation of a wide range of responses, including overt responses (e.g., moving in a particular way) and covert responses (e.g., initiating a memory search).

response threshold The quantity of information or activation needed to trigger a response.

response time (RT) The amount of time (usually measured in milliseconds) needed for a person to respond to a particular event (such as a question or a cue to press a specific button).

retention interval The amount of time that passes between the initial learning of some material and the subsequent memory *retrieval* of that material.

retina The light-sensitive tissue that lines the back of the eyeball.

retrieval The process of locating information in memory and activating that information for use.

retrieval block A circumstance in which a person seems unable to retrieve a bit of information that he or she knows reasonably well.

retrieval cue An instruction or stimulus input, provided at the time of *recall*, that can potentially guide recall and help the person to retrieve the target memory.

retrieval failure A mechanism that probably contributes to a great deal of forgetting. Retrieval failure occurs when a memory is, in fact, in long-term storage but the person is unable to locate that memory when trying to retrieve it.

retrieval path A connection (or series of connections) that can lead to a sought-after memory in long-term storage.

retrograde amnesia An inability to remember experiences that occurred *before* the event that triggered the memory disruption. Often contrasted with *anterograde amnesia*.

review article A scholarly report that summarizes the results of many different research papers, seeking to synthesize those results into a coherent pattern.

risk aversion A tendency toward avoiding risk. People tend to be risk averse when contemplating gains, choosing instead to hold tight to what they already have. Often contrasted with *risk seeking*.

risk seeking A tendency toward seeking out risk. People tend to be risk seeking when contemplating losses, presumably because they are willing to gamble in hopes of avoiding (or diminishing) their losses. Often contrasted with *risk aversion*.

rod A *photoreceptor* that is sensitive to very low light levels but that is unable to discriminate hues and that has relatively poor *acuity*. Often contrasted with *cone*.

sample The subset of the population that an investigator studies to learn about the population at large.

savant syndrome A pattern of traits in a developmentally disabled person such that the person has some remarkable talent that contrasts with his or her very low level of *general intelligence*.

schema (pl. schemata) Knowledge describing what is typical or frequent in a particular situation. For example, a "kitchen schema" would stipulate that a stove and refrigerator are likely to be present, whereas a coffeemaker may be or may not be present, and a piano is likely not to be present.

selection task An experimental procedure, commonly used to study reasoning, in which a person is presented with four cards with certain information on either side of the card. The person is also given a rule that may describe the cards, and the person's task is to decide which cards must be turned over to find out if the rule describes the cards or not. Also called the *four-card task*.

selective attention The skill through which a person focuses on one input or one task while ignoring other stimuli that are also on the scene.

self-reference effect The tendency to have better memory for information that is relevant to oneself than for other sorts of material.

self-report data A form of evidence in which the person is asked directly about his or her own thoughts or experiences.

self-schema The set of interwoven beliefs and memories that constitute one's knowledge about oneself.

self-selected group A group of participants who are in a particular condition within a study because they put themselves in that condition. In some cases, participants choose which condition to be in. In other cases, they have some trait (e.g., showing up late; arriving only in the evening) that causes them to be put into a particular condition. In all cases, there is a risk that these participants are, from the start of the experiment, different from those in the other conditions. If so, then any differences observed within the experiment are ambiguous: These differences might be the result of the experimental manipulation but might also be the lingering effect of some preexisting difference. See also *random assignment*.

semantic bootstrapping An important process in language learning in which a person (usually a child) uses knowledge of semantic relationships as a basis for figuring out the *syntax* of the language.

semantic priming A process in which activation of an idea in memory causes activation to spread to other ideas related to the first in meaning.

sentence A sequence of words that conforms to the rules of *syntax* (and so has the right constituents in the right sequence).

sentence verification task An experimental procedure used for studying memory in which participants are given simple *sentences* (e.g., "Cats are animals") and must respond as quickly as possible whether the sentence is true or false.

sequential lineup A procedure used for eyewitness identification in which the witness sees faces one by one and cannot see the next face until he or she has made a yes/no decision about the face currently in view.

serial position A data pattern summarizing the relationship between some performance measure (often, likelihood of *recall*) and the order in which the test materials were presented (i.e., where the materials were located within the series). In

memory studies, the serial position curve tends to be U-shaped, with people being best able to recall the first-presented items (the *primacy effect*) and also the last-presented items (the *recency effect*).

serial processing A system in which only one step happens at a time (and so the steps go on in a series). Usually contrasted with *parallel processing*.

7 plus-or-minus 2 A number often offered as an estimate of the holding capacity of *working memory*.

shadowing A task in which research participants are required to repeat back a verbal input, word for word, as they hear it.

shallow processing A mode of thinking about material in which one pays attention only to appearances and other superficial aspects of the material; shallow processing typically leads to poor memory retention. Often contrasted with *deep processing*.

shape constancy The achievement of perceiving the constant shape of objects in the world despite changes in the shape of the retinal image that result from variations in viewing angle.

short-term memory An older term for what is now called *working memory*.

simultaneous multiple constraint satisfaction An attribute of much of our thinking, in which we seem able to find solutions to problems, or answers to questions, that satisfy several requirements ("multiple constraints") by using a search process that seems to be guided by all of these requirements at the same time.

single-cell recording A technique for recording the moment-by-moment *activation level* of an individual *neuron* within a healthy, normally functioning brain.

size constancy The achievement of perceiving the constant size of objects in the world despite

changes in the size of the retinal image that result from variations in viewing distance.

somatic markers States of the body used in decision making. For example, a tight stomach and an accelerated heart rate when a person is thinking about a particular option can signal to the person that the option has risk associated with it.

source confusion A memory error in which one misremembers where a bit of information was learned or where a particular stimulus was last encountered.

source memory A form of memory that enables a person to recollect the episode in which learning took place or the time and place in which a particular stimulus was encountered.

source monitoring The process of keeping track of when and where one encountered some bit of information (i.e., keeping track of the source of that information).

spaced learning A memorization strategy in which a person works on memorizing for a while, then does something else, then returns to memorizing, then does something else, and so on. Often contrasted with *massed learning*.

span test A procedure used for measuring *working memory*'s holding capacity. In newer studies, the *operation span* test is used.

spatial attention The mechanism through which a person allocates processing resources to particular positions in space, so that he or she more efficiently processes any inputs from that region in space.

specific language impairment A syndrome in which individuals seem to have normal intelligence but experience problems in learning the rules of language.

speech segmentation The process through which a stream of speech is "sliced" into its constituent words and, within words, into the constituent *phonemes*.

spreading activation A process through which activation travels from one *node* to another, via *associative links*. As each node becomes activated, it serves as a source for further activation, spreading onward through the network.

stereotype threat A mechanism through which a person's performance is influenced by the perception that his or her score will confirm stereotypes about his or her group.

storage The state in which a memory, once acquired, remains until it is retrieved. Many people understand storage to be a "dormant" process, so that the memory remains unchanged while it is in storage. Modern theories, however, describe a more dynamic form of storage, in which older memories are integrated with (and sometimes replaced by) newer knowledge.

Stroop interference A classic demonstration of *automaticity* in which research participants are asked to name the color of ink used to print a word, and the word itself is a different color name. For example, participants might see the word "yellow" printed in blue ink and be required to say "blue." Considerable interference is observed in this task, with participants apparently being unable to ignore the word's content even though it is irrelevant to their task.

subcortical Beneath the surface (i.e., beneath the cortex).

subjective utility A measure of how valuable a state of affairs would be for a person. This notion is central to "utility theory" accounts of decision making, on the idea that the person tries to select the option that will lead to the greatest subjective utility.

subliminal prime A *prime* that is presented so quickly that it is not consciously detected; such primes nonetheless can have an impact on subsequent perceptions or thoughts.

subthreshold activation Activation levels below *response threshold*. Subthreshold activation, by definition, will not trigger a response; nonetheless, this activation is important because it can accumulate, leading eventually to an *activation level* that exceeds the response threshold.

subvocalization Covert speech in which one goes through the motions of speaking, or perhaps forms a detailed motor plan for speech movements, but without making any sound.

sufficient condition A condition that, if satisfied, guarantees that a certain consequence will occur. However, sufficient conditions may not be necessary for that consequence (since the same consequence might occur for some other reasons). Often contrasted with *necessary condition*.

summation The addition of two or more separate inputs so that the effect of the combined inputs is greater than the effect of any one of the inputs by itself.

surface structure The representation of a *sentence* that is actually expressed in speech. In some treatments, this structure is referred to as "s-structure." Often contrasted with *underlying structure*.

synapse The area that includes the *presynaptic membrane* of one *neuron*, the *postsynaptic membrane* of another neuron, and the tiny gap between them. The presynaptic membrane releases a small amount of *neurotransmitter* that drifts across the gap and stimulates the postsynaptic membrane.

syntax Rules governing the sequences and combinations of words in the formation of phrases and *sentences*.

systematic data collection Recording of *all* the evidence or at least the collection of evidence in a fashion carefully designed to be independent of the hypothesis being considered; hence, neither biased toward the hypothesis nor against it.

tachistoscope A device that allows the presentation of stimuli for precisely controlled amounts of time, including very brief presentations.

temporal lobe The lobe of the *cortex* lying inward and down from the temples. The temporal lobe in each *cerebral hemisphere* includes the primary auditory projection area, *Wernicke's area*, and, subcortically, the *amygdala* and *hippocampus*.

testable hypothesis A supposition about the facts that has been formulated clearly enough to delineate what observations would confirm the supposition and what would challenge it.

test-retest reliability An assessment of whether a test is consistent in what it measures, determined by asking whether the test's results on one occasion are *correlated* with results from the same test (or a close variant on it) on another occasion.

thalamus A part of the lower portion of the *forebrain* that serves as a major relay and integration center for sensory information.

third-variable problem The possibility that two observations are *correlated*, not because either one is causing the other but because both are the result of some other (third) factor. The third-variable problem is one of the reasons why a *correlation* (e.g., the finding that cell-phone use and accidents are correlated) cannot, on its own, show *causation* (e.g., the idea that cell-phone use causes accidents).

threshold The activity level at which a cell or *detector* responds, or *fires*.

TMS See *transcranial magnetic stimulation*.

token node A *node* that represents a specific example or instance of a category and therefore is used in propositions concerned with specific events and individuals. Often contrasted with *type node*.

top-down influences The term given to factors arising from a person's knowledge and expectations, and shaping his or her processing of the stimulus input.

top-down processing See *concept-driven processing*.

TOT phenomenon An often-observed effect in which people are unable to remember a particular word, even though they are certain that the word (typically identified via its definition) is in their vocabulary. People in this state often can remember the starting letter for the word and its number of syllables, and they insist that the word is on the "tip of their tongue" (hence, the "TOT" label).

transcendental method A type of theorizing first proposed by the philosopher Immanuel Kant. To use this method, an investigator first observes the effects or consequences of a process and then asks: What must the process have been to bring about these effects?

transcranial magnetic stimulation (TMS) A technique in which a series of strong magnetic pulses at a specific location on the scalp causes temporary disruption in the brain region directly underneath this scalp area.

tree structure A style of depiction often used to indicate hierarchical relationships, such as the relationships (specified by *phrase structure rules*) among the words in a phrase or *sentence*.

Type 1 A commonly used name for judgment and reasoning strategies that are fast and effortless, but prone to error.

Type 2 A commonly used name for judgment and reasoning strategies that are slower and require more effort than Type 1 strategies, but are less prone to error.

type node A *node* that represents a general category and therefore is embedded in propositions that are true for the entire category. Often contrasted with *token node*.

typicality The degree to which a particular case (an object, situation, or event) is typical for its kind.

unattended channel A stimulus (or group of stimuli) that a person is not trying to perceive. Ordinarily, little information is understood or remembered from the unattended channel. Often contrasted with *attended channel*.

unconscious inference The hypothesized steps that perceivers follow in order to take one aspect of the visual scene (e.g., viewing distance) into account in judging another aspect (e.g., size).

underlying structure An abstract representation of the *sentence* to be expressed; sometimes called "deep structure" (or "d-structure"). Often contrasted with *surface structure*.

unilateral neglect syndrome A pattern of symptoms in which affected individuals ignore all inputs coming from one side of space. Individuals with this syndrome put only one of their arms into their jackets, eat food from only half of their plates, read only half of words (e.g., they might read "blouse" as "use"), and so on.

utility A measure of the subjective value that an individual puts on a particular outcome; this measure can then be used to compare various outcomes, allowing choices to be based on these comparisons.

utility maximization The proposal that people make decisions by selecting the option that has the greatest *utility*.

V1 See *Area V1*.

valid syllogism A syllogism for which the conclusion follows from the *premise*, in accord with the rules of logic.

validity The extent to which a method or procedure measures what it is supposed to measure. Validity is assessed in a variety of ways, including through *predictive validity*.

verb phrase (VP) One of the constituents of a phrase structure that defines a *sentence*.

verification One of the four steps that are commonly hypothesized as part of creative *problem solving*; in this step, the problem solver confirms that a new idea really does lead to a problem solution, and then he or she works out the details. (The other steps are *preparation, incubation,* and *illumination*.)

viewpoint-dependent recognition A process in which the ease or success of *recognition* depends on the perceiver's particular viewing angle or distance with regard to the target object.

viewpoint-independent recognition A process in which the ease or success of *recognition* does *not* depend on the perceiver's particular viewing angle or distance with regard to the target object.

visual acuity A measure of one's ability to see fine detail.

visual features The constituents of a visual pattern—vertical lines, curves, diagonals, and so on—that, together, form the overall pattern.

visual search task A commonly used laboratory task in which research participants are asked to search for a specific target (e.g., a shape, or a shape of a certain color) within a field of other stimuli; usually, the researcher is interested in how quickly the participants can locate the target.

visuospatial buffer One of the low-level assistants used as part of the *working-memory system*. This buffer plays an important role in storing visual or spatial representations, including visual images.

voice-onset time (VOT) The time that elapses between the start of a speech sound and the onset of *voicing*. VOT is the main feature distinguishing "voiced" consonants (such as [b], with a near-zero VOT) and "unvoiced" consonants (such as [p], with a VOT of approximately 60 ms).

voicing One of the properties that distinguishes different categories of speech sounds. A sound is considered "voiced" if the vocal folds are vibrating while the sound is produced. If the vocal folds start vibrating sometime after the sound begins (i.e., with a long *voice-onset time*), the sound is considered "unvoiced."

weapon-focus effect A pattern, often alleged for witnesses to violent crimes, in which one pays close attention to some crucial detail (such as the weapon within a crime scene) to the exclusion of much else.

well-defined problem A problem for which the *goal state* is clearly specified at the start and the operators available for reaching that goal are clearly identified. Often contrasted with *ill-defined problem*.

Wernicke's area An area in the left *frontal lobe* of the brain; damage here typically causes *fluent aphasia*.

what system The system of visual circuits and pathways leading from the visual *cortex* to the *temporal lobe* and especially involved in object recognition. Often contrasted with the *where system*.

where system The system of visual circuits and pathways leading from the visual *cortex* to the *parietal lobe* and especially involved in the spatial localization of objects and in the coordination of movements. Often contrasted with the *what system*.

word-stem completion A task in which research participants are given the beginning of a word (e.g., "TOM") and must provide a word that starts with the letters provided. In some versions of the task, only one solution is possible, so performance is measured by counting the number of words completed. In other versions of the task, several solutions are possible for each stem, and performance is assessed by determining which responses fulfill some other criterion.

word-superiority effect The data pattern in which research participants are more accurate and more efficient in recognizing words (and wordlike letter strings) than they are in recognizing individual letters.

working memory The storage system in which information is held while that information is being worked on. All indications are that working memory is a system, not a single entity, and that information is held here via active processes, not via some sort of passive storage. Formerly called *short-term memory*.

working-memory system A system of mental resources used for holding information in an easily accessible form. The *central executive* is at the heart of this system, and the executive then relies on a number of low-level assistants, including the *visuospatial buffer* and the *articulatory rehearsal loop*.

References

Ackerman, P. L., Beier, M. E., & Boyle, M. O. (2002). Individual differences in working memory within a nomological network of cognitive and perceptual speed abilities. *Journal of Experimental Psychology: General, 131*, 567–589.

Aggleton, J. P., & Brown, M. W. (2006). Interleaving brain systems for episodic and recognition memory. *Trends in Cognitive Sciences, 10*, 455–463.

Akers, K. G., Martinez-Canabal, A., Restivo, L., Yiu, A. P., De Cristofaro, A., Hsiang, H. L., Wheeler, A. L., Guskjolen, A., Niibori, Y., Shoji, H., Ohira, K., Richards, B. A., Miyakawa, T., Josselyn, S. A., & Frankland, P. W. (2014, May 9). Hippocampal neurogenesis regulates forgetting during adulthood and infancy. *Science, 344*(6184), 598–602.

Alberts, A. M., Kok, P., Toni, I., Dijkerman, H. C., & de Lange, F. P. (2013). Shared representations for working memory and mental imagery in early visual cortex. *Current Biology, 23*, 1427–1431.

Alexander, K. W., Quas, J. A., Goodman, G. S., Ghetti, S., Edelstein, R. S., Redlich, A. D., et al. (2005). Traumatic impact predicts long-term memory for documented child sexual abuse. *Psychological Science, 16*, 33–40.

Alkire, M., Hudetz, A., & Tononi, G. (2008). Consciousness and anesthesia. *Science, 322*, 876–880.

Allport, A. (1989). Visual attention. In M. Posner (Ed.), *Foundations of cognitive science* (pp. 631–682). Cambridge, MA: MIT Press.

Allport, D., Antonis, B., & Reynolds, P. (1972). On the division of attention: A disproof of the single channel hypothesis. *Quarterly Journal of Experimental Psychology, 24*, 225–235.

Almor, A., & Sloman, S. A. (2000). Reasoning versus text processing in the Wason selection task: A non-deontic perspective on perspective effects. *Memory & Cognition, 28*, 1060–1070.

Alter, A. L., & Oppenheimer, D. M. (2006). Predicting stock price fluctuations using processing fluency. *Proceedings of the National Academy of Sciences, 103*(24), 9369–9372.

Altmann, E. M., & Schunn, C. D. (2012). Decay versus interference: A new look at an old interaction. *Psychological Science, 23*, 1435–1437.

Amishav, R., & Kimchi, R. (2010). Perceptual integrality of componential and configural information in faces. *Psychonomic Bulletin & Review, 17*, 743–748.

Anderson, J. R. (1976). *Language, memory, and thought.* Hillsdale, NJ: Erlbaum.

Anderson, J. R. (1980). *Cognitive psychology and its implications.* San Francisco, CA: Freeman.

Anderson, J. R. (1993). Problem solving and learning. *American Psychologist, 48*, 35–44.

Anderson, J. R., & Bower, G. H. (1973). *Human associative memory.* Washington, DC: Winston.

Anderson, M. C., & Bell, T. (2001). Forgetting our facts: The role of inhibitory processes in the loss of propositional knowledge. *Journal of Experimental Psychology: General, 130*, 544–570.

Anderson, R., & Helstrup, T. (1993). Visual discovery in mind and on paper. *Memory & Cognition, 21*, 283–293.

Antonio, L. Z., Nielsen, T. A., & Donderi, D. C. (1998). Prevalance of auditory, olfactory and gustatory experiences in home dreams. *Perceptual and Motor Skills, 87*, 819-826.

Ariely, D. (2009). *Predictably irrational.* New York, NY: Harper.

Arkes, H. (1991). Costs and benefits of judgment errors: Implications for debiasing. *Psychological Bulletin, 110*, 486–498.

Arkes, H., & Harkness, A. (1983). Estimates of contingency between two dichotomous variables. *Journal of Experimental Psychology: General, 112*, 117–135.

Armstrong, S. L., Gleitman, L. R., & Gleitman, H. (1983). What some concepts might not be. *Cognition, 13*, 263–308.

Arnau, R. C., & Thompson, B. (2000). Second-order confirmatory factor analysis of the Wais-III. *Assessment, 7*, 237–246.

Aron, A. (2008). Progress in executive-function research. *Current Directions in Psychological Science, 17*, 124–129.

Arrigo, J. M., & Pezdek, K. (1997). Lessons from the study of psychogenic amnesia. *Current Directions in Psychological Science, 6*, 148–152.

Ash, I. K., & Wiley, J. (2006). The nature of restructuring in insight: An individual-differences approach. *Psychonomic Bulletin & Review, 13*, 66–73.

Ashbridge, E., Walsh, V., & Cowey, A. (1997). Temporal aspects of visual search studied by transcranial magnetic stimulation. *Neuropsychologia, 35*, 1121–1131.

Asher, E. J. (1935). The inadequacy of current intelligence tests for testing Kentucky Mountain children. *Journal of Genetic Psychology, 46*, 480–486.

Aslin, R. N., Saffran, J. R., & Newport, E. L. (1998). Computation of conditional probability statistics by 8-month-old infants. *Psychological Science, 9*, 321–324.

Atkinson, A. P., Thomas, M. S. C., & Cleeremans, A. (2000). Consciousness: Mapping the theoretical landscape. *Trends in Cognitive Sciences, 4*, 372–382.

Atkinson, R. C., & Shiffrin, R. M. (1968). Human memory: A proposed system and its control processes. In K. W. S. Spence & J. T. Spence (Eds.), *The psychology of learning and motivation* (pp. 89–105). New York, NY: Academic Press.

Atran, S. (1990). *Cognitive foundations of natural history*. New York, NY: Cambridge University Press.

Attneave, F. (1953). Psychological probability as a function of experienced frequency. *Journal of Experimental Psychology, 46*, 81–86.

Awh, E., & Pashler, H. (2000). Evidence for split attentional foci. *Journal of Experimental Psychology: Human Perception and Performance, 26*, 834–846.

Baars, B. J. (2005). Global workspace theory of consciousness: Toward a cognitive neuroscience of human experience. *Progress in Brain Research, 150*, 45–53.

Baars, B. J., & Franklin, S. (2003). How conscious experience and working memory interact. *Trends in Cognitive Sciences, 7*, 166–172.

Baddeley, A. (2000). The episodic buffer: A new component of working memory? *Trends in Cognitive Sciences, 4*, 417–423.

Baddeley, A. D. (1986). *Working memory*. Oxford, England: Clarendon.

Baddeley, A. D. (1992). Is working memory working? The fifteenth Bartlett lecture. *Quarterly Journal of Experimental Psychology, 44A*, 1–31.

Baddeley, A. D. (1996). Exploring the central executive. *Quarterly Journal of Experimental Psychology: Human Experimental Psychology, 49A*, 5–28.

Baddeley, A. D. (2012). Working memory: Theories, models, and controversies. *Annual Review of Psychology, 63*, 1–12.

Baddeley, A. D., Aggleton, J. P., & Conway, M. A. (Eds.). (2002). *Episodic memory: New directions in research*. New York, NY: Oxford University Press.

Baddeley, A. D., Gathercole, S., & Papagno, C. (1998). The phonological loop as a language learning device. *Psychological Review, 105*, 158–173.

Baddeley, A. D., & Hitch, G. (1974). Working memory. In G. Bower (Ed.), *Recent advances in learning and motivation* (pp. 47–90). New York, NY: Academic Press.

Baddeley, A. D., & Hitch, G. (1977). Recency re-examined. In S. Dornic (Ed.), *Attention and performance VI* (pp. 646–667). Hillsdale, NJ: Erlbaum.

Bahrick, H. (1984). Semantic memory content in permastore: 50 years of memory for Spanish learned in school. *Journal of Experimental Psychology: General, 113*, 1–29.

Bahrick, H., Bahrick, P. O., & Wittlinger, R. P. (1975). Fifty years of memory for names and faces: A cross-sectional approach. *Journal of Experimental Psychology: General, 104*, 54–75.

Bahrick, H., & Hall, L. (1991). Lifetime maintenance of high school mathematics content. *Journal of Experimental Psychology: General, 120*, 20–33.

Bahrick, H., Hall, L. K., & Berger, S. A. (1996). Accuracy and distortion in memory for high school grades. *Psychological Science, 7*, 265–271.

Baird, B., Smallwood, J., Mrazek, M. D., Kam, J. W. Y., Franklin, M. S., & Schooler, J. W. (2012). Inspired by distraction: Mind wandering facilitates creative incubation. *Psychological Science, 23*, 1117–1122.

Balch, W., Bowman, K., & Mohler, L. (1992). Music-dependent memory in immediate and delayed word recall. *Memory & Cognition, 20*, 21–28.

Bang, M., Medin, D., & Atran, S. (2007). Cultural mosaics and mental models of nature. *Proceedings of the National Academy of Sciences. 104*, 13868–13874.

Baratgin, J., & Noveck, I. A. (2000). Not only base rates are neglected in the engineer-lawyer problem: An investigation of reasoners' underutilization of complementarity. *Memory & Cognition, 28*, 79–91.

Barclay, J., Bransford, J., Franks, J., McCarrell, N., & Nitsch, K. (1974). Comprehension and semantic flexibility. *Journal of Verbal Learning & Verbal Behavior, 13*, 471–481.

Bargh, J. B. (2005). Toward demystifying the nonconscious control of social behavior. In R. Hasslin, J. Uleman, & J. A. Bargh (Eds.), *The new unconscious* (pp. 37–58). New York, NY: Oxford University Press.

Barkley, R. A., Murphy, K. R., & Fischer, M. (2008). *ADHD in adults: What the science says.* New York, NY: Guilford.

Baron, J. (1988). *Thinking and reasoning.* Cambridge, England: Cambridge University Press.

Baron, J. (1998). *Judgment misguided: Intuition and error in public decision making.* New York, NY: Oxford University Press.

Barsalou, L. (1983). Ad hoc categories. *Memory and Cognition, 11,* 211–227.

Barsalou, L. (1985). Ideals, central tendency, and frequency of instantiation. *Journal of Experimental Psychology: Learning, Memory, & Cognition, 11,* 629–654.

Barsalou, L. (1988). The content and organization of autobiographical memories. In U. Neisser & E. Winograd (Eds.), *Remembering reconsidered* (pp. 193–243). Cambridge, England: Cambridge University Press.

Barsalou, L., & Sewell, D. R. (1985). Contrasting the representation of scripts and categories. *Journal of Memory and Language, 24,* 646–665.

Bartlett, F. C. (1932). *Remembering: A study in experimental and social psychology.* Cambridge, England: Cambridge University Press.

Barrett, L. F., Tugade, M. M., & Engle, R. W. (2004). Individual differences in working memory capacity and dual-process theories of the mind. *Psychological Bulletin, 130,* 553–573.

Bartolomeo, P., Bachoud-Levi, A-C., De Gelder, B., Denes, G., Barba, G. D., Brugieres, P., et al. (1998). Multiple-domain dissociation between impaired visual perception and preserved mental imagery in a patient with bilateral extrastriate lesions. *Neuropsychologia, 36*(3), 239–249.

Bassok, M. (1996). Using content to interpret structure: Effects on analogical transfer. *Current Directions in Psychological Science, 5,* 54–57.

Bassok, M., & Novick, L. R. (2012). Problem solving. In K. J. Holyoak & R. G. Morrison (Eds.), *The Oxford handbook of thinking and reasoning* (pp. 413–432). New York, NY: Oxford University Press.

Bates, T. C., Lewis, G. J., & Weiss, A. (2013). Childhood socioeconomic status amplifies genetic effects on adult intelligence. *Psychological Science, 24,* 2111–2116.

Bates, T. C., & Shieles, A. (2003). Crystallized intelligence as a product of speed and drive for experience: The relationship of inspection time and openness to *g* and *Gc. Intelligence, 31,* 275–287.

Bauer, P. J. (2007). *Remembering the times of our lives: Memory in infancy and beyond.* Mahwah, NJ: Erlbaum.

Beach, C. M. (1991). The interpretation of prosodic patterns at points of syntactic structural ambiguity: Evidence for cue trading relations. *Journal of Memory and Language, 30,* 644–663.

Beaty, R. E., Silvia, P. J., Nusbaum, E. C., Jauk, E., & Benedek, M. (2014). The roles of associative and executive processes in creative cognition. *Memory & Cognition, 42,* 1186–1197.

Bechara, A., Damasio, H., & Damasio, A. R. (2003). Role of the amygdala in decision-making. *Annals of the New York Academy of Sciences, 985,* 356–369.

Bechara, A., Damasio, H., Tranel, D., & Damasio, A. R. (2005). The Iowa Gambling Task and the somatic marker hypothesis: Some questions and answers. *Trends in Cognitive Sciences, 9,* 159–162.

Bechara, A., Tranel, D., Damasio, H., Adolphs, R., Rockland, C., & Damasio, A. (1995). Double dissociation of conditioning and declarative knowledge relative to the amygdala and hippocampus in humans. *Science, 269,* 1115–1118.

Bédard, J., & Chi, M. (1992). Expertise. *Current Directions in Psychological Science, 1,* 135–139.

Begg, I., Anas, A., & Farinacci, S. (1992). Dissociation of processes in belief: Source recollection, statement familiarity, and the illusion of truth. *Journal of Experimental Psychology: General, 121,* 446–458.

Begg, I., Armour, V., & Kerr, T. (1985). On believing what we remember. *Canadian Journal of Behavioral Science, 17,* 199–214.

Behrmann, M. (2000). The mind's eye mapped onto the brain's matter. *Current Directions in Psychological Science, 9,* 50–54.

Behrmann, M., & Avidan, G. (2005). Congenital prosopagnosia: Face-blind from birth. *Trends in Cognitive Sciences, 9,* 180–187.

Behrmann, M., Peterson, M. A., Moscovitch, M., & Suzuki, S. (2006). Independent representation of parts and relations between them: Evidence from integrative agnosia. *Journal of Experimental Psychology: Human Perception and Performance, 32,* 1169–1184.

Behrmann, M., & Tipper, S. (1999). Attention accesses multiple reference frames: Evidence from visual neglect. *Journal of Experimental Psychology: Human Perception and Performance, 25,* 83–101.

Bekerian, D. A., & Baddeley, A. D. (1980). Saturation advertising and the repetition effect. *Journal of Verbal Learning & Verbal Behavior, 19,* 17–25.

Belli, R. B. (Ed.). (2012). *True and false recovered memories: Toward a reconciliation of the debate.* New York, NY: Springer.

Benjamin, L. (2008). *A history of psychology.* New York: Wiley-Blackwell.

Benyamin B., Pourcain B., Davis, O. S, Davies, G., Hansell, N. K., Brion, M. J., Kirkpatrick, R. M., Cents, R. A., Franić, S., Miller, M. B., Haworth, C. M., Meaburn, E., Price, T. S., Evans, D. M., Timpson, N., Kemp, J., Ring, S., McArdle, W., Medland, S. E., Yang, J., Harris, S. E., Liewald, D. C., Scheet, P., Xiao, X., Hudziak, J. J., de Geus, E. J., Jaddoe, V. W., Starr, J. M., Verhulst, F. C., Pennell, C., Tiemeier,

H., Iacono, W. G., Palmer, L. J., Montgomery, G. W., Martin, N. G., Boomsma, D. I., Posthuma, D., McGue, M., Wright, M. J., Davey Smith, G., Deary, I. J., Plomin, R., & Visscher, P. M. (2013). Childhood intelligence is heritable, highly polygenic and associated with FNBP1L. *Molecular Psychiatry, 19,* 253–258.

Bergen, B., Medeiros-Ward, N., Wheeler, K., Drews, F., & Strayer, D. (2013). The crosstalk hypothesis: Why language interferes with driving. *Journal of Experimental Psychology: General, 142,* 119–130.

Berger, S. A., Hall, L. K., & Bahrick, H. P. (1999). Stabilizing access to marginal and submarginal knowledge. *Journal of Experimental Psychology: Applied, 5,* 438–447.

Berko, J. (1958). The child's learning of English morphology. *Word, 14,* 150–177.

Besken, M., & Mulligan, N. W. (2014). Perceptual fluency, auditory generation, and metamemory: Analyzing the perceptual fluency hypothesis in the auditory modality. *Journal of Experimental Psychology: Learning, Memory, & Cognition, 40*(2), 429–440.

Besner, D., & Stolz, J. A. (1999a). Unconsciously controlled processing: The Stroop effect reconsidered. *Psychonomic Bulletin & Review, 6,* 449–455.

Besner, D., & Stolz, J. A. (1999b). What kind of attention modulates the Stroop effect? *Psychonomic Bulletin & Review, 6,* 99–104.

Bever, T. (1970). The cognitive basis for linguistic structures. In J. R. Hayes (Ed.), *Cognition and the development of language* (pp. 279–362). New York, NY: Wiley.

Bialystok, E., Craik, F., Green, D., & Gollan, T. (2009). Bilingual minds. *Psychological Science in the Public Interest, 10,* 89–129.

Biederman, I. (1987). Recognition by components: A theory of human image understanding. *Psychological Review, 94,* 115–147.

Biederman, I. (1990). Higher-level vision. In D. Osherson, S. Kosslyn, & J. Hollerbach (Eds.), *An invitation to cognitive science: Visual cognition and action* (Vol. 2, pp. 41–72). Cambridge, MA: MIT Press.

Bilalić, M., McLeod, P., & Gobet, F. (2010). The mechanism of the Einstellung (set) effect: A pervasive source of cognitive bias. *Current Directions in Psychological Science, 19,* 111–115.

Billock, V. A., & Tsou, B. H. (2012). Elementary visual hallucinations and their relationships to neural pattern-forming mechanisms. *Psychological Bulletin, 138,* 744–774.

Bindemann, M., Brown, C., Koyas, T., & Russ, A. (2012). Individual differences in face identification postdict eyewitness accuracy. *Journal of Applied Research in Memory & Cognition, 1,* 96–103.

Binder, J., & Desai, R. (2011). The neurobiology of semantic memory. *Trends in Cognitive Sciences, 15,* 527–536.

Bishop, D., & Norbury, C. F. (2008). Speech and language disorders. In M. Rutter, D. Bishop, D. Pine, S. Scott, J. Stevenson, E. Taylor, & A. Thapar (Eds.). *Rutter's child and adolescent psychiatry* (pp. 782–801). Oxford, England: Blackwell.

Bisiach, E., & Luzzatti, C. (1978). Unilateral neglect of representational space. *Cortex, 14,* 129–133.

Bisiach, E., Luzzatti, C., & Perani, D. (1979). Unilateral neglect, representational schema, and consciousness. *Brain, 102,* 609–618.

Blinkhorn, S. (2005). A gender bender. *Nature, 438,* 31–32.

Block, N. (1997). Biology vs. computation in the study of consciousness. *Behavioral and Brain Sciences, 20,* 1.

Block, N. (2005). Two neural correlates of consciousness. *Trends in Cognitive Sciences, 9,* 46–52.

Block, N., Carmel, D., Fleming, S. M., Kentridge, R. W., Koch, C., Lamme, V. A. F., Lau, H., & Rosenthal, D. (2014). Consciousness science: Real progress and lingering misconceptions. *Trends in Cognitive Sciences, 18,* 556–557.

Blount, G. (1986). Dangerousness of patients with Capgras Syndrome. *Nebraska Medical Journal, 71,* 207.

Bobrow, S., & Bower, G. H. (1969). Comprehension and recall of sentences. *Journal of Experimental Psychology, 80,* 455–461.

Bogen, J. E. (1995). On the neurophysiology of consciousness: I. An overview. *Consciousness & Cognition: An International Journal, 4,* 52–62.

Boole, G. (1854). *An investigation of the laws of thought, on which are founded the mathematical theories of logic and probabilities.* London, England: Maberly.

Borges, J. L. (1964). *Labyrinths.* New York, NY: New Directions.

Bornstein, B. (1963). Prosopagnosia. In L. Halpern (Ed.), *Problems of dynamic neurology* (pp. 283–318). Jerusalem, Israel: Hadassah Medical Organization.

Bornstein, B., Sroka, H., & Munitz, H. (1969). Prosopagnosia with animal face agnosia. *Cortex, 5,* 164–169.

Boroditsky, L. (2001). Does language shape thought? Mandarin and English speakers' conceptions of time. *Cognitive Psychology, 43,* 1–22.

Boroditsky, L. (2011, February). How language shapes thought. *Scientific American,* 63–65.

Borst, G., Thompson, W., & Kosslyn, S. (2011). Understanding the dorsal and ventral systems of the human cerebral cortex. *American Psychologist, 66,* 624–632.

Botvinick, M. M., Cohen, J. D., & Carter, C. S. (2004). Conflict monitoring and anterior cingulate cortex: An update. *Trends in Cognitive Sciences, 8,* 539–546.

Bouchard, T. J., Jr., Lykken, D. T., McGue, M., Segal, N. L., & Tellegen, A. (1990). Sources of human psychological differences: The Minnesota study of twins reared apart. *Science, 250,* 223–250.

Bouchard, T. J., Jr., & McGue, M. (1981). Familial studies of intelligence: A review. *Science, 212,* 1055–1059.

Bourke, P. A., & Duncan, J. (2005). Effect of template complexity on visual search and dual-task performance. *Psychological Science, 16*, 208–213.

Bowden, E., Jung-Beeman, M., Fleck, J., & Kounios, J. (2005). New approaches to demystifying insight. *Trends in Cognitive Sciences, 9*, 322–328.

Bower, G. H. (1970). Analysis of a mnemonic device. *American Scientist, 58*, 496–510.

Bower, G. H. (1972). Mental imagery and associative learning. In L. W. Gregg (Ed.), *Cognition in learning and memory* (pp. 51–88). New York, NY: Wiley.

Bower, G. H., Karlin, M. B., & Dueck, A. (1975). Comprehension and memory for pictures. *Memory & Cognition, 3*, 216–220.

Bower, G. H., & Reitman, J. S. (1972). Mnemonic elaboration in multilist learning. *Journal of Verbal Learning and Verbal Behavior, 11*, 478–485.

Bower, G. H., & Winzenz, D. (1970). Comparison of associative learning strategies. *Psychonomic Science, 20*, 119–120.

Bower, J. M., & Parsons, L. M. (2003, August). Rethinking the "lesser brain." *Scientific American, 289*, 50–57.

Bowles, B., Crupi, C., Mirsattari, S. M., Pigott, S. E., Parent, A. G., Pruessner, J. C., Yonelinas, A., & Köhler, S. (2007). Impaired familiarity with preserved recollection after anterior temporal-lobe resection that spares the hippocampus. *Proceedings of the National Academy of Sciences, 104*, 16382–16387.

Brackett, M. A., & Mayer, J. D. (2003). Convergent, discriminant, and incremental validity of competing measures of emotional intelligence. *Personality and Social Psychology Bulletin, 29*, 1147–1158.

Brand, M., & Markowitsch, H. J. (2010). Aspects of forgetting in psychogenic amnesia. In S. Della Sala (Ed.), *Forgetting* (pp. 239–251). New York, NY: Taylor & Francis.

Bransford, J. (1979). *Human cognition: Learning, understanding and remembering.* Belmont, CA: Wadsworth.

Bransford, J., & Franks, J. J. (1971). The abstraction of linguistic ideas. *Cognitive Psychology, 2*, 331–350.

Bransford, J., & Johnson, M. K. (1972). Contextual prerequisites for understanding: Some investigations of comprehension and recall. *Journal of Verbal Learning and Verbal Behavior, 11*, 717–726.

Brase, G. (2008). Frequency interpretation of ambiguous statistical information facilitates Bayesian reasoning. *Psychonomic Bulletin & Review, 15*, 284–289.

Brewer, J., Zhao, Z., Desmond, J., Glover, G., & Gabrieli, J. (1998). Making memories: Brain activity that predicts how well visual experience will be remembered. *Science, 281*, 1185–1187.

Brewer, W., & Treyens, J. C. (1981). Role of schemata in memory for places. *Cognitive Psychology, 13*, 207–230.

Brewin, C. R., & Andrews, B. (2014). Why it is scientifically respectable to believe in repression: A response to Patithis, Ho, Tingen, Lilienfeld, and Loftus. *Psychological Science, 25*, 1964–1966.

Brigham, J., & Cairns, D. L. (1988). The effect of mugshot inspections on eyewitness identification accuracy. *Journal of Applied Social Psychology, 18*, 1394–1410.

Brigham, J., & Wolfskiel, M. P. (1983). Opinions of attorneys and law enforcement personnel on the accuracy of eyewitness identification. *Law and Human Behavior, 7*, 337–349.

Broadbent, D. E. (1958). *Perception and communication.* London, England: Pergamon.

Bronfman, Z. Z., Brezis, N., Jacobson, H., & Usher, M. (2014). We see more than we can report: "Cost free" color phenomenality outside focal attention. *Psychological Science, 25*, 1394–1403.

Brooks, L., Norman, G., & Allen, S. (1991). Role of specific similarity in a medical diagnostic task. *Journal of Experimental Psychology: General, 120*, 278–287.

Brown, A. S. (1991). A review of the tip-of-the-tongue experience. *Psychological Bulletin, 109*, 204–223.

Brown, A. S. (2002). Consolidation theory and retrograde amnesia in humans. *Psychonomic Bulletin & Review, 9*, 403–425.

Brown, A. S., & Halliday, H. E. (1990, November). *Multiple-choice tests: Pondering incorrect alternatives can be hazardous to your knowledge.* Paper presented at the meeting of the Psychonomic Society, New Orleans, LA.

Brown, A. S., & Marsh, E. (2008). Evoking false beliefs about autobiographical experience. *Psychonomic Bulletin & Review, 15*, 186–190.

Brown, E., Deffenbacher, K., & Sturgill, W. (1977). Memory for faces and the circumstances of encounter. *Journal of Applied Psychology, 62*, 311–318.

Brown, J., Reynolds, J., & Braver, T. (2007). A computational model of fractionated conflict-control mechanisms in task-switching. *Cognitive Psychology, 55*, 37–85

Brown, R. (1958). *Words and things.* New York, NY: Free Press, Macmillan.

Brown, R., & Kulik, J. (1977). Flashbulb memories. *Cognition, 5*, 73–99.

Brown, R., & McNeill, D. (1966). The "tip of the tongue" phenomenon. *Journal of Verbal Learning and Verbal Behavior, 5*, 325–337.

Bruce, V., & Young, A. W. (1986). Understanding face recognition. *British Journal of Psychology, 77*, 305–327.

Bruck, M., & Ceci, S. J. (1999). The suggestibility of children's memory. *Annual Review of Psychology, 50*, 419–440.

Bruck, M., & Ceci, S. J. (2009). Developmental science in the courtroom. In S. Lilienfeld and J. Skeem (Eds.),

Psychological science in the courtroom: Controversies and consensus. New York, NY: Guilford.

Bruner, J. S. (1973). *Beyond the information given*. New York, NY: Norton.

Buchanan, T. W. (2007). Retrieval of emotional memories. *Psychological Bulletin, 133*, 761–779.

Buchanan, T. W., & Adolphs, R. (2004). The neuroanatomy of emotional memory in humans. In D. Reisberg & P. Hertel (Eds.), *Memory and emotion* (pp. 42–75). New York, NY: Oxford University Press.

Bukach, C., Gauthier, I., & Tarr, M. J. (2006). Beyond faces and modularity: The power of an expertise framework. *Trends in Cognitive Sciences, 10*, 159–166.

Bullock, T. H., Bennett, M. V., Johnston, D., Josephson, R., Marder, E., & Fields, R. D. (2005). The neuron doctrine, redux. *Science, 310*, 791–793.

Bundesen, C., Kyllingsbaek, S., & Larsen, A. (2003). Independent encoding of colors and shapes from two stimuli. *Psychonomic Bulletin & Review, 10*, 474–479.

Burgess, G. C., Braver, T. S., Conway, A. R. A., & Gray, J. R. (2011). Neural mechanisms of interference control underlie the relationship between fluid intelligence and working memory span. *Journal of Experimental Psychology: General, 140*, 674–692.

Burton, A. M., Jenkins, R., & Schweinberg, S. R. (2011). Mental representations of familiar faces. *British Journal of Psychology, 102*, 943–958.

Burton, A. M., Young, A., Bruce, V., Johnston, R., & Ellis, A. (1991). Understanding covert recognition. *Cognition, 39*, 129–166.

Buschman, T. J., & Miller, E. K. (2007). Top-down and bottom-up control of attention in the prefrontal and posterior parietal cortices. *Science, 315*, 1860.

Busey, T. A., Tunnicliff, J., Loftus, G. R., & Loftus, E. F. (2000). Accounts of the confidence-accuracy relation in recognition memory. *Memory & Cognition, 7*, 26–48.

Butler, K., Arrington, C., & Weywadt, C. (2011). Working memory capacity modulates task performance but has little influence on task choice. *Memory & Cognition, 39*, 708–724.

Buzsáki, G., & Draguhn, A. (2004). Neuronal oscillations in cortical networks. *Science, 304*, 1926–1929.

Byron, K., & Khazanchi, S. (2012). Rewards and creative performance: A meta-analytic test of theoretically derived hypotheses. *Psychological Bulletin, 138*, 809–830.

Cabeza, R., Ciaramelli, E., Olson, I. R., & Moscovitch, M. (2008). The parietal cortex and episodic memory: An attentional account. *Nature Reviews Neuroscience, 9*(8), 613–625.

Cabeza, R., & Moscovitch, M. (2012). Memory systems, processing modes, and components: Functional neuroimaging evidence. *Perspective on Psychological Science, 8*, 49–55.

Cabeza, R., & Nyberg, L. (2000). Imaging cognition II: An empirical review of 275 PET and fMRI studies. *Journal of Cognitive Neuroscience, 12*, 1–47.

Cabeza, R., & St. Jacques, P. (2007). Functional neuroimaging of autobiographical memory. *Trends in Cognitive Sciences, 11*, 219–227.

Calvo, A., & Bialystok, E. (2013). Independent effects of bilingualism and socioeconomic status on language ability and executive functioning. *Cognition, 130*, 278–288.

Campitelli, G., & Gobet, F. (2011). Deliberate practice: Necessary but not sufficient. *Current Directions in Psychological Science. 20*, 280–285.

Cann, A., & Ross, D. A. (1989). Olfactory stimuli as context cues in human memory. *American Journal of Psychology, 102*, 91–102.

Capgras, J., & Reboul-Lachaux, J. (1923). L'illusion des "sosies" dans un déliré systématisé chronique. *Bulletine de Société Clinique de Medicine Mentale, 11*, 6–16.

Caramazza, A., & Shelton, J. (1998). Domain-specific knowledge systems in the brain: The animate-inanimate distinction. *Journal of Cognitive Neuroscience, 10*, 1–34.

Carmichael, L. C., Hogan, H. P., & Walters, A. A. (1932). An experimental study of the effect of language on the reproduction of visually perceived form. *Journal of Experimental Psychology, 15*, 73–86.

Carpenter, P., & Eisenberg, P. (1978). Mental rotation and the frame of reference in blind and sighted individuals. *Perception & Psychophysics, 23*, 117–124.

Carpenter, P. A., et al. (1999). Graded functional activation in the visuospatial system and the amount of task demand. *Journal of Cognitive Neuroscience, 11*, 14.

Carpenter, S., Pashler, H., & Cepeda, N. (2009). Using tests to enhance 8th grade students' retention of U.S. history facts. *Applied Cognitive Psychology, 23*, 760–771.

Carrasco, M., & Ridout, J. B. (1997). Olfactory perception and olfactory imagery: A multidimensional analysis. *Journal of Experimental Psychology: Human Perception of Performance, 19*, 287–301.

Carrasco, M., Ling, S., & Read, S. (2004). Attention alters appearance. *Nature Neuroscience, 7*, 308–313.

Carrasco, M., Penpeci-Talgar, C., & Eckstein, M. (2000). Spatial covert attention increases contrast sensitivity across the CSF: Support for signal enhancement. *Vision Research, 40*, 1203–1215.

Carreiras, M., Armstrong, B. C., Perea, M., & Frost, R. (2014). The what, when, where, and how of visual word recognition. *Trends in Cognitive Sciences, 18*, 90–98.

Carroll, J. B. (1993). *Human cognitive abilities: A survey of factor-analytic studies*. New York, NY: Cambridge University Press.

Carroll, J. B. (2005). The three-stratum theory of cognitive abilities. In D. P. Flanagan & P. L. Harrison (Eds.), *Contemporary intellectual assessment: Theories, tests, and issues* (2nd ed., pp. 69–76). New York, NY: Guilford.

Carson, S., Peterson, J. B., & Higgins, D. M. (2005). Reliability, validity, and factor structure of the Creative Achievement Questionnaire. *Creativity Research Journal, 17,* 37–50.

Castel, A. D., Vendetti, M., & Holyoak, K. J. (2012). Fire drill: Inattentional blindness and amnesia for the location of fire extinguishers. *Attention, Perception and Psychophysics, 74,* 1391–1396.

Catrambone, R. (1998). The subgoal learning model: Creating better examples so that students can solve novel problems. *Journal of Experimental Psychology: General, 127,* 355–376.

Catrambone, R., Craig, D., & Nersessian, N. (2006). The role of perceptually represented structure in analogical problem solving. *Memory & Cognition, 34,* 1126–1132.

Cattell, J. M. (1885). Über die Zeit der Erkennung and Benennung von Schriftzeichen, Bildern and Farben. *Philosophische Studien, 2,* 635–650.

Cave, K. R. (2012). Spatial attention. In D. Reisberg (Ed.), *The Oxford handbook of cognitive psychology.* New York, NY: Oxford University Press.

Cave, R. (2013). Spatial attention. In D. Reisberg (Ed.), *The Oxford handbook of cognitive psychology* (pp. 117–130). New York, NY: Oxford University Press.

Ceci, S. J., & Williams, W. M. (1997). Schooling, intelligence, and income. *American Psychologist, 52,* 1051–1058.

Chabris, C., & Simons, D. (2010). *The invisible gorilla: How our intuitions deceive us.* New York, NY: Crown Archetype.

Chajut, E., Caspi, A., Chen, R., Hod, M., & Ariely, D. (2014). In pain thou shalt bring forth children: The peak-and-end rule in recall of labor pain. *Psychological Science, 25,* 2266–2271.

Chalmers, D. (1998). What is a neural correlate of consciousness? In T. Metzinger (Ed.), *Neural correlates of consciousness: Empirical and conceptual issues* (pp. 17–39). Cambridge, MA: MIT Press.

Chalmers, D. (1996). *The conscious mind.* New York, NY: Oxford University Press.

Chambers, D., & Reisberg, D. (1985). Can mental images be ambiguous? *Journal of Experimental Psychology: Human Perception and Performance, 11,* 317–328.

Chan, J., Paletz, S. B., & Schunn, C. D. (2012). Analogy as a strategy for supporting complex problem solving under uncertainty. *Memory & Cognition, 40,* 1352–1365.

Chan, J., Thomas, A., & Bulevich, J. (2009). Recalling a witnessed event increases eyewitness suggestibility: The reversed testing effect. *Psychological Science, 20,* 66–73.

Chao, L., Weisberg, J., & Martin, A. (2002). Experience-dependent modulation of category related cortical activity. *Cerebral Cortex, 12,* 545–551.

Chapman, J., & Chapman, L. J. (1959). Atmosphere effect re-examined. *Journal of Experimental Psychology, 58,* 220–226.

Chapman, L. J., & Chapman, J. (1971). Test results are what you think they are. *Psychology Today, 5,* 106–110.

Charniak, E. (1972). *Toward a model of children's story comprehension.* Unpublished doctoral dissertation, Massachusetts Institute of Technology, Cambridge, MA.

Chase, W., & Ericsson, K. A. (1982). Skill and working memory. In G. H. Bower (Ed.), *The psychology of learning and motivation* (pp. 1–58). New York, NY: Academic Press.

Chase, W., & Simon, H. (1973). Perception in chess. *Cognitive Psychology, 4,* 55–81.

Chen, J.-Y. (2007). Do Chinese and English speakers think about time differently? Failure of replicating Boroditsky (2001). *Cognition, 104,* 427–436.

Chen, Z., & Cave, K. R. (2006). Reinstating object-based attention under positional certainty: The importance of subjective parsing. *Perception and Psychophysics, 68,* 992–1003.

Chen, Z., & Daehler, M. W. (2000). External and internal instantiation of abstract information facilitates transfer in insight problem solving. *Contemporary Educational Psychology, 25,* 423–449.

Cheng, P., & Holyoak, K. J. (1985). Pragmatic reasoning schemas. *Cognitive Psychology, 17,* 391–416.

Cheng, P., Holyoak, K. J., Nisbett, R. E., & Oliver, L. M. (1986). Pragmatic versus syntactic approaches to training deductive reasoning. *Cognitive Psychology, 18,* 293–328.

Cherry, E. C. (1953). Some experiments on the recognition of speech with one and with two ears. *Journal of the Acoustical Society of America, 25,* 975–979.

Chi, M. (1976). Short-term memory limitations in children: Capacity or processing deficits? *Memory & Cognition, 4,* 559–572.

Chi, M., Feltovich, P., & Glaser, R. (1981). Categorization and representation of physics problems by experts and novices. *Cognitive Science, 5,* 121–152.

Chincotta, D., & Underwood, G. (1997). Digit span and articulatory suppression: A cross-linguistic comparison. *European Journal of Cognitive Psychology, 9,* 89–96.

Chomsky, N., & Halle, M. (1968). *The sound pattern of English.* New York, NY: Harper & Row.

Christen, F., & Bjork, R. A. (1976). *On updating the loci in the method of loci.* Paper presented at the meeting of the Psychonomic Society, St. Louis, MO.

Christensen, B. T., & Schunn, C. D. (2005). Spontaneous access and analogical incubation effects. *Creativity Research Journal, 17,* 207–220.

Christiaansen, R., Sweeney, J., & Ochalek, K. (1983). Influencing eyewitness descriptions. *Law and Human Behavior, 7,* 59–65.

Chrobak, Q. M., & Zaragoza, M. S. (2008). Inventing stories: Forcing witnesses to fabricate entire fictitious events leads to freely reported false memories. *Psychonomics Bulletin and Review, 15,* 1190–1195.

Chronicle, E. P., MacGregor, J. N., & Ormerod, T. C. (2004). What makes an insight problem? The roles of heuristics, goal conception, and solution recoding in knowledge-lean problems. *Journal of Experimental Psychology: Learning, Memory, & Cognition, 30,* 14–27.

Chuderiski, A., & Necka, E. (2012). The contribution of working memory to fluid reasoning. *Journal of Experimental Psychology: Learning, Memory, & Cognition, 38,* 1689–1710.

Chun, W. Y., & Kruglanski, A. W. (2006). The role of task demands and processing resources in the use of base-rate and individuating information. *Journal of Personality and Social Psychology, 91,* 205–217.

Claparède, E. (1951). Reconnaissance et moitié. In D. Rapaport (Ed.), *Organization and pathology of thought* (pp. 58–75). New York, NY: Columbia University Press. (Original work published in 1911.)

Coates, S. L., Butler, L. T., & Berry, D. C. (2006). Implicit memory and consumer choice: The mediating role of brand familiarity. *Applied Cognitive Psychology 20*(8), 1101–1116.

Cohen, G. L., Garcia, J., Apfel, N., & Master, A. (2006). Reducing the racial achievement gap: A social-psychological intervention. *Science, 313,* 1307–1310.

Cohen, G. L., Garcia, J., Purdie-Vaughns, V., Apfel, N., & Brzustoski, P. (2009). Recursive processes in self-affirmation: Intervening to close the minority achievement gap. *Science, 324,* 400–403.

Cohen, M., Cavanagh, P, Chun, M., & Nakayama, K. (2012). The attentional requirements of consciousness. *Trends in Cognitive Sciences, 16,* 418–426.

Cohen, M., & Dennett, D. (2011). Consciousness cannot be separated from function. *Trends in Cognitive Sciences, 15,* 358–364.

Cohen, M. R. (2012). When attention wanders. *Science, 338,* 58–59.

Cohen, N. J., & Squire, L. R. (1980). Preserved learning and retention of pattern analyzing skill in amnesics: Dissociation of knowing how and knowing that. *Science, 210,* 207–210.

Coley, J. D., Medin, D. L., & Atran, S. (1997). Does rank have its privilege? Inductive inferences within folk-biological taxonomies. *Cognition, 64,* 73–112.

Collins, A. M., & Quillian, M. R. (1969). Retrieval time from semantic memory. *Journal of Verbal Learning and Verbal Behavior, 8,* 240–247.

Conrad, C. (1972). Cognitive economy in semantic memory. *Journal of Experimental Psychology, 92,* 149–154.

Conway, A. R., Cowan, N., & Bunting, M. F. (2001). The cocktail party phenomenon revisited: The importance of working memory capacity. *Psychonomic Bulletin & Review, 8,* 331–335.

Conway, A. R., Kane, M. J., Bunting, M., Hambrick, D., Wilhelm, O., & Engle, R. (2005). Working memory span tasks: A methodological review and user's guide. *Psychonomic Bulletin & Review, 12,* 769–786.

Conway, M., Anderson, S., Larsen, S., Donnelly, C., McDaniel, M., McClelland, A. G. R., et al. (1994). The formation of flashbulb memories. *Memory & Cognition, 22,* 326–343.

Conway, M., Cohen, G., & Stanhope, N. (1991). On the very long-term retention of knowledge acquired through formal education: Twelve years of cognitive psychology. *Journal of Experimental Psychology: General, 120,* 395–409.

Conway, M., Cohen, G., & Stanhope, N. (1992). Why is it that university grades do not predict very long term retention? *Journal of Experimental Psychology: General, 121,* 382–384.

Conway, M., & Fthenaki, K. (1999). Disruption and loss of autobiographical memory. In L. S. Cermak (Ed.), *Handbook of neuropsychology: Memory.* Amsterdam, Netherlands: Elsevier.

Conway, M., & Haque, S. (1999). Overshadowing the reminiscence bump: Memories of a struggle for independence. *Journal of Adult Development, 6,* 35–43.

Conway, M., & Holmes, A. (2004). Psychosocial stages and the accessibility of autobiographical memories across the life cycle. *Journal of Personality, 72,* 461–480.

Conway, M., & Pleydell-Pearce, C. W. (2000). The construction of autobiographical memories in the self-memory system. *Psychological Review, 107,* 261–288.

Conway, M., & Ross, M. (1984). Getting what you want by revising what you had. *Journal of Personality and Social Psychology, 39,* 406–415.

Conway, M. A., Wang, Q., Hanyu, K., & Haque, S. (2005). A cross-cultural investigation of autobiographical memory. *Journal of Cross-Cultural Psychology, 36,* 739–749.

Cooney, J. W., & Gazzaniga, M. S. (2003). Neurological disorders and the structure of human consciousness. *Trends in Cognitive Sciences, 7,* 161–165.

Cooper, L., & Shepard, R. N. (1973). Chronometric studies of the rotation of mental images. In W. G. Chase (Ed.), *Visual information processing* (pp. 75–176). New York, NY: Academic Press.

Corbetta, M., & Shulman, G. L. (2002). Control of goal-directed and stimulus-driven attention in the brain. *Nature Reviews Neuroscience, 3*(3), 201–215.

Corbetta, M., & Shulman, G. L. (2011). Spatial neglect and attention networks. *Annual Review of Neuroscience, 34,* 569–599.

Coricelli, G., Dolan, R., & Sirigu, A. (2007). Brain, emotion and decision making: The paradigmatic example of regret. *Trends in Cognitive Sciences, 11,* 258–265.

Corkin, S. (2013). *Permanent present tense: The unforgettable life of the amnesic patient, H. M.* New York, NY: Basic Books.

Corter, J., & Gluck, M. (1992). Explaining basic categories: Feature predictability and information. *Psychological Bulletin, 111,* 291–303.

Cosmides, L. (1989). The logic of social exchange: Has natural selection shaped how humans reason? Studies with the Wason selection task. *Cognition, 31,* 187–276.

Cosmides, L., & Tooby, J. (1996). Are humans good intuitive statisticians after all? Rethinking some conclusions from the literature on judgment. *Cognition, 58,* 1–73.

Costa, A., Hernández, M., Costa-Faidella, J., & Sebastián-Galés, N. (2009). On the bilingual advantage in conflict processing: Now you see it, now you don't. *Cognition, 113,* 135–149.

Courtney, S. M., Petit, L., Maisog, J. M., Ungerleider, L. G., & Haxby, J. V. (1998). An area specialized for spatial working memory in human frontal cortex. *Science, 279,* 1347–1351.

Cowan, N. (2010). The magical mystery four: How is working memory capacity limited, and why? *Current Directions in Psychological Science, 19,* 51–57.

Cowan, R., & Carney, D. (2006). Calendrical savants: Exceptionality and practice. *Cognition, 100,* B1–B9.

Coyle, T., Pillow, D., Snyder, A., & Kochunov, P. (2011). Processing speed mediates the development of general intelligence (g) in adolescence. *Psychological Science, 22,* 1265–1269.

Craik, F. I. M., & Lockhart, R. S. (1972). Levels of processing: A framework for memory research. *Journal of Verbal Learning and Verbal Behavior, 11,* 671–684.

Craik, F. I. M., & Tulving, E. (1975). Depth of processing and the retention of words in episodic memory. *Journal of Experimental Psychology: General, 104,* 269–294.

Craik, F. I. M., & Watkins, M. J. (1973). The role of rehearsal in short-term memory. *Journal of Verbal Learning and Verbal Behavior, 12,* 599–607.

Crick, F., & Koch, C. (1995). Are we aware of neural activity in primary visual cortex? *Nature, 375,* 121–123.

Crick, F., & Koch, C. (2003). A framework for consciousness. *Nature Neuroscience, 6,* 119–126.

Crombag, H. F. M., Wagenaar, W. A., & van Koppen, P. J. (1996). Crashing memories and the problem of "source monitoring." *Applied Cognitive Psychology, 10,* 95–104.

Csibra, G., Davis, G., Spratling, M. W., & Johnson, M. H. (2000). Gamma oscillations and object processing in the infant brain. *Science, 290,* 1582–1585.

Cui, X., Jeter, C., Yang, D., Montague, P. R., & Eagleman, D. M. (2006). Vividness of mental imagery: Individual variability can be measured objectively. *Vision Research, 47,* 474–478.

Cummins, D. (1992). Role of analogical reasoning in induction of problem categories. *Journal of Experimental Psychology: Learning, Memory, & Cognition, 18,* 1103–1124.

Cummins, D. (2004). The evolution of reasoning. In J. P. Leighton & R. J. Sternberg (Eds.), *The nature of reasoning* (pp. 339–374). New York, NY: Cambridge University Press.

Cummins, D., & Allen, C. (Eds.). (1998). *The evolution of mind.* New York, NY: Oxford University Press.

Custers, R., & Aarts, H. (2010). The unconscious will: How the pursuit of goals operates outside of conscious awareness. *Science, 329,* 47–50.

Cutler, B. L., Penrod, S. D., & Dexter, H. R. (1990). Juror sensitivity to eyewitness identification evidence. *Law and Human Behavior, 14,* 185–191.

Dalenberg, C. J., Brand, B. L., Gleaves, D. H., Dorahy, M. J., Loewenstein, R. J., Cardeña, E., Frewen, P. A., Carlson, E. B., & Spiegel, D. (2012, March 12). Evaluation of the evidence for the trauma and fantasy models of dissociation. *Psychological Bulletin, 138,* 550–588.

Daley, T. C., Whaley, S. E., Sigman, M. D., Espinosa, M. P., & Neumann, C. (2003). IQ on the rise: The Flynn effect in rural Kenyan children. *Psychological Science, 14,* 215–219.

Dalton, P., & Fraenkel, N. (2012). Gorillas we have missed: Sustained inattentional deafness for dynamic events. *Cognition, 124,* 367–372.

Damasio, A. R. (1985). Disorders of complex visual processing. In M.-M. Mesulam (Ed.), *Principles of behavioral neurology.* Philadelphia, PA: Davis.

Damasio, A. R., Damasio, H., & Van Hoesen, G. W. (1982). Prosopagnosia: Anatomic basis and behavioral mechanisms. *Neurology, 32,* 331–341.

Damasio, A. R., Tranel, D., & Damasio, H. (1989). Disorders of visual recognition. In H. Goodglass & A. R. Damasio (Eds.), *Handbook of neuropsychology* (Vol. 2, pp. 317–332). New York, NY: Elsevier.

Damasio, A. R., Tranel, D., & Damasio, H. (1990). Face agnosia and the neural substrates of memory. *Annual Review of Neuroscience, 13,* 89–109.

Damasio, H., Grabowski, T., Tranel, D., Hichwa, R. D., & Damasio, A. R. (1996). A neural basis for lexical retrieval. *Nature, 380,* 499–505.

Daneman, M., & Hannon, B. (2001). Using working memory theory to investigate the construct validity of multiple-choice reading comprehension tests such as the SAT. *Journal of Experimental Psychology: General, 130,* 208–223.

Daniloff, R., & Hammarberg, R. (1973). On defining coarticulation. *Journal of Phonetics, 1,* 185–194.

Danthiir, V., Roberts, R. D., Schulze, R., & Wilhelm, O. (2005). Mental speed: On frameworks, paradigms, and a platform for the future. In O. Wilhelm & R. W. Engle (Eds.), *Handbook of understanding and measuring intelligence* (pp. 27–46). Thousand Oaks, CA: Sage.

Dar-Nimrod, I., & Heine, S. (2006). Exposure to scientific theories affects women's math performance. *Science, 314,* 435.

Davachi, L., & Dobbins, I. (2008). Declarative memory. *Current Directions in Psychological Science, 17,* 112–118.

Davachi, L., Mitchell, J., & Wagner, A. (2003). Multiple routes to memory: Distinct medial temporal lobe processes build item and source memories. *Proceedings of the National Academy of Science, 100,* 2157–2162.

Davis, D., Loftus, E., Vanous, S., & Cucciare, M. (2008). "Unconscious transference" can be an instance of "change blindness." *Applied Cognitive Psychology, 22,* 605–623.

Davis, O. S. P., Haworth, C. M. A., & Plomin, R. (2009). Dramatic increase in heritability of cognitive development from early to middle childhood: An 8-year longitudinal study of 8,700 pairs of twins. *Psychological Science, 20,* 1301–1308.

Dawes, R. M. (1988). *Rational choice in an uncertain world.* San Diego, CA: Harcourt Brace Jovanovich.

de Bruin, A., Treccani, B., & Della Salla, S. (2015). Cognitive advantage in bilingualism: An example of publication bias? *Psychological Science, 26,* 99–107.

de Gelder, B. (2010, May). Uncanny sight in the blind. *Scientific American,* 60–64.

de Groot, A. (1965). *Thought and choice in chess.* The Hague, Netherlands: Mouton.

de Groot, A. (1966). Perception and memory versus thought: Some old ideas and recent findings. In B. Kleinmuntz (Ed.), *Problem solving* (pp. 19–50). New York, NY: Wiley.

de Haan, E., & Cowey, A. (2011). On the usefulness of "what" and "where" pathways in vision. *Trends in Cognitive Sciences, 15,* 460–466.

De Neys, W. (2006). Dual processing in reasoning: Two systems but one reasoner. *Psychological Science, 17,* 428–433.

De Neys, W., & Bonnefon, J.-F. (2013). The "whys" and "whens" of individual differences in thinking biases. *Trends in Cognitive Sciences, 17,* 172–178.

De Neys, W., Vartanian, O., & Goel, V. (2008). Smarter than we think: When our brains detect that we are biased. *Psychological Science, 19,* 483–489.

De Renzi, E., Faglioni, P., Grossi, D., & Nichelli, P. (1991). Apperceptive and associative forms of prosopagnosia. *Cortex, 27,* 213–221.

Deary, I. J. (2012). Intelligence. *Annual Review of Psychology, 63,* 453–482.

Deary, I. J. (2014). The stability of intelligence from childhood to old age. *Current Directions in Psychological Science, 23,* 239–245.

Deary, I. J., & Derr, G. (2005). Reaction time explains IQ's association with death. *Psychological Science, 16,* 64–69.

Deary, I. J., Pattie, A., & Starr, J. M. (2013). The stability of intelligence from age 11 to age 90: The Lothian birth cohort of 1921. *Psychological Science, 24,* 2361–2368.

Deary, I. J., Weiss, A., & Batty, G. D. (2010). Intelligence and personality as predictors of illness and death: How researchers in differential psychology and chronic disease epidemiology are collaborating to understand and address health inequalities. *Psychological Science in the Public Interest, 11,* 53–79.

Deese, J. (1957). Serial organization in the recall of disconnected items. *Psychological Reports, 3,* 577–582.

Deese, J., & Kaufman, R. A. (1957). Serial effects in recall of unorganized and sequentially organized verbal material. *Journal of Experimental Psychology, 54,* 180–187.

DeGutis, J., Wilmer, J., Mercado, R., & Cohan, S. (2013). Using regression to measure holistic face processing reveals a strong link with face recognition ability. *Cognition, 126,* 87–100.

DeHaan, R. L. (2011). Teaching creative science thinking. *Science, 334,* 1499–1500.

Dehaene, S., Artiges, E., Naccache, L., Martelli, C., Viard, A., Schurhoff, F., et al. (2003). Conscious and subliminal conflicts in normal subjects and patients with schizophrenia: The role of the anterior cingulate. *Proceedings of the National Academy of Sciences, USA, 100,* 13722–13727.

Dehaene, S., & Changeux, J. (2004). Neural mechanisms for access consciousness. In M. Gazzaniga (Ed.), *The cognitive neurosciences III.* Cambridge, MA: MIT Press.

Dehaene S., & Changeux, J. (2011). Experimental and theoretical approaches to conscious processing. *Neuron, 70,* 200–227.

Dehaene, S., & Naccache, L. (2001). Toward a cognitive neuroscience of consciousness: Basic evidence and a workspace framework. *Cognition, 79,* 1–37.

Dehaene, S., Sergent, C., & Changeux, J. (2003). A neuronal network model linking subjective reports and objective physiological data during conscious perception. *Proceedings of the National Academy of Science, USA, 100,* 8520–8525.

Della Sala, S. (Ed.). (2010). *Forgetting.* New York, NY: Taylor & Francis.

Demonet, J. F., Wise, R. A., & Frackowiak, R. S. J. (1993). Language functions explored in normal subjects by positron emission tomography: A critical review. *Human Brain Mapping, 1,* 39–47.

Dempster, F. N. (1981). Memory span: Sources of individual and developmental differences. *Psychological Bulletin, 89,* 63–100.

Dennett, D. (1992). *Consciousness explained.* Boston, MA: Little, Brown.

DePaulo, B., Lindsay, J., Malone, B., Muhlenbruck, L., Charlton, K., & Cooper, H. (2003). Cues to deception. *Psychological Bulletin, 129,* 74–118.

Dewar, M., Cowan, N., & Della Salla, S. (2010). Forgetting due to retroactive interference in amnesia. In S. Della Sala (Ed.), *Forgetting* (pp. 185–209). New York, NY: Taylor & Francis.

Diamond, A. (2013). Executive functions. *Annual Review of Psychology, 64,* 135–168.

Diamond, A., & Lee, K. (2011). Interventions shown to aid executive function development in children from 4 to 12 years old. *Science, 333,* 959–964.

Diana, R., Yonelinas, A., & Ranganath, C. (2007). Imaging recollection and familiarity in the medial temporal lobe: A three-component model. *Trends in Cognitive Sciences, 11,* 379–386.

Dickens, W. T., & Flynn, J. R. (2001). Heritability estimates versus large environmental effects: The IQ paradox resolved. *Psychological Review, 108(2),* 346–369.

Dickens, W. T., & Flynn, J. R. (2006). Black Americans reduce the racial IQ gap: Evidence from standardization samples. *Psychological Science, 17,* 913–920.

Dickson, R., Pillemer, D., & Bruehl, E. (2011). The reminiscence bump for salient personal memories: Is a cultural life script required? *Memory & Cognition, 39,* 977–991.

Dobbins, I. G., Foley, H., Wagner, A. D., & Schacter, D. L. (2002). Executive control during episodic retrieval: Multiple prefrontal processes subserve source memory. *Neuron, 35,* 989–996.

Dodds, R. A., Ward, T. B., & Smith, S. M. (2007). A review of the experimental literature on incubation in problem solving and creativity. In M. Runco (Ed.), *Creative research handbook* (3rd ed.). Cresskill, NJ: Hampton.

Dodds, R. A., Ward, T. B., & Smith, S. M. (2012). A review of experimental literature on incubation in problem solving and creativity. In M. A. Runco (Ed.), *Creativity research handbook* (Vol. 3). Cresskill, NJ: Hampton Press.

Donnelly, C. M., & McDaniel, M. A. (1993). Use of analogy in learning scientific concepts. *Journal of Experimental Psychology: Learning, Memory, & Cognition, 19,* 975–986.

Douglas, A., Neuschatz, J., Imrich, J., & Wilkinson, M. (2010). Does post identification feedback affect evaluations of eyewitness testimony and identification procedures? *Law & Human Behavior, 34,* 282–294.

Downs, J., & Shafir, E. (1999). Why some are perceived as more confident and more insecure, more reckless and more cautious, more trusting and more suspicious, than others: Enriched and impoverished options in social judgment. *Psychonomic Bulletin & Review, 6,* 598–610.

Drew, T., Võ, M. H., & Wolfe, J. M. (2013). The invisible gorilla strikes again: Sustained inattentional blindness in expert observers. *Psychological Science, 24,* 1848–1853.

Drews, F. A., Pasupathi, M., & Strayer, D. L. (2008). Passenger and cell phone conversations in simulated driving. *Journal of Experimental Psychology: Applied, 14,* 392–400.

Dronkers, N., Wilkins, D., Van Valin, R., Redefern, B., & Jaeger, J. (2004). Lesion analysis of the brain areas involved in language comprehension. *Cognition, 92,* 145–177.

Dror, I. E., & Charlton, D. (2006). Why experts make errors. *Journal of Forensic Identification, 56(4),* 600–616.

Drummond, P. D. (1995). Effect of imagining and actual tasting a sour taste on one side of the tongue *Physiology & Behavior, 57,* 373–376.

Duchaine, B. C., & Nakayama, K. (2006). Developmental prosopagnosia: A window to content-specific face processing. *Current Opinion in Neurobiology, 16,* 166–173.

Dudai, Y. (2004). The neurobiology of consolidations, or, how stable is the engram. *Annual Review of Psychology, 55,* 51–86.

Duncan, G. J., Yeung, W. J., Brooks-Gunn, J., & Smith, J. R. (1998). How much does childhood poverty affect the life chances of children? *American Sociological Review, 63,* 406–423.

Duncan, J. (1994). Attention, intelligence, and the frontal lobes. In M. Gazzaniga (Ed.), *The cognitive neurosciences.* Cambridge, MA: MIT Press.

Duncan, J., Parr, A., Woolgar, A., Thompson, R., Bright, P., Cox, S., Bishop, S., & Nimmo-Smith, I. (2008). Goal neglect and Spearman's g: Competing parts of a complex task. *Journal of Experimental Psychology: General, 137,* 131–148.

Duncan, J., Schramm, M., Thompson, R., & Dumontheil, I. (2012). Task rules, working memory, and fluid intelligence. *Psychonomic Bulletin and Review, 19,* 864–870.

Duncker, K. (1945). *On problem-solving* (Psychological Monographs: General and Applied, Vol. 58, No. 5 [whole no. 270]). Washington, DC: American Psychological Association.

Dunlosky, J., & Bjork, R. A. (Eds.) (2008). *Handbook of metamemory and memory.* New York, NY: Psychology Press.

Dunn, B., Galton, H., Morgan, R., Evans, D., Oliver, C., Meyer, M., et al. (2010). Listening to your heart: How interoception shapes emotion experience and intuitive decision making. *Psychological Science, 21,* 1835–1844.

Dunning, D., & Parpal, M. (1989). Mental addition versus subtraction in counterfactual reasoning. *Journal of Personality and Social Psychology, 57*, 5–15.

Dunning, D., & Perretta, S. (2002). Automaticity and eyewitness accuracy: A 10- to 12-second rule for distinguishing accurate from inaccurate positive identifications. *Journal of Applied Psychology, 87*, 951–962.

Durgin, F. H. (2000). The reverse Stroop effect. *Psychonomic Bulletin & Review, 7*, 121–125.

Duyme, M., Dumaret, A. C., & Tomkiewicz, S. (1999). How can we boost IQs of "dull children"? A late adoption study. *Proceedings of the National Academy of Sciences, 96*, 8790–8794.

Easterbrook, J. A. (1959). The effect of emotion on cue utilization and the organization of behavior. *Psychological Review, 66*, 183–201.

Eberhard, K. M., Spivey-Knowlton, M. J., Sedivy, J. C., & Tanenhaus, M. K. (1995). Eye movements as a window into real-time spoken language comprehension in natural contexts. *Journal of Psycholinguistic Research, 24*, 409–436.

Eddy, D. M. (1982). Probabilistic reasoning in clinical medicine: Problems and opportunities. In D. Kahneman, P. Slovic, & A. Tversky (Eds.), *Judgment under uncertainty: Heuristics and biases* (pp. 249–267). Cambridge, England: Cambridge University Press.

Edelson, M., Sharon, T., Dolan, R., & Dudai, Y. (2011). Following the crowd: Brain substrates of long-term memory conformity. *Science, 333*, 108–111.

Edelstyn, N. M. J., & Oyebode, F. (1999). A review of the phenomenology and cognitive neuropsychological origins of the Capgras Syndrome. *International Journal of Geriatric Psychiatry, 14*, 48–59.

Egan, D., & Schwartz, B. (1979). Chunking in the recall of symbolic drawings. *Memory & Cognition, 7*, 149–158.

Eich, J. E. (1980). The cue-dependent nature of state dependent retrieval. *Memory & Cognition, 8*, 157–173.

Elliott, M. A., & Müller, H. J. (2000). Evidence for 40-Hz oscillatory short-term visual memory revealed by human reaction-time measurements. *Journal of Experimental Psychology: Learning, Memory, & Cognition, 26*, 7093–7718.

Ellis, H. D., & De Pauw, K. W. (1994). The cognitive neuropsychiatric origins of the Capgras delusion. In A. S. David & J. C. Cutting (Eds.), *The neuropsychology of schizophrenia* (pp. 317–335). Hillsdale, NJ: Erlbaum.

Ellis, H. D., & Lewis, M. B. (2001). Capgras delusion: A window on face recognition. *Trends in Cognitive Sciences, 5*, 149–156.

Ellis, H. D., & Young, A. (1990). Accounting for delusional misidentifications. *British Journal of Psychiatry, 157*, 239–248.

Elstein, A., Holzman, G., Ravitch, M., Metheny, W., Holmes, M., Hoppe, R., et al. (1986). Comparison of physicians' decisions regarding estrogen replacement therapy for menopausal women and decisions derived from a decision analytic model. *American Journal of Medicine, 80*, 246–258.

Engel, A. K., & Singer, W. (2001). Temporal binding and the neural correlates of sensory awareness. *Trends in Cognitive Sciences, 5*, 16–25.

Engel de Abreu, P. M. J., Cruz-Santos, A., Tourinho, C. J., Martion, R., & Bialystok, E. (2012). Bilingualism enriches the poor: Enhanced cognitive control in low-income minority children. *Psychological Science 23*, 1364–1371.

Engle, R. W., & Kane, M. J. (2004). Executive attention, working memory capacity, and a two-factor theory of cognitive control. In B. Ross (Ed.), *The psychology of learning and motivation 44* (pp. 145–199). New York, NY: Elsevier.

Ericsson, K. A. (2003). Exceptional memorizers: Made, not born. *Trends in Cognitive Sciences, 7*, 233–235.

Ericsson, K. A. (2005). Recent advances in expertise research: A commentary on the contributions to the special issue. *Applied Cognitive Psychology, 19*, 233–241.

Ericsson, K. A., & Towne, T. J. (2012). Experts and their superior performance. In D. Reisberg (Ed.), *The Oxford handbook of cognitive psychology*. New York, NY: Oxford University Press.

Ericsson, K. A., & Ward, P. (2007). Capturing the naturally occurring superior performance of experts in the laboratory: Toward a science of expert and exceptional performance. *Current Directions in Psychological Science, 16*, 346–350.

Ernest, C. (1977). Imagery ability and cognition: A critical review. *Journal of Mental Imagery, 2*, 181–216.

Ervin-Tripp, S. (1993). Conversational discourse. In J. B. Gleason & N. B. Ratner (Eds.), *Psycholinguistics* (pp. 237–270). New York, NY: Harcourt Brace Jovanovich.

Estes, Z. (2003). Domain differences in the structure of artifactual and natural categories. *Memory & Cognition, 31*, 199–214.

Evans, J. S. B. T. (1982). *The psychology of deductive reasoning*. London, England: Routledge & Kegan Paul.

Evans, J. S. B. T. (1989). *Bias in human reasoning*. Hillsdale, NJ: Erlbaum.

Evans, J. S. B. T. (2003). In two minds: Dual-process accounts of reasoning. *Trends in Cognitive Sciences, 7*, 454–459.

Evans, J. S. B. T. (2006). The heuristic-analytic theory of reasoning: Extension and evaluation. *Psychonomics Bulletin & Review, 13*, 378–395.

Evans, J. S. B. T. (2008). Dual-processing accounts of reasoning, judgment, and social cognition. *Annual Review of Psychology, 59*, 255–278.

Evans, J. S. B. T. (2012a). Dual-process theories of deductive reasoning: Facts and fallacies. In K. J. Holyoak & R. G. Morrison (Eds.), *The Oxford handbook of thinking and reasoning* (pp. 115–133). New York, NY: Oxford University Press.

Evans, J. S. B. T. (2012b). Reasoning. In D. Reisberg (Ed.), *The Oxford handbook of cognitive psychology*. New York, NY: Oxford University Press.

Evans, J. S. B. T., & Feeney, A. (2004). The role of prior belief in reasoning. In J. P. Leighton & R. J. Sternberg (Eds.), *The nature of reasoning* (pp. 78–102). New York, NY: Cambridge University Press.

Evans, J. S. B. T., Handley, S. J., Perham, N., Over, D. E., & Thompson, V. A. (2000). Frequency versus probability formats in statistical word problems. *Cognition, 77*, 197–213.

Evans, J. S. B. T., Newstead, S. E., & Byrne, R. M. J. (1993). *Human reasoning: The psychology of deduction*. London, England: Erlbaum.

Evans, J. S. B. T., & Stanovich, K. E. (2013). Dual-process theories of higher cognition: Advancing the debate. *Perspectives on Psychological Science, 8*, 223–241.

Eysenck, M. W. (1982). *Attention and arousal: Cognition and performance*. Berlin, Germany: Springer.

Eysenck, H. J. (1986). Toward a new model of intelligence. *Personality and Individual Differences, 7*(5), 731–736.

Farah, M. J. (1990). *Visual agnosia: Disorders of object recognition and what they tell us about normal vision*. Cambridge, MA: MIT Press.

Farah, M. J., Hammond, K. M., Levine, D. N., & Calvanio, R. (1988). Visual and spatial mental imagery: Dissociable systems of representation. *Cognitive Psychology, 20*, 439–462.

Farah, M. J., Shera, D. M., Savage, J. H., Betancourt, L., Gianetta, J. M., Brodsky, N. L., et al. (2006). Childhood poverty: Specific associations with neurocognitive development. *Brain Research, 1110*, 166–174.

Farah, M. J., & Smith, A. (1983). Perceptual interference and facilitation with auditory imagery. *Perception & Psychophysics, 33*, 475–478.

Farah, M. J., Soso, M., & Dasheiff, R. (1992). Visual angle of the mind's eye before and after unilateral occipital lobectomy. *Journal of Experimental Psychology: Human Perception and Performance, 18*, 241–246.

Feldman, H., Goldin-Meadow, S., & Gleitman, L. (1978). Beyond Herodotus: The creation of language by linguistically deprived deaf children. In A. Lock (Ed.), *Action, gesture and symbol: The emergence of language* (pp. 351–414). New York, NY: Academic Press.

Fendrich, R., Wessinger, C. M., & Gazzaniga, M. S. (1992). Residual vision in a scotoma: Implications for blindsight. *Science, 258*, 1489–1491.

Fenske, M. J., Raymond, J. E., Kessler, K., Westoby, N., & Tipper, S. P. (2005). Attentional inhibition has social-emotional consequences for unfamiliar faces. *Psychological Science, 16*, 753–758.

Ferreira, M. B., Garcia-Marques, L., Sherman, S. J., & Sherman, J. W. (2006). Automatic and controlled components of judgment and decision making. *Journal of Personality & Social Psychology, 91*, 797–813.

Fiedler, K., Brinkmann, B., Betsch, T., & Wild, B. (2000). A sampling approach to biases in conditional probability judgments: Beyond base rate neglect and statistical format. *Journal of Experimental Psychology: General, 129*, 399–418.

Fiedler, K., Walther, E., Armbruster, T., Fay, D., & Naumann, U. (1996). Do you really know what you have seen? Intrusion errors and presuppositions effects on constructive memory. *Journal of Experimental Social Psychology, 2*, 484–511.

Finke, R., & Kosslyn, S. M. (1980). Mental imagery acuity in the peripheral visual field. *Journal of Experimental Psychology: Human Perception and Performance, 6*, 126–139.

Finke, R., & Pinker, S. (1982). Spontaneous imagery scanning in mental extrapolation. *Journal of Experimental Psychology: Learning, Memory, & Cognition, 8*, 142–147.

Finucane, M. L., Alhakami, A., Slovic, P., & Johnson, S. M. (2000). The affect heuristic in judgments of risks and benefits. *Journal of Behavioral Decision Making, 13*, 1–17.

Fischhoff, B., Slovic, P., & Lichtenstein, S. (1978). Fault trees: Sensitivity of estimated failure probabilities to problem representation. *Journal of Experimental Psychology: Human Perception & Performance, 4*, 330–344.

Fisher, R., & Schreiber, N. (2007). Interview protocols to improve eyewitness memory. In M. P. Toglia et al. (Eds.), *Handbook of eyewitness psychology*. Mahwah, NJ: Erlbaum.

Fitousi, D. (2013). Mutual information, perceptual independence, and holistic face perception. *Attention, Perception, & Psychophysics, 75*, 983–1000.

Flanagan, D. P., McGrew, K. S., & Ortiz, S. (2000). *The Wechsler Intelligence Scales and Gf-Gc Theory: A contemporary approach to interpretation*. Boston, MA: Allyn & Bacon.

Flavell, J. H. (1979). Metacognition and cognitive monitoring. A new area of cognitive-development inquiry. *American Psychologist, 34*(10), 906–911.

Fleck, J. I., Beeman, M., & Kounios, J. (2012) Insight. In D. Reisberg (Ed.), *The Oxford handbook of cognitive psychology*. New York, NY: Oxford University Press.

Fleck, J. I., & Weisberg, R. W. (2004). The use of verbal protocols as data: An analysis of insight in the candle problem. *Memory & Cognition, 32*, 990–1006.

Flynn, J. R. (1984). The mean IQ of Americans: Massive gains 1932 to 1978. *Psychological Bulletin, 95*, 29–51.

Flynn, J. R. (1987). Massive IQ gains in 14 nations: What IQ tests really measure. *Psychological Bulletin, 101*, 171–191.

Flynn, J. R. (1999). Searching for justice: The discovery of IQ gains over time. *American Psychologist, 54*, 5–20.

Flynn, J. R. (2009). Requiem for nutrition as a cause of IQ gains: Raven's gains in Britain 1938–2008. *Economics & Human Biology, 7*, 18–27.

Fong, G., Krantz, D., & Nisbett, R. (1986). The effects of statistical training on thinking about everyday problems. *Cognitive Psychology, 18*, 253–292.

Fong, G., & Nisbett, R. (1991). Immediate and delayed transfer of training effects in statistical reasoning. *Journal of Experimental Psychology: General, 120*, 34–45.

Forgas, J., & East, R. (2003). Affective influences on social judgments and decisions: Implicit and explicit processes. In J. P. Forgas and K. D. Williams (Eds.), *Social judgments: Implicit and explicit processes* (pp. 198–226). New York, NY: Cambridge University Press.

Fox, C. R. (2006). The availability heuristic in the classroom: How soliciting more criticism can boost your course ratings. *Judgment and Decision Making, 1*, 86–90.

Fox, M. C., & Mitchum, A. L. (2013). A knowledge-based theory of rising scores on "cultural-free" tests. *Journal of Experimental Psychology: General, 142*, 979–1000.

Franconeri, S. L. (2013). The nature and status of visual resources. In D. Reisberg (Ed.), *The Oxford handbook of cognitive psychology* (pp. 147–162). New York, NY: Oxford University Press.

Franconeri, S. L., Alvarez, G. A., & Cavanagh, P. (2013). Flexible cognitive resources: Competitive content maps for attention & memory. *Trends in Cognitive Sciences, 17*, 134–141.

Fredrickson, B. L. (2000). Extracting meaning from past affective experiences: The importance of peaks, ends, and specific emotions. *Cognition & Emotion, 14*(4), 577–606.

Frenda, S. J., Nichols, R. M., & Loftus, E. F. (2011). Current issues and advances in misinformation research. *Current Directions in Psychological Science, 20*, 20–23.

Freyd, J. J. (1996). *Betrayal trauma: The logic of forgetting childhood abuse.* Cambridge, MA: Harvard University Press.

Freyd, J. J. (1998). Science in the memory debate. *Ethics & Behavior, 8*, 101–113.

Friedman, A. (1979). Framing pictures: The role of knowledge in automatized encoding and memory for gist. *Journal of Experimental Psychology: General, 108*, 316–355.

Friedman, A., & Brown, N. R. (2000a). Reasoning about geography. *Journal of Experimental Psychology: General, 129*, 193–219.

Friedman, A., & Brown, N. R. (2000b). Updating geographical knowledge: Principles of coherence and inertia. *Journal of Experimental Psychology: Learning, Memory, & Cognition, 26*, 900–914.

Fries, P., Reynolds, J. H., Rorie, A. E., & Desimone, R. (2001). Modulation of oscillatory neural synchronization by selective visual attention. *Science, 291*, 1560–1563.

Frings, C., & Wühr, P. (2014). Top-down deactivation of interference from irrelevant spatial or verbal stimulus features. *Attention, Perception, & Psychophysics, 76*, 2360–2374.

Frost, P. (2000). The quality of false memory over time: Is memory for misinformation "remembered" or "known"? *Psychonomic Bulletin & Review, 7*, 531–536.

Fukuda, K., Vogel, E., Mayr, U., & Awh, E. (2011). Quantity, not quality: The relationship between fluid intelligence and working memory capacity. *Psychonomic Bulletin & Review, 17*, 673–679.

Gable, P. A., & Harmon-Jones, E. (2008). Approach-motivated positive affect reduces breadth of attention. *Psychological Science, 19*, 476–482.

Gallo, D. A. (2010). False memories and fantastic beliefs: 15 years of the DRM illusion. *Memory & Cognition, 38*, 833–848.

Gallo, D. A., Roberts, M. J., & Seamon, J. G. (1997). Remembering words not presented in lists: Can we avoid creating false memories? *Psychonomic Bulletin & Review, 4*, 271–276.

Gallo, V., & Chitajullu, R. (2001). Unwrapping glial cells from the synapse: What lies inside? *Science, 292*, 872–873.

Galton, F. (1883). *Inquiries into human faculty.* London, England: Dent.

Gardiner, J. M. (1988). Functional aspects of recollective experience. *Memory & Cognition, 16*, 309–313.

Gardner, H. (1974). *The shattered mind: The person after brain damage.* New York, NY: Vintage.

Gardner, H. (1983). *Frames of mind: The theory of multiple intelligences.* New York, NY: Basic Books.

Gardner, H. (2006). *Multiple intelligences: New horizons in theory and practice.* New York, NY: Basic Books.

Garrett, B. (2011). *Convicting the innocent: Where criminal prosecutions go wrong.* Cambridge, MA: Harvard University Press.

Garrison, T. M., & Williams, C. C. (2013). Impact of relevance and distraction on driving performance and visual attention in a simulated driving environment. *Applied Cognitive Psychology, 27*, 396–405.

Garry, M., Manning, C. G., Loftus, E. F., & Sherman, S. J. (1996). Imagination inflation: Imagining a childhood event inflates confidence that it occurred. *Psychonomic Bulletin & Review, 3,* 208–214.

Gaspar, J. G., Street, W. N., Windsor, M. B., Carbonari, R., Kaczmarski, H., Kramer, A. F., & Mathewson, K. E. (2014). Providing views of the driving scene to drivers' conversation partners mitigates cell phone-related distraction. *Psychological Science, 25,* 2136–2146.

Gathercole, S. E., & Pickering, S. J. (2000). Assessment of working memory in six- and seven-year-old children. *Journal of Educational Psychology, 92,* 377–390.

Gathercole, S. E., Service, E., Hitch, G. J., Adams, A.-M., & Martin, A. J. (1999). Phonological short-term memory and vocabulary development: Further evidence on the nature of the relationship. *Applied Cognitive Psychology, 13,* 65–77.

Gauthier, I. L., Skudlarski, P., Gore, J. C., & Anderson, A. W. (2000). Expertise for cars and birds recruits brain areas involved in face recognition. *Nature Neuroscience, 3,* 191–197.

Gazzaniga, M. S., Fendrich, R., & Wessinger, C. M. (1994). Blindsight reconsidered. *Current Directions in Psychological Science 3,* 93–96.

Gazzaniga, M. S., Ivry, R. B., & Mangun, G. R. (2014). *Cognitive neuroscience: The biology of the mind* (4th ed.). New York, NY: Norton.

Gelman, S., & Wellman, H. (1991). Insides and essences: Early understandings of the non-obvious. *Cognition, 38,* 213–244.

Gentner, D., & Smith, L. A. (2012). Analogical learning and reasoning. In D. Reisberg (Ed.), *The Oxford handbook of cognitive psychology.* New York, NY: Oxford University Press.

Geraerts, E., Bernstein, D., Merckelbach, H., Linders, C., Raymaekers, L., & Loftus, E. F. (2008). Lasting false beliefs and their behavioral consequences. *Psychological Science, 19,* 749–753.

Geraerts, E., Lindsay, D. S., Merckelbach, H., Jelicic, M., Raymaekers, L., Arnold, M. M., et al. (2009). Cognitive mechanisms underlying recovered-memory experiences of childhood sexual abuse. *Psychological Science, 20,* 92–99.

Geraerts, E., Schooler, J. W., Merckelbach, H., Jelicic, M., Hauer, B., & Ambadar, Z. (2007). The reality of recovered memories: Corroborating continuous and discontinuous memories of child sexual abuse. *Psychological Science, 18,* 564–568.

Gerlach, C., Law, I., & Paulson, O. B. (2002). When action turns into words. Activation of motor-based knowledge during categorization of manipulable objects. *Journal of Cognitive Neuroscience, 14,* 1230–1239.

German, T., & Barrett, H. C. (2005). Functional fixedness in a technologically sparse culture. *Psychological Science, 16,* 1–5.

Geschwind, N. (1970). The organization of language and the brain. *Science, 170,* 940–944.

Ghetti, S., Edelstein, R. S., Goodman, G. S., Cordon, I. M., Quas, J. A., Alexander, K. W., et al. (2006). What can subjective forgetting tell us about memory for childhood trauma? *Memory & Cognition, 34,* 1011–1025.

Gibson, E. (2006). The interaction of top-down and bottom-up statistics in the resolution of syntactic category ambiguity. *Journal of Memory & Language, 54,* 363–388.

Gibson, E., Bishop, C., Schiff, W., & Smith, J. (1964). Comparison of meaningfulness and pronounceability as grouping principles in the perception and retention of verbal material. *Journal of Experimental Psychology, 67,* 173–182.

Gibson, J. J. (1950). *The perception of the visual world.* Boston, MA: Houghton Mifflin.

Gibson, J. J. (1966). *The senses considered as perceptual systems.* Boston, MA: Houghton Mifflin.

Gibson, J. J. (1979). *The ecological approach to visual perception.* Boston, MA: Houghton Mifflin.

Gick, M., & Holyoak, K. J. (1980). Analogical problem solving. *Cognitive Psychology, 12,* 306–355.

Giesbrecht, T., Lynn, S. J., Lilienfeld, S., & Merckelbach, H. (2008). Cognitive processes in dissociation: An analysis of core theoretical assumptions. *Psychological Bulletin, 134,* 617–647.

Gigerenzer, G. (1991). From tools to theories: A heuristic of discovery in cognitive psychology. *Psychological Review, 98,* 254–267.

Gigerenzer, G., Gaissmaier, W., Kurz-Milcke, E., Schwartz, L. M., & Woloshin, S. (2008). Helping doctors and patients make sense of health statistics. *Psychological Science in the Public Interest, 8,* 53–96.

Gigerenzer, G., Hell, W., & Blank, H. (1988). Presentation and content: The use of base rates as a continuous variable. *Journal of Experimental Psychology: Human Perception and Performance, 14,* 513–525.

Gigerenzer, G., & Hoffrage, U. (1995). How to improve Bayesian reasoning without instruction: Frequency formats. *Psychological Review, 102,* 684–704.

Gigerenzer, G., & Hug, K. (1992). Domain-specific reasoning: Social contracts, cheating and perspective change. *Cognition, 43,* 127–172.

Gilbert, D. T. (1989). Thinking lightly about others: Automatic components of the social inference process. In J. S. Uleman & J. A. Bargh (Eds.), *Unintended thought* (pp. 189–211). New York, NY: Guilford.

Gilbert, D. T. (2006). *Stumbling on happiness.* New York, NY: Random House.

Gilbert, D. T., & Ebert, J. E. J. (2002). Decisions and revisions: The affective forecasting of changeable-outcomes. *Journal of Personality and Social Psychology, 82,* 503–514.

Gilbert, D. T., Morewedge, C. K., Risen, J. L., & Wilson, T. D. (2004). Looking forward to looking backward. *Psychological Science, 15,* 346–350.

Gilbert, S. J., & Shallice, T. (2002). Task switching: A PDP model. *Cognitive Psychology, 44,* 297–337.

Gilhooly, K. J., Georgiou, G. J., Garrison, J., Reston, J. D., & Sirota, M. (2012). Don't wait to incubate: Immediate versus delayed incubation in divergent thinking. *Memory & Cognition, 40,* 966–975.

Gilovich, T. (1983). Biased evaluation and persistence in gambling. *Journal of Personality & Social Psychology, 44,* 1110–1126.

Gilovich, T. (1991). *How we know what isn't so.* New York, NY: Free Press.

Gilovich, T., & Douglas, C. (1986). Biased evaluations of randomly determined gambling outcomes. *Journal of Experimental Social Psychology, 22,* 228–241.

Girotto, V. (2004). Task understanding. In J. P. Leighton & R. J. Sternberg (Eds.), *The nature of reasoning* (pp. 103–128). New York, NY: Cambridge University Press.

Girotto, V., & Gonzalez, M. (2001). Solving probabilistic and statistical problems: A matter of information structure and question form. *Cognition, 78,* 247–276.

Giudice, N. A., Betty, M. R., & Loomis, J. M. (2011). Functional equivalence of spatial images from touch and vision: Evidence from spatial updating in blind and sighted individuals. *Journal of Experimental Psychology: Learning Memory, & Cognition, 37,* 621–634.

Gladwell, B. (2007). *Blink: The power of thinking without thinking.* New York, NY: Back Bay Books.

Glanzer, M., & Cunitz, A. R. (1966). Two storage mechanisms in free recall. *Journal of Verbal Learning and Verbal Behavior, 5,* 351–360.

Gleitman, H., Gross, J., & Reisberg, D. *Psychology* (8th ed.). New York, NY: Norton.

Gleitman, L., & Papafragou, A. (2012). Relations between language and thought. In D. Reisberg (Ed.), *The Oxford handbook of cognitive psychology.* New York, NY: Oxford University Press.

Glisky, E. L., Polster, M. R., & Routhieaux, B. C. (1995). Double dissociation between item and source memory. *Neuropsychology, 9,* 229–235.

Godden, D. R., & Baddeley, A. D. (1975). Context-dependent memory in two natural environments: On land and underwater. *British Journal of Psychology, 66,* 325–332.

Goebel, R., Khorram-Sefat, D., Muckli, L., Hacker, H., & Singer, W. (1998). The constructive nature of vision: Direct evidence from functional magnetic resonance imaging studies of apparent motion and motion imagery. *European Journal of Neuroscience, 10,* 1563–1573.

Goldenberg, G., Müllbacher, W., & Nowak, A. (1995). Imagery without perception—A case study of anosognosia for cortical blindness. *Neuropsychologia, 33,* 1373–1382.

Goldenberg, J., Mazursky, D., & Solomon, S. (1999). Creative sparks. *Science, 285,* 1495–1496.

Goldin-Meadow, S. (2003). *The resilience of language: What gesture creation in deaf children can tell us about how all children learn language.* New York, NY: Psychology Press.

Goldman-Rakic, P. S. (1987). Development of cortical circuitry and cognitive function. *Child Development, 58,* 601–622.

Goldman-Rakic, P. S. (1998). The prefrontal landscape: Implications of functional architecture for understanding human mentation and the central executive. In A. C. Roberts & T. W. Robbins (Eds.), *The prefrontal cortex: Executive and cognitive functions* (pp. 87–102). New York, NY: Oxford University Press.

Goldstone, R. L, & Son, J. Y. (2012). Similarity. In K. J. Holyoak & R. G. Morrison (Eds.), *The Oxford handbook of thinking and reasoning* (pp. 155–176). New York, NY: Oxford University Press.

Goodale, M. A. (1995). The cortical organization of visual perception and visuomotor control. In S. M. Kosslyn & D. Osherson (Eds.), *Visual cognition: An invitation to cognitive science* (2nd ed., pp. 167–213). Cambridge, MA: MIT Press.

Goodale, M. A., & Milner, A. D. (2004). *Sight unseen.* New York, NY: Oxford University Press.

Goodale, M. A., Milner, A. D., Jacobson, L. S., & Carey, D. P. (1991). A neurological dissociation between perceiving objects and grasping them. *Nature, 349,* 154–156.

Goodman, G. S., Ghetti, S., Quas, J. A., Edelstein, R. S., Alexander, K. W., Redlich, A. D., et al. (2003). A prospective study of memory for child sexual abuse: New findings relevant to the repressed-memory controversy. *Psychological Science, 14,* 113–118.

Goodman, N. (1972). Seven strictures on similarity. In N. Goodman (Ed.), *Problems and projects* (pp. 437–446). New York, NY: Bobbs-Merrill.

Gordon, H. (1923). Mental and scholastic tests among retarded children. *Educational pamphlet, no. 44.* London, England: Board of Education.

Gordon, R. D. (2006). Selective attention during scene perception: Evidence from negative priming. *Memory & Cognition, 34,* 1484–1494.

Gottfredson, L. S. (1997a). Mainstream science on intelligence: An editorial with 52 signatories, history, and bibliography. *Intelligence, 24,* 13–23.

Gottfredson, L. S. (1997b). Why *g* matters: The complexity of everyday life. *Intelligence, 24,* 79–132.

Gottfredson, L. S. (2003). Dissecting practical intelligence theory: Its claims and evidence. *Intelligence, 31,* 343–397.

Gottfredson, L. S. (2004). Intelligence: Is it the epidemiologists' elusive "fundamental cause" of social class inequalities in health? *Journal of Personality and Social Psychology, 86,* 174–199.

Graesser, A. C., Millis, K. K., & Zwaan, R. A. (1997). Discourse comprehension. *Annual Review of Psychology, 48*, 163–189.

Graf, P., Mandler, G., & Haden, P. E. (1982). Simulating amnesic symptoms in normals. *Science, 218*, 1243–1244.

Graf, P., & Schacter, D. L. (1985). Implicit and explicit memory for new associations in normal and amnesic subjects. *Journal of Experimental Psychology: Learning, Memory, & Cognition, 11*, 501–518.

Grainger, J., Rey, A., & Dufau, S. (2008). Letter perception: From pixels to pandemonium. *Trends in Cognitive Sciences, 12*, 381–387.

Grainger, J., & Whitney, C. (2004). Does the huamn mnid raed wrods as a wlohe? *Trends in Cognitive Sciences, 8*, 58–59.

Grant, H. M., Bredahl, L. C., Clay, J., Ferrie, J., Groves, J. E., McDorman, T. A., et al. (1998). Context-dependent memory for meaningful material: Information for students. *Applied Cognitive Psychology, 12*, 617–623.

Gray, J. R., Chabris, C. F., & Braver, T. S. (2003). Neural mechanisms of general fluid intelligence. *Nature Neuroscience, 6*, 316–322.

Green, R. L., Hoffman, L. T., Morse, R., Hayes, M. E. B., & Morgan, R. F. (1964). *The educational status of children in a district without public schools.* Cooperative Research Project No. 23211. Washington, DC: Office of Education, U.S. Department of Health, Education, and Welfare.

Greenberg, D. L., & Knowlton, B. J. (2014). The role of visual imagery in autobiographical memory. *Memory & Cognition, 42*, 922–934.

Greenfield, P. M. (2009). Technology and informal education: What is taught, what is learned. *Science, 323*, 69–71.

Gregg, M. K., & Samuel, A. G. (2008). Change deafness and the organizational properties of sounds. *Journal of Experimental Psychology: Human Perception & Performance, 34*, 974–991.

Grewal, D., & Salovey, P. (2005). Feeling smart: The science of emotional intelligence. *American Scientist, 93*, 330–339.

Griffin, D. W., Gonzalez, R., Koehler, D. J., & Gilovich, T. (2012). Judgmental heuristics: A historical overview. In K. J. Holyoak & R. G. Morrison (Eds.), *The Oxford handbook of thinking and reasoning* (pp. 322–345). New York, NY: Oxford University Press.

Griggs, R., & Cox, J. R. (1982). The elusive thematic-materials effect in Wason's selection task. *British Journal of Psychology, 73*, 407–420.

Grigorenko, E. L., Jarvin, I., & Sternberg, R. J. (2002). School-based tests of the triarchic theory of intelligence. *Contemporary Educational Psychology, 27*, 167–208.

Grill-Spector, K., Knouf, N., & Kanwisher, N. (2004). The fusiform face area subserves face perception, not generic within-category identification. *Nature Neuroscience, 7*, 555–562.

Grodner, D., & Gibson, E. (2005). Consequences of the serial nature of linguistic input. *Cognitive Science, 29*, 261–291.

Grotzer, T. A., & Perkins, D. N. (2000). Teaching intelligence: A performance conception. In R. J. Sternberg (Ed.), *Handbook of intelligence* (pp. 492–515). Cambridge, England: Cambridge University Press.

Gruber, H. E. (1981). *Darwin on man: A psychological study of scientific creativity* (2nd ed.). Chicago, IL: University of Chicago Press.

Guilford, J. (1967). *The nature of human intelligence.* New York, NY: Scribner.

Guilford, J. (1979). Some incubated thoughts on incubation. *Journal of Creative Behavior, 13*, 1–8.

Haber, R. N. (1969). Eidetic images. *Scientific American, 220*, 36–44.

Haber, R. N., & Haber, L. (1988). The characteristics of eidetic imagery. In D. Fein & L. Obler (Eds.), *The exceptional brain* (pp. 218–241). New York, NY: Guilford.

Hackman, D., & Farah, M. (2009). Socioeconomic status and the developing brain. *Trends in Cognitive Sciences, 13*, 65–73.

Hadar, L., & Sood, S. (2014). When knowledge is demotivating: Subjective knowledge and choice overload. *Psychological Science, 25*, 1739–1747.

Hafstad, G. S., Memon, A., & Logie, R. H. (2004). Post-identification feedback, confidence, and recollections of witnessing conditions in child witnesses. *Applied Cognitive Psychology, 18*, 901–912.

Hahn, B., Ross, T. J., & Stein, E. A. (2006). Neuroanatomical dissociation between bottom-up and top-down processes of visuospatial selective attention. *NeuroImage, 32*, 842–853.

Hahn, U., Prat-Sala, M., Pothos, E. M., & Brumby, D. P. (2010) Exemplar similarity and rule application. *Cognition, 114*, 1–18.

Halamish, V., & Bjork, R. (2011). When does testing enhance retention? A distribution-based interpretation of retrieval as a memory modifier. *Journal of Experimental Psychology: Learning, Memory, & Cognition, 37*, 801–812.

Halberstadt, J., & Rhodes, G. (2003). It's not just average faces that are attractive: Computer-manipulated averageness makes birds, fish, and automobiles attractive. *Psychonomic Bulletin & Review, 10*, 149–156.

Halle, M. (1990). Phonology. In D. Osherson & H. Lasnik (Eds.), *Language: An invitation to cognitive science* (pp. 43–68). Cambridge, MA: MIT Press.

Halpern, D. (1984). *Thought and knowledge: An introduction to critical thinking.* Hillsdale, NJ: Erlbaum.

Hamann, S. (2001). Cognitive and neural mechanisms of emotional memory. *Trends in Cognitive Sciences, 5,* 394–400.

Hamill, R., Wilson, T. D., & Nisbett, R. E. (1980). Insensitivity to sample bias: Generalizing from atypical cases. *Journal of Personality and Social Psychology, 39,* 578–589.

Hampshire, A., Duncan, J., & Owen, A. M. (2007). Selective tuning of the blood oxygenation level-dependent response during simple target detection dissociates human frontoparietal subregions. *Journal of Neuroscience, 27*(23), 6219–6223.

Hanako, Y., & Smith, L. B. (2005). Linguistic cues enhance the learning of perceptual cues. *Psychological Science, 16,* 90–95.

Handel, S. (1989). *Listening: An introduction to the perception of auditory events.* Cambridge, MA: MIT Press.

Handley, S. J., Newstead, S. E., & Trippas, D. (2011). Logic, beliefs, and instruction: A test of the default interventionist account of belief bias. *Journal of Experimental Psychology: Learning, Memory, & Cognition, 37,* 28–43.

Hardt, O., Einarsson, E., & Nader, K. (2010). A bridge over troubled water: Reconsolidation as a link between cognitive and neuroscientific memory research traditions. *Annual Review of Psychology, 61,* 141–168.

Hardt, O., Nader, K., & Nadel, L. (2013). Decay happens: The role of active forgetting in memory. *Trends in Cognitive Sciences, 17,* 111–120.

Harinck, F., Van Dijk, E., Van Beest, I., & Mersmann, P. (2007). When gains loom larger than losses: Reversed loss aversion for small amounts of money. *Psychological Science, 18,* 1099–1105.

Harley, T. A., & Bown, H. E. (1998). What causes a tip-of-the-tongue state? Evidence for lexical neighbourhood effects in speech production. *British Journal of Psychology, 89*(1), 151–174.

Harmon-Jones, E., Gable, P. A., & Price, T. F. (2013). Does negative affect always narrow and positive affect always broaden the mind? *Current Directions in Psychological Science, 22,* 301–307.

Harvey, L. O., Jr., & Leibowitz, H. (1967). Effects of exposure duration, cue reduction, and temporary monocularity on size matching at short distances. *Journal of the Optical Society of America, 57,* 249–253.

Harwood, D. G., Barker, W. W., Ownby, R. L., & Duara, R. (1999). Prevalence and correlates of Capgras syndrome in Alzheimer's disease. *International Journal of Geriatric Psychiatry, 14,* 415–420.

Hasel, L. E., & Kassin, S. M. (2009). On the presumption of evidentiary independence: Can confessions corrupt eyewitness identifications? *Psychological Science, 20,* 122–126.

Hasselmo, M. E. (1999). Neuromodulation: Acetylcholine and memory consolidation. *Trends in Cognitive Sciences, 6,* 351–359.

Hassin, R. R. (2013). Yes it can: On the functional abilities of the human unconscious. *Perspectives on Psychological Science, 8,* 195–207.

Hayes, J., & Simon, H. (1977). Psychological differences among problem solving isomorphs. In N. Castellan, D. Pisoni, & G. Potts (Eds.), *Cognitive theory* (pp. 21–42). Hillsdale, NJ: Erlbaum.

Hayne, H. (2004). Infant memory development: Implications for childhood amnesia. *Developmental Review, 24,* 33–73.

Hayward, W., & Williams, P. (2000). Viewpoint dependence and object discriminability. *Psychological Science, 11,* 7–12.

Heathcote, A., Freeman, E., Etherington, J., Tonkin, J., & Bora, B. (2009). A dissociation between similarity effects in episodic face recognition. *Psychonomic Bulletin & Review, 16,* 824–831.

Heckman, J. J. (2006). Skill formation and the economics of investing in disadvantaged children. *Science, 312,* 1900–1902.

Hegarty, M. (2004). Mechanical reasoning by mental simulation. *Trends in Cognitive Sciences, 8,* 280–285.

Hegarty, M., & Stull, A. T. (2012). Visuospatial thinking. In K. J. Holyoak & R. G. Morrison (Eds.), *The Oxford handbook of thinking and reasoning* (pp. 606–630). New York, NY: Oxford University Press.

Heil, M., Rösler, F., & Hennighausen, E. (1993). Imagery-perception interaction depends on the shape of the image: A reply to Farah. *Journal of Experimental Psychology: Human Perception and Performance, 19,* 1313–1319.

Heil, M., Rösler, F., & Hennighausen, E. (1994). Dynamics of activation in long-term memory: The retrieval of verbal, pictorial, spatial and color information. *Journal of Experimental Psychology: Learning, Memory, & Cognition, 20,* 169–184.

Heit, E. (2000). Properties of inductive reasoning. *Psychonomic Bulletin & Review, 7,* 569–592.

Heit, E., & Bott, L. (2000). Knowledge selection in category learning. In D. L. Medin (Ed.), *The psychology of learning and motivation: Advances in research and theory* (Vol. 39, pp. 163–199). San Diego, CA: Academic Press.

Heit, E., & Feeney, A. (2005). Relations between premise similarity and inductive strength. *Psychonomic Bulletin & Review, 12,* 340–344.

Hélie, S., & Sun, R. (2010). Incubation, insight, and creative problem solving: A unified theory and a connectionist model. *Psychological Review, 117,* 994–1024.

Heller, J., & Reif, F. (1984). Prescribing effective human problem-solving processes: Problem description in physics. *Cognition and Instruction, 1,* 177–216.

Heller, M. A., & Gentaz, E. (2014). *Psychology of touch and blindness*. New York, NY: Taylor & Francis.

Helmholtz, H. (1909). *Wissenschaftliche Abhandlungen, II* (pp. 764–843). Leipzig, Germany: Barth.

Helmuth, L. (2001). Boosting brain activity from the outside in. *Science, 292,* 1284–1286.

Henderson, J. M. (2013). Eye movements. In D. Reisberg (Ed.), *The Oxford handbook of cognitive psychology* (pp. 69–82). New York, NY: Oxford University Press.

Henderson, J. M., & Hollingworth, A. (2003). Global transsaccadic change blindness during scene perception. *Psychological Science, 14,* 493–497.

Henle, M. (1962). On the relation between logic and thinking. *Psychological Review, 69,* 366–378.

Henle, M. (1978). Foreword. In R. Revlin & R. Mayer (Eds.), *Human reasoning* (pp. xiii–xviii). New York, NY: Wiley.

Hennessey, B., & Amabile, A. (2010). Creativity. *Annual Review of Psychology, 61,* 569–598.

Hermer-Vazquez, L., Spelke, E. S., & Katsnelson, A. S. (1999). Sources of flexibility in human cognition: Dual-task studies of space and language. *Cognitive Psychology, 39,* 3–36.

Hernández, M., Costa, A., & Humphreys, G. (2012). Escaping caption: Bilingualism modulates distraction from working memory. *Cognition, 122,* 37–50.

Hertwig, R., Herzog, S. M., Schooler, L. J., & Reimer, T. (2008). Fluency heuristic: A model of how the mind exploits a by-product of information retrieval. *Journal of Experimental Psychology: Learning, Memory, & Cognition, 34,* 1191–1206.

Hertwig, R., & Ortmann, A. (2003). Economists' and psychologists' experimental practices: How they differ, why they differ, and how they could converge. In I. Brocas & J. D. Carrillo (Eds.), *The psychology of economic decisions: Rationality and well-being* (Vol. 1, pp. 253–272). New York, NY: Oxford University Press.

Hicks, J. L., & Marsh, R. L. (1999). Remember-Know judgments can depend on how memory is tested. *Psychonomic Bulletin & Review, 6,* 117–122.

Higbee, K. L. (1977). *Your memory: How it works and how to improve it*. Englewood Cliffs, NJ: Prentice-Hall.

Hilchey, M., & Klein, R. (2011). Are there bilingual advantages on nonlinguistic interference tasks? Implications for the plasticity of executive control processes. *Psychonomic Bulletin & Review, 18,* 625–658.

Hill, A. L. (1978). Savants: Mentally retarded individuals with specific skills. In N. R. Ellis (Ed.), *International review of research in mental retardation* (Vol. 9). New York: Academic Press.

Hillyard, S. A., Vogel, E. K., & Luck, S. J. (1998). Sensory gain control (amplification) as a mechanism of selective attention: Electrophysiological and neuroimaging evidence. *Philosophical Transactions of the Royal Society: Biological Sciences, 353,* 1257–1270.

Hilton, D. J. (1995). The social context of reasoning: Conversational inference and rational judgment. *Psychological Bulletin, 118,* 248–271.

Hilton, D. J. (2003). Psychology and the financial markets: Applications to understanding and remedying irrational decision-making. In I. Brocas & J. D. Carrillo (Eds.), *The psychology of economic decisions: Rationality and well-being* (Vol. 1, pp. 273–297). New York, NY: Oxford University Press.

Hilts, P. J. (1995). *Memory's ghost: The strange tale of Mr. M and the nature of memory*. New York, NY: Simon & Schuster.

Hirst, W., Phelps, E., Buckner, R., Budson, A., Cuc, A., et al. (2009). Long-term memory for the terrorist attack of September 11: Flashbulb memories, event memories, and the factors that influence their retention. *Journal of Experimental Psychology: General, 138,* 161–176.

Hirst, W., Spelke, E., Reaves, C., Caharack, G., & Neisser, U. (1980). Dividing attention without alternation or automaticity. *Journal of Experimental Psychology: General, 109,* 98–117.

Hodges, J. R., & Graham, K. S. (2001). Episodic memory: Insights from semantic dementia. In A. D. Baddeley, J. P. Aggleton, & M. A. Conway (Eds.), *Episodic memory: New directions in research* (pp. 132–152). New York, NY: Oxford University Press.

Holland, J. H., Holyoak, K. F., Nisbett, R. E., & Thagard, P. R. (1986). *Induction*. Cambridge, MA: MIT Press.

Holmberg, D., & Homes, J. G. (1994). Reconstruction of relationship memories: A mental models approach. In N. Schwarz & S. Sudman (Eds.), *Autobiographical memory and the validity of retrospective reports* (pp. 267–288). New York, NY: Springer.

Holmes, J. B., Waters, H. S., & Rajaram, S. (1998). The phenomenology of false memories: Episodic content and confidence. *Journal of Experimental Psychology: Learning, Memory, & Cognition, 24,* 1026–1040.

Holway, A. F., & Boring, E. G. (1947). Determinants of apparent visual size with distance variant. *American Journal of Psychology, 54,* 21–37.

Holyoak, K. (2012). Analogy and relational reasoning. In K. J. Holyoak & R. G. Morrison (Eds.), *The Oxford handbook of thinking and reasoning* (pp. 234–259). New York, NY: Oxford University Press.

Homa, D., Dunbar, S., & Nohre, L. (1991). Instance frequency, categorization, and the modulating effect of experience. *Journal of Experimental Psychology: Learning, Memory, & Cognition, 17,* 444–458.

Hon, N., Epstein, R. A., Owen, A. M., & Duncan, J. (2006). Frontoparietal activity with minimal decision and control. *Journal of Neuroscience, 26*(38), 9805–9809.

Horn, J. L. (1985). Remodeling old models of intelligence. In B. B. Wolman (Ed.), Handbook of intelligence: Theories, measurements, and applications (pp. 267–300). New York: Wiley.

Horn, J. L., & Blankson, N. (2005). Foundations for better understanding of cognitive abilities. In D. Flanagan & P. Harrison (Eds.), *Contemporary intellectual assessment: Theories, tests, and issues* (2nd ed., pp. 41-68). New York: Guilford.

Horn, J. L., & Noll, J. (1994). A system for understanding cognitive capabilities: A theory and the evidence on which it is based. In D. K. Detterman (Ed.), *Current topics in human intelligence* (Vol. 4, *Theories of intelligence*). Norwood, NJ: Ablex.

Hornby, P. (1974). Surface structure and presupposition. *Journal of Verbal Learning and Verbal Behavior, 13,* 530–538.

Hoschedidt, S. M., Dongaonkar, B., Payne, J., & Nadel, L. (2012). Emotion, stress and memory. In D. Reisberg (Ed.), *The Oxford handbook of cognitive psychology.* New York, NY: Oxford University Press.

Howe, M. L. (2011). The adaptive nature of memory and its illusions. *Current Directions in Psychological Science, 20,* 312–315.

Howe, M. L., Courage M. L., and Rooksby, M. (2009). The genesis and development of autobiographical memory. In M. L. Courage & N. Cowan (Eds.), *The development of memory in infancy and childhood* (pp. 177–196). Hove, England: Psychology Press.

Hsee, C. K., & Hastie, R. (2005). Decision and experience: Why don't we choose what makes us happy? *Trends in Cognitive Sciences, 10,* 31–37.

Hsee, C. K., Hastie, R., & Chen, J. (2008). Hedonomics: Bridging decision research with happiness research. *Perspectives on Psychological Science, 3,* 224–243.

Hubel, D. (1963, November). The visual cortex of the brain. *Scientific American, 209,* 54–62.

Hubel, D., & Wiesel, T. (1959). Receptive fields of single neurones in the cat's visual cortex. *Journal of Physiology, 148,* 574–591.

Hubel, D., & Wiesel, T. (1968). Receptive fields and functional architecture of monkey striate cortex. *Journal of Physiology, 195,* 215–243.

Huey, E. D., Krueger, F., & Grafman, J. (2006). Representations in the human prefrontal cortex. *Current Directions in Psychological Science, 5,* 167–171.

Hummel, J. E. (2013). Object recognition. In D. Reisberg (Ed.), *The Oxford handbook of cognitive psychology* (pp. 32–45). New York, NY: Oxford University Press.

Hummel, J. E., & Biederman, I. (1992). Dynamic binding in a neural network for shape recognition. *Psychological Review, 99,* 480–517.

Humphreys, G., & Riddoch, J. (2014). *A case study in visual agnosia: To see but not to see.* New York, NY: Psychology Press.

Hung, J., Driver, J., & Walsh, V. (2005). Visual selection and posterior parietal cortex: Effects of repetitive transcranial magnetic stimulation on partial report analyzed by Bundesen's theory of visual attention. *Journal of Neuroscience, 25*(42), 9602–9612.

Hunt, E. (1995). *Will we be smart enough? A cognitive analysis of the coming workforce.* New York, NY: Russell Sage Foundation.

Hunt, R., & Ellis, H. D. (1974). Recognition memory and degree of semantic contextual change. *Journal of Experimental Psychology, 103,* 1153–1159.

Huntsinger, J. R. (2012). Does positive affect broaden and negative affect narrow attentional scope? A new answer to an old question. *Journal of Experimental Psychology: General, 141,* 595–600.

Huntsinger, J. R. (2013). Does emotion directly tune the scope of attention? *Current Directions in Psychological Science, 22,* 265–270.

Husserl, E. (1931). *Ideas.* New York, NY: Collier.

Hutchison, K. A. (2003). Is semantic priming due to association strength or feature overlap? A *micro* analytic review. *Psychonomic Bulletin & Review, 10,* 785–813.

Hyde, T. S., & Jenkins, J. J. (1969). Differential effects of incidental tasks on the organization of recall of a list of highly associated words. *Journal of Experimental Psychology, 82,* 472–481.

Hyde, T. S., & Jenkins, J. J. (1973). Recall for words as a function of semantic, graphic, and syntactic orienting tasks. *Journal of Verbal Learning and Verbal Behavior, 12,* 471–480.

Hyman, I., Boss, M., Wise, B., McKenzie, K., & Caggiano, J. (2010). Did you see the unicycling clown? Inattentional blindness while walking and talking on a cell phone. *Applied Cognitive Psychology, 24,* 597–607.

Hyman, I. E., Jr. (2000). Creating false autobiographical memories: Why people believe their memory errors. In E. Winograd, R. Fivush, & W. Hirst (Eds.), *Ecological approaches to cognition: Essays in honor of Ulric Neisser.* Hillsdale, NJ: Erlbaum.

Hyman, I. E., Jr., Husband, T. H., & Billings, F. J. (1995). False memories of childhood experiences. *Applied Cognitive Psychology, 9,* 181–197.

Intons-Peterson, M. J. (1983). Imagery paradigms: How vulnerable are they to experimenters' expectations? *Journal of Experimental Psychology: Human Perception & Performance, 9,* 394–412.

Intons-Peterson, M. J. (1999). Comments and caveats about "scanning visual mental images." *Cahiers de Psychologie Cognitive, 18,* 534–540.

Intons-Peterson, M. J., & White, A. (1981). Experimenter naiveté and imaginal judgments. *Journal of Experimental Psychology: Human Perception and Performance, 7,* 833–843.

Intraub, H., & Bodamer, J. (1993). Boundary extension: Fundamental aspect of pictorial representation or encoding artifact? *Journal of Experimental*

Psychology: Learning, Memory, & Cognition, 19, 1387–1397.

Intraub, H., & Dickinson, C. A. (2008). False memory 1/20th of a second later. *Psychological Science, 19*, 1007–1014.

Intraub, H., Gottesman, C. V., & Bills, A. J. (1998). Effects of perceiving and imagining scenes on memory for pictures. *Journal of Experimental Psychology: Learning, Memory, & Cognition, 24*, 1–16.

Intraub, H., Hoffman, J. E., Wetherhold, C. J., & Stoehs, S.-A. (2006). More than meets the eye: The effect of planned fixations on scene representation. *Perception and Psychophysics, 68*, 759–769.

Intraub, H., & Richardson, M. (1989). Wide-angle memories of close-up scenes. *Journal of Experimental Psychology: Learning, Memory, & Cognition, 15*, 179–187.

Isha, A., & Sagi, D. (1995). Common mechanisms of visual imagery and perception. *Science, 268*, 1772–1774.

Jackendoff, R. (1972). *Semantic interpretation in generative grammar.* Cambridge, MA: MIT Press.

Jacoby, L. L. (1978). On interpreting the effects of repetition: Solving a problem versus remembering a solution. *Journal of Verbal Learning and Verbal Behavior, 17*, 649–667.

Jacoby, L. L. (1983). Remembering the data: Analyzing interactive processes in reading. *Journal of Verbal Learning and Verbal Behavior, 22*, 485–508.

Jacoby, L. L., & Dallas, M. (1981). On the relationship between autobiographical memory and perceptual learning. *Journal of Experimental Psychology: General, 3*, 306–340.

Jacoby, L. L., Jones, T. C., & Dolan, P. O. (1998). Two effects of repetition: Support for a dual process model of know judgments and exclusion errors. *Psychonomic Bulletin & Review, 5*, 705–509.

Jacoby, L. L., Kelley, C. M., Brown, J., & Jasechko, J. (1989). Becoming famous overnight: Limits on the ability to avoid unconscious influences of the past. *Journal of Personality and Social Psychology, 56*, 326–338.

Jacoby, L. L., Lindsay, D. S., & Hessels, S. (2003). Item-specific control of automatic processes: Stroop process dissociations. *Psychonomic Bulletin & Review, 10*, 638–644.

Jacoby, L. L., & Whitehouse, K. (1989). An illusion of memory: False recognition influenced by unconscious perception. *Journal of Experimental Psychology: General, 118*, 126–135.

Jacoby, L. L., & Witherspoon, D. (1982). Remembering without awareness. *Canadian Journal of Psychology, 36*, 300–324.

James, L. E., & Burke, D. M. (2000). Phonological priming effects on word retrieval and tip-of-the-tongue experiences in young and older adults. *Journal of Experimental Psychology: Learning, Memory, & Cognition, 26*, 1378–1391.

James, W. (1890). *The principles of psychology* (Vol. 2). New York, NY: Dover.

January, D., & Kako, E. (2007). Re-evaluating evidence for linguistic relativity: Reply to Boroditsky (2001). *Cognition, 104*, 417–426.

Jeffries, R., Polson, P., Razran, L., & Atwood, M. (1977). A process model for missionaries-cannibals and other river-crossing problems. *Cognitive Psychology, 9*, 412–440.

Jelicic, M., Smeets, T., Peters, M., Candel, I., Horselenberg, R., & Merckelbach, H. (2006). Assassination of a controversial politician: Remembering details from another non-existent film. *Applied Cognitive Psychology, 20*, 591–596.

Jencks, C., & Phillips, M. (Eds). (1998). *The Black-White test score gap.* Washington, DC: Brookings Institution.

Jenkins, R., Lavie, N., & Driver, J. (2005). Recognition memory for distractor faces depends on attentional load at exposure. *Psychological Bulletin & Review, 12*, 314–320.

Jennings, D. L., Amabile, T. M., & Ross, L. (1982). Informal covariation assessment: Data-based versus theory-based judgments. In D. Kahneman, P. Slovic, & A. Tversky (Eds.), *Judgments under uncertainty: Heuristics and biases* (pp. 211–230). Cambridge, England: Cambridge University Press.

Jensen, A. R. (1985). The nature of the black-white difference on various psychometric tests: Spearman's hypothesis. *Behavioral and Brain Sciences, 8*, 193–263.

Jepson, D., Krantz, D., & Nisbett, R. (1983). Inductive reasoning: Competence or skill? *Behavioral and Brain Sciences, 6*, 494–501.

Joels, M., Fernandez, G., & Roosendaal, B. (2011). Stress and emotional memory: A matter of timing. *Trends in Cognitive Sciences, 15*, 280–288.

Johnson, H., & Seifert, C. (1994). Sources of the continued influence effect: When misinformation affects later inferences. *Journal of Experimental Psychology: Learning, Memory, & Cognition, 20*, 1420–1436.

Johnson, M. K. (1988). Reality monitoring: An experimental phenomenological approach. *Journal of Experimental Psychology: General, 117*, 390–394.

Johnson, M. K., Hashtroudi, S., & Lindsay, S. (1993). Source monitoring. *Psychological Bulletin, 114*, 3–28.

Johnson, S. K., & Anderson, M. C. (2004). The role of inhibitory control in forgetting semantic knowledge. *Psychological Science, 15*, 448–453.

Johnson, W., Carothers, A., & Deary, I. J. (2008). Sex differences in variability in general intelligence. *Perspectives on Psychological Science, 3*, 518–531.

Johnson, W., Nijenhuis, J., & Bouchard, T. (2007). Replication of the hierarchical visual-perceptual-image rotation model in de Wolff and Buiten's (1963) battery of 46 tests of mental ability. *Intelligence, 35,* 69–81.

Johnson, W., Segal, N. L., & Bouchard, T. J., Jr. (2008). Heritability of fluctuating asymmetry in a human twin sample: The effect of trait aggregation. *American Journal of Human Biology, 20,* 651–658.

Johnson-Laird, P. N. (1988). A computational analysis of consciousness. In A. Marcel & E. Bisiach (Eds.), *Consciousness in contemporary science* (pp. 357–368). Oxford, England: Oxford University Press.

Johnston, J., & McClelland, J. (1973). Visual factors in word perception. *Perception & Psychophysics, 14,* 365–370.

Jones, G. (2003). Testing two cognitive theories of insight. *Journal of Experimental Psychology: Learning, Memor, & Cognition, 29,* 1017–1027.

Jones, J. L., Esber, G. R., McDannald, M. A., Gruber, A. J., Hernandez, A., Mirenzi, A., & Schoenbaum, G. (2012). Orbitofrontal cortex supports behavior and learning using inferred but not cached values. *Science, 338,* 953–956.

Jones, T. C., & Bartlett, J. C. (2009). When false recognition is out of control: The case of facial conjunctions. *Memory & Cognition, 37,* 143–157.

Jonides, J., Kahn, R., & Rozin, P. (1975). Imagery instructions improve memory in blind subjects. *Bulletin of the Psychonomic Society, 5,* 424–426.

Jonides, J., Lacey, S. C., & Nee, D. E. (2005). Processes of working memory in mind and brain. *Current Directions in Psychological Science, 14,* 2–5.

Jonides, J., Lewis, R., Nee, D. E., Lustig, C. A., Berman, M. G., & Moore, K. S. (2008). The mind and brain of short-term memory. *Annual Review of Psychology, 59,* 193–224.

Jung, R., & Haier, R. (2007). The parieto-frontal integration theory (P-FIT) of intelligence: Converging neuroimaging evidence. *Behavioral and Brain Sciences, 30,* 135–154.

Just, M., Carpenter, P. A., & Hemphill, D. D. (1996). Constraints on processing capacity: Architectural or implementational? In D. Steier & T. Mitchell (Eds.), *Mind matters: A tribute to Allen Newell* (pp. 141–178). Mahwah, NJ: Erlbaum.

Kahneman, D. (1973). *Attention and effort.* Englewood Cliffs, NJ: Prentice-Hall.

Kahneman, D. (2003). A perspective on judgment and choice: Mapping bounded rationality. *American Psychologist, 58,* 697–720.

Kahneman, D. (2011). *Thinking, fast and slow.* New York, NY: Farrar, Straus and Giroux.

Kahneman, D., Frederickson, B. L., Schreiber, C. A., & Redelmeier, D. A. (1993). When more pain is preferred to less: Adding a better end. *Psychological Science, 4,* 401–405.

Kahneman, D., & Klein, G. (2009). Conditions for intuitive expertise: A failure to disagree. *American Psychologist, 64,* 515–526.

Kahneman, D., & Snell, J. (1992). Predicting a changing taste: Do people know what they will like? *Journal of Behavioral Decision Making, 5,* 187–200.

Kahneman, D., & Tversky, A. (1973). On the psychology of prediction. *Psychological Review, 80,* 237–251.

Kahney, H. (1986). *Problem solving: A cognitive approach.* Milton Keynes, England: Open University Press.

Kamin, L. (1974). *The science and politics of IQ.* Potomac, MD: Erlbaum.

Kanaya, T., Scullin, M. H., & Ceci, S. (2003). The Flynn effect and U.S. policies: The impact of rising IQ scores on American society via mental retardation diagnoses. *American Psychologist, 58,* 778–790.

Kane, M. J., Conway, A., Hambrick, D., & Engle, R. (2007). Variation in working memory capacity as variation in executive attention and control. In A. Conway, K. Jarrold, M. Kane, A. Miyake, & J. Towse (Eds.), *Variation in working memory* (pp. 21–46). New York, NY: Oxford University Press.

Kane, M. J., & Engle, R. W. (2003). Working-memory capacity and the control of attention: The contributions of goal neglect, response competition, and task set to Stroop interference. *Journal of Experimental Psychology: General, 132,* 47–70.

Kane, M. J., & McVay, J. C. (2012). What mind wandering reveals about executive-control abilities and failures. *Current Directions in Psychological Science, 21,* 348–354.

Kanwisher, N. (2006). What's in a face? *Science, 311,* 617–618.

Kanwisher, N., McDermott, J., & Chun, M. M. (1997). The fusiform face area: A module in human extrastriate cortex specialized for face perception. *Journal of Neuroscience, 17,* 4302–4311.

Kanwisher, N., & Yovel, G. (2006). The fusiform face area: A cortical region specialized for the perception of faces. *Philosophical Transactions of the Royal Society of London B, 361,* 2109–2128.

Kaplan, A. S., & Murphy, G. L. (2000). Category learning with minimal prior knowledge. *Journal of Experimental Psychology: Learning, Memory, & Cognition, 26,* 829–846.

Karpicke, J., & Blunt, J. (2011). Retrieval practice produces more learning than elaborative studying with concept mapping. *Science, 331,* 772–775.

Karpicke, J. D. (2012). Retrieval-based learning: Active retrieval promotes meaningful learning. *Current Directions in Psychological Science, 21,* 157–163.

Kassin, S., Bogart, D., & Kerner, J. (2012). Confessions that corrupt: Evidence from the DNA exoneration cases. *Psychological Science, 23,* 1–5.

Kassin, S., Drizin, S., Grisso, T., Gudjonsson, G., Leo, R., & Redlich, A. (2010). Police-induced confessions: Risk factors and recommendations. *Law & Human Behavior, 34,* 3–38.

Katona, G. (1940). *Organizing and memorizing*. New York, NY: Columbia University Press.

Katz, A. (1983). What does it mean to be a high imager? In J. Yuille (Ed.), *Imagery, memory and cognition* (pp. 39–63). Hillsdale, NJ: Erlbaum.

Kaufman, A. S., & Kaufman, N. L. (2004). *Manual for Kaufman Assessment Battery for Children—Second Edition (KABC-II)—Comprehensive Form*. Circle Pines, MN: American Guidance Service.

Kaufman, J. C., Kaufman, S. B., & Plucker, J. (2012). Contemporary theories of intelligence. In D. Reisberg (Ed.), *The Oxford handbook of cognitive psychology*. New York, NY: Oxford University Press.

Kay, P., & Regier, T. (2007). Color naming universals: The case of Berinmo. *Cognition, 102,* 289–298.

Keil, F. C. (1986). The acquisition of natural-kind and artifact terms. In W. Demopoulos & A. Marras (Eds.), *Language, learning, and concept acquisition* (pp. 133–153). Norwood, NJ: Ablex.

Keil, F. C. (1989). *Concepts, kinds, and cognitive development*. Cambridge, MA: MIT Press.

Keil, F. C. (2003). Folkscience: Coarse interpretations of a complex reality. *Trends in Cognitive Sciences, 7,* 368–373.

Kellenbach, M. L., Brett, M., & Patterson, K. (2003). Actions speak louder than functions: The importance of manipulability and action in tool representation. *Journal of Cognitive Neuroscience, 15,* 30–46.

Kelley, W. M., Macrae, C. N, Wyland, C. L., Cagalar, S., Inatai, S., & Heatherton, T. F. (2002). Finding the self? An event-related fMRI study. *Journal of Cognitive Neuroscience, 14,* 785–794.

Kensinger, E. (2007). Negative emotion enhances memory accuracy. *Current Directions in Psychological Science, 16,* 213–218.

Keogh, R., & Pearson, J. (2011). Mental imagery and visual working memory. *PLoS ONE, 6,* e29221.

Kermer, D., Driver-Linn, E., Wilson, T., & Gilbert, D. (2006). Loss aversion is an effective forecasting error. *Psychological Science, 17,* 649–653.

Kerr, N. H. (1983). The role of vision in "visual imagery" experiments: Evidence from the congenitally blind. *Journal of Experimental Psychology: General, 112,* 265–277.

Kerr, N. H., & Domhoff, G. W. (2004). Do the blind literally "see" in their dreams? A critique of a recent claim that they do. *Dreaming, 14,* 230–233.

Kershaw, T. C., & Ohlsson, S. (2004). Multiple causes of difficulty in insight: The case of the nine-dot problem. *Journal of Experimental Psychology: Learning, Memory, & Cognition, 30,* 3–13.

Keys, D., & Schwartz, B. (2007). "Leaky" rationality: How research on behavioral decision making challenges normative standards of rationality. *Perspectives on Psychological Science, 2,* 162–180.

Keysers, C., Cohen, J., Donald, M., Guth, W., John, E., et al. (2008). Explicit and implicit strategies in decision making. In C. Engel & W. Singer (Eds.), *Better than conscious? Decision making, the human mind, and implications for institutions* (pp. 225–258). Cambridge, MA: MIT Press.

Khlemani, S., & Johnson-Laird, P. N. (2012). Theories of the syllogism: A meta-analysis. *Psychological Bulletin, 138,* 427–457.

Kihlstrom, J. F. (2006). Trauma and memory revisited. In B. Uttl, N. Ohta, & A. Siegenthaler (Eds.), *Memory and emotion: Interdisciplinary perspectives* (pp. 259–291). Malden, MA: Blackwell.

Kihlstrom, J. F., & Schacter, D. L. (2000). Functional amnesia. In F. Boller & J. Grafman (Eds.), *Handbook of neuropsychology* (2nd ed., Vol. 2, pp. 409–427). Amsterdam, Netherlands: Elsevier.

Kim, C.-Y., & Blake, R. (2005). Psychophysical magic: Rendering the visible "invisible." *Trends in Cognitive Sciences, 9,* 381–388.

Kimberg, D. Y., D'Esposito, M., & Farah, M. J. (1998). Cognitive functions in the prefrontal cortex in working memory and executive control. *Current Directions in Psychological Science, 6,* 185–192.

King, R. N., & Koehler, D. J. (2000). Illusory correlations in graphological inference. *Journal of Experimental Psychology: Applied, 6,* 336–348.

Klahr, D., & Simon, H. A. (2001). What have psychologists (and others) discovered about the process of scientific discovery? *Current Directions in Psychological Science, 10,* 75–79.

Klauer, K. C., Musch, J., & Naumer, B. (2000). On belief bias in syllogistic reasoning. *Psychological Review, 107,* 852–884.

Klauer, K. C., & Zhao, Z. (2004). Double dissociations in visual and spatial short-term memory. *Journal of Experimental Psychology: General, 133,* 355–381.

Klayman, J., & Brown, K. (1993). Debias the environment instead of the judge: An alternative approach to reducing error in diagnostic (and other) judgment. *Cognition, 49,* 97–122.

Klein, G. (2013). *Seeing what others don't: The remarkable ways we gain insights*. New York, NY: PublicAffairs.

Knoblich, G., Ohlsson, S., & Raney, G. E. (2001). An eye movement study of insight problem solving. *Memory & Cognition, 29,* 1000–1009.

Knowlton, B., & Foerde, K. (2008). Neural representations of nondeclarative memories. *Current Directions in Psychological Science, 17,* 107–111.

Koch, C. (2008). The neuroscience of consciousness. In L. R. Squire, F. E. Bloom, N. C. Spiter, S. du Lac, A. Ghosh, & D. Berg (Eds.), *Fundamental neuroscience* (3rd ed., pp. 1223–1236). Burlington, MA: Academic Press.

Koehler, D. J., Brenner, L., & Griffin, D. W. (2002). The calibration of expert judgment: Heuristics and biases beyond the laboratory. In T. Gilovich, D. Griffin, & D. Kahneman (Eds.), *Heuristics and biases: The psychology of intuitive judgment* (pp. 686–715). New York, NY: Cambridge University Press.

Kohler, W. (1969). *The task of Gestalt psychology.* Princeton, NJ: Princeton University Press.

Kolb, B., & Whishaw, I. Q. (2008). *Fundamentals of human neuropsychology.* New York, NY: Worth.

Kopelman, M. D., & Kapur, N. (2001). The loss of episodic memories in retrograde amnesia: Single-case and group studies. In A. D. Baddeley, J. P. Aggleton, & M. A. Conway (Eds.), *Episodic memory: New directions in research* (pp. 110–131). New York, NY: Oxford University Press.

Kosslyn, S. M. (1976). Can imagery be distinguished from other forms of internal representation? Evidence from studies of information retrieval times. *Memory & Cognition, 4,* 291–297.

Kosslyn, S. M. (1980). *Image and mind.* Cambridge, MA: Harvard University Press.

Kosslyn, S. M. (1983). *Ghosts in the mind's machine.* New York, NY: Norton.

Kosslyn, S. M. (1994). *Image and brain: The resolution of the imagery debate.* Cambridge, MA: MIT Press.

Kosslyn, S. M., Ball, T. M., & Reiser, B. J. (1978). Visual images preserve metric spatial information: Evidence from studies of image scanning. *Journal of Experimental Psychology: Human Perception and Performance, 4,* 1–20.

Kosslyn, S. M., Pascual-Leone, A., Felician, O., Camposano, S., Keenan, J. P., Thompson, W. L., et al. (1999). The role of area 17 in visual imagery: Convergent evidence from PET and rTMS. *Science, 284,* 167–170.

Kosslyn, S. M., & Thompson, W. L. (1999). Shared mechanisms in visual imagery and visual perception: Insights from cognitive neuroscience. In M. S. Gazzaniga (Ed.), *The new cognitive neurosciences* (pp. 975–986). Cambridge, MA: MIT Press.

Kosslyn, S. M., & Thompson, W. L. (2003). When is early visual cortex activated during mental imagery? *Psychological Bulletin, 129,* 723–746.

Koulder, S., de Gardelle, V., Sackur, J., & Dupoux, E. (2010). How rich is consciousness? The partial awareness hypothesis. *Trends in Cognitive Sciences, 14,* 301–307.

Kounios, J., & Beeman, M. (2014). The cognitive neuroscience of insight. *Annual Review of Psychology, 65,* 71–93.

Kovelman, I., Shalinsky, M. H., Berens, M. S., & Petitto, L. (2008). Shining new light on the brain's "bilingual signature": A functional Near Infrared Spectroscopy investigation of semantic processing. *Neuroimage, 39,* 1457–1471.

Kozhevnikov, M., Kosslyn, S., & Shephard, J. (2005). Spatial versus object visualizers: A new characterization of visual cognitive style. *Memory & Cognition, 33,* 710–726.

Kraha, A., Talarico, J. M., & Boals, A. (2014). Unexpected positive events do not result in flashbulb memories. *Applied Cognitive Psychology, 28,* 579–589.

Kroll, J. F., Bobb, S. C., & Hoshino, N. (2014). Two languages in mind: Bilingualism as a tool to investigate language, cognition, and the brain. *Current Directions in Psychological Science, 23,* 159–163.

Kroll, J. F., & Potter, M. C. (1984). Recognizing words, pictures, and concepts: A comparison of lexical, object, and reality decisions. *Journal of Verbal Learning and Verbal Behavior, 23,* 39–66.

Kruglanski, A., & Orehek, E. (2007). Partitioning the domain of social inference: Dual mode and systems models and their alternatives. *Annual Review of Psychology, 58,* 291–316.

Kumon-Nakamura, S., Glucksberg, S., & Brown, M. (1995). How about another piece of pie: The allusional pretense theory of discourse irony. *Journal of Experimental Psychology: General, 124,* 3–21.

Kunar, M., Carter, R., Cohen, M., & Horowitz, T. (2008). Telephone conversation impairs sustained visual attention via a central bottleneck. *Psychonomic Bulletin & Review, 15,* 1135–1140.

Kuncel, N. R., Hezlett, S. A., & Ones, D. S. (2004). Academic performance, career potential, creativity, and job performance: Can one construct predict them all? *Journal of Personality and Social Psychology, 86,* 148–161.

Kunda, Z., & Nisbett, R. E. (1986). The psychometrics of everyday life. *Cognitive Psychology, 18,* 195–224.

Küpper, C. S., Benoid, R. G., Dalgleish, T., & Anderson, M. C. (2014). Direct suppression as a mechanism for controlling unpleasant memories in daily life. *Journal of Experimental Psychology: General, 143,* 1443–1449.

Kurtz, K., & Loewenstein, J. (2007). Converging on a new role for analogy in problem solving and retrieval: When two problems are better than one. *Memory & Cognition, 35,* 334–341.

LaBar, K. (2007). Beyond fear: Emotional memory mechanisms in the human brain. *Current Directions in Psychological Science, 16,* 173–177.

LaBar, K., & Cabeza, R. (2006). Cognitive neuroscience of emotional memory. *Nature Reviews Neuroscience, 7,* 54–64.

Labov, B. (2007). Transmission and diffusion. *Language, 83,* 344–387.

Lai, C. S., Fisher, S. E., Hurst, J. A., Vargha-Khadem, F., & Monaco, A. P. (2001). A forkhead-domain gene is mutated in a severe speech and language disorder. *Nature, 413,* 519–522.

Lakoff, G. (1987). Cognitive models and prototype theory. In U. Neisser (Ed.), *Concepts and conceptual development* (pp. 63–100). Cambridge, England: Cambridge University Press.

Lamble, D., Kauranen, T., Laakso, M., & Summala, H. (1999). Cognitive load and detection thresholds in car following situations: Safety implications for using mobile (cellular) telephones while driving. *Accident Analysis & Prevention, 31,* 617–623.

Lampinen, J., Meier, C., Arnal, J., & Leding, J. (2005). Compelling untruths: Content borrowing and vivid false memories. *Journal of Experimental Psychology: Learning, Memory, & Cognition, 31,* 954–963.

Lane, S. M., & Schooler, J. W. (2004). Skimming the surface: Verbal overshadowing of analogical retrieval. *Psychological Science, 15,* 715–719.

Laney, C. (2012). The sources of memory errors. In D. Reisberg (Ed.), *The Oxford handbook of cognitive psychology.* New York, NY: Oxford University Press.

Laney, C., & Loftus, E. F. (2010). False memory. In J. Brown & E. Campbell (Eds.), *The Cambridge handbook of forensic psychology* (pp. 187–194). Cambridge, England: Cambridge University Press.

Laney, C., Morris, E., Bernstein, D., Wakefield, B., & Loftus, E. F. (2008). Asparagus: A love story: Healthier eating could be just a false memory away. *Experimental Psychology, 55,* 291–300.

Langer, E. (1989). *Mindfulness.* Reading, MA: Addison-Wesley.

Lanska, M., Old, J. M., & Westerman, D. L. (2013). Fluency effects in recognition memory: Are perceptual fluency and conceptual fluency interchangeable? *Journal of Experimental Psychology: Learning, Memory, & Cognition, 40,* 1–11.

Lapate, R. C., Rokers, B., Li, T., & Davidson, R. J. (2014). Nonconscious emotional activation colors first impressions: A regulatory role for conscious awareness. *Psychological Science, 25,* 349–357.

Lassiter, G. D., & Meissner, C. (2010). Police interrogations and false confessions. Washington, DC: American Psychological Assocation.

Lau, H., & Rosenthal, D. (2011). Empirical support for higher-order theories of conscious awareness. *Trends in Cognitive Sciences, 15,* 365–373.

Laureys, S. (2005). The neural correlate of (un)awareness: Lessons from the vegetative state. *Trends in Cognitive Sciences, 9,* 556–559.

Lavie, N. (2001). Capacity limits in selective attention: Behavioral evidence and implications for neural activity. In J. Braun, C. Koch, & J. L. Davis (Eds.), *Visual attention and cortical circuits* (pp. 49–68). Cambridge, MA: MIT Press.

Lavie, N. (2005). Distracted and confused? Selective attention under load. *Trends in Cognitive Sciences, 9,* 75–82.

Lavie, N., Lin, Z., Zokaei, N., & Thoma, V. (2009). The role of perceptual load in object recognition. *Journal of Experimental Psychology: Human Perception & Performance, 35,* 1346–1358.

Layard, R. (2010). Measuring subjective well being. *Science, 327,* 534–535.

LeBoeuf, R. A., & Shafir, E. (2012). Decision making. In K. J. Holyoak & R. G. Morrison (Eds.), *The Oxford handbook of thinking and reasoning* (pp. 301–321). New York, NY: Oxford University Press.

Leh, S. E., Johansen-Berg, H., & Ptito, A. (2006). Unconscious vision: New insights into the neuronal correlate of blindsight using diffusion tractography. *Brain, 129,* 1822–1832.

Lehman, D. R., & Nisbett, R. (1990). A longitudinal study of the effects of undergraduate education on reasoning. *Developmental Psychology, 26,* 952–960.

Leo, R. (2008). *Police interrogations and American justice.* Cambridge, MA: Harvard University Press.

Levin, D., Takarae, Y., Miner, A., & Keil, F. (2001). Efficient visual search by category: Specifying the features that mark the difference between artifacts and animals in preattentive vision. *Perception and Psychophysics, 63,* 676–697.

Levin, D. T., & Simons, D. J. (1997). Failure to detect changes to attended objects in motion pictures. *Psychonomic Bulletin and Review, 4,* 501–506.

Levin, I., & Gaeth, G. (1988). How consumers are affected by the framing of attribute information before and after consuming the product. *Journal of Consumer Research, 15,* 374–378.

Levin, I., Schnittjer, S., & Thee, S. (1988). Information framing effects in social and personal decisions. *Journal of Experimental Social Psychology, 24,* 520–529.

Levine, L. J. (1997). Reconstructing memory for emotions. *Journal of Experimental Psychology: General, 126,* 165–177.

Levine, L. J., & Edelstein, R. S. (2009). Emotion and memory narrowing: A review and goal relevance approach. *Cognition and Emotion, 23,* 833–875.

Levy, B. J., Kuhl, B. A., & Wagner, A. D. (2010). The functional neuroimaging of forgetting. In S. Della Sala (Ed.), *Forgetting* (pp. 135–163). New York, NY: Taylor & Francis.

Levy, J., & Pashler, H. (2008). Task prioritisation in multitasking during driving: Opportunity to abort a concurrent task does not insulate braking responses from dual-task slowing. *Applied Cognitive Psychology, 22,* 507–525.

Lewis, C., & Keren, G. (1999). On the difficulties underlying Bayesian reasoning: A comment on Gigerenzer and Hoffrage. *Psychological Review, 106,* 411–416.

Li, P., Abarbanell, L., Gleitman, L., & Papafragou, A. (2011). Spatial reasoning in Tenejapan Mayans. *Cognition, 120,* 33–53.

Li, P., & Gleitman, L. R. (2002). Turning the tables: Language and spatial reasoning. *Cognition, 83,* 265–294.

Liberman, A. (1970). The grammars of speech and language. *Cognitive Psychology, 1,* 301–323.

Liberman, A., Harris, K., Hoffman, H., & Griffith, B. (1957). The discrimination of speech sounds within and across phoneme boundaries. *Journal of Experimental Psychology, 54,* 358–368.

Lichtenstein, S., & Slovic, P. (2006). *The construction of preference.* New York, NY: Cambridge University Press.

Lichtenstein, S., Slovic, P., Fischhoff, B., Layman, M., & Combs, B. (1978). Judged frequency of lethal events. *Journal of Experimental Psychology: Human Learning and Memory, 4,* 551–578.

Liesefeld, H. R., & Zimmer, H. D. (2013). Think spatial: The representation in mental rotation is nonvisual. *Journal of Experimental Psychology: Learning, Memory, & Cognition, 39,* 167–182.

Light, L. L., & Carter-Sobell, L. (1970). Effects of changed semantic context on recognition memory. *Journal of Verbal Learning and Verbal Behavior, 9,* 1–11.

Lindsay, D. S., Hagen, L., Read, J. D., Wade, K. A., & Garry, M. (2004). True photographs and false memories. *Psychological Science, 15,* 149–154.

Lindsay, R. C. L., Semmler, C., Weber, N., Brewer, N., & Lindsay, M. R. (2008). How variations in distance affect eyewitness reports and identification accuracy. *Law and Human Behavior, 32,* 526–535.

Lisker, L., & Abramson, A. (1970). *The voicing dimension: Some experiments in comparative phonetics.* Paper presented at the Proceedings of the Sixth International Congress of Phonetic Sciences, Prague.

Lockhart, R. S., Craik, F. I. M., & Jacoby, L. (1976). Depth of processing, recall, and recognition. In J. Brown (Ed.), *Recall and recognition* (pp. 75–102). New York, NY: Wiley.

Loehlin, J. C., Lindzey, G., & Spuhler, J. N. (1975). *Race difference in intelligence.* San Francisco, CA: Freeman.

Loewenstein, G., & Schkade, D. (1999). Wouldn't it be nice? Predicting future feelings. In D. Kahneman, E. Diener, & N. Schwarz (Eds.), *Well-being: The foundations of hedonic psychology* (pp. 85–105). New York, NY: Russell Sage Foundation.

Loewenstein, G., Weber, E. U., Hsee, C. K., & Welch, N. (2001). Risk as feelings. *Psychological Bulletin, 127,* 267–286.

Loftus, E. F. (1979). *Eyewitness testimony.* Cambridge, MA: Harvard University Press.

Loftus, E. F. (2003). Make-believe memories. *American Psychologist, 58,* 867–873.

Loftus, E. F. (2004). Memories of things unseen. *Current Directions in Psychological Science, 13,* 145–147.

Loftus, E. F., & Guyer, M. J. (2002). Who abused Jane Doe? The hazards of the single case history. *Skeptical Inquirer, 26,* 24–32.

Loftus, G. R. & Harley, E. M. (2004). Why is it easier to identify someone close than far away? *Psychonomic Bulletin & Review, 12,* 43–65.

Loftus, E. F., & Palmer, J. C. (1974). Reconstruction of automobile destruction: An example of the interaction between language and memory. *Journal of Verbal Learning and Verbal Behavior, 13,* 585–589.

Logie, R. H. (2012). Disorders of attention. In D. Reisberg (Ed.), *The Oxford handbook of cognitive psychology.* New York, NY: Oxford University Press.

Logie, R. H., & Della Salla, S. (2005). Disorders of visuospatial working memory. In P. Shah & A. Miyake (Eds.), *The Cambridge handbook of visuospatial thinking* (pp. 81–120). New York, NY: Cambridge University Press.

Lopes, P. N., Salovey, P., Côté, S., & Beers, M. (2005). Emotion regulation ability and the quality of social interaction. *Emotion, 5,* 113–118.

Lubinski, D. (2004). Introduction to the special section on cognitive abilities: 100 years after Spearman's (1904) "'General intelligence,' objectively determined and measured." *Journal of Personality and Social Psychology, 86,* 96–111.

Lucas, M. (2000). Semantic priming without association: A meta-analytic review. *Psychonomic Bulletin & Review, 7,* 618–630.

Luchins, A. (1942). *Mechanization in problem solving: The effect of Einstellung.* (Psychological Monographs, Vol. 54, No. 6 [whole no. 248]). Evanston, IL: American Psychological Association.

Luchins, A., & Luchins, E. (1950). New experimental attempts at preventing mechanization in problem solving. *Journal of General Psychology, 42,* 279–297.

Luchins, A., & Luchins, E. (1959). *Rigidity of behavior: A variational approach to the effects of Einstellung.* Eugene: University of Oregon Books.

Luminet, O., & Curci, A. (Eds.). (2009). *Flashbulb memories: New issues and new perspectives.* New York, NY: Psychology Press.

Luria, A. R. (1966). *Higher cortical functions in man.* New York, NY: Basic Books.

Luria, A. R. (1968). *The mind of a mnemonist: A little book about a vast memory.* New York, NY: Basic Books.

Lyman. B. J. & McDaniel, M. A. (1986). Memory for odors and odor names. *Quartelry Journal of Experimental Psychology, 38A,* 753–765.

Lynn, S., Neuschatz, J., Fite, R., & Rhue, J. (2001). Hypnosis and memory: Implications for the courtroom and psychotherapy. In M. Eisen & G. Goodman (Eds.), *Memory, suggestion, and the forensic interview.* New York, NY: Guilford Press.

Lynn, S. J., Lilienfeld, S. O., Merckelbach, H., Giesbrecht, T., McNally, R. J., Loftus, E. F., Bruck, M., Garry, M., & Malaktaris, A. (2014). The trauma model of dissociation: Inconvenient truths and stubborn fictions. Comment on Dalenberg et al., 2012. *Psychological Bulletin, 140,* 896–910.

Macdonald, G. (Ed.). (1995). *Connectionism: Debates on psychological explanation.* Oxford, England: Blackwell.

MacDonald, J., & Lavie, N. (2008). Load induced blindness. *Journal of Experimental Psychology: Human Perception & Performance, 34,* 1078–1091.

MacDonald, M., Pearlmutter, N., & Seidenberg, M. (1994). The lexical nature of syntactic ambiguity. *Psychological Review, 101*, 676–703.

MacGregor, J. N., Ormerod, T. C., & Chronicle, E. P. (2001). Information processing and insight: A process model of performance on the 9-dot and related problems. *Journal of Experimental Psychology: Learning, Memory, & Cognition, 27*, 176–201.

Mack, A. (2003). Inattentional blindness: Looking without seeing. *Current Directions in Psychological Science, 12*, 180–184.

Mack, A., & Rock, I. (1998). *Inattentional blindness*. Cambridge, MA: MIT Press.

Mahon, B., & Caramazza, A. (2009). Concepts and categories: A cognitive neuropsychological perspective. *Annual Review of Psychology, 60*, 27–51.

Mahoney, M., & DeMonbreun, B. (1978). Problem-solving bias in scientists. *Cognitive Therapy and Research, 1*, 229–238.

Maia, T. V., & Cleeremans, A. (2005). Consciousness: Converging insights from connectionist modeling and neuroscience. *Trends in Cognitive Sciences, 9*, 397–404.

Maia, T. V., & McClelland, J. L. (2005). The somatic marker hypothesis: Still many questions but no answers. *Trends in Cognitive Sciences, 9*, 162–164.

Majerus, S., Poncelet, M., Elsen, B., & van der Linden, M. (2006). Exploring the relationship between new word learning and short-term memory for serial order recall, item recall, and item recognition. *European Journal of Cognitive Psychology, 18*, 848–873.

Majid, A., Bowerman, M., Kita, S., Haun, D. B. M., & Levinson, S. (2004). Can language restructure cognition? The case for space. *Trends in Cognitive Sciences, 8*, 108–114.

Malone, J. C. (2009). *Psychology: Pythagoras to present*. Cambridge, MA: MIT Press.

Malt, B. C., & Smith, E. E. (1984). Correlated properties in natural categories. *Journal of Verbal Learning and Verbal Behavior, 23*, 250–269.

Mandel, D. R. (2014). Do framing effects reveal irrational choice? *Journal of Experimental Psychology: General, 143*, 1185–1198.

Mandler, G. (2011). *A history of modern experimental psychology*. Cambridge, MA: MIT Press.

Mandler, J. M., & Ritchey, G. H. (1977). Long-term memory for pictures. *Journal of Experimental Psychology: Human Learning and Memory, 3*, 386–396.

Marcus, G. B. (1986). Stability and change in political attitudes: Observe, recall, and "explain." *Political Behavior, 8*, 21–44.

Marcus, G. F. (2001). *The algebraic mind: Integrating connectionism and cognitive science (learning, development, and conceptual change)*. Cambridge, MA: MIT Press.

Marcus, G. F., Pinker, S., Ullman, M., Hollander, M., Rosen, T., & Xu, F. (1992). Overregularization in *language acquisition* (Monographs of the Society for Research in Child Development, Vol. 57, No. 4 [serial no. 228]). Chicago, IL: University of Chicago Press.

Marcus, G. F., Vijayan, S., Rao, S. B., & Vishton, P. M. (1999). Rule learning by seven-month-old infants. *Science, 283*, 77–80.

Markman, A. B., & Gentner, D. (2001). Thinking. *Annual Review of Psychology, 52*, 223–247.

Markman, A. B., & Rein, J. R. (2013). The nature of mental concepts. In D. Reisberg (Ed.), *The Oxford handbook of cognitive psychology* (pp. 321–329). New York, NY: Oxford University Press.

Marks, D. (1983). Mental imagery and consciousness: A theoretical review. In A. Sheikh (Ed.), *Imagery: Current theory, research and application* (pp. 96–130). New York, NY: Wiley.

Marmor, G. S., & Zabeck, L. A. (1976). Mental rotation by the blind: Does mental rotation depend on visual imagery? *Journal of Experimental Psychology: Human Perception and Performance, 2*, 515–521.

Marslen-Wilson, W. D., & Teuber, H. L. (1975). Memory for remote events in anterograde amnesia: Recognition of public figures from news photographs. *Neuropsychologia, 13*, 353–364.

Martin, R. C. (2003). Language processing: Functional organization and neuroanatomical basis. *Annual Review of Psychology, 54*, 55–89.

Martinez, M. E. (2000). *Education as the cultivation of intelligence*. Mahwah, NJ: Erlbaum.

Massimini, M., Ferrarelli, F., Huber, R., Esser, S., Singh, H., & Tononi, G. (2005). Breakdown of cortical effective connectivity during sleep. *Science, 309*, 2228–2232.

Mather, M., Shafir, E., & Johnson, M. K. (2000). Misremembrance of options past: Source monitoring and choice. *Psychological Science, 11*, 132–138.

Mattys, S. (2012). Speech perception. In D. Reisberg, (Ed.), *The Oxford handbook of cognitive psychology*. New York, NY: Oxford University Press.

Mayer, J. D., Roberts, R. D., & Barsade, S. G. (2008). Human abilities: Emotional intelligence. *Annual Review of Psychology, 59*, 507–536.

Mayer, R. E. (2012). Problem solving. In D. Reisberg (Ed.), *The Oxford handbook of cognitive psychology*. New York, NY: Oxford University Press.

Mayr, U. (2004). Conflict, consciousness, and control. *Trends in Cognitive Sciences, 8*, 145–148.

Mazzoni, G., Loftus, E. F., & Kirsch, I. (2001). Changing beliefs about implausible autobiographical events. *Journal of Experimental Psychology: Applied, 7*, 51–59.

Mazzoni, G., & Lynn, S. (2007). Using hypnosis in eyewitness memory. In D. Ross, M. Toglia, R. Lindsay, & D. Read (Eds.), *Handbook of eyewitness memory* (Vol. 1, *Memory for events*). Mahwah, NJ: Erlbaum.

Mazzoni, G., & Memon, A. (2003). Imagination can create false autobiographical memories. *Psychological Science, 14*, 186–188.

McAdams, C., & Reid, R. (2005). Attention modulates the responses of simple cells in the monkey visual cortex. *Journal of Neuroscience, 25*, 11022–11033.

McCaffrey, T. (2012). Innovation relies on the obscure: A key to overcoming the classic problem of functional fixedness. *Psychological Science, 23*, 215–218.

McCann, R., & Johnston, J. (1992). Locus of the single-channel bottleneck in dual-task interference. *Journal of Experimental Psychology: Human Perception and Performance, 18*, 471–484.

McClelland, J. L., & Rumelhart, D. E. (1981). An interactive model of context effects in letter perception. Part 1: An account of basic findings. *Psychological Review, 88*, 375–407.

McCloskey, M., & Glucksberg, S. (1978). Natural categories: Well-defined or fuzzy sets? *Memory & Cognition, 6*, 462–472.

McDaniel, M., Anderson, J., Derbish, M., & Morrisette, N. (2007). Testing the testing effect in the classroom. *European Journal of Cognitive Psychology, 19*, 494–513.

McDermott, K. B., Agarwal, P. K., D'Antonio, L., Roediger, H. L., & McDaniel, M. A. (2014). Both multiple-choice and short-answer quizzes enhance later exam performance in middle and high school classes. *Journal of Experimental Psychology: Applied, 20*, 3–21.

McDermott, K. B., & Roediger, H. (1994). Effects of imagery on perceptual implicit memory tests. *Journal of Experimental Psychology: Learning, Memory, & Cognition, 20*, 1379–1390.

McDermott, K. B., & Roediger, H. (1998). False recognition of associates can be resistant to an explicit warning to subjects and an immediate recognition probe. *Journal of Memory & Language, 39*, 508–520.

McDunn, B. A., Siddiqui, A. P., & Brown, J. M. (2014). Seeking the boundary of boundary extension. *Psychonomic Bulletin & Review, 21*, 370–375.

McFarland, C., & Buehler, R. (2012). Negative moods and the motivated remembering of past selves: The role of implicit theories of personal stability. *Journal of Personality and Social Psychology, 102*, 242–263.

McGaugh, J. L. (2000). Memory—A century of consolidation. *Science, 287*, 248–251.

McGaugh, J. L., & LePort, A. (2014, February). Remembrance of all things past. *Scientific American*, 41–45.

McGrew, K. (2009). CHC theory and the human cognitive abilities project: Standing on the shoulders of the giants of psychometric intelligence research. *Intelligence, 37*, 1–10.

McGue, M., Bouchard, T. J., Jr., Iacono, W. G., & Lykken, D. T. (1993). Behavioral genetics of cognitive ability: A life span perspective. In R. Plomin & G. E. McClearn (Eds.), *Nature, nurture and psychology*

(pp. 59–76). Washington, DC: American Psychological Association.

McIntosh, A. R., Rajah, M. N., & Lobaugh, N. J. (1999). Interactions of prefrontal cortex in relation to awareness in sensory learning. *Science, 284*, 1531–1533.

McKelvie, S. (1995). The VVIQ as a psychometric test of individual differences in visual imagery vividness: A critical quantitative review and plea for direction. *Journal of Mental Imagery, 19*(3&4), 1–106.

McNally, R. J. (2003). Recovering memories of trauma: A view from the laboratory. *Current Directions in Psychological Science, 12*, 32–35.

McNally, R. J., Lasko, N., Clancy, S. A., Macklin, M. L., Pitman, R. K., & Orr, S. P. (2004). Psychophysiological responding during script-driven imagery in people reporting abduction by space aliens. *Psychological Science, 15*, 493–497.

McRae, K., & Jones, M. (2012). Semantic memory. In D. Reisberg (Ed.), *The Oxford handbook of cognitive psychology*. New York, NY: Oxford University Press.

Meadows, J. C. (1974). Disturbed perception of colours associated with localized cerebral lesions. *Brain, 97*, 615–632.

Medin, D. L. (1989). Concepts and conceptual structure. *American Psychologist, 44*, 1469–1481.

Medin, D. L., Coley, J. D., Storms, G., & Hayes, B. K. (2003). A relevance theory of induction. *Psychonomic Bulletin & Review, 10*, 517–532.

Medin, D. L., Goldstone, R., & Gentner, D. (1993). Respects for similarity. *Psychological Review, 100*, 254–278.

Medin, D. L., & Ortony, A. (1989). Psychological essentialism. In S. Vosniadou & A. Ortony (Eds.), *Similarity and analogical reasoning* (pp. 179–195). New York, NY: Cambridge University Press.

Medin, D. L., Schwartz, H., Blok, S. V., & Birnbaum, L. A. (1999). The semantic side of decision making. *Psychonomic Bulletin & Review, 6*, 562–569.

Mednick, S. (1962). The associative basis of the creative process. *Psychological Review, 69*, 220–232.

Mednick, S., & Mednick, M. (1967). *Examiner's manual, Remote Associates Test*. Boston, MA: Houghton Mifflin.

Mellers, B., Chang, S.-J., Birnbaum, M., & Ordóñez, L. (1992). Preferences, prices, and ratings in risky decision making. *Journal of Experimental Psychology: Human Perception and Performance, 18*, 347–361.

Mellers, B., Hertwig, R., & Kahneman, D. (2001). Do frequency representations eliminate conjunction effects? An exercise in adversarial collaboration. *Psychological Science, 12*, 269–275.

Mervis, C. B., Catlin, J., & Rosch, E. (1976). Relationships among goodness-of-example, category norms and word frequency. *Bulletin of the Psychonomic Society, 7*, 268–284.

Metcalfe, J. (1986). Premonitions of insight predict impending error. *Journal of Experimental Psychology: Learning, Memory, & Cognition, 12,* 623–634.

Metcalfe, J., & Weibe, D. (1987). Intuition in insight and noninsight problem solving. *Memory & Cognition, 15,* 238–246.

Meyer, D. E., & Schvaneveldt, R. W. (1971). Facilitation in recognizing pairs of words: Evidence of a dependence between retrieval operations. *Journal of Experimental Psychology, 90,* 227–234.

Meyer, D. E., Schvaneveldt, R. W., & Ruddy, M. G. (1974). Functions of graphemic and phonemic codes in visual word recognition. *Memory & Cognition, 2,* 309–321.

Michel, C., Rossion, B., Han, J., Chung, C.-S., & Caldara, R. (2006). Holistic processing is finely tumed for faces of one's own race. *Psychological Science, 17,* 608–615.

Mill, J. S. (1874). *A system of logic* (8th ed.). New York, NY: Harper.

Miller, A. (1986). *Imagery in scientific thought.* Cambridge, MA: MIT Press.

Miller, D. I., & Halpern, D. F. (2013). The new science of cognitive sex differences. *Trends in Cognitive Sciences, 18*(1), 37–45.

Miller, E. K., & Cohen, J. D. (2001). An integrative theory of prefrontal cortex function. *Annual Review of Neuroscience, 24,* 167–202.

Miller, E. M. (1994). Intelligence and brain myelination: A hypothesis. *Personality and Individual Differences, 17,* 803–832.

Miller, G. A. (1951). *Language and communication.* New York, NY: McGraw-Hill.

Miller, G. A. (1956). The magical number seven plus or minus two: Some limits on our capacity for processing information. *Psychological Review, 63,* 81–97.

Miller, G. A. (1962). *Psychology: The science of mental life.* New York, NY: Harper & Row.

Miller, G. A. (1991). *The science of words.* New York, NY: Freeman.

Miller, G. A., Bruner, J. S., & Postman, L. (1954). Familiarity of letter sequences and tachistoscopic identification. *Journal of General Psychology, 50,* 129–139.

Miller, G. A., Galanter, E., & Pribram, K. (1960). *Plans and the structure of behavior.* New York, NY: Holt, Rinehart and Winston.

Miller, L. K. (1999). The Savant Syndrome: Intellectual impairment and exceptional skill. *Psychological Bulletin, 125,* 31–46.

Miller, M. B., van Horn, J. D., Wolford, G. L., Handy, T. C., Valsangkar-Smyth, M., Inati, S., et al. (2002). Extensive individual differences in brain activations associated with episodic retrieval are reliable over time. *Journal of Cognitive Neuroscience, 14,* 1200–1214.

Milner, B. (1966). Amnesia following operation on the temporal lobes. In C. W. M. Whitty & O. L. Zangwill (Eds.), *Amnesia* (pp. 109–133). London, England: Butterworths.

Milner, B. (1970). Memory and the medial temporal regions of the brain. In K. H. Pribram & D. E. Broadbent (Eds.), *Biology of memory* (pp. 29–48). New York, NY: Academic Press.

Minda, J. P., & Smith, J. D. (2001). Prototypes in category learning: The effects of category size, category structure and stimulus complexity. *Journal of Experimental Psychology: Learning, Memory, & Cognition, 27,* 775–799.

Mitroff, I. (1981). Scientists and confirmation bias. In R. Tweney, M. Doherty, & C. Mynatt (Eds.), *On scientific thinking* (pp. 170–175). New York, NY: Columbia University Press.

Miyake, A., & Friedman, N. (2012). The nature and organization of individual differences in executive functions: Four general conclusions. *Current Directions in Psychological Science, 21,* 8–14.

Miyashita, Y. (1995). How the brain creates imagery: Projection to primary visual cortex. *Science, 268,* 1719–1720.

Molden, D. C., & Higgins, E. T. (2012). Motivated thinking. In K. J. Holyoak & R. G. Morrison (Eds.), *The Oxford handbook of thinking and reasoning* (pp. 390–412). New York, NY: Oxford University Press.

Moons, W. G., Mackie, D. M., & Garcia-Marques, T. (2009). The impact of repetition-induced familarity on agreement with weak and strong arguments. *Journal of Personality & Social Psychology, 96,* 32–44.

Moore, C. M., & Egeth, H. (1997). Perception without attention: Evidence of grouping under conditions of inattention. *Journal of Experimental Psychology: Human Perception and Performance, 23,* 339–352.

Moors, A., & De Houwer, J. (2006). Automaticity: A theoretical and conceptual analysis. *Psychological Bulletin, 132,* 297–326.

Morawetz, C., Holz, P., Baudewig, J., Treue S., & Dechent, P. (2007). Split of attentional resources in human visual cortex. *Visual Neuroscience, 24,* 817–826.

Moray, N. (1959). Attention in dichotic listening: Affective cues and the influence of instructions. *Quarterly Journal of Experimental Psychology, 11,* 56–60.

Morrison, C., & Conway, M. (2010). First words and first memories. *Cognition, 116,* 23–32.

Morsella, E., & Bargh, J. (2011). Unconscious action tendencies: Sources of "unintegrated" action. In J. Cacioppo & J. Decety (Eds.), *The handbook of social neuroscience* (pp. 335–347). New York, NY: Oxford University Press.

Morsella, E., Krieger, S., & Bargh, J. (2010). Minimal neuroanatomy for a conscious brain: Homing in on the networks constituting consciousness. *Neural Networks, 23,* 14–15.

Moscovitch, M. (1982). Multiple dissociations of function in amnesia. In L. S. Cermak (Ed.), *Human memory and amnesia* (pp. 337–370). Hillsdale, NJ: Erlbaum.

Most, S. B., Simons, D. J., Scholl, B. J., Jimenez, R., Clifford, E., & Chabris, C. F. (2001). How not to be seen: The contribution of similarity and selective ignoring to sustained inattentional blindness. *Psychological Science, 12,* 9–17.

Mudrik, L., Faivre, N., & Koch, C. (2014). Information integration without awareness. *Trends in Cognitive Sciences, 18,* 488–496.

Mumford, M., & Antes, A. (2007). Debates about the "general" picture: Cognition and creative achievement. *Creativity Research Journal, 19,* 367–374.

Murdock, B. B., Jr. (1962). The serial position effect of free recall. *Journal of Experimental Psychology, 64,* 482–488.

Murphy, G. L. (2003). *The big book of concepts.* Cambridge, MA: MIT Press.

Murphy, G. L., & Medin, D. L. (1985). The role of theories in conceptual coherence. *Psychological Review, 92,* 289–316.

Murphy, G. L., & Ross, B. H. (2005). The two faces of typicality in category-based induction. *Cognition, 95,* 175–200.

Murphy, S. T. (2001). Feeling without thinking: Affective primacy and the nonconscious processing of emotion. In J. A. Bargh & D. K. Apsley (Eds.), *Unraveling the complexities of social life: A festschrift in honor of Robert B. Zajonc* (pp. 39–53). Washington, DC: American Psychological Association.

Murray, C., Pattie, A., Starr, J. M., & Deary, I. J. (2012). Does cognitive ability predict mortality in the ninth decade? The Lothian birth cohort 1921. *Intelligence, 40,* 490–498.

Mynatt, C., Doherty, M., & Tweney, R. (1977). Confirmation bias in a simulated research environment: An experimental study of scientific inference. *Quarterly Journal of Experimental Psychology, 29,* 85–95.

Mynatt, C., Doherty, M., & Tweney, R. (1978). Consequences of confirmation and disconfirmation in a simulated research environment. *Quarterly Journal of Experimental Psychology, 30,* 395–406.

Nadel, L., & Moscovitch, M. (2001). The hippocampal complex and long-term memory revisited. *Trends in Cognitive Sciences, 5,* 228–230.

Naghavi, H. R., & Nyberg, L. (2005). Common frontoparietal activity in attention, memory, and consciousness: Shared demands on integration? *Conscious Cognition, 13,* 390–425.

Naqvi, N., Shiv, B., & Bechara, A. (2006). The role of emotion in decision making. *Current Directions in Psychological Science, 15,* 260–264.

Nasar, J., Hecht, P., & Wener, R. (2008). Mobile telephones, distracted attention, and pedestrian safety. *Accident Analysis and Prevention, 4,* 69–75.

Nee, D., Berman, M., Moore, K., & Jonides, J. (2008). Neuroscientific evidence about the distinction between short- and long-term memory. *Current Directions in Psychological Science, 17,* 102–106.

Needham, D., & Begg, I. (1991). Problem-oriented training promotes spontaneous analogical transfer: Memory-oriented training promotes memory for training. *Memory & Cognition, 19,* 543–557.

Neisser, U. (1967). *Cognitive psychology.* New York, NY: Appleton-Century-Crofts.

Neisser, U., & Becklen, R. (1975). Selective looking: Attending to visually significant events. *Cognitive Psychology, 7,* 480–494.

Neisser, U., Boodoo, G., Bouchard, T. J., Jr., Boykin, A. W., Brody, N., Ceci, S. J., et al. (1996). Intelligence: Knowns and unknowns. *American Psychologist, 51*(2), 77–101.

Neisser, U., & Harsch, N. (1992). Phantom flashbulbs: False recollections of hearing the news about *Challenger.* In E. Winograd & U. Neisser (Eds.), *Affect and accuracy in recall: Studies of "flashbulb" memories* (pp. 9–31). Cambridge, England: Cambridge University Press.

Neisser, U., Winograd, E., & Weldon, M. S. (1991, November). *Remembering the earthquake: "What I experienced" vs. "How I heard the news."* Paper presented at the meeting of the Psychonomic Society, San Francisco, CA.

Nelson, T. O., & Narens, L. (1990). Metamemory: A theoretical framework and new findings. *Psychology of Learning and Motivation, 26,* 125–173.

Nettelbeck, T. (2003). Inspection time and g. In H. Nyborg (Ed.), *The scientific study of general intelligence: A tribute to Arthur Jensen* (pp. 77–92). New York, NY: Elsevier.

Newcombe, F., Ratcliff, G., & Damasio, H. (1987). Dissociable visual and spatial impairments following right posterior cerebral lesions: Clinical, neuropsychological and anatomical evidence. *Neuropsychologia, 25,* 149–161.

Newell, A., & Simon, H. (1972). *Human problem solving.* Englewood Cliffs, NJ: Prentice-Hall.

Nickerson, R. S., & Adams, M. J. (1979). Long-term memory for a common object. *Cognitive Psychology, 11,* 287–307.

Nisbett, R. E. (Ed.). (1993). *Rules for reasoning.* Hillsdale, NJ: Erlbaum.

Nisbett, R. E. (2009). *Intelligence and how to get it.* New York, NY: Norton.

Nisbett, R. E., Krantz, D. H., Jepson, C., & Kunda, Z. (1983). The use of statistical heuristics in everyday inductive reasoning. *Psychological Review, 90,* 339–363.

Nisbett, R. E., & Ross, L. (1980). *Human inference: Strategies and shortcomings of social judgment.* Englewood Cliffs, NJ: Prentice-Hall.

Nisbett, R. E., & Schachter, S. (1966). Cognitive manipulation of pain. *Journal of Experimental Social Psychology, 2,* 277–236.

Nisbett, R. E., & Wilson, T. (1977). Telling more than we can know: Verbal reports on mental processes. *Psychological Review, 84*, 231–259.

Nisbett, R. E., Aronson, J., Blair, C., Dickens, W., Flynn, J., Halpern, D. F., & Turkheimer, E. (2012a). Group differences in IQ are best understood as environmental in origin. *American Psychologist, 67*, 503–504.

Nisbett, R. E., Aronson, J., Blair, C., Dickens, W., Flynn, J., Halpern, D. F., & Turkheimer, E. (2012b). Intelligence: New findings and theoretical developments. *American Psychologist, 67*, 130–159.

Norman, D. (1981). Categorization of action slips. *Psychological Review, 88*, 1–15.

Norman, D., Rumelhart, D. E., & Group, T. L. R. (1975). *Explorations in cognition.* San Francisco, CA: Freeman.

Norman, D., & Shallice, T. (1986). Attention to action: Willed and automatic control of behavior. In R. Davidson, G. Schwartz, & D. Shapiro (Eds.), *Consciousness and self-regulation* (pp. 1–18). New York, NY: Plenum.

Northup, T., & Mulligan, N. (2013). Conceptual implicit memory in advertising research. *Applied Cognitive Psychology, 27*, 127–136.

Northup, T., & Mulligan, N. (2014). Online advertisements and conceptual implicit memory: Advances in theory and methodology. *Applied Cognitive Psychology, 28*, 66–78.

Noveck, I., & Reboul, A. (2008). Experimental pragmatics: A Gricean turn in the study of language. *Trends in Cognitive Sciences, 12*, 425–431.

Noveck, J., & Sperber, D. (2005). *Experimental pragmatics.* New York, NY: Oxford University Press.

Novick, L., & Holyoak, K. (1991). Mathematical problem solving by analogy. *Journal of Experimental Psychology: Learning, Memory, & Cognition, 17*, 398–415.

O'Connor, D., Fukui, M., Pinsk, M., & Kastner, S. (2002). Attention modulates responses in the human lateral geniculate nucleus. *Nature Neuroscience, 5*, 1203–1209.

O'Connor, M., Walbridge, M., Sandson, T., & Alexander, M. (1996). A neuropsychological analysis of Capgras syndrome. *Neuropsychiatry, Neuropsychology, and Behavioral Neurology, 9*, 265–271.

O'Craven, K. M., & Kanwisher, N. (2000). Mental imagery of faces and places activates corresponding stimulus-specific brain regions. *Journal of Cognitive Neuroscience, 12*, 1013–1023.

O'Kane, G., Kensinger, E. A., & Corkin, S. (2004). Evidence for semantic learning in profound amnesia: An investigation with patient H.M. *Hippocampus, 14*(4), 417–425.

Oaksford, M., & Chater, N. (1995). Information gain explains relevance, which explains the selection task. *Cognition, 57*, 97–108.

Oberauer, K., & Hein, L. (2012). Attention to information in working memory. *Current Directions in Psychological Science, 21*, 164–169.

Obrecht, N., Chapman, G., & Gelman, R. (2009). An encounter frequency account of how experience affects likelihood estimation. *Memory & Cognition, 37*, 632–643.

Ochsner, K. N., & Schacter, D. L. (2000). A social cognitive neuroscience approach to emotion and memory. In J. C. Borod (Ed.), *The neuropsychology of emotion* (pp. 163–193). New York, NY: Oxford University Press.

Öhman, A. (2002). Automaticity and the amygdala: Nonconscious responses to emotional faces. *Current Directions in Psychological Science, 11*, 62–66.

Oldfield, R. (1963). Individual vocabulary and semantic currency: A preliminary study. *British Journal of Social and Clinical Psychology, 2*, 122–130.

Oliphant, G. W. (1983). Repetition and recency effects in word recognition. *Australian Journal of Psychology, 35*, 393–403.

Öllinger, M., Jones, G., Faber, A. H., & Knoblich, G. (2013). Cognitive mechanisms of insight: The role of heuristics and representational change in solving the eight-coin problem. *Journal of Experimental Psychology: Learning, Memory, & Cognition, 39*, 931–939.

Oppenheimer, D. M. (2004). Spontaneous discounting of availability in frequency judgment tasks. *Psychological Science, 15*, 100–105.

Oppenheimer, D. M. (2005). Consequences of erudite vernacular utilized irrespective of necessity: Problems with using long words needlessly. *Applied Cognitive Psychology, 20*(2), 139–156.

Oppenheimer, D. M. (2008). The secret life of fluency. *Trends in Cognitive Sciences, 12*, 237–241.

Oppenheimer, D. M., & Alter A. L. (2014). The search for moderators in disfluency research. *Applied Cognitive Psychology, 28*, 502–504.

Oppenheimer, D. M., & Frank, M. C. (2007). A rose in any other font wouldn't smell as sweet: Fluency effects in categorization. *Cognition, 106*, 1178–1194.

Osman, M. (2004). An evaluation of dual-process theories of reasoning. *Psychonomic Bulletin & Review, 11*, 988–1010.

Ost, J., Vrij, A., Costall, A., & Bull, R. (2002). Crashing memories and reality monitoring: Distinguishing between perceptions, imaginations and "false memories." *Applied Cognitive Psychology, 16*, 125–134.

Overton, D. (1985). Contextual stimulus effects of drugs and internal states. In P. D. Balsam & A. Tomie (Eds.), *Context and learning* (pp. 357–384). Hillsdale, NJ: Erlbaum.

Owens, J., Bower, G. H., & Black, J. B. (1979). The "soap opera" effect in story recall. *Memory & Cognition, 7*, 185–191.

Özgen, E. (2004). Language, learning, and color perception. *Current Directions in Psychological Science, 13*, 95–98.

Özgen, E., & Davies, I. R. L. (2002). Acquisition of categorical color perception: A perceptual learning approach to the linguistic relativity hypothesis. *Journal of Experimental Psychology: General, 131*, 477–493.

Pachur, T., Hertwig, R., & Steinmann, F. (2012). How do people judge risks: Availability heuristic, affect heuristic, or both? *Journal of Experimental Psychology: Applied, 18*, 314–330.

Paivio, A. (1969). Mental imagery in associative learning and memory. *Psychological Review, 76*, 241–263.

Paivio, A. (1971). *Imagery and verbal processes.* New York, NY: Holt, Rinehart & Winston.

Paivio, A., & Okovita, H. W. (1971). Word imagery modalities and associative learning in blind and sighted subjects. *Journal of Verbal Learning and Verbal Behavior, 10*, 506–510.

Paivio, A., Smythe, P. C., & Yuille, J. C. (1968). Imagery versus meaningfulness of nouns in paired-associate learning. *Canadian Journal of Psychology, 22*, 427–441.

Paivio, A., Yuille, J. C., & Madigan, S. (1968). *Concreteness, imagery, and meaningfulness values for 925 nouns.* [Monograph supplement]. *Journal of Experimental Psychology, 76*(1), Pt. 2. Washington, DC: American Psychological Association.

Paller, K. A., & Suzuki, S. (2014). Response to Block et al.: First-person perspectives are both necessary and troublesome for consciousness science. *Trends in Cognitive Sciences, 18*, 557–558.

Palmer, S., Schreiber, C., & Fox, C. (1991, November). *Remembering the earthquake: "Flashbulb" memory for experienced vs. reported events.* Paper presented at the meeting of the Psychonomic Society, San Francisco, CA.

Pansky, A., & Koriat, A. (2004). The basic-level convergence effect in memory distortions. *Psychological Science, 15*, 52–59.

Papafragou, A., Li, P., Choi, Y., & Han, C-h. (2007). Evidentiality in language and cognition. *Cognition, 103*, 253–299.

Parker, E. S., Cahill, L., & McGaugh, J. L. (2006, February). A case of unusual autobiographical remembering. *Neurocase, 12*(1): 35–49.

Parkin, A. J. (1984). Levels of processing, context, and facilitation of pronunciation. *Acta Psychologia, 55*, 19–29.

Pashler, H. (1991). Dual-task interference and elementary mental mechanisms. In D. E. Meyer & S. Kornblum (Eds.), *Attention and performance XIV* (pp. 245–264). Hillsdale, NJ: Erlbaum.

Pashler, H. (1992). Attentional limitations in doing two tasks at the same time. *Current Directions in Psychological Science, 1*, 44–47.

Pashler, H. (1996). Structures, processes and the flow of information. In E. Bjork & R. Bjork (Eds.), *Handbook of perception and cognition* (2nd ed., Vol. 10: *Memory*, pp. 3–29). San Diego, CA: Academic Press.

Pashler, H., & Johnston, J. (1989). Interference between temporally overlapping tasks: Chronometric evidence for central postponement with or without response grouping. *Quarterly Journal of Experimental Psychology, 41A*, 19–45.

Pashler, H., Rohrer, D., Cepeda, N., & Carpenter, S. (2007). Enhancing learning and retarding forgetting: Choices and consequences. *Psychonomic Bulletin & Review, 14*, 187–193.

Paterson, H. M., & Kemp, R. I. (2006). Comparing methods of encountering post-event information: The power of co-witness suggestion. *Applied Cognitive Psychology, 20*, 1083–1099.

Patihis, L., Frenda, S. J., LePort, A. K. R., Petersen, N., Nichols, R. M., Stark, C. E. L., McGaugh, J. L., & Loftus, E. F. (2013). False memories in highly superior autobiographical memory individuals. *Proceedings of the National Academy of Sciences, 110*(52), 20947–20952.

Patihis, L., Lilienfeld, S. O., Ho, L., & Loftus, E. F. (2014). Unconscious repressed memory is scientifically questionable. *Psychological Science, 25*, 197–198.

Payne, J. D., Nadel, L., Britton, W. B., & Jacobs, W. J. (2004). The bio-psychology of trauma and memory. In D. Reisberg & P. Hertel (Eds.), *Memory and emotion* (pp. 76–128). New York, NY: Oxford University Press.

Payne, L., & Sekuler, R. (2014). The importance of ignoring: Alpha oscillations protect selectivity. *Current Directions in Psychological Science, 23*, 171–177.

Payton, A. (2009). The impact of genetic research on our understanding of normal cognitive aging: 1995 to 2009. *Neuropsychology Review, 19*, 451–477.

Paz-Alonso, P., & Goodman, G. (2008). Trauma and memory: Effects of post-event misinformation, retrieval order, and retention interval. *Memory, 16*, 58–75.

Peace, K. A., & Porter, S. (2004). A longitudinal investigation of the reliability of memories for trauma and other emotional experiences. *Applied Cognitive Psychology, 18*, 143–159.

Pearson, J. (2014). New directions in mental-imagery research: The binocular-rivalry technique and decoding fMRI patterns. *Current Directions in Psychological Science, 23*, 178–183.

Pearson, J., Clifford, C. W. G., & Tong, F. (2008). The functional impact of mental imagery on conscious perception. *Current Biology, 18*, 982–986.

Pederson, E., Danziger, E., Wilkins, D., Levinson, S., Kita, S., & Senft, G. (1998). Semantic typology and spatial conceptualization. *Language, 74*, 557–589.

Pedrone, R., Hummel, J. E., & Holyoak, K. J. (2001). The use of diagrams in analogical problem solving. *Memory & Cognition, 29*, 214–221.

Peissig, J., & Tarr, M. J. (2007). Visual object recognition: Do we know more now than we did 20 years ago? *Annual Review of Psychology, 58*, 75–96.

Pelham, S., & Abrams, L. (2014). Cognitive advantages and disadvantages in early and late bilinguals. *Journal of Experimental Psychology: Learning, Memory, & Cognition, 40*(2), 313–325.

Penke, L., Muñoz Maniega, S., Bastin, M. E., Valdés Hernández, M. C., Murray, C., Royle, N. A., Starr, J. M., Wardlaw, J. M., & Deary, I. J. (2012). Brain white matter tract integrity as a neural foundation for general intelligence. *Molecular Psychiatry, 17*, 1026–1030.

Pennycook, G., Trippas, D., Hadley, S. J., & Thompson, V. A. (2014). Base rates: Both neglected and intuitive. *Journal of Experimental Psychology: Learning, Memory, & Cognition, 40*, 544–554.

Peru, A., & Avesani, R. (2008). To know what it is for, but not how it is: Semantic dissociations in a case of visual agnosia. *Neurocase, 14*, 249–263.

Peterson, M., Kihlstrom, J. F., Rose, P., & Glisky, M. (1992). Mental images can be ambiguous: Reconstruals and reference-frame reversals. *Memory & Cognition, 20*, 107–123.

Pezdek, K., Blandon-Gitlin, I., & Gabbay, P. (2006). Imagination and memory: Does imagining implausible events lead to false autobiographical memories? *Psychonomic Bulletin & Review, 13*, 764–769.

Pfordresher, P. Q., & Halpern, A. R. (2013). Auditory imagery and the poor-pitch singer. *Psychonomic Bulletin & Review, 20*, 747–753.

Phelps, E. (2004). Human emotion and memory: Interactions of the amygdala and hippocampal complex. *Current Opinion in Neurobiology, 14*, 198–202.

Phillips, J. A., Noppeney, U., Humphreys, G. W., & Price, C. J. (2002). Can segregation within the semantic system account for category-specific deficits? *Brain, 125*, 2067–2080.

Piaget, J. (1952). *The origins of intelligence in children.* New York, NY: International Universities Press.

Pillemer, D. B. (1984). Flashbulb memories of the assassination attempt on President Reagan. *Cognition, 16*, 63–80.

Pinker, S. (1987). The bootstrapping problem in language acquisition. In B. MacWhinney (Ed.), *Mechanisms of language acquisition* (pp. 339–441). Hillsdale, NJ: Erlbaum.

Pinker, S. (1994). *The language instinct: How the mind creates language.* New York, NY: Harper Perennial.

Plomin, R., Fulker, D. W., Corley, R., & DeFries, J. C. (1997). Nature, nurture, and cognitive development from 1 to 16 years: A parent-offspring adoption study. *Psychological Science, 8*, 442–447.

Plomin, R., Haworth, C., Meaburn, E., Price, T. S., et al. (2013). Common DNA markers can account for more than half of the genetic influence on cognitive abilities. *Psychological Science, 24*, 562–568.

Plomin, R., & Spinath, F. M. (2004). Intelligence: Genetics, genes, and genomics. *Journal of Personality and Social Psychology, 86*, 112–129.

Poeppel, D., & Hickok, G. (2004). Towards a new functional anatomy of language. *Cognition, 92*, 1–12.

Polk, T., & Newell, A. (1995). Deduction as verbal reasoning. *Psychological Review, 102*, 533–566.

Poole, D. A., & Lindsay, D. S. (2001). Children's eyewitness reports after exposure to misinformation from parents. *Journal of Experimental Psychology: Applied, 7*, 27–50.

Popper, K. (1934). *The logic of scientific discovery.* London, England: Routledge.

Porter, S., & Peace, K. A. (2007). The scars of memory: A prospective, longitudinal investigation of the consistency of traumatic and positive emotional memories in adulthood. *Psychological Science, 18*(5), 435–441.

Posner, M., & Rothbart, M., (2007). Research on attention networks as a model for the integration of psychological science. *Annual Review of Psychology, 58*, 1–23.

Posner, M., & Snyder, C. (1975). Facilitation and inhibition in the processing of signals. In P. Rabbitt & S. Dornic (Eds.), *Attention and performance V* (pp. 669–682). New York, NY: Academic Press.

Posner, M., Snyder, C., & Davidson, B. (1980). Attention and the detection of signals. *Journal of Experimental Psychology: General, 109*, 160–174.

Postman, L., & Phillips, L. W. (1965). Short-term temporal changes in free recall. *Quarterly Journal of Experimental Psychology, 17*, 132–138.

Pretz, J. (2008). Intuition versus analysis: Strategy and experience in complex everyday problem solving. *Memory & Cognition, 36*, 554–566.

Protzko, J., Aronson, J., & Blair, C. (2012). How to make a young child smarter: Evidence from the Database of Raising Intelligence. *Perspective on Psychological Science, 8*, 25–40.

Pylyshyn, Z. (1981). The imagery debate: Analogue media versus tacit knowledge. In N. Block (Ed.), *Imagery* (pp. 151–206). Cambridge, MA: MIT Press.

Quinlan, P. T. (2003). Visual feature integration theory: Past, present and future. *Psychological Bulletin, 129*, 643–673.

Radel, R., Davaranche, K., Fournier, M., & Dietrich, A. (2015). The role of (dis)inhibition in creativity: Decreased inhibition improves idea generation. *Cognition, 134*, 110–120.

Radoeva, P. D., Prasad, S., Brainard, D. H., & Aguirre, G. K. (2008). Neural activity within area V1 reflects unconscious visual performance in a case of blindsight. *Journal of Cognitive Neuroscience, 20*(11), 1927–1939.

Rae, C., Digney, A. L., McEwan, S. R., & Bates, T. C. (2003). Oral creatine monohydrate supplementation improves brain performance: A double-blind, placebo-controlled, cross-over trial. *Proceedings of the Royal Society of London, Series B: Biological Sciences, 270*, 2147–2150.

Raghubir, P., & Menon, G. (2005). When and why is ease of retrieval informative? *Memory & Cognition, 33*, 821–832.

Raizada, R., & Kishiyama, M. (2010). Effects of socioeconomic status on brain development. *Frontiers in Human Neuroscience, 5*, 1–18.

Rakover, S. (2013). Explaining the face-inversion effect: The face-scheme incompatibility (FSI) model. *Psychonomic Bulletin & Review, 20*, 665–692.

Ramachandran, V. S., & Blakeslee, S. (1998). *Phantoms in the brain.* New York, NY: Morrow.

Ramsden, S., Richdson, F., Josse, G., Thomas, M., Ellis, C., Shakeshaft, C., Seghier, M., & Price, C. (2011). Verbal and nonverbal intelligence changes in the teenage brain. *Nature, 479*, 113–116.

Ranganath, C., & Blumenfeld, R. S. (2005). Doubts about double dissociations between short- and long-term memory. *Trends in Cognitive Sciences, 9*, 374–380.

Ranganath, C., Yonelinas, A. P., Cohen, M. X., Dy, C. J., Tom, S., & D'Esposito, M. (2003). Dissociable correlates for familiarity and recollection within the medial temporal lobes. *Neuropsychologia, 42*, 2–13.

Rao, G. A., Larkin, E. C., & Derr, R. F. (1986). Biologic effects of chronic ethanol consumption related to a deficient intake of carbohydrates. *Alcohol and Alcoholism, 21*, 369–373.

Rathbone, C. J., Moulin, C. J. A., & Conway, M. A. (2008). Self-centered memories: The reminiscence bump and the self. *Memory & Cognition, 36*, 1403–1414.

Raven, J., & Raven, J. (Eds.). (2008). *Uses and abuses of intelligence: Studies advancing Spearman and Raven's quest for non-arbitrary metrics.* Unionville, NY: Royal Fireworks Tests.

Ravenzwaaij, D. V., Brown, S., & Wagenmakers, E.-J. (2011). An integrated perspective on the relation between response speed and intelligence. *Cognition, 119*, 381–393.

Rayner, K., & Pollatsek, A. (2011). Basic processes in reading. In D. Reisberg (Ed.), *Handbook of cognitive psychology.* New York, NY: Oxford University Press.

Reason, J. T. (1990). *Human error.* Cambridge, England: Cambridge University Press.

Redelmeier, D., & Shafir, E. (1995). Medical decision making in situations that offer multiple alternatives. *Journal of the American Medical Association, 273*(4), 302–305.

Redelmeier, D., & Tversky, A. (1996). On the belief that arthritis pain is related to the weather. *Proceedings of the National Academic of Sciences, USA, 93*, 2895–2896.

Redick, T. S., Shipstead, Z., Harrison, T. L., Hicks, K. L., Fried, D. E., Hambrich, D. Z., Kane, M. J., & Engle, R. W. (2013). No evidence of intelligence improvement after working memory training: A randomized, placebo-controlled study. *Journal of Experimental Psychology: General, 142*, 359–379.

Reed, S. (1993). Imagery and discovery. In B. Roskos-Ewoldsen, M. J. Intons-Peterson, & R. Anderson (Eds.), *Imagery, creativity, and discovery: A cognitive perspective* (pp. 287–312). New York, NY: North-Holland.

Rees, G., Kreiman, G., & Koch, C. (2002). Neural correlates of consciousness in humans. *Nature Reviews Neuroscience, 3*, 261–270.

Rehder, B., & Hastie, R. (2004). Category coherence and category-based property induction. *Cognition, 91*, 113–153.

Rehder, B., & Ross, B. H. (2001). Abstract coherent categories. *Journal of Experimental Psychology: Learning, Memory, & Cognition, 27*, 1261–1275.

Reicher, G. M. (1969). Perceptual recognition as a function of meaningfulness of stimulus material. *Journal of Experimental Psychology, 81*, 275–280.

Reisberg, D. (1996). The non-ambiguity of mental images. In C. Cornold, R. H. Logie, M. Brandimonte, G. Kaufmann, & D. Reisberg (Eds.), *Stretching the imagination: Representation and transformation in mental imagery* (pp. 119–171). New York, NY: Oxford University Press.

Reisberg, D. (2000). The detachment gain: The advantage of thinking out loud. In B. Landau, J. Sabini, E. Newport, & J. Jonides (Eds.), *Perception, cognition and language: Essays in honor of Henry and Lila Gleitman* (pp. 139–156). Cambridge, MA: MIT Press.

Reisberg, D. (2014). *The science of perception and memory: A pragmatic guide for the justice system.* New York, NY: Oxford University Press.

Reisberg, D., & Heuer, F. (2004). Memory for emotional events. In D. Reisberg & P. Hertel (Eds.), *Memory and emotion* (pp. 3–41). New York, NY: Oxford University Press.

Rensink, R. A. (2002). Change detection. *Annual Review of Psychology, 53*, 245–277.

Rensink, R. A. (2012). Perception and attention. In D. Reisberg (Ed.), *Handbook of cognitive psychology.* New York, NY: Oxford University Press.

Rensink, R. A., O'Regan, J. K., & Clark, J. J. (1997). To see or not to see: The need for attention to perceive changes in scenes. *Psychological Science, 8*, 368–373.

Repovš, G., & Baddeley, A. (2006). The multicomponent model of working memory: Explorations in experimental cognitive psychology. *Neuroscience, 139*, 5–21.

Repp, B. (1992). Perceptual restoration of a "missing" speech sound: Auditory induction or illusion? *Perception & Psychophysics, 51*, 14–32.

Reynolds, C. R., Chastain, R. L., Kaufman, A. S., & McLean, J. E. (1987). Demographic characteristics and IQ among adults: Analysis of the WAIS-R standardization sample as a function of the stratification variables. *Journal of School Psychology, 25*(4), 323–342.

Reynolds, J. H., Pasternak, T., & Desimone, R. (2000). Attention increases sensitivity of V4 neurons. *Neuron, 26,* 703–714.

Rhodes, G. (2012). Face recognition. In D. Reisberg (Ed.), *Handbook of cognitive psychology.* New York, NY: Oxford University Press.

Rhodes, G., Brake, S., & Atkinson, A. (1993). What's lost in inverted faces? *Cognition, 47,* 25–57.

Riccio, D. C., Millin, P. M., & Gisquet-Verrier, P. (2003). Retrograde amnesia: Forgetting back. *Current Directions in Psychological Science, 12,* 41–44.

Richard, A. M., Lee, H., & Vecera, S. P. (2008). Attentional spreading in object-based attention. *Journal of Experimental Psychology: Human Perception & Performance, 34,* 842–853.

Richardson, J. (1980). *Mental imagery and human memory.* New York, NY: St. Martin's Press.

Richler, J. J., & Gauthier, I. (2014). A meta-analysis and review of holistic face processing. *Psychological Bulletin, 140,* 1281–1302.

Riesenhuber, M., & Poggio, T. (1999). Hierarchical models of object recognition in cortex. *Nature Neuroscience, 2,* 1019–1025.

Riesenhuber, M., & Poggio, T. (2002). Neural mechanisms of object recognition. *Current Opinion in Neurobiology, 12,* 162–168.

Rinck, M. (1999). Memory for everyday objects: Where are the digits on numerical keypads? *Applied Cognitive Psychology, 13,* 329–350.

Rips, L. (1975). Inductive judgements about natural categories. *Journal of Verbal Learning and Verbal Behavior, 14,* 665–681.

Rips, L. (1990). Reasoning. *Annual Review of Psychology, 41,* 321–353.

Rips, L. J., Smith, E. E., & Medin, D. L. (2012). Concepts and categories: Memory, meaning, and metaphysics. In K. J. Holyoak & R. G. Morrison (Eds.), *The Oxford handbook of thinking and reasoning* (pp. 177–209). New York, NY: Oxford University Press.

Ritchie, J. M. (1985). The aliphatic alcohols. In A. G. Gilman, L. S. Goodman, T. W. Rall, & F. Murad (Eds.), *The pharmacological basis of therapeutics* (pp. 372–386). New York, NY: Macmillan.

Rizzi, T., & Posthuma, D. (2012). Genes and intelligence. In D. Reisberg (Ed.), *The Oxford handbook of cognitive psychology.* New York, NY: Oxford University Press.

Roberson, D., Davies, I., & Davidoff, J. (2000). Color categories are not universal: Replications and new evidence from a stone-age culture. *Journal of Experimental Psychology: General, 129,* 369–398.

Robertson, L., Treisman, A., Friedman-Hill, S., & Grabowecky, M. (1997). The interaction of spatial and object pathways: Evidence from Balint's syndrome. *Journal of Cognitive Neuroscience, 9,* 295–317.

Roediger, H. L. (1980). The effectiveness of four mnemonics in ordering recall. *Journal of Experimental Psychology: Human Learning and Memory, 6,* 558–567.

Roediger, H. L., & McDermott, K. (1995). Creating false memories: Remembering words not presented in lists. *Journal of Experimental Psychology: Learning, Memory, & Cognition, 21,* 803–814.

Roediger, H. L., & McDermott, K. (2000). Tricks of memory. *Current Directions in Psychological Science, 9,* 123–127.

Rogers, T. T., & McClelland, J. L. (2014). Parallel distributed processing at 25: Further explorations in the microstructure of cognition. *Cognitive Science, 6,* 1024–1077.

Rogers, T. T., & Patterson, K. (2007). Object categorization: Reversals and explanations of the basic-level advantage. *Journal of Experimental Psychology: General, 136,* 451–469.

Roid, G. (2003). *Stanford-Binet Fifth Edition.* Itasca, IL: Riverside.

Rosch, E. (1973). On the internal structure of perceptual and semantic categories. In T. E. Moore (Ed.), *Cognitive development and the acquisition of language* (pp. 111–144). New York, NY: Academic Press.

Rosch, E. (1975). Cognitive representations of semantic categories. *Journal of Experimental Psychology: General, 104,* 192–233.

Rosch, E. (1978). Principles of categorization. In E. Rosch & B. B. Lloyd (Eds.), *Cognition and categorization* (pp. 27–48). Hillsdale, NJ: Erlbaum.

Rosch, E., & Mervis, C. B. (1975). Family resemblances: Studies in the internal structure of categories. *Cognitive Psychology, 7,* 573–605.

Rosch, E., Mervis, C. B., Gray, W., Johnson, D., & Boyes-Braem, P. (1976). Basic objects in natural categories. *Cognitive Psychology, 3,* 382–439.

Roser, M., & Gazzaniga, M. S. (2004). Automatic brains—Interpretive minds. *Current Directions in Psychological Science, 13,* 56–59.

Ross, B. (1984). Remindings and their effects in learning a cognitive skill. *Cognitive Psychology, 16,* 371–416.

Ross, B. (1987). This is like that: The use of earlier problems and the separation and similarity effects. *Journal of Experimental Psychology: Learning, Memory, & Cognition, 13,* 629–639.

Ross, B. (1989). Distinguishing types of superficial similarities: Different effects on the access and use of earlier problems. *Journal of Experimental Psychology: Learning, Memory, & Cognition, 15,* 456–468.

Ross, J., & Lawrence, K. A. (1968). Some observations on memory artifice. *Psychonomic Science, 13*, 107–108.

Ross, L., & Anderson, C. (1982). Shortcomings in the attribution process: On the origins and maintenance of erroneous social assessments. In D. Kahneman, P. Slovic, & A. Tversky (Eds.), *Judgment under uncertainty: Heuristics and biases* (pp. 129–152). New York, NY: Cambridge University Press.

Ross, L., Lepper, M., & Hubbard, M. (1975). Perseverance in self perception and social perception: Biased attributional processes in the debriefing paradigm. *Journal of Personality and Social Psychology, 32*, 880–892.

Ross, M., & Wilson, A. E. (2003). Autobiographical memory and conceptions of self: Getting better all the time. *Current Directions in Psychological Science, 12*, 66–69.

Rouder, J. N., & Ratcliff, R. (2006). Comparing exemplar- and rule-based theories of categorization. *Current Directions in Psychological Science, 5*, 9–13.

Rowland, C. A. (2014). The effect of testing versus restudy on retention: A meta-analytic review of the testing effect. *Psychological Bulletin, 140*, 1432–1463.

Rubin, D. C., & Kontis, T. S. (1983). A schema for common cents. *Memory & Cognition, 11*, 335–341.

Rubin, D. C., & Kozin, M. (1984). Vivid memories. *Cognition, 16*, 81–95.

Rubin, D., C. & Talarico, J. (2007). Flashbulb memories are special after all; in phenomology, not accuracy. *Applied Cognitive Psychology, 21*, 557–558.

Rubin, E. (1915). *Synoplevede figuren.* Copenhagen, Denmark: Gyldendalske.

Rubin, E. (1921). *Visuell wahrgenommene figuren.* Copenhagen, Denmark: Gyldendalske.

Rueckl, J. G., & Oden, G. C. (1986). The integration of contextual and featural information during word identification. *Journal of Memory and Language, 25*, 445–460.

Rugg, M. D., & Curran, T. (2007). Event-related potentials and recognition memory. *Trends in Cognitive Sciences, 11*, 251–257.

Rugg, M. D., & Yonelinas, A. P. (2003). Human recognition memory: A cognitive neuroscience perspective. *Trends in Cognitive Sciences, 7*, 313–319.

Rumelhart, D. E., & Siple, P. (1974). Process of recognizing tachistoscopically presented words. *Psychological Review, 81*, 99–118.

Rundus, D. (1971). Analysis of rehearsal processes in free recall. *Journal of Experimental Psychology, 89*, 63–77.

Rushton, J. P., & Jensen, A. R. (2005). Thirty years of research on race differences in cognitive ability. *Psychology, Public Policy, and Law, 11*, 235–294.

Russell, R., Duchaine, B., & Nakayama, K. (2009). Super-recognizers: People with extraordinary face recognition ability. *Psychonomic Bulletin and Review, 16*, 252–257.

Ruthruff, E., Johnston, J. C., & Remington, R. W. (2009). How strategic is the central bottleneck: Can it be overcome by trying harder? *Journal of Experimental Psychology: Human Perception & Performance, 35*, 1368–1384.

Saalmann, Y., Pigarev, I., & Vidyasagar, T. (2007). Neural mechanisms of visual attention: How top-down feedback highlights relevant locations. *Science, 316*, 1612–1615.

Sackett, P., Borneman, M., & Connelly, B. (2008). High-stakes testing in higher education and employment: Appraising the evidence for validity and fairness. *American Psychologist, 63*, 215–227.

Sacks, O. (1985). *The man who mistook his wife for a hat and other clinical tales.* New York, NY: Harper & Row.

Saffran, J. R. (2003). Statistical language learning: Mechanisms and constraints. *Current Directions in Psychological Science, 12*, 110–114.

Saj, A., Fuhrman, O., Vuilleumier, P., & Boroditsky, L. (2014). Patients with left spatial neglect also neglect the "left side" of time. *Psychological Science, 25*, 207–214.

Salazar, R. F., Dotson, N. M., Bressler, S. L., & Gray, C. M. (2012). Content-specific fronto-parietal synchronization during visual working memory. *Science, 338*, 1097–1100.

Salthouse, T. A. (2004). What and when of cognitive aging. *Current Directions in Psychological Science, 13*, 140–144.

Salthouse, T. A. (2012). Consequences of age-related cognitive declines. *Annual Review of Psychology, 63*, 201–226.

Salthouse, T., & Pink, J. (2008). Why is working memory related to fluid intelligence? *Psychonomic Bulletin & Review, 15*, 364–371.

Sampaio, C., & Brewer, W. (2009). The role of unconscious memory errors in judgments of confidence for sentence recognition. *Memory & Cognition, 37*, 158–163.

Samuel, A. G. (1987). Lexical uniqueness effects on phonemic restoration. *Journal of Memory and Language, 26*, 36–56.

Samuel, A. G. (1991). A further examination of attentional effects in the phonemic restoration illusion. *Quarterly Journal of Experimental Psychology: Human Experimental Psychology, 43*, 679–699.

Savage-Rumbaugh, E. S., & Fields, W. (2000). Linguistic, cultural and cognitive capacities of bonobos (*Pan paniscus*). *Culture & Psychology, 6*, 131–153.

Savage-Rumbaugh, S., & Lewin, R. (1994). *Kanzi, the ape at the brink of the human mind.* New York, NY: Wiley.

Savova, V., Roy, D., Schmidt, L., & Tenenbaum, J. (2007). Discovering syntactic hierarchies. Proceedings of the Twenty-Ninth Annual Conference of the Cognitive Science Society, Nashville, TN.

Sawyer, R. K. (2006). *Explaining creativity: The science of human innovation*. New York, NY: Oxford University Press.

Schab, F. (1990). Odors and the remembrance of things past. *Journal of Experimental Psychology: Learning, Memory, & Cognition, 16*, 648–655.

Schacter, D. (1996). *Searching for memory: The brain, the mind, and the past*. New York, NY: Basic Books.

Schacter, D., Guerin, S., & St. Jacques, P. (2011). Memory distortion: an adaptive perspective. *Trends in Cognitive Sciences, 15*, 467–474.

Schacter, D., & Tulving, E. (1982). Amnesia and memory research. In L. S. Cermak (Ed.), *Human memory and amnesia* (pp. 1–32). Hillsdale, NJ: Erlbaum.

Schacter, D., Tulving, E., & Wang, P. (1981). *Source amnesia: New methods and illustrative data*. Paper presented at the meeting of the International Neuropsychological Society, Atlanta, GA.

Schenk, T., Ellison, A., Rice, N., & Milner, A. D. (2005). The role of V5/MT+ in the control of catching movements: An rTMS study. *Neuropsychologia, 43*, 189–198.

Schlegel, A., Kohler, P. J., Fogelson, S. V., Alexander, P., Konuthula, D., & Tse, P. U. (2013). Network structure and dynamics of the mental workspace. *Proceeds of the National Academy of Sciences, USA, 110*, 16277–16282.

Schmidt, F. L., & Hunter, E. (1998). The validity and utility of selection methods in personnel psychology: Practical and theoretical implications of 85 years of research findings. *Psychological Bulletin, 124*, 262–274.

Schmidt, F. L., & Hunter, E. (2004). General mental ability in the world of work: Occupational attainment and job performance. *Journal of Personality and Social Psychology, 86*, 162–173.

Schmidt, S. R. (2012). *Extraordinary memories for exceptional events*. New York, NY: Taylor & Francis.

Schneider, S. (1992). Framing and conflict: Aspiration level contingency, the status quo, and current theories of risky choice. *Journal of Experimental Psychology: Learning, Memory, & Cognition, 18*, 1040–1057.

Schraw, G., Dunkle, M., & Bendixen, L. (1995). Cognitive processes in well-defined and ill-defined problem solving. *Applied Cognitive Psychology, 9*, 523–538.

Schulz-Hardt, S., Frey, D., Lüthgens, C., & Moscovici, S. (2000). Biased information search in group decision making. *Journal of Personality and Social Psychology, 78*, 655–669.

Schunn, C. D., & Anderson, J. R. (1999). The generality/specificity of expertise in scientific reasoning. *Cognitive Science, 23*, 337–370.

Schustack, M., & Sternberg, R. (1981). Evaluation of evidence in causal inference. *Journal of Experimental Psychology: General, 110*, 101–120.

Schwartz, B. (2003). *The paradox of choice*. New York, NY: Ecco.

Schwartz, B. L., & Metcalfe, J. (2011). Tip-of-the-tongue (TOT) states: Retrieval, behavior, and experience. *Memory & Cognition 39*, 737–749.

Schwartz, J., Chapman, G., & Brewer, N. (2004). The effects of accountability on bias in physician decision making: Going from bad to worse. *Psychonomic Bulletin & Review, 11*, 173–178.

Schwarz, N. (1998). Accessible content and accessibility experiences: The interplay of declarative and experiential information in judgments. *Personality and Social Psychology Review, 2*, 87–99.

Schwarz, N. (1999). Self-reports: How the questions shape the answers. *American Psychologist, 54*, 93–105.

Schwarz, N., Bless, H., Strack, F., Klumpp, G., Rittenauer-Schatka, H., & Simons, A. (1991). Ease of retrieval as information: Another look at the availability heuristic. *Journal of Personality & Social Psychology, 61*, 195–202.

Scoboria, A., Mazzoni, G., Kirsch, I., & Jimenez, S. (2006). The effects of prevalence and script information on plausibility, belief, and memory of autobiographical events. *Applied Cognitive Psychology, 20*, 1049–1064.

Seamon, J. G., Philbin, M. M., & Harrison, L. G. (2006). Do you remember proposing marriage to the Pepsi machine? False recollections from a campus walk. *Psychonomic Bulletin & Review, 13*, 752–755.

Sedivy, J. C., Tanenhaus, M. K., Chambers, C. G., & Carlson, G. N. (1999). Achieving incremental semantic interpretation through contextual representation. *Cognition, 71*, 109–147.

Seegmiller, J. K., Watson, J. M., & Strayer, D. L. (2011). Individual differences in susceptibility to inattentional blindness. *Journal of Experimental Psychology: Learning, Memory, & Cognition, 37*, 785–791.

Segal, E. (2004). Incubation in insight problem solving. *Creative Research Journal, 16*, 141–148.

Segal, S., & Fusella, V. (1970). Influence of imaged pictures and sounds in detection of visual and auditory signals. *Journal of Experimental Psychology, 83*, 458–474.

Segal, S., & Fusella, V. (1971). Effect of images in six sense modalities on detection of visual signal from noise. *Psychonomic Science, 24*, 55–56.

Selfridge, O. (1955). *Pattern recognition and modern computers*. Proceedings of the Western Joint Computer Conference, Los Angeles, CA.

Selfridge, O. (1959). Pandemonium: A paradigm for learning. In D. Blake & A. Uttley (Eds.), *The mechanisation of thought processes: Proceedings of a symposium held at the National Physics Laboratory* (pp. 511–529). London, England: H. M. Stationery Office.

Seltzer, B., & Benson, D. F. (1974). The temporal pattern of retrograde amnesia in Korsakoff's Disease. *Neurology, 24*, 527–530.

Semmler, C., & Brewer, N. (2006). Postidentification feedback effects on face recognition confidence: Evidence for metacognitive influences. *Applied Cognitive Psychology, 20,* 895–916.

Senghas, A., Román, D., & Mavillapalli, S. (2006). *Simply unique.* London: Leonard Cheshire International.

Servos, P., & Goodale, M. A. (1995). Preserved visual imagery in visual form agnosia. *Neuropsychologia, 33,* 1383–1394.

Sevdalis, N., & Harvey, N. (2007). Biased forecasting of postdecisional affect. *Psychological Science, 18,* 678–681.

Shafir, E. (1993). Choosing versus rejecting: Why some options are both better and worse than others. *Memory & Cognition, 21,* 546–556.

Shafir, E., & LeBoeuf, R. A. (2002). Rationality. *Annual Review of Psychology, 53,* 491–517.

Shaklee, H., & Mims, M. (1982). Sources of error in judging event covariations. *Journal of Experimental Psychology: Learning, Memory, & Cognition, 8,* 208–224.

Sharman, S. J., & Barnier, A. J. (2008). Imagining nice and nasty events in the distant or recent past: Recent positive events show the most imagination inflation. *Acta Psychologica, 129,* 228–233.

Sharman, S. J., Manning, C., & Garry, M. (2005). Explain this: Explaining childhood events inflates confidence for those events. *Applied Cognitive Psychology, 19,* 67–74.

Shepard, R. N. (1988). The imagination of the scientist. In K. Egan & D. Nadaner (Eds.), *Imagination and education* (pp. 153–185). New York, NY: Teachers College Press.

Shepard, R. N., & Cooper, L. A. (1982). *Mental images and their transformations.* Cambridge, MA: MIT Press.

Shepard, R. N., & Metzler, J. (1971). Mental rotation of three-dimensional objects. *Science, 171,* 701–703.

Sheppard, L. D. (2008). Intelligence and speed information-processing: A review of 50 years of research. *Personality and Individual Differences, 44,* 535–551.

Shidlovski, D., Schul, Y., & Mayo, R. (2014). If I imagine it, then it happened: The implicit truth value of imaginary representations. *Cognition, 133,* 517–529.

Shiffrin, R. M., & Schneider, W. (1977). Controlled and automatic human information processing: II. Perceptual learning, automatic attending, and a general theory. *Psychological Review, 84,* 127–190.

Shin, H., & Kominski, R. (2010). *Language use in the United States, 2007.* Washington, DC: U.S. Dept. of Commerce Economics and Statistics Administration, U.S. Census Bureau.

Shore, D. I., & Klein, R. M. (2000). The effects of scene inversion on change blindness. *Journal of General Psychology, 127,* 27–43.

Sieroff, E., Pollatsek, A., & Posner, M. I. (1988). Recognition of visual letter strings following injury to the posterior visual spatial attention system. *Cognitive Neuropsychology, 5,* 427–450.

Silbersweig, D. A., Stern, E., Frith, C., Cahill, C., Holmes, A., Grootoonk, S., et al. (1995). A functional neuro-anatomy of hallucinations in schizophrenia. *Nature, 378,* 176–179.

Simon, H. (1973). The structure of ill-defined problems. *Artificial Intelligence, 4,* 181–201.

Simons, D. J., & Ambinder, M. S. (2005). Change blindness: Theory and consequences. *Current Directions in Psychological Science, 14,* 44–48.

Simons, D. J., & Chabris, C. F. (1999). Gorillas in our midst: Sustained inattentional blindness for dynamic events. *Perception, 28,* 1059–1074.

Simons, D. J., & Rensink, R. A. (2005). Change blindness: Past, present, and future. *Trends in Cognitive Sciences, 9,* 1–20.

Simonton, D. K. (2003). Scientific creativity as constrained stochastic behavior: The integration of product, person, and process perspectives. *Psychological Bulletin, 129,* 475–494.

Simonton, D. K. (2009). Creativity as a Darwinian phenomenon: The blind-variation and selective-retention model. In M. Krausz, D. Dutton, & K. Bardsley (Eds.), *The idea of creativity* (2nd ed., pp. 63–81). Leiden, Netherlands: Brill.

Simonton, D. K. (2011). Creativity and discovery as blind variation: Campbell's (1960) BVSR model after the half-century mark. *Review of General Psychology, 15,* 158–174.

Simonton, D. K., & Damian, R. D. (2012). Creativity. In D. Reisberg (Ed.), *The Oxford handbook of cognitive psychology.* New York, NY: Oxford University Press.

Sio, U. N., & Ormerod, T. C. (2009). Does incubation enhance problem solving? A meta-analytic review. *Psychological Bulletin, 135,* 94–120.

Skotko, B. G., Kensinger, E. A., Locascio, J. J., Einstein, G., Rubin, D. C., Tupler, L. A., et al. (2004). Puzzling thoughts for H.M.: Can new semantic information be anchored to old semantic memories? *Neuropsychology, 18*(4), 756–769.

Skotko, B. G., Rubin, D., & Tupler, L. (2008). H.M.'s personal crossword puzzles. *Memory, 16,* 89–96.

Slamecka, N. J., & Graf, P. (1978). The generation effect: Delineation of a phenomenon. *Journal of Experimental Psychology: Human Learning and Memory, 4,* 592–604.

Slobin, D. (1966). Grammatical transformations and sentence comprehension in childhood and adulthood. *Journal of Verbal Learning and Verbal Behavior, 5,* 219–227.

Slovic, P., Finucane, M., Peters, E., & MacGregor, D. G. (2002). The affect heuristic. In T. Gilovich, D. Griffin, & D. Kahneman (Eds.), *Heuristics and biases* (pp. 397–420). New York, NY: Cambridge University Press.

Slovic, P., & Peters, E. (2010). Risk perception and affect. *Current Directions in Psychological Science, 15,* 322–325.

Smedslund, J. (1963). The concept of correlation in adults. *Scandinavian Journal of Psychology, 4,* 165–173.

Smeets, T., Jelicic, M., Peters, M. J. V., Candel, I., Horselenberg, R., & Merckelbach, H. (2006). "Of course I remember seeing that film"—How ambiguous questions generate crashing memories. *Applied Cognitive Psychology, 20,* 779–789.

Smith, E. E., Rips, L. J., & Shoben, E. J. (1974). Structure and process in semantic memory: A featural model for semantic decisions. *Psychological Review, 81,* 214–241.

Smith, E. R., & Miller, F. (1978). Limits on perception of cognitive processes: A reply to Nisbett & Wilson. *Psychological Review, 85,* 355–362.

Smith, J. D. (2002). Exemplar theory's predicted typicality gradient can be tested and disconfirmed. *Psychological Science, 13,* 437–442.

Smith, J. D. (2014). Prototypes, exemplars, and the natural history of categorization. *Psychonomic Bulletin & Review, 21,* 312–331.

Smith, K. A., Huber, D. E., & Vul, E. (2013). Multiply constrained semantic search in the Remote Associates Test. *Cognition, 128,* 64–75.

Smith, S. M. (1979). Remembering in and out of context. *Journal of Experimental Psychology: Human Learning and Memory, 5,* 460–471.

Smith, S. M. (1985). Background music and context-dependent memory. *American Journal of Psychology, 6,* 591–603.

Smith, S. M., & Blankenship, S. E. (1989). Incubation effects. *Bulletin of the Psychonomic Society, 27,* 311–314.

Smith, S. M., & Blankenship, S. E. (1991). Incubation and the persistence of fixation in problem solving. *American Journal of Psychology, 104,* 61–87.

Smith, S. M., Glenberg, A., & Bjork, R. A. (1978). Environmental context and human memory. *Memory & Cognition, 6,* 342–353.

Smith, S. M., & Vela, E. (2001). Environmental context-dependent memory: A review and meta-analysis. *Psychonomic Bulletin & Review, 8,* 203–220.

Smith, S. M., & Ward, T. B. (2012). Cognition and the creation of ideas. In K. J. Holyoak & R. G. Morrison (Eds.), *The Oxford handbook of thinking and reasoning* (pp. 456–474). New York, NY: Oxford University Press.

Snow, R. E. (1994). Abilities in academic tasks. In R. J. Sternberg & R. K. Wagner (Eds.), *Mind in context: Interactionist perspectives on human intelligence* (pp. 3–37). Cambridge, England: Cambridge University Press.

Snow, R. E. (1996). Aptitude development and education. *Psychology, Public Policy, and Law, 2,* 536–560.

Soto, D., & Silvanto, J. (2014). Reappraising the relationship between working memory and conscious awareness. *Trends in Cognitive Sciences, 18,* 520–525.

Spearman, C. (1904). "General intelligence," objectively determined and measured. *American Journal of Psychology, 15,* 201–293.

Spearman, C. (1927). *The abilities of man.* New York, NY: Macmillan.

Speekenbrink, M., & Shanks, D. (2012). Decision making. In D. Reisberg (Ed.), *The Oxford handbook of cognitive psychology.* New York, NY: Oxford University Press.

Spelke, E., Hirst, W., & Neisser, U. (1976). Skills of divided attention. *Cognition, 4,* 215–230.

Spellman, B. A., Holyoak, K. J., & Morrison, R. G. (2001). Analogical priming via semantic relations. *Memory & Cognition, 29,* 383–393.

Sperber, D., Cara, F., & Girotto, V. (1995). Relevance theory explains the selection task. *Cognition, 57,* 31–95.

Spiegel, D. (1995). Hypnosis and suggestion. In D. L. Schacter, J. T. Coyle, G. D. Fischbach, M.-M. Mesulam, & L. E. Sullivan (Eds.), *Memory distortion: How minds, brains and societies reconstruct the past* (pp. 129–149). Cambridge, MA: Harvard University Press.

Sporer, S. (1988). Long-term improvement of facial recognition through visual rehearsal. In M. Gruneberg, P. Morris, & R. Sykes (Eds.), *Practical aspects of memory: Current research and issues* (pp. 182–188). New York, NY: Wiley.

Sporer, S., Penrod, S., Read, D., & Cutler, B. (1995). Choosing, confidence, and accuracy: A meta-analysis of the confidence-accuracy relation in eyewitness identification studies. *Psychological Bulletin, 118,* 315–327.

Squire, L., & McKee, R. (1993). Declarative and nondeclarative memory in opposition: When prior events influence amnesic patients more than normal subjects. *Memory & Cognition, 21,* 424–430.

Stangor, C., & McMillan, D. (1992). Memory for expectancy-congruent and expectancy-incongruent information: A review of the social and social developmental literatures. *Psychological Bulletin, 111,* 42–61.

Stanovich, K. E. (2009). *What intelligence tests miss: The psychology of rational thought.* New Haven, CT: Yale University Press.

Stanovich, K. E. (2012). On the distinction between rationality and intelligence: Implications for understanding individual differences in reasoning. In K. J. Holyoak & R. G. Morrison (Eds.), *The Oxford handbook of thinking and reasoning* (pp. 433–455). New York, NY: Oxford University Press.

Stanovich, K. E., & West, R. F. (2000). Individual differences in reasoning: Implications for the rationality debate. *Behavioral and Brain Sciences, 23,* 645–665.

Stanovich, K. E., West, R. F., & Toplak, M. E. (2013). Myside bias, rational thinking, and intelligence.

Current Directions in Psychological Science, 22, 259–264.

Stapel, D., & Semin, G. (2007). The magic spell of language: Linguistic categories and their perceptual consequences. *Journal of Personality and Social Psychology, 93,* 23–33.

Steblay, N. J. (1992). A meta-analytic review of the weapon focus effect. *Law and Human Behavior, 16,* 413–424.

Steele, C. (2010). *Whistling Vivaldi: And other clues to how stereotypes affect us.* New York, NY: Norton.

Steele, C. M., & Aronson, J. (1995). Stereotype threat and the intellectual test performance of African Americans. *Journal of Personality and Social Psychology, 69(5),* 797–811.

Sternberg, R. J., & Grigorenko, E. L. (2004). Successful intelligence in the classroom. *Theory into Practice, 43,* 274–280.

Sternberg, R. J., Kaufman, J. C., & Grigorenko, E. L. (2008). *Applied intelligence.* New York, NY: Cambridge University Press.

Stevens, A., & Coupe, P. (1978). Distortions in judged spatial relations. *Cognitive Psychology, 10,* 422–437.

Storm, B., Angello, G., & Bjork, E. (2011). Thinking can cause forgetting: Memory dynamics in creative problem solving. *Journal of Experimental Psychology: Learning, Memory, & Cognition, 37,* 1287–1293.

Storm, B. C., & Patel, T. N. (2014). Forgetting as a consequence and enabler of creative thinking. *Journal of Experimental Psychology: Learning, Memory & Cognition, 40,* 1594–1609.

Strayer, D. L., & Drews, F. A. (2007). Cell phone–induced driver distraction. *Current Directions in Psychological Science, 16,* 128–131.

Strayer, D. L., Drews, F. A., & Johnston, W. A. (2003). Cell phone–induced failures of visual attention during simulated driving. *Journal of Experimental Psychology: Applied, 9,* 23–32.

Strayer, D. L., & Johnston, W. A. (2001). Driven to distraction: Dual-task studies of simulated driving and conversing on a cellular phone. *Psychological Science, 12,* 462–466.

Strenze, T. (2007). Intelligence and socioeconomic success: A meta-analytic review of longitudinal research. *Intelligence, 35,* 401–426.

Stromeyer, C. (1982). *An adult eidetiker.* In U. Neisser (Ed.), *Memory observed* (pp. 399–404). New York, NY: Freeman.

Stroop, J. R. (1935). Studies of interference in serial verbal reaction. *Journal of Experimental Psychology, 18,* 643–662.

Stuss, D. T., & Alexander, M. P. (2007). Is there a dysexecutive syndrome? *Philosophical Transactions of the Royal Society of London, Series B, Biological Sciences, 362,* 901–915.

Stuss, D. T., & Levine, B. (2002). Adult clinical neuropsychology: Lessons from studies of the frontal lobes. *Annual Review of Psychology, 53,* 401–433.

Sulin, R. A., & Dooling, D. J. (1974). Intrusion of a thematic idea in retention of prose. *Journal of Experimental Psychology, 103,* 255–262.

Sumby, W. H. (1963). Word frequency and serial position effects. *Journal of Verbal Learning and Verbal Behavior, 1,* 443–450.

Sundet, J., Eriksen, W., & Tambs, K. (2008). Intelligence correlations between brothers decrease with increasing age difference: Evidence for shared environmental effects in young adults. *Psychological Science, 19,* 843–847.

Svartik, J. (1966). *On voice in the English verb.* The Hague, Netherlands: Mouton.

Swanson, J., Posner, M. I., Cantwell, D., Wigal, S., Crinella, F., Filipek, P., Emerson, J., Tucker, D., & Nalcioglu, O. (1998). Attention Deficit/Hyperactivity Disorder: Symptom domain, cognitive processes and neural networks. In R. Parasuraman (Ed.), *The attentive brain* (pp. 445–460). Cambridge, MA: MIT Press.

Symons, C. S., & Johnson, B. T. (1997). The self-reference effect in memory: A meta-analysis. *Psychological Bulletin, 121,* 371–394.

Tabachnick, B., & Brotsky, S. (1976). Free recall and complexity of pictorial stimuli. *Memory & Cognition, 4,* 466–470.

Talarico, J. M., & Rubin, D. C. (2003). Confidence, not consistency, characterizes flashbulb memories. *Psychological Science, 14,* 455–461.

Talmi, D. (2013). Enhanced emotional memory: Cognitive and neural mechanisms. *Current Directions in Psychological Science, 22,* 430–436.

Talmi, D., Grady, C. L., Goshen-Gottstein, Y., & Moscovitch, M. (2005). Neuroimaging the serial position curve: A test of single-store versus dual-store models. *Psychological Science, 16,* 716–723.

Tamietto, M., et al. (2010). Collicular vision guides nonconscious behavior. *Journal of Cognitive Neuroscience, 22,* 888–902.

Tanenhaus, M. K., & Spivey-Knowlton, M. J. (1996). Eye-tracking. *Language & Cognitive Processes, 11,* 583–588.

Tanenhaus, M. K., & Trueswell, J. C. (2006). Eye movements and spoken language comprehension. In M. J. Traxler & M. A. Gernsbacher (Eds.), *Handbook of psycholinguistics* (2nd ed.). Amsterdam, Netherlands: Elsevier.

Tarr, M. (1995). Rotating objects to recognize them: A case study on the role of viewpoint dependency in the recognition of three-dimensional objects. *Psychonomic Bulletin & Review, 2,* 55–82.

Tarr, M. (1999). News on views: Pandemonium revisited. *Nature Neuroscience, 2,* 932–935.

Tarr, M., & Bülthoff, H. (1998). Image-based object recognition in man, monkey and machine. *Cognition, 67,* 1–208.

Tattersall, I., & DeSalle, R. (2011). *Race? Debunking a scientific myth.* College Station: Texas A&M University Press.

Taylor, J., Roehrig, A., Hensler, B., Connor, C., & Schatschneider, C. (2010). Teacher quality moderates the genetic effects on early reading. *Science, 328,* 512–514.

Terr, L. C. (1991). Acute responses to external events and posttraumatic stress disorders. In M. Lewis (Ed.), *Child and adolescent psychiatry: A comprehensive textbook* (pp. 755–763). Baltimore, MD: Williams & Wilkins.

Terr, L. C. (1994). *Unchained memories: The stories of traumatic memories, lost and found.* New York, NY: Basic Books.

Thaler, R., & Sunstein, C. (2009). Nudge: Improving decisions about health, wealth, and happiness. New York, NY: Penguin.

Thioux, M., Stark, D. E., Klaiman, C., & Shultz, R. T. (2006). The day of the week when you were born in 700 ms: Calendar computation in an autistic savant. *Journal of Experimental Psychology: Human Perception and Performance, 32,* 1155–1168.

Thirion, B., Duchesnay, E., Hubbard, E., Dubois, J., Poline, J.-B., Lebihan, D., & Dehaene, S. (2006). Inverse retinotopy: Inferring the visual content of images from brain activation patterns. *Neuroimage, 33,* 1104–1116.

Thomas, A. K., & Loftus, E. F. (2002). Creating bizarre false memories through imagination. *Memory & Cognition, 30,* 423–431.

Thomas, J. (1974). An analysis of behavior in the Hobbits-Orcs problem. *Cognitive Psychology, 6,* 257–269.

Thompson, E., & Varela, F. J. (2001). Radical embodiment: Neural dynamics and consciousness. *Trends in Cognitive Sciences, 5,* 418–425.

Thompson, P. (1980). Margaret Thatcher: A new illusion. *Perception, 9,* 483–484.

Thompson, W. L., & Kosslyn, S. M. (2000). Neural systems activated during visual mental imagery: A review and meta-analyses. In J. Mazziotta & A. Toga (Eds.), *Brain mapping II: The applications* (pp. 535–560). New York, NY: Academic Press.

Thompson, W. L., Kosslyn, S. M., Hoffman, M. S., & Kooij, K. v. d. (2008). Inspecting visual mental images: Can people "see" implicit properties as easily in imagery and perception? *Memory & Cognition, 36,* 1024–1032.

Thompson, W. L., Slotnick, S., Burrage, M., & Kosslyn, S. (2009). Two forms of spatial imagery: Neuroimaging evidence. *Psychological Science, 20,* 1245–1253.

Thomsen, D. K., & Berntsen, D. (2009). The long-term impact of emotionally stressful events on memory characteristics and life story. *Applied Cognitive Psychology, 23,* 579–598.

Thomson, D., Milliken, B., & Smilek, D. (2010). Long-term conceptual implicit memory: A decade of evidence. *Memory & Cognition, 38,* 42–46.

Tinti, C., Schmidt, S., Sotgiu, I., Testa, S., & Curci, A. (2009). The role of importance/consequentiality appraisal in flashbulb memory formation: The case of the death of Pope John Paul II. *Applied Cognitive Psychology, 23,* 236–253.

Tinti, C., Schmidt, S., Testa, S., & Levine, L. J. (2014). Distinct processes shape flashbulb and event memories. *Memory and Cognition, 42,* 539–551.

Todd, P. M., & Gigerenzer, G. (2007). Environments that make us smart. *Current Directions in Psychological Science, 16,* 167–171.

Tombu, M., & Jolicoeur, P. (2003). A central capacity sharing model of dual-task performance. *Journal of Experimental Psychology: Human Perception & Performance, 29,* 3–18.

Tononi, G., & Cirelli, C. (2013). New hypothesis explains why we sleep. *Scientific American, 309*(2).

Topolinski, S., & Reber, R. (2010). Gaining insight into the "Aha" experience. *Current Directions in Psychological Science, 19,* 402–405.

Trahan, L. H., Stuebing, K. K., Fletcher, J. M., & Hiscock, M. (2014). The Flynn effect: A meta-analysis. *Psychological Bulletin, 140,* 1332–1360.

Treffert, D. A. (2014, August). Accidental genius. *Scientific American,* 52–57.

Treisman, A. (1964). Verbal cues, language, and meaning in selective attention. *American Journal of Psychology, 77,* 206–219.

Treisman, A., & Gelade, G. (1980). A feature-integration theory of attention. *Cognitive Psychology, 12,* 97–136.

Treisman, A., Sykes, M., & Gelade, G. (1977). Selective attention and stimulus integration. In S. Dornic (Ed.), *Attention and performance VI* (pp. 333–361). Hillsdale, NJ: Erlbaum.

Trippas, D., Handley, S. J., & Verde, M. F. (2013). The SDT model of belief bias: Complexity, time, and cognitive ability mediate the effects of believability. *Journal of Experimental Psychology: Learning, Memory, & Cognition, 39,* 1939–1402.

Trippas, D., Verde, M. F., & Handley, S. J. (2014). Using forced choice to test belief bias in syllogistic reasoning. *Cognition, 133,* 586–600.

Trueswell, J. C., Tanenhaus, M.K., & Garnsey, S. M. (1994). Semantic influences on parsing: Use of thematic role information in syntactic ambiguity resolution. *Journal of Memory and Language, 33,* 285–318.

Tsai, C., & Thomas, M. (2011). When does feeling of fluency matter? How abstract and concrete thinking influence fluency effects. *Psychological Science, 22,* 348–354.

Tsushima, Y., Sasaki, Y., & Watanabe, T. (2006). Greater disruption due to failure of inhibitory control on an ambiguous distractor. *Science, 314,* 1786–1788.

Tucker-Drob, E. M., Rhemtulla, M., Harden, K. P., Turkheimer, E., & Fask, D. (2011). Emergence of a gene x socioeconomic status interaction on infant mental ability between 10 months and 2 years. *Psychological Science, 22*, 125–133.

Tuffiash, M., Roring, R., & Ericsson, K. A. (2007). Expert performance in SCRABBLE: Implications for the study of the structure and acquisition of complex skills. *Journal of Experimental Psychology: Applied, 13*, 124–134.

Tulving, E. (1983). *Elements of episodic memory.* Oxford, England: Oxford University Press.

Tulving, E. (1993). What is episodic memory? *Current Directions in Psychological Science, 2*, 67–70.

Tulving, E. (2002). Episodic memory: From mind to brain. *Annual Review of Psychology, 53*, 1–25.

Tulving, E., & Gold, C. (1963). Stimulus information and contextual information as determinants of tachistoscopic recognition of words. *Journal of Experimental Psychology, 92*, 319–327.

Tulving, E., Mandler, G., & Baumal, R. (1964). Interaction of two sources of information in tachistoscopic word recognition. *Canadian Journal of Psychology, 18*, 62–71.

Turkheimer, E., Haley, A., Waldron, M., D'Onofrio, B., & Gottesman, I. I. (2003). Socioeconomic status modifies heritability of IQ in young children. *Psychological Science, 14*, 623–628.

Tversky, A., & Kahneman, D. (1973). Availability: A heuristic for judging frequency and probability. *Cognitive Psychology, 5*, 207–232.

Tversky, A., & Kahneman, D. (1974). Judgments under uncertainty: Heuristics and biases. *Science, 185*, 1124–1131.

Tversky, A., & Kahneman, D. (1982). Evidential impact of base rates. In D. Kahneman, P. Slovic, & A. Tversky (Eds.), *Judgment under uncertainty: Heuristics and biases* (pp. 153–160). New York, NY: Cambridge University Press.

Tversky, A., & Kahneman, D. (1987). Rational choice and the framing of decisions. In R. Hogarth & M. Reder (Eds.), *Rational choice: The contrast between economics and psychology* (pp. 67–94). Chicago, IL: University of Chicago Press.

Tweney, R. D., Doherty, M. E., & Mynatt, C. R. (1981). *On scientific thinking.* New York, NY: Columbia University Press.

Ullman, S. (2007). Object recognition and segmentation by a fragment-based hierarchy. *Trends in Cognitive Sciences, 11*, 58–64.

Ungerleider, L. G., & Haxby, J. V. (1994). "What" and "where" in the human brain. *Current Opinions in Neurobiology, 4*, 157–165.

Ungerleider, L. G., & Mishkin, M. (1982). Two cortical visual systems. In D. J. Ingle, M. A. Goodale, & R. J. W. Mansfield (Eds.), *Analysis of visual behavior* (pp. 549–586). Cambridge, MA: MIT Press.

Unkelbach, C. (2007). Reversing the truth effect: Learning the interpretation of processing fluency in judgments of truth. *Journal of Experimental Psychology: Learning, Memory, & Cognition, 33*, 219–230.

Unsworth, N., & Engle, R. (2007). The nature of individual differences in working memory capacity: Active maintenance in primary memory and controlled search in secondary memory. *Psychological Review, 114*, 104–132.

Valentine, T. (1988). Upside-down faces: A review of the effects of inversion upon face recognition. *British Journal of Psychology, 79*, 471–491.

Vallar, G., & Cappa, S. F. (1987). Articulation and verbal short-term memory: Evidence from anarthria. *Cognitive Neuropsychology, 4*, 55–78.

Van der Lely, H. K. J. (2005). Domain-specific cognitive systems: Insight from grammatical-SLI. *Trends in Cognitive Sciences, 9*, 53–59.

Van der Lely, H. K. J., & Pinker, S. (2014). The biological basis for language: Insight from developmental grammatical impairments. *Trends in Cognitive Sciences*, 586–595.

Van Essen, D. C., & DeYoe, E. A. (1995). Concurrent processing in the primate visual cortex. In M. S. Gazzaniga (Ed.), *The cognitive neurosciences* (pp. 383–400). Cambridge, MA: MIT Press.

Van Steenburgh, J. J., Fleck, J. I., Beeman, M., & Kounios, J. (2012). Insight. In K. J. Holyoak & R. G. Morrison (Eds.), *The Oxford handbook of thinking and reasoning* (pp. 475–491). New York, NY: Oxford University Press.

Van Veen, V., & Carter, C. S. (2006). Conflict and cognitive control in the brain. *Current Directions in Psychological Science, 15*, 237–240.

Vandierendonck, A., Liefooghe, B., & Verbruggen, F. (2010). Task switching: Interplay of reconfiguration and interference control. *Psychological Bulletin, 136*, 601–626.

Vanpaemel, W., & Storms, G. (2008). In search of abstraction: The varying abstraction model of categorization, *Psychonomic Bulletin & Review, 15*, 732–749.

Vargha-Khadem, F., Gadian, D. G., Copp, A., & Mishkin, M. (2005). FOXP2 and the neuroanatomy of speech and language. *Nature Reviews Neuroscience, 32*, 131–138.

Vartanian, O., Martindale, C., & Matthews, J. (2009). Divergent thinking ability is related to faster relatedness judgments. *Psychology of Aesthetics, Creativity, and the Arts, 3*, 99–103.

Vergauwe, E., Barrouillet, P., & Camos, V. (2010). Do mental processes share a domain-general resource? *Psychological Science, 21*, 384–390.

Vernon, P. A. (Ed.). (1987). *Speed of information processing and intelligence.* Canada: Ablex.

Verstijnen, I. M., Hennessey, J. M., van Leeuwen, C., Hamel, R., & Goldschmidt, G. (1998). Sketching and creative discovery. *Design Studies, 19*, 519–546.

Verstijnen, I. M., van Leeuwen, C., Goldschmidt, G., Hamel, R., & Hennessey, J. M. (1998). Creative discovery in imagery and perception: Combining is relatively easy, restructuring takes a sketch. *Acta Psychologica, 99*, 177–200.

Vinkhuyzen, A. A., van der Sluis, S., & Posthuma, D. (2011). Life events moderate variation in cognitive ability (g) in adults. *Molecular Psychiatry, 16*(1), 4–6.

Visser, B., Ashton, M., & Vernon, P. (2006). Beyond "g": Putting multiple intelligences theory to the test. *Intelligence, 34*, 487–502.

Vitevitch, M. S. (2003). Change deafness: The inability to detect changes between two voices. *Journal of Experimental Psychology: Human Perception and Performance, 29*, 333–342.

Võ, M. L.-H., & Henderson, J. M. (2009) Does gravity matter? Effects of semantic and syntactic inconsistencies on the allocation of attention during scene perception. *Journal of Vision, 9*(3), 24, 1–15.

von Neumann, J., & Morgenstern, O. (1947). *Theory of games and economic behavior*. Princeton, NJ: Princeton University Press.

Vul, E., & Pashler, H. (2007). Incubation benefits only after people have been misdirected. *Memory & Cognition, 35*, 701–710.

Vuong, Q. C., & Tarr, M. (2004). Rotation direction affects object recognition. *Vision Research, 44*, 1717–1730.

Wade, K. A., Garry, M., Read, J. D., & Lindsay, D. S. (2002). A picture is worth a thousand lies: Using false photographs to create false childhood memories. *Psychonomic Bulletin & Review, 9*, 597–603.

Wagenaar, W. A., & Groeneweg, J. (1990). The memory of concentration camp survivors. *Applied Cognitive Psychology, 4*, 77–88.

Wagner, A. D., Koutstaal, W., & Schacter, D. L. (1999). When encoding yields remembering: Insights from event-related neuroimaging. *Philosophical Transactions of the Royal Society of London, Biology, 354*, 1307–1324.

Wagner, A. D., Schacter, D. L., Rotte, M., Koutstaal, W., Maril, A., Dale, A., et al. (1998). Building memories: Remembering and forgetting of verbal experiences as predicted by brain activity. *Science, 281*, 1188–1191.

Wagner, A. D., Shannon, B., Kahn, I., & Buckner, R. (2005). Parietal lobe contributions to episodic memory retrieval. *Trends in Cognitive Sciences, 9*, 445–453.

Wagner, R. K. (2000). Practical intelligence. In R. J. Sternberg (Ed.), *Handbook of human intelligence* (pp. 380–395). New York, NY: Cambridge University Press.

Wai, J., Putallaz, M., & Makel, M. C. (2012). Studying intellectual outliers: Are there sex differences, and are the smart getting smarter? *Current Directions in Psychological Science, 21*, 382–390.

Wallas, G. (1926). *The art of thought*. New York, NY: Harcourt, Brace.

Wallis, G., & Bülthoff, H. (1999). Learning to recognize objects. *Trends in Cognitive Sciences, 3*, 22–31.

Walton, G., & Spencer, S. (2009). Latent ability: Grades and test scores systematically underestimate the intellectual ability of negatively stereotyped students. *Psychological Science, 20*, 1132–1139.

Wang, R., Li, J., Fang, H., Tian, M., & Liu, J. (2012). Individual differences in holistic processing predict face recognition ability. *Psychological Science, 23*, 169–177.

Wang, S. H., & Morris, R. G. (2010). Hippocampal-neocortical interactions in memory formation, consolidation, and reconsolidation. *Annual Review of Psychology, 61*, 49–79.

Warrington, E. K., & Shallice, T. (1984). Category specific semantic impairments. *Brain, 107*, 829–854.

Wason, P. (1966). Reasoning. In B. Foss (Ed.), *New horizons in psychology* (pp. 135–151). Middlesex, England: Penguin.

Wason, P. (1968). Reasoning about a rule. *Quarterly Journal of Experimental Psychology, 20*, 273–281.

Wason, P., & Johnson-Laird, P. (1972). *Psychology of reasoning: Structure and content*. Cambridge, MA: Harvard University Press.

Watkins, M., Wilson, S., Kotz, K., Carbone, M., & Babula, T. (2006). Factor structure of the Wechsler Intelligence Scale for Children—Fourth edition among referred students. *Educational and Psychological Measurement, 66*, 975–983.

Watkins, M. J. (1977). The intricacy of memory span. *Memory & Cognition, 5*, 529–534.

Wattenmaker, W. D., Dewey, G. I., Murphy, T. D., & Medin, D. L. (1986). Linear separability and concept learning: Context, relational properties, and concept naturalness. *Cognitive Psychology, 18*, 158–194.

Waugh, N. C., & Norman, D. A. (1965). Primary memory. *Psychological Review, 72*, 89–104.

Wearing, D. (2011). *Forever today: A memoir of love and amnesia*. New York, NY: Doubleday.

Weaver, C. (1993). Do you need a "flash" to form a flashbulb memory? *Journal of Experimental Psychology: General, 122*, 39–46.

Weber, E., & Johnson, E. (2009). Mindful judgment and decision making. *Annual Review of Psychology, 60*, 53–85.

Weber, N., Brewer, N., Wells, G., Semmler, C., & Keast, A. (2004). Eyewitness identification accuracy and response latency: The unruly 10–12-second rule. *Journal of Experimental Psychology: Applied, 10*, 139–147.

Wechsler, D. (2003). *Wechsler Intelligence Scale for Children—Fourth edition*. San Antonio, TX: Psychological Corporation.

Wegner, D., Wenzlaff, R., Kerker, R., & Beattie, A. (1981). Incrimination through innuendo: Can media questions become public answers? *Journal of Personality and Social Psychology, 40,* 822–832.

Weiner, K. S., & Grill-Spector, K. (2013). The improbable simplicity of the fusiform face area. *Trends in Cognitive Sciences, 16,* 251–254.

Weisberg, R. W. (1986). *Creativity: Genius and other myths.* New York, NY: Freeman.

Weisberg, R. W. (2006). *Creativity: Understanding innovation in problem solving, science, invention and the arts.* New York, NY: Wiley.

Weisberg, R., & Alba, J. (1981). An examination of the alleged role of "fixation" in the solution of several "insight" problems. *Journal of Experimental Psychology: General, 110,* 169–192.

Weisberg, R., DiCamillo, M., & Phillips, D. (1978). Transferring old associations to new problems: A nonautomatic process. *Journal of Verbal Learning and Verbal Behavior, 17,* 219–228.

Weiskrantz, L. (1986). *Blindsight: A case study and implications.* New York, NY: Oxford University Press.

Weiskrantz, L. (1997). *Consciousness lost and found.* New York, NY: Oxford University Press.

Wells, G. L., & Bradfield, A. L. (1998). "Good, you identified the suspect": Feedback to eyewitnesses distorts their reports of the witnessed experience. *Journal of Applied Psychology, 83,* 360–376.

Wells, G. L., Lindsay, R. C. L., & Ferguson, T. J. (1979). Accuracy, confidence, and juror perceptions in eyewitness identification. *Journal of Applied Psychology, 64,* 440–448.

Wells, G. L., Olson, E. A., & Charman, S. D. (2002). The confidence of eyewitnesses in their identifications from lineups. *Current Directions in Psychological Science, 11,* 151–154.

Wells, G. L., Olson, E. A., & Charman, S. D. (2003). Distorted retrospective eyewitness reports as functions of feedback and delay. *Journal of Experimental Psychology: Applied, 9,* 42–51.

Wells, G. L., & Quinlivan, D. S. (2009). Suggestive eyewitness identification procedures and the Supreme Court's reliability test in light of eyewitness science: 30 years later. *Law and Human Behavior, 33,* 1–24.

Westmacott, R., & Moscovitch, M. (2003). The contribution of autobiographical significance to semantic memory. *Memory & Cognition, 31,* 761–774.

Wharton, C., Holyoak, K., Downing, P., & Lange, T. (1994). Below the surface: Analogical similarity and retrieval competition in reminding. *Cognitive Psychology, 26,* 64–101.

Wheeler, D. (1970). Processes in word recognition. *Cognitive Psychology, 1,* 59–85.

Wheeler, M. E., Petersen, S. E., & Buckner, R. L. (2000). Memory's echo: Vivid remembering reactivates sensory-specific cortex. *Proceedings of the National Academy of Sciences, USA, 97,* 11125–11129.

White, J. (2008). Illusory intelligences? *Journal of Philosophy of Education, 42,* 611–630.

White, P. (1988). Knowing more than we can tell: "Introspective access" and causal report accuracy 10 years later. *British Journal of Psychology, 79,* 13–45.

Whitney, C. (2001). How the brain encodes the order of letters in a printed word: The SERIOL model and selective literature review. *Psychonomic Bulletin & Review, 8,* 221–243.

Whittlesea, B. W. A. (2002). False memory and the discrepancy-attribution hypothesis: The prototype-familiarity illusion. *Journal of Experimental Psychology: General, 131,* 96–115.

Whittlesea, B. W. A., Jacoby, L., & Girard, K. (1990). Illusions of immediate memory: Evidence of an attributional basis for feelings of familiarity and perceptual quality. *Journal of Memory and Language, 29,* 716–732.

Whorf, B. L. (1956). *Language, thought, and reality.* Cambridge, England: Technology Press.

Willemsen, M., Böckenholt, U., & Johnson, E. (2011). Choice by value encoding and value construction: Processes of loss aversion. *Journal of Experimental Psychology: General, 140,* 303–324.

Williams, L. M., Liddell, B. J., Kemp, A. H., Bryant, R. A., Meares, R. A., Peduto, A. S., & Gordon, E. (2006). Amygdala-prefrontal dissociation of subliminal and supraliminal fear. *Human Brain Mapping 27*(8), 652–661.

Wilson, T. D. (2002). *Strangers to ourselves: Discovering the adaptive unconscious.* Cambridge, MA: Harvard University Press.

Wilson, T. D., & Dunn, E. W. (2004). Self-knowledge: Its limits, value, and potential for improvement. *Annual Review of Psychology, 55,* 493–518.

Wilson, T. D., Wheatley, T., Meyers, J. M., Gilbert, D., & Axsom, D. (2000). Focalism: A source of durability bias in affective forecasting. *Journal of Personality and Social Psychology, 78,* 821–836.

Winkielman, P., & Schwarz, N. (2001). How pleasant was your childhood? Beliefs about memory shape inferences from experienced difficulty of recall. *Psychological Science, 12,* 176–179.

Winnick, W., & Daniel, S. (1970). Two kinds of response priming in tachistoscopic recognition. *Journal of Experimental Psychology, 84,* 74–81.

Winograd, E., & Neisser, U. (Eds.). (1993). *Affect and accuracy in recall: Studies of "flashbulb" memories.* New York, NY: Cambridge University Press.

Wiseman, S., & Neisser, U. (1974). Perceptual organization as a determinant of visual recognition memory. *American Journal of Psychology, 87,* 675–681.

Wittgenstein, L. (1953). *Philosophical investigations* (G. E. M. Anscombe, Trans.). Oxford, England: Blackwell.

Wixted, J. (2004). The psychology and neuroscience of forgetting. *Annual Review of Psychology, 55*, 235–269.

Wolfe, J. M. (1999). Inattentional amnesia. In V. Coltheart (Ed.), *Fleeting memories* (pp. 71–94). Cambridge, MA: MIT Press.

Wollen, K. A., Weber, A., & Lowry, D. (1972). Bizarreness versus interaction of mental images as determinants of learning. *Cognitive Psychology, 3*, 518–523.

Womelsdorf, T., Schoffelen, J.-M., Oostenveld, R., Singer, W., Desimone, R., Engel, A., & Fries, P. (2007). Modulation of neuronal interactions through neuronal synchronization. *Science, 316*, 1609–1612.

Wood, N., & Cowan, N. (1995). The cocktail party phenomenon revisited: How frequent are attention shifts to one's name in an irrelevant auditory channel? *Journal of Experimental Psychology: Learning, Memory, & Cognition, 21*, 255–260.

Wright, D., & Skagerberg, E. (2007). Postidentification feedback affects real eyewitnesses. *Psychological Science, 18*, 172–177.

Wright, R. D., & Ward, L. M. (2008). *Orienting of attention*. New York, NY: Oxford University Press.

Xu, F., & Garcia, V. (2008). Intuitive statistics by 8-month-old infants. *Proceedings of the National Academy of Sciences, 105*, 5012–5015.

Yamaguchi, M., & Proctor, R. (2011). Automaticity without extensive training: The role of memory retrieval in implementation of task-defined rules. *Psychonomic Bulletin and Review, 18*, 347–354.

Yantis, S. (2008). The neural basis of selective attention: Cortical sources and targets of attentional modulation. *Current Directions in Psychological Science, 17*, 86–90.

Yates, F. A. (1966). *The art of memory*. London, England: Routledge and Kegan Paul.

Yeni-Komshian, G. (1993). Speech perception. In J. B. Gleason & N. B. Ratner (Eds.), *Psycholinguistics* (pp. 90–133). New York, NY: Harcourt Brace Jovanovich.

Yin, R. (1969). Looking at upside-down faces. *Journal of Experimental Psychology, 81*, 141–145.

Yonelinas, A., & Jacoby, L. (2012). The process-dissociation approach two decades later: Convergence, boundary conditions, and new direction. *Memory & Cognition, 40*, 663–680.

Young, A. W., Hellawell, D., & Hay, D. C. (1987). Configurational information in face perception. *Perception, 16*, 747–759.

Zaragoza, M. S., Payment, K. E., Ackil, J. K., Drivdahl, S. B., & Beck, M. (2001). Interviewing witnesses: Forced confabulation and confirmatory feedback increases false memories. *Psychological Science, 12*, 473–477.

Zechmeister, E. B., Chronis, A. M., Cull, W. L., D'Anna, C. A., & Healy, N. A. (1995). Growth of a functionally important lexicon. *Journal of Reading Behavior, 27*(2), 201–212.

Zeki, S. (1991). Cerebral akinetopsia (visual motion blindness): A review. *Brain, 114*, 811–824.

Zelazo, P. D. (2006). The dimensional change card sort (DCCS): A method of assessing executive function in children. *Nature Protocols, 1*, 297–301.

Zillmer, E. A., Spiers, M. V., & Culbertson, W. C. (2008). *Principles of neuropsychology*. Belmont, CA: Wadsworth.

Zimler, J., & Keenan, J. M. (1983). Imagery in the congenitally blind: How visual are visual images? *Journal of Experimental Psychology: Learning, Memory, & Cognition, 9*, 269–282.

Credits

Photographs

Stephen Lovekin/Getty Images; **p. 136:** M. Bar, K. S. Kassam, A. S. Ghuman, J. Boshyan, A. M. Schmid, A. M. Dale, M. S. Hamalainen, K. Markinkovic, D. L. Schacter, B. R. Rosen, and E. Halgren, "Top-Down Facilitation of Visual Recognition," *PNAS* 103, no. 2 (January 10, 2006): 449–454. © 2006 Proceedings of the National Academy of Science of the United States of America; **p. 137:** Fuse/Thinkstock; **(Chapter 5) pp. 140–141:** Paul Bradbury/Getty Image; **p. 144 (all):** Courtesy of Daniel J. Simons and Christopher Chabris; **p. 145:** Javier Pierini/Getty Images; **p. 147:** iStockphoto; **p. 148 (top two):** Galina Barskaya | Dreamstime.com; **(bottom two):** Titania1980 | Dreamstime.com; **p. 149 (all):** Daniel T. Levin and Daniel J. Simons, "Failure to Detect Changes to Attended Objects in Motion Pictures," *Psychonomic Bulletin and Review* 4, no. 4 (1997): 501–506, Figure 1; **p. 159:** Rykoff Collection/Corbis; **p. 162 (both):** M. Corbetta and G. L. Shulman, "Control of Goal-Directed and Stimulus-Driven Attention in the Brain," *Nature Reviews Neuroscience* 3, no. 3 (March 2002): 201–215; **p. 163:** D. Y. Kimberg, M. D'Esposito, and M. J. Farah, "Cognitive Functions in the Prefrontal Cortex-Working Memory and Executive Control," *Current Directions in Psychological Science* 6, no. 6 (1997): 186; **p. 169:** The Granger Collection; **p. 173:** AP Photo/Marshall Gorby, Springfield News-Sun; **p. 180:** Paul Bradbury/Getty Images; **(Chapter 6) pp. 184–185:** Digital Vision/Getty Images; **p. 186 (top):** Ros Drinkwater/Alamy; **(bottom):** © Jiri Rezac; **p. 195:** Talmi et al., "Neuroimaging the Serial Position Curve," *Psychoogical Science* 16, no. 9 (September 2005): 716–723; **p. 202:** Alberto Pomares/Getty Images; **p. 208 (left):** Imagic Chicago/Alamy; **(right):** Stuart Black/Alamy; **p. 211:** Mnesmosyne, 1881 (oil on canvas); Rossetti, Dante Gabriel Charles (1828-1882)/Delaware Art Museum, Wilmington, USA/Samuel and Mary R. Bancroft Memorial/Bridgeman Images; p.212: ScienceCartoonsPlus.com; **p. 217:** S. Wiseman and U. Neisser, "Perceptual Organization as a Determinant of Visual Recognition Memory," *American Journal of Psychology* 87, no. 4 (1974): 675–681; **p. 219:** Blend Images/Getty Images; **(Chapter 7) pp. 222–223:** Tim Macpherson/Cultura/Getty Images; **p. 225:** Photo by Project Neuron, University of Illinois at Urbana-Champaign; **p. 230 (all, except bottom right):** Wheeler et al., "Memory Echo: Vivid Remembering Reactivates Sensory-Specific Cortex," *Proceedings of the National Academy of Sciences* 97, no. 20 (September 26, 2000): 11125–11129; **(bottom right):** Jason LaVeris/FimMagic/Getty Images; **p. 238 (left):** Dave J. Hogan/Getty Images; **(center left):** Steve Granitz/Wire Image/Getty Images; **(center):** Barry King/Film Magic/Getty Images; **(center right):** John Shearer/Wire Image/Getty Images; **(right):** Jon Kopaloff Film Magic/Getty Images; **p. 239 (both):** Ranganath et al., "Dissociable Correlates of Recollection and Familiarity within the Medial Temporal Lobes," *Neuropsychologia* 42, no. 1 (2004): 2–13. © 2003 Elsevier Ltd. All rights reserved; **p. 245 (all):** Courtesy of Daniel Reisberg; **p. 250:** Junko Kimura/

Getty Images; **p. 254:** The Canadian Press/Helen Branswell; **p. 255 (both):** Corkin et al., "H.M.'s Medial Temporal Lobe Lesion: Findings from Magnetic Resonance Imaging," *The Journal of Neuroscience* 17, no. 10 (May 15, 1997): 3964–3979. © 1997 Society of Neuroscience; **p. 259:** Paul Doyle/Alamy; **(Chapter 8) pp. 262–263:** Ryan McVay/Getty Images; **p. 266:** W. F. Brewer and J. C. Treyens, "Role of Schemata in Memory for Places," *Cognitive Psychology* 13, no. 2 (April 1981): 207–230; **p. 274:** Eric Kayne/Houston Chronicle; **p. 278 (both):** K. A. Wade, M. Garry, J. D. Read, and D. S. Lindsay, "A Picture Is Worth a Thousand Lies: Using False Photographs to Create False Childhood Memories," *Psychonomic Bulletin & Review* 9, no. 3 (September 2002): 597–603; **p. 279:** D. S. Lindsay et al., "True Photographs and False Memories," *Psychological Science* 15, no. 3 (March 2004): 149–154; **p. 280:** Robyn Mackenzie/Shutterstock; **p. 286 (both):** M. T. Orne, "The Nature of Hypnosis: Artifact and Essence," *Journal of Abnormal and Social Psychology* 58 (1959): 277–299; **p. 289:** Kelley et al., "Finding the Self? An Event-Related fMRI Study," *Journal of Cognitive Neuroscience* 14 (2002): 785–794. © 2002, Massachusetts Institute of Technology; **p. 294 (left):** Bettmann/Corbis; **(center):** Reuters; **(right):** Joel Ryan/AP Photo; **p. 302:** Will & Deni McIntyre/Corbis; **(Chapter 9) pp. 306–307:** Gozooma/Gallery Stock; **p. 310:** Tierfotoagentur/Alamy; **p. 313 (top left):** GK Hart/Vikki Hart/Getty Images; **(all, except top left):** Eric Issel/Dreamstime.com; **p. 315:** Adrian Lewart/Dreamstime.com; **p. 317 (top):** Rick & Nora Bowers/Alamy; **(bottom left):** Photoshot Holdings Ltd/Alamy; **(bottom right):** Hiroya Minakuchi/Getty Images; **p. 318:** Emilio Ereza/age fotostock; **p. 320:** EPA European PressPhoto Agency B.V./Alamy; **p. 322:** Look and Learn/Bridgeman Art Library; **p. 324:** © Sidney Harris/Science CartoonsPlus.com; **p. 326:** age fotostock/Superstock; **p. 328:** Courtesy of Robert Malseed; **p. 330:** Courtesy of Daniel Reisberg; **p. 341:** Bubbles Photolibrary/Alamy; **(Chapter 10) pp. 344–345:** Photosindia/age fotostock; **p. 351:** Courtney Leigh Rubin/Creators Syndicate, Inc.; **p. 353:** iStockphoto; **p. 358:** Lebrecht Music & Arts/Corbis; **p. 360:** Hulton-Deutsch Collection/Corbis; **p. 361:** Paramount Television/The Kobal Collection/Art Resource; **p. 363:** © Sidney Harris; **p. 372:** N. F. Dronkers et al., "Paul Brocas Historic Cases," *Brain* 130, no. 5 (2007): 1436, Figure 3a. By permission of Oxford University Press; **p. 375:** Stu Porter/Alamy; **p. 376 (left):** Rolls Press/Popperfoto/Getty Images; **(right):** Hulton Archive/Getty Images; **p. 378:** ColsTravel/Alamy; **p. 383:** Marmaduke St. John/Alamy; **(Chapter 11) pp. 386–387:** Friderike Heuer; **p. 396:** Adapted by Marcel Just from P. A. Carpenter, M. A. Just, T. A. Keller, et al., "Graded Functional Activation in the Visuospatial System and the Amount of Task Demand," *Journal of Cognitive Neuroscience* 11, no. 1 (January 1999): 14, doi:10.1162/089892999563210. © 1999 Massachusetts Institute of Technology; **p. 398:** Comstock/Getty Images; **p. 401 (all):** K. O'Craven and N. Kanwisher, "Mental

Imagery of Faces and Places Activates Corresponding Stimulus-Specific Brain Regions," *Journal of Cognitive Neuroscience* 12, no. 6 (2000): 1013–1023; **p. 403:** Atlantide Phototravel/Corbis; **p. 405:** W. L. Thompson and S. D. Slotnick, "Two Forms of Spatial Imagery: Neuroimaging Evidence," *Psychological Science* 20, no. 10 (October 2009): 1245–1253; **p. 409:** John Tenniel (1820–1914)/Private Collection/The Bridgeman Art Library; **p. 411:** The National Portrait Gallery; **p. 412:** Kellydt/Dreamstime.com; **p. 420:** H. Intraub and M. Richardson, "Wide-Angle Memories of Close-Up Scenes," *J Exp Psychol Learn* 15 (1989): 179–187; **p. 423:** Phanie/Alamy; **(Chapter 12) pp. 426–427:** Sean Justice/Getty Images; **p. 429:** Paul Wicks/Wikimedia Commons; **p. 434:** Corbis; **p. 441:** POM Wonderful poster, *The Guardian*, April 8, 2009; **p. 442 (all):** W. De Neys and V. Goel, "Heuristics and Biases in the Brain: Dual Neural Pathways for Decision Making," in *Neuroscience of Decision Making*, ed. O. Vartanian and D. R. Mandel (Hove, UK: Psychology Press, in press); **p. 448:** © Sidney Harris/Cartoonstock.com; **p. 453:** © Sidney Harris/ScienceCartoonsPlus.com; **p. 468:** Mark Parisi/www.offthemark.com; **p. 470:** Ulrich Baumgarten via Getty Images; **(Chapter 13) pp. 474–475:** Lucidio Studio, Inc./Getty Images; **p. 493:** Sam Gross/The New Yorker Collection/www.cartoonbank.com; **p. 498 (both):** J. Kounios and M. Beeman, "The Aha! Moment: The Cognitive Neuroscience of Insight," *Current Directions*

in Psychological Science 18, no. 4 (August 2009): 210–216; **p. 504:** Sample item similar to those in the *Wechsler Adult Intelligence Scale*, 4th ed. (WAIS-IV). © 2008 NCS Pearson, Inc. Reproduced with permission. All rights reserved. Wechsler Adult Intelligence Scale (WAIS) and Ravens Progressive Matrices are trademarks, in the United States and/or other countries, of Pearson Education, Inc. or its affiliates(s); **p. 511:** R. E. Jung and R. J. Haier, "The Parieto-Frontal Integration Theory (P-FIT) of Intelligence: Converging Neuroimaging Evidence," *Behavioral and Brain Sciences* 30, no. 2 (April 2007): 135–154. Courtesy Brain and Behavioral Associates, P.C.; **p. 514:** L. Selfe, *Nadia: A Case of Extraordinary Drawing Ability in an Autistic Child* (New York: Academic Press, 1977). Reproduced by permission of Academic Press and Lorna Selfe; **p. 515:** Michael Parmlelee/NBC/NBCU Photo Bank via Getty Images; **p. 517 (both):** Gary Parker/Science Source; **p. 523:** Robert Churchill/Getty Images; **p. 526:** Mark Scott/Getty Images; **(Chapter 14) pp. 530–531:** Sarah Wilmer/Gallery Stock; **p. 539:** Joel W. Rogers/Corbis; **p. 541:** © John Caldwell; **p. 549:** Jupiterimages/Getty Images; **p. 555:** Naotsugu Tsuchiya and Ralph Adolphs, "Emotion and Consciousness," *Trends in Cognitive Sciences* 11, no. 4 (April 2007): 158–167, doi:10.1016/j.tics.2007.01 .005. © 2007 Elsevier Ltd. All rights reserved; **p. 561:** John Springer Collection/Corbis; **p. 563:** Inmagine Asia/Corbis.

Figures

Figure 4.3 (p. 106): Figure 3 from, O. G. Selfridge, "Pattern Recognition and Modern Computers." AFIPS '55 (Western) Proceedings of the March 1–3, 1955, western joint computer conference. Copyright © 1955 by the Association for Computing Machinery, Inc. doi:10.1145/1455292.1455310. Reprinted by permission; **Figure 4.11 (p. 123):** Figure 3 from James L. McClelland and David E. Rumelhart, "An Interactive Model of Context Effects in Letter Perception," *Psychological Review* 88, no. 5 (September 1981): 375–407. Copyright © 1981 by the American Psychological Association. Reprinted with permission; **Figure 5.6 (p. 151):** Figure 6.7A–B from Purves, Cabeza, Huettel, LaBar, Platt, and Woldorff, *Principles of Cognitive Neuroscience,* 2nd ed. Used by permission of Sinauer Associates, Inc.; **Figure 6.6 (p. 198):** Figure 7 from R. Cabeza and L. Nyberg, "Imaging Cognition II: An Empirical Review of 275 PET and fMRI Studies," *Journal of Cognitive Neuroscience* 12, no. 1 (January 2000): 1–47. Copyright © 2000 by the Massachusetts Institute of Technology. Reprinted by permission of MIT Press Journals; **Figure 8.14 (p. 298):** Figure 1 from Martin A. Conway, Gillian Cohen, and Nicole Stanhope, "On the

Very Long-Term Retention of Knowledge Acquired through Formal Education: Twelve Years of Cognitive Psychology," *Journal of Experimental Psychology* 120, no. 4 (December 1991): 395–409. Copyright © 1991 by the American Psychological Association. Reprinted with permission; **Figure 8.15 (p. 300):** Figure 2: "Life-Span Retrieval Curves from Five Countries" from Martin A. Conway, Qi Wang, Kazunori Hanyu, and Shamsul Haque, "A Cross-Cultural Investigation of Autobiographical Memory," *Journal of Cross-Cultural Psychology* 36, no. 6 (November 2005): 739–749. Copyright © 2005 by SAGE Publications. Reprinted by permission of SAGE Publications; **Figure 10.10a–b (p. 365):** Figure from T. F. Munte, H. J. Heinze, and G. R. Mangun, "Dissociation of Brain Activity Related to Syntactic and Semantic Aspects of Language," *Journal of Cognitive Neuroscience* 5, no. 3 (Summer 1993): 335–344. Copyright © 1993 by the Massachusetts Institute of Technology. Reprinted by permission of MIT Press Journals; **Figure 10.12 (p. 368):** Figure 1 from Peter Hagoort, Lea Hald, Marcel Bastiaansen, and Karl Magnus Petersson, "Integration of World Meaning World Knowledge in Language Comprehension," *Science* 304, no. 5669 (April 2004): 438–441. Copyright © 2004, American Association for the Advancement of Science. Reprinted with permission from AAAS; **Figure 11.4a–c (p. 395):** Figure 1 from Roger N. Shepard and Jaqueline Metzler, "Mental Rotation of Three-Dimensional Objects," *Science* 171, no. 3972 (February 1971): 701–703. Copyright © 1971, American Association for the Advancement of Science. Reprinted with permission from AAAS; **Figure 12.4 (p. 446):** Figure 1 from R. E. Nisbett, D. H. Krantz, C. Jepson, and Z. Kunda, "The Use of Statistical Heuristics in Everyday Inductive Reasoning," *Psychological Review* 90, no. 4 (October 1983): 339–363. Copyright © 1983 by the American Psychological Association. Reprinted with permission; **Figure 12.5 (p. 447):** Figure 2 from Geoffrey T. Fong and Richard E. Nisbett, "Immediate and Delayed Transfer of Training Effects in Statistical Reasoning," *Journal of Experimental Psychology: General* 120, no. 1 (March 1991): 34–45. Copyright © 1991 by the American Psychological Association. Reprinted with permission; **Figure 12.12 (p. 459):** Problem 5 from A. Tversky and D. Kahneman, "Rational Choice and the Framing of Decisions," *Journal of Business* 59, no. 4 (October 1986): Part 2, S251–S278. Copyright © 1986 by the University of Chicago Press. Reprinted by permission; **Figure 12.17 (p. 466):** Figure 14.20A from Purves, Cabeza, Huettel, LaBar, Platt, and Woldorff, *Principles of Cognitive Neuroscience*, 2nd ed. Used by permission of Sinauer Associates, Inc.; **Figure 12.18 (p. 467):** Figure 13.10: Results of Kermer et al.'s experiment republished with permission of Cengage Learning, from E. Bruce Goldstein, *Cognitive Psychology*, 3rd ed., p. 378. Copyright © 2011 Cengage Learning. Permission conveyed through Copyright Clearance Center; **Figure 13.8a–c (p. 487):** Figure 8.15 from R. Bootzin, *Psychology Today: An Introduction*, 4th ed. Copyright © 1979 McGraw-Hill Education. Reprinted with permission.

Author Index

Frost, P., 282
Frost, R., 112
Fthenaki, K., 253
Fuhrman, O., 418
Fukuda, K., 510
Fukui, M., 152
Fulker, D. W., 516
Fusella, V., 398, 399

Gabbay, P., 276
Gable, P. A., 292
Gabrieli, J., 203
Gadian, D. G., 375
Gaeth, G., 462
Gaissmaier, W., 446
Galanter, E., 15
Gallo, D. A., 269
Gallo, V., 53
Galton, F., 390, 391, 406, 407
Garcia, J., 524, 526
Garcia, V., 374
Garcia-Marques, L., 442
Garcia-Marques, T., 244
Gardiner, J. M., 238
Gardner, H., 371, 514, 515
Garnsey, S. M., 366
Garrett, B., 246, 274
Garrison, J., 498
Garrison, T. M., 171
Garry, M., 276, 278, 282
Gaspar, J. G., 171
Gathercole, S., 24, 171
Gauthier, I. L., 131, 132
Gazzaniga, M. S., 78, 540, 542, 552, 553
Gelade, G., 80, 167
Gelman, R., 432
Gelman, S., 323
Gentaz, E., 214
Gentner, D., 325, 327, 483
Georgiou, G. J., 498
Geraerts, E., 277, 280, 296
Gerlach, C., 331
German, T., 323
Geschwind, N., 371
Ghetti, S., 296
Gibson, E., 112, 364, 366
Gibson, J. J., 96, 97
Gick, M., 483
Giesbrecht, T., 296
Gigerenzer, G., 444, 446, 447, 457
Gilbert, D., 468
Gilbert, D. T., 443, 467, 468, 469
Gilbert, S. J., 173, 175

Gilhooly, K. J., 498
Gilovich, T., 251, 431, 438, 440, 441, 449, 450, 558
Girard, K., 251
Girotto, V., 444, 457
Gisquet-Verrier, P., 253
Giudice, N. A., 404
Gladwell, B., 443
Glanzer, M., 191, 193
Glaser, R., 486
Gleitman, H., 321, 555
Gleitman, L. R., 321, 373, 381
Glenberg, A., 227
Glisky, E. L., 34
Glisky, M., 411
Glover, G., 203
Gluck, M., 316
Glucksberg, S., 370
Gobet, F., 449, 488
Godden, D. R., 226, 228
Goebel, R., 401
Goel, V., 442
Gold, C., 134
Goldenberg, G., 404
Goldenberg, J., 501
Goldin-Meadow, S., 373
Goldman-Rakic, P. S., 174, 553
Goldschmidt, G., 412
Goldstone, R., 325
Gollan, T., 381
Gonzalez, M., 444
Gonzalez, R., 251, 431, 558
Goodale, M. A., 77, 78, 404, 543, 559
Goodman, G., 295, 299
Goodman, N., 325
Gordon, H., 518
Gordon, R. D., 287
Gore, J. C., 131
Goshen-Gottstein, Y., 194
Gottesman, C. V., 419
Gottesman, I. I., 521
Gottfredson, L. S., 503, 505, 506, 513
Grabowecky, M., 80, 108
Grabowski, T., 332
Grady, C. L., 194
Graesser, A. C., 370
Graf, P., 207, 241, 256, 559
Grafman, J., 175
Graham, K. S., 289
Grainger, J., 115
Grant, H. M., 227
Gray, C. M., 551
Gray, J. R., 199, 510

Gray, W., 312
Green, D., 381
Green, R. L., 518
Greenberg, D. L., 408
Gregg, M. K., 149
Grewal, D., 513
Griffin, D. W., 251, 431, 440, 558
Griffith, B., 355
Griggs, R., 456
Grigorenko, E. L., 513
Grill-Spector, K., 131
Grodner, D., 364
Groeneweg, J., 293
Gross, J., 555
Grossi, D., 129
Grotzer, T. A., 519
Group, T. L. R., 336
Gruber, H. E., 500
Guerin, S., 288
Guilford, J., 501

Haber, L., 408
Haber, R. N., 408, 409
Hacker, H., 401
Hackman, D., 521
Hadar, L., 463
Haden, P. E., 241, 559
Hafstad, G. S., 281
Hagen, L., 278
Hahn, B., 156
Hahn, U., 485
Haier, R., 511
Halamish, V., 287, 302
Halberstadt, J., 317
Haley, A., 521
Hall, L. K., 297, 301
Halle, M., 350, 355
Halliday, H. E., 244
Halpern, A. R., 389
Halpern, D. F., 488, 519, 522
Hamann, S., 291, 295
Hambrick, D., 173
Hamel, R., 412
Hamill, R., 435
Hammarberg, R., 352
Hammond, K. M., 406
Hampshire, A., 162
Han, C-h., 318
Han, J., 134
Hanako, Y., 381
Handel, S., 355
Handley, S. J., 440, 444, 454
Hannon, B., 199
Hanyu, K., 299

Subject Index

(*Note:* Italicized page numbers indicate figures; notes and tables are denoted with "n" and "t" next to the page numbers.)

Attention
    as achievement, 168
    automaticity and, 176–177
    brain sites in, 160–161, *160*
    chronometric studies and,
        157–159
    deep processing and, *206*, 207,
        208, 221
    dichotic listening and, 143–144,
        144
    divided, 169–175, 182
    emotion and, 292
    executive control and, 173–175
    feature binding and, 166–168, *167*
    focus of, *4*
    general resources identification
        and, 171–172, *172*
    generality of resources and,
        171–172
    limits on, 177–179
    limits on cognitive capacity and,
        145–152
    movement of, 160
    neural activity and, *553*
    object-based, 163–165, *163*, *164*
    practice and, 175–179
    selective. *See* selective attention
    selective priming and, 152–157,
        154t, *155*, *156*
    shifting, 160–161
    space-based, 163–165, *163*, *164*
    spatial, 157–159, *158*
    specificity of resources and,
        169–170, *170*
    as spotlight, 159–162
    Stroop interference, 177, *178*
    summary, 181–182
    synchrony and, 80
    unattended inputs and, 144–145
    of witnesses, 179–181
Attention deficit disorder, 141
Attention deficit hyperactivity
    disorder (ADHD), 141, 161,
    161t
Attractiveness, typicality and, *317*
Attribute substitution, 430–431,
    431t
Auditory projection area, *51*
Autistic savants, 476–477, 514, *514*
Autobiographical memory
    defined, 288
    emotion and, 290–292, *291*
    errors in, 288–299, *299*
    flashbulb memories and, 292–294,
        293, *294*

long, long-term remembering and,
    296–299, *297*, *298*
overview of, 288–289
the self and, 289–290, *289*
summary, 303–304
See also Memory
Automatic tasks, 177
Automaticity, 176–177
Availability heuristic
    abuse of, *434*
    defined, 431
    range of effects, 432–433
    summary of, 471
    See also Judgment
Awareness
    brain activity and, *46*
    content of consciousness and, 550
    See also Attention; Consciousness
Axons, *54*, 55

Background knowledge
    as guide to parsing, 366–367, *367*
    thinking and, 445–447, *446*, *447*
Base rates
    defined, 439
    example of, 439–440, 439t
    frequencies, 444
    importance of, 439, 439t
    sensitivity to, 444
    summary, 472
Basic-level categorization, 315–316,
    316
Behaviorism, 11–13, 13n, 27
Behaviorist theory, 11
Belief bias, 453–454
Belief preservation, 450–452
"Betsy and Jacob" story, 5–6,
    5, 12
Big-C Creativity, 494–495
Bigram detectors, 114, *115*
Bilabial sounds, 349
Bilingualism, 381–382, 385
Binding problem, 79, 101, 166–168,
    167
Binocular disparity, 93–95, *94*, *95*
Binocular rivalry, 400
Bipolar cells, 68
Blind sight
    amnesia and, 542–543, *543*, 564
    defined, 532, 542
    patients with, 532–533
Blindness
    change, 147–149, *148*, *149*
    color, 78n

conscious seeing and, *543*
inattentional, 145–147, *146*
Bodily-kinesthetic intelligence, 514
Bookworm problem, 481–482, *482*
Bottom-up processes, 106
Boundary extension, 419–421, *420*
Brain
    Area MT, 74
    Area V1, 74, *75*, 402
    Area V4, 74
    central fissure, *32*, 38
    cerebellum, *32*, 37
    cerebral cortex, 37, 49–53
    cerebral hemisphere, 37
    convolutions, 37
    dual-process models and, *442*
    forebrain, 37
    frontal lobes, *32*, 37–38
    fusiform face area (FFA), 46, *46*
    glial cells, 35–38
    hindbrain, 37
    lateral fissure, *32*, 38
    lateralization, 39–40
    lobes, *32*, *32*
    localization of function, 47–49, *48*
    longitudinal fissure, 37
    midbrain, 37
    neurons, 43–45
    occipital lobes, *32*, 38
    parietal lobes, *32*, 38
    rhythm, 79
    self-referencing and, *289*
    structures of, 37–40, 59
    study of, 35–38
    subcortical structures, 38–39, *38*
    temporal lobes, *32*, 38
    visual imagery and, 400–413
Brain activity
    awareness and, *46*
    electrical recording, 43–45, *44*
    in mental rotation, *396*
    sentence parsing and, *368*
Brain areas
    categorization and, 331, *332*
    for consciousness, 548–550, *549*,
        550
    for language, *372*
    for visual and spatial tasks, 404,
        405
Brain cells, 53–55, *54*
Brain damage
    agnosias and, 52, 77, *103*, 128, 130
    anomias and, *332*
    aphasias and, 53, 345–346, 371
    Capgras syndrome and, 29–30

diversity of, 331
exemplar. *See* exemplars
explanatory theories, 327–329, *328*
family resemblance and, 311–312, *311*, 342
inferences based on theories and, 329–330, *330*
knowledge network and, 333–339
legal, 340–341
prototypes and typicality effects and, 312–316
representation of, 342
summary, 339–340, 342
as theories, 327–332
typicality versus categorization and, 321–324, 321t, *322*, *323*
understanding, 309–312, *310*, *311*
Conceptual mental maps, *416*
Concurrent articulation
articulatory loop and, *20*
defined, 19
effect on span, 20, *20*
effects of, *19*
sound-alike errors and, 21
Conditional statements, 455
Cones, 66–68, *66*
Confidence
malleability, *281*
memory, 280–282, *281*
Confirmation and disconfirmation, 448–452, *448*, *449*
Confirmation bias
defined, 438, 449
demonstration of, 450
forms of, *449*
in police investigations, 469–471, *470*
power of, *470*
summary, 472
Confusion, recovery from, 115–117, *116*
Conjunction errors, 80
Connection weights, 339
Connectionist networks, 338
Connections
among ideas, 217
creativity as ability to find, 501, *502*
excitatory, 123, *123*
formation of, 221
importance of, *208*
inhibitory, 123, *123*

McClelland and Rumelhart model, 122–124, *123*
meaning and, 207–210, *208*, *210*, 229
memory error and, 287
in memory retrieval, 208–209, *208*
multiple, 214
retrieval paths, 210
See also Memory
Conscious products, 534–535
Conscious seeing, *543*
Conscious thought, 425
Consciousness
aspects of, *549*
brain areas, 548–550, *549*, *550*
cognitive neuroscience of, 548–555
content of, 549, 550
defined, 533
degree of awareness and, 550
executive control and, 544–548, *545*, *546*
as justification for action, 558–560, 564
neuronal workspace and, 550–555, *552*, *555*, 564
phenomenal, 555–560, 564
processes versus products in, 534–535
processing fluency and, 556–558
qualia and, 556, *557*
study of, 533
summary, 564
unconscious guides and, 540–541, *541*, 564
variations in, 550, *550*
what is left unsaid, 560–562
Consolidation, memory, 290–291
Constancy
brightness, 87
illusions and, 91–92, *91*, *92*, *93*
perceptual, 87
shape, 87, *89*
size, 87, *88*
summary, 101
unconscious interference and, 87–90, *90*
See also Visual system
Context
extralinguistic, 367–369, *369*
object recognition in, 134–135
perception and, 106, *106*
reinstatement, 228, 233–234, *234*, 236

Context-dependent learning
defined, 226
experiment, 226–228, *228*
experiment design, 226, *227*
Contralateral control, 49
Contrast effect, 92
Control
executive, 544–548, *545*, *546*
prerequisites of, 547
role of, 546–547
Controlled tasks, 177
Conversation, remembering, 382–384
Convolutions, *32*
Cornea, 65–66, *65*
Corpus callosum, 39
Correlational data, neuroimaging, 46
Cortex
anterior cingulate, 554
association, 52–53, 59–60
defined, *32*
prefrontal, 33
Covariation
base rates in, 439–440, 439t, 472
confirmation bias and, 438
detecting, 437–440
illusions of, 438
importance of, 437
summary of, 471–472
See also Judgment
Creativity
Big-C Creativity and, 494–495
case studies of, 494–495
as divergent thinking, 501, *501*
as finding new connections, 501, *502*
illumination in, 496
incubation in, 495, 498–499, *500*
insight problems and, 496, 497, *498*
moment of illumination in, 495–496, *497*, *498*
nature of, 499–502, *501*, *502*
personality traits and, 500
preparation in, 495
summary, 527
verification in, 496
See also Problem solving
Crystallized intelligence, 509–510, *509*, 528
CT scans. *See* Computerized axial tomography

Evidence
  disconfirming, reinterpreting, 450
  framing of, 461–462, *462*
  memory errors and, 277–279,
    278, 279
  of schematic knowledge, 271–273,
    272
  for working-memory system,
    18–24, *19, 20, 23*
Excitatory connections, 123, *123*
Executive control
  action slips and, 545
  consciousness and, 544–548, *545,
    546*
  defined, 173
  diminished, 173–174
  goal neglect and, 174–175, *174*
  metacognition and, 547–548
  neuronal workspace and,
    554–555, *555*
  perseveration error and, 174
  prerequisites of, 547
  processes, 201
  role of, 546–547
Exemplar-based reasoning, 317–318
Exemplars
  analogies from, 316–318
  approach, 316–318
  prototypes and, 319–320, *320*
  summary, 342
  typicality and, 318–319, *319*
Expectation-driven priming, 153,
  157
Experience
  conscious, *553, 564*
  judgment and, 430
  phenomenal, *555–560*
  in problem solving, 482–488
Expert problem solvers, 486, *487*,
  527
Expertise, 499, 527
Explanatory theories, 327–328, *328*
Explicit memory
  defined, 241
  implicit memory and, 257–258,
    257
  learning and, 261
  subcategories, 251
Extralinguistic context, 367–369,
  369
Eyes
  cones, 66–68, *66*
  cornea, 65–66, *65*
  fovea, *65*, 68
  lens, 65–66, *65*

  retina, 65–68, *65*
  rods, 66, *66*
  See also Visual system
Eyewitness errors, 274
Eyewitness testimony, 98–100

Face recognition
  brain areas for, *132*
  composite effect in, 132, *133*
  criminal justice system and, 134
  inversion effect and, 129, *129*
  prosopagnosia and, 128, 130
  upside-down, 129–130, *130*
Faces, imagery in brain, *401*
Factor analysis, 507
False fame test, 241–243
False memories
  leading questions and, 275, *275*
  misinformation effect and, 277, 303
  outside laboratory, 279–280
  planting, 274–280, *278, 279, 280*
  summary, 303
  See also Memory
Familiarity
  chain of events leading to, *249*
  illusion of, 251
  implicit memory and, *248*,
    249–251, *249*
  nature of, 249–251, *249*
  source memory and, 237–240,
    238, 239, 421
  specialness as, 248
  spelling and, *248*
Family resemblance, 311–312, *311*,
  342
Feature binding, 166–168, *167*
Feature nets
  ambiguous inputs and, 117–118
  defined, 113
  descendants of, 122–128
  design of, 112–114, *113*
  distributed knowledge and,
    120–121
  efficiency versus accuracy and,
    121–122
  implementation of, 139
  McClelland and Rumelhart
    model, 122–124, *123*
  recognition by components and,
    124–126, *125*
  recognition errors and, 118–120,
    119
  recognition via multiple views
    and, 126–127, *127, 128*

  recovery from confusion and,
    115–117, *116*
  summary, 139
  top-down influences and,
    134–136, 139
  well-formedness and, 114–115
  word recognition and, 112–122
Features
  combination of, 168
  form perception and, 85–87, *85, 86*
  in object recognition, 107–108, *108*
  priority in perception, 166
Feedback, 535–536, *537*
FFA (fusiform face area), 131
Figure ground organization, 82
Filters, 145
Fires, 55, 231
Fixation target, 146, *146*
Flashbulb memories, 292–294, *293,
  294, 304*
Fluency, processing of, 246–248, *248*
Fluent aphasia, 371
Fluid intelligence, 509–510, *509*, 528
Flynn effect, 519–520, *520*
fMRI. *See* Functional magnetic
  resonance imaging
Food supplements, 58–59, *58*
Forebrain, *32*
Forgetting
  avoiding, 287
  causes of, 282–284, *283, 285*
  curve, *283*
  decay and, 283
  hypnosis and, 285–286, *286*
  interference theory and, 283, 284,
    285
  from interfering events, 284, *285*
  retrieval failure and, 283, 284, *285*
  TOT phonomenon and, 284
  undoing, 285–287, *286*
  See also Memory errors
Form perception
  figure ground organization and, 82
  Gestalt principles and, 82–85, *83, 84*
  "information gathering" step, 85
  "interpretation" step, 85
  Necker cube, 81, *81*
  organization and "features" and,
    85–87, *85, 86*
  overview of, 80–82
  proximity and, 84
  similarity and, 84
  stimuli and, 82, *82*
  summary, 101
  See also Visual system

Four-card task
   defined, 455
   easier version of, 456, *456*
   illustrated, *455*
   rationale in, 457, *457*
   summary, 472
Fovea, *65*, 68
Frame, decision, 541
Framing
   defined, 460
   in monetary choices, 460–461, *460*
   negative frame, *459*
   of outcomes, 458–461, *459*, *460*
   positive frame, *459*
   of questions and evidence, 461–462, *462*
   risk aversion and, 461
   risk seeking and, 461
   See also Decision-making
Fraternal twins, 516, *517*
Free recall, 190, *191*
Frequency estimation, 430
Frequency principle, 114
Frontal lobe, *32*, 37–38
Functional fixedness, 489–490, *489*, *490*
Functional magnetic resonance imaging (fMRI)
   Capgras syndrome and, 33, *33*
   defined, 41
   results of, 42, 45
Fusiform face area (FFA), 46, *46*, 131

Ganglion cells, 68
Garden-path sentences, 363–364
General intelligence, 506–507, 528
General resources, 171–172, *172*
Generality
   of memory principles, 299–301
   of resources, 171–172
Generativity, of language, 357
Genetics and intelligence
   dizygotic (DZ) twins and, 516, *517*
   interaction among environment and, 520–522, *521*, 528
   monozygotic (MZ) twins and, 516, *517*
   relatedness and, *518*
   summary, 528
   See also Intelligence
Geons, 125–126, *125*

Gestalt principles, 82–85, *83*, *84*
Gingko biloba, 58–59, *58*
Glial cells, 35–38, 60
Goal neglect, 174–175, *174*
Goal-derived categories, 331
Graded membership, 312–313, *313*

H. M. (amnesia case), 6–7, *7*, 254–255
Happiness research, 468–469
Heuristics
   availability, 431, 432–433, *434*, 471
   defined, 432
   representativeness, 431, 433–437, *436*, 471
   summary, 471
Hierarchical model of intelligence, 507–508, *508*
Hierarchical structure of language, 347, *347*
Hill-climbing strategy, 480
Hindbrain, 37
Hints, 261
Hippocampus
   damage to, 257–258, *257*
   memory consolidation and, 291
Hobbits and Orcs problem, 478–480, *478*, *479*
Holistic recognition, 131–134, *132*, *133*
Homogeneity, category, 434–435, *436*
Hyperthymesia, 263–264
Hypnosis, 285–286
Hypnotic age regression, *286*
Hypothalamus, 38, *38*
Hypotheses, testing, 14, 15

Iconic memory, 188
Identical twins, 516, *517*
Ill-defined problems, 488–489
Illumination
   in creativity, 495–496, *497*, *498*
   defined, 496
   insight problem and, 496, *497*, *498*
   moment of, 495–496
Illusion of truth, 243–244
Illusions, constancy and, 91–93, *91*, *92*, *93*
Image files, in long-term memory, 414, 424

Images
   creating, 413, 424
   as depictions, 394–395
   dual coding and, 418
   introspections about, 390–391
   in long-term memory, 413–414, *414*
   memory and, 417–421, *420*
   mental rotation and, 395–397, *395*, *396*
   pictures versus, 409–413, *410*, *411*, *412*
   spatial versus visual, 403–406, *405*, 424
   See also Visual imagery
Image-scanning procedure, 392, 393–394, *393*
Implicit memory
   attributing to wrong source, 244–246, *245*
   defined, 241
   explicit memory and, 251, 257–258, *257*
   false fame test and, 241–243
   familiarity and, *248*, 249–251, *249*
   fluency processing and, 246–248, *248*
   illusion of truth and, 243–244
   source confusion and, 245–246, *245*
   subcategories, 251, *252*
   summary, 261
   theoretical treatments of, 246–251
   without awareness, *242*
Inattentional blindness, 145–147, *146*
Incidental learning, 206
Incubation
   benefit from simple forgetting, *500*
   in creativity, 495, 498–499
   defined, 495
Indirect memory testing, 241
Induction, 448, *448*
Inference, in unconscious reasoning, 536–537
Inhibitory connections, 123, *123*
Inner ear, 22
Inner hand, 23, *24*
Inner speech, 22
Inner voice, 22, 23, *24*
Inputs
   ambiguous, 117–118
   unattended, 144–145, 181
Insight problems, 496, *497*, *498*
Inspection time, 510

Integrative agnosia, 108
Intelligence
    across lifespan, 509, *509*
    American Whites and American
        Blacks and, 522–524, 528
    beyond IQ tests, 511–515, *514, 515*
    bodily-kinesthetic, 514
    brain basis for, 512
    building blocks of, 510, *511*
    comparison of groups in,
        522–524, *523*
    crystallized, 509–510, *509*, 528
    defining, 503–506, *504, 506t*
    emotional, 513–514
    environmental influences on,
        517–520, *519, 520*, 528
    factor analysis, 507
    fluid, 509–510, *509*, 528
    general, 506–507, 528
    genetic influences on, 516–517,
        517, 518, 528
    hierarchical model of, 507–508, *508*
    inspection time and, 510
    interaction among genetics and
        environment and, 520–522,
        521, 528
    interpersonal, 514
    intrapersonal, 514
    as life outcome predicator, 524
    measurement of, 475, 503–506,
        504, 506t
    multiple, 514
    musical, 514
    naturalistic, 514
    overview of, 502
    performance improvement,
        525–526
    P-FIT model and, 510, *511, 512*
    poverty and, 521
    practical, 511–513
    rationality and, 513
    roots of, 516–524
    savant syndrome and, *514*
    specialized, 506–507
    summary, 528
    tests. *See* IQ tests
    working memory and, 24
    working-memory capacity
        (WMC) and, 510
Intentional learning, 206
Interference theory, 283, 284, *285*
Interpersonal intelligence, 514
Interpolated activity, impact on
    recency effect, 193, *194*
Interposition, *95, 96*

Interpretation
    perception and, 83, *83*, 91
    of situations, 12
    in unconscious reasoning, 536–537
Interrogations, 383
Intrapersonal intelligence, 514
Introspection
    consciousness researchers and, 533
    defined, 9
    limits of, 8–10
    mistaken, 538–540, *539*
Intrusion errors, 268
Invalid syllogisms, 453
Inversion effect, 129, *129*
Inverted spectrum, *557*
Invisible causes, 14, 27
IQ tests
    intelligence beyond, 511–515,
        514, 515
    items, *504*
    poverty and, 521
    reliability, 503–506, *504*
    scores, 505–506, 528
    scores between American Whites
        and American blacks,
        522–524, 528
    scores between men and women,
        522
    stereotype threat, 523
    validity, 503–506, *504*
    See also Intelligence

Judgment
    attribute substitution and,
        430–431, 431t
    availability heuristic, 431,
        432–433, *434*, 471
    covariation and, 437–440, 439t,
        471–472
    dual-process models and, 440–447
    errors in, 440–447, 472
    experience and, 430
    frequency estimation and, 430
    heuristics, 431, 432–437, *434,
        436*, 471
    prerequisites of, 342
    representativeness heuristic, 431,
        433–437, *436*, 471
    of resemblance, 325
    summary of, 471–472
    typicality versus categorization
        and, 321, 323
Justification for action, consciousness
    and, 558–560, 564

Knowledge
    background, 366–367, *367*
    distributed, 120–121
    diversity of, 421–422
    essential properties, 342
    locally represented, 121
    memory structure for, *334*
    representations, 333, *335*, 338
    retrieval, 333–336, *334, 335*
    schematic, 270–273, *272*, 287–288
    storage, 342
    summary, 342
    visual, 386–424
Knowledge networks
    connection weights, 339
    connectionist, 338
    distributed processing, 338–339
    propositional, 336–337, *337*
    representations, *335*
    in retrieval, 333–336, *334, 335*
Korsakoff's syndrome, 223–224,
    255, 256, 258

Labiodental sounds, 349
Language
    animal, 375–376, *375*
    aphasias and, 371–373, *372*
    bilingualism and, 381–382, 385
    biological roots of, 371–377, 385
    brain areas for, *372*
    colors in, *379*
    generativity of, 357
    hierarchical structure of, 347, *347*
    learning biology, 373
    learning processes, 373–375, 385
    linguistic relativity and, 377–381,
        379
    organization of, 346–348, *347*
    phonemes combining, 355
    phonology. *See* phonology
    pragmatics and, 370, 371
    prescriptive rules, 359–360, *360*
    production, 345, 348–350, *349*
    prosody and, 370, 371
    sentence parsing, 362–371, *363,
        365, 367, 368, 369*
    speech perception, 350–355, *350,
        351, 353, 354*
    summary, 384–385
    syntax. *See* syntax
    thought and, 377–382, *378, 379*,
        385
    use of, 370–371
Late selection, 150–151, *150*

Neuropsychology, 22, 40–41
Neurotransmitters, 55, 56, 57
Neutral trials, 156
Nine-dot problem, 492, *492*
Nodes, network
    activation from two sources, *233*, 261
    defined, 231
    response threshold, *233*
Non-conscious states, *555*
Nonfluent aphasia, 371
Noun phrases, *359*

Object model, 126
Object recognition
    bottom-up processes and, 106
    early considerations in, 106–108, *108*
    example of, 103–105, *104*, *105*
    feature nets and, *128*
    importance of features in, 107–108, *108*
    larger contexts and, 134–135
    summary, 138–139
    systems, 128–134
    top-down influences on, 134–136
    top-down processes and, 107
    See also Recognition
Object-based attention, 163–165, *163*, *164*
Occipital lobes, *32*, 38
Operation span, 198–200, *198*, *200*
Optic flow, 97
Optic nerve, 68
Optimal learning, 258–259
Organization
    in form perception, 85–87, *85*, *86*
    Gestalt principles of, 84, *84*
    of language, 346–348, *347*
    memory acquisition and, 210–216
    phrase structure, 361, *361*
Orientation-specific visual fields, 73, *73*
Orthography, 356
Outcomes, framing of, 458–461, *459*, *460*
Overregularization errors, 374

P cells, 76
Parallel distributed processing (PDP), 338
Parallel processing, visual system, 74–78, *75*, *76*, *77*, 100–101

Parietal lobes, *32*, 38
Parvocellular cells, 76
Passive-voice sentences, 365
Paying attention, 140–182, 402, 563, *563*
PDP (parallel distributed processing), 338
Peg-word systems, 211–212
Perception
    brain damage and, 402
    categorical, 353–355, *353*, *354*
    context and, 106, *106*
    of depth, 93–98
    form, 80–87
    holistic, 131–134, *132*, *133*
    interpretation and, 83, *83*, 91
    limits on, 150
    mental resources for, 181
    speech, 350–355, *350*, *351*, *353*, *354*, 384
    unconscious, *150*
    of upside-down faces, *30*, 129–130
    visual imagery and, 398–400, *399*, 423–424
Percepts, 410
Perceptual constancy, 87
Perceptual learning, *252*
Perseveration error, 174
Perspectives
    multiple, in learning, 258–259
    spatial, 260
PET scans. *See* Positron emission tomography
P-FIT model, 510, *511*, *512*
Phenomenal consciousness
    as justification for action, 558–560
    overview of, 555
    processing fluency and, 556–558
    qualia and, *556*, *557*
    role of, *555*–560
    summary, 564
Phonemes, 384
    assembly, 348
    combining, 355
    defined, 347
    in linguistic hierarchy, 347
Phonemic restoration effect, 352
Phonological buffer, 17
Phonology
    categorical perception, 353–355, *353*, *354*
    complexity of speech perception, 350–355, *350*, *351*, *353*, *354*

phonemes combining, 355
    production of speech, 345, 348–350, *349*
    speech perception aids, 352–353
    See also Language
Photoreceptors, 65–68, *65*, *66*
Phrase structure
    ambiguity, 362, *362*
    descriptive rules, 360
    function of, 360–361, *361*, *362*
    noun phrase, *359*
    organization, 361, *361*
    prescriptive rules, 359–360, *360*
    rules, 358–360, *360*
    tree, *359*
    verb phrase, *359*
    See also Syntax
Phrases
    in linguistic hierarchy, *347*
    noun, *359*
    verb, *359*
Pictorial cues, 95–96, *95*, *96*
Pictures
    boundary extension and, 419–421, *420*
    images versus, 409–413, *410*, *411*, *412*
    memory for, *217*, 218, 418–421, *421*, 424
    in problem solving, 480–482, *481*, *482*, 527
    summary, 412–413
Place of articulation, 349
Places, imagery in brain, *401*
Positron emission tomography (PET scans)
    defined, 41
    illustrated, *42*
    results of, 42, 45
    use of, 41
Postsynaptic membrane, 55, 56
Poverty, intellectual development and, 521
Practice
    automaticity and, 176–177
    effects of, 175
    limits and, 177–179, *178*
    resource demand and, 176
    See also Attention
Pragmatics, 370, 371
Predictive validity, 505
Prefrontal area, damage to, 53, 60
Prefrontal cortex, 33
Preparation, in creativity, 495
Prescriptive rules, 359–360, *360*

Presynaptic membrane, 55, 56
Primacy effect
  defined, 191
  explaining, 192
  in free recall, 191
  testing claims about, 193–194
Primary motor projection areas, 49, 50, 59
Primary sensory projection areas, 49, 50, 59
Primed trials, 154, 154t
Primes, 110
Priming
  biological mechanisms for, 156–157, 156
  effects on stimulus processing, 155
  expectation-driven, 153, 157
  as implicit memory, 252
  large contexts and, 135
  relationship between levels of, 121
  repetition, 110, 114, 240
  selective, 152–157
  semantic, 234–236, 236
  types of, 153
Problem definition
  Einstellung and, 491–494, 491
  functional fixedness and, 489–490, 489, 490
  ill-defined, 488–489
  overview of, 488
  summary, 527
  well-defined, 489
Problem solving
  creativity and, 494–502, 527
  defined, 477
  defining the problem in, 488–494, 527
  from experience, 482–488
  expert, 486, 487, 527
  general methods of, 477–482
  heuristics, 480, 481
  hill-climbing strategy, 480
  means-end analysis, 480, 481
  pictures and diagrams in, 480–482, 481, 482, 527
  as search, 478–480, 478, 479, 527
  subgoals, 486–488, 487
  summary, 527
  thinking outside the box and, 492–494, 492, 493
  via analogy, 482–485, 483, 484, 527
Problem space, 478, 479
Problem-solving set, 491–492, 491

Procedural memory, 252
Processing fluency, 247–248, 556–558
Processing pathway, 247
Production of speech, 345, 348–350, 349
Production task, 314
Profiles, for different concepts, 330–332, 332
Propositional networks, 336, 337
Prosody, 370, 371
Prosopagnosia, 128, 130
Prototypes
  basic versus superordinate labeling and, 315, 315
  basic-level categories, 315–316, 315, 342
  defined, 312
  exemplars and, 319–320, 320
  graded membership and, 312–313, 313
  "ideal," 312
  notion, testing, 313–315, 314t
  production task and, 314
  rating tasks and, 315
  sentence verification task and, 313–314
Proximity, 84

Qualia, 556, 557
Questions, framing of, 461–462, 462

Rating tasks, 315
Rationality, intelligence and, 513
Reason-based choices, 463
Reasoning
  about syllogisms, 452–454, 452, 453, 454
  belief bias and, 453–454
  belief preservation and, 450–452
  conditional statements and, 455
  confirmation and disconfirmation and, 448–452, 448
  confirmation bias and, 449–450, 449, 472
  in decision-making, 458–469, 472
  exemplar-based, 317–318
  four-card task and, 455–457, 455, 466, 472, 477
  logic and, 452–457, 472
  reinterpreting disconfirming evidence and, 450
  summary of, 472
  unconscious, 535–538, 537

Recall
  defined, 237
  imagery in, 424
  retention intervals and, 299
  schemata and, 270
Recency effect
  defined, 191
  explaining, 191–192
  in free recall, 191
  impact of interpolated activity on, 193, 194
  testing claims about, 193–194, 194
Recency principle, 114
Receptive fields, 71–73, 72, 73
Recognition
  by components, 124–126, 125
  early considerations, 106–108
  errors, 118–120, 119
  of faces, 128–131
  holistic, 131–134
  from memory, 237
  by multiple views, 126–127, 127, 128
  viewpoint-dependent, 126, 128
  viewpoint-independent, 126
  word, 108–112, 138
  See also Object recognition
Reconstructions, after-the-fact, 539–540
Recovered memories, 295–296
Recovery from confusion, 115–117, 116
Redundancy, in perception of depth, 97–98, 98
Rehearsal
  articulatory, 24–25
  maintenance, 202, 221
  memory and, 192, 202–203, 204
  relational, 202
  working memory, 23
Rehearsal loop, 17, 18, 18, 20
Relational categories, 331
Relational rehearsal, 202
Reliability
  defined, 503
  intelligence test, 503–506
  test-retest, 503
Remembering
  conversation, 382–384
  false memories and, 274–280, 275, 278, 279, 280
  hyperthymesia and, 263–264
  imagery in, 424
  long, long-term, 296–299, 297, 298
  memory errors and, 264–282
  number of propositions, 269t

Remember/know distinction, 238
Reminiscence bump, 299, *300*
Repetition priming, 110, 114, 240
Representativeness heuristic
  defined, 431
  functioning of, 433–434
  homogeneity, 434–435, *436*
  reasoning from single case to entire population, 435–437
  summary of, 471
Repressed memories, 295, 296
Research
  in cognitive psychology, 15–25
  diverse methods, 15–25
  on happiness, 468–469
Resemblance
  categorization via, 320–326, 321t, *322, 326*
  family, concepts and, 311–312, *311,* 342
  judgment of, 325
  from shared properties, 325–326
Resources
  demand, 177–178
  general, 171–172, *172*
  generality of, 171–172
  practice and, 176
  specificity of, 169–170, *170*
Response selector, 172
Response speed, memory, 282
Response threshold, 113, 231
Response times (RTs), 153
Retention intervals, 282, *283,* 297, 299
Reticular activating system, 549
Retina, 65–68, *65*
Retrieval. *See* Memory retrieval
Retrieval cues, 232–233, *233*
Retrieval failure, 283, 284, 303
Retrieval paths
  connections as, 267, 303
  defined, 210, *225*
  role of, 225–226
Retrograde amnesia, 252, *253*
Reversible figures, *81*
Risk aversion, 461
Risk seeking, 461
Rods, 66, *66*
RTs (response times), 153

Salt-passing behavior, 12–13, *13*
Savant syndrome, *514*
Schema (schemata), 270

Schematic knowledge
  defined, 270
  evidence of, 271–273, *272*
  overview of, 270–271
  reliance on, 287–288
Search, problem solving as, 478–480, *478, 479,* 527
Selection task. *See* Four-card task
Selective attention
  alerting system, 161
  chronometric studies and, 157–159
  costs and benefits of, *167*
  dichotic listening and, 143–144, *144*
  executive system, 161
  feature binding and, 166–168, *167*
  limits on cognitive capacity and, 145–152
  object-based versus space-based, 163–165, *163, 164*
  orienting system, 160–161
  selective priming and, 152–157, 154t, *155, 156*
  spatial attention and, 157–159, *158*
  as spotlight, 159–162
  unattentive inputs and, 144–145
  visual cortex activation, 162, *162*
  See also Attention
Selective priming, 152–157, 154t, *155, 156*
Self-referencing, *289*
Self-report data, 390
Self-schema, 290
Semantic bootstrapping, 375
Semantic expectations, *365*
Semantic facts verification, *335*
Semantic memory, 251, 253, *254*
Semantic priming, 234–236, *236*
Sensory areas, 50–52, *51*
Sensory maps, 50–51
Sensory memory, 188–189
Sentence parsing
  background knowledge as guide, 366–367, *367*
  brain activity and, *368*
  defined, 363
  extralinguistic context in, 367–369, *369*
  summary, 385
  syntax as guide, 364–366, *365*
Sentence verification task, 313–314, 333

Sentences
  active-voice, 365
  defined, 347
  garden-path, 363–364
  interpreting, 366–367, *367*
  in linguistic hierarchy, 347
  passive-voice, 365
  semantic expectations and, *365*
  syntactic expectations and, *365*
  temporary ambiguity, 364
Serial processing, 74
Serial-position effect, 191, *195*
"7 plus-or-minus 2," 197
Shadowing, 143, 170
Shallow processing, 207
Shape constancy, 87, *89*
Short-term memory. *See* Working memory
Similarity, complexity of, 324–326, *326*
Similarity principle, 84
Single-cell recording, 70–71, 100
Size constancy, 87, *88*
Skin conductance response (SCR), 257
SLI (specific language impairment), 373
Somatic markers, 428, 465
Somatosensory area, 51
Sound-alike errors, 18, 21
Sounds
  alveolar, 350
  bilabial, 349
  labiodental, 349
  manner of production, 348
  place of articulation, 349
  of speech, 348–350
  voiced versus unvoiced, 349
  word, 356
Source confusion, 245–246, *245*
Source memory
  defined, 237
  familiarity and, 237–240, *239,* 421
Space-based attention, 163–165, *163, 164*
Spaced learning, 219
Span test
  concurrent articulation and, 20, *20*
  defined, 16
  sound-alike errors in, 18
Spatial attention, 157–159, *158*
Spatial images, 403–406, *405,* 424
Spatial position, 79
Specialized intelligence, 506–507